Bipolar Disorder

Kostas N. Fountoulakis

Bipolar Disorder

An Evidence-Based Guide to Manic Depression

Springer

Kostas N. Fountoulakis
Division of Neurosciences
3rd Department of Psychiatry
Aristotle University of Thessaloniki
School of Medicine
Thessaloniki
Greece

ISBN 978-3-642-37215-5 ISBN 978-3-642-37216-2 (eBook)
DOI 10.1007/978-3-642-37216-2
Springer Heidelberg New York Dordrecht London

Library of Congress Control Number: 2014956965

Printed on acid-free paper

Springer is part of Springer Science+Business Media (www.springer.com)

To Katerina
My sons Nickolas and Ioannis
My parents Nick and Olga and parents-in-law Ioannis and Zoumboulia
For without their enduring support, this book would not have been possible to author

Foreword

During the latter part of the twentieth century, manic depression emerged as a new focus of research that over time came to achieve an equal status with schizophrenia and depression among mental health professionals. Indeed, because of its complexity and high cost and its flamboyant symptomatology, it now tends to enjoy a privileged status, especially in the minds of those working in the arts and sciences.

Manic depression has a number of impressive characteristics. First, it has become almost fashionable to admit that one suffers from this mental disease. Second, there is a widespread belief that it is strongly correlated with creativity. Many famous people announce publicly that they suffer from it, while historical and biographical data suggest that other renowned personalities from the past have been afflicted with the illness. Third, manic depression is one of the very few medical conditions that respond to treatment with a single simple natural element: lithium. This is extraordinary, and the way in which this happens is unique in medicine.

This book is a single-authored work. This is rather unusual today, when multi-authored books are the rule. An extremely large amount of work is needed to accomplish such a task, especially when the purpose is to systematically review the literature and try to follow the rules of evidence-based medicine to the extent that the literature permits it. The result, however, is a comprehensive, solid book and not a heterogeneous compilation of book chapters.

The various chapters of this book address distinct aspects of the disease, from traditional ones such as the historical perspective to modern approaches like staging. Especially the chapter on biological therapies utilizes a precise methodology in the collecting and ranking of data and agents and thereby provides the reader with the state of the art in a comprehensive way which can rarely be found in a book. I strongly believe that the book will satisfy the most discriminating of readers, including both those seeking an update on a specific aspect of the illness and those whose need is a comprehensive reference.

I have no doubt that this book will have a significant impact on the field and will constitute a very important resource for teaching, training and research and provide guidance for everyday clinical practice.

The hope is that it will also help to upgrade the status of bipolar disorder on the agenda of policy makers and promote awareness of the illness so that the needed resources are allocated both for further research in the field and for the targeted treatment and care of patients and their families.

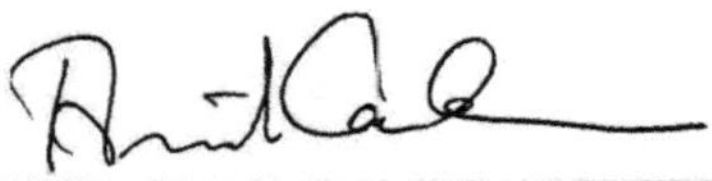

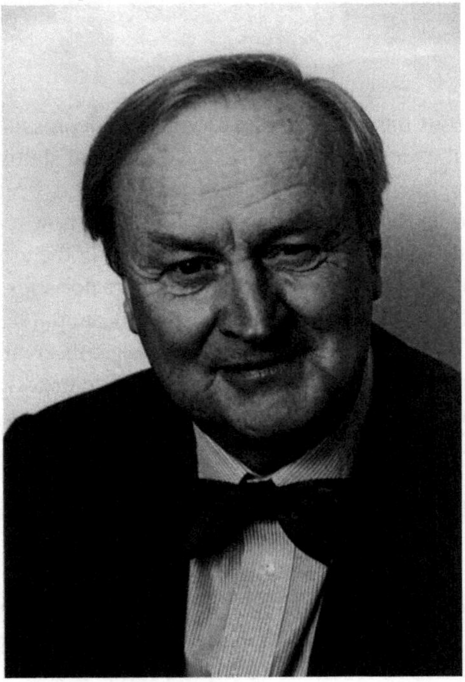

Gothenburg, Sweden
October 2014

Arvid Carlsson
Nobel laureate in medicine 2000
Emeritus Professor of Pharmacology
Sahlgrenska Academy,
University of Gothenburg,
Gothenburg,
Sweden

Contents

Introduction

Since nearly 3,000 years, mood disorders have been described in the medical literature, and the terms mania and melancholia are the oldest in psychiatry and also among the oldest in medicine. Although they are considered to constitute one of the most common group diseases of humanity, accompanied by heavy burden, disability, mortality and cost, only recently the major public health interest focused on them. Since the 1990s, the World Health Organization has ranked them among the most disabling medical conditions and among the most urgent health problems worldwide.

From Hippocrates to Aretaeus of Cappadocia, to Kraepelin, Aubrey Lewis and Sir Martin Roth, to Fred Goodwin, Hagop Akiskal and other prominent researchers, our understanding of bipolar disorder (BD) evolved from an episodic disorder with little disability and good prognosis to a probably developmental, chronic, disabling disease with significant burden, mortality and global cost for the society (Goodwin and Jamison 1990; Aretaeus of Cappadocia 1856; Kraepelin 1921). With the introduction of modern classification systems and the advancement of the evidence-based movement in medicine and psychiatry, our approach is reshaped and our knowledge and data are scrutinized and re-evaluated.

Still many questions remain to be answered. One of them concerns the existence of a spectrum of mood disorders which includes many conditions previously diagnosed as schizophrenia, personality disorder, or neurosis. This implies the presence of a clinical continuum, and it is in sharp contrast to the categorical approach of classification systems. Another question concerns the possible role and place of juvenile mood disorders (Poznanski and Zrull 1970; Puig-Antich 1987; Weller et al. 1995; Carlson and Strober 1978; Akiskal et al. 1985). One of the most cardinal issues is how to reduce overall mortality in general and suicidality in particular, since mood disorders underlie nearly two-thirds of suicide attempts (Isometsa et al. 1994; Luoma et al. 2002; Rihmer et al. 2002; Rihmer 2007), and therefore early identification and correct treatment is important.

Bipolar disorder (BD) was previously called manic–depressive psychosis, and its clinical picture consists of at least one hypomanic, manic, or mixed episode and one or more depressive episodes. Euphoric mania was the classic feature of BD, but today we know that mixed and agitated depression or dysphoric manic states are more prevalent. Also, recent data suggest the existence of a spectrum of milder, short-duration and ambulatory mood states that alternate. Comorbidity patterns include high rates of panic, obsessive–compulsive disorder, social phobia, and alcohol and stimulants abuse. Somatic illness is also highly prevalent, and vascular brain disease might relate to a specific type of late-onset BD. In many ways, the old term 'manic depression' seems much more appropriate than the modern 'bipolar disorder'.

The aetiopathogenesis might include genetic, neurodevelopmental and psychosocial factors with neurobiological factors being predominant. Since antiquity, temperament was considered to constitute a vulnerability factor for the development of mood disorders. During the last few decades, the concept of temperament has been refined and redefined and specific variations, possibly hereditary to a significant degree, have been described (Akiskal and McKinney 1973; Akiskal 1995). Women might be at higher risk, but the specific sex-related factors leading to this increased vulnerability are unknown (Nazroo et al. 1997; Parry 1989).

However, a family environment with parents suffering from overt mood disorders or having personality or temperament features that predispose to mood disorders is often characterized by conflicts, bereavement, divorce and suicide, but often it is also characterized by creativity and openness. This is often the environment where a child with a genetic vulnerability to mood disorders is born and raised. The interaction between adverse life events and genetic vulnerability might further increase the risk for the development of mood disorders (Kendler and Karkowski-Shuman 1997).

More than a century has already passed since Frederik Lange in the late nineteenth century (Lange 1894) used lithium for the first time. Also more than half a century has passed since John Cade used it for the treatment of affective patients (Cade 1949, 1970; Bech 2006) and since Jean Delay and Pierre Deniker used an antipsychotic for the first time most likely in agitated manic patients (Delay and Deniker 1955). Psychopharmacology reshaped the way we view and treat mental disorders, including BD. It 'medicalized' psychiatry because one needs to be competent in medicine in order to use medication properly and adequately. It is widely accepted that BD requires prolonged somatic treatment in order to achieve remission of symptomatology and return of functioning. Polypharmacy might be the rule rather than the exception, and this issue requires caution and further research. Psychosocial therapy by skilled clinicians can provide support, combat demoralization, change maladaptive behaviours and improve functioning. It can provide relief and support not only to patients but also to caregivers and families.

It is disappointing that any advances that have occurred in our understanding of BD do not appear to have improved the morbidity and mortality of BD patients and their long-term prognosis to the extent it was anticipated. On the other hand, it is a difficult task for the average clinician to keep abreast of the advances in the field, and it is even more difficult to carry these advances into everyday clinical practice.

The current book aims at carrying these advances from the research literature to the everyday diagnostic and therapeutic practice, in a concise, comprehensive and operationalized way, for the ultimate benefit of the patients and their families.

It is not easy nowadays to write and publish a single-authored book. The challenge was great for me, and I would dare to say that this is the most challenging invitation I have ever received. It took me almost three years to complete the writing, and it was a fascinating journey with hot interactions between my personal clinical experience and research and the literature.

My driving thought was to write a book as much evidence-based as possible. Eventually, this was possible for almost all chapters which were based on an in-depth systematic review of the literature updated through the year 2014. More than 3,700 references are included in the book, and many times this number were the references that were screened and rejected.

The text includes a balanced view of conflicting approaches, but this is not done in a neutral or uncritical manner. The conclusions are evidenced-based, after a critical systematic review of the literature, and only on rare occasions my own clinical perspective or opinion leads to the conclusions.

At this point, I would like to thank two eminent people who guided, assisted and supported me through my journey into the science of psychiatry all these years. I have the pleasure to call them my mentors and the privilege to consider them friends.

It is Hagop S. Akiskal who over the last 15 years has introduced me to and helped me with the modern concepts and understanding of mood disorders, while it is Hans-Jurgen Moeller who has guided me for more than a decade in the difficult pathways of modern psychopharmacology and trusted me with important initiatives in the field. Without their unconditional support, my journey in the international arena of science wouldn't have been possible. Of course, the current book reflects my personal view on the topic of manic depression, and I am the only one to assume full responsibility for the content of the text.

I also would like to thank Professor Arvid Carlsson, Nobel Laureate in Medicine for the year 2000, for accepting to write a prologue for the book. His kind words are a great honour and ethical satisfaction for my efforts, and since I met him for the first time some 10 years ago, his figure serves as an ideal paradigm for my journey through the wandering rocks of science (only to quote his words).

Finally, I would like to thank all my colleagues in my research team through the last 15 years. They worked hard, accepted me and my peculiarities and demands, and together we tried to contribute to the development of the field through the accumulation of evidence. I also want to thank my colleagues in the 3rd Department of Psychiatry for their continuous support and understanding.

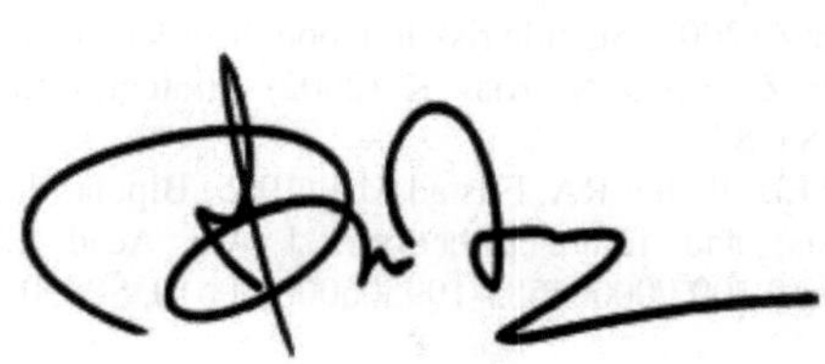

Thessaloniki, Greece
10 September 2014

Kostas N. Fountoulakis, MD, PhD

References

Akiskal HS (1995) Toward a temperament-based approach to depression: implications for neurobiologic research. Adv Biochem Psychopharmacol 49:99–112

Akiskal HS, McKinney WT Jr (1973) Depressive disorders: toward a unified hypothesis. Science 182(4107):20–29

Akiskal HS, Downs J, Jordan P, Watson S, Daugherty D, Pruitt DB (1985) Affective disorders in referred children and younger siblings of manic-depressives. Mode of onset and prospective course. Arch Gen Psychiatry 42 (10):996–1003

Aretaeus of Cappadocia (1856) The extant works of Aretaeus, the Cappadocian. Sydenham Society, London

Bech P (2006) The full story of lithium. A tribute to Mogens Schou (1918–2005). Psychother Psychosom 75(5):265–269

Cade J (1949) Lithium salts in the treatment of psychotic excitement. Med J Aust 36:349–352

Cade J (1970) The story of lithium. In: Ayd F, Blackwell B (eds) Discoveries in biological psychiatry. Lippincott, Philadelphia

Carlson GA, Strober M (1978) Manic-depressive illness in early adolescence. A study of clinical and diagnostic characteristics in six cases. J Am Acad Child Psychiatry 17(1):138–153

Delay J, Deniker P (1955) Neuroleptic effects of chlorpromazine in therapeutics of neuropsychiatry. J Clin Exp Psychopathol 16(2):104–112

Goodwin F, Jamison K (1990) Manic-depressive illness. Oxford University Press, New York

Isometsa E, Henriksson M, Aro H, Heikkinen M, Kuoppasalmi K, Lonnqvist J (1994) Suicide in psychotic major depression. J Affect Disord 31(3):187–191

Kendler KS, Karkowski-Shuman L (1997) Stressful life events and genetic liability to major depression: genetic control of exposure to the environment? Psychol Med 27(3):539–547

Kraepelin E (1921) Manic-depressive insanity and paranoia. Livingstone, Edinburgh

Lange F (1894) De vigtigste Sindssygdomme (The most important Pychiatric disorders). Gyldendal, Copenhagen

Luoma JB, Martin CE, Pearson JL (2002) Contact with mental health and primary care providers before suicide: a review of the evidence. Am J Psychiatry 159(6):909–916

Nazroo JY, Edwards AC, Brown GW (1997) Gender differences in the onset of depression following a shared life event: a study of couples. Psychol Med 27(1):9–19

Parry BL (1989) Reproductive factors affecting the course of affective illness in women. Psychiatr Clin North Am 12(1):207–220

Poznanski E, Zrull JP (1970) Childhood depression. Clinical characteristics of overtly depressed children. Arch Gen Psychiatry 23(1):8–15

Puig-Antich J (1987) Affective disorders in children and adolescents. In: Meltzer H (ed) Psychopharmacology: the third generation of progress. Raven, New York

Rihmer Z (2007) Suicide risk in mood disorders. Curr Opin Psychiatry 20(1):17–22

Rihmer Z, Belso N, Kiss K (2002) Strategies for suicide prevention. Curr Opin Psychiat 15:83–87

Weller EB, Weller RA, Fristad MA (1995) Bipolar disorder in children: misdiagnosis, underdiagnosis, and future directions. J Am Acad Child Adolesc Psychiatry 34(6):709–714. doi:10.1097/00004583-199506000-00010, S0890-8567(09)63568-1 [pii]

Historical Perspective

1

1.1 Antiquity

The history of mood disorders and specifically of bipolar disorder (BD) is dated as back as 3000 BC in ancient Egypt, when depression and bipolarity were mentioned in Ebers papyrus (book of the heart; Fig. 1.1) but described as heart diseases, not mental disorders (Okasha and Okasha 2000). In most contemporary societies, mental illness was attributed to magical forces, malevolent deities or demons, and 'treatment' was exercised by priests in the form of religious or magical rituals. Hippocrates (460–370 BC; Fig. 1.2), Galen (131–201 AD; Fig. 1.3) and Aretaeus of Cappadocia (Fig. 1.4) were the first to describe manic–depressive illness as mental illnesses.

The Hippocratic texts (today is believed to be the work of unknown authors) introduced the concept of the four essential body humours (phlegm, yellow bile, black bile and blood), secreted by different organs, possess different qualities and vary with the seasons. Early versions of this theory might had existed in ancient Egypt or Mesopotamia, but the essence of this approach is ascribed to the school of Cos and to Polybus which was a pupil and son-in-law to Hippocrates (fourth century BC) and author of the book Περί φύσεως αιvθρώπου (Peri physeos anthropou meaning 'On the Nature of Man'). This theory is in fact a microcosmic form of the macrocosmic theory of the four elements (earth, water, air, fire) and the four qualities (dry, wet, cold, hot) as first proposed by Empedocles (fifth century BC). Essentially it was a model with two factors: humidity and temperature.

In the Hippocratic texts it is mentioned that yellow bile causes manic rage, while black bile (which was under the influence of the planet Saturn and related to autumn) caused melancholia (in ancient Greek melan = black, choli = bile), and this constitutes the very first biological model of a mental disorder. It is also important that they believed that the black bile causes melancholia because it influences the brain. Long-lasting anxiety, fear and moodiness were described as core characteristics of melancholia. Concerning mania, they believed that it is caused by excess of blood. Different patterns of body fluids was believed to underlie different idiosyncrasies (in Greek ιδιοσυγκρασίες meaning unique or characteristic admixtures of elements,

K.N. Fountoulakis, *Bipolar Disorder: An Evidence-Based Guide to Manic Depression*, DOI 10.1007/978-3-642-37216-2_1

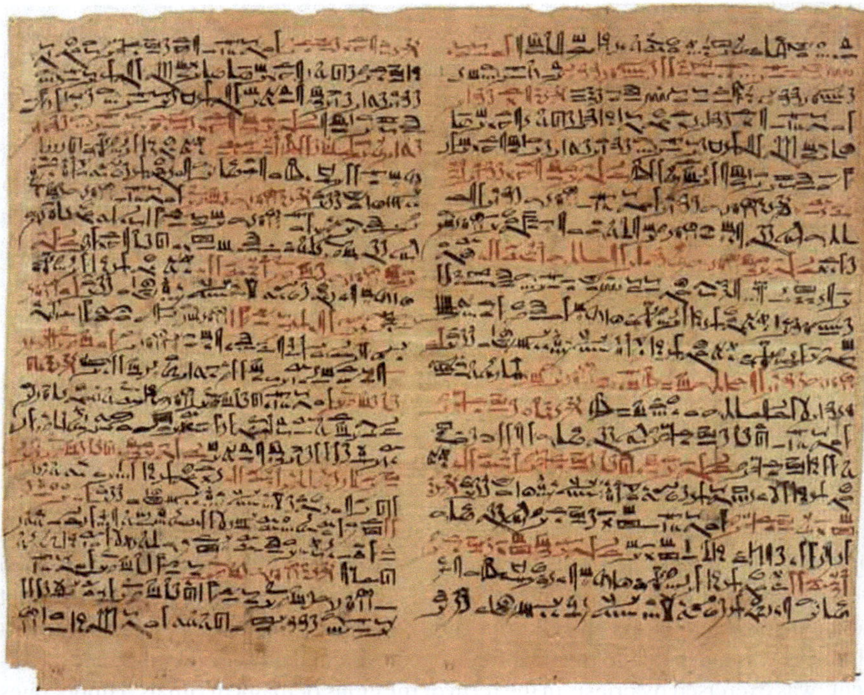

Fig. 1.1 Ebers Papyrus (book of the heart); Egypt c. 3000 BC

temperaments). It is interesting to mention that it was thought that yellow bile was responsible for the choleric temperament (irritable, hostile and given to rage) while phlegm for the phlegmatic (indolent, irresolute and timid).

These authors described and classified mania and melancholia for the first time. These two concepts are the oldest ones in psychiatry. Their view of mania probably corresponds to what we consider 'excited psychoses' today, while melancholia corresponds to anxious fearful depression rather than what we today consider 'melancholic features'.

The etymology of the word 'mania' is interesting since it reflects the early concepts for this condition. It has the same root with the Greek words μένος (menos) and μήνις (minis) which both mean anger. It is also related to the verb μένω (meno = stay) and thus reflects a condition in which the state of the mind is stalled because of the intrusion of anger and intense emotions. Interestingly, in ancient Greek the word μήνις, which is related to the Latin word *mens* (=mind), also means crescent and thus relates the states of the mind with the phases of the moon. The Greek word for month (which corresponds to moon phases) is μήνας (minas), while the Latin word is *mensis*. This group includes also the words 'menses' and 'menstrual', and thus they possess both a temporal/cyclical and an emotional meaning. The word μαινάς (=maenad) used for women who participated in the orgiastic rites of God Dionysus and μηνίσκος (meniscus of the knee) have a similar etymology. Peculiarly, in his book 'On acute diseases' the Roman physician Caelius Aurelianus, which

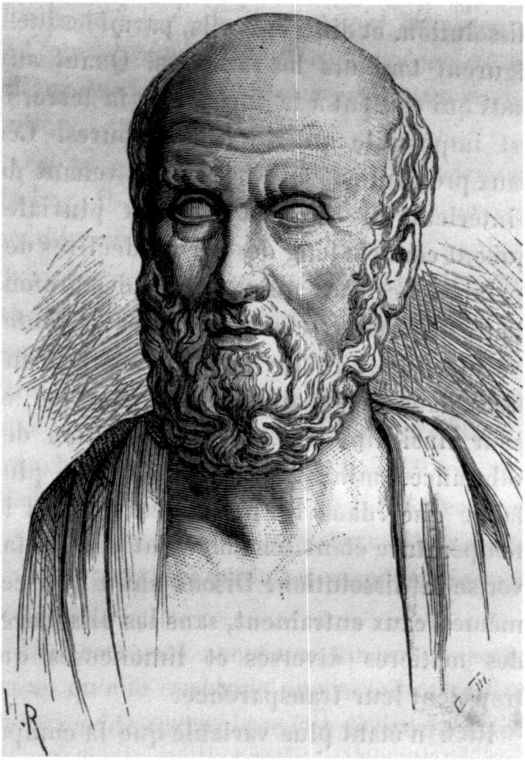

Fig. 1.2 Hippocrates (460–370 BC)

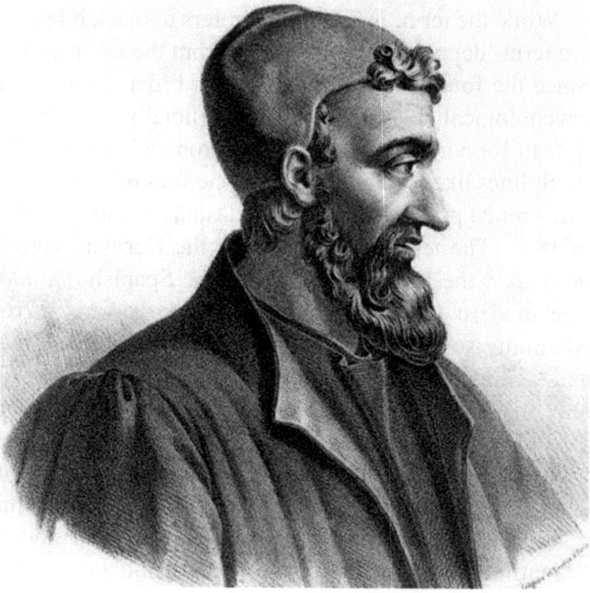

Fig. 1.3 Galen (131–201 AD)

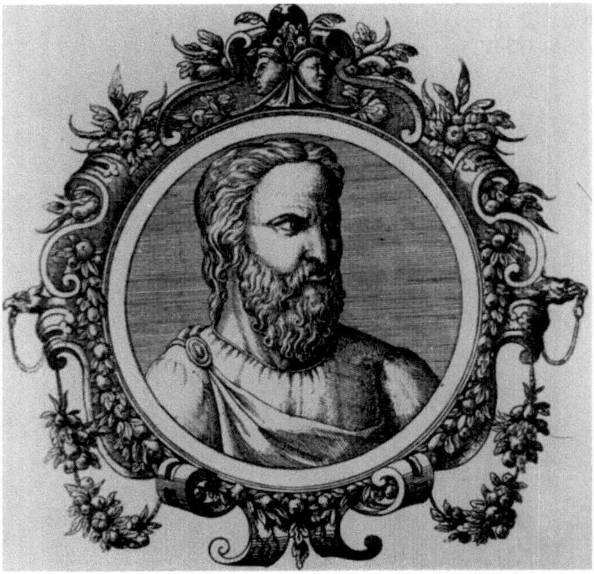

Fig. 1.4 Aretaeus of Cappadocia (second century AD)

was a student of Soranus of Ephesus and member of the Methodist school, suggested several different etymologies. One of them relates mania to the Greek word ανία (ania = dysphoric boredom), while another to the word λυμαίνειν (lymainin = devastate, defile). The other options include variations like μονούσθαι (monousthae = seeks solitude) or υπομονετικός (ypomonetikos = having patience). It is obvious that the term 'mania' belongs to a group of words coming from the Ancient Greek language and refers to mind and its states, intense emotions and especially anger, crescent and phases of the moon, loneliness and patience.

While the term 'melancholia' refers to black bile (as mentioned above), the modern term 'depression' was derived from the Latin verb *deprimere* (=to press down). Since the fourteenth century, the word 'depression' was used to denote a negative psychological state, and this was officially done in written language for the first time in 1665 in Richard Baker's 'Chronicle'. The term is also used in other scientific disciplines like physiology and economics (e.g. 'the great depression' of the 1930s). The French psychiatrist Louis Delasiauve (1804–1893) was the first to use the term in 1856. The term is equivalent to the German word *niedergedruckt*, the English *downcast*, the French *abattement*, the Spanish *abatido* and the Italian *essere giu*. The modern Greek translation of depression is κατάθλιψη (katathlipsi = overwhelming sorrow). The word κατά means among others 'overwhelming', 'down' and 'against', while it is to be noted that in Greek the verb θλίβω (thlivo) means not only that I cause sorrow but also that I break into pieces. In this sense, the word κατάθλιψη also means 'total breaking' and 'destruction'.

Ancient Greeks described melancholia as a state of aversion to food, despondency, sleeplessness, irritability and restlessness, and they also recognized the close relationship between depression and anxiety. Also they were the first to recommend 'scientific', 'non-metaphysical' therapeutic interventions, like personal hygiene,

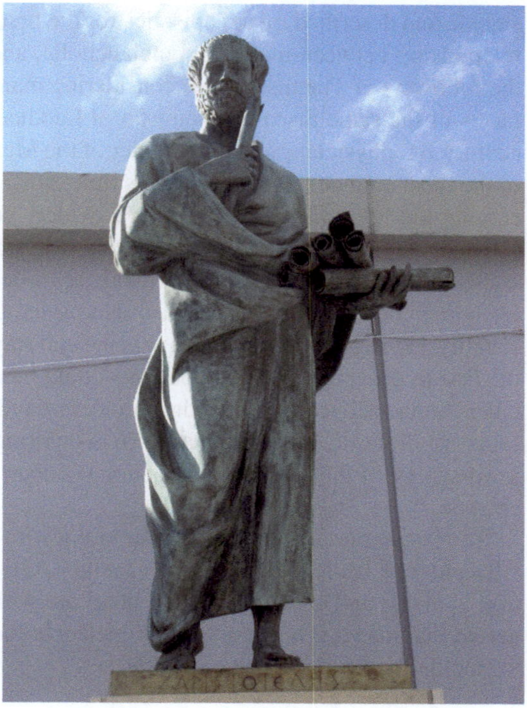

Fig. 1.5 Aristotle (384–322 BC). Statue in the campus of the Aristotle University of Thessaloniki, Greece

bathing and dieting so as to keep the humours in balance. They also used purgatives, cathartics and bleeding as a more aggressive attempt to reset the balance of humours in more difficult or emergency cases. At that period, psychological treatments were also available, including the interpretation of dreams as well as talking to encourage, console and understanding of the illness (Plato's dialectics).

In general, during the times of ancient Greece and the Roman Empire, religion, science and philosophy were interplexed in the way mental illness was conceived. The psychological vs. somatic approach has its roots in that time period, and essentially it derives from the differences in the philosophical views of Plato (424–348 BC) vs. Aristotle (384–322 BC) (Fig. 1.5). Aristotle was the first to describe accurately the affections of desire, anger, fear, courage, envy, joy, hatred and pity. He was the first to suggest a predisposition to develop melancholia in those who possess an excess of black bile (melancholic temperament), and additionally in his writings we find the first mentioning of a relationship between creativity and melancholic temperament.

Latter, Galen's treatise 'On Melancholia' influenced medical thinking for almost 15 centuries. In its treatise, Galen (131–201 AD) makes a description of fear and aggression inherent in the pathophysiology of depression. Galen proposed that mania could be either primary or secondary to other diseases, and his most important contribution in the field was the elaboration of the theory of humours. According to Aurelianus, his contemporary Soranus of Ephesus (first to second century AD) refereed to the episodic nature of depression, linked depression and aggression to suicide and described mixed episodes for the first time. Soranus probably rejected a relationship between mania and melancholia, and in his writings he mentions that the followers of Themison were considering mania and melancholia to be different facets of the same disease. Themison of Laodicea (modern-day Syria) was a first-century BC physician, was the founder of the Methodic school of medicine and one of the most eminent physicians of his time; however, we know almost nothing concerning his life and works. Thus, it is widely considered that it was Aretaeus of Cappadocia (second century AD) the one who strongly connected melancholy with mania and made a description of manic episodes very close to modern approach, including comorbid personality disorder, psychotic features, alcohol abuse and seasonality. He suggested that mania was the end stage of melancholia, and he was also the first to observe that manic patients could be either euphoric or aggressive–irritable. Aretaeus lived in Alexandria (modern-day Egypt) and was a prominent representative of the school of Eclectics. In his writings he considers mania to represent a worsening of the disease (melancholia) rather than a distinct type of disorder or episode.

The last important physician of antiquity who studied mania and depression was Alexander of Tralles in Lydia (sixth century AD) who wrote on the cyclical alternation of mania and melancholia, and in accord with Aretaeus of Cappadocia, he suggested that mania is a worse form of melancholia and that melancholia predisposes to suicidality but also to homicidality.

1.2 Middle Ages

After the fall of the Greco-Roman world, science and particularly medicine retreated in front of religious–metaphysical approaches and priests, and the church took over health and particularly mental health in Europe. Thus, during the tenth and eleventh century AD, Arab scholars dominated medicine. Avicenna (980–1037) further developed the theory of the temperaments (Fig. 1.6). He also observed that the emergence of anger, restlessness and violence marked the transition from melancholia to mania. Ishaq Ibn Imran developed an early bio-psychosocial model by suggesting that melancholia is caused by 'damaged father's sperm' in interaction with temperament and circadian rhythms.

In Europe in 1486 two monks, Henry Kramer (1430–1505) and James Sprenger (1436–1495), published the Malleus Maleficarum which resulted in the persecution of mental patients as being witches. Later, Paracelsus (ca. 1493–1541) rejected the theory of body humours, but his medical ideas were often confused, contradictory and influenced by philosophy, astrology, magic and myths (Fig. 1.7). During the late Middle Ages, science and medicine gradually gain ground, and eventually in the early seventeenth century, empirical scientific approaches, free of metaphysical and religious influences, start appearing again in Europe.

In 1602 Felix Platter (1536–1614) published his classification of mental diseases, but he failed to connect mania with depression. In 1621, Robert Burton (1577–1640) wrote the first English-speaking text on the field of mood disorders,

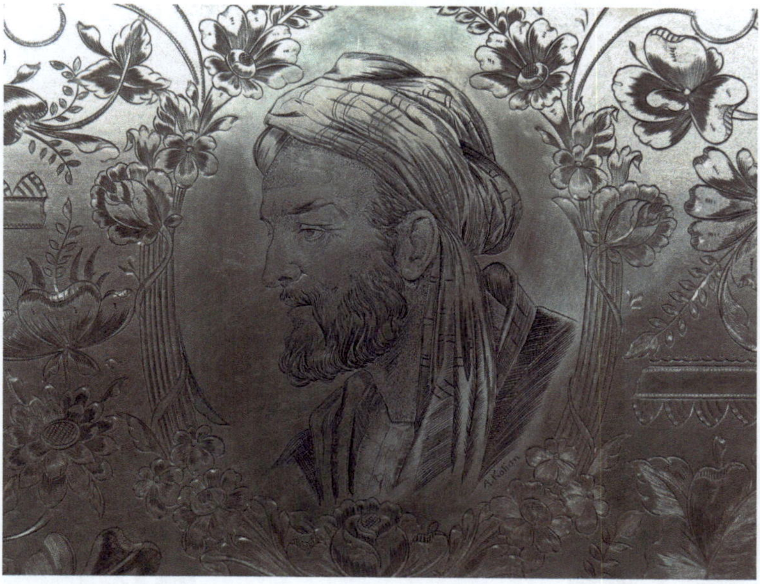

Fig. 1.6 Avicenna (980–1037) Portrait on Silver Tea Tray – Museum at BuAli Sina (Avicenna) Mausoleum, Hamadan, Western Iran

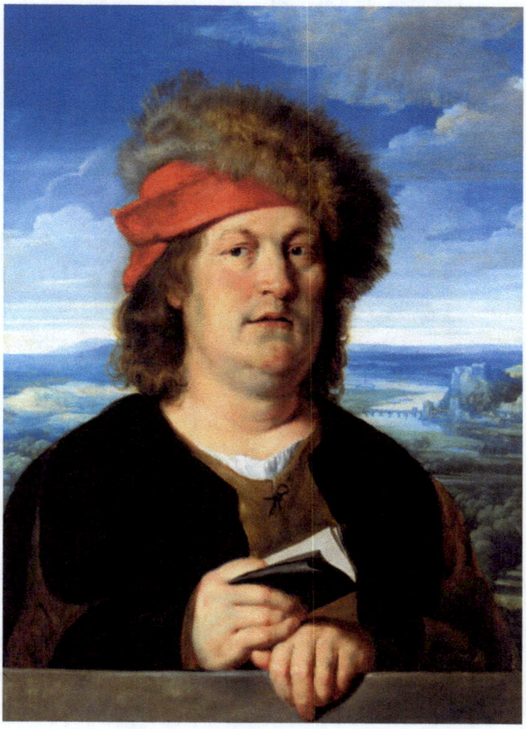

Fig. 1.7 Paracelsus (ca. 1493–1541). Portrait by Quentin Massys

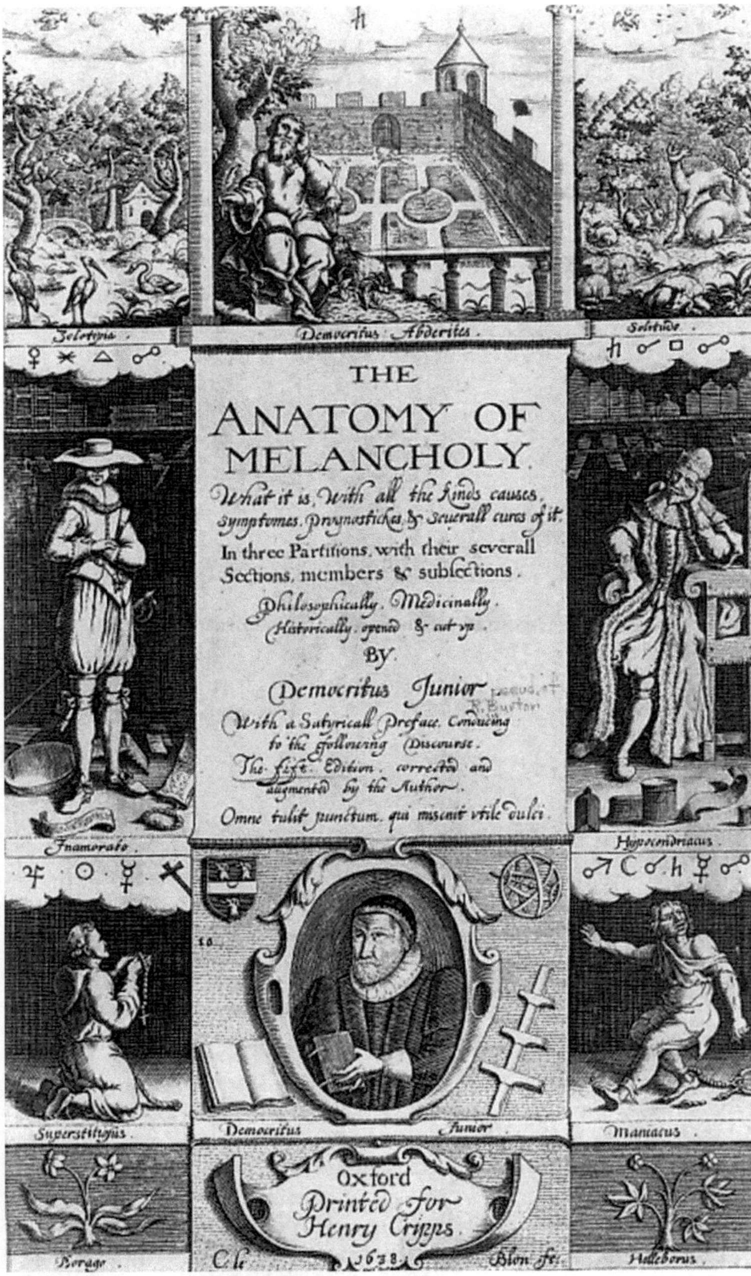

Fig. 1.8 Robert Burton's (1577–1640) 'Anatomy of Melancholy' cover page

the 'Anatomy of Melancholy' (Fig. 1.8), which was a scholarly review of medical and philosophical wisdom accumulated in the past. Among other things, Burton created a list of causes of melancholia (including among others the influence of planet Saturn, autumn, heredity, diet, alcohol, biological rhythms and intense love) but also mentioned the existence of 'causeless' melancholias. Interestingly, like others before him he considered men to be at a higher risk, and also he made an early reference to mixed depressive episodes and to BD-II by suggesting that both melancholic and sanguine temperaments are responsible for the emergence of depression.

A pivotal moment in the history of modern psychiatry and neurosciences is the suggestion of mind–body dichotomy (Cartesian dualism) by René Descartes (1596–1650) in his books 'The Description of the Human Body' (1647) and 'Passions of the Soul' (1649). This assumption suggested that mind was distinct from matter, but could influence matter (through an unknown way). This was essentially a compromise between the Catholic Church and the scientific community, allowing medicine to progress in issues pertaining to the physical body, but the same time kept the realm of human behaviour (and mental health) still in the 'jurisdiction' of religion.

It seems that the first modern description of a mixed state was made by the seventeenth-century physician Brouchier in 1679 and concerned one of his patients, namely, Lady Grenville (Goodwin and Jamison 2007).

1.3 Modern Era

Andrés Piquer-Arrufat (1711–1772) described the alternation of manic and depressive episodes in King Ferdinand VI of Spain (in 1759). He considered them both to constitute a single diagnostic entity. He also described mixed states, seasonality and rapid cycling and included his approach in a medical textbook he published in 1764 (Perez et al. 2011). At that time, the need for gathering and organizing the various independent observations and reports into a comprehensive classification system was evident for medicine. It was the work of Carl Linnaeus (1707–1778), the Swedish father of modern taxonomy, whose book 'Species Plantarum' published in 1753 is considered to be the starting point of modern botanical nomenclature, who created a scientific earthquake and pushed physicians towards a similar direction.

William Cullen (1710–1790) repeats the suggestions of Aretaeus of Cappadocia, and in his book 'First Lines of the Practice of Physic' (repeated editions through the years 1777–1784), he writes that the same state of brain dysfunction when moderate causes melancholia and when extreme it causes mania. Benjamin Rush (1745–1813), the father of American psychiatry, described 'tristimania' (from Latin *tristis* = sorrow) as a form of melancholia with sadness as the predominant feature (Fig. 1.9). Jean-Philippe Esquirol (1772–1840) was the first to clearly point that melancholia was a disorder of the mood (of 'passions') with 'partial insanity' (monomania) (Fig. 1.10). He used the word 'lypemania' (from Greek λύπη = sorrow) to describe a kind of depressive insanity. Thus both Rush and Esquirol used the term 'mania' to denote insanity and not elevated mood. Johann Christian August Heinroth (1773–1843) classified mental disorders into 'hyperthymias', 'asthenias' and 'hypo-asthenias'. In 'hyperthymias' he included 'melancholia erotica', 'melancholia metamorphosis' and 'melancholia saltans'. Clearly mixed states dominate

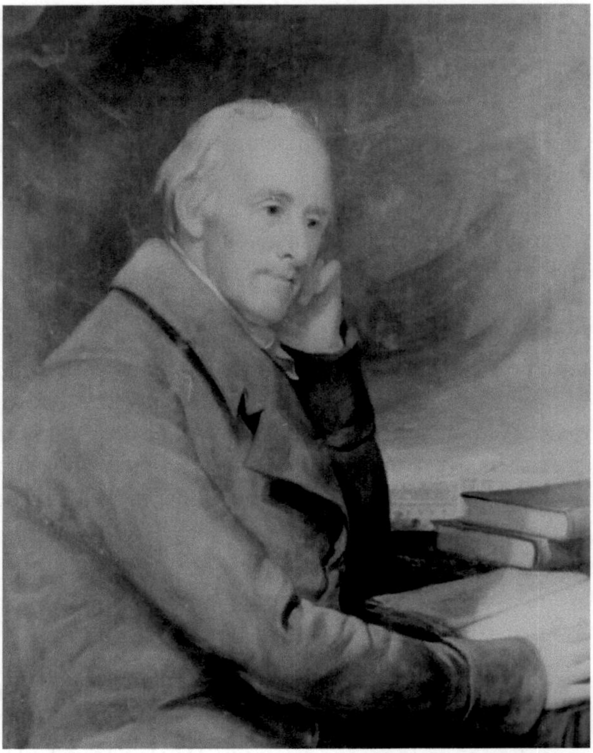

Fig. 1.9 Benjamin Rush (1745–1813)

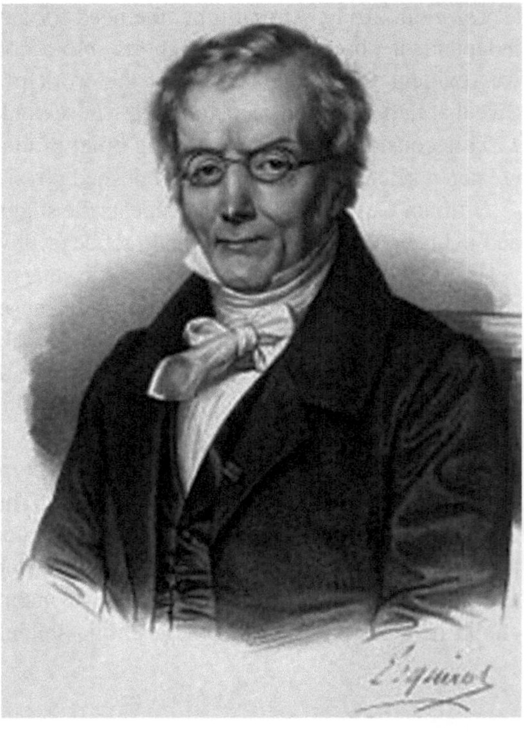

Fig. 1.10 Jean-Philippe Esquirol (1772–1840)

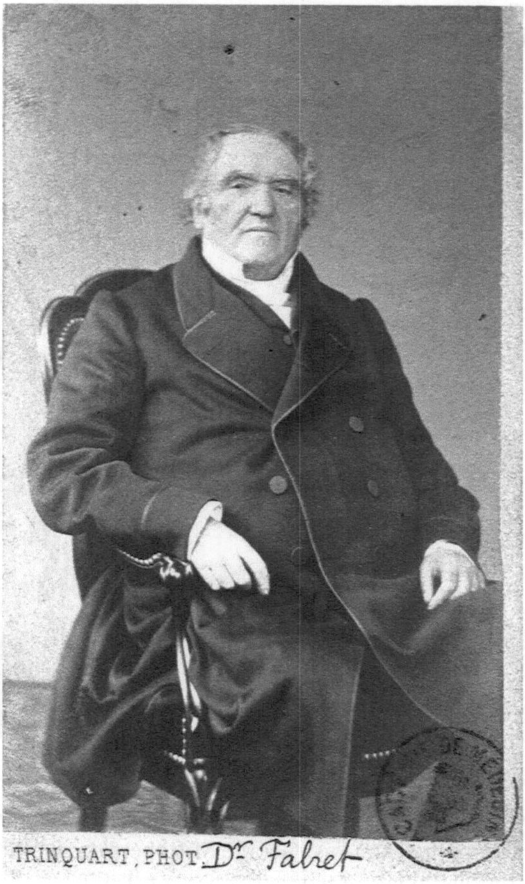

Fig. 1.11 Jean-Pierre Falret (1794–1870)

his works, and this is also the case in the writings of Joseph Guislain (1797–1860). Jean-Pierre Falret (1794–1870) (Fig. 1.11) and Jules Gabriel Francois Baillarger (1809–1890) (Fig. 1.12) established the connection between depression and mania. Jean-Pierre Falret (Fig. 1.11) in 1851 defined it as an illness and gave it a name ('folie circulaire' or 'folie à double forme'). In 1858 Frank Richarz introduced the term 'agitated depression'. Following them Henry Maudsley (1835–1918) coined the term 'affective disorder' to describe milder forms of melancholia without psychotic features.

During the middle of the nineteenth century, the 'unitary psychosis theory' (einheitspsychose), appeared in the works of Joseph Guislain (1797–1860), Ernst Albrecht von Zeller (1804–1877), Wilhelm Griesinger (1817–1868) and Heinrich Neumann (1814–1888) (Angst 2002; Berrios and Beer 1994; Moller 2008).

Karl Ludwig Kahlbaum (1828–1899) and especially his pupil Ewald Hecker (1843–1909) developed the concepts of hebephrenia and cyclothymia and proposed the existence of more than one discrete psychiatric disorder, in sharp contrast to the concept of 'unitary psychosis', thus preparing the way for the separation between schizophrenia and manic depression. Emanuel Mendel (1839–1907) was the first to officially describe hypomania in 1881, as a milder form of mania, and this was in

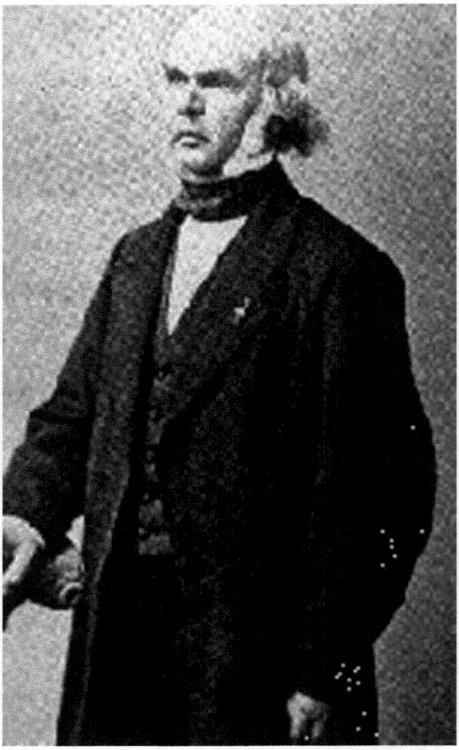

Fig. 1.12 Jules Baillarger (1809–1890)

sharp contrast to the previous traditions which were focusing on chronic patients with poor prognosis. George M Robertson in 1890 described the 'hilarious' and the 'furious' types of mania (Robertson 1890).

Finally, Emil Kraepelin (1856–1926; Fig. 1.13) in his sixth but in more details in the eighth edition of his textbook of psychiatry in 1899 established manic–depressive illness as a distinct nosological entity and separated it from schizophrenia, on the basis of heredity, longitudinal follow-up and a supposed favourable outcome (Kraepelin 1921). In clinical terms, Kraepelin suggested that depression is characterized by lowered mood and physical and psychomotor retardation, while on the contrary, mania is characterized by elevation and acceleration of these processes. He also described 'involutional melancholia' as a form of agitated mixed state. His pupil Wilhelm Weygandt (1870–1939) published the first book on mixed clinical states (Weygandt 1899). Weygandt considered stupor to be the most important element of mixed state.

Kraepelin conceptualized three basic dimensions (fundamental symptoms) of BD. These concern mood (euphoria vs. depression), cognition (flight of ideas vs. thought slowing) and physical activity (hyperactivity vs. inhibition). He proposed that these three dimensions fluctuate independently, and the combination of their phases could thus produce six different types of affective episodes: (a) depressive or anxious mania (depressed affect with flight of ideas and hyperactivity), (b) excited

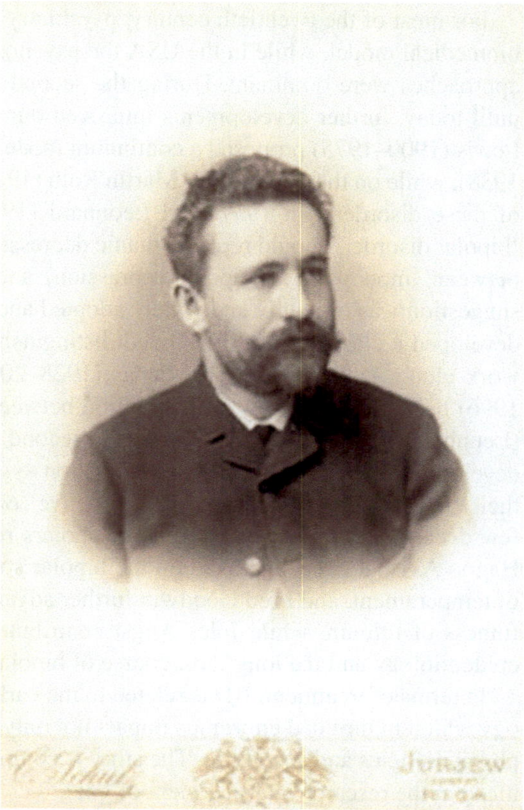

Fig. 1.13 Emil Kraepelin (1856–1926)

depression (depressed affect with thought poverty and hyperactivity), (c) mania with thought poverty (manic affect with thought poverty and hyperactivity), (d) manic stupor (manic affect with thought poverty and inhibition), (e) depression with flight of ideas (depressed affect with flight of ideas and inhibition) and (f) inhibited mania (manic affect with flight of ideas and inhibition).

Following a similar line of thinking, and in spite of some important objections to the Kraepelinian approach, Karl Jaspers (1883–1969) described aspects of mixed depressive states which he named 'querulant mania', 'nagging depression' or 'wailing melancholia'(Jaspers 1913).

Eugen Bleuler coined the term 'affective illness', and in this way he broadened the concept of manic depression. He also pointed to the relationship between schizophrenia and manic depression and suggested they lie on a continuum.

During the same period, Ernst Kretschmer (1888–1964) and William H. Sheldon (1899–1977) proposed that body types correlate with personality, temperament and mental health. They suggested that thin, asthenic individuals are prone to introversion, schizoid tendencies and schizophrenia, while short and round individuals are extrovert and with cyclothymic personalities and manic depression. Their theories are not of academic value anymore, but continue to influence lay people.

For most of the twentieth century, psychiatry in Europe continued to follow the biomedical model, while in the USA the psychosocial model and psychoanalytical approaches were dominant. During the second half of the twentieth century and until today, further developments improved our understanding of BD. Sir Aubrey Lewis (1900–1975) proposed a continuum model from anxiety to psychosis (Lewis 1938), while on the contrary Sir Martin Roth (1917–2006) suggested categorization of these disorders. In 1957 Karl Leonhard (1902–1988) proposed that the term 'bipolar disorder' should replace 'manic depression', and he also made a distinction between 'monopolar' (unipolar depression) and 'bipolar' illness. Eventually his suggestion was officially and widely adopted and included in the DSM-III. He also developed a classification of BD and distinguished it from cycloid psychoses. His work along with that of Carlo Perris (1928–2000) and George Winokur (1925–1996) helped establishing the distinction between unipolar and bipolar depression (Leonhard 1957a, b, 1979). During the second half of the twentieth century, the development of the two major classification systems (DSM and ICD), in spite of their shortcomings, confirmed the 'objective' orientation of diagnosis. In the last few decades, a number of prominent scholars reshaped the concept of bipolarity. Hagop Akiskal conceptualized on the bipolar spectrum and elaborated on the role of temperament, and Fred Goodwin further advanced our understanding of the usefulness of lithium, while Jules Angst contributed valuable long-term data on the epidemiology and the long-term course of bipolar illness.

In terms of treatment, BD is related to the earliest progress in psychopharmacology which in turn had enormous impact not only on psychiatry but also on philosophy, ideologies and social life. The story is complex and involves also the advances made in the research and treatment of gout.

In 1847 Alfred Baring Garrod (1819–1907) announced that he had discovered uric acid in the blood of gouty patients. Since at least in the laboratory, lithium could dissolve uric acid crystals isolated from the kidneys, using lithium to dissolve urate in the body seemed a logical step. Garrod discovered that gouty uric acid deposits in finger joints are soluble in vitro in a lithium solution, and Alexander Ure (early nineteenth century to 1866) in 1843 introduced lithium into medicine by showing that in vitro a uric acid bladder stone lost weight in a lithium carbonate solution. It is interesting that according to the works of Armand Trousseau (1801–1867) in France and Alexander Haig in the UK, mania and depression are related to the uric acid nosology (brain gout). Although Garrod made lithium treatment of gout widely known in 1859, unfortunately it was proven that the levels of lithium needed to dissolve urate in the body were toxic (Marmol 2008; Shorter 2009; Johnson and Amdisen 1983; Strobusch and Jefferson 1980). Following these observations and suggestions, a number of beverages included lithium as their component in the late nineteenth and early twentieth century. Charles Leiper Grigg (1868–1940) introduced a lemon–lime soft drink in 1929 under the label 'Bib-Label Lithiated Lemon-Lime Soda' which soon changed to 7 Up. However by 1948 lithium has been removed from all beverages because of cases of toxicity, and its free marketing was prohibited (Marmol 2008). In parallel, a number of remedies with lithium were marketed in the early twentieth century and were mostly indicated for the control of renal calculi and 'uric acid diathesis' (Shorter 2009).

Fig. 1.14 Carl Georg Lange (1834–1900)

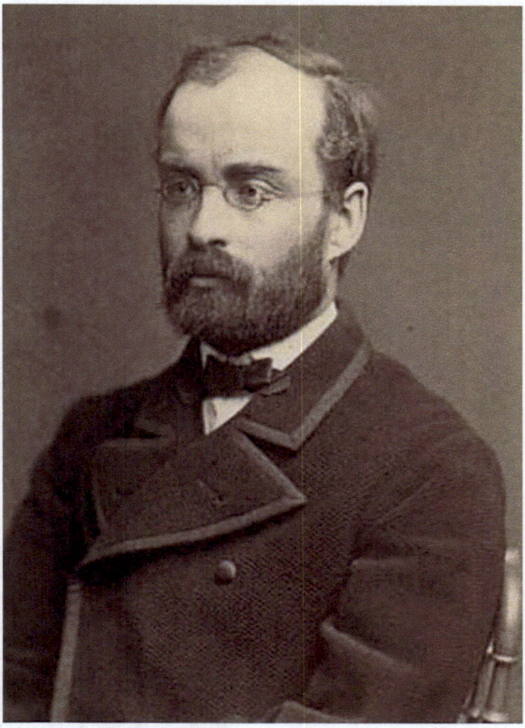

The first psychiatric indication for lithium came from Silas Weir Mitchell (1829–1914), a neurologist from Philadelphia, in 1870. Mitchell recommended lithium as anticonvulsant and hypnotic (Mitchell 1870) and letter for 'general nervousness' (Mitchell 1877). Already in 1871, William Alexander Hammond (1828–1900) was maybe the first to prescribe a modern and effective psychotropic agent, and this was lithium (Mitchell and Hadzi-Pavlovic 2000). At that time he was professor of Diseases of the Mind and Nervous System at the Bellevue Hospital Medical College in New York. The Danish psychiatrist Carl Lange (1834–1900) (Fig. 1.14) used lithium in the treatment of recurrent brief depression in 1886, while his brother Frederik Lange (1842–1907) used lithium in the treatment of 35 melancholic depressive patients (including some milder forms of BD) in 1894 (Lenox and Watson 1994).

However in spite of encouraging results, by the turn of the twentieth century, the 'brain gout' theory of mood disorders disappeared as a medical entity, and the use of lithium in psychiatry was abandoned.

Just before WWII, the Italians Ugo Cerletti (1877–1963) and Lucio Bini (1908–1964) developed electroconvulsive therapy (ECT) for the treatment of mental disorders. ECT continues to constitute a valuable tool especially in refractory bipolar cases.

After the WWII, in 1949 in the Bundoora Repatriation Hospital, a veterans hospital in a suburb of Melbourne, the Australian John Cade (1912–1980) injected

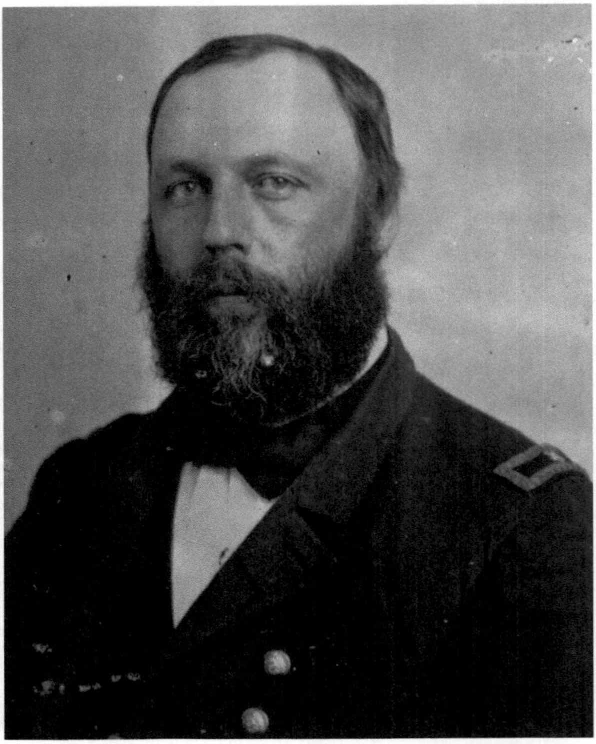

Fig. 1.15 William Alexander Hammond (1828–1900)

urine from patients with schizophrenia to guinea pigs to test the hypothesis that mania is caused by intoxication by a normal body element circulating in excess, while melancholia is the corresponding deprative condition. He used lithium urate as control and observed it and caused the rodents to be tranquilized. In fact it is possible that the animals were lethargic because of lithium toxicity, and this seems to be the case with the patients of William Alexander Hammond, since the dosages reported by both researchers lead to lithium intoxication (Fig. 1.15). In 1949 Cade reported positive results from the treatment of 10 acutely manic patients (Cade 1949, 2000); however, 2 years later he reported the first death because of lithium toxicity in a patient whose bipolar illness otherwise responded extremely well to treatment (Fig. 1.16). Subsequent research with other ions (rubidium, cesium, lanthanum, neodymium and strontium) gave no positive results.

During the 1950s several researchers studied lithium and its usefulness in BD (Noack and Trautner 1951). However the important contribution that made the difference came from Denmark again in 1952, when Erik Stromgren (1909–1993), head of the Aarhus University psychiatric clinic in Risskov at that time, asked Mogens Schou (1918–2005) (Fig. 1.17) to undertake a randomized controlled trial of lithium in mania (Bech 2006). Mogens Schou was not a psychiatrist but a physician specialized in clinical chemistry and had observed a dramatic therapeutic effect of long-term lithium treatment in his younger brother. Schou randomized acutely manic patients with a flip of a coin to lithium or placebo, and in 1954 he published the results which made a significant impact (Schou et al. 1954). However lithium was still difficult to administer and blood levels a matter of guesswork. The

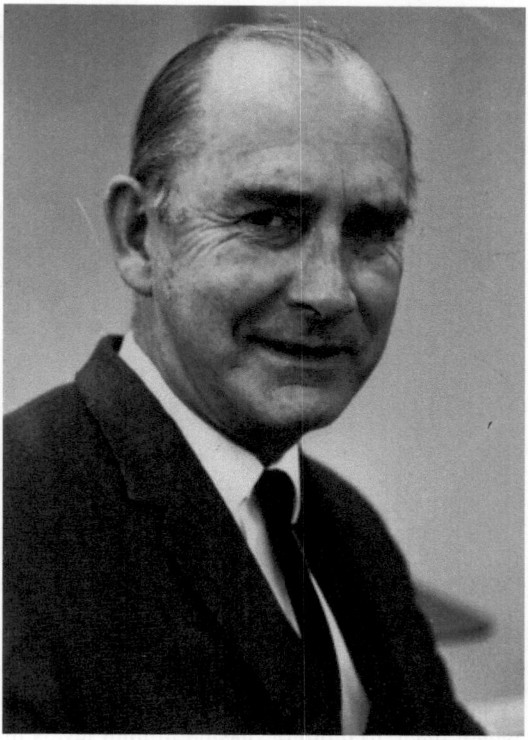

Fig. 1.16 John Cade (1912–1980)

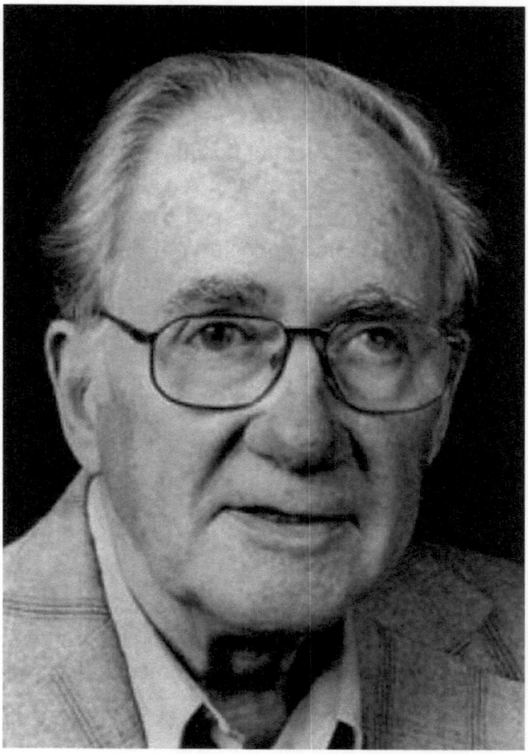

Fig. 1.17 Mogens Schou (1918–2005)

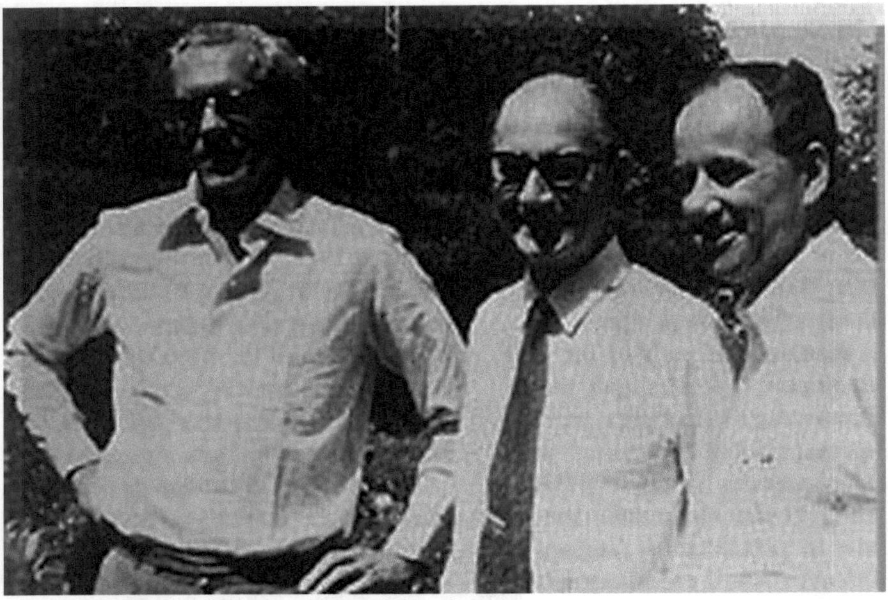

Fig. 1.18 John Cade, Mogens Schou and Paul Christian Baastrup

situation changed with the introduction of the Coleman flame photometer in 1958 which made to monitor plasma lithium levels much more precisely in comparison to the previously used Beckman photometer.

It was, however, the Danish psychiatrist Poul Christian Baastrup (1918–2002) who demonstrated in 1964 the efficacy of lithium for the maintenance phase (Baastrup 1964) (Fig. 1.18). In the USA in 1960, Samuel Gershon joined the Schizophrenia and Psycho- pharmacology Joint Research Project of the University of Michigan at the mental hospital in Ypsilanti, Michigan, and the same year along with Arthur Yuwiler, also at Ypsilanti, they published the first North American paper on lithium (Gershon and Yuwiler 1960). For the next few years, there was significant academic opposition to the use of lithium as the standard treatment for BD, and much emphasis was given to its toxicity. Aubrey Lewis (1900–1975), professor of psychiatry and head of the Maudsley, considered lithium treatment 'dangerous nonsense', and Michael Shepherd (1923–1995) was also extremely negative towards it and suggested that lithium was toxic in mania and that claims of efficacy for it in preventing depression rested on 'dubious scientific methodology' (Blackwell and Shepherd 1968; Shepherd 1970; Blackwell 1969, 1970, 1971, 1972). However later studies established lithium and robustly linked it to the treatment of all phases of (Schou et al. 1970; Angst et al. 1969, 1970; Baastrup et al. 1970; Baastrup and Schou 1967; Bech 2006; Schioldann 1999, 2006, 2011; Johnstone et al. 1988; Mitchell and Hadzi-Pavlovic 2000). Latter Fred Goodwin suggested it could be also useful in the treatment of depression as add-on to antidepressants (Goodwin et al. 1969a, b, 1972; 2003; Goodwin 2002; Goodwin and Zis 1979). The recommended serum lithium levels were determined with certainty in 1976 (Bech et al. 1976). The

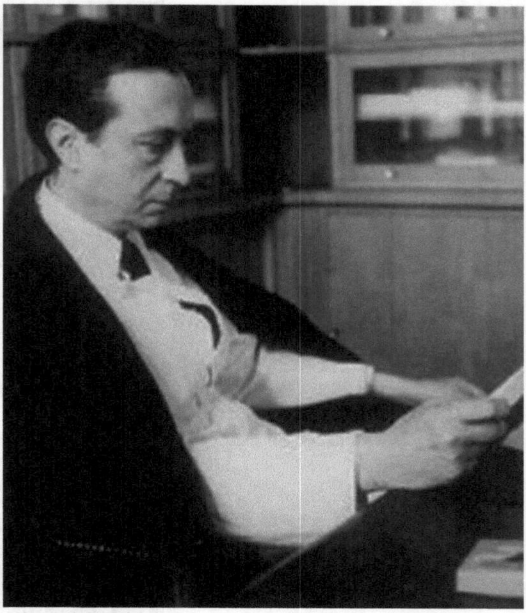

Fig. 1.19 Jean Delay (1907–1987)

term 'mood normalizer' was proposed by Mogens Schou for lithium (Schou 1963) after the term 'mood stabilizer', which was used during the 1950s to refer to a combination of amphetamine and a barbiturate to treat patients with neurotic instability but not patients with BD.

Lithium treatment for BD was approved in 1961 in France, in 1966 in the UK, in 1967 in Germany and in 1970 in Italy and the USA. In 1974, this application was extended to its use as a preventive agent for manic–depressive illness (Mitchell and Hadzi-Pavlovic 2000).

Following the success with lithium treatment, valproate was introduced in 1966 (Lambert et al. 1966) and later carbamazepine (Okuma et al. 1979). Antipsychotics were introduced by Jean Delay (1907–1987) (Fig. 1.19) and Pierre Deniker (1917–1999) (Fig. 1.20) in 1955, and probably many of their patients were bipolar suffering from acute mania (Delay and Deniker 1955). Though widely prescribed, antipsychotics were 'academically' accepted only after 2000 mostly because second-generation agents carry a low incidence of tardive dyskinesia. Benzodiazepines were introduced by Leo Henryk Sternbach (1908–2005) in 1956. In 1958 Roland Kuhn (1912–2005) (Fig. 1.21) reported on the efficacy of the first antidepressant, imipramine (Kuhn 1958).

There were several reports in the 1970s suggesting that the use of antidepressants might induce mania, mixed episodes and rapid cycling. In 1994 the first detailed operational treatment guidelines were published by the American Psychiatric Association, and after 2000 there was a systematic industry-sponsored study of second-generation antipsychotics (SGAs) and haloperidol. Also, during this period the first meta-analytic studies emerged, and the evidence-based medicine principles gained ground in the treatment recommendations (Table 1.1).

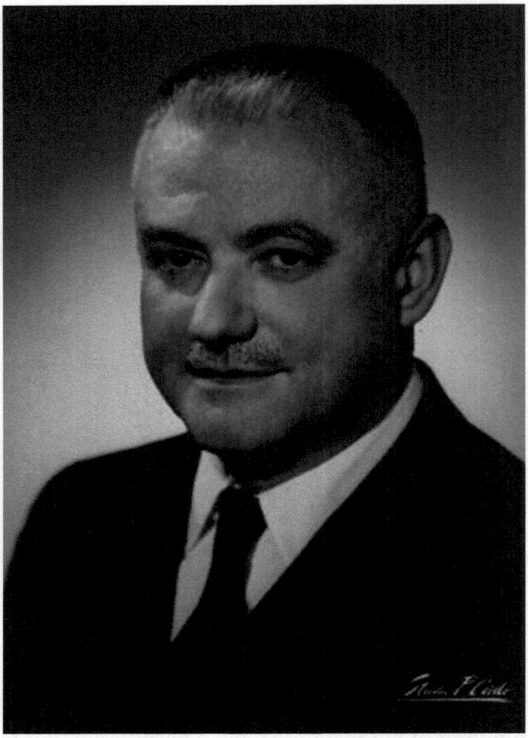

Fig. 1.20 Pierre Deniker (1917–1999)

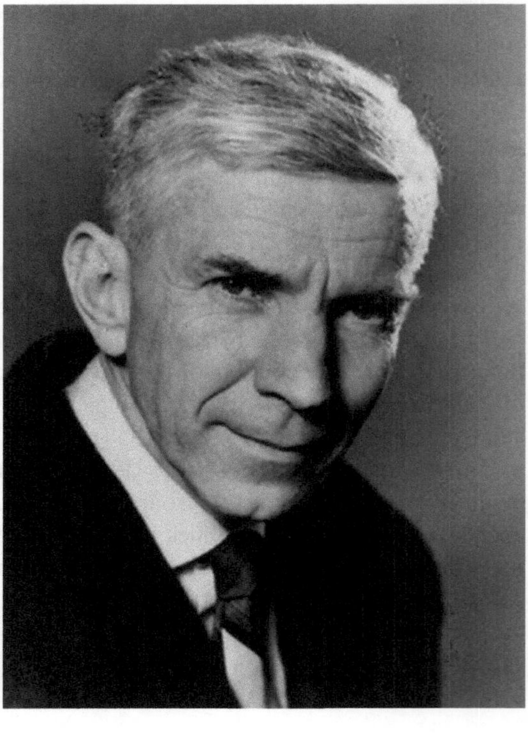

Fig. 1.21 Roland Kuhn (1912–2005)

Table 1.1 Chronological chart of the most important developments in the understanding of bipolar disorder

Person or event	Country	Contribution
Hippocrates of Cos (ca 460–370 BC) and Polybus	Greece	The 4 humours theory
Plato (424–348 BC)	Greece	Interpretation of and psychotherapeutic techniques, e.g. talking to encourage, console and understanding of the illness (Plato's dialectics)
Aristotle (384–322 BC)	Greece	Described the affections of desire, anger, fear, courage, envy, joy, hatred and pity. Related creativity to melancholy
Galen of Pergamum (131–201 AD)	Greek Asia Minor during the Roman Empire period	Elaborated on the thoughts of Hippocrates, Plato and Aristotle. His approach determined medical thinking for the next 15 centuries
Soranus of Ephesus (first to second century AD)	Rome and Alexandria during the Roman Empire period	Episodic nature of depression, linked depression and aggression to suicide and described mixed episodes for the first time
Aretaeus of Cappadocia (second century AD)	Alexandria during the Roman Empire period	Strongly connected melancholy with mania. Described manic episodes including comorbid personality disorder, psychotic features, alcohol abuse and seasonality
Avicenna (980–1037)	Persia	Wrote the Canon of Medicine; further developed the theory of temperaments
Paracelsus (ca. 1493–1541)	Switzerland	Rejected the theory of body humours, but his medical ideas were often confused, contradictory and influenced by philosophy, astrology, magic and myths
Robert Burton (1577–1640)	England	The 'Anatomy of Melancholy', a scholarly review of medical and philosophical wisdom. It included a list of causes of melancholia but also mentioned the existence of 'causeless' melancholias. Mentioned temperaments and mixed states
Benjamin Rush (1745–1813)	US	Described 'tristimania' as a form of melancholia with sadness as the predominant feature
Jean-Philippe Esquirol (1772–1840)	France	Was the first to clearly point that melancholia was a disorder of the mood with 'partial insanity'. He used the word 'lypemania' to describe a kind of depressive insanity
Johann Christian August Heinroth (1773–1843)	Germany	He classified mental disorders into 'hyperthymias', 'asthenias' and 'hypo-asthenias'. Clearly mixed states dominate his works

(continued)

Table 1.1 (continued)

Person or event	Country	Contribution
Jean-Pierre Falret (1794–1870) and Jules Baillarger (1809–1890)	France	Baillarger and Falret called bipolar disorder 'double insanity' and 'circular insanity'
Armand Trousseau (1801–1867), Alexander Haig, Alexander Ure and Sir Alfred Baring Garrod (1819–1907)	France, UK	They suggested that mania and depression are related to the uric acid nosology and introduced lithium into medicine
Joseph Guislain (1797–1860), Ernst Albrecht von Zeller (1804–1877), Wilhelm Griesinger (1817–1868) and Heinrich Neumann (1814–1888)	Belgium and Germany	Unitary psychosis theory (einheitspsychose)
Karl Ludwig Kahlbaum (1828–1899) and Ewald Hecker (1843–1909)	Germany	Developed the concepts of hebephrenia and cyclothymia and proposed the existence of more than one discrete psychiatric disorder, in sharp contrast to the concept of 'unitary psychosis' (einheitspsychose)
Carl Georg Lange (1834–1900), Frederik Lange (1842–1907) and William Alexander Hammond (1828–1900)	Denmark, USA	They used lithium in depression and bipolar disorder in the late nineteenth century
Emil Kraepelin (1856–1926)	Germany	The major psychoses were divided into two groups: dementia precox, later named schizophrenia, and manic–depressive psychosis, on the basis of long-term outcome. Identified three major components of mood episodes: affect, cognition and activity
Wilhelm Weygandt (1870–1939)	Germany	Published the first book on mixed clinical states
Ernst Kretschmer (1888–1964) and William H. Sheldon (1899–1977)	Germany, USA	Kretschmer and Sheldon suggested the relationship of body types to personality, temperament and mental health
Ugo Cerletti (1877–1963) and Lucio Bini (1908–1964)	Italy	Electroconvulsive therapy (ECT)
International Classification of Diseases	WHO	In 1948 the World Health Organization (WHO) adopted the ICD which eventually evolved into adopting operationalized criteria for the diagnosis of mental disorders
John Cade (1912–1980)	Australia	Reported the treatment of 10 manic patients in 1949. Reported the first death from lithium toxaemia

Table 1.1 (continued)

Person or event	Country	Contribution
Diagnostic and Statistical Manual for Mental Disorders	USA	In 1952 the DSM-I was published by the American Psychiatric Association. It eventually evolved into adopting operationalized criteria for the diagnosis of mental disorders
Mogens Schou (1918–2005)	Denmark	In 1954 he conducted the first double-blind study in psychiatry and it concerned lithium
Jean Delay (1907–1987) and Pierre Deniker (1917–1999)	France	Introduced antipsychotics (chlorpromazine) in 1955. Probably most of their early psychotic patients were bipolar in acute mania
Leo Henryk Sternbach (1908–2005)	USA	Introduced benzodiazepines in 1956
Karl Leonhard (1904–1988)	Germany	In 1957 he proposed that the term 'bipolar disorder' should replace 'manic depression'. Eventually his suggestion was officially and widely adopted
Roland Kuhn (1912–2005)	Switzerland	In 1958 he reported on the efficacy of the first antidepressant, imipramine
Karl Leonhard (1904–1988), Carlo Perris (1928–2000) and George Winokur (1925–1996)	USA	Established the distinction between unipolar and bipolar depression
Hagop Akiskal	USA	The role of temperament, development of the concept of the bipolar spectrum, attempts for a unified theory for mood disorders
Frederik Goodwin	USA	Lithium in the treatment of depression
Jules Angst	Switzerland	Epidemiology of bipolarity

References

Angst J (2002) Historical aspects of the dichotomy between manic-depressive disorders and schizophrenia. Schizophr Res 57(1):5–13, doi:S0920996402003286 [pii]

Angst J, Grof P, Schou M (1969) Lithium. Lancet 1(7605):1097

Angst J, Weis P, Grof P, Baastrup PC, Schou M (1970) Lithium prophylaxis in recurrent affective disorders. Br J Psychiatry 116(535):604–614

Baastrup PC (1964) The use of lithium in manic-depressive psychosis. Compr Psychiatry 5(6):396–408

Baastrup PC, Schou M (1967) Lithium as a prophylactic agents. Its effect against recurrent depressions and manic-depressive psychosis. Arch Gen Psychiatry 16(2):162–172

Baastrup PC, Poulsen JC, Schou M, Thomsen K, Amdisen A (1970) Prophylactic lithium: double blind discontinuation in manic-depressive and recurrent-depressive disorders. Lancet 2(7668):326–330

Bech P (2006) The full story of lithium. A tribute to Mogens Schou (1918–2005). Psychother Psychosom 75(5):265–269. doi:10.1159/000093947

Bech P, Vendsborg PB, Rafaelsen OJ (1976) Lithium maintenance treatment of manic-melancholic patients: its role in the daily routine. Acta Psychiatr Scand 53(1):70–81
Berrios GE, Beer D (1994) The notion of a unitary psychosis: a conceptual history. Hist Psychiatry 5(17 Pt 1):13–36
Blackwell B (1969) Need for careful evaluation of lithium. Am J Psychiatry 125(8):1131
Blackwell B (1970) Lithium. Lancet 2(7678):875–876
Blackwell B (1971) Lithium prophylaxis in recurrent affective disorders. Br J Psychiatry 118(542):131–132
Blackwell B (1972) Prophylactic lithium: science or science fiction? Am Heart J 83(1):139–141
Blackwell B, Shepherd M (1968) Prophylactic lithium: another therapeutic myth? An examination of the evidence to date. Lancet 1(7549):968–971
Cade J (1949) Lithium salts in the treatment of psychotic excitement. Med J Aust 36:349–352
Cade JF (2000) Lithium salts in the treatment of psychotic excitement. 1949. Bull World Health Organ 78(4):518–520
Delay J, Deniker P (1955) Neuroleptic effects of chlorpromazine in therapeutics of neuropsychiatry. J Clin Exp Psychopathol 16(2):104–112
Gershon S, Yuwiler A (1960) Lithium ion: a specific psychopharmacological approach to the treatment of mania. J Neuropsychiatry 1:229–241
Goodwin FK (2002) Rationale for long-term treatment of bipolar disorder and evidence for long-term lithium treatment. J Clin Psychiatry 63(Suppl 10):5–12
Goodwin F, Jamison K (2007) Manic-depressive illness, 2nd edn. Oxford University Press, New York
Goodwin FK, Zis AP (1979) Lithium in the treatment of mania: comparisons with neuroleptics. Arch Gen Psychiatry 36(8 Spec No):840–844
Goodwin FK, Murphy DL, Bunney WE Jr (1969a) Lithium. Lancet 2(7613):212–213
Goodwin FK, Murphy DL, Bunney WE Jr (1969b) Lithium-carbonate treatment in depression and mania. A longitudinal double-blind study. Arch Gen Psychiatry 21(4):486–496
Goodwin FK, Murphy DL, Dunner DL, Bunney WE Jr (1972) Lithium response in unipolar versus bipolar depression. Am J Psychiatry 129(1):44–47
Goodwin FK, Fireman B, Simon GE, Hunkeler EM, Lee J, Revicki D (2003) Suicide risk in bipolar disorder during treatment with lithium and divalproex. JAMA 290(11):1467–1473. doi:10.1001/jama.290.11.1467, 290/11/1467 [pii]
Jaspers K (1913) General psychopathology (trans: Hoenig J, Hamilton M). The Johns Hopkins University Press (1997), Chicago
Johnson FN, Amdisen A (1983) The first era of lithium in medicine. An historical note. Pharmacopsychiatria 16(2):61–63. doi:10.1055/s-2007-1017450
Johnstone EC, Crow TJ, Frith CD, Owens DG (1988) The Northwick Park "functional" psychosis study: diagnosis and treatment response. Lancet 2(8603):119–125
Kraepelin E (1921) Manic-depressive insanity and paranoia. Livingstone, Edinburgh
Kuhn R (1958) The treatment of depressive states with G 22355 (imipramine hydrochloride). Am J Psychiatry 115(5):459–464
Lambert PA, Carraz G, Borselli S, Carbel S (1966) Neuropsychotropic action of a new anti-epileptic agent: depamide. Ann Med Psychol (Paris) 124(5):707–710
Lenox RH, Watson DG (1994) Lithium and the brain: a psychopharmacological strategy to a molecular basis for manic depressive illness. Clin Chem 40(2):309–314
Leonhard K (1957a) Cycloid psychoses, often erroneously considered as schizophrenia. Psychiatr Neurol Med Psychol (Leipz) 9(12):359–365
Leonhard K (1957b) Pathogenesis of manic-depressive disease. Nervenarzt 28(6):271–272
Leonhard K (1979) The classification of endogenous psychoses, 5th edn. Irvington, New York
Lewis A (1938) States of depression: their clinical and aetiological differentiation. Br Med J2:875
Marmol F (2008) Lithium: bipolar disorder and neurodegenerative diseases possible cellular mechanisms of the therapeutic effects of lithium. Prog Neuropsychopharmacol Biol Psychiatry 32(8):1761–1771. doi:10.1016/j.pnpbp.2008.08.012

Mitchell S (1870) On the use of bromide of lithium. Am J Med Sci 60:443–445

Mitchell S (1877) Clinical lecture on nervousness in the male. Med News 35:177–184

Mitchell PB, Hadzi-Pavlovic D (2000) Lithium treatment for bipolar disorder. Bull World Health Organ 78(4):515–517

Moller HJ (2008) Systematic of psychiatric disorders between categorical and dimensional approaches: Kraepelin's dichotomy and beyond. Eur Arch Psychiatry Clin Neurosci 258(Suppl 2):48–73. doi:10.1007/s00406-008-2004-3

Noack CH, Trautner EM (1951) The lithium treatment of maniacal psychosis. Med J Aust 2(7):219–222

Okasha A, Okasha T (2000) Notes on mental disorders in pharaonic Egypt. Hist Psychiatry XI:413–424

Okuma T, Inanaga K, Otsuki S, Sarai K, Takahashi R, Hazama H, Mori A, Watanabe M (1979) Comparison of the antimanic efficacy of carbamazepine and chlorpromazine: a double-blind controlled study. Psychopharmacology (Berl) 66(3):211–217

Perez J, Baldessarini RJ, Cruz N, Salvatore P, Vieta E (2011) Andres Piquer-Arrufat (1711–1772): contributions of an eighteenth-century spanish physician to the concept of manic-depressive illness. Harv Rev Psychiatry 19(2):68–77. doi:10.3109/10673229.2011.565251

Robertson G (1890) Does mania include two distinct varieties of insanity, and should it be subdivided? J Nerv Ment Dis 36:338–347

Schioldann J (1999) John Cade's seminal lithium paper turns fifty. Acta Psychiatr Scand 100(6):403–405

Schioldann J (2006) Obituary: Mogens Abelin Schou (1918–2005) – half a century with lithium. Hist Psychiatry 17(2):247–252

Schioldann J (2011) 'On periodical depressions and their pathogenesis' by Carl Lange (1886). Hist Psychiatry 22(85 Pt 1):108–130

Schou M (1963) Normothymotics, "mood-normalizers": are lithium and the imipramine drugs specific for affective disorders? Br J Psychiatry 109:803–809

Schou M, Juel-Nielsen N, Stromgren E, Voldby H (1954) The treatment of manic psychoses by the administration of lithium salts. J Neurol Neurosurg Psychiatry 17(4):250–260

Schou M, Baastrup PC, Grof P, Weis P, Angst J (1970) Pharmacological and clinical problems of lithium prophylaxis. Br J Psychiatry 116(535):615–619

Shepherd M (1970) A prophylactic myth. Int J Psychiatry 9:423–425

Shorter E (2009) The history of lithium therapy. Bipolar Disord 11(Suppl 2):4–9. doi:10.1111/j.1399-5618.2009.00706.x

Strobusch AD, Jefferson JW (1980) The checkered history of lithium in medicine. Pharm Hist 22(2):72–76

Weygandt W (1899) Uber die mischzustande des manisch-depressiven irreseins. JF Lechman, Munich

Clinical Description 2

2.1 Normal Emotions, Neurobiology and Ethological Considerations

Modern approach distinguishes between 'mood' which is the long-lasting internal emotional tone and largely characteristic of the individual; 'affect' which is the general emotional status during the last few days or weeks, and it is observable through the individual's behaviour; and 'emotion' which corresponds to the transient emotional state which also manifests itself through motor behaviours (face mimics, body movements, complex behaviours, etc.). Mood has an enduring nature, tends to be unfocused and diffused, involves expectation of the future and is manifested in subtle ways, while, in contrast, emotions tend to be short lived and to have a clear focus.

In terms of etymology, the word 'mood' comes from Proto-Germanic 'modaz' and is related to the old high German 'muot' (in German: Mut) and the old Saxon mod (in Dutch: moed). Similar words exist in Scandinavian languages, and they mean 'anger' and 'emotion'. The ancient Greek word μῶθαι (mothai) and the Latin *mos* (=mores) come from the same Indo-European root. The word 'affect' comes from the middle French word 'affecter' which in turn derived from the Latin *afficere* (*ad+ facere* which means 'to act upon', 'influence', 'attack with disease'). It seems that it had entered the English language in the fourteenth century and it is first recorded in Geoffrey Chaucer's 'Troilus and Cressida'. 'Emotion' comes from the French word 'émouvoir' which is based on the Latin *emovere* (e-movere means 'without move'). Thus, the original meanings of these terms relate to anger and to the tendency to act or remain still. It is interesting that one of the etymological approaches to the word 'mania' suggests it comes from the Greek word μένω which means 'remain still' (also see Chap. 1).

Aristotle's concept of affect is 'that which leads one's condition to become so transformed that his judgment is affected, and which is accompanied by pleasure and pain' (Aristotle, 'Rhetoric' 6). While he was the first to elaborate on human affective states and various terms can be found in his works, in Greek the word for

K.N. Fountoulakis, *Bipolar Disorder: An Evidence-Based Guide to Manic Depression*, DOI 10.1007/978-3-642-37216-2_2

mood is διάθεση (diathesi=disposition, tendency, availability), for affect is συναίσθημα (synaesthima= complex or combined feelings, sentiment) and for emotion is αίσθημα (aesthima=feeling)

Affects and emotions serve two main aims. The first concerns the internal functioning of the individual and provides the individual with fast decisions which serve the survival of the individual but also of the species. Some of these decisions are easy to understand (e.g. fear of animals), but others are incomprehensible in principal (aesthetics and attraction to the opposite sex). In the same frame, emotions provide feedback concerning the behaviour of the individual, and in this way they enhance the expression of the specific behaviour or preclude its future manifestations. For example, sadness constitutes the emotional response to loss, defeat, disappointment or other adversities. Its adaptive function includes permitting withdrawal to conserve resources, asking for support from significant others and the autonomic arousal which might be present facilitates the search for the lost object or an appropriate substitute.

The second aim is to communicate the internal emotional state of the individual to others, and this is achieved with facial expressions, gestures, bodily moves and posture and voice verbal and nonverbal elements. These ways of communicating emotions vary between cultures, but most of the repertoire is universal for human beings. They constitute a main source for the interaction with others, since the emotions of an individual influence the emotions, thoughts and behaviours of others, produce positive or negative feedback and give birth to circles of future interactions and reciprocal influence.

The feelings of one individual evoke feelings in the others by 'emotion contagion' (i.e. others tend to automatically and unconsciously mimic behaviours) and 'emotion interpretation' (i.e. others perceive the individual's emotions and react with complementary or any kind of appropriate emotions). It is interesting that positive affect promotes social interaction and activity and is related to high functional support. How and why this happens is unknown, but it is likely to be mediated through the induction of positive feelings and pleasant emotional states to others.

In the early 1970s, Paul Ekman (Ekman and Friesen 1971) classified emotions into the basic: anger, disgust, fear, happiness, sadness and surprise, and the in the early 1980s Robert Plutchik (1927–2006) (Plutchik 2002) developed the 'wheel (or cone) of emotions' (Fig. 2.1), by proposing the existence of four bipols with eight emotions (joy vs. sadness, anger vs. fear, trust vs. distrust and surprise vs. anticipation) corresponding to situations of promoting or rejecting behaviour, fight or flight, social interaction and expectation. Combinations of these basic emotions might produce other feelings human beings experience. Plutchik suggested that basic emotions relate in specific ways and the existence of one modifies the possibility for the coexistence of another. However, it has not been proven that the existence of one pole precludes the existence of another (e.g. that anger and fear cannot coexist). It still remains controversial whether affective (or emotional) states should include emotional experiences related to bodily functions (e.g. hunger, sex, etc.).

The first modern neurobiological theory of emotions was independently developed in the 1880s by William James (1842–1910) and Carl Lange (1834–1900).

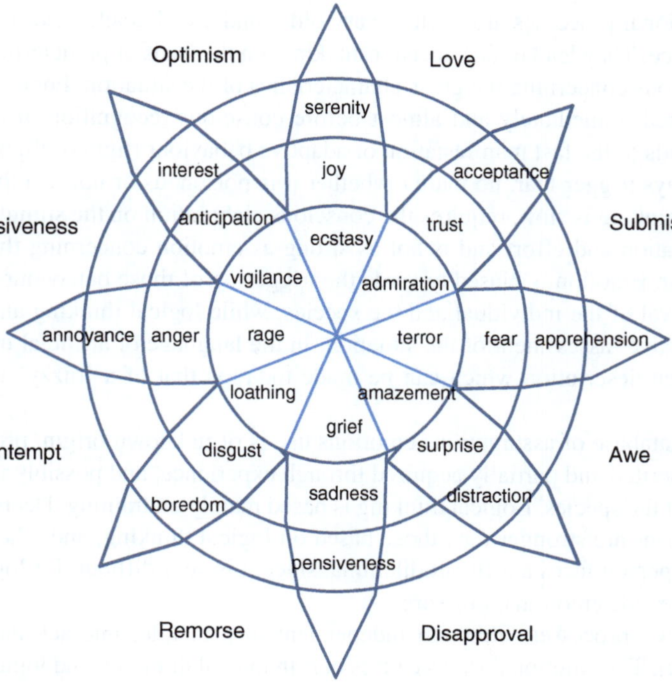

Fig. 2.1 The 'wheel (cone) of emotions' according to Robert Plutchik

That theory proposed that emotions are the result of changes in the physiology of the body caused by a stimulus and not the result of the stimulus directly.

A modern approach to the issue goes through a basic approach to brain function which could suggest that there are two distinct mental processes: logical thinking and emotions. While emotions are present also in animals, logical thinking is present primarily in humans, while some elements are also evident in the behaviour of primates.

Traditionally, the left hemisphere is considered to be the site of logical thinking, while the right hemisphere serves the creation of emotions. Although this assumption is supported by some neuropsychological data, especially in neurosurgical patients and head injury, it is almost certain that complete and opposite lateralization of logic and emotions does not exist. A consequence of the above assumption is that the dysfunctions leading to schizophrenia are supposed to be localized in the left hemisphere, while those leading to depression are localized in the right.

A very simplified neurobiological model may propose that 'mood' derives probably from processes largely taking part in the amygdala and the insula, while 'emotion' is generated mainly in the anterior cingulate cortex (ACC) and more specifically in area 25. However, its effortful regulation is likely to implicate area 24 and the dorsolateral prefrontal cortex (DLPFC). In the middle between 'mood' and 'emotion' lies the 'affect' which is at least partially generated in the ACC and partially in other brain areas including the prefrontal cortex (PFC) (Phillips et al. 2003).

Emotional processes are evolutionary older and are characterized by speed and dominance. They lead to fast decision-making, on the basis of predetermined strong assumptions concerning the gross characteristics of the situation. For example, fear is triggered immediately and almost before conscious recognition of the stimuli, and it leads to the fast manifestation of adaptive behaviour (fight or flight). A snake will always trigger fear, no matter whether it is poisonous or not. On the contrary, logical thinking is slow, requires the conscious elaboration on the stimuli, demands concentration and effort and is not as strong as emotion concerning the effect on behaviour. Emotion is biased towards the triggering of those behaviours that serve the survival of the individual and the species, while logical thinking aims towards an 'objective' assessment of the situation. In the language of artificial intelligence, the closest description which can be made today is that of a 'fuzzy' vs. 'digital' systems.

The database of assumptions emotions use is of unknown origin, probably partially inherited and partially acquired through experience, and possibly it is characteristic of the species. Logical thinking is based mainly on training. Decisions based on emotions are stronger than those based on logical thinking, and when they collide, the person faces a difficult dilemma, since it is very difficult for logical thinking to override emotional pressure.

The two processes, although independent in principle, interact and influence each other. The emotional status causes bias in logical thinking, and logical analysis triggers emotions depending on the positive or negative outcome. This interaction is likely to happen at multiple levels (e.g. selective memory recall, reinforcement through new analysis, biased selection of possible solutions, etc.).

Normal mental functioning includes low emotional condition, called 'grief' in response to significant separations and losses (e.g. death, divorce, romantic disappointment, bereavement, various catastrophes), and high emotional condition called 'elation' in response to significant positive events (e.g. success and achievement). Sometimes it is neither uncommon nor abnormal for the individual to manifest a paradoxical reaction, which is low emotion as response to positive events or high emotion as response to negative events. These paradoxical emotional experiences are usually the result of hidden threats in the positive events or stem out of complex dynamic intrapsychic processes aiming to protect the person from experiencing grief.

As previously mentioned, according to current ethological theories, the expression of emotions through physical behaviour communicates to others information concerning the individual's emotional state, and this is considered to be one of the most important elements in social behaviour and interaction with others.

Interest in emotions from an evolutionary perspective was triggered by the publication of the book *The Expression of the Emotions in Man and Animals* by Charles Darwin (1809–1882) in 1872. In that book, Darwin stresses the universal nature of emotions and the connection of mental states to the neurological organization of movement. Central to his understanding was a shared human and animal ancestry in sharp contrast to the contemporary claims that there were divinely created human muscles to express uniquely human feelings. Darwin's original suggestion was that emotions evolved via natural selection and therefore have cross-culturally universal counterparts, a proposal confirmed almost a century later by the works of Paul Ekman. Furthermore, animals undergo emotions comparable to those of humans.

2.2 The Conceptualization of Bipolar Disorder

Normal affects and emotions are characterized by their correspondence in terms of intensity and duration to the respected stimuli which had triggered them. Intensity depends on the significance of the stimuli and the threat they constitute for the person, while duration is related to the duration of exposure plus some time the individual needs to regain internal homeostasis. However, eventually, affects and emotions disappear (after the stimulus disappears first), and the individual returns to its normal steady affective state. However, in contrast, pathological affects are characterized by intensity which is disproportional (higher or lower) to the triggering stimuli, inappropriate duration (too short or prolonged) and possibly problematic nature (emotions are inappropriate, alternate or coexist). The 'quality' is often similar between 'normal' and 'pathological' affects and emotions, and only in the more severe cases pathological affect obtains a 'difference in quality' which is often difficult to describe accurately and possibly reflects a collapse in the ways affects and emotions are behaviourally expressed. It is also possible that this difference in 'quality' merely reflects the impact of more severe pathological affect on other mental processes including insight, judgment and overall functioning. Another abnormal element which suggests a 'qualitative' difference is that pathological affects and emotions, especially when very severe, might be independent of environmental events, either positive or negative, congruent or incongruent to the affective state of the person. Although the term 'endogenous' is often used to denote that the mood episode is occurring in the absence of precipitants, many authors prefer the term 'endoreactive' which denotes that once the episode is triggered, it tends to persist in an autonomous way. The homeostatic dyscontrol of mood, which is part of a more pervasive mood dysregulation, resists reversal to the habitual baseline affective tone.

Normal mood permits the normal function of affective and emotional processes in response to environmental cues. Grief or elation rarely leads to depression or mania, with maybe the exception of major catastrophes and very traumatic events. However, bereaved persons exhibit many depressive-like symptoms during the first 1–2 years after their loss, but only 5 % of them progress to clinical depression. Severity of grief might be predictive of future depression especially if features like marked psychomotor retardation and thoughts of guilt of commission are present. Grief might constitute a severe medical condition, and it is not uncommon for elderly people to die within a few months of the death of their spouse.

However, pathological mood disrupts these functions and has a pervasive impact on the individual. The result of pathological mood is pathological affect and emotions which characterize a group of mental disorders under the collective label of 'mood disorders'. It is indeed problematic that until today there are no pathophysiological methods identified and no biochemical laboratory tests developed to assist the diagnosis and to distinguish 'normal' from 'abnormal' mood and affect. Because of this failure, the diagnostic decision is based on intensity, severity and maybe the presence of some 'qualitative' differences. Of course the words 'intensity', 'severity' and 'quality' have intrinsically problematic definitions when it comes to behaviour and internal experience. This is a major drawback concerning the adoption of the biomedical model vs. the psychosocial model. The former has always been dominant in Europe, while the second was dominant in the USA for most of the twentieth century. Another problematic area was the adoption of a categorical diagnostic model vs. a dimensional model. It is interesting that while Emil Kraepelin strongly endorsed the categorical distinction between schizophrenia and manic–depressive illness, Eugen Bleuler, on the contrary, suggested that both illnesses lie on a continuum with no sharp line of demarcation. According to Bleuler, a patient could be conceptualized as being predominantly schizophrenic or predominantly manic–depressive, and additionally, his position on the continuum between the two illnesses was not considered to be stable but ever changing during the course of the illness. Currently, the categorical model, which is closer to the mentality of the biomedical model and more 'user-friendly' for the average clinician, is utilized in most clinical and research approaches. In the past the term 'affective' disorders was used, but today the term 'mood' disorders is preferred, and this is because it refers to more enduring and deeply rooted emotional states.

The World Health Organization's tenth edition of the International Statistical Classification of Diseases and Related Health Problems (ICD-10) includes such a chapter; however, the American Psychiatric Association's fifth edition of the Diagnostic and Statistical Manual of Mental Disorders (DSM-5) includes a separate chapter for bipolar disorders and a separate for unipolar depressions. In details the classification systems (American Psychiatric Association 2013; WHO 1992) are described in Chap. 12 of the current book. Both systems include a number of personality disorder diagnostic categories with strong emotional components. Also they both include 'not-otherwise-specified' categories.

The core concept for the diagnosis of these disorders is the polarity, intensity, duration and frequency of change of affects and their correspondence and appropriateness, relation and autonomicity with respect to stimuli. In terms of polarity, (hypo)manic and dysthymic/depressive states denote the presence of high or low affect, respectively. Both classification systems consider that BD consists of at least one manic or mixed episode and a depressive episode. DSM distinguishes two types of the presence of manic (BD-I) or hypomanic (BD-II) episodes. However, apart from these hallmarks of clinical picture, BD is a highly complex disorder with many facets, aspects and special issues in its clinical picture (Table 2.1).

It is both interesting and important to look at the literature which predates the psychopharmacology era, that is, the nineteenth century and the first half of the twentieth century. This literature is important not only because patients were experiencing the 'natural' course of the illness without the 'contamination' of psychopharmacotherapy but also because at that time, nosological categories had not been identified and distinguished yet and authors were describing the clinical picture with less

Table 2.1 List of the multiple clinical aspects of manic–depressive illness

1. Manic episodes
2. Depressive episodes
3. Mixed episodes
4. Subthreshold manic symptoms
5. Subthreshold depressive symptoms
6. 'Mixed' states and 'roughening'
7. Mood lability/cyclothymia/'personality-like' behaviour
8. Predominant polarity
9. Frequency of episodes/rapid cycling
10. Psychotic features
11. Neurocognitive disorder
12. Functional deficit and disability
13. Drug/alcohol abuse
14. Comorbid anxiety and other mental disorders
15. Self-destructive behaviour and suicidality

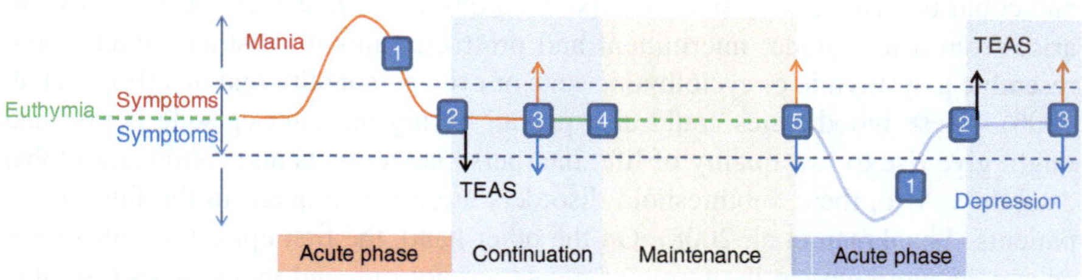

Fig. 2.2 Graphic representation of the alteration of types of mood episodes and the course of bipolar disorder. *1* Response, *2* remission, *3* relapse, *4* recovery, *5* recurrence. *TEAS* treatment emergent affective switch

channelling and top-down bias. On the other hand, one should bear in mind that in these times, physicians were confronting with the most severe group of patients, and their observations were based mainly on chronic institutionalized patients, often distorted by personal issues and philosophical and often religious and political influences.

Unfortunately, more than a century after the first modern nosology was formulated, the boundaries between personality, temperament, grief and mood disorder, mood-congruent and mood-incongruent psychotic features and, even worse, the schizophrenic group of disorders and mood disorders remain unresolved.

The definition of bipolar disorder (BD, previously called manic–depressive psychosis) as conceptualized by Emil Kraepelin a century ago suggests that this disorder is characterized by the presence and alteration of manic and depressive episodes (mixed episodes are usually considered to be a variation of manic) with a return to premorbid level of functioning between the episodes and a favourable outcome in comparison to schizophrenia (Kraepelin 1921). A graphic chart of this prototypical concept is shown in Fig. 2.2. Today we know that this is not always the case (Tohen et al. 1990). The Kraepelinian concept largely corresponds to BD type I (BD-I) according to DSM-5 (American Psychiatric Association 2013). Another type, BD-II, is officially recognized as a bipolar illness subtype, and it is characterized by the presence of hypomanic instead of manic episodes. It was first proposed as a subtype by the group of Fred Goodwin at the NIMH (Dunner et al. 1976). However, it is important to note that according to DSM-5 hypomania is defined mainly in terms of a shorter duration and lower severity of the episode. BD-II is more prevalent than BD-I. Today we also know that the categorical distinction between manic and depressive episodes in the frame of BD is not as clear as previously thought, since 94 % of acutely manic or hypomanic patients and 70 % of depressed patients also manifest symptoms of the opposite pole at a clinically significant level. Even more important is the observation that these symptoms correlate positively and not inversely to each other (Bauer et al. 2005). In this frame, it seems more important to focus on the coexistence of the two poles, the transitional phases between them as well as their fluctuating nature rather than to insist on the description and treatment of the rigid 'classical' and pure clinical pictures of either pole.

The first mood episode typically begins in late adolescence, the 20s or the 30s and could be manic, depressive or mixed. Its onset could be acute or insidious and arise from a low-grade, intermittent and protracted mood substrate which could resemble a dysthymic or cyclothymic state or even personality features (Fogel et al. 2006). These mood states could also prevail during the inter-episode period and might give rise to low quality of life, interpersonal conflicts and significant global disability. Also, these subthreshold disorders are quite frequent in the families of patients (Shankman et al. 2008). On the other hand, the first episodes with severe psychotic symptoms in the frame of mania are not rare and many times resemble schizophreniform episodes. Frequently the correct diagnosis is put after several years because the first episode is psychotic like or depressive, and the diagnosis is put only after a manic or mixed episode emerges. It has been estimated that more than half of patients originally manifesting a depressive episode will turn out to be bipolars in the next 20 years (Angst et al. 2005). Also, it seems that patients spend more time during depressive episodes than manic ones (Mitchell and Malhi 2004). More, subsyndromal depressive symptoms are usually present during the interepisode period (Judd et al. 2002). An additional problem for the diagnosis is that patients usually experience hypomania as a recovery from depression and almost always as a pleasant ego-syntonic mood state, and they, as well as their families, often fail to report these hypomanic episodes and tend to consider them as normothymic recovery periods. This has profound implications concerning the treatment and its overall efficacy. On average, manic episodes predominate in youth, and depressive episodes predominate in later years. Although the overall sex ratio is approximately 1:1, men, on average, undergo more manic episodes, and women experience more mixed and depressive episodes.

The term 'rapid cycling' refers to patients suffering from at least four mood episodes in a year. It seems that females are more often rapid cyclers as well as higher social class subjects. In essence, these patients tend to be symptomatic most of their life and are considered to be refractory to lithium. The diagnosis might elude for prolonged periods of time and the patients can receive the diagnosis of a personality disorder or cyclothymia. Their treatment is based on a complex, delicate and difficult to design multiple pharmacotherapy which includes atypical antipsychotics, anticonvulsants and even antidepressants, although the latter are believed to induce rapid cycling (Bauer et al. 1994a).

It is of outmost importance for both clinicians and researchers to create a biographical chart with the patient's course over time. This was first introduced by Kraepelin who used colours to mark the polarity of episodes and was further developed by Robert Post at the NIMH. This biographical chart should include any important event in the developmental history of the patient, the main events and hallmarks of his/her life and his full psychiatric and medical history. The use of such charts is of great importance not only for mood patients but for all psychiatric patients, since it clarifies both the diagnosis and the course of the disease and response to therapeutic interventions.

2.3 Bipolar Depression

Depressive episodes are considered to be a diagnostic pillar of BD. However, in contrast to manic episodes which lead to the diagnosis of BD immediately, depressive episodes pose a dilemma to the clinician whether he faces a unipolar depression of a BD. This is an important dilemma to solve since the treatment is different between these disorders.

The data suggest that more often the first episode of BD is depressive, especially in females (Angst et al. 2005; Perlis et al. 2005). In 15 % of patients, depressive episodes appear abruptly (Winokur et al. 1969) and are characterized by a constellation of symptoms and signs, with depressed mood and anhedonia being the most characteristic. As mentioned above, depressed mood is the pathological equivalent of grief and mourning and is characterized by a painful negative emotion, which is typically experienced as worse than severe physical pain. This experience is out of proportion and out of frame of existing stimuli and is characterized by groundless apprehensions with severe inner turmoil and torment. The suffering is persistent although in milder cases spontaneous fluctuation even during the same day can occur (typically in the morning or in the afternoon). It is paradoxical that although depressed patients experience a hypervigilant state with heightened perception of pain, many also experience an inability to experience emotions, and they are even unable to cry. Previous opinions that anxiety and hypervigilance and anhedonia are more or less mutually exclusive were not confirmed by empirical research which showed higher levels of anxiety in those patients with more severe form of depression and melancholia (Regier et al. 1998). Anhedonia does not simply mean the patient has lost the sense of pleasure. It also means that has abandoned previously enjoyed pastimes. In milder cases, anhedonia manifests itself by decreased interest in hobbies and life, but in most severe cases it leads the patient to lose feelings for loved significant ones (kids, spouse) and to be cut off from other people and the world in general. Patients typically describe their environment as without any colours, as if everything is black and with shades of grey. This is a quite odd experience which alienates patients from others and from the environment. Depersonalization and derealization might follow and often the experience has a psychotic-like quality, with impairment of the patient's judgment. This lack of feeling emotions in severely depressed patients is itself painful, and in this way it differs from flat affect experienced by patients with schizophrenia and constricted affect experienced by obsessive–convulsive patients. It is important to note that often the interviewer cannot assess the depth and the severity of depression on the basis of its outward expression. Often tears are present on a motionless face, and the patient seems calm and indifferent, where in other instances a smile, expression of sardonic humour or even elements of joy might accompany the verbal expression of self-accusation or self-derogatory thoughts. In the majority of patients (64–72 %), there is significant diurnal variation of mood (Casper et al. 1985; Winokur et al. 1969).

Two-thirds of bipolar depressed patients present with multiple physical pains and complains (e.g. headache, epigastric pain, precordial distress, etc.) in the absence of any physical illness (Winokur et al. 1969) especially in primary care. These patients also might deny the experience of depressed mood. These conditions have been described as masked depression, but current classification systems do not recognize such a syndrome, mostly because lack of depressive mood is not complete and there is significant overlap with undiagnosed or difficult to diagnose medical conditions.

Irritability is pervasive in BD patients and is manifested by almost 75 % of them (Winokur et al. 1969). The picture includes also psychomotor disorder with the form of either agitation or retardation. These terms correspond to changes in the motor expression of mental and emotional activity. Agitation is easily observed since it includes commission of behaviours (increased speech, restlessness, increased gesturing, hand wringing, nail biting, hair pulling, etc.). On the contrary psychomotor retardation is characterized by the lowing of psychomotor activity and lack of spontaneous behaviours which are usually included in the usual 'every minute' activity of the individual (e.g. lack of the usual body posture, visual exploration of the environment or usual gestures during speech, etc.). Thus, patients with psychomotor retardation manifest a slumped posture, downcast gaze, fatigue, poor concentration and effortful thinking and indecisiveness. Additionally, they don't speak much and often discussion and interview is difficult. Sometimes psychomotor slowing is so extreme that in elderly patients gives the impression of organic confusion or dementia-like syndrome, while in younger patients it might evolve into a stupor with patients being unable to participate even in basic everyday functions, such as feeding themselves or going to the toilet.

Activity and behaviour become slower during periods of depression. Patients move and walk slowly and react sluggishly, their movements are restricted to the absolutely necessary ones, the whole body and especially the face lack muscle tone and vitality, and the eyes are dull and reflect the inner retardation, often with a faraway unnatural stare. Fatigue and psychomotor retardation dominate the clinical picture in 75 % of patients (Carlson and Strober 1978; Winokur et al. 1969). It is important to note that in most patients features of both agitation and retardation seem to coexist. In gross clinical observation, retardation rather than agitation is more characteristic for depression, and the presence of overt agitation poses a question of diagnosis, whether the episode is in fact mixed. Some authors suggest that retardation constitutes the core problem in depression since mental slowness leads to inertia and makes the patients unable to act physically and mentally. They also suggest psychomotor retardation is the main cause for the high disability related to depression.

Although depression is characterized by depressed mood, an important feature in its psychopathology is depressive thought content. Thought disorder is also called 'cognitive disorder', and this term should be distinguished from 'neurocognitive disorder' which refers to disorders of concentration, memory, executive function, etc. (this distinction is not mandatory, however, and many authors use both terms in a confusing way). The fundamental depressive thoughts are negative evaluations of the self, the world and the future (the negative triad) which according to cognitive theory are central to the aetiopathogenesis of depression. However, it is equally likely that the depressed mood biases thought process towards a negativistic way of thinking. To the author's opinion, our neurobiological and ethological understanding of emotion and logical thinking does not support the possibility that negative thoughts induce depressed affect in such a pervasive and enduring way. It is more reasonable to consider the cognitive disorder as being part of the psychopathological manifestations of depression.

The essential characteristic of depressive thinking is that the patient views everything in an extremely negative light. In line with Kurt Schneider's theory on humankind's four basic insecurities (health, financial status, moral worth and relationship to others), thought disorder includes, among others, ideas of deprivation and loss; low self-esteem and self-confidence; ideas of poverty and disaster; self-reproach and pathological guilt; helplessness, hopelessness and pessimism; hypochondriacal thoughts; and recurrent thoughts of death and suicide. It is as if the patients are actively looking for the negative and unpleasant aspect in everything. These negative thoughts are typically unjustified or are blown out of proportion and sometimes could be truly delusional. Sometimes extreme impairment because of psychomotor retardation might trigger thoughts of low self-esteem which although seem exaggerated and almost delusional, in fact they accurately reflect the perception the patient has concerning his disability.

When depressive thoughts acquire delusional proportions, then delusions of worthlessness and sinfulness, reference, infidelity and persecution appear (often in the form of prosecutor). Delusions are present in 12–66 % of bipolar depressed patients (Black and Nasrallah 1989; Carlson and Strober 1978; Rosenthal et al. 1980; Winokur et al. 1969). Other delusions include delusions of poverty, disaster and ill health (suffering from an occult illness, like cancer or AIDS). A special form is nihilistic delusions, which include thoughts that parts of the body are missing, also known as Cotard's syndrome after Jules Cotard (1840–1889) who described it for the first time in 1880. Under the influence of delusional depression, not only suicide but also homicide can occur, usually with an 'altruistic' motive. For example, under delusions of poverty, disaster or moral decay, a father might kill his children in order to 'save' and 'protect' them and afterwards commits suicide. Another not unusual scenario is infanticide by mothers with psychotic depression during the postpartum period.

The above-mentioned delusions are mood-congruent, that is, they are in line with the depressed mood. However, mood-incongruent delusions can be also present (e.g. persecutory delusions which cannot be considered in the frame of the depressed mood); however, if bizarre delusions are present, then the diagnosis of schizoaffective disorder should be considered.

Psychotic symptoms during bipolar depressive episodes include also hallucinations, most often auditory. They are less frequent (8–50 %) in comparison to acute mania (Baethge et al. 2005; Black and Nasrallah 1989; Carlson and Strober 1978; Rosenthal et al. 1980; Winokur et al. 1969). Typically they are extremely unpleasant, and their content is in accord with depressed mood and delusional ideation. They can be mood-congruent (e.g. accusatory or derogatory) or mood-incongruent (e.g. two voices discussing without any reference to the patient). It has been reported that depressed patients with psychotic symptoms are more often turned to be bipolars than those without (Akiskal et al. 1983). Also, it is believed that psychotic features constitute a stable trait which tends to repeat itself across episodes, although the studies suggesting this use a mixture of bipolar and unipolar patients and generalizability is problematic (Helms and Smith 1983; Nelson et al. 1984; Aronson et al. 1988a, b).

Overall, psychotic symptoms are more frequent in bipolar in comparison to unipolar depression (Goes et al. 2007).

Suicide is the worst outcome of depression. Often suicidal thoughts are present during the whole course of the disease. Attempts may happen, but the majority of patients do not commit suicide in spite of the continuous presence of suicidal ideation. It seems that the risk of suicide is less pronounced during acute severe depression, and traditionally, the suggestion made by Emil Kraepelin that when psychomotor activity starts improving, but still mood and thinking are still severely depressive, at that particular period the patient has the combination of ideation and energy to commit the suicide. This often happens in an unpredictable impulsive way. According to Aaron Beck hopelessness is the specific symptom that should alert the clinician concerning high suicidal risk. Empirical research rejected the hypothesis that inquiring about suicide provokes it. On the contrary, patients are often relieved that the physician appreciates the magnitude of their suffering. Suicidal ideation is commonly expressed indirectly (e.g. in a wish not to wake up or to die from a malignant disease), while it is not unusual the patients to conceal their suicidal ideation behind a joyful behaviour. Some depressed persons are tormented with suicidal obsessions and are constantly resisting unwanted urges or impulses to destroy themselves. Others might yield to such urges passively (e.g. by careless driving or by walking into high-speed traffic). A third group harbours elaborate plans, carefully preparing a will and taking out insurance. Deliberate planning indicates a high suicidal risk.

Since antiquity, depression was linked to the disturbance of a number of somatic functions including appetite, circadian rhythms, sleep and sex. Typically depression is related to a reduction in the quantity of these functions (insomnia, loss of appetite and weight, loss of libido); however, there is a subgroup of patients experiencing an increase (overeating, oversleeping and maybe increase of sexual activity). This latter group is also characterized by higher anxiety, personality psychopathology, mood reactivity, fatigue and long-term sensitivity to rejection. It is interesting that this latter symptom is then only one in DSM-5 Axis I which resembles more the personality disorder criteria of Axis II rather than the criteria of mood disorders.

Depending on the study sample composition, changes in appetite for food are seen in almost all patients (Winokur et al. 1969), with one-fourth manifesting overeating and one-fourth losing significant weight (Casper et al. 1985). Women are especially vulnerable to manifest these symptoms and signs (Kawa et al. 2005). Anorexia and weight loss could be a core independent symptom of depression, but it can also be secondary to blunted olfactory or taste sensations or a decreased enjoyment of food. Anorexia should be distinguished from avoidance of food, for example, because of a delusional belief that it is poisoned. Especially in elderly persons, it can lead to malnutrition and electrolyte disturbances which both represent medical emergencies. On the contrary, overeating especially in combination might result in weight gain which in turn increases the burden of overall morbidity and mortality especially in middle-aged patients, especially if diabetes mellitus, hypertension or coronary artery disease coexists.

Sleep disturbance constitutes a cardinal (although non-specific) sign of depression. Almost all bipolar depressed patients experience some kind of sleep problem (Winokur et al. 1969; Casper et al. 1985). It has been described as abnormally deep or abnormally light. It includes difficulty to fall asleep, multiple awakenings during the night and especially in the early hours of the morning and often early morning awakening. Not only quantity but also quality of sleep seems to be disordered with deep stages of sleep (III and IV) being decreased or deficient. In this frame, some patients try to self-medicate them with alcohol or sedative–hypnotic medication, which may initially succeed but ultimately aggravates the sleep patterns and insomnia because in the long term they further diminish stage III and stage IV sleep. Dreams are typically vivid, restless and anxious. On the contrary, a subgroup of bipolar depressed patients (up to 25 %) often exhibit excessive sleep and have difficulty getting up in the morning (Winokur et al. 1969). Often these patients are failed to be diagnosed properly, and it is supposed to be 'laziness' or 'character disorder'.

Decreased sexual desire is seen in more than 75 % of patients (Casper et al. 1985; Winokur et al. 1969) and concerns both sexes. Some women experience temporary interruption of their menses while male experience erectile dysfunction. Both conditions might lead the patient to seek expert opinion from endocrinologists, urologists or gynaecologists. Disruption of sexual life might cause marital problems especially when the patient is female. In turn, marital problems fuel depression, and many therapists focus on the problems within the couple's relationship rather than the causal element which is depression. Especially sexual dysfunction and the resulting marital problems might delay the correct assessment of the problem and the appropriate therapy. Especially problematic is that most of antidepressant agents might worsen the problem, while the use of agents like sildenafil is not always successful. It is not common for depressed patients to manifest hypersexuality. In these cases the presence of a mixed episode should be considered.

Until now there were a lot of efforts to describe and classify depressive symptomatology in detail. Essentially these efforts do not distinguish between unipolar and bipolar depression. The core concept in almost all classifications was the psychological vs. biological aetiopathogenesis and concern depression as a syndrome without distinguishing between unipolar and bipolar. Kraepelin believed that the two types (psychological and biological) were naturally divided (Kraepelin and Johnstone 2010), and in 1896, he accepted the aetiological classification of 'exogenous' and 'endogenous' diseases by Paul Julius Möbius (1853–1907). This was in part the source of the nature/nurture split in the conceptualization of psychiatric disorders and led to an unfortunate link between phenomenology and aetiology bypassing the syndrome notion of Thomas Sydenham (1624–1689). Gillespie (Gillespie 1926) further contributed to the confusion between phenomenology and aetiology since the main difference of the depressive types he proposed was reactivity of mood. On the contrary, Aubrey Julian Lewis (1900–1975) suggested in 1934 that reactive and endogenous depressions could not be separated. A more pragmatic approach is reflected in the thoughts of Raymond Bernard Cattell (1905–1998) (Cattell 1943) who strongly supported the separation of nosology from aetiology.

Kraepelin described 'melancholia gravis' as a more severe form of depression with psychotic features. He also proposed the term 'fantastic melancholia' for even more severe forms with more pronounced psychotic symptoms, alternation of agitation with stupor and clouding of consciousness. According to Kraepelin the most severe form of depression is 'delirious melancholia' with very severe and almost 'schizophrenic-like' delusions and hallucinations. In these cases, clouding of consciousness dominates the clinical picture (Kraepelin 1921).

Most classification systems include a subtype who is melancholic like under several different names, like 'endogenous depression' (Roth 1959), 'vital depression' (Van Praag et al. 1965), 'retarded depression' (Overall et al. 1966), etc. Diagnostic operationalizations of the melancholic (endogenous) concept are found in all DSM editions after the third one, in the ICD-10, the Research Diagnostic Criteria (Spitzer et al. 1978), the World Health Organization Depression Scale (Bech et al. 1980) and the Newcastle Scales (Carney et al. 1965; Roth et al. 1983). The most usual profile all these systems describe for melancholic patients is a constellation of symptoms which includes psychomotor retardation, late insomnia, early morning worsening, weight loss, psychomotor agitation and guilt. The most frequently specified non-symptom clinical feature is normal personality. Several reviews of the literature have been published on this matter (Davidson et al. 1984; Mendels and Cochrane 1968; Nelson and Charney 1981; Parker et al. 1989; Rush and Weissenburger 1994).

Most classification efforts also include a pole opposite to the 'endogenous/melancholic'. This pole has received various names like 'reactive' or 'neurotic'; however, the most recent label given was that of 'atypical depression' and has been the focus of research during the last few decades, but it was not recognized by official classification systems until DSM-IV (American Psychiatric Association 2000).

Originally, this category has been proposed to describe depressed patients who respond poorly to tricyclics (TCAs) and well to monoamine oxidase inhibitors (MAOIs) (West and Dally 1959; Dally and Rohde 1961; Liebowitz et al. 1988); however, subsequent research suggested that these patients are refractory to all classes of antidepressants. It is not yet clear how best to define the subtype (Davidson et al. 1982; Thase 2007; Fountoulakis et al. 1999), and very little are known concerning its reliability, prevalence, relationship to other subtypes of depression and the performance characteristics of various possible defining items (Rabkin et al. 1996). The Columbia definition (Liebowitz et al. 1984) has been the most advanced and the predecessor of the DSM definition. These patients generally have laboratory testing similar to control subjects.

The terms 'endogenous depression', 'neurotic depression', 'anxious depression', 'involutional melancholia' and 'psychotic depressive reaction' are not included in modern classification systems for a variety of reasons. The term 'neurasthenia' is maintained in ICD-10, but its meaning is vague.

A term used in the past to denote this particular group of patients was 'hysteroid dysphoria' which combined reverse vegetative signs (overeating and oversleeping) with giddy behaviour in romantic affairs and intensive dysphoria with anxiety, anger and suicidality as a response to romantic disappointment. Craving for chocolate and sweets as well as impaired anticipatory pleasure but preserved consummatory reward have been also described in these patients. Anticipatory pleasure is more closely linked to motivation and goal-directed behaviour, leading one to have the experience of wanting more, and that consummatory pleasure is more closely linked to satiation or a resolution of desire (Klein 1984; Depue and Collins 1999; Morrone-Strupinsky and Depue 2004). The term 'hysteroid' denotes the presence of a biologically based character-like pathology. Clinically it seems that hysteroid dysphoria is probably a variant of BD-II with cyclothymic and irritable temperament traits.

The question whether melancholic features are merely a severity dimension cannot yet be answered. Studies on the stability of depressive subtypes across episodes of depression revealed that 'non-endogenous' depressions may develop endogenous features during subsequent episodes, but endogenous depressions are likely to remain that way (Kendell 1974; Paykel et al. 1976; Coryell et al. 1994). Reports on ways of defining melancholia without the confounding effect of severity (Parker et al. 1990) are not convincing. The question on the true nature of melancholic features is complicated by methodological problems concerning all the spectrum of the research methodology used (Zimmerman et al. 1990; Everitt 1981) and particularly by the poor definition of depression severity. The lack of data specifically for bipolar depression confuses the picture even more.

To date, there is no satisfactory definition for severity. If one relies on the number of symptoms, then a circular reasoning leads to the conclusion that melancholia is a more severe form of depression and no difference in quality exists between melancholic and non-melancholic depressives. A different approach would be to take into consideration the degree of disability as an index of severity. But again, often the definition of disability, e.g. in the General Assessment of Functioning Scale (American Psychiatric Association 1994), is related to specific symptoms like suicidal ideation, anhedonia or fatigue, so reasoning may again be circular. Biochemical evidence provided no way out from this problem.

Unfortunately, the recognition of the disorder might delay by as much as 8–10 years, mainly because manic or hypomanic episodes appear late in the course of the illness (Angst 2007). As mentioned before, maybe more than half of hospitalized patients originally manifesting a depressive episode will turn out to be bipolars in the next 20 years (Angst et al. 2005). We can divide these patients into two groups: the 'false unipolars' that is those patients who turn eventually to be bipolars but do not manifest any manic or bipolar characteristic during depressive episodes and before the manifestation of a full manic or hypomanic episode, and the 'pseudounipolars', that is, those patients with subthreshold or subtle symptoms and signs belonging to the manic pole. It seems that the belief that the chances of a patient being bipolar instead of unipolar decreases by successive depressive episode is not true and the chances remain relatively stable thought the course of depressive disorder (Goodwin and Jamison 2007). According to DSM-5 both groups of patients are considered to be unipolar.

There is a large literature on the possibility to distinguish unipolar from false unipolar and pseudounipolar depressives. Karl Leonhard had already since 1957 noted that bipolar depressives manifest greater variability in their symptomatology across episodes (Leonhard 1957). Later this was confirmed mainly concerning BD-II depressives (Hantouche and Akiskal 2005). Overall it is believed that bipolar depressives manifest less anxiety, somatic complaints, psychomotor agitation, appetite and weight loss and early insomnia and more tension, fearfulness, psychomotor retardation, atypical features, variability across episodes, mood lability within an episode, late insomnia and hypersomnia, postpartum appearance, psychotic features and substance abuse (Goodwin and Jamison 2007).

Pseudounipolar patients often manifest agitation during a depressive episode. This 'agitated depression' has also named 'depressive mixed state' (Koukopoulos 1999). These patients, when assessed carefully, are reported to manifest additional manic-like features (Maj et al. 2003) and more frequently family history of BD (Maj et al. 2006). Up to 70 % of depressed were reported to have had significant manic symptoms but without fulfilling the definition of a mixed episode (Bauer et al. 2005). Since agitation and irritability are frequent symptoms during the course of a depressive episode (Serretti and Olgiati 2005), there are concerns whether 'agitated depressions' and 'depressive mixed states' should be included in the bipolar spectrum or whether such an inclusion will cause important problems in the conceptualization of BD. In accord with this concern, DSM-5 kept this condition in the chapter of (unipolar) depressive disorders.

Unipolar depressed patients who later 'convert' to BD over time, as well as bipolar depressives, manifest more frequently 'atypical' depressive features (hypersomnia, hyperphagia, leaden paralysis, long-term interpersonal rejection sensitivity) (Perugi et al. 1998), psychomotor retardation, psychotic features, pathological guilt and mood lability. Especially those who convert to BD-I (by manifesting mania) are characterized by early age at onset and pleomorphic psychopathology beyond the usual affective realm, high rates of substance abuse;

Table 2.2 Signs and symptoms which could assist in the differentiation between unipolar and bipolar depression

In comparison to unipolar, bipolar depression is characterized by:
Younger age at onset
Presence of either agitation or retardation
Less
Anxiety
Somatic complaints
Appetite and weight loss
Early insomnia
More
Irritability
Tension
Fearfulness
Atypical features
Late insomnia
Hypersomnia
Frequent postpartum appearance
Frequent psychotic features
Substance abuse
Variability in symptomatology across episodes
Mood lability within an episode
Family history

educational, marital and occupational disruption; and minor antisocial behaviour (Akiskal et al. 1995). BD patients also tend to have younger age of onset, more prior episodes of depression, shorter depressive episodes and family history of BD (Mitchell et al. 2008; Akiskal and Benazzi 2008; Rao et al. 1995; Geller et al. 1994, 2001). The latter is a strong predictor of bipolarity even in children and adolescents (Geller et al. 1994).

The clinical features more common in bipolar depression are summarized in Table 2.2. The characteristics could be useful in the prediction of a future manic or hypomanic episode in false unipolar or pseudounipolar depression.

The above clearly point to the fact that 'melancholic' features as defined by DSM are not useful in this differentiation. Atypical features, on the other hand, seem to be a better predictor and might even constitute the 'bridge' between unipolar and BD-II cases (Akiskal and Benazzi 2005, 2006), although some data dispute this relationship (Parker et al. 2005). Atypical depression puts forward also the question concerning the relationship between bipolar illness and personality disorders. Clinically they are often inseparable, but it is generally preferable in most cases to diagnose mood disorders at the expense of a diagnosis of personality disorders.

There seems to be some differences between BD-I and BD-II patients in terms of their depressions. BD-II patients tend to be female, with less but more chronic episodes of lower severity, less frequently psychotic features and with more atypical features and anxiety (Goodwin and Jamison 2007).

2.4 Mania

Acute manic episodes constitute the second diagnostic pillar of BD and they put the diagnosis of bipolarity in a definite way. Typically, acute mania develops over a period of 1–2 weeks although both more protracted and more sudden onsets have also been described. Its major feature is a distinct period characterized by elevated or irritable mood or both, which clearly represents an observable and significant change from the normal behaviour, mood and functioning of the individual.

In general, the clinical features of classic mania are the opposite of those of depression. Thus, classic mania is characterized by elevated mood, rush of ideas, greater energy, psychomotor acceleration, impulsivity and ideas of grandiosity. However, there are features that can be seen both in depression and in mania, like irritability, anger, insomnia and agitation, even hypersexuality, although the exaggerated presence of them suggests the diagnosis of a mixed episode rather than that of a depressive or manic. Classic acute mania (i.e. without mixed features) is relatively easy to recognize, in spite of the fact that more severe cases with psychotic features might be misdiagnosed as schizophrenia, while milder cases might be misdiagnosed as personality disorders (especially borderline, narcissistic and antisocial personality disorders).

The patient's mood during acute mania is characteristically elated with euphoria, jubilation, laughing, punning and gesturing. Euphoria is observed in 30–97 % of patients during acute mania (Abrams and Taylor 1976; Beigel and Murphy 1971; Carlson and Goodwin 1973; Clayton and Pitts 1965; Taylor and Abrams 1973, 1977; Winokur et al. 1969; Winokur and Tsuang 1975; Leff et al. 1976; Loudon et al. 1977; Cassidy et al. 1998b). Mood is unrestrained and expansive in the majority of patients (44–66 %) (Loudon et al. 1977; Taylor and Abrams 1973, 1977) and typically lifts that of the observer, especially in cases of classic euphoric mania. Elevated mood, jokes, gestures and overall behaviour cheer up the others and often the patient is at the centre of fun. A deep feeling of general well-being is present. However, in cases of dysphoric mania or anger, or even in cases of very 'silly' or dramatic behaviour, the result could be irritating for the others. This is in contrast to the indifferent or cold emotional feeling induced by patients with schizophrenia to those observing or examining them. The prevailing positive mood in mania is often not stable and brief intrusions of crying and tears are common. Additionally, acceleration and expansion are so excessive that many patients experience high levels of anxiety, tension and nervousness. Patients are dissatisfied and intolerant and the vast majority manifests mood lability and instability (42–95 %) (Abrams and Taylor 1976; Carlson and Goodwin 1973; Cassidy et al. 1998b; Loudon et al. 1977; Taylor and Abrams 1977; Winokur et al. 1969). Lability seems to be a dominant feature with only a few patients being free of it and often resembles a 'personality-like' feature, being capricious and intense. Irritability is also very frequent (51–100 %) (Carlson and Goodwin 1973; Cassidy et al. 1998b; Serretti and Olgiati 2005; Winokur et al. 1969; Taylor and Abrams 1973, 1977; Winokur and Tsuang 1975; Abrams and Taylor 1976; Loudon et al. 1977). Thus, irritability seems to be an inherent component of manic mood. Since also omnipotent thoughts are often present, when crossed, these patients might become irritable, hostile (with verbal as well as physical aggressiveness) and even dangerous. However, even significant depressive symptoms are experienced by as many as 29–100 % of acutely manic patients (Beigel and Murphy 1971; Carlson and Goodwin 1973; Cassidy et al. 1998b; Kotin and Goodwin 1972; Loudon et al. 1977; Murphy and Beigel 1974; Prien et al. 1988; Winokur et al. 1969). This intrusion of depressed features during an acute manic episode seems to be more frequent and significant in females (Winokur et al. 1969). When excessive they give rise to dysphoric or mixed mania. This is not identical to a mixed episode. In at least a significant proportion of patients, the ratings of depressive symptoms are higher during their acute mania periods in comparison to their acute depressive periods (Kotin and Goodwin 1972). During periods of dysphoric mania, irritability, anger, panic attacks, agitation, suicidal ideation, severe insomnia and persecutory delusions often coexist with more classic manic symptoms.

It has been proposed that acute mania starts with increased activity accompanied by euphoria or mild irritability, while thinking remains coherent (stage I), then progresses to the experience of dysphoria and the manifestation of open hostility and anger and disorganization (stage II) and finally to an undifferentiated psychotic state with dysphoria, severe disorganization and psychotic features (stage III). The episode disappears in the reverse order, from stage III to stage I and normality (Carlson and Goodwin 1973).

However, 'pure' affective states are rare. It has been reported that 94 % of DSM-IV manic patients had significant depressive but without fulfilling the definition of a mixed episode (Bauer et al. 2005). That study suggested that mixed pictures are more frequent than pure ones, and interestingly, they reported (in accord to an earlier study) a positive correlation between manic and depressed symptoms in contrast to what common sense would have predicted (Bauer et al. 2005; Kotin and Goodwin 1972).

Accelerated psychomotor activity, which constitutes the hallmark of mania, is characterized by overabundant energy, activity and rapid, pressured speech, which is fast and often witty. It is observed in the vast majority of patients (56–100 %) (Abrams and Taylor 1976; Carlson and Goodwin 1973; Carlson and Strober 1978; Cassidy et al. 1998a, b; Leff et al. 1976; Loudon et al. 1977; Serretti and Olgiati 2005; Taylor and Abrams 1973; Winokur et al. 1969). Pressured speech is observed in almost all patients (Abrams and Taylor 1976; Carlson and Goodwin 1973; Cassidy et al. 1998a; Clayton and Pitts 1965; Loudon et al. 1977; Serretti and Olgiati 2005; Taylor and Abrams 1973; Winokur et al. 1969; Carlson and Strober 1978; Leff et al. 1976). Subjectively, the patient experiences an unusual sense of well-being and physical and mental strength. Increase in goal-directed activity is characteristic of the situation, with patients starting multiple unrelated tasks simultaneously and often continue with new tasks before completing the previous ones, and in spite of the fact that it is obvious, they will be unable to cope with them. These tasks vary from simple everyday works (cleaning, cooking, painting the house, etc.) to complex ambitious enterprise (opening multiple new businesses, etc.). Pressured writing leads to the production of a large number of declarations, poems and various texts or a combination of text and some kind of drawing. Handwriting becomes irregular and often peculiar. Often the risk associated with these multiple goals is significant both in financial and in physical terms. It is to be noted that although an appetite disorder is not present in manic patients, often they lose weight due to excess physical activity and neglect of nutrition.

Thought disorder in manic patients includes problems with abstract thinking, conceptualization and coherence. Thought disorder should be separated from speech disorder, although the two concepts as well as clinical pictures relate to each other and overlap. Most studies reported that there is no 'quantitative' difference (Harrow et al. 1982, 1986; Breakey and Goodell 1972), although others find a slightly better thought functioning in manic patients in comparison to patients with schizophrenia (Resnick and Oltmanns 1984). However, there seems to be a qualitative difference with manic patients having more disordered structure, with a dominance of extravagance, playfulness and humour, over inclusion, tangentiality, circumstantiality and incoherence, while patients with schizophrenia have more disordered thought content with underinclusiveness, poverty of content, idiosyncratic and autistic thinking, conceptual deficit, tangentiality, peculiar and fluid ideas and unstable structure and disorganization (Simpson and Davis 1985; Daniels et al. 1988; Solovay et al. 1987; Andreasen and Powers 1975; Jampala et al. 1989). It is interesting also that this thought disorder is reversible in a significant proportion of BD patients, and this improvement is greater in comparison to schizophrenia, although a surprisingly high number of them (up to one-third) show severe thought disturbance which cannot be attributed to the presence of psychotic features alone (Harrow et al. 1986; Grossman et al. 1986).

A number of studies reported that manic patients have more complex speech and more overall quantity in comparison to patients with schizophrenia (Morice and Igram 1983; Morice and McNicol 1986; Docherty et al. 1996; Thomas et al. 1996; Lott et al. 2002). It is reported that the speech in manic patients is mainly because of shifting from one discourse to another. In comparison, patients with schizophrenia have significant difficulty in elaborating any discourse (Hoffman et al. 1986). Furthermore, the speech of manic patients is more complex in terms of syntax and with fewer errors (Lott et al. 2002; Thomas et al. 1996), less predictable in comparison to controls but more in comparison to that in schizophrenia (Ragin and Oltmanns 1983). Speech analysis alone seems to be able to identify up to 80 % of BD patients and normal controls (Fraser et al. 1986).

Pressured writing is characteristic of acute mania and leads to the production of an astonishing number of various texts, from poems to political manifesto. In milder cases these writings could be impressive; however, with increasing severity they become incoherent and the style becomes bizarre.

The content of thoughts is dominated by inflated self-esteem, ideas of grandiose, high confidence and a sense of very important achievements. Thinking is excessively positive, optimistic and expansive. Insight and judgment are impaired and transient. The line between nonpsychotic manic thought content and psychotic is very thin, and for many authors it does not exist at all. These mean that clinicians should routinely obtain clinically relevant information concerning the previous psychiatric history of the patient from significant others, and often the hospitalization is arranged on an involuntary basis. The thinking process is accelerated, and it is subjectively experienced as flight of ideas. Thinking and perception are unusually sharp; however, creativity is facilitated only in very mild cases. Sharpening is usually accompanied by instability thus leading to easy distraction by irrelevant stimuli and inability to differentiate between unimportant and important stimuli. It is not unusual that the examiner has difficulty to interrupt and ask a question. The patient may speak with such pressure that associations are difficult to follow. Often hoarseness develops, but this usually does not have a significant effect on the pressure to speak. In more severe cases the patient might 'jump' from one topic to another with loose associations or even his speech becomes completely incomprehensive. 'Clang' associations often based on rhyming or chance perceptions might appear. This puts the possibility of schizophrenia or gives the impression of organic confusion and even of some type of aphasia. To make things more complex, the patients might experience periods of amnesia (hours or days) when their mental activity is extremely accelerated because of inability to register any memories at that particular time period. This often covers much of the manic episode itself, and as a result the patients cannot recall and report it to the examiner.

'Delirious' mania constitutes an extremely severe expression of mania. It is also known as Bell's mania after Luther Bell (1806–1862) who first described it in 1849, and today it is very rare. It has an abrupt onset, ranging from hours to days, and it involves extreme physical activity with loss of appetite, insomnia, confusion, paranoia, confabulations and extremely bizarre hallucinations and delusions. Patients often run nude in the street, or on the contrary they isolate themselves inside their house, lock doors and shut windows. It constitutes a life-threatening medical emergency since fever, tachycardia, hypertension and rapid breathing often exist. During episodes of delirious mania, mood shifts rapidly between extreme mania and severe depression, suggesting a possible link to mixed states. Speech follows this shifting and logorrhoea alternates with mutism. A number of symptoms and signs which are unusual during mood episodes, like negativism, stereotypical movements, posturing, echolalia and echopraxia, are prominent. Typically, the presence of these symptoms and signs should be used in the differential diagnosis between schizophrenia and mood disorders, but Bell's mania constitutes an exception. Bell's mania responds to standard antimanic treatment although the use of typical antipsychotics might led to clinical worsening especially when given in combination with anticholinergic drugs (Fink 1999; Bipeta and Khan 2012; Bond 1980; Friedman et al. 2003; Jacobowski et al. 2013; Jarvie and Hood 1952; Karmacharya et al. 2008; Lee et al. 2012; Swartz et al. 1982).

The overall behaviour in mania is characterized by impulsivity and disinhibition. Patients act impulsively and show interest in every new activity that strikes their fancy. Judgment is thus impaired, and they engage in various activities which are often embarrassing, problematic or even dangerous in many ways and can lead to long-term problems (physical, personal, financial) that persist in the life of the patient long after the remission of the episode. Typical examples include dancing in the street; flirting indiscretionally; paying the bills of total strangers in bars; abusing phone calls; buying cars, jewellery or other unnecessary expensive items; giving away property; gambling; engaging in risky business venture, etc. Also, manic patients are meddlesome; they show abnormal familiarity with total strangers and are intrusive and with increased involvement with others. This embarrasses family, friends and colleagues. On the other hand, manic patients are often violent and interpersonally aggressive because of low tolerance to confrontation, paranoid tendencies and impulsivity.

One of the most problematic behaviours is hypersexuality which usually leads to sexual indiscretion and marital problems. It is present in 25–80 % of patients (Allison and Wilson 1960; Carlson and Goodwin 1973; Carlson and Strober 1978; Clayton and Pitts 1965; Leff et al. 1976; Loudon et al. 1977; Winokur et al. 1969). Typically women have provocative and embarrassing sexual affairs, while males spend large amounts of money on prostitutes and other sex-related activities. The risks because of hypersexuality in combination with poor judgment and impulsivity include disasters in personal life, financial problems and sexually transmitted diseases (e.g. AIDS).

During periods of acute mania, patients show a characteristic decreased need for sleep (hyposomnia). This is present in 63–100 % of patients (Carlson and Strober 1978; Cassidy et al. 1998a; Clayton and Pitts 1965; Leff et al. 1976; Loudon et al. 1977; Serretti and Olgiati 2005; Winokur et al. 1969), and in spite of the fact that they sleep only for a few hours (or even not at all of several nights in the row), they feel fresh, full of strength and energy on awakening. Some patients may actually go sleepless for several days. Severe hyposomnia worsens manic symptomatology and especially excitation, while the same time precludes resting, thus leading to physical exhaustion.

As mentioned above, the line between manic thought content (e.g. inflated self-esteem and grandiose ideas accompanied with impaired judgment and insight) and delusional beliefs is very thin, and some authors suggest that manic thought content is 'psychotic' by definition. However, formally, milder cases of increased self-esteem and ideas of superiority can be considered as stemming out of the heightened mood and being extreme manifestations of normal human thoughts. However, the rule rather than the exception is that during an acute manic episode, patients experience ideas of delusional quality and intensity (exceptional mental and physical fitness and talent, wealth, power, influence or affiliation, aristocratic ancestry). Delusions of reference and persecution are common, usually embedded on the on the belief that others envy them because of their special abilities or talents. Often delusional thinking is bizarre, e.g. patients might adopt a different grandiose identity, or they think they possess supernatural powers. Auditory and visual hallucinations are also very often experienced and typically are congruent with the elevated mood (e.g. voice of the God or the angels). Non-congruent delusions or hallucinations are less often experienced, and in these cases the diagnosis of schizoaffective disorder should be considered.

Although an early report by Lange, on the basis of study of 700 patients, suggested that psychotic symptoms are rare and present in less than 10 % of manic patients (Lange 1922), the rest of the literature supports the conclusion that overall, psychotic features are common in bipolar patients, and thus acute mania should be considered primarily a psychotic state (Koukopoulos 2006). Probably 33–96 % of acutely manic patients manifest psychotic features (Black and Nasrallah 1989; Carlson and Strober 1978; Rosenthal et al. 1980; Winokur et al. 1969). Although older studies suggested that a younger age at onset is related to more frequent and florid psychotic symptoms (Rosen et al. 1983), it is possible that this finding was because of confusion of bipolar disorder with schizoaffective especially since more recent studies did not find such a relationship (Perugi et al. 2000; Toni et al. 2001; Baethge et al. 2005). It is almost certain that the presence, quality and intensity of psychotic features correlates with the overall severity of manic symptoms (Abrams and Taylor 1976; Carlson and Goodwin 1973; Young et al. 1983; Baethge et al. 2005)

Delusions are present in 24–96 % of bipolar patients, and it is interesting that persecutory is equally frequent with grandiose (Rennie 1942; Carlson and Goodwin 1973; Carlson and Strober 1978; Clayton and Pitts 1965; Leff et al. 1976; Winokur et al. 1969; Winokur 1984; Black and Nasrallah 1989; Serretti et al. 2002; Keck et al. 2003; Bowman and Raymond 1932; Astrup et al. 1959; Abrams and Taylor 1976; Beigel and Murphy 1971; Loudon et al. 1977; Murphy and Beigel 1974; Taylor and Abrams 1973, 1977; Rosenthal et al. 1980; Goodwin and Jamison 2007). The main difference of delusions in BD patients in comparison to schizophrenia is that in BD they have a changing nature, they usually are appropriate to the patient's mood, and they are not systematized, but they tend to be more wish fulfilling, while in schizophrenia they tend to isolate the patient from the others (Goodwin and Jamison 2007). Delusions of grandiose can be so intense and severe that the term 'manic dementia' was coined by Emil Kraepelin.

Hallucinations are less frequent and present in 13–66 %; they can either be congruent or non-congruent, with auditory, visual and olfactory being almost equally frequent (Goodwin and Jamison 2007; Abrams and Taylor 1976; Astrup et al. 1959; Bowman and Raymond 1932; Carlson and Strober 1978; Lange 1922; Rosenthal et al. 1980; Taylor and Abrams 1973, 1977; Winokur et al. 1969; Black and Nasrallah 1989; Keck et al. 2003; Serretti et al. 2002; Winokur 1984). They are more frequent in females (Baethge et al. 2005), and according to some authors their quality resembles more that of organic psychoses than schizophrenia, including the presence of better insight concerning them (Bowman and Raymond 1932; Lowe 1973; Silberman et al. 1985). Often they are in close relationship with a specific delusion, and thus they are unstable and changing (Winokur et al. 1969). Sixty-one percent of BD patients experience some type of psychotic symptoms at least once in their lifetime with 17 % experiencing first-rank symptoms (Goodwin and Jamison 2007). Almost one-third of acutely manic patients are 'confused', 46–75 % are violent (Abrams and Taylor 1976; Carlson and Goodwin 1973; Cassidy et al. 1998a; Taylor and Abrams 1973, 1977), 23–33 % have significant sexual exposure (Abrams and Taylor 1976; Taylor and Abrams 1973, 1977), and 10–20 % have fetal incontinence (Abrams and Taylor 1976; Taylor and Abrams 1973, 1977). As many as 14–56 % manifest severe regression, catatonia, posturing and negativism often making differential diagnosis from schizophrenia difficult (Carlson and Goodwin 1973;

Carlson and Strober 1978; Kruger et al. 2003; Lange 1922; Taylor and Abrams 1973, 1977; Abrams and Taylor 1981; Braunig et al. 1998). The frequent presence of catatonia is recognized also by the DSM-5.

Unfortunately, the detection of psychotic symptoms is problematic with relatives reporting them accurately in less than 20 % of cases (Orvaschel et al. 1982; Thompson et al. 1982; Price et al. 1984), while very often their detection makes the diagnosis of mood disorder less likely, in favour of schizophrenia (Pope and Lipinski 1978).

The pattern of symptoms seems to be relatively stable from episode to episode at least in the short term in the same patient (Beigel and Murphy 1971; Cassidy et al. 2002) although the progression of the illness changes both its polarity and its dominant clinical manifestations in the long term.

All the studies which analyzed the factorial structure of mania agree that there is a mood component, a psychomotor component (mostly activation) and a component corresponding to irritability and aggression and another one related to psychotic features. It is possible that none of these components is primary and homogenous. Not even the mood component is such, since euphoria and dysphoria does not seem to be mutually exclusive but often coexist (Murphy and Beigel 1974; Double 1991; Cassidy et al. 1998a, 2001; Dilsaver et al. 1999; Swann et al. 2001; Sato et al. 2002; Akiskal et al. 2003; Gonzalez-Pinto et al. 2003). What seems to derive from these factorial studies is that psychomotor activation is the core feature of mania (Bauer et al. 1994b; Akiskal et al. 2001) although this is not in direct accord with the concept of acute mania neither in the way it is defined by contemporary classification systems nor in the way most psychiatrists perceive it.

Two special topics concern chronic and unipolar mania. Around 5 % of BD patients have chronic mania (Akiskal 2000). Technically it is difficult if not impossible to make a distinction between true chronic mania and ultrarapid cycling. It is characterized by lack of adherence to treatment and reduced mental as well as general activity. Mood is often 'silly' rather than euphoric, and there seems as if the finest emotions have disappeared and only the coarser enjoyments still exist (Kraepelin 1921). 'Unipolar mania' is reported in 5–28 % of mood patients in some studies; however, there is much concern on the duration of follow-up and the methods used to identify depressive episodes. A 20-year follow-up study from the NIMH suggested that not more than 4 % of 'bipolar' patients can be considered to suffer from unipolar mania (Solomon et al. 2003). According to an original suggestion by Koukopoulos, mania is primary and depression is a consequence (mania is the fire and depression the ashes) (Koukopoulos 2006). This theory has not been confirmed, and a problem is that under the umbrella of the term 'mania', many states characterized by excitement, agitation and irritability are included. However, it might suit a subgroup of patients, especially those whose illness starts with a manic episode. Of course these patients constitute a minority, manifest also a predominant manic polarity, have a better overall course and outcome and respond very well to lithium, especially the MDI type (mania–depression-free interval).

Secondary mania is another interesting topic. Acute mania in patients without prior bipolar illness and with a characteristically low family history load could be triggered during postpartum, in the course of various somatic illnesses like thyrotoxicosis, systemic lupus erythematosus, rheumatic chorea, multiple sclerosis, Huntington's disease, cerebrovascular disease, brain tumours, head trauma, complex partial seizures, syphilis and AIDS, or it could be a consequence of their treatment. Although some authors support the concept of 'reactive' mania as a consequence of life events, there are no positive data in support of it.

2.5 Hypomania

Formally, those episodes with manic symptoms but less pronounced in terms of severity and with shorter duration are labelled 'hypomanic'. However, it can also be defined as distinct periods of at least a few days characterized by mild elevation of mood; increase in cheerfulness and jocularity; sharpened and positive thinking; increased self-confidence, optimism, gregariousness, talkativeness and people seeking; greater interest in sex; decreased inhibitions and decreased need for sleep accompanied by increased energy and activity levels. There is no impairment which characterizes full-blown manic episodes, and in this frame it cannot be considered to be merely a milder form of mania. The presence of psychotic symptoms, although in lower frequency in comparison to mania, supports this. Hypomania often heralds the end of a depressive episode (in the form of a rebound relief), and in this case it lasts only 1–2 days.

Hypomania is much more common than mania but its recognition is mostly achieved mainly by interviewing significant others and not the patient. It is distinguished from normal happiness because it tends to recur in an 'endogenous' way and cyclicity and often can be triggered by stimulants, caffeine abuse or antidepressants. If chronic, it can constitute the habitual baseline of a hyperthymic temperament.

Hypomanic episodes cause mild or no impairment at all, and on the contrary, in some cases, they may even contribute to success in business, leadership roles and the arts. Patients often experience the hypomanic episodes as ego-syntonic and pleasant, might not recognize them at all as abnormal or tend to deny them. Often these periods are considered as periods of perfect functioning and recovering from depression. In some cases, hypomanic episodes might be irritable or dysphoric, and in these patients the misdiagnosis of a personality or characterological disorder is usual. Psychotic symptoms are less frequent (around 20 %) in comparison to full-blown manic episodes, but they do occur (Mazzarini et al. 2010). However, in the long term, the recurrence of hypomanic episodes accumulates burden and adverse consequences because of a behaviour which is essentially abnormal and probably dysfunctional in the long term and thus poses the individual at risk at the personal, financial and physical level. The elated mood, although not overtly manic, is related to over optimism, overestimation of abilities, impulsivity and a degree of judgment and insight impairment, while the presence of irritable or dysphoric features causes impairment in occupational and interpersonal functioning over time.

2.6 Mixed States

In spite of the fact that the definition of BD is based on the alteration between two separate and distinct poles, 'pure' affective states are rare. It has been reported that 94 % of DSM-IV manic patients and 70 % of depressed had significant symptoms of the opposite pole, but without fulfilling the definition of a mixed episode (Bauer et al. 2005). That study suggested that mixed pictures are more frequent than pure ones, and interestingly, (in accord with an earlier study) they reported a positive correlation between manic and depressed symptoms in contrast to what common sense would had predicted (Bauer et al. 2005; Kotin and Goodwin 1972).

In this frame, mixed episodes are also considered to be part of the BD picture and clinically are defined as the coexistence of both depressive and manic symptoms. Although as mentioned before, manic and depressive symptoms almost always coexist, the concept of mixed episodes has been proposed to describe cases where this coexistence is profound. Earlier suggestions included also ultrarapid cycling cases. This kind of episodes might appear as a short transitional phase (transitional forms) between the two poles or as independent episodes (autonomic forms) (Kraepelin 1921; Weygandt 1899; Akiskal and Benazzi 2004). The presence of a limited number of depressive symptoms during a full-blown manic episode gives rise to dysphoric mania (Kotin and Goodwin 1972; McElroy et al. 1992; Prien et al. 1988), while similarly, the presence of a limited number of manic symptoms during a full-blown depressive episode leads to mixed agitated depression (Himmelhoch et al. 1976; Koukopoulos and Tundo 1992; Perugi et al. 1997; Cassidy et al. 1998a, b; Dilsaver et al. 1994).

Earlier approaches considered stupor to be a core characteristic of mixed states (Weygandt 1899), but currently psychomotor activation with irritability and mood lability seems to be more important (Winokur et al. 1969; Akiskal and Mallya 1987; Koukopoulos 1999; Sato et al. 2005). In mixed episodes the rate of psychotic symptoms is probably similar to that of manic ones and approximately 40 % (Mantere et al. 2004).

DSM-IV demanded the presence of both full-blown depressive and manic episodes in order to allow the label of a 'mixed' episode, in accord with the approach by Winokur et al. (1969), Evans and Nemeroff (1983) and Strakowski et al. (1992), but DSM-5 included mixed features as a specifier only. Both classification systems classify ultrarapid cases within the mixed pictures domain rather than rapid cycling. Essentially, ultrarapid cycling is the only way full-blown manic/hypomanic and depressive episodes can coexist as DSM-IV required.

The DSM-5 demands the presence of a full-blown episode of either pole together with at least three symptoms of the opposite pole being present in order to allow the label of 'mixed features' specifier. This is largely in accord with the proposals of Susan L. McElroy (McElroy et al. 1992, 1995), while other authors had proposed that the presence of only two (Akiskal et al. 1998) or even only one criterion (Swann et al. 1997) should be sufficient. The proportion of mixed episodes depends both on the study sample and on the definition utilized (McElroy et al. 1992) and varies from 5 % to 70 % (Himmelhoch et al. 1976; Kotin and Goodwin 1972; Winokur et al. 1969; Murphy and Beigel 1974; Carlson and Goodwin 1973; Keller 1988; Keller et al. 1986; Nunn 1979; Strakowski et al. 1992; Cassidy et al. 1998b, 2001; Dell'Osso et al. 1991; Dilsaver et al. 1999; Gonzalez-Pinto et al. 2003; Kruger et al. 2003; McElroy et al. 1995; Perugi et al. 1997; Post et al. 1989; Prien et al. 1988; Sato et al. 2002; Secunda et al. 1987; Akiskal et al. 1998). When using the definition with the three or more criteria, mixed episodes are more often diagnosed in females, and the disease is more likely to begin with a mixed episode and characterized by fewer episodes of longer duration (McElroy et al. 1995).

Often the criteria for a mixed features specifier are not fulfilled. A special case is the coexistence of hypomanic features or even of a fully blown hypomanic episode in the frame either of type II BD (BD-II) or even unipolar depression. Although full hypomanic episodes are rare (2.8 %), at least three were registered in 28.5 % of unipolar depressed patients. The respective rate was 48.7 % for BD-II patients during a depressed phase (Benazzi 2000; Benazzi and Akiskal 2001).

Sometimes there is an admixture of a number of manic and depressive symptoms in a combination which does not fulfil the specific DSM criteria for a manic or depressive episode; thus, the only possible diagnosis is that of a not-otherwise-specified (NOS) mood episode (Akiskal et al. 1998; Akiskal 1996). There seems to be a constellation of types of affective episodes which are not part of the official classification, and they are so prevalent in real-life clinical practice that many authors consider them to be the rule rather than the exception.

Mixed episodes are also considered to be part of the BD picture and according to DSM-IV-TR are defined as the coexistence of both depressive and manic symptoms to the extent that the criteria for both manic and depressed episodes are fulfilled (Akiskal and Benazzi 2004). In DSM-5 the definition was softened, and instead of 'mixed episodes' a 'mixed features specifier' was included. Alterations in mood characterize several other DSM disorders which have a bipolar character. These include cyclothymic disorder and borderline personality disorder. However, there is a constellation of types of affective episodes which are not part of the official classification, and they are so prevalent in real-life clinical practice that many authors consider them to be the rule rather than the exception.

Frequently the manic symptoms can go unnoticed by the clinician because instead of being hyperthymic, the mood is irritable, and it is diluted in the presence of depressed thought content and suicidal ideation, leading the clinician to the diagnosis of anxious or agitated depression, or worse, of a personality disorder, instead of a mixed or mixed-NOS mood episode. Frequently, this irritable mood can lead the person to manifest aggressive behaviour especially if confronted or rejected while having grandiose and paranoid delusions, and these patients are maybe the most aggressive seen in the emergency room (Maj et al. 2003; Sato et al. 2005).

Although clinically manic and depressive symptoms appear simply to coexist, there are a number of observations suggesting that there is a deeper and complex interplay of various factors which gives rise to mixed episodes. Originally Kraepelin (1921) and Weygandt (1899) proposed the existence of three separate components which fluctuate independently from each other: mood, cognition and psychomotor activity. The combination of their phases could thus produce six different types of affective episodes: (a)

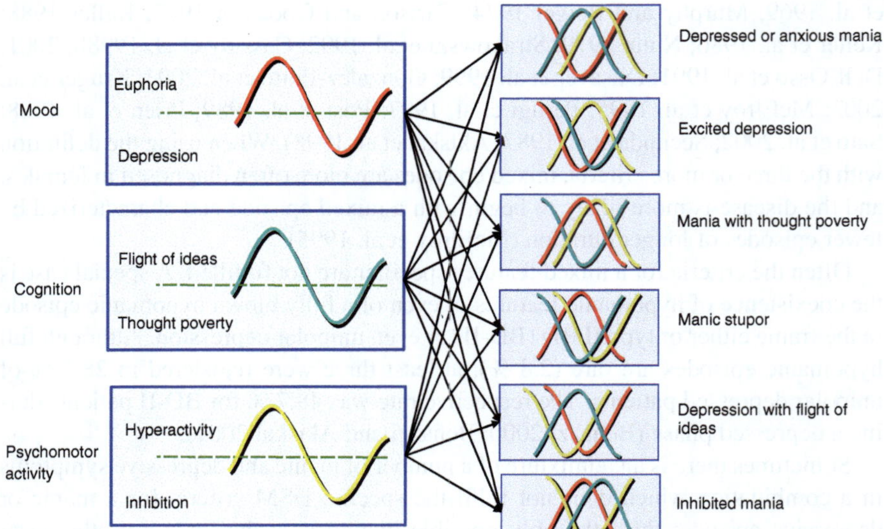

Fig. 2.3 Graphic representation of the three separate components of mood episodes (mood, cognition and psychomotor activity) and their independent fluctuation which gives rise to six different types of mood episodes

depressive or anxious mania (depressed affect with flight of ideas and hyperactivity), (b) excited depression (depressed affect with thought poverty and hyperactivity), (c) mania with thought poverty (manic affect with thought poverty and hyperactivity), (d) manic stupor (manic affect with thought poverty and inhibition), (e) depression with flight of ideas (depressed affect with flight of ideas and inhibition) and (f) inhibited mania (manic affect with flight of ideas and inhibition) (Fig. 2.3).

A more or less similar approach suggests that the superimposition of an affective episode on a temperament of opposite polarity (pointing to a conflict between the components of affect and mood) might explain better the complex psychopathology and quality of patients with mixed episodes (Akiskal 1992). In support of such a distinct quality in psychopathology of mixed patients is the observed mood liability and higher frequency of non-congruent psychotic features (Akiskal and Mallya 1987; Perugi et al. 1997; Akiskal et al. 1998; Winokur et al. 1969; Kotin and Goodwin 1972; Himmelhoch et al. 1976; Post et al. 1989; Strakowski et al. 1992). In accord is also the observation that patients who experience a mixed episode tend to experience only such episodes in the future (Dell'Osso et al. 1991) and that mixed patients tend to have neuropsychiatric abnormalities more often than classic manic patients (Himmelhoch and Garfinkel 1986).

As mentioned before, the admixture of manic and depressive elements may give two 'mirror' clinical pictures, that is, 'dysphoric mania' (Kotin and Goodwin 1972; McElroy et al. 1992; Prien et al. 1988) and 'mixed agitated depression' (Himmelhoch et al. 1976; Koukopoulos and Tundo 1992; Perugi et al. 1997; Cassidy et al. 1998a, b; Dilsaver et al. 1994).

In agitated depression, depressed mood, anxiety, inner tension, unrest and agitation dominate the clinical picture. Anhedonia is also marked, and suicidality is frequently present, although not to the same degree as in unipolar patients (Angst et al. 2002). Typically, there is no speech retardation, and although there is usually an increased overall physical activity, the purposeful activity is significantly reduced. In more severe cases, there is total lack of purposeful activity. It has been reported that mental excitement might be more pronounced in the lack of marked physical agitation. Thoughts are typically fast and overcrowded (Akiskal and Mallya 1987; Koukopoulos 1999; Benazzi and Akiskal 2001). However, in contrast to mania, where mental speed is generally reflected in pressured speech, in agitated depression this is not the case. On the contrary, although these patients experience crowded or racing thoughts, their speech is normal or even retarded and monotonous. 'Racing thoughts' are observed in approximately one-third of hospitalized depressive patients (Braden and Qualls 1979), and they differ from 'flight of ideas' in the sense that the former do not express themselves in the patient's speech directly, and their content torments the patient (in contrast to the flight of ideas whose content is usually joyful). They also differ from 'depressive ruminations' which are clearly depressed thoughts which tend to recur but without high speed and do not completely fill the mind. The content of racing thoughts is not always depressive; it can include also trivial issues. However, this unusual number of thoughts is disturbing and painful, and this experience poses a significant burden on the individual (Koukopoulos et al. 2005).

There is evidence that a development of an excited/irritable state could happen when antidepressants, especially dual action ones, are used. Many patients will not develop a classic manic episode in response; many will either develop a full-blown mixed episode or more likely a DSM-subthreshold mixed-NOS episode with the presence of a small number of manic symptoms in combination with depression, especially agitation, and this state could persist and worsen if more aggressive antidepressant treatment is tried.

At least 50 % of BD patients experience a mixed manic state with two to four depressive symptoms in the frame of a full-blown manic episode. Mixed episodes seem to last longer than manic ones, but it is unclear whether they manifest any difference in the age of onset (Keller et al. 1986; Dell'Osso et al. 1991). While during acute mania suicidality is almost absent, the presence of mixed features induces it in up to 14–55% of patients (Dilsaver et al. 1994; Strakowski et al. 1996; Marneros et al. 2004; Kotin and Goodwin 1972; Winokur et al. 1969). Psychotic and catatonic symptoms are also frequent, and in the case of mixed episodes, they are associated with greater severity and poor prognosis (Kruger et al. 2003). Mixed episodes by themselves do not seem to correlate with severity of illness and rapid cycling (Himmelhoch et al. 1976) although the outcome seems to be poorer.

There is some but not concluding evidence that a development of an excited/irritable state could happen when antidepressants, especially dual action ones, are used. Many patients will not develop a classic manic episode in response; many will either develop a full-blown mixed episode or more likely a DSM-subthreshold mixed-NOS episode with the presence of a small number of manic symptoms in combination with depression, especially agitation, and this state could persist and worsen if more aggressive antidepressant treatment is tried.

2.7 Psychotic Features

Although psychotic features were described in previous parts of the current chapter in the frame of specific mood episodes, it is important to summarize the knowledge concerning them, since psychosis in BD constitutes an important element with profound consequences for the treatment, prognosis and overall outcome of the patients. However, in spite of the fact that psychosis is very frequent in BD patients, unfortunately the detection of psychotic symptoms is problematic with relatives reporting them accurately in less than 20 % of cases (Orvaschel et al. 1982; Thompson et al. 1982; Price et al. 1984), while very often their detection makes the diagnosis of mood disorder less likely, in favour of schizophrenia (Pope and Lipinski 1978).

Psychotic features may include delusions or hallucinations of any sensory modality, and they can either be congruent or non-congruent, and both could occur in the context of any type of episode, but more often during acute manic and mixed episodes. Sixty-one percent of BD patients experience some type of psychotic symptoms at least once in their lifetime with 17 % experiencing first-rank symptoms (Goodwin and Jamison 2007). Almost one-third of acutely manic patients are 'confused', 46–75 % are violent (Abrams and Taylor 1976; Carlson and Goodwin 1973; Cassidy et al. 1998a; Taylor and Abrams 1973, 1977), and 10–20 % have fetal incontinence (Abrams and Taylor 1976; Taylor and Abrams 1973, 1977). As many as 14–56 % manifest severe regression, catatonia, posturing and negativism often making differential diagnosis from schizophrenia difficult (Carlson and Goodwin 1973; Carlson and Strober 1978; Kruger et al. 2003; Lange 1922; Taylor and Abrams 1973, 1977; Abrams and Taylor 1981; Braunig et al. 1998). It is important to note that catatonia is recognized by the DSM-5 as part of the bipolar clinical picture and not exclusively of schizophrenia.

This often creates a diagnostic dilemma; however, in order to put the diagnosis of schizoaffective disorder according to DSM-5, there must be a psychotic episode of at least 2 weeks duration in the absence of mood symptoms of sufficient intensity to qualify for a major mood episode. In ICD-10 this diagnostic boundary is vague and differential classification is often difficult. In DSM-5 bipolar disorders were included in a separate chapter between the chapters of schizophrenia and depressive disorders so as to stress their position as a bridge between the other two. It has been argued that psychotic features constitute a stable trait which tends to repeat itself across episodes, although the studies which suggest this use a mixture of bipolar and unipolar patients, and therefore, generalizability is problematic (Helms and Smith 1983; Nelson et al. 1984; Aronson et al. 1988a, b).

Psychotic features in BD patients are usually in accord with mood. Thus, not only they differ between acute mania and acute depression but also fluctuate as mood fluctuates, and they are less fixated in comparison to schizophrenia. In BD patients psychotic features have a self-fulfilling quality rather than being part of a fixed system of beliefs. They present in 9–66 % during periods of acute bipolar depression and probably in 33–96 % of acutely manic patients manifest psychotic features (Black and Nasrallah 1989; Carlson and Strober 1978; Rosenthal et al. 1980; Winokur et al. 1969; Mantere et al. 2004; Goes et al. 2007). In mixed episodes the rate is probably similar to that of manic ones (Mantere et al. 2004). Thus, it seems that psychotic features are somewhat more frequent during acute mania, but this difference is not overwhelming. They are more frequent in bipolar than in unipolar depression (Goes et al. 2007).

During periods of depression, delusions are present in 12–66 % of patients (Black and Nasrallah 1989; Carlson and Strober 1978; Rosenthal et al. 1980; Winokur et al. 1969). They include mood-congruent delusions of worthlessness and sinfulness, reference, infidelity and persecution (often in the form of prosecutor); poverty, disaster or ill health appears (suffering from an occult illness, like cancer or AIDS). A special type is nihilistic delusions (Cotard's syndrome after Jules Cotard; 1840–1889) which include thoughts that parts of the body are missing. Under the influence of depressive delusions, not only suicide but also homicide can occur, usually with an 'altruistic' motive (e.g. under delusions of poverty, disaster or moral decay, a father might kill his children in order to 'save' and 'protect' them and afterwards commits suicide; mothers with psychotic depression during the postpartum period could commit infanticide). Mood-incongruent delusions can be also present (e.g. persecutory delusions which cannot be considered in the frame of the depressed mood); however, if bizarre delusions are present, then the diagnosis of schizoaffective disorder should be considered.

Several authors suggest that manic thought content is 'psychotic' by definition (Koukopoulos 2006). Delusions are present in 24–96 % of acutely manic patients, and it is interesting that persecutory is equally frequent with grandiose (Rennie 1942; Carlson and Goodwin 1973; Carlson and Strober 1978; Clayton and Pitts 1965; Leff et al. 1976; Winokur et al. 1969; Winokur 1984; Black and Nasrallah 1989; Serretti et al. 2002; Keck et al. 2003; Bowman and Raymond 1932; Astrup et al. 1959; Abrams and Taylor 1976; Beigel and Murphy 1971; Loudon et al. 1977; Murphy and Beigel 1974; Taylor and Abrams 1973, 1977; Rosenthal et al. 1980; Goodwin and Jamison 2007). Almost always patients experience ideas of delusional quality and intensity (exceptional mental and physical fitness and talent, wealth, power, influence or affiliation, aristocratic ancestry). Delusions of reference and persecution are common, usually embedded on the belief that others envy them because of their special abilities or talents. Often delusional thinking is bizarre, e.g. patients might adopt a different grandiose identity, or they think they possess supernatural powers and frequently non-mood-congruent. It is almost certain that the presence, quality and intensity of psychotic features correlate with the overall severity of manic symptoms (Abrams and Taylor 1976; Carlson and Goodwin 1973; Young et al. 1983; Baethge et al. 2005).

The main difference of delusions in manic patients in comparison to schizophrenia is that in BD they have a changing nature, they usually are appropriate to the patient's mood, and they are not systematized, but they tend to be more wish fulfilling, while in schizophrenia they tend to isolate the patient from the others (Goodwin and Jamison 2007).

During acute bipolar depression hallucinations are less frequent (8–50 %) in comparison to acute mania (Baethge et al. 2005; Black and Nasrallah 1989; Carlson and Strober 1978; Rosenthal et al. 1980; Winokur et al. 1969) and are most often auditory (Black and Nasrallah 1989; Carlson and Strober 1978; Rosenthal et al. 1980; Winokur et al. 1969; Mantere et al. 2004). Typically they are extremely unpleasant, and their content is in accord with depressed mood and delusional ideation. They can be mood-congruent (e.g. accusatory or derogatory) or mood-incongruent (e.g. two voices discussing without any reference to the patient). Often they are so schizophrenia like that they pose a diagnostic dilemma.

Hallucinations in mania are present in 13–66 %; they can either be congruent or non-congruent, with auditory, visual and olfactory being almost equally frequent (Goodwin and Jamison 2007; Abrams and Taylor 1976; Astrup et al. 1959; Bowman and Raymond 1932; Carlson and Strober 1978; Lange 1922; Rosenthal et al. 1980; Taylor and Abrams 1973, 1977; Winokur et al. 1969; Black and Nasrallah 1989; Keck et al. 2003; Serretti et al. 2002; Winokur 1984). They are more frequent in females (Baethge et al. 2005), and according to some authors their quality resembles more that of organic psychoses than schizophrenia, including the presence of better insight concerning them (Bowman and Raymond 1932; Lowe 1973; Silberman et al. 1985). Often they are in close relationship with a specific delusion, and thus, they are unstable and changing (Winokur et al. 1969).

Already since the earlier attempts for the creation of the modern era nosological classification, specific severe psychotic clinical pictures had been identified and described in BD patients. Kraepelin described 'melancholia gravis' as a more severe form of depression with psychotic features and 'fantastic melancholia' for even more severe forms with more pronounced psychotic symptoms, alternation of agitation with stupor and clouding of consciousness. According to Kraepelin the most severe form of depression is 'delirious melancholia' with very severe and almost 'schizophrenic-like' delusions and hallucinations. In these cases, clouding of consciousness dominates the clinical picture (Kraepelin 1921). Kraepelin also coined the term 'manic dementia' for those cases of acute mania in which the delusions of grandiose were extremely intense and severe.

Even before Kraepelin, in 1849, Luther Bell (1806–1862) had coined the term 'delirious' mania for cases of extremely severe expression of mania. It is also known as Bell's mania and today it is very rare. It has an abrupt onset, ranging from hours to days, and it involves extreme physical activity with loss of appetite, insomnia, confusion, paranoia, confabulations and extremely bizarre hallucinations and delusions. Patients often run nude in the street, or on the contrary they isolate themselves inside their house, lock doors and shut windows. It constitutes a life-threatening medical emergency since fever, tachycardia, hypertension and rapid breathing often exist. During episodes of delirious mania, mood shifts rapidly between extreme mania and severe depression, suggesting a possible link to mixed states. Speech follows this shifting and logorrhoea alternates with mutism. A number of symptoms and signs which are unusual during mood episodes, like negativism, stereotypical movements, posturing, echolalia and echopraxia are prominent. Typically the presence of these symptoms and signs should be used in the differential diagnosis between schizophrenia and mood disorders, but Bell's mania constitutes an exception. Bell's mania responds to standard antimanic treatment although the use of typical antipsychotics might led to clinical worsening especially when given in combination with anticholinergic drugs (Fink 1999; Bipeta and Khan 2012; Bond 1980; Friedman et al. 2003; Jacobowski et al. 2013; Jarvie and Hood 1952; Karmacharya et al. 2008; Lee et al. 2012; Swartz et al. 1982).

2.8 Other Clinical Issues

Frequently the correct diagnosis is put only after several years have passed since onset because the first episode is often psychotic like or depressive and the diagnosis is put correctly only after a manic or mixed episode emerges. It has been estimated that more than half of hospitalized patients originally manifesting a depressive episode will turn out to be bipolars in the next 20 years (Angst et al. 2005). This has profound implications concerning the treatment and its overall efficacy. An additional problem for the diagnosis is that patients usually experience hypomania as a recovery from depression and almost always as a pleasant ego-syntonic mood state.

The clinical picture of BD includes a number of symptoms and syndromes which according to contemporary classification systems constitute comorbid conditions, but historically one can argue that they constitute core features of BD itself and not separate or semi-separate disorders. In the current textbook they will be discussed in detail in the chapter dedicated to comorbidity and other specifically dedicated chapters. Of special interest are also the neurocognitive impairment which is reported to exist in both BD-I and BD-II patients, although more so in the bipolar I group, and this is true even during the euthymic period (Dixon et al. 2004; Malhi et al. 2004; Sole et al. 2011) and the psychosocial impairment which seems to be significant and present even when patients are euthymic. It is reported that only a minority achieves complete functional recovery (Goldberg et al. 1995a, b; Keck et al. 1998; Strakowski et al. 1998; Martinez-Aran et al. 2007; Mur et al. 2007; Daban et al. 2006). It is reported that in 69.6 % of cases the course resembles that of a recurrent episodic illness, while in 25 % of cases there is a chronic course without clear remissions between episodes. In only 5.4 % there is a single episode of mania. Suicidal ideation is present in 78.6 % of cases at some time in their life. Alcohol and drug abuse/dependence is present in 32.1 %. Around 84.8 % of patients have at least one contact with any health services during the previous year (Morgan et al. 2005). It seems that in the long term at least one-third of patients are symptomatic with depressed episodes manifesting three times more than manic/hypomanic (De Dios et al. 2009).

Clinicians and researchers together often neglect the fact that although mania is the key diagnostic feature of BP, it is depression that is mainly responsible for the burden of the disease (Judd et al. 2002, 2003; Goodwin and Jamison 2007). Bipolar depression is more refractory than unipolar and has poor response to antidepressants, and only limited options for its treatment are available (Fountoulakis et al. 2008, 2011; Fountoulakis and Vieta 2008; Fountoulakis 2009). Subsyndromal depressive symptoms are usual, they cause significant disability (Judd and Akiskal 2003), and they put the patient at a three-time higher risk to relapse (Judd et al. 2008). On the other hand, potentially insufficient or wrong aggressive monotherapy with antidepressants might worsen the long-term outcome of the illness and put the patient at a higher risk for suicide.

The most frequent comorbid mental disorders are alcohol and drug use and abuse, anxiety disorders, obsessive–compulsive disorder, social phobia, personality disorders, post-traumatic stress disorder, eating disorders and migraine (Altamura et al. 2011; Boylan et al. 2004; Chen and Dilsaver 1995; Fasmer 2001; Kessler et al. 1999; Low et al. 2003; Mahmood et al. 1999; McElroy et al. 2006; Merikangas et al. 2007; Otto et al. 2004; Regier et al. 1990; Simon et al. 2007; Strakowski et al. 1992). Alcohol abuse could be present in more than half of patients and frequently represents self-medication efforts, and it is particularly problematic during adolescence and early adulthood. The drug abuse pattern of BD patients concerns mainly stimulant drugs (Winokur et al. 1998).

Approximately one-third of BP-I patients suffer from one or more general medical conditions, and BP-I constitutes an important risk factor for 7 of 11 general medical conditions (Perron et al. 2009a; b). The most prevalent conditions are cardiovascular (e.g. hypertension, present in 35 %), endocrine (e.g. hyperlipidaemia, 23 %; diabetes, 17 % vs. 15 % for controls), alcohol use disorder (25 %), hepatitis C (5.9 % vs. 1.1 % of controls), lower back pain (15.4 % vs. 10.6 % of controls) and pulmonary conditions (e.g. COPD: 10.6 % vs. 9.4 % of controls) (Goldstein et al. 2008, 2009, 2011; Kilbourne 2005; Kilbourne et al. 2004; Soreca et al. 2008, 2009).

2.9 The Subjective Experience of Manic–Depressive Patients

Hearing what patients can say to describe their experience of living with the illness is important. It is also of value to take into consideration their narrations so as to better understand the nature and the whole spectrum of illness manifestations. Unfortunately, the value of these narrations is problematic because of their subjective nature, the limitations of the language when it comes to the description of unusual inner experiences and the large variability in the experience itself among patients. However, these narrations still constitute the only means to comprehend not only the negative but also the positive aspects of manic depression and its treatment (Jamison 1993; Jamison et al. 1980), the burden and the attitudes towards the illness and treatment with special focus on the subjective experience of adverse effects and the influence of religious, popular and philosophical beliefs. Most narrations share a pattern of tempestuous emotions, religious and/or mystical experience, paranoia, violence, impulsivity and periodicity. In order to understand the inner experience it is important to realize that existential issues are of prime importance. Religious and mystical themes often dominate the patients' existence. In this frame, both the positive and the negative consequences of the illness make sense as they are embedded in the life of the patient.

As mentioned above, depressed mood is the pathological equivalent of grief and mourning and is characterized by a painful negative emotion, which is typically experienced as worse than severe physical pain. This experience is out of proportion and out of frame of existing stimuli and is characterized by groundless apprehensions with severe inner turmoil and torment. The suffering is persistent although in milder cases spontaneous fluctuation even during the same day can occur (typically worse in the morning or in the afternoon). It is paradoxical that although depressed patients experience a hypervigilant state with heightened perception of pain, many also experience an inability to experience emotions, and they are even unable to cry. Anhedonia makes the patient to abandon previously enjoyed pastimes. In milder cases, it is manifested by decreased interest in hobbies and life, but in most severe cases it leads the patient to lose feelings for loved significant ones (kids, spouse). Patients typically describe their environment as without any colours, as if everything is black and with shades of grey. This is a quite odd experience which alienates patients from others and from the environment. Depersonalization and derealization might follow and often the experience has a psychotic-like quality.

Depressed patients usually experience a form of lethargy, mental and physical paralysis and suffocation. Often they experience a tearing of their chest and internal organs as a form of tearing of existence and self. Trivial things and senses could be painful for no reason. Casual and irrelevant memories could be dreadful and horrifying. Even pleasant events and beautiful things trigger despair because of the realization of inability to feel joy. Patients cannot find peace and cannot rest. Sleep is equal to losing consciousness without rest. Cognitive slowing and difficulty in concentration might lead to indecisiveness and feelings of inefficiency. The difficulty in thinking makes patients tied to the actual consciousness of the moment. Depression triggers the dark and negative side of existential dilemmas and fears, including sense of purpose, life and death, values and morality and religious beliefs, thus making internal experience unbearable. Pain, lack of motivation and psychomotor retardation makes even everyday basic casual activities an effort and trigger a vicious cycle of emotional downfall.

During periods of mania, patients experience a pervasive sense of well-being which acts as background for all their experiences and decisions during this period. They often feel that nothing is beyond their abilities. They have a time urgency, their creativity and learning ability are somewhat increased during the mild phase of the episode, and they tend to make notes of everything. Their omnipotent feelings make them feel that money is not important and there are no consequences concerning any risky or compulsive behaviour they take (Goodwin and Jamison 2007).

Often this well-being is accompanied by pleasurable or stimulating somatic sensations, like tingling of the spinal cord or the solar plexus. The experience of somatic sensations changes, and the patients are able to withstand extreme situations like running naked and barefooted on the streets in the cold or on the snow. They often have a 'heightened sense of reality' (Henderson and Gillespie 1956) which makes them feel in intimate contact with the universe, all the creatures and God. Sometimes they might feel fused with them, identify with them, and almost they lose identity. Senses become more acute, perception increases, and this leads to a complete change in the awareness of the environment. Although this is not related to psychotic phenomena per se, the increased awareness of details, the emotional investment of them and on trivial things as well as the simultaneous perception of different objects and situations make the whole experience outside the range of sanity. It is similar in many ways to the experiences induced by psychomimetic substances and in the past might had been considered mystical religious or spiritual trance conditions.

The subjective experience of patients during a mixed episode is reported to be far worse in comparison to a depressive one. Mixed episodes are characterized by the experience of extreme anguish and mental pain as a result of the combination of depression with acceleration, psychoticism and confusion.

2.10 List and Definitions of Symptoms and Signs

It is important to have a list of signs and symptoms along with their description readily available. The following list serves the purpose of a short encyclopaedic lexicon of the most basic and important clinical terms used in the study of manic depression. The list is organized in domains (mood, psychomotor disorder, neurocognitive disorder, thought disorder, psychotic symptoms, somatic and neurovegetative symptoms and behavioural disorder).

A list of comparison of symptoms between depression and mania organized in hypothetical bipols is shown in Table 2.3.

2.10.1 Mood

1. *Euthymia* refers to the normal range of mood and the absence of any disorder.
2. *Mourning* refers to the experience of sadness as a consequence of a loss of a loved one. It includes crying, sadness and preoccupation with the lost person and related memories.
3. *Depressed mood* means that the patient experiences a 'negative' and unpleasant affect, and in Western cultures and languages, the words (or their linguistic equivalents) 'depressed', 'anguished', 'mournful', 'sad', 'anxious' and 'blues' are used. The word 'depressed' is increasingly used because of the higher information (partially because of the Internet) the public has today on depression. The way and the words the patient uses to describe this experience depend on the cultural and educational background and can focus on bodily function or on existential and interpersonal dysphoria and difficulties. Somatic complains are more prominent in milder cases usually seen in the primary care setting in patients with anxious depression. These cases were considered to suffer from 'masked' depression.
4. *Anhedonia* refers to the inability to experience normal emotions. Frequently, patients with anhedonia are incapable of even feeling the depressed affect, and they can't even cry. The patient abandons activities which in the past were a source of joy and gives up interest in life. Patients with more severe depression

Table 2.3 List of manic and depressive bipols of symptoms and signs. Almost any combination is possible in real-life clinical practice and especially in the frame of mixed mood states

Depressive episode	Manic episode
Mood	
Dysphoria	Euphoria
Depressed mood	Mood elevation
Anhedonia	Excessive interest in pleasurable activities
Indifference/irritability	Irritability
Mood lability	Mood lability
Passivity	Anger
Thought disorder	
Crowded thoughts	
Racing thoughts	Racing thoughts
Slow thinking	Flight of ideas
Concentration difficulties	Distractibility
Difficulty in thinking	Sharpened or unusually creative thinking
Low self-esteem	Inflated self-esteem or grandiosity
Depressive thought content	Manic thought content
Hopelessness/helplessness	Omnipotency
Feelings of guilt	Expansive attitude/impulsivity
Somatic symptoms	
Insomnia or hypersomnia	Decreased need for sleep (hyposomnia)
Loss of libido	Increased sexual activity
Tiredness/fatigue/leaden paralysis	High energy level
Weight/appetite changes	Loss of weight due to hyperactivity
Psychomotor change	
Inertia	Full of vitality
Decreased speech	More talkative than usual or pressure to keep talking, articulate and jocular
Decrease in goal-directed activity	Increase in goal-directed activity
Psychomotor slowing/retardation	Psychomotor acceleration
Psychomotor agitation	Psychomotor agitation
Passive behaviour	Verbal/physical aggressiveness
Stupor/catatonia	Stupor/catatonia
Psychotic features	
Delusions	Delusions
Hallucinations	Hallucinations
Sociality	
Psychosocial withdrawal	Increased sociability
	Loss of social inhibitions
	Impulsive behaviour/disinhibition
Others	
Logorrhoea	Mutism

(continued)

Table 2.3 (continued)

Depressive episode	Manic episode
Suicidal thoughts/attempts	Omnipotent thoughts
Anxiety	Anxiety
Indecisiveness	Impulsivity
Relative preservation of insight	Lack of insight

are indifferent even concerning their kids or spouse and isolate themselves. The difference from the flat (blunted) affect seen in schizophrenia is that anhedonia is itself painful. As depression starts remitting, anhedonia is one of the first symptoms to remit.

5. The term *elevated mood* refers to a state of elation, overconfidence and enjoyment, with the person being cheerful, laughing, punning and making happy and expressive gestures. It is not always pathological.
6. *Euphoria* refers to a pathologically too much elevated mood that is inappropriate to real events. It is considered to constitute the opposite pole of 'depressed mood' with 'normality' in the middle. It is interesting and important that experiencing a euphoric mood is pleasant; thus, patients are reluctant to receive treatment.
7. *Euthymia*: Although the original Greek word clearly suggests an elevated mood (in good spirits, a bit lower than during euphoria), the term is used currently in the international literature to denote a normothymic condition.
8. *Expansive mood* is a condition with the patient expressing his feelings without restraint and control, and behaviour is usually coloured by thoughts of grandiose.
9. *Emotional lability* refers to unstable and rapidly changing emotions often because of hyperreactivity to environmental stimuli. It is not always pathological.
10. *Irritable mood* is a state in which the person is easily annoyed by external stimuli and expresses anger and hostility at a low threshold. The presence of an irritable mood is often the cause for misdiagnosis of the patient, especially in combination with lability and mixed states.

2.10.2 Psychomotor Disorder

11. *Flight of ideas* refers to an acceleration of the thinking processes, which almost always manifests itself through rapid speaking. Speech could be coherent and thoughts unusually sharp; however, when speed is excessively high, they both become incoherent and fragmented with content changing abruptly. Associations could be based on rhyme or chance perceptions.
12. *Racing thoughts* refer to the experience of thoughts running fast inside the mind, but this is not evident in speech which is normal or even retarded and monotonous or in behaviour. The content of these thoughts could be manic and depressive but also trivial.

13. *Crowded thoughts*: A large number of thoughts pilling inside the brain, without racing or flying. The patient experiences a large number of them simultaneously occupying his consciousness without moving from the front stage, but instead they tend to accumulate and push each other for space in consciousness. They are seen mainly in depression, and their content could be depressive or trivial.
14. *Psychomotor acceleration* is considered to be the hallmark of mania, characterized by excessive activity which is goal directed, high energy and endurance as well as rapid, pressured speech.
15. In comparison, *psychomotor agitation* also refers to both mental and physical overactivity (pressured speech, restlessness, motor behaviour) usually accompanied by a feeling of an inner turmoil or severe anxiety, with the intensity being so great that in spite of the fact that the patient has normal arousal, most if not all of this activity is purposeless.
16. *Psychomotor slowing* means that the patient is inert and slow, both physically and mentally, but this does not always have an effect on overall performance although everything is done with much effort.
17. When psychomotor slowing is excessive, then *psychomotor retardation* appears, and it includes reduction or disappearance of spontaneous motor activity, slumped posture and gaze, reduced and slow speech and great fatigue.
18. *Stupor* appears in younger patients when the psychomotor retardation is so extreme that they are unable to function even concerning basic everyday needs. In more severe cases, motor immobility appears. It often constitutes an acute medical emergency. Essentially, the patient regresses to a primitive infantile functioning level, with inability to control even basic bodily functions. Physical health is greatly endangered because of immobility, bad nutrition and weight loss, constipation, circulation problems, etc. There is immobility and a strong resistance to all attempts at movements, or on the contrary there is so much muscle relaxation that the body parts can be moulded onto any position and remain there, no matter how inconvenient the position is. Although in most patients there is clouding of consciousness, most of them are able to recall their experience during periods of stupor and the great distress that accompanies it.
19. *Catatonia* is defined as a complex condition which can include diverse symptoms and signs like motor immobility or on the contrary excessive purposeless motor activity not influenced by external stimuli, motiveless negativism, mutism, peculiar or stereotyped movements, mannerisms, grimacing and sometimes echolalia or echopraxia.
20. *Fatigue* is a common problem in all mental disorders but especially in mood disorders and includes feeling tired or weak, sleepy and sometimes irritable.

2.10.3 Neurocognitive Disorder

21. The term *neurocognitive* is often used with reference to higher cognitive function, like attention, concentration, memory, praxis, etc., and in psychiatry

in contrast to the term *cognitive* which often is used with reference to the thought content or style and relates to cognitive therapy. Bipolar patients constitute a clinically heterogenous group; however, they seem to perform poorly on most neuropsychological tests in comparison to healthy controls. They seem to suffer from deficits especially related to attention, inhibitory control, spatial working memory, semantic verbal fluency, verbal learning and memory and maybe executive function, especially when considering the more severe and psychotic end of the bipolar spectrum. Verbal memory and probably executive function impairments may represent a trait rather than a state marker.

22. In extreme cases, neurocognitive disorder is so severe, especially in elderly patients that the picture resembles that of a dementing disease, thus is called *pseudodementia*. However, it seems that at least half of these patients do in fact suffer from a dementing process at its early stages, and later they manifest a formal dementia syndrome. If one looks at the problem from another point of view, depression with mild cognitive disorder may be either the first manifestation or a risk factor for the development of dementia, especially when combined with a family history of dementia.

2.10.4 Thought Disorder

23. *Depressive thought content*: Depressed patients are characterized by a negative evaluation of the self, the world and the future (the negative cognitive triad). In this frame, the depressive thought content includes pessimism, low self-esteem and low self-confidence, ideas of loss, deprivation and guilt, helplessness and hopelessness and ultimately thoughts of death and suicide. The extent to which this negative way of thinking is primary or secondary is a matter of debate.
24. *Clang association*: It refers to the condition when the patient's thought association and subsequently the speech are directed by the sound of a word rather than by its meaning. Thus, words are not connected in a logical way and punning and rhyming serve as the drive.
25. *Thoughts of guilt* concern self-reproach, self-accusing and feeling the need for punishment. Thoughts and feelings of guilt are largely normal, and they could appear during a mood disorder because of the disability the disorder causes and the inability of the patient to fulfil his/her obligations towards significant others. In this frame patients might also feel shame. However, when the intensity and the content are excessive or even inappropriate, then thoughts of guilt should be considered to be part of the symptoms, and in more severe cases these thoughts could obtain a delusional character.
26. *Thoughts of death*: Thoughts of death are particularly important because they might eventually lead to suicidal behaviour. The common belief that inquiring about such thoughts provokes suicidal behaviour has no scientific basis. On the contrary, patients are often relieved this way. These thoughts include thoughts

that the person will die and often the wish to die in some way so as to leave the suffering behind; this way they lead to suicidal ideation.

27. *Suicidal ideation* refers to specific thoughts of killing oneself. It has many different forms, ranging from indirect expression (e.g. in a wish not to wake up or to die from a disease or an accident) to suicidal obsessions (urges or impulses to destroy oneself) and finally to elaborate planning of suicide. Some patients behave in a passive self-destructing way (e.g. careless driving or walking), while others plan their death in detail leaving notes and making sure no help will come on time.
28. *Manic thinking* is excessively positive and optimistic. It is characterized by inflated self-esteem, grandiose sense (concerning importance, power, knowledge or identity), overconfidence and sense of high achievements and abilities. Manic patients are refractory to explanations and confrontation, and to a significant extent they lack self-examination and insight; because of this lack of insight, mania nearly always, sooner or later, acquires a delusional character.

2.10.5 Psychotic Features

29. *Mood-congruent depressive delusions*: Often depressed thoughts could acquire a delusional severity and delusions congruent with depressive mood appear. Their content concerns inappropriate or over-exaggerated thoughts of guilt, sin, worthlessness, poverty and somatic health. Nihilistic delusions constitute a special kind under which the patient believes that parts of his/her body are missing. Delusions concerning persecution and jealousy, although seemingly non-congruent, could be mood-congruent also, if they can be explained by or strongly related to thoughts of sin, guilt, jealousy or worthlessness. This kind of delusional thought makes a parent kill his/her family so as to save them from moral or physical corruption, and then he/she commits suicide.
30. *Nihilistic delusions (Cotard's delusion or Cotard's syndrome, negation delusion)*: This special kind of delusions is related to depressive mood and concerns the delusional belief that all or parts of the patient's body are missing or rotten or decomposing; their internal organs are rotten or solidifying or even are actually dead; the world and everything related to it have ceased to exist.
31. *Mood-congruent manic delusions*: During manic episodes usually the thought content becomes delusional and includes delusions of exceptional mental and physical fitness or special talents. It also may include delusions of wealth, some kind of grandiose identity or importance. Sometimes the delusion can be so excessive that the identity itself changes (e.g. the patient believes that he is incarnation of a messiah or a prophet, etc.). Delusions of reference and persecution are considered to be mood-congruent on the basis of the belief that jealousy of the others at their special abilities is the cause of problems.
32. *Mood-incongruent delusions*: Various delusional ideas seemingly non-congruent (e.g. ideas of persecution or reference) could eventually be understood

as arising from the grandiose sense of self and the belief of the patient that this importance causes the others to envy. However, sometimes there are delusions whose content has no association to current mood (e.g. bizarre delusions without contextual relationship to mood). Sometimes a mixed mood episode can manifest itself with 'mood-incongruent' delusions, e.g. grandiose delusions in the presence of depressed mood.

33. *Depressive mood-congruent hallucinations* are hallucinations whose content is depressed (e.g. voices accusing or humiliating). Depressive mood-congruent hallucinations have an unpleasant content, and they cause significant additional distress to the patient. Sometimes they command the patient to commit suicide and even dictate the method.
34. *Manic mood-congruent hallucinations*: Sometimes it is considered that the intense experience of a mood episode, especially a manic one is characterized, causes such a vivid internal experience that the patients feel they can hear or see their thoughts (e.g. hear hymns or live in the paradise).
35. *Mood-incongruent hallucinations*: These are hallucinations unrelated to the current mood state.
36. *Insight*: Classically, usually the depressive episodes are characterized by a fair degree of insight with the exception of the severer psychotic cases. On the contrary, manic episodes are routinely characterized by a significant lack of insight, and thus clinicians must routinely obtain basic information from significant others. This lack of insight might lead to refusal of any treatment and to the need for an involuntary admission to a hospital.

2.10.6 Somatic and Neurovegetative Symptoms

37. *Anorexia and weight loss*: Anorexia and weight loss are considered to be reliable signs of depression. They can both be considered in the frame of a generalized inability to enjoy things (anhedonia). Weight loss is seen sometimes in paranoid patients who are afraid that food is poisoned, and this should not be confused with anorexia and weight loss in the frame of depression. Weight loss is also frequent in cases of malignant disease so a full medical investigation should accompany any patient with changes in appetite or weight.
38. *Weight gain* has been relatively recently recognized as a depressive feature and could be the result of overeating, decreased activity or both. Apart from its devastating effect on the self-confidence and self-image, it can worsen the general somatic health especially in patients that become obese and suffer from metabolic syndrome.
39. *Insomnia* is one of the hallmarks of depression and one of its most disturbing features. There are many types of insomnia, that is, difficulty falling asleep (initial insomnia), multiple awakenings during the night (middle insomnia) or early morning awakening (terminal insomnia). Insomnia prolongs the depressive agony round the clock. Some patients try to self-medicate and solve the

problem by alcohol or drug abuse (sedatives or hypnotics), but both eventually worsen the problem partially because of tolerance and dependence problems and partially because they both further destroy the architecture of sleep. Unipolar depressed patients tend to exhibit insomnia stereotypically episode after episode, and characteristically in spite of extreme fatigue, they rarely oversleep.

40. *Hyposomnia*: The term suggests a decreased need for sleep. That is, the patient feels energetic on awakening even though he slept for short periods. Some patients feel fresh and energetic even though they haven't slept for days. This condition is usually seen during manic episodes, and sometimes it heralds the beginning of such an episode. It is not synonymous to insomnia.
41. *Hypersomnia*: Some patients, especially younger ones and females, often sleep too much and find it difficult to get up from the bed in the morning. Along with the other atypical features, it is considered to be a marker for an underlying bipolar illness even in case no other bipolar feature is present. This condition should be differentially diagnosed from a number of medical conditions including narcolepsy and the Klein–Levin syndrome. In spite of prolonged sleep, depressed patients are characteristically tired in the morning, meaning that even prolonged sleep is not refreshing for them. The change in the pattern of sleep disruption with insomnia alternating with hypersomnia or hyposomnia suggests the presence of a bipolar illness rather than a unipolar depression.
42. *Circadian dysregulation*: Although many circadian functions could be disrupted in depressed patients, mainly the disturbance of sleep rhythms has been adequately studied. This disturbance includes deficits in delta sleep and more intense rapid eye movement (REM) activity during the first third of the night. A marked shortening of REM latency (i.e. the time from the onset of sleep to the first REM period) is considered to be characteristic for depression of any type and seen even in remitted depressive patients and their healthy relatives.
43. *Seasonality*: Seasonal (especially autumn–winter) emergence or worsening of depression has been recognized since antiquity, and mood has been related to the period of the year. Most patients seem to experience increased energy and activation during spring and the opposite during the fall and winter. Usually patients with strong seasonality also have reverse neurovegetative symptoms (fatigue, crave sugars, overeat and oversleep). In some patients seasonality is so concrete and important that modern classification includes a seasonal pattern for mood disorders.
44. *Sexual dysfunction*: Depressed patients classically report a decreased sexual desire and activity, while additionally some women manifest a temporary interruption of their menses. Sexual dysfunction especially in females could lead to marital conflict and a psychodynamic/psychotherapeutically oriented therapist could mistakenly ascribe depression to the marital conflict with profound negative effects on the therapeutic outcome. Treating the sexual dysfunction or its consequences and leaving depression untreated is not uncommon and includes even surgical or unusual therapeutic interventions. An additional problem is that treatment with antidepressants often has sexual dysfunction as an adverse

effect. The recent emergence of agents that treat impotence (e.g. sildenafil, tadalafil) could add a new method to treat this problematic symptom, but this should never move the focus of treatment away from depression.

45. *Increased sexual desire and activity*: This is typical for manic episodes, but also a subgroup of depressed patients may manifest increased sexual drive or activity, and usually they also manifest other atypical or 'reversed' features. Thus, if seen in the frame of depression, it heralds the presence of a depressive mixed episode. The increased sexual appetite usually leads to sexual indiscretion accompanied by a risky sexual life, often leading to marital problems, multiple separations or divorces, alcohol and drug abuse, gambling and sexually transmitted diseases like AIDS.

2.10.7 Behavioural Disorder

46. *Logorrhoea*: It refers to pressured, excessive and not always coherent speech, which is often uncontrollable. It is observed during manic episodes. Speech could be completely uncomprehending, with destroyed syntax and loose associations, often posing diagnostic dilemmas (e.g. from stroke). Other similar terms used are tachylogia, verbomania and volubility.
47. *Impulsive behaviour*: During mood episodes, either manic, depressive or mixed, patients tend to exhibit impulsive behaviour. Especially during manic episodes they tend to be impulsive, disinhibited and meddlesome. They are intrusive with increased involvement with others, have poor social judgment and engage in a variety of activities without control or restrain (including aggression, sex, gambling, drug and alcohol abuse, spending, making gifts, risk taking, travelling, etc.). Impulsive behaviour is the part of symptomatology that causes most problems and especially financial and interpersonal. In some cases even suicide could be acted on an impulsive basis.

References

Abrams R, Taylor MA (1976) Mania and schizo-affective disorder, main type: a comparison. Am J Psychiatry 133(12):445–447

Abrams R, Taylor MA (1981) Importance of schizophrenic symptoms in the diagnosis of mania. Am J Psychiatry 138(5):658–661

Akiskal HS (1992) The distinctive mixed states of bipolar I, II, and III. Clin Neuropharmacol 15(Suppl 1 Pt A):632A–633A

Akiskal HS (1996) The prevalent clinical spectrum of bipolar disorders: beyond DSM-IV. J Clin Psychopharmacol 16(2 Suppl 1):4S–14S

Akiskal H (2000) Mood disorders. In: Sadock B, Sadock V (eds) Comprehensive textbook of psychiatry, vol I. Lippincott Williams & Wilkins, Philadelphia, pp 1338–1377

Akiskal HS, Benazzi F (2004) Validating Kraepelin's two types of depressive mixed states: "depression with flight of ideas" and "excited depression". World J Biol Psychiatry 5(2):107–113

Akiskal HS, Benazzi F (2005) Atypical depression: a variant of bipolar II or a bridge between unipolar and bipolar II? J Affect Disord 84(2–3):209–217
Akiskal HS, Benazzi F (2006) The DSM-IV and ICD-10 categories of recurrent [major] depressive and bipolar II disorders: evidence that they lie on a dimensional spectrum. J Affect Disord 92(1):45–54. doi:10.1016/j.jad.2005.12.035, S0165-0327(05)00403-9 [pii]
Akiskal HS, Benazzi F (2008) Continuous distribution of atypical depressive symptoms between major depressive and bipolar II disorders: dose-response relationship with bipolar family history. Psychopathology 41(1):39–42
Akiskal HS, Mallya G (1987) Criteria for the "soft" bipolar spectrum: treatment implications. Psychopharmacol Bull 23(1):68–73
Akiskal HS, Walker P, Puzantian VR, King D, Rosenthal TL, Dranon M (1983) Bipolar outcome in the course of depressive illness. Phenomenologic, familial, and pharmacologic predictors. J Affect Disord 5(2):115–128
Akiskal HS, Maser JD, Zeller PJ, Endicott J, Coryell W, Keller M, Warshaw M, Clayton P, Goodwin F (1995) Switching from 'unipolar' to bipolar II. An 11-year prospective study of clinical and temperamental predictors in 559 patients. Arch Gen Psychiatry 52(2): 114–123
Akiskal HS, Hantouche EG, Bourgeois ML, Azorin JM, Sechter D, Allilaire JF, Lancrenon S, Fraud JP, Chatenet-Duchene L (1998) Gender, temperament, and the clinical picture in dysphoric mixed mania: findings from a French national study (EPIMAN). J Affect Disord 50(2–3):175–186
Akiskal HS, Hantouche EG, Bourgeois ML, Azorin JM, Sechter D, Allilaire JF, Chatenet-Duchene L, Lancrenon S (2001) Toward a refined phenomenology of mania: combining clinician-assessment and self-report in the French EPIMAN study. J Affect Disord 67(1–3):89–96. doi:S0165032701004414 [pii]
Akiskal HS, Azorin JM, Hantouche EG (2003) Proposed multidimensional structure of mania: beyond the euphoric-dysphoric dichotomy. J Affect Disord 73(1–2):7–18. doi:S016503270200318X [pii]
Allison JB, Wilson WP (1960) Sexual behavior of manic patients: a preliminary report. South Med J 53:870–874
Altamura AC, Serati M, Albano A, Paoli RA, Glick ID, Dell'Osso B (2011) An epidemiologic and clinical overview of medical and psychopathological comorbidities in major psychoses. Eur Arch Psychiatry Clin Neurosci 261(7):489–508. doi:10.1007/s00406-011-0196-4
American Psychiatric Association (1994) Diagnostic and statistical manual of mental disorders, 4th edn, DSM-IV. American Psychiatric Press, Washington, DC
American Psychiatric Association (2000) Diagnostic and statistical manual of mental disorders, 4th edn, Text Revision, DSM-IV-TR. American Psychiatric Publishing, Washington, DC
American Psychiatric Association (2013) Diagnostic and statistical manual of mental disorders, 5th edn, DSM-5. American Psychiatric Association, Washington, DC
Andreasen NJ, Powers PS (1975) Creativity and psychosis. An examination of conceptual style. Arch Gen Psychiatry 32(1):70–73
Angst J (2007) The bipolar spectrum. Br J Psychiatry 190:189–191. doi:10.1192/bjp.bp.106.030957, 190/3/189 [pii]
Angst F, Stassen HH, Clayton PJ, Angst J (2002) Mortality of patients with mood disorders: follow-up over 34–38 years. J Affect Disord 68(2–3):167–181. doi:S0165032701003779 [pii]
Angst J, Sellaro R, Stassen HH, Gamma A (2005) Diagnostic conversion from depression to bipolar disorders: results of a long-term prospective study of hospital admissions. J Affect Disord 84(2–3):149–157. doi:10.1016/S0165-0327(03)00195-2, S0165032703001952 [pii]
Aronson TA, Shukla S, Gujavarty K, Hoff A, DiBuono M, Khan E (1988a) Relapse in delusional depression: a retrospective study of the course of treatment. Compr Psychiatry 29(1):12–21
Aronson TA, Shukla S, Hoff A, Cook B (1988b) Proposed delusional depression subtypes: preliminary evidence from a retrospective study of phenomenology and treatment course. J Affect Disord 14(1):69–74
Astrup C, Fossum A, Holmboe R (1959) A follow-up of 270 patients with acute affective psychoses. Acta Psychiatr Scand Suppl 34(135):1–65

Baethge C, Baldessarini RJ, Freudenthal K, Streeruwitz A, Bauer M, Bschor T (2005) Hallucinations in bipolar disorder: characteristics and comparison to unipolar depression and schizophrenia. Bipolar Disord 7(2):136–145. doi:10.1111/j.1399-5618.2004.00175.x, BDI175 [pii]
Bauer MS, Calabrese J, Dunner DL, Post R, Whybrow PC, Gyulai L, Tay LK, Younkin SR, Bynum D, Lavori P et al (1994a) Multisite data reanalysis of the validity of rapid cycling as a course modifier for bipolar disorder in DSM-IV. Am J Psychiatry 151(4):506–515
Bauer MS, Whybrow PC, Gyulai L, Gonnel J, Yeh HS (1994b) Testing definitions of dysphoric mania and hypomania: prevalence, clinical characteristics and inter-episode stability. J Affect Disord 32(3):201–211
Bauer MS, Simon GE, Ludman E, Unutzer J (2005) 'Bipolarity' in bipolar disorder: distribution of manic and depressive symptoms in a treated population. Br J Psychiatry 187:87–88. doi:10.1192/bjp.187.1.87, 187/1/87 [pii]
Bech P, Gram LF, Reisby N, Rafaelsen OJ (1980) The WHO depression scale. Relationship to the Newcastle scales. Acta Psychiatr Scand 62(2):140–153
Beigel A, Murphy DL (1971) Assessing clinical characteristics of the manic state. Am J Psychiatry 128(6):688–694
Benazzi F (2000) Depressive mixed states: unipolar and bipolar II. Eur Arch Psychiatry Clin Neurosci 250(5):249–253
Benazzi F, Akiskal HS (2001) Delineating bipolar II mixed states in the Ravenna-San Diego collaborative study: the relative prevalence and diagnostic significance of hypomanic features during major depressive episodes. J Affect Disord 67(1–3):115–122. doi:S016503270100444X [pii]
Bipeta R, Khan MA (2012) Delirious mania: can we get away with this concept? A case report and review of the literature. Case Rep Psychiatry 2012:720354. doi:10.1155/2012/720354
Black DW, Nasrallah A (1989) Hallucinations and delusions in 1,715 patients with unipolar and bipolar affective disorders. Psychopathology 22(1):28–34
Bond TC (1980) Recognition of acute delirious mania. Arch Gen Psychiatry 37(5):553–554
Bowman K, Raymond A (1932) A statistical study of delusions in the manic-depressive psychoses. Am J Psychiatry 88:111–121
Boylan KR, Bieling PJ, Marriott M, Begin H, Young LT, MacQueen GM (2004) Impact of comorbid anxiety disorders on outcome in a cohort of patients with bipolar disorder. J Clin Psychiatry 65(8):1106–1113
Braden W, Qualls CB (1979) Racing thoughts in depressed patients. J Clin Psychiatry 40(8): 336–339
Braunig P, Kruger S, Shugar G (1998) Prevalence and clinical significance of catatonic symptoms in mania. Compr Psychiatry 39(1):35–46. doi:S0010-440X(98)90030-X [pii]
Breakey WR, Goodell H (1972) Thought disorder in mania and schizophrenia evaluated by Bannister's grid test for schizophrenic thought disorder. Br J Psychiatry 120(557): 391–395
Carlson GA, Goodwin FK (1973) The stages of mania. A longitudinal analysis of the manic episode. Arch Gen Psychiatry 28(2):221–228
Carlson GA, Strober M (1978) Affective disorder in adolescence: issues in misdiagnosis. J Clin Psychiatry 39(1):59–66
Carney MW, Roth M, Garside RF (1965) The diagnosis of depressive syndromes and the prediction of E.C.T. Response. Br J Psychiatry 111:659–674
Casper RC, Redmond DE Jr, Katz MM, Schaffer CB, Davis JM, Koslow SH (1985) Somatic symptoms in primary affective disorder. Presence and relationship to the classification of depression. Arch Gen Psychiatry 42(11):1098–1104
Cassidy F, Forest K, Murry E, Carroll BJ (1998a) A factor analysis of the signs and symptoms of mania. Arch Gen Psychiatry 55(1):27–32
Cassidy F, Murry E, Forest K, Carroll BJ (1998b) Signs and symptoms of mania in pure and mixed episodes. J Affect Disord 50(2–3):187–201. doi:S0165-0327(98)00016-0 [pii]
Cassidy F, McEvoy JP, Yang YK, Wilson WH (2001) Insight is greater in mixed than in pure manic episodes of bipolar I disorder. J Nerv Ment Dis 189(6):398–399
Cassidy F, Ahearn EP, Carroll BJ (2002) Symptom profile consistency in recurrent manic episodes. Compr Psychiatry 43(3):179–181. doi:S0010440X02465121 [pii]

Cattell R (1943) The description of personality, I: foundations of trait measurement. Psychol Rev 50:559–594

Chen YW, Dilsaver SC (1995) Comorbidity of panic disorder in bipolar illness: evidence from the Epidemiologic Catchment Area Survey. Am J Psychiatry 152(2):280–282

Clayton PJ, Pitts FN Jr (1965) Affect disorder. IV. Mania. Compr Psychiatry 6(5):313–322

Coryell W, Winokur G, Shea T, Maser JD, Endicott J, Akiskal HS (1994) The long-term stability of depressive subtypes. Am J Psychiatry 151(2):199–204

Daban C, Martinez-Aran A, Torrent C, Tabares-Seisdedos R, Balanza-Martinez V, Salazar-Fraile J, Selva-Vera G, Vieta E (2006) Specificity of cognitive deficits in bipolar disorder versus schizophrenia. A systematic review. Psychother Psychosom 75(2):72–84

Dally PJ, Rohde P (1961) Comparison of antidepressant drugs in depressive illnesses. Lancet 1(7167):18–20

Daniels EK, Shenton ME, Holzman PS, Benowitz LI, Coleman M, Levin S, Levine D (1988) Patterns of thought disorder associated with right cortical damage, schizophrenia, and mania. Am J Psychiatry 145(8):944–949

Davidson JR, Miller RD, Turnbull CD, Sullivan JL (1982) Atypical depression. Arch Gen Psychiatry 39(5):527–534

Davidson J, Turnbull C, Strickland R, Belyea M (1984) Comparative diagnostic criteria for melancholia and endogenous depression. Arch Gen Psychiatry 41(5):506–511

De Dios C, Ezquiaga E, Garcia A, Soler B, Vieta E (2009) Time spent with symptoms in a cohort of bipolar disorder outpatients in Spain: a prospective, 18-month follow-up study. J Affect Disord 125(1–3):74–81. doi:10.1016/j.jad.2009.12.006, S0165-0327(09)00539-4 [pii]

Dell'Osso L, Placidi GF, Nassi R, Freer P, Cassano GB, Akiskal HS (1991) The manic-depressive mixed state: familial, temperamental and psychopathologic characteristics in 108 female inpatients. Eur Arch Psychiatry Clin Neurosci 240(4–5):234–239

Depue RA, Collins PF (1999) Neurobiology of the structure of personality: dopamine, facilitation of incentive motivation, and extraversion. Behav Brain Sci 22(3):491–517; discussion 518–569

Dilsaver SC, Chen YW, Swann AC, Shoaib AM, Krajewski KJ (1994) Suicidality in patients with pure and depressive mania. Am J Psychiatry 151(9):1312–1315

Dilsaver SC, Chen YR, Shoaib AM, Swann AC (1999) Phenomenology of mania: evidence for distinct depressed, dysphoric, and euphoric presentations. Am J Psychiatry 156(3):426–430

Dixon T, Kravariti E, Frith C, Murray RM, McGuire PK (2004) Effect of symptoms on executive function in bipolar illness. Psychol Med 34(5):811–821

Docherty NM, DeRosa M, Andreasen NC (1996) Communication disturbances in schizophrenia and mania. Arch Gen Psychiatry 53(4):358–364

Double DB (1991) A cluster analysis of manic states. Compr Psychiatry 32(3):187–194. doi:0010-440X(91)90039-F [pii]

Dunner DL, Gershon ES, Goodwin FK (1976) Heritable factors in the severity of affective illness. Biol Psychiatry 11(1):31–42

Ekman P, Friesen W (1971) Constants across cultures in the face and emotion. J Pers Soc Psychol 17(2):124–129

Evans DL, Nemeroff CB (1983) The dexamethasone suppression test in mixed bipolar disorder. Am J Psychiatry 140(5):615–617

Everitt BS (1981) Bimodality and the nature of depression. Br J Psychiatry 138:336–339

Fasmer OB (2001) The prevalence of migraine in patients with bipolar and unipolar affective disorders. Cephalalgia 21(9):894–899. doi:279 [pii]

Fink M (1999) Delirious mania. Bipolar Disord 1(1):54–60

Fogel J, Eaton WW, Ford DE (2006) Minor depression as a predictor of the first onset of major depressive disorder over a 15-year follow-up. Acta Psychiatr Scand 113:36–43. doi:10.1111/j.1600-0447.2005.00654.x, ACP654 [pii]

Fountoulakis KN (2009) An update of evidence-based treatment of bipolar depression: where do we stand? Curr Opin Psychiatry 23(1):19–24. doi:10.1097/YCO.0b013e328333e132

Fountoulakis KN, Vieta E (2008) Treatment of bipolar disorder: a systematic review of available data and clinical perspectives. Int J Neuropsychopharmacol 11(7):999–1029. doi:10.1017/S1461145708009231, S1461145708009231 [pii]

Fountoulakis KN, Iacovides A, Nimatoudis I, Kaprinis G, Ierodiakonou C (1999) Comparison of the diagnosis of melancholic and atypical features according to DSM-IV and somatic syndrome according to ICD-10 in patients suffering from major depression. Eur Psychiatry 14(8):426–433
Fountoulakis KN, Grunze H, Panagiotidis P, Kaprinis G (2008) Treatment of bipolar depression: an update. J Affect Disord 109(1–2):21–34. doi:10.1016/j.jad.2007.10.016, S0165-0327(07)00378-3 [pii]
Fountoulakis KN, Kelsoe JR, Akiskal H (2011) Receptor targets for antidepressant therapy in bipolar disorder: an overview. J Affect Disord 138(3):222–238. doi:10.1016/j.jad.2011.04.043, S0165-0327(11)00210-2 [pii]
Fraser WI, King KM, Thomas P, Kendell RE (1986) The diagnosis of schizophrenia by language analysis. Br J Psychiatry 148:275–278
Friedman RS, Mufson MJ, Eisenberg TD, Patel MR (2003) Medically and psychiatrically ill: the challenge of delirious mania. Harv Rev Psychiatry 11(2):91–98
Geller B, Fox LW, Clark KA (1994) Rate and predictors of prepubertal bipolarity during follow-up of 6- to 12-year-old depressed children. J Am Acad Child Adolesc Psychiatry 33(4):461–468
Geller B, Zimerman B, Williams M, Bolhofner K, Craney JL (2001) Bipolar disorder at prospective follow-up of adults who had prepubertal major depressive disorder. Am J Psychiatry 158(1):125–127
Gillespie R (1926) Discussion on manic-depressive psychosis. BMJ 2:878–879
Goes FS, Sadler B, Toolan J, Zamoiski RD, Mondimore FM, Mackinnon DF, Schweizer B, Raymond Depaulo J Jr, Potash JB (2007) Psychotic features in bipolar and unipolar depression. Bipolar Disord 9(8):901–906. doi:10.1111/j.1399-5618.2007.00460.x, BDI460 [pii]
Goldberg JF, Harrow M, Grossman LS (1995a) Course and outcome in bipolar affective disorder: a longitudinal follow-up study. Am J Psychiatry 152(3):379–384
Goldberg JF, Harrow M, Grossman LS (1995b) Recurrent affective syndromes in bipolar and unipolar mood disorders at follow-up. Br J Psychiatry 166(3):382–385
Goldstein BI, Birmaher B, Axelson DA, Goldstein TR, Esposito-Smythers C, Strober MA, Hunt J, Leonard H, Gill MK, Iyengar S, Grimm C, Yang M, Ryan ND, Keller MB (2008) Preliminary findings regarding overweight and obesity in pediatric bipolar disorder. J Clin Psychiatry 69(12):1953–1959. doi:ej07m03953 [pii]
Goldstein BI, Fagiolini A, Houck P, Kupfer DJ (2009) Cardiovascular disease and hypertension among adults with bipolar I disorder in the United States. Bipolar Disord 11(6):657–662. doi:10.1111/j.1399-5618.2009.00735.x, BDI735 [pii]
Goldstein BI, Liu SM, Zivkovic N, Schaffer A, Chien LC, Blanco C (2011) The burden of obesity among adults with bipolar disorder in the United States. Bipolar Disord 13(4):387–395. doi:10.1111/j.1399-5618.2011.00932.x
Gonzalez-Pinto A, Ballesteros J, Aldama A, Perez de Heredia JL, Gutierrez M, Mosquera F (2003) Principal components of mania. J Affect Disord 76(1–3):95–102. doi:S0165032702000708 [pii]
Goodwin F, Jamison K (2007) Manic-depressive illness, 2nd edn. Oxford University Press, New York
Grossman LS, Harrow M, Sands JR (1986) Features associated with thought disorder in manic patients at 2–4-year follow-up. Am J Psychiatry 143(3):306–311
Hantouche EG, Akiskal HS (2005) Bipolar II vs. unipolar depression: psychopathologic differentiation by dimensional measures. J Affect Disord 84(2–3):127–132. doi:10.1016/j.jad.2004.01.017, S0165032704001429 [pii]
Harrow M, Grossman LS, Silverstein ML, Meltzer HY (1982) Thought pathology in manic and schizophrenic patients. Its occurrence at hospital admission and seven weeks later. Arch Gen Psychiatry 39(6):665–671
Harrow M, Grossman LS, Silverstein ML, Meltzer HY, Kettering RL (1986) A longitudinal study of thought disorder in manic patients. Arch Gen Psychiatry 43(8):781–785
Helms PM, Smith RE (1983) Recurrent psychotic depression. Evidence of diagnostic stability. J Affect Disord 5(1):51–54

Henderson D, Gillespie R (1956) A textbook of psychiatry for students and practitioners, 8th edn. Oxford University Press, London

Himmelhoch JM, Garfinkel ME (1986) Sources of lithium resistance in mixed mania. Psychopharmacol Bull 22(3):613–620

Himmelhoch J, Mulla D, Neil J, Detre T, Kupfer D (1976) Incidence and significance of mixed affective states in a bipolar population. Arch Gen Psychiatry 33:1062–1066

Hoffman RE, Stopek S, Andreasen NC (1986) A comparative study of manic vs schizophrenic speech disorganization. Arch Gen Psychiatry 43(9):831–838

Jacobowski NL, Heckers S, Bobo WV (2013) Delirious mania: detection, diagnosis, and clinical management in the acute setting. J Psychiatr Pract 19(1):15–28. doi:10.1097/01.pra.0000426324.67322.0600131746-201301000-00003 [pii]

Jamison K (1993) Touched with fire: manic-depressive illness and the artistic temperament. Free Press, New York

Jamison KR, Gerner RH, Hammen C, Padesky C (1980) Clouds and silver linings: positive experiences associated with primary affective disorders. Am J Psychiatry 137(2):198–202

Jampala VC, Taylor MA, Abrams R (1989) The diagnostic implications of formal thought disorder in mania and schizophrenia: a reassessment. Am J Psychiatry 146(4):459–463

Jarvie HF, Hood MC (1952) Acute delirious mania. Am J Psychiatry 108(10):758–763

Judd LL, Akiskal HS (2003) The prevalence and disability of bipolar spectrum disorders in the US population: re-analysis of the ECA database taking into account subthreshold cases. J Affect Disord 73(1–2):123–131

Judd LL, Akiskal HS, Schettler PJ, Endicott J, Maser J, Solomon DA, Leon AC, Rice JA, Keller MB (2002) The long-term natural history of the weekly symptomatic status of bipolar I disorder. Arch Gen Psychiatry 59(6):530–537. doi:yoa20425 [pii]

Judd LL, Akiskal HS, Schettler PJ, Coryell W, Endicott J, Maser JD, Solomon DA, Leon AC, Keller MB (2003) A prospective investigation of the natural history of the long-term weekly symptomatic status of bipolar II disorder. Arch Gen Psychiatry 60(3):261–269. doi:yoa20225 [pii]

Judd LL, Schettler PJ, Akiskal HS, Coryell W, Leon AC, Maser JD, Solomon DA (2008) Residual symptom recovery from major affective episodes in bipolar disorders and rapid episode relapse/recurrence. Arch Gen Psychiatry 65(4):386–394. doi:10.1001/archpsyc.65.4.386, 65/4/386 [pii]

Karmacharya R, England ML, Ongur D (2008) Delirious mania: clinical features and treatment response. J Affect Disord 109(3):312–316. doi:10.1016/j.jad.2007.12.001, S0165-0327(07)00420-X [pii]

Kawa I, Carter JD, Joyce PR, Doughty CJ, Frampton CM, Wells JE, Walsh AE, Olds RJ (2005) Gender differences in bipolar disorder: age of onset, course, comorbidity, and symptom presentation. Bipolar Disord 7(2):119–125. doi:10.1111/j.1399-5618.2004.00180.x, BDI180 [pii]

Keck PE Jr, McElroy SL, Strakowski SM, West SA, Sax KW, Hawkins JM, Bourne ML, Haggard P (1998) 12-month outcome of patients with bipolar disorder following hospitalization for a manic or mixed episode. Am J Psychiatry 155(5):646–652

Keck PE Jr, McElroy SL, Havens JR, Altshuler LL, Nolen WA, Frye MA, Suppes T, Denicoff KD, Kupka R, Leverich GS, Rush AJ, Post RM (2003) Psychosis in bipolar disorder: phenomenology and impact on morbidity and course of illness. Compr Psychiatry 44(4):263–269. doi:10.1016/S0010-440X(03)00089-0, S0010440X03000890 [pii]

Keller MB (1988) The course of manic-depressive illness. J Clin Psychiatry 49(Suppl):4–7

Keller MB, Lavori PW, Coryell W, Andreasen NC, Endicott J, Clayton PJ, Klerman GL, Hirschfeld RM (1986) Differential outcome of pure manic, mixed/cycling, and pure depressive episodes in patients with bipolar illness. JAMA 255(22):3138–3142

Kendell RE (1974) The stability of psychiatric diagnosis. Br J Psychiatry 124:352–356

Kessler RC, Stang P, Wittchen HU, Stein M, Walters EE (1999) Lifetime co-morbidities between social phobia and mood disorders in the US National Comorbidity Survey. Psychol Med 29(3):555–567

Kilbourne AM (2005) The burden of general medical conditions in patients with bipolar disorder. Curr Psychiatry Rep 7(6):471–477

Kilbourne AM, Cornelius JR, Han X, Pincus HA, Shad M, Salloum I, Conigliaro J, Haas GL (2004) Burden of general medical conditions among individuals with bipolar disorder. Bipolar Disord 6(5):368–373. doi:10.1111/j.1399-5618.2004.00138.x, BDI138 [pii]

Klein D (1984) Depression and anhedonia. In: Clark D, Fawcett J (eds) Anhedonia and affective deficit states. PMA Publishing, New York, pp 1–14

Kotin J, Goodwin FK (1972) Depression during mania: clinical observations and theoretical implications. Am J Psychiatry 129(6):679–686

Koukopoulos A (1999) Agitated depression as a mixed state and the problem of melancholia. Psychiatr Clin N Am 22(3):547–564

Koukopoulos A (2006) The primacy of mania. Bipolar psychopharmacology: caring for the patient. Wiley, New York

Koukopoulos A, Tundo A (1992) A mixed depressive syndrome. Clin Neuropharmacol 15(Suppl 1 Pt A):626A–627A

Koukopoulos A, Sani G, Albert M, Minnai G, Koukopoulos A (2005) Agitated depression: spontaneous and induced. In: Marneros A, Goodwin F (eds) Bipolar disord. Cambridge University Press, New York

Kraepelin E (1921) Manic-depressive insanity and paranoia. Livingstone, Edinburgh

Kraepelin E, Johnstone T (2010) Lectures on clinical psychiatry. Nabu Press

Kruger S, Cooke RG, Spegg CC, Braunig P (2003) Relevance of the catatonic syndrome to the mixed manic episode. J Affect Disord 74(3):279–285. doi:S0165032702000885 [pii]

Lange J (1922) Katatonische erscheinungen im rahmen manischer erkrankungen. Julius Springer, Berlin

Lee BS, Huang SS, Hsu WY, Chiu NY (2012) Clinical features of delirious mania: a series of five cases and a brief literature review. BMC Psychiatry 12:65. doi:10.1186/1471-244X-12-65, 1471-244X-12-65 [pii]

Leff JP, Fischer M, Bertelsen A (1976) A cross-national epidemiological study of mania. Br J Psychiatry 129:428–442

Leonhard K (1957) Pathogenesis of manic-depressive disease. Nervenarzt 28(6):271–272

Liebowitz MR, Quitkin FM, Stewart JW, McGrath PJ, Harrison W, Rabkin J, Tricamo E, Markowitz JS, Klein DF (1984) Phenelzine v imipramine in atypical depression. A preliminary report. Arch Gen Psychiatry 41(7):669–677

Liebowitz MR, Quitkin FM, Stewart JW, McGrath PJ, Harrison WM, Markowitz JS, Rabkin JG, Tricamo E, Goetz DM, Klein DF (1988) Antidepressant specificity in atypical depression. Arch Gen Psychiatry 45(2):129–137

Lott PR, Guggenbuhl S, Schneeberger A, Pulver AE, Stassen HH (2002) Linguistic analysis of the speech output of schizophrenic, bipolar, and depressive patients. Psychopathology 35(4):220–227. doi:63831 [pii] 63831

Loudon JB, Blackburn IM, Ashworth CM (1977) A study of the symptomatology and course of manic illness using a new scale. Psychol Med 7(4):723–729

Low NC, Du Fort GG, Cervantes P (2003) Prevalence, clinical correlates, and treatment of migraine in bipolar disorder. Headache 43(9):940–949. doi:03184 [pii]

Lowe GR (1973) The phenomenology of hallucinations as an aid to differential diagnosis. Br J Psychiatry 123(577):621–633

Mahmood T, Romans S, Silverstone T (1999) Prevalence of migraine in bipolar disorder. J Affect Disord 52(1–3):239–241

Maj M, Pirozzi R, Magliano L, Bartoli L (2003) Agitated depression in bipolar I disorder: prevalence, phenomenology, and outcome. Am J Psychiatry 160(12):2134–2140

Maj M, Pirozzi R, Magliano L, Fiorillo A, Bartoli L (2006) Agitated "unipolar" major depression: prevalence, phenomenology, and outcome. J Clin Psychiatry 67(5):712–719

Malhi GS, Ivanovski B, Szekeres V, Olley A (2004) Bipolar disorder: it's all in your mind? The neuropsychological profile of a biological disorder. Can J Psychiatr 49(12):813–819

Mantere O, Suominen K, Leppamaki S, Valtonen H, Arvilommi P, Isometsa E (2004) The clinical characteristics of DSM-IV bipolar I and II disorders: baseline findings from the Jorvi Bipolar

Study (JoBS). Bipolar Disord 6(5):395–405. doi:10.1111/j.1399-5618.2004.00140.x, BDI140 [pii]

Marneros A, Rottig S, Wenzel A, Bloink R, Brieger P (2004) Affective and schizoaffective mixed states. Eur Arch Psychiatry Clin Neurosci 254(2):76–81. doi:10.1007/s00406-004-0462-9

Martinez-Aran A, Vieta E, Torrent C, Sanchez-Moreno J, Goikolea JM, Salamero M, Malhi GS, Gonzalez-Pinto A, Daban C, Alvarez-Grandi S, Fountoulakis K, Kaprinis G, Tabares-Seisdedos R, Ayuso-Mateos JL (2007) Functional outcome in bipolar disorder: the role of clinical and cognitive factors. Bipolar Disord 9(1–2):103–113

Mazzarini L, Colom F, Pacchiarotti I, Nivoli AM, Murru A, Bonnin CM, Cruz N, Sanchez-Moreno J, Kotzalidis GD, Girardi P, Tatarelli R, Vieta E (2010) Psychotic versus non-psychotic bipolar II disorder. J Affect Disord 126(1–2):55–60. doi:10.1016/j.jad.2010.03.028, S0165-0327(10)00321-6 [pii]

McElroy SL, Keck PE Jr, Pope HG Jr, Hudson JI, Faedda GL, Swann AC (1992) Clinical and research implications of the diagnosis of dysphoric or mixed mania or hypomania. Am J Psychiatry 149(12):1633–1644

McElroy SL, Strakowski SM, Keck PE Jr, Tugrul KL, West SA, Lonczak HS (1995) Differences and similarities in mixed and pure mania. Compr Psychiatry 36(3):187–194. doi:0010-440X(95)90080-F [pii]

McElroy SL, Kotwal R, Keck PE Jr (2006) Comorbidity of eating disorders with bipolar disorder andtreatmentimplications.BipolarDisord8(6):686–695.doi:10.1111/j.1399-5618.2006.00401.x, BDI401 [pii]

Mendels J, Cochrane C (1968) The nosology of depression: the endogenous-reactive concept. Am J Psychiatry 124(11):1–11

Merikangas KR, Akiskal HS, Angst J, Greenberg PE, Hirschfeld RM, Petukhova M, Kessler RC (2007) Lifetime and 12-month prevalence of bipolar spectrum disorder in the National Comorbidity Survey replication. Arch Gen Psychiatry 64(5):543–552. doi:10.1001/archpsyc.64.5.543, 64/5/543 [pii]

Mitchell PB, Malhi GS (2004) Bipolar depression: phenomenological overview and clinical characteristics. Bipolar Disord 6(6):530–539

Mitchell PB, Goodwin GM, Johnson GF, Hirschfeld RM (2008) Diagnostic guidelines for bipolar depression: a probabilistic approach. Bipolar Disord 10(1 Pt 2):144–152

Morgan VA, Mitchell PB, Jablensky AV (2005) The epidemiology of bipolar disorder: sociodemographic, disability and service utilization data from the Australian National Study of Low Prevalence (Psychotic) Disorders. Bipolar Disord 7(4):326–337. doi:10.1111/j.1399-5618.2005.00229.x, BDI229 [pii]

Morice RD, Igram JC (1983) Language complexity and age of onset of schizophrenia. Psychiatry Res 9(3):233–242

Morice R, McNicol D (1986) Language changes in schizophrenia: a limited replication. Schizophr Bull 12(2):239–251

Morrone-Strupinsky J, Depue R (2004) Differential relation of two distinct, film-induced positive emotional states to affiliative and agentic extraversion. Personal Individ Differ 36:1109–1126

Mur M, Portella MJ, Martinez-Aran A, Pifarre J, Vieta E (2007) Persistent neuropsychological deficit in euthymic bipolar patients: executive function as a core deficit. J Clin Psychiatry 68(7):1078–1086

Murphy DL, Beigel A (1974) Depression, elation, and lithium carbonate responses in manic patient subgroups. Arch Gen Psychiatry 31(5):643–648

Nelson JC, Charney DS (1981) The symptoms of major depressive illness. Am J Psychiatry 138(1):1–13

Nelson WH, Khan A, Orr WW Jr (1984) Delusional depression. Phenomenology, neuroendocrine function, and tricyclic antidepressant response. J Affect Disord 6(3–4):297–306

Nunn CM (1979) Mixed affective states and the natural history of manic-depressive psychosis. Br J Psychiatry 134:153–156

Orvaschel H, Thompson WD, Belanger A, Prusoff BA, Kidd KK (1982) Comparison of the family history method to direct interview. Factors affecting the diagnosis of depression. J Affect Disord 4(1):49–59

Otto MW, Perlman CA, Wernicke R, Reese HE, Bauer MS, Pollack MH (2004) Posttraumatic stress disorder in patients with bipolar disorder: a review of prevalence, correlates, and treatment strategies. Bipolar Disord 6(6):470–479. doi:10.1111/j.1399-5618.2004.00151.x, BDI151 [pii]

Overall J, Hollister L, Johnson M (1966) Nosology of depression and differential response to drugs. JAMA 195:946–950

Parker G, Hadzi-Pavlovic D, Boyce P (1989) Endogenous depression as a construct: a quantitative analysis of the literature and a study of clinician judgements. Aust N Z J Psychiatry 23(3): 357–368

Parker G, Hadzi-Pavlovic D, Boyce P, Wilhelm K, Brodaty H, Mitchell P, Hickie I, Eyers K (1990) Classifying depression by mental state signs. Br J Psychiatry 157:55–65

Parker G, Parker K, Mitchell P, Wilhelm K (2005) Atypical depression: Australian and US studies in accord. Curr Opin Psychiatry 18(1):1–5

Paykel ES, Prusoff BA, Tanner J (1976) Temporal stability of symptom patterns in depression. Br J Psychiatry 128:369–374

Perlis RH, Delbello MP, Miyahara S, Wisniewski SR, Sachs GS, Nierenberg AA (2005) Revisiting depressive-prone bipolar disorder: polarity of initial mood episode and disease course among bipolar I systematic treatment enhancement program for bipolar disorder participants. Biol Psychiatry 58(7):549–553. doi:10.1016/j.biopsych.2005.07.029, S0006-3223(05)00918-2 [pii]

Perron BE, Bohnert AS, Vaughn MG, Bauer MS, Kilbourne AM (2009a) Profiles of disability among adults with bipolar spectrum disorders. Soc Psychiatry Psychiatr Epidemiol 45(12):1125–1134. doi:10.1007/s00127-009-0153-y

Perron BE, Howard MO, Nienhuis JK, Bauer MS, Woodward AT, Kilbourne AM (2009b) Prevalence and burden of general medical conditions among adults with bipolar I disorder: results from the National Epidemiologic Survey on alcohol and related conditions. J Clin Psychiatry 70(10):1407–1415. doi:10.4088/JCP.08m04586yel

Perugi G, Akiskal HS, Micheli C, Musetti L, Paiano A, Quilici C, Rossi L, Cassano GB (1997) Clinical subtypes of bipolar mixed states: validating a broader European definition in 143 cases. J Affect Disord 43(3):169–180. doi:S0165-0327(97)01446-8 [pii]

Perugi G, Akiskal HS, Lattanzi L, Cecconi D, Mastrocinque C, Patronelli A, Vignoli S, Bemi E (1998) The high prevalence of "soft" bipolar (II) features in atypical depression. Compr Psychiatry 39(2):63–71. doi:S0010-440X(98)90080-3 [pii]

Perugi G, Micheli C, Akiskal HS, Madaro D, Socci C, Quilici C, Musetti L (2000) Polarity of the first episode, clinical characteristics, and course of manic depressive illness: a systematic retrospective investigation of 320 bipolar I patients. Compr Psychiatry 41(1):13–18. doi:S0010-440X(00)90125-1 [pii]

Phillips ML, Drevets WC, Rauch SL, Lane R (2003) Neurobiology of emotion perception II: implications for major psychiatric disorders. Biol Psychiatry 54(5):515–528

Plutchik R (2002) Nature of emotions. Am Sci 89:349

Pope HG Jr, Lipinski JF Jr (1978) Diagnosis in schizophrenia and manic-depressive illness: a reassessment of the specificity of 'schizophrenic' symptoms in the light of current research. Arch Gen Psychiatry 35(7):811–828

Post RM, Rubinow DR, Uhde TW, Roy-Byrne PP, Linnoila M, Rosoff A, Cowdry R (1989) Dysphoric mania. Clinical and biological correlates. Arch Gen Psychiatry 46(4):353–358

Price LH, Nelson JC, Charney DS, Quinlan DM (1984) Family history in delusional depression. J Affect Disord 6(1):109–114

Prien RF, Himmelhoch JM, Kupfer DJ (1988) Treatment of mixed mania. J Affect Disord 15(1):9–15

Rabkin J, Stewart J, Quitkin F, McGrath P, Harrison W, Klein D (1996) Should atypical depression be included in DSM-IV? In: Widiger TA, Frances AJ, Pincus HA, Ross R, First MB, Davis WW (eds) DSM-IV Sourcebook, vol 2. American Psychiatric Association, pp 239–260

Ragin AB, Oltmanns TF (1983) Predictability as an index of impaired verbal communication in schizophrenic and affective disorders. Br J Psychiatry 143:578–583

Rao U, Ryan ND, Birmaher B, Dahl RE, Williamson DE, Kaufman J, Rao R, Nelson B (1995) Unipolar depression in adolescents: clinical outcome in adulthood. J Am Acad Child Adolesc Psychiatry 34(5):566–578. doi:10.1097/00004583-199505000-00009, S0890-8567(09)63541-3 [pii]

Regier DA, Farmer ME, Rae DS, Locke BZ, Keith SJ, Judd LL, Goodwin FK (1990) Comorbidity of mental disorders with alcohol and other drug abuse. Results from the Epidemiologic Catchment Area (ECA) Study. JAMA 264(19):2511–2518

Regier DA, Rae DS, Narrow WE, Kaelber CT, Schatzberg AF (1998) Prevalence of anxiety disorders and their comorbidity with mood and addictive disorders. Br J Psychiatry Suppl 34:24–28

Rennie T (1942) Prognosis in manic-depressive psychosis. Am J Psychiatry 98:801–814

Resnick HS, Oltmanns TF (1984) Hesitation patterns in the speech of thought-disordered schizophrenic and manic patients. J Abnorm Psychol 93(1):80–86

Rosen LN, Rosenthal NE, Van Dusen PH, Dunner DL, Fieve RR (1983) Age at onset and number of psychotic symptoms in bipolar I and schizoaffective disorder. Am J Psychiatry 140(11):1523–1524

Rosenthal NE, Rosenthal LN, Stallone F, Dunner DL, Fieve RR (1980) Toward the validation of RDC schizoaffective disorder. Arch Gen Psychiatry 37(7):804–810

Roth M (1959) The phenomenology of depressive states. Can Psychiatr Assoc J 1959(4 (suppl)):32–52

Roth M, Gurney C, Mountjoy CQ (1983) The Newcastle rating scales. Acta Psychiatr Scand Suppl 310:42–54

Rush AJ, Weissenburger JE (1994) Melancholic symptom features and DSM-IV. Am J Psychiatry 151(4):489–498

Sato T, Bottlender R, Kleindienst N, Moller HJ (2002) Syndromes and phenomenological subtypes underlying acute mania: a factor analytic study of 576 manic patients. Am J Psychiatry 159(6):968–974

Sato T, Bottlender R, Kleindienst N, Moller HJ (2005) Irritable psychomotor elation in depressed inpatients: a factor validation of mixed depression. J Affect Disord 84(2–3):187–196. doi:10.1016/S0165-0327(02)00172-6, S0165032702001726 [pii]

Secunda SK, Swann A, Katz MM, Koslow SH, Croughan J, Chang S (1987) Diagnosis and treatment of mixed mania. Am J Psychiatry 144(1):96–98

Serretti A, Olgiati P (2005) Profiles of "manic" symptoms in bipolar I, bipolar II and major depressive disorders. J Affect Disord 84(2–3):159–166. doi:10.1016/j.jad.2003.09.011, S016503270300257X [pii]

Serretti A, Mandelli L, Lattuada E, Cusin C, Smeraldi E (2002) Clinical and demographic features of mood disorder subtypes. Psychiatry Res 112(3):195–210. doi:S0165178102002275 [pii]

Shankman SA, Klein DN, Lewinsohn PM, Seeley JR, Small JW (2008) Family study of subthreshold psychopathology in a community sample. Psychol Med 38(2):187–198. doi:10.1017/S0033291707001857, S0033291707001857 [pii]

Silberman EK, Post RM, Nurnberger J, Theodore W, Boulenger JP (1985) Transient sensory, cognitive and affective phenomena in affective illness. A comparison with complex partial epilepsy. Br J Psychiatry 146:81–89

Simon GE, Hunkeler E, Fireman B, Lee JY, Savarino J (2007) Risk of suicide attempt and suicide death in patients treated for bipolar disorder. Bipolar Disord 9(5):526–530. doi:10.1111/j.1399-5618.2007.00408.x, BDI408 [pii]

Simpson DM, Davis GC (1985) Measuring thought disorder with clinical rating scales in schizophrenic and nonschizophrenic patients. Psychiatry Res 15(4):313–318. doi:0165-1781(85)90068-X [pii]

Sole B, Martinez-Aran A, Torrent C, Bonnin CM, Reinares M, Popovic D, Sanchez-Moreno J, Vieta E (2011) Are bipolar II patients cognitively impaired? A systematic review. Psychol Med 41(9):1791–1803. doi:10.1017/S0033291711000018, S0033291711000018 [pii]

Solomon DA, Leon AC, Endicott J, Coryell WH, Mueller TI, Posternak MA, Keller MB (2003) Unipolar mania over the course of a 20-year follow-up study. Am J Psychiatry 160(11): 2049–2051

Solovay MR, Shenton ME, Holzman PS (1987) Comparative studies of thought disorders. I. Mania and schizophrenia. Arch Gen Psychiatry 44(1):13–20

Soreca I, Fagiolini A, Frank E, Houck PR, Thompson WK, Kupfer DJ (2008) Relationship of general medical burden, duration of illness and age in patients with bipolar I disorder. J Psychiatr Res 42(11):956–961. doi:10.1016/j.jpsychires.2007.10.009, S0022-3956(07)00183-5 [pii]

Soreca I, Frank E, Kupfer DJ (2009) The phenomenology of bipolar disorder: what drives the high rate of medical burden and determines long-term prognosis? Depress Anxiety 26(1):73–82. doi:10.1002/da.20521

Spitzer RL, Endicott J, Robins E (1978) Research diagnostic criteria: rationale and reliability. Arch Gen Psychiatry 35(6):773–782

Strakowski SM, Tohen M, Stoll AL, Faedda GL, Goodwin DC (1992) Comorbidity in mania at first hospitalization. Am J Psychiatry 149(4):554–556

Strakowski SM, McElroy SL, Keck PE Jr, West SA (1996) Suicidality among patients with mixed and manic bipolar disorder. Am J Psychiatry 153(5):674–676

Strakowski SM, Keck PE Jr, McElroy SL, West SA, Sax KW, Hawkins JM, Kmetz GF, Upadhyaya VH, Tugrul KC, Bourne ML (1998) Twelve-month outcome after a first hospitalization for affective psychosis. Arch Gen Psychiatry 55(1):49–55

Swann AC, Bowden CL, Morris D, Calabrese JR, Petty F, Small J, Dilsaver SC, Davis JM (1997) Depression during mania. Treatment response to lithium or divalproex. Arch Gen Psychiatry 54(1):37–42

Swann AC, Janicak PL, Calabrese JR, Bowden CL, Dilsaver SC, Morris DD, Petty F, Davis JM (2001) Structure of mania: depressive, irritable, and psychotic clusters with different retrospectively-assessed course patterns of illness in randomized clinical trial participants. J Affect Disord 67(1–3):123–132. doi:S0165032701004475 [pii]

Swartz MS, Henschen GM, Cavenar JO Jr, Hammett EB (1982) A case of intermittent delirious mania. Am J Psychiatry 139(10):1357–1358

Taylor MA, Abrams R (1973) The phenomenology of mania. A new look at some old patients. Arch Gen Psychiatry 29(4):520–522

Taylor MA, Abrams R (1977) Catatonia. Prevalence and importance in the manic phase of manic-depressive illness. Arch Gen Psychiatry 34(10):1223–1225

Thase ME (2007) Recognition and diagnosis of atypical depression. J Clin Psychiatry 68(Suppl 8): 11–16

Thomas P, Kearney G, Napier E, Ellis E, Leuder I, Johnson M (1996) Speech and language in first onset psychosis differences between people with schizophrenia, mania, and controls. Br J Psychiatry 168(3):337–343

Thompson WD, Orvaschel H, Prusoff BA, Kidd KK (1982) An evaluation of the family history method for ascertaining psychiatric disorders. Arch Gen Psychiatry 39(1):53–58

Tohen M, Waternaux CM, Tsuang MT (1990) Outcome in Mania. A 4-year prospective follow-up of 75 patients utilizing survival analysis. Arch Gen Psychiatry 47(12):1106–1111

Toni C, Perugi G, Mata B, Madaro D, Maremmani I, Akiskal HS (2001) Is mood-incongruent manic psychosis a distinct subtype? Eur Arch Psychiatry Clin Neurosci 251(1):12–17

Van Praag H, Uleman A, Spitz J (1965) The vital syndrome interview. Psychiatr Neurol Neurochir 68:329–349

West ED, Dally PJ (1959) Effects of iproniazid in depressive syndromes. Br Med J 1(5136):1491–1494

Weygandt W (1899) Uber die mischzustande des manisch-depressiven irreseins. JF Lechman, Munich

WHO (1992) The ICD-10 classification of mental and behavioural disorders – clinical descriptions and diagnostic guidelines. World Health Organization, Geneva

Winokur G (1984) Psychosis in bipolar and unipolar affective illness with special reference to schizo-affective disorder. Br J Psychiatry 145:236–242

Winokur G, Tsuang MT (1975) Elation versus irritability in mania. Compr Psychiatry 16(5):435–436. doi:0010-440X(75)90032-2 [pii]

Winokur G, Clayton P, Reich T (1969) Manic depressive illness. CV Mosby, Saint Louis

Winokur G, Turvey C, Akiskal H, Coryell W, Solomon D, Leon A, Mueller T, Endicott J, Maser J, Keller M (1998) Alcoholism and drug abuse in three groups–bipolar I, unipolars and their acquaintances. J Affect Disord 50(2–3):81–89

Young RC, Schreiber MT, Nysewander RW (1983) Psychotic mania. Biol Psychiatry 18(10): 1167–1173

Zimmerman M, Coryell WH, Black DW (1990) Variability in the application of contemporary diagnostic criteria: endogenous depression as an example. Am J Psychiatry 147(9):1173–1179

Long-Term Course 3

3.1 Predominant Polarity

Historically, the first note on polarity was made in the early 1960s when Leonhard reported that 17.9 % of patients had a manic and 25.6 % had a depressive predominant polarity, while the rest of the patients had similar occurrence of the two poles (Leonhard 1963). However, the concept was formulated by Jules Angst (1978).

Recently, the concept of predominant polarity has been introduced to further characterize the subtypes of bipolar disorders, especially in terms of long-term prognosis, and to assist clinicians in the long-term therapeutical design (Judd et al. 2003; Colom et al. 2006; Quitkin et al. 1986). Several attempts to develop an operationalized concept have been published (Rosa et al. 2008; Vieta et al. 2009; Pacchiarotti et al. 2013; Osher et al. 2000; Daban et al. 2006; Baldessarini et al. 2012b). Some authors suggested that having more lifetime episodes of a given polarity would be sufficient to determine the predominant polarity (Henry et al. 1999; Osher et al. 2000; Colom et al. 2006; Forty et al. 2009; Gonzalez-Pinto et al. 2010a). Eventually it has been suggested that a reliable definition of predominant polarity should demand that at least two-thirds of episodes belong to one of the poles (Colom et al. 2006). Further research confirmed the validity of this approach (Baldessarini et al. 2012b; Rosa et al. 2008; Vieta et al. 2009; Pacchiarotti et al. 2013; Nivoli et al. 2011b; Garcia-Lopez et al. 2009; Mazzarini et al. 2009). This definition has been accepted by the International Society for Bipolar Disorders (ISBD) Task Force report on the nomenclature of the course and outcome in bipolar disorders (Tohen et al. 2009). Even before research had recognized it, naturalistic data suggest that predominant polarity seems to be a major factor in determining the long-term treatment of BD patients in clinical practice (Nivoli et al. 2012). In this frame, it had been proposed to be included as a course specifier in DSM-5 (Colom and Vieta 2009), but this did not happen.

Two types of bipolar predominant polarity have been described: the depressive and the manic. Currently there are not enough data to support the presence of a third type of predominant polarity on the basis of the presence of mixed episodes (Tohen

K.N. Fountoulakis, *Bipolar Disorder: An Evidence-Based Guide to Manic Depression*, DOI 10.1007/978-3-642-37216-2_3

et al. 2009). Patients with predominant depressive polarity tend to experience depressive episodes at a frequency of at least 2:1 in comparison to manic episodes, while patients with predominant manic polarity experience the opposite pattern.

Almost half of the BD patients manifest a predominant polarity (Rosa et al. 2008; Baldessarini et al. 2012b; Mazzarini et al. 2009; Vieta et al. 2009); however, it seems that this percentage depends on the method and the sample (especially the stage of the illness). Of those with predominant polarity present, the majority (two-thirds) are classified as having depressive polarity vs. one-third with a manic polarity (Rosa et al. 2008; Nivoli et al. 2011b; Gonzalez-Pinto et al. 2010a; Colom et al. 2006; Mazzarini et al. 2009; Vieta et al. 2009). Other studies report a 50–50 ratio (Gonzalez-Pinto et al. 2010b; Rosa et al. 2008). The studies that included BD-II patients report a higher prevalence of the depressive predominant polarity (Rosa et al. 2008; Colom et al. 2006; Goikolea et al. 2007; Popovic and Vieta 2013), while those which incorporated samples of exclusively type I BD patients report a higher prevalence of the manic predominant polarity (Osher et al. 2000; Baldessarini et al. 2012a, b; Pacchiarotti et al. 2013; Mazzarini et al. 2009). Also, the studies that included a broader spectrum of BD patients tended to report a higher prevalence of the depressive predominant polarity (Alessandra et al. 2013; Garcia-Lopez et al. 2009; Popovic and Vieta 2013). This difference in percentages is probably caused by differences in the quality of the samples between studies reflecting the fact that later in the long-term course of BD depression prevails (especially in a chronic form) while mania is attenuated. It is interesting that a study from Israel is the only one to have reported a clear predominance of the manic pole (Osher et al. 2000).

A list of studies which report rates of predominant polarity in BD patients is shown in Table 3.1. It is not possible to calculate a weighted average since many publications probably have overlapping samples.

It should be noted however that if the number of days spent in a specific type of episodes is used to define the predominant polarity instead of the number of episodes, then the vast majority of BD patients will be classified as predominantly depressed (Judd et al. 2003; Perlis et al. 2005).

Depressive predominant polarity is related to more frequent ECT, longer latency time to correct the diagnosis since the first episode was more frequently depressive or mixed, more suicide attempts, more Axis-II comorbidity, history of mixed states, ever married and female sex (Rosa et al. 2008; Baldessarini et al. 2012b; Gonzalez-Pinto et al. 2010a; Nivoli et al. 2011a). In patients with a depressive predominant polarity, the depressive are both the first mood episode (Baldessarini et al. 2012b; Popovic et al. 2013; Rosa et al. 2008; Forty et al. 2009; Etain et al. 2012; Colom et al. 2006) as well as the index mood episode (Colom et al. 2006; Baldessarini et al. 2012b). A mixed onset of illness is also associated with a depressive predominant polarity (Baldessarini et al. 2012b), and more mixed episodes are observed in patients with depressive predominant polarity (Baldessarini et al. 2012b; Colom et al. 2006; Pacchiarotti et al. 2011, 2013). Melancholic features are very frequent (Daban et al. 2006). These patients also have a lifetime history with higher number of stressful life events, more suicide attempts (Colom et al. 2006; Baldessarini et al. 2012b; Gonzalez-Pinto et al. 2010b; Rosa et al. 2008) and more family history of affective disorders (Gonzalez-Pinto et al. 2010b).

Table 3.1 List of papers reporting rates of predominant polarity in BD patients. It is not possible to calculate a weighted average since many publications probably have overlapping samples

Publication	Sample size *N*	DPP *N* (%)	MPP *N* (%)	Definition of PP	Comments
Daban et al. (2006)	300	128 (42.7 %)		>50 %	
Colom et al. (2006)	224	135 (60.3 %)	89 (39.7 %)	≥2/3	Pts with predominant polarity only
Osher et al. (2000)	71	12 (16.9 %)	39 (54.9 %)	>50 %	BD-I only
Goikolea et al. (2007)	325	65 (20.0 %)	48 (14.8 %)	≥2/3	Prospective 10-year follow-up
Rosa et al. (2008)	149	45 (30.2 %)	47 (31.5 %)	≥2/3	
Forty et al. (2009)	552	238 (43.1 %)	215 (38.9 %)	>50 %	BD-I only
Garcia-Lopez et al. (2009)	296	71 (23.9 %)	65 (21.9 %)	≥2/3	Prospective follow-up time: 1–4 years
Mazzarini et al. (2009)	124	22 (17.7 %)	47 (37.9 %)	≥2/3	BD-I only
Vieta et al. (2009)	788	269 (34.1 %)	98 (12.4 %)	≥2/3	BD-I only
González-Pinto et al. (2010a, b)	169	51 (30.1 %)	44 (26.0 %)	>50 %	Prospective BD-I
Koyuncu et al. (2010)	70	30 (42.9 %)	27 (38.6 %)	>50 %	
Nivoli et al. (2011a, b)	604	143 (23.7 %)	114 (18.9 %)	≥2/3	
Pacchiarotti et al. (2011)	134	28 (21.1 %)	50 (37.3 %)	≥2/3	BD-I
Baldessarini et al. (2012a, b)	928	199 (21.4 %)	290 (31.3 %)	≥2/3	BD-I
Pacchiarotti et al. (2013)	187	18 (9.6 %)	30 (16.0 %)	≥2/3	BD-I inpatients
Popovic et al. (2013); Nivoli et al. (2013)	604	143 (55.6 %)	114 (44.4 %)	≥2/3	

DPP depressive predominant polarity, *MPP* manic predominant polarity, *PP* predominant polarity, *>50 %* PP defined as higher rate of either pole, *≥2/3* PP defined as at least 2/3 of episodes belonging to a specific pole

On the contrary, the predominant manic polarity is associated with an earlier age at onset, initial manic episodes and psychotic episodes, more frequent psychotic symptoms, cognitive impairment, more drug abuse, higher education and more family psychiatric history studies (Baldessarini et al. 2012b; Popovic et al. 2013; Forty et al. 2009; Gonzalez-Pinto et al. 2010a; Colom et al. 2006; Daban et al. 2006; Martinez-Aran et al. 2004; Post et al. 2003). Also in the beginning the manic predominant polarity is related to more hospitalizations, although this seems to reverse later in the course of the illness (Gonzalez-Pinto et al. 2010b). One study suggested that the manic predominant polarity is associated with rapid cycling (Vieta et al. 2009); however, subsequent studies rejected this suggestion (Nivoli et al. 2013; Vieta et al. 2009; Baldessarini et al. 2012b; Rosa et al. 2008; Popovic et al. 2013). Similarly, there does not seem to be any relationship of polarity and seasonality (Goikolea et al. 2007; Colom et al. 2006; Popovic et al. 2013).

There does not seem to exist any differences between the two types of predominant polarity concerning the psychiatric comorbidity (Colom et al. 2006; Popovic et al. 2013; Baldessarini et al. 2012b; Nivoli et al. 2013; Murru et al. 2011; Koyuncu et al. 2010; Mazzarini et al. 2009). It is interesting to note that some authors reported that the depressive predominant polarity is associated with the female gender (Nivoli et al. 2011a; Baldessarini et al. 2012b) and the manic with male (Popovic et al. 2013) although other studies did not confirm this finding (Baldessarini et al. 2012b; Vieta et al. 2009; Colom et al. 2006; Osher et al. 2000; Rosa et al. 2008; Gonzalez-Pinto et al. 2010a; Mazzarini et al. 2009). The depressive predominant polarity group has been associated with a greater likelihood of having been married (Gonzalez-Pinto et al. 2010a; Baldessarini et al. 2012b).

There are no clear differences between the manic and depressive groups in the long-term alcohol abuse or other substance abuse although there seems to be a tendency for the manic group to do better, especially in the long term (Gonzalez-Pinto et al. 2010a, b). A history of substance abuse preceding the first episode has been reported to correlate with a manic predominant polarity (Colom et al. 2006; Popovic et al. 2013).

Disability does not seem to differ between the two groups either (Colom et al. 2006), although in general the predominantly depressive group has a worse prognosis (Gonzalez-Pinto et al. 2010b) including the response to treatment of the acute bipolar depression phase (Vieta et al. 2009). Probably, the depressive predominant polarity is associated with a higher number of suicide attempts (Baldessarini et al. 2012b; Colom et al. 2006; Gonzalez-Pinto et al. 2010a; Popovic et al. 2013; Mazzarini et al. 2009), but one study suggested that a 'mixed episode polarity' is considerably more related to suicidality (Baldessarini et al. 2012b).

3.2 Seasonality

Seasonality is a classic rhythmic disturbance in mood disorders. It is generally believed that autumn and winter are related to depression and spring and summer to mania. Some relationship of seasonality to atypical features of depression is also believed to exist, especially concerning the manifestation of fatigue in combination with craving for carbohydrates and oversleeping in winter (Simonsen et al. 2011; Shin et al. 2005).

Somewhere between 15 % and 50 % of bipolar patients are reported to manifest some type of seasonal variation of symptomatology, with 25 % being the most probable percentage (Faedda et al. 1993; Goikolea et al. 2007; Hunt et al. 1992; Shand et al. 2011). Even a genetic marker has been proposed with genetic variants in the NF1A gene region predisposing to seasonal pattern of mania (Lee et al. 2012).

Two seasonal variations, which are opposing, have been described: fall–winter depression with or without spring–summer mania or hypomania and spring–summer depression with or without fall–winter mania or hypomania (Faedda et al. 1993). Most studies support the first subtype (Lee et al. 2007; Clarke et al. 1999; Murray et al. 2011; Partonen and Lonnqvist 1996; Peck 1990; Walter 1977; Parker and Walter 1982; Mulder et al. 1990), but some authors suggest that seasonality is purely idiosyncratic and no universal patterns can be traced across patients (Hunt et al. 1992; Bauer et al. 2009; Eastwood and Stiasny 1978).

It is reported also that lithium levels in plasma peak in summer (Cusin et al. 2002; Wilting et al. 2007), especially in males (D'Mello et al. 1995), and this difference could be up to 25 % (Medhi et al. 2008). It seems this phenomenon is part of a larger seasonal variation in the metabolism of electrolytes (Mellerup and Mellerup 1984).

Although it has been reported that there are no demographic differences between BD patients with seasonality and those without (Goikolea et al. 2007), certain subtypes of BD patients are reported to manifest specific seasonality in aspects of symptoms, like younger patients having trouble with the law mainly between August and January (London and Taylor 1981). However, an opposite pattern concerning aggression has also been reported (D'Mello et al. 1995; Volpe et al. 2008), and suicidality might be more often in winter (Volpe et al. 2008). Also, seasonal BD patients are reported to be more often BD-II with depressive predominant polarity (Goikolea et al. 2007); however, the fact that BD-II patients tend to be chronically depressed often seems to attenuate any seasonal effect (Friedman et al. 2006).

It is well known that females experience premenstrual changes in mood and behaviour, and these changes might be more pronounced in mood disorder patients. BD female patients are reported to experience seasonal and premenstrual changes in mood and behaviour regardless of their mood episodes (Choi et al. 2011). Depression during autumn–winter is the most reported seasonality trend among females (Murray et al. 2011) with admission to hospital with mania being more frequent in late summer and early autumn (Symonds and Williams 1976). A seasonal trend is also reported for admissions for depression with the highest peak in November for women and in April for men (Morken et al. 2002). However, other reports suggest that women demonstrated a bimodal seasonal distribution, with peak admission rates in spring and fall, while among men, the admission rate peaked in the springtime (D'Mello et al. 1995). Premenstrual and mood symptoms are associated with each other and are more pronounced in BD-II in comparison to BD-I (Choi et al. 2011). A significant elevation of lithium plasma levels in summer was reported for males alone (D'Mello et al. 1995); however, a more recent study suggested the same for females alone (Cusin et al. 2002). There are also negative reports on the relationship of gender with seasonality (Myers and Davies 1978; Walter 1977).

It is interesting that lithium might induce subsensitivity to light since it was reported to significantly raise the dark adaptation threshold which is a measure of night vision (Carney et al. 1988b). Of course, it is unlikely that lithium exerts its antimanic effect through this mechanism.

It has also been reported that exposure to natural light appears to have a substantial effect on well-being in twins with BD (Hakkarainen et al. 2003), while admission rates because of acute mania were reported to be higher in the sunnier months and in months with a greater average day length (Carney et al. 1988a).

Also such an exposure was reported to reduce hospital stay in bipolar depression (Benedetti et al. 2001), although another study reported no correlation of depressive symptoms to sunshine and cloudiness. That latter study reported a strong correlation of depression with temperature (Christensen et al. 2008).

Although there is one negative (Dauphinais et al. 2012) and one positive trial (Deltito et al. 1991) on the usefulness of light therapy against bipolar depression, there are also reports on mania or hypomania induced by light therapy (Kantor et al. 1991; Labbate et al. 1994; Pande 1985; Chan et al. 1994).

Concerning location, there are three major zones: the northern and the southern hemispheres and the tropics. There are no differences between the northern and southern hemispheres when taking into consideration the reversed seasonality. Comparing studies from the two hemispheres helps in controlling for confounding variables such as public holidays.

In the USA, admissions to hospital (irrespective of type of episode) are reported to peak in summer (Myers and Davies 1978) or in spring (D'Mello et al. 1995). Manic episodes seem to peak in early spring, with a nadir in late fall. Mixed episodes might peak in late summer with a nadir in November (Cassidy and Carroll 2002). In Norway admissions specifically for bipolar depression had the highest peak in November for women and for men in April (Morken et al. 2002). A study from Finland reported that there was no seasonal variation concerning admissions; however, the first admission for a depressive compared with a manic episode occurred significantly more often in the autumn (Partonen and Lonnqvist 1996). One study from Hungary (Rihmer 1980) and one from Greece (Frangos et al. 1980) reported that hospitalizations for mania might happen more often in spring and autumn and for depression mainly in summer and winter. In Israel admission rates were higher during spring and summer (Shapira et al. 2004). In Canada there was no statistically significant seasonal pattern of admissions, but for mixed state admissions peaked in the summer (Whitney et al. 1999). In the UK there was a peak of admissions for mania only concerning females during August–September (Symonds and Williams 1976), where an analysis of the Wales data suggested a peak during spring–summer (Walter 1977). The STEP-BD study provided some but rather unclear data concerning a greater prevalence of bipolar depression in northern vs. southern study sites. Seasonal peak prevalence rates of depression differ by region (Friedman et al. 2006).

Studies reporting data from countries located in the southern hemisphere reported a spring–summer peak of admissions for mania (Sayer et al. 1991; Jones et al. 1995; Mulder et al. 1990; Parker and Walter 1982), but there was significant variability and heterogeneity of the results.

Studies comparing data coming from different hemispheres suggest there is no difference between them and also that no real seasonality was present (Bauer et al. 2009; Silverstone et al. 1995). One of them suggested an autumn preponderance of depressive episodes in both hemispheres (Silverstone et al. 1995).

The studies reporting data from the tropical zone mostly do not suggest the presence of a seasonal trend (Abdul-Rahim et al. 1992; Daniels et al. 2000; Jain et al. 1992). One study from Taiwan suggested the presence of a typical seasonal pattern with winter depression and summer manias (Lee et al. 2007).

Meteorological conditions have been studied in order to identify possible causative factors responsible for a seasonal pattern in BD. Light was a probable candidate factor, and supersensitivity to light has been proposed as a trait marker for BD (Lewy et al. 1985). Data from Korea suggested that the mean monthly hours of sunshine and sunlight radiation correlated significantly with manic episodes (Lee et al. 2002). Two papers from Brazil correlate symptoms not with seasons but with climate variables, with sunshine, temperature, rainfall and humidity being more important for manic episodes (Volpe et al. 2010; Volpe and Del Porto 2006). Humidity, barometric pressure and atmospheric ionization were the factors identified in a study from the UK (Mawson and Smith 1981).

Taken together, the above studies suggest that there are some data suggesting a peak of episodes and hospital admissions because of mania during spring to autumn and because of depression during the cold period of the year, but this was not consistent across studies. It is even more interesting that the data from the southern hemisphere report similar seasonal distribution. This is supported also by the reports from the tropical zone, where a similar seasonality pattern seems to exist, while in that zone the climate changes are not great between seasons.

3.3 Rapid Cycling

Although as early as 1911, Eugen Bleuler described a 50-h cycle in a mood patient (Zis and Goodwin 1979), and Emil Kraepelin commented on the relationship between cycle length and illness progression in 1921 (Kraepelin 1921), the concept of rapid cycling appeared for the first time in the 1970s in a landmark paper by Dunner and Fieve (1974). These authors also gave a definition of rapid cycling which includes the occurrence of at least four major depressive, manic, hypomanic or mixed episodes during a 12-month period, and this approach stands until today. Since then, several authors have discussed and disputed this definition, and they also described subpopulations of patients with even higher frequency of episodes. In general, the classic rapid cycling includes cycles of weeks to months of duration. Ultrarapid cycling is reported when mood cycling has frequency of weeks to days and ultradian cycling when there is significant mood variation within a 24-h period

(Kramlinger and Post 1996). Other terms include 'ultra-ultrarapid' and 'ultradian rapid' and refer to weekly or daily cycling which is not uncommon in BD patients (Kramlinger and Post 1996). So far, however, the data are limited and do not permit definite conclusions on the clinical phenomenology and nature of these mood swings (Barrios et al. 2001; Kramlinger and Post 1996; Maggini et al. 2000; Tillman and Geller 2003).

It is extremely interesting that a retrospective study which analysed 570 patient records from the 1960s, 1970s and 1980s reported that very rapid mood fluctuations were absent among bipolar patients in 1960s but were evident in the 1970s and the 1980s (Wolpert et al. 1990). However, this is not entirely true. Apart from Eugen Bleuler's report, during the last couple of centuries, there were many case reports, mainly of a 48-h cycle (Bunney et al. 1965; Jenner et al. 1967).

Recognition of this condition might be difficult especially for clinicians without this nosological entity embedded in their mind. This is because the higher the frequency, the lower the possibility patients are free of symptoms for prolonged periods. Essentially rapid cycling patients might not ever achieve complete remission during the interepisode intervals, and this leads to significant disability, but also often leads to a personality-like clinical picture. The correct diagnosis might elude for prolonged periods of time the diagnosis of a personality disorder is often put, and as a consequence treatment is inappropriate. This might be one of the reasons rapid cycling was rarely put as a diagnosis before its 'official' recognition in the mid-1970s, while today up to one-tenth or one-third of inpatients might be diagnosed as manifesting it.

Even today much confusion still exists. For example, both classification systems classify ultrarapid cases within the mixed episode category rather than rapid cycling. Essentially ultrarapid cycling is the only way a full-blown manic/hypomanic together with a full depressive episode can coexist in the same patient during the same time period, as classification systems require. This is in sharp contrast to the Kraepelinian proposal concerning the three independent factors underlying mood episodes (mood, cognition and physical activity; see the 'mixed episodes' part of this book). Even when the correct diagnosis is put, treatment is complex and difficult and requires advanced skills from the side of the therapist (Bauer et al. 1994; Fountoulakis et al. 2012).

Taking into consideration the orientation of the US National Institute of Mental Health (NIMH) to develop neurobiologically based Research Domain Criteria (RDoC) (Insel et al. 2010) and thus integrating genetic, environment, biological and experiential components in the classification (Cuthbert and Insel 2013), RC could serve as a model. Eventually this approach will lead to 'personalized psychiatry', also known as 'stratified psychiatry' (Schumann et al. 2013). However, there are no sufficient data yet to specifically utilize RC in order to develop such an advanced classification approach (Valenti et al. 2012; Mahon et al. 2013; Rovai et al. 2013).

The exact proportion of bipolar patients manifesting a rapid cycling course is not known. In the first ever study, Dunner and Fieve (1974) reported a prevalence of 13 %. In accord with this, data from most subsequent studies suggest a 5–33.3 % cross-sectional prevalence (Azorin et al. 2008; Coryell et al. 1992; Cruz et al. 2008;

Garcia-Amador et al. 2009; Kukopulos et al. 1980; Nurnberger et al. 1988; Schneck et al. 2004, 2008; Lee et al. 2010) and a 25.8–43 % lifetime prevalence (Coryell et al. 2003; Dittmann et al. 2002; Hajek et al. 2008; Yildiz and Sachs 2004; Lee et al. 2010). However, both lower and higher rates have been reported by a significant number of papers. These rates are as low as 4 % (Avasthi et al. 1999), and the higher ones distribute smoothly up to more than 50 %. Depending on the site of the research and probably the study sample, methodology and definition, rates of 25.8 % (Coryell et al. 2003), 30 % for 'frequent mood episodes' (Wells et al. 2010), 40 % (Dittmann et al. 2002), 33.3 % for primary care and 26.9 % for tertiary care samples (Hajek et al. 2008), 43 % for tertiary care (Yildiz and Sachs 2004), 33.3 % for lifetime and 40 % for year prevalence (Lee et al. 2010) and 56 % in a convenient clinical sample (Cowdry et al. 1983) have been published. In the multinational WAVE-BD study, prevalence rates ranged from 6.6 % (Romania) to 28.7 % (Turkey) (Vieta et al. 2013a).

One analysis from the National Comorbidity Survey Replication (NCS-R) study suggested a prevalence of 44 % (MacKinnon et al. 2003a), while another calculation on the basis of the same data reported 33.3 % lifetime and 50 % year prevalence of rapid cycling (Nierenberg et al. 2010). Probably this last estimation is closer to the reality at least for the bipolar population as shaped during the most recent decade. It is also interesting to note that in convenient clinical samples under follow-up, there seems to be a gradual improvement which contaminates epidemiological data. In one study it has been found that 32 % of the patients were manifesting rapid cycling at entry but only 5 % after 1 year (Schneck et al. 2008).

As mentioned above, the relationship between cycle length and illness progression was discussed for the first time by Emil Kraepelin (1921). Later the shortening of the cycle by passing the years and accumulation of episodes has been documented (Roy-Byrne et al. 1985; Angst 1981). Although it has been proposed that there is a ceiling effect and the frequency of the cycle might stabilize after four to six episodes (Goodwin and Jamison 1990), the data from the Stanley Bipolar Treatment Network suggest that rapid cycling characteristics are continuously increasing without any indication of a ceiling effect (Kupka et al. 2003). More recent studies suggest that rapid cycling constitutes a worsening of BD and develops later in the course of illness (Calabrese et al. 2001) possibly following a sensitization process triggered by antidepressant use or thyroid dysfunction, in patients with a depression–mania-free interval course and cyclothymic temperament (Azorin et al. 2008). At least in some patients, rapid cyclicity, spontaneous or induced, once established, becomes for many years a stable rhythm linked more to endogenous and to a lesser degree to environmental factors (Koukopoulos et al. 2003). In contrast to the above, apart from episode frequency, there are no solid data to support rapid cycling patients as a specific subgroup and suggest that in many cases rapid cycling is a transient phenomenon and not the final and stable stage of the illness (Bauer et al. 2008; Coryell 2005; Coryell et al. 1992, 2003; Kilzieh and Akiskal 1999).

Depression seems to relate very closely to rapid cycling in a variety of ways. There is a bulk of data suggesting that in most patients, rapid cycling is developed from an index episode of depression (Wehr et al. 1988; Roy-Byrne et al. 1985;

Perugi et al. 2000), and patients with depressive onset of bipolar illness are at higher risk to develop a rapid cycling course later (Garcia-Amador et al. 2009; Azorin et al. 2008; Perugi et al. 2000). Additionally, it is reported that depression often dominates the long-term clinical picture (Coryell et al. 2003; Goldberg et al. 2004; Lee et al. 2010; Schneck et al. 2004), although a manic predominance has also been reported (Kupka et al. 2005). The reason behind this relationship between depression and rapid cycling is not well understood; however, treatment with antidepressants and female gender might act as mediators (Ernst and Goldberg 2004; Schneck et al. 2008). It is well known that women are more likely to manifest a predominant depressive polarity (Nivoli et al. 2011a; Baldessarini et al. 2012b; Rosa et al. 2008), which in turn increases the likelihood of antidepressant treatment, and this creates a complex relationship with no clear cause and effect (Kilzieh and Akiskal 1999).

A closer look on the available data suggests an even more complex picture. In rapid cycling patients, more frequent cycling between depression and hypomania within the index episode has been reported (Coryell et al. 1992), and salient manic features are often present during depressive episodes (Goldberg et al. 2004, 2009). This puts forward the question whether at least some of these episodes are essentially mixed, although they might not fulfil standard diagnostic criteria (Vieta and Valenti 2013a). Conflicting reports and suggestions on this issue have been published with one paper suggesting that patients with a mixed episode at onset are highly unlikely to develop rapid cycling (Perugi et al. 2000) and several (with authors overlapping) suggesting the opposite (Azorin et al. 2008, 2009, 2012; Perugi et al. 1997). The failure of the recently released DSM-5 to capture the essence of mixed depressive states (e.g. agitated depression) significantly adds to the diagnostic and therapeutic uncertainties (Koukopoulos and Sani 2013; Koukopoulos et al. 2013).

Labile emotion is very frequent in rapid cycling patients and often might take the form of a soft ultrarapid pattern (Coryell et al. 1992). In this later case when the cycle lasts less than 24 h, the majority of switches (two-thirds) occur between morning and evening, and they usually follow a pattern from depression into mania/hypomania or euthymia, while only the remaining one-third follows the opposite direction. Likewise, switches that occur following the evening to the next morning pattern are correspondingly opposite (Feldman-Naim et al. 1997; Wilk and Hegerl 2010). On the other hand when the cycle lasts more than 24 h, the previously mentioned parameters (time of the day plus polarity of the episode) do not follow a systematic pattern anymore (Wilk and Hegerl 2010).

Although there is a general impression that rapid cycling is related to BD-II (Baek et al. 2011; Calabrese et al. 2001; Hajek et al. 2008; Kilzieh and Akiskal 1999; Baldessarini et al. 2000; Bauer et al. 1994; Coryell et al. 1992; Kukopulos et al. 1980; Perugi et al. 2000), the data from the Stanley Bipolar Treatment Network suggest that on the contrary it is weakly related to BD-I subtype (Kupka et al. 2003, 2005), and other studies suggest there is no preference (Garcia-Amador et al. 2009; Mackin 2005; Maj et al. 1994).

The literature on the clinical correlates of rapid cycling is rather consistent and suggests it is related to a greater number of total episodes and greater number of hospitalizations (Avasthi et al. 1999; Bauer et al. 1994; Coryell 2005; Kupka et al.

2005), with no symptom-free intervals between episodes and cyclothymic temperament (Azorin et al. 2008), worst long-term course (Mackin 2005; Coryell 2005; Kilzieh and Akiskal 1999), higher overall comorbidity (MacKinnon et al. 2003a, b; Hajek et al. 2008; Lee et al. 2010) and more severe disability (Hajek et al. 2005; Lee et al. 2010; Schneck et al. 2004; Wells et al. 2010), although there is one study suggesting no relationship to increased comorbidity (Wells et al. 2010). Most data reported so far agree that rapid cycling patients manifest onset of their illness at a younger age (Azorin et al. 2008; Bowden et al. 1999; Ernst and Goldberg 2004; Hajek et al. 2008; Lee et al. 2010; Lin et al. 2006; MacKinnon et al. 2003a; Schneck et al. 2004; Wells et al. 2010; Fountoulakis 2012) even before the age of 17 (Coryell et al. 2003). Two papers report later age at onset for rapid cycling patients (Baldessarini et al. 2000; Serretti et al. 2002) and some others no difference in age of onset (Bauer et al. 1994; Coryell et al. 1992; Kukopulos et al. 1980; Maj et al. 1994; Perugi et al. 2000; Schneck et al. 2008). In children and adolescents BD very often follows a rapid or ultrarapid course (Geller et al. 1998; Findling et al. 2001), and this might mean that there is great heterogeneity concerning the age-of-onset effect in the development of rapid cycling. One paper reports that the duration of illness is not longer in rapid cyclers, thus disputing the earlier onset of bipolar illness suggestion (Yildiz and Sachs 2004).

Alcohol and drug abuse are consistently reported to be more frequent in this group (Cruz et al. 2008; Kupka et al. 2003, 2005; MacKinnon et al. 2003a). One paper suggests the more frequent presence of history of childhood physical or sexual abuse (Kupka et al. 2005). Rapid cycling patients also manifest more suicide attempts (Azorin et al. 2008, 2010; Coryell et al. 2003; Cruz et al. 2008; Goldberg et al. 2004; Hajek et al. 2008), but this might be because of more frequent and more severe attempts in the same percentage of persons in comparison to non-rapid cyclers (Garcia-Amador et al. 2009). A limited number of papers suggest such a correlation with suicidality does not exist (Kilzieh and Akiskal 1999; MacKinnon et al. 2003a; Wells et al. 2010).

Overall, close relationship to depression could be the cause of all of the above. But also, at least partially the above characteristics could be explained by the fact that probably because of earlier onset of bipolar illness, rapid cycling patients manifest longer duration of illness in comparison to the same age patients without rapid cycling, and this overloads them in a variety of ways (Azorin et al. 2008; Avasthi et al. 1999; Maj et al. 1994; Berk et al. 2011; Vieta et al. 2013b).

Emotional lability and soft ultrarapid cycling within rapid cycling are not uncommon (Coryell et al. 1992). In cases of ultrarapid cycling with cycle length less than 24 h, two-thirds of switches occurring between morning and evening are from depression into mania/hypomania or euthymia and one-third in the opposite direction. Similarly, switches occurring between evening and the next morning are, respectively, opposite (Feldman-Naim et al. 1997; Wilk and Hegerl 2010). When the cycle length is greater than 24 h, the time of the day and the polarity of the episode seem to be random (Wilk and Hegerl 2010).

More severe forms of premenstrual tension syndrome, when present, might accelerate cycling in female BD patients (Price and DiMarzio 1986). In retrospective studies of rapid cycling, the presence of severe premenstrual syndrome might constitute a confounding variable (Dias et al. 2011). It is reported that rapid cycling is found more often during the menopause (Dunner and Fieve 1974); however, most data do not support any relationship between the female reproducing cycle and phase and rapid cycling (Bauer et al. 1994; Leibenluft et al. 1999).

The outcome of rapid cycling BD is variable. It is well known that a subgroup of mood patients becomes 'sensitized', after repeated mood episodes, and the threshold for the manifestation of new episodes becomes progressively lower leading to more frequent relapses. Eventually the episodes are triggered spontaneously. This 'kindling' phenomenon is considered to be analogous to that observed in epilepsy (Post et al. 1986; Post 1992). Some authors suggest that rapid cycling is the result of a 'kindling' mechanism which results in shorter cycles and higher frequency of episodes after the experiencing of repeated episodes (Cutler and Post 1982; Goldberg and Harrow 1994; Post 1992; Zis and Goodwin 1979); however, there are some data against such an assumption, suggesting no relationship of rapid cycling to number of previous episodes (Turvey et al. 1999; Hammen and Gitlin 1997).

It is reported that one-third of patients manifest complete remission for at least the past year, 40 % continue being rapid cyclers with severe episodes, while 14 % remain rapid cycling but with attenuated episodes. A significant proportion of patients (13 %) might become long cyclers (Koukopoulos et al. 2003). However, as already mentioned before, in many cases rapid cycling is a transient phenomenon rather than the final and stable stage of the illness (Bauer et al. 2008; Coryell 2005; Coryell et al. 1992, 2003; Kilzieh and Akiskal 1999). Maybe patients with an initial cycle pattern of depression–mania/hypomania-free interval have a worse outcome, while patients with an initial cycle pattern of mania/hypomania–depression-free interval might do better (Koukopoulos et al. 2003). This pattern was not observed in other studies, and it is a matter of debate (Bauer et al. 1994; Coryell et al. 1992; Maj et al. 1994).

A robust finding in the literature is that females constitute the majority of patients with rapid cycling (Arnold 2003; Bauer et al. 1994; Cruz et al. 2008; Schneck et al. 2004; Tondo and Baldessarini 1998; Wehr et al. 1988; Yildiz and Sachs 2004), with their proportion to be reported as high as 92 % (Wehr et al. 1988). However, the most realistic estimations suggest that it averages around 72 % (Bauer et al. 1994). The true risk is somewhat different and is reported to be inconsistently higher among women (29.6 %) than among men (16.5 %) (Tondo and Baldessarini 1998). This was confirmed by a recent meta-analysis (Kupka et al. 2003). Only one study has reported a higher prevalence in males (Joffe et al. 1988), and some other reported equal rates between males and females (Maj et al. 1994; Baldassano et al. 2005; Serretti et al. 2002; Joffe et al. 1988). In one of them the study populations suffered from a too large proportion of males (Baldassano et al. 2005). In another study, the proportion of women was greater than the proportion of men only among patients with eight or more episodes per year (Kupka et al. 2005).

This correlation between rapid cycling and female gender might stem from a variety of factors, including the menstrual cycle and the higher risk of hypothyroidism in females. Also there is a circular correlation of female gender with a number

Table 3.2 Prevalence of rapid cycling in BD patients

Publication	Prevalence	Sample size *N*	Rapid cycling *N* (%)	Comments
Kukopulos et al. (1980)	Current	434	86 (20 %)	
Nurnberger et al. (1988)	Current	195	29 (15 %)	
Coryell et al. (1992)	Current	919	46 (5 %)	
Schneck et al. (2004)	Current	456	91 (20 %)	STEP-BD
Azorin et al. (2008)	Current	1,090	86 (9 %)	
Cruz et al. (2008)	Current	3,089	535 (17.3 %)	EMBLEM
Garcia-Amador et al. (2009)	Current	305	55 (18 %)	
Coryell et al. (2003)	Lifetime	345	89 (25.8 %)	13.7 (±6.1) years follow-up
Dittmann et al. (2002)	Lifetime	152	41 (27 %)	2.5 years follow-up
Hajek et al. (2008)	Lifetime	240	80 (33.3 %)	Primary care sample
Yildiz and Sachs (2004)	Lifetime	197	84 (43 %)	Tertiary care sample
Schneck et al. (2008)	Current	1,742	562 (32 %)	STEP-BD
Total current		**8,230**	**1,490 (18.10 %)**	
Total lifetime		**934**	**294 (31.48 %)**	

of factors, including depression and cyclothymic temperament (Kilzieh and Akiskal 1999) as well as a more deleterious effect of antidepressant treatment in females specifically (Yildiz and Sachs 2003). The role of the bipolar type seems controversial since the gender effect was reported to be stronger in the BD-I type (Schneck et al. 2004; Yildiz and Sachs 2004), although BD-II is strongly related to female gender. Overall the mean weighted by sample size, annual/current prevalence rate is 18.10 %, while the lifetime prevalence is estimated to be 31.48 % (Table 3.2).

A variety of medical conditions might cause rapid cycling BD in previously mentally healthy individuals. These include subarachnoid haemorrhage (Blackwell 1991), closed head injury (Zwil et al. 1993) or focal temporal pole damage (Murai and Fujimoto 2003). Other conditions related to rapid cycling include homocystinuria (Awara et al. 2012), mild immune activation which seems to normalize with lithium treatment (Rapaport et al. 1999) and the effect of environmental temperature and its changes (Boker et al. 2008). One study correlated rapid cycling in BD-II to changes in the ventromedial prefrontal cortex (Narita et al. 2011).

The first report on the possible relationship between hypothyroidism and rapid cycling appeared in 1979 and was an observation that patients receiving lithium and thyroid substitution therapy were more prone to become rapid cyclers (Cho et al. 1979).

Today, hypothyroidism is considered by many authors to correlate with rapid cycling with around half of rapid cycling patients manifesting it (Cowdry et al. 1983; Bauer et al. 1990; Bauer and Whybrow 1990; Azorin et al. 2008; Kusalic 1992).

However, there are a number of methodological considerations including the medication status, recruitment bias, definition of hypothyroidism as well as the comparison groups. Also several authors report that no such a correlation exists (Joffe et al. 1988; Post et al. 1997; Maj et al. 1994; Bartalena et al. 1990; Coryell et al. 1992; Kupka et al. 2002; Oomen et al. 1996; Wehr et al. 1988), and this is supported by a meta-analysis (Kupka et al. 2003). On this basis thyroid augmentation is not recommended for the treatment of rapid cycling BD patients (Kilzieh and Akiskal 1999) although there are some but limited data in support of its efficacy (Kusalic 1992).

Although previous treatment with lithium was considered to be the cause of hypothyroidism in many cases, there seems to be at least some rapid cycling patients for whom this explanation is not valid (Bauer and Whybrow 1990; Fountoulakis et al. 2013; Bauer et al. 1990). However, the relationship between lithium treatment, female gender, hypothyroidism and rapid cycling (Bauer and Whybrow 1990; Cowdry et al. 1983; Fountoulakis et al. 2008; Bauer et al. 1990) seems to be more complex, since even in euthyroid rapid cycling patients but not in controls, short-term lithium treatment might cause grade III hypothyroidism (Gyulai et al. 2003). Also an association between the occurrence of thyroperoxidase antibodies and a history of rapid cycling has been reported (Oomen et al. 1996). However, another study disputed the presence of even this latent hypothyroidism (Joffe et al. 1988).

Conclusively, there are not sufficient data to support a direct link between rapid cycling and hypothyroidism. More research is needed especially in patients who have never received lithium.

It is widely accepted among clinicians that treatment of antidepressants, apart from the induction of the manic pole, might also cause cycle acceleration. However, this has not been solidly proven. The first case report of a possible antidepressant-induced rapid cycling appeared in 1956 and concerned the monoamine oxidase inhibitor iproniazid (Crane 1956). For the first time this issue was put forward systematically in the seminal paper of Wehr and Goodwin (1979). Since then many studies addressed this question both retrospectively and prospectively. A major problem is that many authors mix induction of the opposite pole by antidepressants with induction of rapid cycling and carry observations from switching to rapid cycling. The conclusions based on such an approach could not be considered to be valid, but often constitute the basis of discussions and reviews.

The classical picture is that rapid cycling may be precipitated by the use of antidepressants in more than 70 % of cases and maintained after their continuation (Wehr et al. 1988). More recent studies reported rates of antidepressant-induced rapid cycling range between 3 % and 50 % (Goodwin and Jamison 1990; Wehr et al. 1988; Yatham et al. 2003), and this wide range is probably because of methodological problems. It is suggested that such an induction happens mostly within the first year of antidepressant initiation (Altshuler et al. 1995). However, the data are rather inconclusive. The data from long-term retrospective studies are conflicting (Wolpert et al. 1990; Angst 1985; Lewis and Winokur 1982, 1987, 1989). All shorter-duration retrospective studies suggest an association between rapid cycling and antidepressant use (Kukopulos et al. 1980; Wehr et al. 1988; Altshuler et al. 1995), while one such study limited this association to female patients only (Yildiz and Sachs 2003).

On the contrary only two prospective studies suggest the presence of such an association (Wehr and Goodwin 1979; Koukopoulos et al. 2003), while three others were negative (Bauer et al. 2005, 2006; Coryell et al. 2003). The clinical profile of those rapid cycling patients supposedly induced by antidepressants is not reported to differ from the rest of rapid cycling population (Bauer et al. 1994) although females (Yildiz and Sachs 2003) and especially female BD-II patients might be overrepresented (Altshuler et al. 1995).

The conclusion of major reviews is that such an association is not supported by the data or it is overvalued (Kilzieh and Akiskal 1999; Coryell 2005; Grunze 2008; Mattes 2006). Also it has been proposed that the relationship of antidepressants with rapid cycling, female gender and possibly BD-II merely probably reflects the predominance of depression in rapid cyclers and consequently the predominance of antidepressant treatment (Coryell et al. 1992; Vieta and Valenti 2013b). Currently there are no data suggesting that other classes of agents (e.g. antipsychotics or antiepileptics) might induce rapid cycling.

Family studies suggest that patients with rapid cycling do not differ from the rest in terms of family load for mood disorders. Although there are some reports suggesting that they might have a stronger family loading of BD (Avasthi et al. 1999; Wehr et al. 1988) and maybe more frequently a relative with rapid cycling (MacKinnon et al. 2003a) and a close relationship to the presence of panic disorder, substance abuse and suicidality in the family (MacKinnon et al. 2003a, b; Vieta et al. 2004), these findings were usually not statistically significant, and essentially most of the data are clearly negative (Bauer et al. 1994; Coryell et al. 1992; Kilzieh and Akiskal 1999; Lish et al. 1993; Nurnberger et al. 1988; Fountoulakis and Akiskal 2008). A meta-analysis confirmed a lack of familial load for rapid cycling bipolar patients (Kupka et al. 2003).

In terms of specific genes, the Val66Met polymorphism (Green et al. 2006; Muller et al. 2006); the SNPs hCV11592756, rs2049045 and GT(n) (Muller et al. 2006) of the brain-derived neurotrophic factor (BDNF); the low activity allele variation in the COMT gene (Kirov et al. 1998; Papolos et al. 1998); the 5-HT transporter gene (Rousseva et al. 2003) and the haplotype GGAC of the circadian gene CRY2 (Sjoholm et al. 2010) have been associated with rapid cycling BD. One study concerning the low activity allele of the COMT gene was negative (Geller and Cook 2000). As a general conclusion from genetic studies, one can say that they are too few, with small study populations, and results need clarification and replication. In the future, it is important to control for a number of confounding factors like exposure to antidepressants, temperament, etc. In this frame, an interesting hypothesis suggests that temperament might act as the determining endophenotype while rapid cycling serves as an intermediate phenotype (Sayin et al. 2007; Mackinnon and Pies 2006; Insel and Cuthbert 2009).

Conclusively, rapid cycling is still an uncharted area. Around one-third of BD patients will experience rapid cycling at some time in their lives. A number of factors, including predominance of depression, treatment with antidepressants, female gender, refractoriness to lithium and hypothyroidism, seem to involve in the aetiopathogenesis or to shape the clinical manifestations and the long-term outcome. The most proper definition of rapid cycling is still not available, since many patients manifest emotional lability which often takes the form of ultra or ultra-ultrarapid cycling, but they are often diagnosed as suffering from mixed episodes or personality disorders according to contemporary classification systems. It is highly likely that rapid cycling represents a worsening of the underlying disorder, which, in turn, leads towards a significant deterioration of clinical outcomes, more severe disability and increased suicidality. There are convincing data that rapid cycling represents a transitory period rather than a stable condition once it manifests. During those rapid cycling periods, patients are difficult to diagnose and to treat especially when the clinical picture resembles a personality disorder (Mackinnon and Pies 2006). Future research should clarify whether rapid cycling represents an exacerbation of emotional endophenotypes (e.g. affective temperaments) linked to disorders associated with affective dysregulation, such as BD.

References

Abdul-Rahim FA, Al-Sabai A, Al-Hamad AR, Bamgboye E (1992) The seasonality of mania: preliminary findings. Ann Saudi Med 12(5):472–475. doi:12-472 [pii]

Alessandra MA, Colom F, Pacchiarotti I, Murru A, Scott J, Valenti M, Mazzarini L, Mar Bonnin CD, Jose SM, Serretti A, Vieta E (2013) Treatment strategies according to clinical features in a naturalistic cohort study of bipolar patients: a principal component analysis of lifetime pharmacological and biophysic treatment options. Eur Neuropsychopharmacol 23(4):263–275

Altshuler LL, Post RM, Leverich GS, Mikalauskas K, Rosoff A, Ackerman L (1995) Antidepressant-induced mania and cycle acceleration: a controversy revisited. Am J Psychiatry 152(8):1130–1138

Angst J (1978) The course of affective disorders. II. Typology of bipolar manic-depressive illness. Arch Psychiatr Nervenkr 226(1):65–73

Angst J (1981) Unsolved problems in the indications for lithium prophylaxis in affective and schizoaffective disorders. Bibliogr Psychiatry (161):32–44

Angst J (1985) Switch from depression to mania–a record study over decades between 1920 and 1982. Psychopathology 18(2–3):140–154

Arnold LM (2003) Gender differences in bipolar disorder. Psychiatr Clin North Am 26(3):595–620

Avasthi A, Sharma A, Malhotra S, Gupta N, Kulhara P (1999) Rapid cycling affective disorder: a descriptive study from North India. J Affect Disord 54(1–2):67–73. doi:S0165-0327(98)00135-9 [pii]

Awara MA, Zahid S, Elnenaei MO (2012) Rapid cycling bipolar affective disorder and recurrent strokes secondary to high blood homocysteine. J Ment Health. doi:10.3109/09638237.2012.670884

Azorin JM, Kaladjian A, Adida M, Hantouche EG, Hameg A, Lancrenon S, Akiskal HS (2008) Factors associated with rapid cycling in bipolar I manic patients: findings from a French national study. CNS Spectr 13(9):780–787

Azorin JM, Aubrun E, Bertsch J, Reed C, Gerard S, Lukasiewicz M (2009) Mixed states vs. pure mania in the French sample of the EMBLEM study: results at baseline and 24 months – European mania in bipolar longitudinal evaluation of medication. BMC Psychiatry 9:33. doi:10.1186/1471-244X-9-33, 1471-244X-9-33 [pii]

Azorin JM, Kaladjian A, Besnier N, Adida M, Hantouche E, Lancrenon S, Akiskal H (2010) Suicidal behaviour in a French Cohort of major depressive patients: characteristics of attempters and nonattempters. J Affect Disord 123(1–3):87–94. doi:10.1016/j.jad.2009.09.004, S0165-0327(09)00422-4 [pii]

Azorin JM, Kaladjian A, Adida M, Fakra E, Belzeaux R, Hantouche E, Lancrenon S (2012) Self-assessment and characteristics of mixed depression in the French national EPIDEP study. J Affect Disord 143(1–3):109–117. doi:10.1016/j.jad.2012.05.036, S0165-0327(12)00391-6 [pii]

Baek JH, Park DY, Choi J, Kim JS, Choi JS, Ha K, Kwon JS, Lee D, Hong KS (2011) Differences between bipolar I and bipolar II disorders in clinical features, comorbidity, and family history. J Affect Disord 131(1–3):59–67. doi:10.1016/j.jad.2010.11.020, S0165-0327(10)00717-2 [pii]

Baldassano CF, Marangell LB, Gyulai L, Ghaemi SN, Joffe H, Kim DR, Sagduyu K, Truman CJ, Wisniewski SR, Sachs GS, Cohen LS (2005) Gender differences in bipolar disorder: retrospective data from the first 500 STEP-BD participants. Bipolar Disord 7(5):465–470. doi:10.1111/j.1399-5618.2005.00237.x, BDI237 [pii]

Baldessarini RJ, Tondo L, Floris G, Hennen J (2000) Effects of rapid cycling on response to lithium maintenance treatment in 360 bipolar I and II disorder patients. J Affect Disord 61(1–2):13–22. doi:S0165-0327(99)00196-2 [pii]

Baldessarini RJ, Salvatore P, Khalsa HM, Imaz-Etxeberria H, Gonzalez-Pinto A, Tohen M (2012a) Episode cycles with increasing recurrences in first-episode bipolar-I disorder patients. J Affect Disord 136(1–2):149–154. doi:10.1016/j.jad.2011.08.037

Baldessarini RJ, Undurraga J, Vazquez GH, Tondo L, Salvatore P, Ha K, Khalsa HM, Lepri B, Ha TH, Chang JS, Tohen M, Vieta E (2012b) Predominant recurrence polarity among 928 adult international bipolar I disorder patients. Acta Psychiatr Scand 125(4):293–302. doi:10.1111/j.1600-0447.2011.01818.x

Barrios C, Chaudhry TA, Goodnick PJ (2001) Rapid cycling bipolar disorder. Expert Opin Pharmacother 2(12):1963–1973. doi:10.1517/14656566.2.12.1963

Bartalena L, Pellegrini L, Meschi M, Antonangeli L, Bogazzi F, Dell'Osso L, Pinchera A, Placidi GF (1990) Evaluation of thyroid function in patients with rapid-cycling and non-rapid-cycling bipolar disorder. Psychiatry Res 34(1):13–17. doi:0165-1781(90)90054-9 [pii]

Bauer MS, Whybrow PC (1990) Rapid cycling bipolar affective disorder. II. Treatment of refractory rapid cycling with high-dose levothyroxine: a preliminary study. Arch Gen Psychiatry 47(5):435–440

Bauer MS, Whybrow PC, Winokur A (1990) Rapid cycling bipolar affective disorder. I. Association with grade I hypothyroidism. Arch Gen Psychiatry 47(5):427–432

Bauer MS, Calabrese J, Dunner DL, Post R, Whybrow PC, Gyulai L, Tay LK, Younkin SR, Bynum D, Lavori P et al (1994) Multisite data reanalysis of the validity of rapid cycling as a course modifier for bipolar disorder in DSM-IV. Am J Psychiatry 151(4):506–515

Bauer M, Rasgon N, Grof P, Altshuler L, Gyulai L, Lapp M, Glenn T, Whybrow PC (2005) Mood changes related to antidepressants: a longitudinal study of patients with bipolar disorder in a naturalistic setting. Psychiatry Res 133(1):73–80. doi:10.1016/j.psychres.2004.08.006, S0165-1781(04)00219-7 [pii]

Bauer M, Rasgon N, Grof P, Glenn T, Lapp M, Marsh W, Munoz R, Suwalska A, Baethge C, Bschor T, Alda M, Whybrow PC (2006) Do antidepressants influence mood patterns? A naturalistic study in bipolar disorder. Eur Psychiatry 21(4):262–269. doi:10.1016/j.eurpsy.2006.04.009, S0924-9338(06)00091-5 [pii]

Bauer M, Beaulieu S, Dunner DL, Lafer B, Kupka R (2008) Rapid cycling bipolar disorder – diagnostic concepts. Bipolar Disord 10(1 Pt 2):153–162. doi:10.1111/j.1399-5618.2007.00560.x, BDI560 [pii]

Bauer M, Glenn T, Grof P, Rasgon NL, Marsh W, Sagduyu K, Alda M, Murray G, Quiroz D, Malliaris Y, Sasse J, Pilhatsch M, Whybrow PC (2009) Relationship among latitude, climate, season and self-reported mood in bipolar disorder. J Affect Disord 116(1–2):152–157. doi:10.1016/j.jad.2008.11.013, S0165-0327(08)00469-2 [pii]

Benedetti F, Colombo C, Barbini B, Campori E, Smeraldi E (2001) Morning sunlight reduces length of hospitalization in bipolar depression. J Affect Disord 62(3):221–223. doi:S016503270000149X [pii]

Berk M, Kapczinski F, Andreazza AC, Dean OM, Giorlando F, Maes M, Yucel M, Gama CS, Dodd S, Dean B, Magalhaes PV, Amminger P, McGorry P, Malhi GS (2011) Pathways underlying neuroprogression in bipolar disorder: focus on inflammation, oxidative stress and neurotrophic factors. Neurosci Biobehav Rev 35(3):804–817. doi:10.1016/j.neubiorev.2010.10.001, S0149-7634(10)00154-5 [pii]

Blackwell MJ (1991) Rapid-cycling manic-depressive illness following subarachnoid haemorrhage. Br J Psychiatry 159:279–280

Boker SM, Leibenluft E, Deboeck PR, Virk G, Postolache TT (2008) Mood oscillations and coupling between mood and weather in patients with rapid cycling bipolar disorder. Int J Child Health Hum Dev 1(2):181–203

Bowden CL, Calabrese JR, McElroy SL, Rhodes LJ, Keck PE Jr, Cookson J, Anderson J, Bolden-Watson C, Ascher J, Monaghan E, Zhou J (1999) The efficacy of lamotrigine in rapid cycling and non-rapid cycling patients with bipolar disorder. Biol Psychiatry 45(8):953–958. doi:S000632239900013X [pii]

Bunney WE Jr, Hartmann EL, Mason JW (1965) Study of a patient with 48-hour manic-depressive cycles. II. Strong positive correlation between endocrine factors and manic defense patterns. Arch Gen Psychiatry 12:619–625

Calabrese JR, Shelton MD, Rapport DJ, Kujawa M, Kimmel SE, Caban S (2001) Current research on rapid cycling bipolar disorder and its treatment. J Affect Disord 67(1–3):241–255. doi:S016503279800161X [pii]

Carney PA, Fitzgerald CT, Monaghan CE (1988a) Influence of climate on the prevalence of mania. Br J Psychiatry 152:820–823

Carney PA, Seggie J, Vojtechovsky M, Parker J, Grof E, Grof P (1988b) Bipolar patients taking lithium have increased dark adaptation threshold compared with controls. Pharmacopsychiatry 21(3):117–120. doi:10.1055/s-2007-1014661

Cassidy F, Carroll BJ (2002) Seasonal variation of mixed and pure episodes of bipolar disorder. J Affect Disord 68(1):25–31. doi:S0165032700003256 [pii]

Chan PK, Lam RW, Perry KF (1994) Mania precipitated by light therapy for patients with SAD. J Clin Psychiatry 55(10):454

Cho JT, Bone S, Dunner DL, Colt E, Fieve RR (1979) The effect of lithium treatment on thyroid function in patients with primary affective disorder. Am J Psychiatry 136(1):115–116

Choi J, Baek JH, Noh J, Kim JS, Choi JS, Ha K, Kwon JS, Hong KS (2011) Association of seasonality and premenstrual symptoms in bipolar I and bipolar II disorders. J Affect Disord 129(1–3): 313–316. doi:10.1016/j.jad.2010.07.030, S0165-0327(10)00512-4 [pii]

Christensen EM, Larsen JK, Gjerris A, Peacock L, Jacobi M, Hassenbalch E (2008) Climatic factors and bipolar affective disorder. Nord J Psychiatry 62(1):55–58. doi:10.1080/08039480801970049, 791409081 [pii]

Clarke M, Moran P, Keogh F, Morris M, Kinsella A, Larkin C, Walsh D, O'Callaghan E (1999) Seasonal influences on admissions for affective disorder and schizophrenia in Ireland: a comparison of first and readmissions. Eur Psychiatry 14(5):251–255. doi:S0924-9338(99)00174-1 [pii]

Colom F, Vieta E (2009) The road to DSM-V. Bipolar disorder episode and course specifiers. Psychopathology 42(4):209–218. doi:10.1159/000218518, 000218518 [pii]

Colom F, Vieta E, Daban C, Pacchiarotti I, Sanchez-Moreno J (2006) Clinical and therapeutic implications of predominant polarity in bipolar disorder. J Affect Disord 93(1–3):13–17

Coryell W (2005) Rapid cycling bipolar disorder: clinical characteristics and treatment options. CNS Drugs 19(7):557–569. doi:1971 [pii]

Coryell W, Endicott J, Keller M (1992) Rapidly cycling affective disorder. Demographics, diagnosis, family history, and course. Arch Gen Psychiatry 49(2):126–131

Coryell W, Solomon D, Turvey C, Keller M, Leon AC, Endicott J, Schettler P, Judd L, Mueller T (2003) The long-term course of rapid-cycling bipolar disorder. Arch Gen Psychiatry 60(9): 914–920. doi:10.1001/archpsyc.60.9.914, 60/9/914 [pii]

Cowdry RW, Wehr TA, Zis AP, Goodwin FK (1983) Thyroid abnormalities associated with rapid-cycling bipolar illness. Arch Gen Psychiatry 40(4):414–420

Crane GE (1956) The psychiatric side-effects of iproniazid. Am J Psychiatry 112(7):494–501

Cruz N, Vieta E, Comes M, Haro JM, Reed C, Bertsch J (2008) Rapid-cycling bipolar I disorder: course and treatment outcome of a large sample across Europe. J Psychiatr Res 42(13):1068–1075. doi:10.1016/j.jpsychires.2007.12.004, S0022-3956(07)00212-9 [pii]

Cusin C, Serretti A, Mandelli L, Lucca A, Smeraldi E (2002) Seasonal variations of lithium plasma levels. Psychiatry Res 111(1):35–41. doi:S0165178102001300 [pii]

Cuthbert BN, Insel TR (2013) Toward the future of psychiatric diagnosis: the seven pillars of RDoC. BMC Med 11:126. doi:10.1186/1741-7015-11-126

Cutler NR, Post RM (1982) Life course of illness in untreated manic-depressive patients. Compr Psychiatry 23(2):101–115. doi:0010-440X(82)90055-4 [pii]
D'Mello DA, McNeil JA, Msibi B (1995) Seasons and bipolar disorder. Ann Clin Psychiatry 7(1):11–18
Daban C, Colom F, Sanchez-Moreno J, Garcia-Amador M, Vieta E (2006) Clinical correlates of first-episode polarity in bipolar disorder. Compr Psychiatry 47(6):433–437. doi:10.1016/j.comppsych.2006.03.009, S0010-440X(06)00051-4 [pii]
Daniels BA, Kirkby KC, Mitchell P, Hay D, Mowry B (2000) Seasonal variation in hospital admission for bipolar disorder, depression and schizophrenia in Tasmania. Acta Psychiatr Scand 102(1):38–43
Dauphinais DR, Rosenthal JZ, Terman M, DiFebo HM, Tuggle C, Rosenthal NE (2012) Controlled trial of safety and efficacy of bright light therapy vs. negative air ions in patients with bipolar depression. Psychiatry Res 196(1):57–61. doi:10.1016/j.psychres.2012.01.015, S0165-1781(12)00045-5 [pii]
Deltito JA, Moline M, Pollak C, Martin LY, Maremmani I (1991) Effects of phototherapy on non-seasonal unipolar and bipolar depressive spectrum disorders. J Affect Disord 23(4):231–237
Dias RS, Lafer B, Russo C, Del Debbio A, Nierenberg AA, Sachs GS, Joffe H (2011) Longitudinal follow-up of bipolar disorder in women with premenstrual exacerbation: findings from STEP-BD. Am J Psychiatry 168(4):386–394. doi:10.1176/appi.ajp.2010.09121816, appi.ajp.2010.09121816 [pii]
Dittmann S, Biedermann NC, Grunze H, Hummel B, Scharer LO, Kleindienst N, Forsthoff A, Matzner N, Walser S, Walden J (2002) The Stanley Foundation Bipolar Network: results of the naturalistic follow-up study after 2.5 years of follow-up in the German centres. Neuropsychobiology 46(Suppl 1):2–9. doi:68018 68018 [pii]
Dunner DL, Fieve RR (1974) Clinical factors in lithium carbonate prophylaxis failure. Arch Gen Psychiatry 30(2):229–233
Eastwood MR, Stiasny S (1978) Psychiatric disorder, hospital admission, and season. Arch Gen Psychiatry 35(6):769–771
Ernst CL, Goldberg JF (2004) Clinical features related to age at onset in bipolar disorder. J Affect Disord 82(1):21–27. doi:10.1016/j.jad.2003.10.002, S0165032703002581 [pii]
Etain B, Lajnef M, Bellivier F, Mathieu F, Raust A, Cochet B, Gard S, M'Bailara K, Kahn JP, Elgrabli O, Cohen R, Jamain S, Vieta E, Leboyer M, Henry C (2012) Clinical expression of bipolar disorder type I as a function of age and polarity at onset: convergent findings in samples from France and the United States. J Clin Psychiatry 73(4):e561–e566
Faedda GL, Tondo L, Teicher MH, Baldessarini RJ, Gelbard HA, Floris GF (1993) Seasonal mood disorders. Patterns of seasonal recurrence in mania and depression. Arch Gen Psychiatry 50(1):17–23
Feldman-Naim S, Turner EH, Leibenluft E (1997) Diurnal variation in the direction of mood switches in patients with rapid-cycling bipolar disorder. J Clin Psychiatry 58(2):79–84
Findling RL, Gracious BL, McNamara NK, Youngstrom EA, Demeter CA, Branicky LA, Calabrese JR (2001) Rapid, continuous cycling and psychiatric co-morbidity in pediatric bipolar I disorder. Bipolar Disord 3(4):202–210. doi:bdi030405 [pii]
Forty L, Jones L, Jones I, Smith DJ, Caesar S, Fraser C, Gordon-Smith K, Hyde S, Craddock N (2009) Polarity at illness onset in bipolar I disorder and clinical course of illness. Bipolar Disord 11(1):82–88
Fountoulakis KN (2012) Introduction–bipolar illness: current understanding and future perspectives. CNS Neurosci Ther 18(3):193. doi:10.1111/j.1755-5949.2012.00298.x
Fountoulakis KN, Akiskal HS (2008) Focus on bipolar illness. CNS Spectr 13(9):762
Fountoulakis KN, Vieta E, Bouras C, Notaridis G, Giannakopoulos P, Kaprinis G, Akiskal H (2008) A systematic review of existing data on long-term lithium therapy: neuroprotective or neurotoxic? Int J Neuropsychopharmacol 11(2):269–287. doi:10.1017/S1461145707007821
Fountoulakis KN, Kontis D, Gonda X, Siamouli M, Yatham LN (2012) Treatment of mixed bipolar states. Int J Neuropsychopharmacol 15(7):1015–1026. doi:10.1017/S1461145711001817
Fountoulakis KN, Kontis D, Gonda X, Yatham LN (2013) A systematic review of the evidence on the treatment of rapid cycling bipolar disorder. Bipolar Disord 15(2):115–137. doi:10.1111/bdi.12045

Frangos E, Athanassenas G, Tsitourides S, Psilolignos P, Robos A, Katsanou N, Bulgaris C (1980) Seasonality of the episodes of recurrent affective psychoses. Possible prophylactic interventions. J Affect Disord 2(4):239–247

Friedman E, Gyulai L, Bhargava M, Landen M, Wisniewski S, Foris J, Ostacher M, Medina R, Thase M (2006) Seasonal changes in clinical status in bipolar disorder: a prospective study in 1000 STEP-BD patients. Acta Psychiatr Scand 113(6):510–517. doi:10.1111/j.1600-0447.2005.00701.x, ACP701 [pii]

Garcia-Amador M, Colom F, Valenti M, Horga G, Vieta E (2009) Suicide risk in rapid cycling bipolar patients. J Affect Disord 117(1–2):74–78. doi:10.1016/j.jad.2008.12.005, S0165-0327(08)00481-3 [pii]

Garcia-Lopez A, De Dios-Perrino C, Ezquiaga E (2009) Polarity of the first episode and predominant polarity in a cohort of bipolar outpatients. Eur Neuropsychopharmacol 19:S571

Geller B, Cook EH Jr (2000) Ultradian rapid cycling in prepubertal and early adolescent bipolarity is not in transmission disequilibrium with val/met COMT alleles. Biol Psychiatry 47(7):605–609. doi:S0006-3223(99)00251-6 [pii]

Geller B, Cooper TB, Sun K, Zimerman B, Frazier J, Williams M, Heath J (1998) Double-blind and placebo-controlled study of lithium for adolescent bipolar disorders with secondary substance dependency. J Am Acad Child Adolesc Psychiatry 37(2):171–178

Goikolea JM, Colom F, Martinez-Aran A, Sanchez-Moreno J, Giordano A, Bulbena A, Vieta E (2007) Clinical and prognostic implications of seasonal pattern in bipolar disorder: a 10-year follow-up of 302 patients. Psychol Med 37(11):1595–1599. doi:10.1017/S0033291707000864, S0033291707000864 [pii]

Goldberg JF, Harrow M (1994) Kindling in bipolar disorders: a longitudinal follow-up study. Biol Psychiatry 35(1):70–72

Goldberg JF, Wankmuller MM, Sutherland KH (2004) Depression with versus without manic features in rapid-cycling bipolar disorder. J Nerv Ment Dis 192(9):602–606. doi:00005053-200409000-00004 [pii]

Goldberg JF, Brooks JO 3rd, Kurita K, Hoblyn JC, Ghaemi SN, Perlis RH, Miklowitz DJ, Ketter TA, Sachs GS, Thase ME (2009) Depressive illness burden associated with complex polypharmacy in patients with bipolar disorder: findings from the STEP-BD. J Clin Psychiatry 70(2):155–162. doi:ej08m04301 [pii]

Gonzalez-Pinto A, Alberich S, Barbeito S, Alonso M, Vieta E, Martinez-Aran A, Saenz M, Lopez P (2010a) Different profile of substance abuse in relation to predominant polarity in bipolar disorder. The Vitoria long-term follow-up study. J Affect Disord 124(3):250–255

Gonzalez-Pinto A, Alberich S, Barbeito S, Alonso M, Vieta E, Martinez-Aran A, Saenz M, Lopez P (2010b) Different profile of substance abuse in relation to predominant polarity in bipolar disorder: the Vitoria long-term follow-up study. J Affect Disord 124(3):250–255. doi:10.1016/j.jad.2009.11.005, S0165-0327(09)00498-4 [pii]

Goodwin F, Jamison K (1990) Manic-depressive illness. Oxford University Press, New York

Green EK, Raybould R, Macgregor S, Hyde S, Young AH, O'Donovan MC, Owen MJ, Kirov G, Jones L, Jones I, Craddock N (2006) Genetic variation of brain-derived neurotrophic factor (BDNF) in bipolar disorder: case-control study of over 3000 individuals from the UK. Br J Psychiatry 188:21–25. doi:10.1192/bjp.BD.105.009969, 188/1/21 [pii]

Grunze HC (2008) Switching, induction of rapid cycling, and increased suicidality with antidepressants in bipolar patients: fact or overinterpretation? CNS Spectr 13(9):790–795

Gyulai L, Bauer M, Bauer MS, Garcia-Espana F, Cnaan A, Whybrow PC (2003) Thyroid hypofunction in patients with rapid-cycling bipolar disorder after lithium challenge. Biol Psychiatry 53(10):899–905. doi:S0006322302015731 [pii]

Hajek T, Slaney C, Garnham J, Ruzickova M, Passmore M, Alda M (2005) Clinical correlates of current level of functioning in primary care-treated bipolar patients. Bipolar Disord 7(3):286–291. doi:10.1111/j.1399-5618.2005.00182.x, BDI182 [pii]

Hajek T, Hahn M, Slaney C, Garnham J, Green J, Ruzickova M, Zvolsky P, Alda M (2008) Rapid cycling bipolar disorders in primary and tertiary care treated patients. Bipolar Disord 10(4):495–502. doi:10.1111/j.1399-5618.2008.00587.x, BDI587 [pii]

Hakkarainen R, Johansson C, Kieseppa T, Partonen T, Koskenvuo M, Kaprio J, Lonnqvist J (2003) Seasonal changes, sleep length and circadian preference among twins with bipolar disorder. BMC Psychiatry 3:6. doi:10.1186/1471-244X-3-6

Hammen C, Gitlin M (1997) Stress reactivity in bipolar patients and its relation to prior history of disorder. Am J Psychiatry 154(6):856–857

Henry C, Lacoste J, Bellivier F, Verdoux H, Bourgeois ML, Leboyer M (1999) Temperament in bipolar illness: impact on prognosis. J Affect Disord 56(2–3):103–108

Hunt N, Sayer H, Silverstone T (1992) Season and manic relapse. Acta Psychiatr Scand 85(2):123–126

Insel TR, Cuthbert BN (2009) Endophenotypes: bridging genomic complexity and disorder heterogeneity. Biol Psychiatry 66(11):988–989. doi:10.1016/j.biopsych.2009.10.008, S0006-3223(09)01208-6 [pii]

Insel T, Cuthbert B, Garvey M, Heinssen R, Pine DS, Quinn K, Sanislow C, Wang P (2010) Research domain criteria (RDoC): toward a new classification framework for research on mental disorders. Am J Psychiatry 167(7):748–751. doi:10.1176/appi.ajp.2010.09091379

Jain S, Kaliaperumal VG, Chatterji S, Rao S, Murthy RS (1992) Climate and admissions for mania in the tropics. J Affect Disord 26(4):247–250

Jenner FA, Gjessing LR, Cox JR, Davies-Jones A, Hullin RP, Hanna SM (1967) A manic depressive psychotic with a persistent forty-eight hour cycle. Br J Psychiatry 113(501):895–910

Joffe RT, Kutcher S, MacDonald C (1988) Thyroid function and bipolar affective disorder. Psychiatry Res 25(2):117–121. doi:0165-1781(88)90042-X [pii]

Jones I, Hornsby H, Hay D (1995) Seasonality of mania: a Tasmanian study. Aust N Z J Psychiatry 29(3):449–453

Judd LL, Akiskal HS, Schettler PJ, Coryell W, Endicott J, Maser JD, Solomon DA, Leon AC, Keller MB (2003) A prospective investigation of the natural history of the long-term weekly symptomatic status of bipolar II disorder. Arch Gen Psychiatry 60(3):261–269. doi:yoa20225 [pii]

Kantor DA, Browne M, Ravindran A, Horn E (1991) Manic-like response to phototherapy. Can J Psychiatry 36(9):697–698

Kilzieh N, Akiskal HS (1999) Rapid-cycling bipolar disorder. An overview of research and clinical experience. Psychiatr Clin North Am 22(3):585–607

Kirov G, Murphy KC, Arranz MJ, Jones I, McCandles F, Kunugi H, Murray RM, McGuffin P, Collier DA, Owen MJ, Craddock N (1998) Low activity allele of catechol-O-methyltransferase gene associated with rapid cycling bipolar disorder. Mol Psychiatry 3(4):342–345

Koukopoulos A, Sani G (2013) DSM-5 criteria for depression with mixed features: a farewell to mixed depression. Acta Psychiatr Scand. doi:10.1111/acps.12140

Koukopoulos A, Sani G, Koukopoulos AE, Minnai GP, Girardi P, Pani L, Albert MJ, Reginaldi D (2003) Duration and stability of the rapid-cycling course: a long-term personal follow-up of 109 patients. J Affect Disord 73(1–2):75–85. doi:S016503270200321X [pii]

Koukopoulos A, Sani G, Ghaemi SN (2013) Mixed features of depression: why DSM-5 is wrong (and so was DSM-IV). Br J Psychiatry 203(1):3–5. doi:10.1192/bjp.BD.112.124404, 203/1/3 [pii]

Koyuncu A, Tukel R, Ozyildirim I, Meteris H, Yazici O (2010) Impact of obsessive-compulsive disorder comorbidity on the sociodemographic and clinical features of patients with bipolar disorder. Compr Psychiatry 51(3):293–297

Kraepelin E (1921) Manic-depressive insanity and paranoia. Livingstone, Edinburgh

Kramlinger KG, Post RM (1996) Ultra-rapid and ultradian cycling in bipolar affective illness. Br J Psychiatry 168(3):314–323

Kukopulos A, Reginaldi D, Laddomada P, Floris G, Serra G, Tondo L (1980) Course of the manic-depressive cycle and changes caused by treatment. Pharmakopsychiatr Neuropsychopharmakol 13(4):156–167. doi:10.1055/s-2007-1019628

Kupka RW, Nolen WA, Post RM, McElroy SL, Altshuler LL, Denicoff KD, Frye MA, Keck PE Jr, Leverich GS, Rush AJ, Suppes T, Pollio C, Drexhage HA (2002) High rate of autoimmune thyroiditis in bipolar disorder: lack of association with lithium exposure. Biol Psychiatry 51(4):305–311. doi:S0006322301012173 [pii]

Kupka RW, Luckenbaugh DA, Post RM, Leverich GS, Nolen WA (2003) Rapid and non-rapid cycling bipolar disorder: a meta-analysis of clinical studies. J Clin Psychiatry 64(12): 1483–1494

Kupka RW, Luckenbaugh DA, Post RM, Suppes T, Altshuler LL, Keck PE Jr, Frye MA, Denicoff KD, Grunze H, Leverich GS, McElroy SL, Walden J, Nolen WA (2005) Comparison of rapid-cycling and non-rapid-cycling bipolar disorder based on prospective mood ratings in 539 outpatients. Am J Psychiatry 162(7):1273–1280. doi:10.1176/appi.ajp.162.7.1273, 162/7/1273 [pii]

Kusalic M (1992) Grade II and grade III hypothyroidism in rapid-cycling bipolar patients. Neuropsychobiology 25(4):177–181. doi:118833 [pii] 118833

Labbate LA, Lafer B, Thibault A, Sachs GS (1994) Side effects induced by bright light treatment for seasonal affective disorder. J Clin Psychiatry 55(5):189–191

Lee HJ, Kim L, Joe SH, Suh KY (2002) Effects of season and climate on the first manic episode of bipolar affective disorder in Korea. Psychiatry Res 113(1–2):151–159. doi:S0165178102002378 [pii]

Lee HC, Tsai SY, Lin HC (2007) Seasonal variations in bipolar disorder admissions and the association with climate: a population-based study. J Affect Disord 97(1–3):61–69. doi:10.1016/j.jad.2006.06.026, S0165-0327(06)00293-X [pii]

Lee S, Tsang A, Kessler RC, Jin R, Sampson N, Andrade L, Karam EG, Mora ME, Merikangas K, Nakane Y, Popovici DG, Posada-Villa J, Sagar R, Wells JE, Zarkov Z, Petukhova M (2010) Rapid-cycling bipolar disorder: cross-national community study. Br J Psychiatry 196(3):217–225. doi:10.1192/bjp.BD.109.067843, 196/3/217 [pii]

Lee HJ, Woo HG, Greenwood TA, Kripke DF, Kelsoe JR (2012) A genome-wide association study of seasonal pattern mania identifies NF1A as a possible susceptibility gene for bipolar disorder. J Affect Disord. doi:10.1016/j.jad.2012.07.032, S0165-0327(12)00563-0 [pii]

Leibenluft E, Ashman SB, Feldman-Naim S, Yonkers KA (1999) Lack of relationship between menstrual cycle phase and mood in a sample of women with rapid cycling bipolar disorder. Biol Psychiatry 46(4):577–580. doi:S0006-3223(99)00023-2 [pii]

Leonhard K (1963) Die prapsychotische Temperamente bei den monopolaren und bipolaren phasischen Psychosen. Psychiatry Neurol (Basel) 146:105–115

Lewis JL, Winokur G (1982) The induction of mania. A natural history study with controls. Arch Gen Psychiatry 39(3):303–306

Lewis JL, Winokur G (1987) The induction of mania: a natural history study with controls. Psychopharmacol Bull 23(1):74–78

Lewis J, Winokur G (1989) Induction of mania by antidepressants. Am J Psychiatry 146(1):126–128

Lewy AJ, Nurnberger JI Jr, Wehr TA, Pack D, Becker LE, Powell RL, Newsome DA (1985) Supersensitivity to light: possible trait marker for manic-depressive illness. Am J Psychiatry 142(6):725–727

Lin PI, McInnis MG, Potash JB, Willour V, MacKinnon DF, DePaulo JR, Zandi PP (2006) Clinical correlates and familial aggregation of age at onset in bipolar disorder. Am J Psychiatry 163(2):240–246. doi:10.1176/appi.ajp.163.2.240, 163/2/240 [pii]

Lish JD, Gyulai L, Resnick SM, Kirtland A, Amsterdam JD, Whybrow PC, Price RA (1993) A family history study of rapid-cycling bipolar disorder. Psychiatry Res 48(1):37–46

London WP, Taylor BM (1981) Seasonality of bipolar disorders in a forensic setting. Psychiatry Res 5(2):139–145. doi:0165-1781(81)90044-5 [pii]

Mackin P (2005) Rapid cycling is equivalently prevalent in bipolar I and bipolar II disorder, and is associated with female gender and greater severity of illness. Evid Based Ment Health 8(2):52. doi:8/2/52 [pii]

Mackinnon DF, Pies R (2006) Affective instability as rapid cycling: theoretical and clinical implications for borderline personality and bipolar spectrum disorders. Bipolar Disord 8(1):1–14. doi:10.1111/j.1399-5618.2006.00283.x, BDI283 [pii]

MacKinnon DF, Zandi PP, Gershon E, Nurnberger JI Jr, Reich T, DePaulo JR (2003a) Rapid switching of mood in families with multiple cases of bipolar disorder. Arch Gen Psychiatry 60(9):921–928. doi:10.1001/archpsyc.60.9.921, 60/9/921 [pii]

MacKinnon DF, Zandi PP, Gershon ES, Nurnberger JI Jr, DePaulo JR Jr (2003b) Association of rapid mood switching with panic disorder and familial panic risk in familial bipolar disorder. Am J Psychiatry 160(9):1696–1698

Maggini C, Salvatore P, Gerhard A, Migone P (2000) Psychopathology of stable and unstable mixed states: a historical view. Compr Psychiatry 41(2):77–82. doi:S0010-440X(00)90136-6 [pii]

Mahon K, Perez-Rodriguez MM, Gunawardane N, Burdick KE (2013) Dimensional endophenotypes in bipolar disorder: affective dysregulation and psychosis proneness. J Affect Disord 151(2):695–701. doi:10.1016/j.jad.2013.08.003

Maj M, Magliano L, Pirozzi R, Marasco C, Guarneri M (1994) Validity of rapid cycling as a course specifier for bipolar disorder. Am J Psychiatry 151(7):1015–1019

Martinez-Aran A, Vieta E, Reinares M, Colom F, Torrent C, Sanchez-Moreno J, Benabarre A, Goikolea JM, Comes M, Salamero M (2004) Cognitive function across manic or hypomanic, depressed, and euthymic states in bipolar disorder. Am J Psychiatry 161(2):262–270

Mattes JA (2006) Antidepressant-induced rapid cycling: another perspective. Ann Clin Psychiatry 18(3):195–199. doi:10.1080/10401230600801242, U40528M04X554240 [pii]

Mawson D, Smith A (1981) Relative humidity and manic admissions in the London area. Br J Psychiatry 138:134–138

Mazzarini L, Pacchiarotti I, Colom F, Sani G, Kotzalidis GD, Rosa AR, Sanna L, De Rossi P, Girardi N, Bonnin CM, Sanchez-Moreno J, Vazquez GH, Gasto C, Tatarelli R, Vieta E (2009) Predominant polarity and temperament in bipolar and unipolar affective disorders. J Affect Disord 119(1–3):28–33. doi:10.1016/j.jad.2009.03.016, S0165-0327(09)00129-3 [pii]

Medhi B, Prakash O, Jose VM, Pradhan B, Chakrabarty S, Pandhi P (2008) Seasonal variation in plasma levels of lithium in the Indian population: is there a need to modify the dose? Singapore Med J 49(9):724–727

Mellerup B, Mellerup ET (1984) Seasonal variation in urinary excretion of calcium, magnesium and phosphate in manic-melancholic patients. Chronobiol Int 1(1):81–86

Morken G, Lilleeng S, Linaker OM (2002) Seasonal variation in suicides and in admissions to hospital for mania and depression. J Affect Disord 69(1–3):39–45. doi:S0165032700003736 [pii]

Mulder RT, Cosgriff JP, Smith AM, Joyce PR (1990) Seasonality of mania in New Zealand. Aust N Z J Psychiatry 24(2):187–190

Muller DJ, de Luca V, Sicard T, King N, Strauss J, Kennedy JL (2006) Brain-derived neurotrophic factor (BDNF) gene and rapid-cycling bipolar disorder: family-based association study. Br J Psychiatry 189:317–323. doi:10.1192/bjp.BD.105.010587, 189/4/317 [pii]

Murai T, Fujimoto S (2003) Rapid cycling bipolar disorder after left temporal polar damage. Brain Inj 17(4):355–358. doi:9UD2D4QQE15824D8 [pii]

Murray G, Lam RW, Beaulieu S, Sharma V, Cervantes P, Parikh SV, Yatham LN (2011) Do symptoms of bipolar disorder exhibit seasonal variation? A multisite prospective investigation. Bipolar Disord 13(7–8):687–695. doi:10.1111/j.1399-5618.2011.00959.x

Murru A, Nivoli AMA, Pacchiarotti I, Popovic D, Vieta E, Colom F (2011) Clinical, functional and therapeutic implications of comorbid personality disorders in a sample of bipolar patients. Eur Neuropsychopharmacol 21:S432–S433

Myers DH, Davies P (1978) The seasonal incidence of mania and its relationship to climatic variables. Psychol Med 8(3):433–440

Narita K, Suda M, Takei Y, Aoyama Y, Majima T, Kameyama M, Kosaka H, Amanuma M, Fukuda M, Mikuni M (2011) Volume reduction of ventromedial prefrontal cortex in bipolar II patients with rapid cycling: a voxel-based morphometric study. Prog Neuropsychopharmacol Biol Psychiatry 35(2):439–445. doi:10.1016/j.pnpBD.2010.11.030, S0278-5846(10)00461-6 [pii]

Nierenberg AA, Akiskal HS, Angst J, Hirschfeld RM, Merikangas KR, Petukhova M, Kessler RC (2010) Bipolar disorder with frequent mood episodes in the national comorbidity survey replication (NCS-R). Mol Psychiatry 15(11):1075–1087. doi:10.1038/mp.2009.61, mp200961 [pii]

Nivoli AM, Pacchiarotti I, Rosa AR, Popovic D, Murru A, Valenti M, Bonnin CM, Grande I, Sanchez-Moreno J, Vieta E, Colom F (2011a) Gender differences in a cohort study of 604 bipolar patients: the role of predominant polarity. J Affect Disord 133(3):443–449. doi:10.1016/j.jad.2011.04.055, S0165-0327(11)00222-9 [pii]

Nivoli AMA, Pacchiarotti I, Rosa AR, Popovic D, Murru A, Valenti M, Bonnin CM, Grande I, Sanchez-Moreno J, Vieta E, Colom F (2011b) Gender differences in a cohort study of 604 bipolar patients: the role of predominant polarity. J Affect Disord 133(3):443–449

Nivoli AM, Colom F, Pacchiarotti I, Murru A, Scott J, Valenti M, Mazzarini L, Del Mar Bonnin C, Sanchez-Moreno J, Serretti A, Vieta E (2012) Treatment strategies according to clinical features in a naturalistic cohort study of bipolar patients: a principal component analysis of lifetime pharmacological and biophysic treatment options. Eur Neuropsychopharmacol. doi:10.1016/j.euroneuro.2012.07.015, S0924-977X(12)00197-6 [pii]

Nivoli AMA, Colom F, Pacchiarotti I, Murru A, Scott J, Valenti M, Mazzarini L, Mar Bonnin CD, Jose SM, Serretti A, Vieta E (2013) Treatment strategies according to clinical features in a naturalistic cohort study of bipolar patients: a principal component analysis of lifetime pharmacological and biophysic treatment options. Eur Neuropsychopharmacol 23(4):263–275

Nurnberger J Jr, Guroff JJ, Hamovit J, Berrettini W, Gershon E (1988) A family study of rapid-cycling bipolar illness. J Affect Disord 15(1):87–91

Oomen HA, Schipperijn AJ, Drexhage HA (1996) The prevalence of affective disorder and in particular of a rapid cycling of bipolar disorder in patients with abnormal thyroid function tests. Clin Endocrinol (Oxf) 45(2):215–223

Osher Y, Yaroslavsky Y, el-Rom R, Belmaker RH (2000) Predominant polarity of bipolar patients in Israel. World J Biol Psychiatry 1(4):187–189

Pacchiarotti I, Mazzarini L, Kotzalidis GD, Valenti M, Nivoli AM, Sani G, Torrent C, Murru A, Sanchez-Moreno J, Patrizi B, Girardi P, Vieta E, Colom F (2011) Mania and depression. Mixed, not stirred. J Affect Disord 133(1–2):105–113. doi:10.1016/j.jad.2011.03.037

Pacchiarotti I, Nivoli AMA, Mazzarini L, Kotzalidis GD, Sani G, Koukopoulos A, Scott J, Strejilevich S, Sanchez-Moreno J, Murru A, Valenti M, Girardi P, Vieta E, Colom F (2013) The symptom structure of bipolar acute episodes: in search for the mixing link. J Affect Disord 149(1–3):56–66

Pande AC (1985) Light-induced hypomania. Am J Psychiatry 142(9):1126

Papolos DF, Veit S, Faedda GL, Saito T, Lachman HM (1998) Ultra-ultra rapid cycling bipolar disorder is associated with the low activity catecholamine-O-methyltransferase allele. Mol Psychiatry 3(4):346–349

Parker G, Walter S (1982) Seasonal variation in depressive disorders and suicidal deaths in New South Wales. Br J Psychiatry 140:626–632

Partonen T, Lonnqvist J (1996) Seasonal variation in bipolar disorder. Br J Psychiatry 169(5):641–646

Peck DF (1990) Climatic variables and admissions for mania: a reanalysis. J Affect Disord 20(4):249–250

Perlis RH, Delbello MP, Miyahara S, Wisniewski SR, Sachs GS, Nierenberg AA (2005) Revisiting depressive-prone bipolar disorder: polarity of initial mood episode and disease course among bipolar I systematic treatment enhancement program for bipolar disorder participants. Biol Psychiatry 58(7):549–553. doi:10.1016/j.biopsych.2005.07.029, S0006-3223(05)00918-2 [pii]

Perugi G, Akiskal HS, Micheli C, Musetti L, Paiano A, Quilici C, Rossi L, Cassano GB (1997) Clinical subtypes of bipolar mixed states: validating a broader European definition in 143 cases. J Affect Disord 43(3):169–180. doi:S0165-0327(97)01446-8 [pii]

Perugi G, Micheli C, Akiskal HS, Madaro D, Socci C, Quilici C, Musetti L (2000) Polarity of the first episode, clinical characteristics, and course of manic depressive illness: a systematic retrospective investigation of 320 bipolar I patients. Compr Psychiatry 41(1):13–18. doi:S0010-440X(00)90125-1 [pii]

Popovic D, Vieta E (2013) Clinical implications of polarity index of drugs in maintenance treatment of bipolar disorder: a naturalistic study. Eur Neuropsychopharmacol 23:S68–S69

Popovic D, Torrent C, Goikolea JM, Cruz N, Sanchez-Moreno J, Gonzalez-Pinto A, Vieta E (2013) Clinical implications of predominant polarity and the polarity index in bipolar disorder: a naturalistic study. Acta Psychiatr Scand 129(5):366–374

Post RM (1992) Transduction of psychosocial stress into the neurobiology of recurrent affective disorder. Am J Psychiatry 149(8):999–1010

Post RM, Rubinow DR, Ballenger JC (1986) Conditioning and sensitisation in the longitudinal course of affective illness. Br J Psychiatry 149:191–201

Post RM, Kramlinger KG, Joffe RT, Roy-Byrne PP, Rosoff A, Frye MA, Huggins T (1997) Rapid cycling bipolar affective disorder: lack of relation to hypothyroidism. Psychiatry Res 72(1): 1–7. doi:S0165-1781(97)00076-0 [pii]

Post RM, Denicoff KD, Leverich GS, Altshuler LL, Frye MA, Suppes TM, Rush AJ, Keck PE Jr, McElroy SL, Luckenbaugh DA, Pollio C, Kupka R, Nolen WA (2003) Morbidity in 258 bipolar outpatients followed for 1 year with daily prospective ratings on the NIMH life chart method. J Clin Psychiatry 64(6):680–690; quiz 738–789

Price WA, DiMarzio L (1986) Premenstrual tension syndrome in rapid-cycling bipolar affective disorder. J Clin Psychiatry 47(8):415–417

Quitkin FM, Rabkin JG, Prien RF (1986) Bipolar disorder: are there manic-prone and depressive-prone forms? J Clin Psychopharmacol 6(3):167–172

Rapaport MH, Guylai L, Whybrow P (1999) Immune parameters in rapid cycling bipolar patients before and after lithium treatment. J Psychiatr Res 33(4):335–340. doi:S0022-3956(99)00007-2 [pii]

Rihmer Z (1980) Season of birth and season of hospital admission in bipolar depressed female patients. Psychiatry Res 3(3):247–251

Rosa AR, Andreazza AC, Kunz M, Gomes F, Santin A, Sanchez-Moreno J, Reinares M, Colom F, Vieta E, Kapczinski F (2008) Predominant polarity in bipolar disorder: diagnostic implications. J Affect Disord 107(1–3):45–51. doi:10.1016/j.jad.2007.07.021, S0165-0327(07)00274-1 [pii]

Rousseva A, Henry C, van den Bulke D, Fournier G, Laplanche JL, Leboyer M, Bellivier F, Aubry JM, Baud P, Boucherie M, Buresi C, Ferrero F, Malafosse A (2003) Antidepressant-induced mania, rapid cycling and the serotonin transporter gene polymorphism. Pharmacogenomics J 3(2):101–104. doi:10.1038/sj.tpj.6500156, 6500156 [pii]

Rovai L, Maremmani AG, Rugani F, Bacciardi S, Pacini M, Dell'osso L, Akiskal HS, Maremmani I (2013) Do Akiskal & Mallya's affective temperaments belong to the domain of pathology or to that of normality? Eur Rev Med Pharmacol Sci 17(15):2065–2079

Roy-Byrne P, Post RM, Uhde TW, Porcu T, Davis D (1985) The longitudinal course of recurrent affective illness: life chart data from research patients at the NIMH. Acta Psychiatr Scand Suppl 317:1–34

Sayer HK, Marshall S, Mellsop GW (1991) Mania and seasonality in the southern hemisphere. J Affect Disord 23(3):151–156. doi:0165-0327(91)90027-P [pii]

Sayin A, Kuruoglu AC, Yazici Gulec M, Aslan S (2007) Relation of temperament and character properties with clinical presentation of bipolar disorder. Compr Psychiatry 48(5):446–451. doi:10.1016/j.comppsych.2007.04.004, S0010-440X(07)00052-1 [pii]

Schneck CD, Miklowitz DJ, Calabrese JR, Allen MH, Thomas MR, Wisniewski SR, Miyahara S, Shelton MD, Ketter TA, Goldberg JF, Bowden CL, Sachs GS (2004) Phenomenology of rapid-cycling bipolar disorder: data from the first 500 participants in the Systematic Treatment Enhancement Program. Am J Psychiatry 161(10):1902–1908. doi:10.1176/appi.ajp.161.10.1902, 161/10/1902 [pii]

Schneck CD, Miklowitz DJ, Miyahara S, Araga M, Wisniewski S, Gyulai L, Allen MH, Thase ME, Sachs GS (2008) The prospective course of rapid-cycling bipolar disorder: findings from the STEP-BD. Am J Psychiatry 165(3):370–377

Schumann G, Binder EB, Holte A, de Kloet ER, Oedegaard KJ, Robbins TW, Walker-Tilley TR, Bitter I, Brown VJ, Buitelaar J, Ciccocioppo R, Cools R, Escera C, Fleischhacker W, Flor H, Frith CD, Heinz A, Johnsen E, Kirschbaum C, Klingberg T, Lesch KP, Lewis S, Maier W, Mann K, Martinot JL, Meyer-Lindenberg A, Muller CP, Muller WE, Nutt DJ, Persico A, Perugi G, Pessiglione M, Preuss UW, Roiser JP, Rossini PM, Rybakowski JK, Sandi C, Stephan KE, Undurraga J, Vieta E, van der Wee N, Wykes T, Haro JM, Wittchen HU (2013) Stratified medicine for mental disorders. Eur Neuropsychopharmacol J Eur Coll Neuropsychopharmacol. doi:10.1016/j.euroneuro.2013.09.010

Serretti A, Mandelli L, Lattuada E, Smeraldi E (2002) Rapid cycling mood disorder: clinical and demographic features. Compr Psychiatry 43(5):336–343. doi:S0010440X02000111 [pii]

Shand AJ, Scott NW, Anderson SM, Eagles JM (2011) The seasonality of bipolar affective disorder: comparison with a primary care sample using the seasonal pattern assessment questionnaire. J Affect Disord 132(1–2):289–292. doi:10.1016/j.jad.2011.02.015, S0165-0327(11)00069-3 [pii]

Shapira A, Shiloh R, Potchter O, Hermesh H, Popper M, Weizman A (2004) Admission rates of bipolar depressed patients increase during spring/summer and correlate with maximal environmental temperature. Bipolar Disord 6(1):90–93. doi:081 [pii]

Shin K, Schaffer A, Levitt AJ, Boyle MH (2005) Seasonality in a community sample of bipolar, unipolar and control subjects. J Affect Disord 86(1):19–25. doi:10.1016/j.jad.2004.11.010, S0165-0327(04)00438-0 [pii]

Silverstone T, Romans S, Hunt N, McPherson H (1995) Is there a seasonal pattern of relapse in bipolar affective disorders? A dual northern and southern hemisphere cohort study. Br J Psychiatry 167(1):58–60

Simonsen H, Shand AJ, Scott NW, Eagles JM (2011) Seasonal symptoms in bipolar and primary care patients. J Affect Disord 132:200–208. doi:10.1016/j.jad.2011.02.018, S0165-0327(11)00072-3 [pii]

Sjoholm LK, Backlund L, Cheteh EH, Ek IR, Frisen L, Schalling M, Osby U, Lavebratt C, Nikamo P (2010) CRY2 is associated with rapid cycling in bipolar disorder patients. PLoS One 5(9):e12632. doi:10.1371/journal.pone.0012632, e12632 [pii]

Symonds RL, Williams P (1976) Seasonal variation in the incidence of mania. Br J Psychiatry 129:45–48

Tillman R, Geller B (2003) Definitions of rapid, ultrarapid, and ultradian cycling and of episode duration in pediatric and adult bipolar disorders: a proposal to distinguish episodes from cycles. J Child Adolesc Psychopharmacol 13(3):267–271. doi:10.1089/104454603322572598

Tohen M, Frank E, Bowden CL, Colom F, Ghaemi SN, Yatham LN, Malhi GS, Calabrese JR, Nolen WA, Vieta E, Kapczinski F, Goodwin GM, Suppes T, Sachs GS, Chengappa KR, Grunze H, Mitchell PB, Kanba S, Berk M (2009) The International Society for Bipolar Disorders (ISBD) Task Force report on the nomenclature of course and outcome in bipolar disorders. Bipolar Disord 11(5):453–473. doi:10.1111/j.1399-5618.2009.00726.x, BDI726 [pii]

Tondo L, Baldessarini RJ (1998) Rapid cycling in women and men with bipolar manic-depressive disorders. Am J Psychiatry 155(10):1434–1436

Turvey CL, Coryell WH, Solomon DA, Leon AC, Endicott J, Keller MB, Akiskal H (1999) Long-term prognosis of bipolar I disorder. Acta Psychiatr Scand 99(2):110–119

Valenti M, Pacchiarotti I, Bonnin CM, Rosa AR, Popovic D, Nivoli AM, Goikolea JM, Murru A, Undurraga J, Colom F, Vieta E (2012) Risk factors for antidepressant-related switch to mania. J Clin Psychiatry 73(2):e271–e276. doi:10.4088/JCP.11m07166

Vieta E, Valenti M (2013a) Mixed states in DSM-5: implications for clinical care, education, and research. J Affect Disord 148(1):28–36. doi:10.1016/j.jad.2013.03.007, S0165-0327(13)00232-2 [pii]

Vieta E, Valenti M (2013b) Pharmacological management of bipolar depression: acute treatment, maintenance, and prophylaxis. CNS Drugs 27(7):515–529. doi:10.1007/s40263-013-0073-y

Vieta E, Calabrese JR, Hennen J, Colom F, Martinez-Aran A, Sanchez-Moreno J, Yatham LN, Tohen M, Baldessarini RJ (2004) Comparison of rapid-cycling and non-rapid-cycling bipolar I manic patients during treatment with olanzapine: analysis of pooled data. J Clin Psychiatry 65(10):1420–1428

Vieta E, Berk M, Wang W, Colom F, Tohen M, Baldessarini RJ (2009) Predominant previous polarity as an outcome predictor in a controlled treatment trial for depression in bipolar I disorder patients. J Affect Disord 119(1–3):22–27. doi:10.1016/j.jad.2009.02.028, S0165-0327(09)00097-4 [pii]

Vieta E, Langosch JM, Figueira ML, Souery D, Blasco-Colmenares E, Medina E, Moreno-Manzanaro M, Gonzalez MA, Bellivier F (2013a) Clinical management and burden of bipolar disorder: results from a multinational longitudinal study (WAVE-bd). Int J Neuropsychopharmacol 16(8):1719–1732. doi:10.1017/S1461145713000278

Vieta E, Popovic D, Rosa AR, Sole B, Grande I, Frey BN, Martinez-Aran A, Sanchez-Moreno J, Balanza-Martinez V, Tabares-Seisdedos R, Kapczinski F (2013b) The clinical implications of cognitive impairment and allostatic load in bipolar disorder. Eur Psychiatry J Assoc Eur Psychiatr 28(1):21–29. doi:10.1016/j.eurpsy.2011.11.007

Volpe FM, Del Porto JA (2006) Seasonality of admissions for mania in a psychiatric hospital of Belo Horizonte, Brazil. J Affect Disord 94(1–3):243–248. doi:10.1016/j.jad.2006.03.025, S0165-0327(06)00173-X [pii]

Volpe FM, Tavares A, Del Porto JA (2008) Seasonality of three dimensions of mania: psychosis, aggression and suicidality. J Affect Disord 108(1–2):95–100. doi:10.1016/j.jad.2007.09.014, S0165-0327(07)00343-6 [pii]

Volpe FM, da Silva EM, dos Santos TN, de Freitas DE (2010) Further evidence of seasonality of mania in the tropics. J Affect Disord 124(1–2):178–182. doi:10.1016/j.jad.2009.11.001, S0165-0327(09)00486-8 [pii]

Walter SD (1977) Seasonality of mania: a reappraisal. Br J Psychiatry 131:345–350

Wehr TA, Goodwin FK (1979) Rapid cycling in manic-depressives induced by tricyclic antidepressants. Arch Gen Psychiatry 36(5):555–559

Wehr TA, Sack DA, Rosenthal NE, Cowdry RW (1988) Rapid cycling affective disorder: contributing factors and treatment responses in 51 patients. Am J Psychiatry 145(2):179–184

Wells JE, McGee MA, Scott KM, Oakley Browne MA (2010) Bipolar disorder with frequent mood episodes in the New Zealand Mental Health Survey. J Affect Disord 126(1–2):65–74. doi:10.1016/j.jad.2010.02.136, S0165-0327(10)00274-0 [pii]

Whitney DK, Sharma V, Kueneman K (1999) Seasonality of manic depressive illness in Canada. J Affect Disord 55(2–3):99–105

Wilk K, Hegerl U (2010) Time of mood switches in ultra-rapid cycling disorder: a brief review. Psychiatry Res 180(1):1–4. doi:10.1016/j.psychres.2009.08.011, S0165-1781(09)00318-7 [pii]

Wilting I, Fase S, Martens EP, Heerdink ER, Nolen WA, Egberts AC (2007) The impact of environmental temperature on lithium serum levels. Bipolar Disord 9(6):603–608. doi:10.1111/j.1399-5618.2007.00438.x, BDI438 [pii]

Wolpert EA, Goldberg JF, Harrow M (1990) Rapid cycling in unipolar and bipolar affective disorders. Am J Psychiatry 147(6):725–728

Yatham LN, Calabrese JR, Kusumakar V (2003) Bipolar depression: criteria for treatment selection, definition of refractoriness, and treatment options. Bipolar Disord 5(2):85–97. doi:019 [pii]

Yildiz A, Sachs GS (2003) Do antidepressants induce rapid cycling? A gender-specific association. J Clin Psychiatry 64(7):814–818

Yildiz A, Sachs GS (2004) Characteristics of rapid cycling bipolar-I patients in a bipolar speciality clinic. J Affect Disord 79(1–3):247–251. doi:10.1016/S0165-0327(02)00350-6, S0165032702003506 [pii]

Zis AP, Goodwin FK (1979) Major affective disorder as a recurrent illness: a critical review. Arch Gen Psychiatry 36(8 Spec No):835–839

Zwil AS, McAllister TW, Cohen I, Halpern LR (1993) Ultra-rapid cycling bipolar affective disorder following a closed-head injury. Brain Inj 7(2):147–152

4 Neurocognitive Functioning in Bipolar Disorder: A Comprehensive Review of Recent Data

The neurocognitive function of BD patients has been the focus of debate for decades. It was unclear whether the observed neurocognitive deficit is because of some kind of iatrogenic or alcohol and/or drug abuse effects, whether it reflects temporary functional changes as a result of mood changes or on the contrary it is the product of degenerative structural brain changes or of some kind of structural changes of a neurodevelopmental origin, or it derives from the same enduring functional brain alterations that cause mood dysregulation. The latest research data suggest that the neurocognitive impairment is an enduring component of BD and represents a core primary characteristic of the illness, rather than being secondary to the mood state or medication. A recent study reported that 84 % of the schizophrenia patients, 58.3 % of psychotic major depression patients and 57.7 % of psychotic BD patients were cognitively impaired (1 SD below healthy controls in at least two domains) (Reichenberg et al. 2009).

Traditionally, BD patients were considered to have higher IQ in comparison to the general population and to be more creative (e.g. artists, scientists etc.) (Andreasen 1987, 2008; Andreasen and Glick 1988; Jamison 1995, 1989). However, recent research revealed the presence of a significant and broad neurocognitive impairment, which seems to be present even before the first manifestation of mood symptoms; it persists across the different phases and even worsens during the course of the illness (Arts et al. 2008; Bora et al. 2009a, 2011; Kurtz and Gerraty 2009; Mann-Wrobel et al. 2011; Robinson et al. 2006). A general impression is that verbal ability is relatively preserved (Mann-Wrobel et al. 2011). The neurocognitive impairment in BD is less pronounced in comparison to schizophrenia, even after controlling for confounding variables, like clinical symptoms, education and social class (Dickerson et al. 2004; Schretlen et al. 2007). Maybe 40 % of BD patients are impaired in one neurocognitive domain, one-third or more are impaired in at least two neurocognitive domains and 22 % are impaired in three or more domains (Gualtieri and Morgan 2008; Martino et al. 2008). This deficit is rather stable and relatively independent from mood changes, probably reflecting trait features of BD (Clark and Goodwin 2004; Quraishi and Frangou 2002; Malhi et al. 2004; Thompson et al. 2005).

K.N. Fountoulakis, *Bipolar Disorder: An Evidence-Based Guide to Manic Depression*, DOI 10.1007/978-3-642-37216-2_4

A number of confounding factors have been identified, including gender, age and education. An additional important confounding variable when comparing the different phases of the illness is that although some of the acutely ill patients might be medication-free during testing, this is not the case with patients in remission. Thus, medication status constitutes a confounding variable which is difficult to control for. Additionally, very severely manic or depressed patients cannot be tested.

An important common limitation in this kind of research is that the performance in most tests is influenced by more than one cognitive process. There are no clear boundaries between neurocognitive processes and no process is independent from the others. Different approaches in their classification and nomenclature have been proposed, adding to the confusion. Especially the domain of executive functions is open to several different approaches and conceptualizations.

A list of neurocognitive domains and the neuropsychological tools usually used for their assessment are shown in Table 4.1.

4.1 General Neurocognitive Functioning and Intelligence Quotient (IQ)

Some studies suggest that BD patients and their families manifest above average IQ and general intellectual functioning (Mason 1956; Woodruff et al. 1968, 1971; Petterson 1977; Waters et al. 1981; Decina et al. 1983; Koenen et al. 2009), or at least they have intelligence similar to healthy controls (Gilvarry et al. 2000; Zammit et al. 2004; Reichenberg et al. 2002; Gooding and Tallent 2001; Seidman et al. 2002). On the other hand, higher functioning and preserved neurocognitive performance during the premorbid phase, as well as higher social class, might push towards a mood disorder diagnosis rather than schizophrenia (Coryell et al. 1989; Woodruff et al. 1971; Morice 1990; Souza et al. 1995; Seidman et al. 2002; Goldberg et al. 1993; Jones et al. 1993; Gard et al. 1999; Gilvarry et al. 2000; Altshuler et al. 2004; Silverstein et al. 1990; Coffman et al. 1990; Fitzgerald et al. 2004; Dittmann et al. 2008b).

Fortunately, today there are enough research data available to elucidate the true relationship between IQ and BD. The literature consistently suggests that BD patients, irrespective of illness phase, show moderate global reduction in their neurocognitive functioning as reflected in their IQ scores and their performance in a number of neuropsychological batteries (Donaldson et al. 2003; Varga et al. 2006; Coffman et al. 1990; Fitzgerald et al. 2004; Glahn et al. 2007). Recent studies suggest that these deficits are milder but maybe qualitatively similar to those of patients with schizophrenia (Schretlen et al. 2007; Czobor et al. 2007). However, the impairment is even more pronounced when psychotic features are present (Seidman et al. 2003), and, in this case, some authors suggest it is comparable to that seen in schizophrenia, especially during the acute manic phase (Dickerson et al. 2001; Zalla et al. 2004; Hoff et al. 1990; Dalby and Williams 1986).

Table 4.1 Neurocognitive domains assessed in the literature and neuropsychological tools used

Domain	Tool
Premorbid IQ	Single-word reading score from the North American Adult Reading Test (NAART)
	Wide Range Achievement Test (WRAT)
	Vocabulary subtest score from the Wechsler Adult Intelligence Scale (WAIS)
Current IQ	Wechsler Adult Intelligence Scale (WAIS)
Psychomotor and mental speed	Digit Symbol Substitution Test (DSST)
	Trail Making Test-A (TMT-A)
	Reaction time tests
Attention	Continuous Performance Test (CPT)
	Digits forward
Working memory	Digits backward
Verbal memory	California Verbal Learning Test (CVLT)
Learning	Rey Auditory Verbal Learning Test (RAVLT)
Short delayed recall	Wechsler Memory Scale-Logical Memory (WMS-LM)
Long delayed recall	Free recall
Recognition	
Nonverbal memory	Rey Complex Figure Test (RCFT)—immediate and delayed recall
	Wechsler Memory Scale-Visual Reproduction (WMS-VR)
Visuospatial function	Block design
	Rey Complex Figure Test (RCFT)—copy
Language/verbal fluency	Controlled Oral Word Association Test (COWA-FAS)
	Animal Naming (AN)
Executive-function	Wisconsin Card Sorting Test (WCST)—categories achieved and perseverative errors
	Stroop Colour–Word Test (SCWT)
	Trail Making Test-B (TMT-B)
Social cognition and theory of mind	Benton Facial Recognition Test (BFRT)
	Faces Test (FT)
	Eyes Test (ET)
	Hinting Task (HT)
	False belief and deception tasks
	Picture sequencing
	Character intention tasks
	Faux pas

One of the most important studies on the topic included one million Swedish men with a mean age of 18.3 years on conscription for military service. It reported data on psychiatric hospital admissions over a mean follow-up period of 22.6 years and suggested a more complex relationship between BD and IQ. That study reported that although BD was indeed related to higher premorbid IQ, further analysis revealed that men with the lowest and the highest IQ (especially verbal or technical ability) had the greatest risk for pure bipolar disorder (without comorbidity) (Gale et al. 2012). It is unclear whether psychotic BD is related to impaired premorbid IQ since one study confirmed this (Badcock et al. 2005), while another one rejected this assumption (Glahn et al. 2006c).

As it is well known, the full IQ is composed of two composite scores: the verbal IQ (VIQ) and the nonverbal or performance IQ (PIQ). The effect size during the manic phase is reported to be equal to 0.06 for PIQ and 0.28 for the VIQ (Hoff et al. 1990). Another study reported an effect size of 0.47 for the full IQ during acute mania (Dalby and Williams 1986). There are no studies of IQ in patients during the acute depressive phase. Since it is possible the premorbid IQ of BD patients is higher in comparison to the normal population, the true magnitude of decline cannot be assessed accurately, and all studies reporting this decline in comparison to population norms underestimate it.

During euthymia, mood patients and particularly BD patients manifest higher VIQ in comparison to PIQ scores according to a meta-analysis (Kluger and Goldberg 1990; McIntosh et al. 2005). This is due to the uniform reduction in all PIQ subtest scores with an accompanying preservation of VIQ scores. It is clear, both from the quality of the deficit which persists during periods of euthymia, as well as from targeted research, that this impairment is not due to the slowing in mental speed which is observed in BD patients (since four PIQ subtests in comparison to one VIQ subtest are timed) (Sackeim et al. 1992). It might be already present during the early stages of the illness (Mojtabai et al. 2000) although more recent data argue against this (Sorensen et al. 2012). Also, although it is largely independent of affective state, marked severity of depression seems to reduce VIQ scores and thus it might diminish the VIQ-PIQ discrepancy (Goodwin and Jamison 2007). It is important to note that this discrepancy does not seem to be present in unipolar depressive patients (Gorlyn et al. 2006).

Although any attempt for a deep understanding of this deficit is risky and premature, it has been suggested that this VIQ-PIQ discrepancy might reflect a specific effect of BD on 'fluid intelligence' (the capacity to think logically and solve problems in novel situations, independently of acquired knowledge) with a simultaneous respect of the 'crystallized intelligence' (the ability to use skills, knowledge and experience; it does rely on long-term memory) (Goodwin and Jamison 2007).

The meta-analytic studies, when taking into consideration all phases of the illness, report effect sizes concerning current IQ reduction, ranging from 0.36 (Krabbendam et al. 2005) to 0.7 (Goodwin and Jamison 2007). For patients in remission the results of meta-analyses are inconclusive. The effect sizes reported range from 0.4 (Bora et al. 2010a) or 0.5 (for PIQ) (Goodwin and Jamison 2007) to lower and within the normal range, that is, 0.16 (Arts et al. 2008) or 0.11 (Mann-Wrobel et al. 2011). A problem is that most meta-analyses report an effect size for the full IQ and not separately for VIQ and PIQ. The effect size of premorbid IQ change in euthymic BD patients is low and not significant (0.04–0.2) (Torres et al. 2007; Bora et al. 2010a).

4.2 Psychomotor and Mental Speed

Much of research in this domain was performed in mixed samples or in samples characterized by psychomotor retardation, and thus, results cannot be carried to the whole population of BD patients in a straightforward way. Mental speed and psychomotor activation are two concepts which overlap but are clearly not identical, and they cover a variety of domains, including reaction time, cognitive and motor speed and manual dexterity. Additionally, most of the neuropsychological tools which are used for the assessment of psychomotor and mental speed also assess other neurocognitive functions, and this is at least partial because in order to measure 'speed', you need to initiate a 'procedure' whose 'speed' is going to be measured.

Reaction time was reported to be prolonged in bipolar depressives (Marvel and Paradiso 2004). Euthymic patients also had prolonged reaction times and more error rates in a visual backward masking test. Burden of illness and especially past history of depressions but not current medication were correlated with reaction time prolongation (MacQueen et al. 2004).

The speed of mental processing was reported to be slower in BD patients irrespective of illness phase and symptom severity (Antila et al. 2009; Chaves et al. 2011; Dittmann et al. 2008a; Hsiao et al. 2009; Langenecker et al. 2010; Martino et al. 2011a; Mur et al. 2007; Basso et al. 2009; Olley et al. 2005; Xu et al. 2012; McIntosh et al. 2005; McGrath et al. 1997; El-Badri et al. 2001; Stoddart et al. 2007; Coffman et al. 1990; Seidman et al. 2002; Fitzgerald et al. 2004; Szoke et al. 2008; Martinez-Aran et al. 2008; Hill et al. 2009; Dittmann et al. 2008b). It is less affected in comparison to patients with schizophrenia (Goldberg et al. 1993; Hawkins et al. 1997; Gard et al. 1999; Mojtabai et al. 2000) in spite of some data suggesting the presence of a similar degree of impairment (Hobart et al. 1999). After correcting for motor speed, bipolar depressives were reported to manifest slower mental speed in comparison to manic and unipolar depressives. In that particular study an interesting feature was that distraction improved the mental speed of BD depressed patients while it adversely influenced the speed of the other two groups (Blackburn 1975).

The impairment is present already during the early stages of BD (Kolur et al. 2006). In individual studies, the magnitude of mental speed impairment in BD is reported to correspond to an effect size as big as 0.82–1.08 (Glahn et al. 2007; Bora et al. 2007; Basso et al. 2009). Meta-analytic studies, when taking into consideration all phases of the illness, suggested an effect size equal to 0.50–0.55 (which is similar to that observed concerning the IQ) (Krabbendam et al. 2005; Goodwin and Jamison 2007). In euthymic BD patients, one meta-analysis reported that the effect size with the use of the TMT-A was 0.52 and with the DSST was 0.59 (Robinson et al. 2006). A second study reported effect sizes of 0.60 and 0.79, respectively (Torres et al. 2007); a third one reported effect sizes equal to 0.64 and 0.76, respectively (Mann-Wrobel et al. 2011); a fourth 0.71 and 0.84, respectively (Arts et al. 2008); and a fifth 0.7 and 07–0.8, respectively (Bora et al. 2010a).

The impairment in processing speed might have a significant confounding effect on the performance in almost all neurocognitive testing, and controlling for it might make any difference between groups concerning other neurocognitive domains disappear (Antila et al. 2011). Additionally, it is reported that global functional impairment is significantly associated with poor performance on a cognitive measure of processing speed (e.g. WAIS Digit Symbol or the TMT) (Burdick et al. 2010; Martino et al. 2011a).

4.3 Attention

The concept of attention includes a number of processes which work together, influence each other or prerequisite each other. These are working memory (the capacity to hold in awareness a limited number of mental objects for a limited duration of time), vigilance (the ability to identify a rarely occurring target among many other stimuli), freedom from distraction or interference and the ability to split or rapidly shift attention. The ability to sustain attention over prolonged periods of time is called concentration. There are a variety of tests, with each of them assessing one of these previously mentioned processes (e.g. Continuous Performance Test assesses vigilance, 'span tasks' assess working memory). However, none of them is free of influence from the other processes. Working memory is often classified as belonging to the executive functions and is often considered in relation to them.

The literature suggests that the attentional deficit is widespread in BD; it covers all related processes. The magnitude of impairment is independent of the phase of the illness and current symptomatology although there is significant variability present (Chaves et al. 2011; Clark et al. 2002, 2005a; Fleck et al. 2005; Liu et al. 2002; Malhi et al. 2007a; Sanchez-Morla et al. 2009; Elshahawi et al. 2011; Strakowski et al. 2004; Rund et al. 1992; Thomas et al. 1996; Harmer et al. 2002a; Zubieta et al. 2001; Seidman et al. 2002; Fitzgerald et al. 2004; Glahn et al. 2007; Hill et al. 2009; Malloy-Diniz et al. 2009; Wilder-Willis et al. 2001; Ali et al. 2000; Asarnow and MacCrimmon 1981). The deficit is present already during the early stages of the disorder (Kolur et al. 2006) and it is less pronounced in comparison to patients with schizophrenia (Goldberg et al. 1993; Addington and Addington 1997; Park and Holzman 1992). However, there are some data suggesting a similar magnitude of impairment between BD and schizophrenia (Hobart et al. 1999; Tam and Liu 2004; Gruzelier et al. 1988). There are only a limited number of negative studies which suggest there is no impairment in attention (Xu et al. 2012; Goswami et al. 2006; Barrett et al. 2009; Tam et al. 1998; Paradiso et al. 1997), and this concerns especially euthymic patients (Swann et al. 2003). Individual studies report effect sizes ranging from 0.36 (Arts et al. 2011) to 0.82 (Glahn et al. 2007; Bora et al. 2007) depending on the domain assessed and the composition of the study sample.

A meta-analysis reported an effect size of 0.64 which is similar to that reported concerning the rest of neurocognitive functions (Goodwin and Jamison 2007). Another meta-analysis suggested that attention is impaired during the acute manic/mixed state ($d=0.79$–0.90), the acute depressed state ($d=0.80$) but also during euthymia ($d=0.41$–0.65) (Kurtz and Gerraty 2009). In euthymic BD patients, a meta-analysis found medium effect sizes (0.48–0.60 depending on the testing condition) (Robinson et al. 2006), while a second one found effect sizes of similar magnitude (0.62 and 0.74 for CPT hits and reaction time, respectively) (Torres et al. 2007). A third meta-analysis

Table 4.2 Effect sizes concerning the various neurocognitive domains during different phases of BD as well as in high-risk relatives (endophenotypes)

Domain	All phases	Acute mania	Acute bipolar depression	Euthymia	Endophenotype
Intelligence quotient (IQ)					
Premorbid IQ	Normal				Normal
Current IQ	0.36–0.70	0.28–0.47		0.11–0.50	0.20
Psychomotor and mental speed	0.50–0.55			0.52–0.80	0.17–0.22
Attention	0.64	0.79–0.90	0.80	0.41–0.80	0.18–0.36
Memory					
Working memory	0.60			0.54–1.02	
Verbal memory					
Immediate	0.43			0.73–0.82	0.33–0.42
Delayed	0.34	1.05	1.20	0.71–0.85	0.27–0.33
Verbal learning	0.91	1.43		0.66–0.90	0.28
Nonverbal memory					
Immediate	0.26			0.73	
Delayed	0.51			0.62–0.80	0.13
Episodic memory				0.62	
Visuospatial function	0.65			0.22–0.57	
Language/verbal fluency	0.63	0.51–0.59	0.93	0.34–0.90	0.27
Executive-function	0.34–0.79	0.64–0.72	0.54–0.75	0.52–0.88	0.24–0.51
Social cognition					
ToM	0.75–0.86				
Emotion recognition	0.35				
Emotion decision-making	Normal				

The range of values reflects heterogeneity in study samples but also heterogeneity because of the different neuropsychological tools used

gave an effect size of 0.58 for CPT and 0.37 for digits forward (Arts et al. 2008) and a fourth reported an effect size equal to 0.8 for CPT (Bora et al. 2010a).

4.4 Learning and Memory

Acquiring and storing new information (learning) and retrieving them later (memory) involve a number of distinct but interrelated and interdependent processes including attention and concentration, encoding and allocation of effort. Different strategies and processes are involved depending on whether a short- or a long-term effect is desirable and also depending on the nature and the quality of the information and the frame it is presented in.

A typical classification of learning and memory structure (Stern and Sackeim 2002) is shown in Table 4.2. Much of research on memory is focused on 'depression' and does not distinguish between unipolar and bipolar cases. Thus, results and conclusions from these studies should be received with reservation and it is uncertain whether they apply to BD and to which extend.

There are several studies reporting impairment in working memory (Barrett et al. 2008; Brown et al. 2007; Dittmann et al. 2008a; Hsiao et al. 2009; Wiegand et al. 2004; Glahn et al. 2006c; Martinez-Aran et al. 2008; Basso et al. 2009; Hill et al. 2009; Simonsen et al. 2011; Dittmann et al. 2008b) and specifically in the visuospatial working memory (Thompson et al. 2006; Green et al. 1994a, b; Gooding and Tallent 2001; McGrath et al. 2001) with psychotic patients doing worse (Glahn et al. 2007). This deficit is reported to be present early in the course of the disorder (Ayres et al. 2007). There are reports suggesting the deficit in working memory concerns acutely manic patients (Hoff et al. 1990; Green et al. 1994a, b). The deficit in visuospatial working memory is also less pronounced in comparison to schizophrenia (Park and Holzman 1992).

Also there are studies suggesting the presence of impairment in the declarative memory (Bearden et al. 2006b) and specifically in its components the semantic (Chang et al. 2011) and the episodic memory (Glahn et al. 2007; Deckersbach et al. 2004b; Malloy-Diniz et al. 2009), verbal learning (Bonnin et al. 2012; Burdick et al. 2005; Dittmann et al. 2008a; Antila et al. 2007a; Cavanagh et al. 2002; Varga et al. 2006; Kaya et al. 2007; Martinez-Aran et al. 2007; Dittmann et al. 2008b; Atre-Vaidya et al. 1998) and verbal memory (Hsiao et al. 2009; Martino et al. 2011a; Sanchez-Morla et al. 2009; Antila et al. 2007a; Cavanagh et al. 2002; Martinez-Aran et al. 2004; Altshuler et al. 2004; Fleck et al. 2003; van Gorp et al. 1998; Goldberg et al. 1993; Ali et al. 2000; Atre-Vaidya et al. 1998). The effect size of the verbal memory deficit was reported to be as high as 0.7–0.9 (Altshuler et al. 2004; Deckersbach et al. 2004b) but less pronounced in comparison to schizophrenia (Verdoux and Liraud 2000), and it seems it cannot be explained by the attentional deficit (Goswami et al. 2006).

Other deficits identified concerned associative learning (Brambilla et al. 2011), delayed memory (Dittmann et al. 2008a; Ha et al. 2012; Zubieta et al. 2001; Seidman et al. 2002; Bora et al. 2007; Martinez-Aran et al. 2008; Basso et al. 2009; Hill et al. 2009; Dittmann et al. 2008b), nonverbal memory (Deckersbach et al. 2004a), visual memory (Langenecker et al. 2010; Sanchez-Morla et al. 2009; Xu et al. 2012; Goldberg et al. 1993; Coffman et al. 1990; Zubieta et al. 2001; Fitzgerald et al. 2004; Ali et al. 2000) and autobiographical (Scott et al. 2000) and prospective memory (Chan et al. 2012).

There is some data which are negative for the presence of a deficit in working memory (Larson et al. 2005; Docherty et al. 1996; Thompson et al. 2007) and spatial working memory (Pirkola et al. 2005) and in verbal learning (Chang et al. 2011) and verbal (Landro et al. 1993; Paradiso et al. 1997; Kerry et al. 1983) and visual memory (Kerry et al. 1983). One study suggested that most of memory deficits are due to the presence of confounding variables except maybe for verbal recall (Malhi et al. 2007a). The possibility that difficulties in semantic clustering or other strategic processing deficits are the cause for the verbal memory impairment has both positive (Ha et al. 2012; Deckersbach et al. 2004b) and negative data (Bearden et al. 2006a, b; Deckersbach et al. 2004a, b).

In meta-analytic studies, when all phases of the illness are taken into consideration, the effect sizes reported were 0.60 for working memory, 0.43 for immediate verbal memory and 0.34 for delayed and 0.26 for immediate visual memory and 0.51 for delayed (Krabbendam et al. 2005). The meta-analysis of short-term memory studies revealed an effect size of 0.58 when span tasks were utilized, without any difference between the nature of the tasks (whether auditory or visual). When verbal learning tasks were used, the effect size was 0.91 (Goodwin and Jamison 2007).

During the acute manic/mixed state, the effect sizes reported were 1.43 for verbal learning and 1.05 for delayed free verbal recall. During the acute depressed state, the effect size for verbal memory was 1.20, while during euthymia the domains impaired were working memory (0.65), verbal learning (0.81), long-delay verbal free recall (0.78), immediate nonverbal memory (0.73) and delayed nonverbal recall (0.80) (Kurtz and Gerraty 2009).

In euthymic patients the average effect size for episodic memory is reported to be equal to 0.62 and for working memory equal to 0.60 (Mann-Wrobel et al. 2011). Again in euthymic BD patients, a large effect size (0.90) is reported for verbal learning and working memory (0.98) and somewhat lower effect sizes for aspects of immediate (0.73) and delayed (0.71) verbal memory (Robinson et al. 2006). A third meta-analysis reported effect sizes of 0.81, 0.54, 0.74 and 0.72, respectively (Torres et al. 2007). Another meta-analysis reported an effect size of 1.02 for working memory. 0.85 for delayed recall, 0.82 for immediate recall and 0.62 for visual memory (Arts et al. 2008). A last one gave an effect size of 0.85 for verbal learning and 0.73 for verbal memory early recall (Bora et al. 2009a, 2010a). It seems there is a publication bias especially concerning verbal learning and after correction for this, the effect size is attenuated (from 0.85 down to 0.66) (Bora et al. 2009a).

Overall, the literature suggests that BD is characterized by a significant impairment in the acquisition of new information, but not in retention, irrespective of illness phase (van Gorp et al. 1999; Altshuler et al. 2004; Goodwin and Jamison 2007; Bearden et al. 2006a; Deckersbach et al. 2004a). In spite of some opposing data, the most probable interpretation which derives from empirical studies is that the attention and concentration deficits impair the acquisition of information and learning by disrupting the engagement of effortful processing which results in a shallow rather than deeper level of processing (e.g. acoustic rather than semantic) (Christensen et al. 1997; Weingartner et al. 1981, Weingartner et al. 1977; Roy-Byrne et al. 1986; el Massioui and Lesevre 1988; Hartlage et al. 1993; Den Hartog et al. 2003; Hammar 2003; Hammar et al. 2003a, b; Bearden et al. 2006a, b).

4.5 Verbal Skills

Usually testing of verbal skills includes mainly verbal fluency. Although verbal skills are reported to be impaired during all phases of BD (Martinez-Aran et al. 2004; Zubieta et al. 2001; Docherty et al. 1996; Kremen et al. 2003; de Almeida Rocca et al. 2008; Martinez-Aran et al. 2008; Simonsen et al. 2011; Atre-Vaidya et al. 1998), there are some papers suggesting that this impairment is not present during euthymia (Zalla et al. 2004; Altshuler et al. 2004) or during the first mood episode (Barrett et al. 2009). Errors in speech are reported during the acute manic state, and they are independent from the coexistence of an attentional deficit (Thomas et al. 1996).

Individual studies report a small effect size (Docherty et al. 1996) and smaller in comparison to that seen in schizophrenia (Mojtabai et al. 2000); however, a higher effect size (0.68–1.73) has been reported in psychotic BD (Gruzelier et al. 1988; Bora et al. 2007; Selva et al. 2007).

One meta-analysis also reports a small effect size, below 0.5 (Goodwin and Jamison 2007). When all phases of the illness are taken into consideration, the effect size is 0.63 (Krabbendam et al. 2005). A meta-analysis suggested that during the acute manic/mixed state, both letter fluency and semantic fluency are impaired with effect sizes equal to 0.51 and 0.59, respectively. During the acute depressed state, phonemic fluency is impaired with an effect size of 0.93, while during euthymia both phonemic and semantic verbal fluency are impaired with effect sizes 0.51 and 0.75, respectively (Kurtz and Gerraty 2009). In euthymic patients the average effect size for verbal fluency was reported to be equal to 0.6–0.9 (Arts et al. 2008; Bora et al. 2010a), or to 0.71 (Torres et al. 2007), but lower estimations also exist, that is, equal to 0.56 (Mann-Wrobel et al. 2011) and even smaller (0.34) for verbal fluency by letter (Robinson et al. 2006).

4.6 Visuospatial Skills

Visuospatial skills are usually assessed with the use of the complex Rey figure or the WAIS-R block design. BD patients and unaffected relatives are reported to manifest an impairment in the visuospatial/constructional abilities (Dittmann et al. 2008b; Atre-Vaidya et al. 1998; Sapin et al. 1987) and visual learning and memory (Ferrier et al. 1999; Sapin et al. 1987). This impairment is reported to be similar in euthymic BD patients and patients with schizophrenia when results are controlled for possible confounding factors (Addington and Addington 1998). In general, the unaffected relatives demonstrated an intermediate level of performance in comparison to the normal control and bipolar group (Frantom et al. 2008). On the contrary, the visual motion integration was reported to be intact in BD patients (Chen et al. 2005). The literature suggests that this impairment is restricted in the acute phase, while these skills might not be affected during remission (Goodwin and Jamison 2007; Altshuler et al. 2004). The overall effect size is reported to be equal to 0.65 (Goodwin and Jamison 2007) and in remitted patients somewhat lower (0.57) (Mann-Wrobel et al. 2011) or almost normal (0.22) (Arts et al. 2008).

4.7 Executive Function

The executive system is thought to be heavily involved in planning or decision-making, error correction or troubleshooting; in situations where responses are not well-rehearsed or contain novel sequences of actions; in situations that are dangerous or technically difficult situations; or in situations requiring the overcoming of a strong habitual response or resisting temptation. 'Controlling of mental and cognitive processes' seems to be the key phrase describing the role of executive functions. Reasoning seems to rely heavily on verbal and linguistic skills and thus in BD patients it might be important to consider it separately from the rest of the executive functions (Goodwin and Jamison 2007).

Significant impairment in executive functions except reasoning is reported to be present during all phases of BD (Elshahawi et al. 2011; Barrett et al. 2009; Frangou et al. 2005a; Frantom et al. 2008; Goswami et al. 2006; Martinez-Aran et al. 2002, 2004, 2007; Hsiao et al. 2009; Martino et al. 2011a; Mur et al. 2007; Rossi et al. 2000; Sanchez-Morla et al. 2009; Torralva et al. 2012; Wolf et al. 2010; Borkowska and Rybakowski 2001; Malhi et al. 2007a; Antila et al. 2007a, 2009; Dittmann et al. 2008a; Basso et al. 2009; Glahn et al. 2007; Zubieta et al. 2001; Tam et al. 1998; Tien et al. 1996; Brambilla et al. 2007; Morice 1990; Coffman et al. 1990; Seidman et al. 2002; Fitzgerald et al. 2004; Bora et al. 2007; Selva et al. 2007; Simonsen et al. 2011; Dittmann et al. 2008b; Malloy-Diniz et al. 2009; Ali et al. 2000; Waddington et al. 1989; Savard et al. 1980; Rubinsztein et al. 2000) and early during the course of the illness (Kolur et al. 2006), but the deficit is less pronounced in comparison to schizophrenia (Goldberg et al. 1993; Tam et al. 1998; Gard et al. 1999; Hobart et al. 1999; Mojtabai et al. 2000; Tam and Liu 2004; Park 1997). However, it seems that at least a subgroup of patients is as severely impaired as patients with schizophrenia (Young et al. 1998; Verdoux and Liraud 2000; Arduini et al. 2003). It is reported that this impairment might be particularly severe concerning interference and inhibitory control (Barbosa et al. 2012; Blumberg et al. 2003; Ferrier et al. 1999; Larson et al. 2005; Varga et al. 2006; Zubieta et al. 2001; McGrath et al. 1997; Kerr et al. 2005; Stoddart et al. 2007; Selva et al. 2007). Also, BD patients might have more risky (Adida et al. 2011) or erratic choices (Yechiam et al. 2008; Chandler et al. 2009) especially when there is a history of alcohol abuse (Kathleen Holmes et al. 2009).

Not all data are straightforward, however. One study reported normal overall executive function (Cavanagh et al. 2002), while another one only prolonged time to complete the test (Rubinsztein et al. 2000). Another study reported a bimodal distribution of the Wisconsin Card Sorting Test (WCST) scores in patients with BD, with some patients at near-control levels and others significantly impaired (Altshuler et al. 2004). According to other authors, the performance on the executive function measures was bimodal among euthymic BD patients (one subgroup with relatively normal and one subgroup with impaired executive functioning) (Altshuler et al. 2004). Some studies report no difference in executive function between BD patients and controls (Paradiso et al. 1997; de Almeida Rocca et al. 2008; Fleck et al. 2008; Olley et al. 2005; Thompson et al. 2007; Friedman et al. 1977), while one study suggested that impairment is present only in the more severe and chronic cases (de Almeida Rocca et al. 2008).

The impairment in executive functions is reported to be independent from illness phase; however, there are reports suggesting aspects of it are related to affective lability (Aminoff et al. 2012), duration of illness, residual mood symptoms and current antipsychotic treatment (Frangou et al. 2005a) and history of psychosis (Glahn et al. 2007). One study related impairment in executive function to the severity of general psychopathology as it is measured by the PANSS (Martinez-Aran et al. 2002). It has also been reported that impaired insight is related to impaired executive functions (Dias et al. 2008).

A meta-analysis reported that when taking all phases of the illness together, the effect size of this impairment when reasoning (which was reported to be intact) is excluded is reported to be equal to 0.79 (Goodwin and Jamison 2007). Another meta-analysis reported an effect size of 0.55 for executive control and 0.34 for concept formation, with no significant effect for current clinical condition (Krabbendam et al. 2005). A different profile in relationship to illness phase was reported by another meta-analysis which suggested that during the acute manic/mixed state, general executive function and speeded set-shifting are impaired with effect sizes equal to 0.72 and 0.64, respectively. During the acute depressed state, speeded set-shifting is impaired (0.64), while during euthymia problem-solving tasks (0.54), verbal interference (0.75) and set-switching tasks (0.73) are impaired (Kurtz and Gerraty 2009). Three recent meta-analytic studies in euthymic patients reported that the effect sizes for executive functioning was equal to 0.80 for the TMT-B, 0.56 for the WCST and 0.80 for the Stroop test (Mann-Wrobel et al. 2011); 0.78, 0.62 and 0.63, respectively, according to the second analysis (Robinson et al. 2006) and 0.55, 0.69 and 0.71, respectively, according to a third meta-analysis (Torres et al. 2007). Another meta-analysis reported an effect size of 0.99 for the TMT-B and 0.88 for the WCST perseverative errors and 0.52 for the WCST categories, 0.73 for the Stroop time and 0.65 for the Stroop correct (Arts et al. 2008). Similarly, another study reported 0.70 for the WCST perseveration score and 0.8 for the TMT-B and the Stroop test (Bora et al. 2009a, 2010a).

4.8 Social Cognition and Theory of Mind (ToM)

The term 'social cognition' is a multidimensional psychological domain which refers to the ability of the person to assume that other people have minds similar to his/hers and to interpret, understand and predict the emotions, desires, intentions, behaviour and speech of others (including nonverbal elements). In this way, social cognition shapes communication and interaction with others thus enabling adaptive social adaptation. It involves a complex set of processes including the representation of internal somatic states, knowledge about the self, perception of others and interpersonal motivations (Amodio and Frith 2006).

There are three main processes within this construct, namely, theory of mind (ToM), emotion processing and affective decision-making. ToM (mentalizing or mindreading) is the ability to attribute mental states (e.g. beliefs, desires and intents) to oneself and others. Emotion processing refers to the ability to identify and discriminate basic emotions. Affective decision-making is crucial for an appropriate social behaviour and concerns weighing up choices in association with reward and punishment (Samame et al. 2012).

The tests utilized to assess the above domains include both verbal (scenario) and nonverbal (pictures). They demand the subject to identify and comprehend the situation, the roles and the interactions and to make appropriate planning. Empirical data so far support the universality of facial emotions. This means that the specific ability to process and identify facial emotions constitutes an essential component of human communication and social interaction, which is independent of culture.

4.8.1 ToM

Most studies report the presence of a deficit concerning ToM and social cognition during all phases of BD (Cusi et al. 2010; Adida et al. 2011; Lahera et al. 2008; Wolf et al. 2010; Bora et al. 2005; Donohoe et al. 2012; Cusi et al. 2012; Martino et al. 2011b; Inoue et al. 2004; Scott et al. 2000). Only a minority of studies is negative (Barrera et al. 2012; Sarfati and Hardy-Bayle 1999). One group of authors reported that BD patients do not differ from controls after controlling for medication and other confounding factors (Martino et al. 2011b). One study reported impaired performance on ToM in acute mania and acute bipolar depression even when memory was controlled for but not in remitted patients (Kerr et al. 2003). Another study reported no impairment in accuracy of responses, but prolonged latency time of response (Kim et al. 2009).

Concerning the various domains, the data are conclusive for the verbal-cognitive part. The literature suggests the presence of a robust deficit in that domain (Montag et al. 2010; Shamay-Tsoory et al. 2009; Adida et al. 2011; Lahera et al. 2012; Olley et al. 2005; Inoue et al. 2004; Bonshtein et al. 2006). Only one study reported subtle deficits (Donohoe et al. 2012) and only one study reported no deficit at all (Rubinow and Post 1992).

4.8.2 Emotion Processing

On the contrary, the data are inconclusive concerning recognition of emotions. There are several studies suggesting an impaired emotion recognition (Brotman et al. 2008; Bozikas et al. 2006; Lennox et al. 2004; Getz et al. 2003; Lembke and Ketter 2002; Loughland et al. 2002; Yurgelun-Todd et al. 2000; Addington and Addington 1998; Rubinow and Post 1992; Donohoe et al. 2012; Derntl et al. 2009; Lahera et al. 2012; Martino et al. 2011b), but also several others report the opposite (Vaskinn et al. 2007; Malhi et al. 2007b; Kucharska-Pietura and David 2003; Bellack et al. 1996; Montag et al. 2010; Olley et al. 2005; Shamay-Tsoory et al. 2009; Robinson et al. 2008; Surguladze et al. 2010). Negative findings are reported especially after controlling for medication and other confounding variables (Martino et al. 2011b).

It has been shown that BD patients do not manifest any impairment in face recognition in general, but they were impaired specifically in the facial affect labelling, even during periods of euthymia (Getz et al. 2003; Venn et al. 2004). The recognition of specific emotions seems to be influenced during specific phases. For example, during acute mania, recognition of fear and disgust is impaired (Lembke and Ketter 2002), while when euthymic, the patients recognized disgust better (Harmer et al. 2002b). Acute bipolar depression and acute mania are reported to be related with reduced and increased biases in emotion recognition, respectively (David and Cutting 1990). Overall, the presence of a mood-congruent bias which is state rather than trait seems to be the core characteristic (Venn et al. 2004; Lennox et al. 2004; Almeida et al. 2010).

4.8.3 Emotional Decision-Making

Four papers report little or no difference of BD patients from controls on the emotional decision-making component (Chandler et al. 2009; Rubinsztein et al. 2000; Adida et al. 2011; Martino et al. 2011b).

4.8.4 Reviews and Meta-analyses

One meta-analysis reported that the effect size concerning ToM was large and equal to 0.75–0.86; concerning emotion processing was small and equal to 0.35, while there was no difference between BD patients and controls concerning the emotional decision-making. That meta-analysis also reported that age, years of education, duration of illness, medication and sex were not associated with ToM or emotion recognition performance (Samame et al. 2012).

From an epistemological and methodological point of view, the recognition of facial affect requires a compilation of attentional, executive and emotional abilities. Thus, it is difficult to determine where exactly the deficit is located within these mechanisms (Yurgelun-Todd et al. 2000).

It is possible that differences among studies pertaining to neuropsychological tools used and the study samples might be the cause of the significant heterogeneity in the results. The specific tests might play an important role since BD patients might perform similar to controls in some aspects of emotion recognition, but other aspects could be impaired or not, depending on the clinical state. For example, stable BD patients might exhibit impaired facial emotion discrimination (Addington and Addington 1998), while depressed patients could be similar to controls in the perception of chimeric faces, and manic patients might judge all chimeric faces as positive (Lior and Nachson 1999). In specific domains, patients might outperform normal controls (e.g. euthymic BD patients in the recognition of disgust) (Harmer et al. 2002b). On the contrary, depressed patients might show impairment only in the most difficult tasks (Loughland et al. 2002). It is important to note, however, that the effect of the clinical state is not consistent across studies and remains controversial (Wolf et al. 2010; Adida et al. 2011).

The reports which identify a deficit in the ToM domain usually suggest it is independent of other cognitive dysfunctions (Bozikas et al. 2006; Wolf et al. 2010) and unrelated to a history of psychotic symptoms (Lahera et al. 2008). However, the opposite opinion exists also and suggests that even in euthymic BD, executive dysfunction and some other cognitive deficits such as basic emotion recognition may be at least partially responsible for the impairment in ToM and social cognition tests (Bora et al. 2005).

This impairment might be predicted by low level of education and family history of BD (Adida et al. 2011). Psychotropic medications, including benzodiazepines, and both use and non-use of antidepressants may have an impact on the perception of emotion. It has been reported than in healthy subjects, benzodiazepines impair the recognition of anger, propranolol increases the reaction time to recognize sadness and citalopram and reboxetine reduce the perception of negative expressions (Venn et al. 2004; Adida et al. 2011).

Overall the literature is suggestive of a ToM deficit in BD, but the available data have important methodological drawbacks (Bora et al. 2009b). Interestingly, the theory concerning a right hemisphere impairment as responsible for the impairment in emotion recognition does not seem to be sufficient (Bearden et al. 2001) and any neurobiological dysfunction is likely to be state-dependent (Rocca et al. 2009).

4.9 Clinical Correlations

Neuropsychological dysfunction in BD may also be related to clinical symptom pattern and severity and has been associated with age, earlier age at onset, medication status as well as with idiosyncratic factors affecting the long-term course.

4.9.1 The Effect of Medication

An important confounding variable when comparing the different phases of the illness is that although some of the acutely ill patients might be medication-free during testing, this is not the case with patients in remission. Thus, medication status constitutes a confounding variable which is difficult to control for and might introduce a bias towards the detection of a worse dysfunction, especially in remitted patients. On the other hand, very severely manic or depressed patients cannot be tested and are rarely free of medication. Since BD is traditionally considered to belong to the 'functional psychoses' and since the attention impairment is traditionally considered to be the core neurocognitive deficit and cause of all the rest, medications are a possible reason why BD patients do poorly on neurocognitive tasks.

Thus, treatment constitutes an important factor, especially given the possible neuroprotective or neurotoxic effect of several agents. For example, while most authors argue that lithium is neuroprotective, a neurotoxic effect is also possible in the long term, even at therapeutic levels, especially in combination with antipsychotics (Fountoulakis et al. 2008b).

Differentiating between the neurocognitive impairment caused by BD itself and a possible medication-induced impairment is of course of prime importance since it determines the long-term therapeutical design and consequently the outcome. Such a differentiation requires a comprehensive assessment, on the basis of knowledge of those neurocognitive domains most affected by specific medications (Goldberg and Chengappa 2009).

It is very interesting and well known that many patients under lithium complain that treatment inhibits their creativity and productivity (Shaw et al. 1986). The reason for this is unknown; however, it has been suggested that it happens possibly because lithium reduces unusual associations (Shaw et al. 1986). On the other hand, it is unclear whether this constitutes a true impairment or it reflects a subjective feeling as a consequence of the transition from the manic/hypomanic to the euthymic state. It is important to note that this loss of creativity might be specifically related to lithium and not divalproex (Stoll et al. 1996). Fortunately, cognitive complaints do not seem to be significant predictors of discontinuation of lithium treatment (Connelly et al. 1982; Maarbjerg et al. 1988).

Apart from reduced creativity, a general negative impact of lithium on neurocognitive function has been reported, especially on memory and psychomotor functioning (Squire et al. 1980; Kocsis et al. 1993; Honig et al. 1999; Lund et al. 1982; Kessing 1998), but fortunately the insult does not seem to be cumulative (Engelsmann et al. 1988). More specifically, lithium impairs both mental and motor speed, short-term memory and verbal or associative fluency, but the deficit is reversible when lithium is withdrawn and re-establishes when lithium is re-administered (Goldberg 2008; Shaw et al. 1987; Kocsis et al. 1993). Lithium also causes a deficit in the long-term recall (retrieval) without having an effect on attention or encoding (Shaw et al. 1987; Squire et al. 1980; Reus et al. 1979; Karniol et al. 1978; Kropf and Muller-Oerlinghausen 1979). This deficit might especially concern verbal memory (Bora et al. 2007; Senturk et al. 2007).

There are limited data which do not support such a negative effect on neurocognitive function because of lithium treatment (Jaeger et al. 2007). These data especially suggest that lithium has no impact on the reaction time (MacQueen et al. 2004) and executive functions (Friedman et al. 1977). In line with this, a longitudinal study failed to detect evidence of neurocognitive decline over a 6-year period in a sample of BD patients treated with lithium (Engelsmann et al. 1988).

The overall effect size related to lithium treatment is small (0.3) (Arts et al. 2008), but could be significant concerning specific domains like psychomotor speed (0.62). However, it is small concerning immediate verbal learning and memory (0.24) and creativity (0.33), while delayed verbal memory, visual memory, attention and executive function might not be affected at all (Wingo et al. 2009).

Reports on antipsychotics and antiepileptics are rare and conflicting (Holmes et al. 2008; Pan et al. 2011; Goldberg and Chengappa 2009). Valproate and carbamazepine may cause attentional difficulties (Thompson and Trimble 1982). It is also important to note the adverse effects of topiramate because although it is not used in the treatment of BD per se, it is often administered in BD patients in order to lose weight or to treat a comorbid substance abuse disorder. It is reported that topiramate impairs attention, verbal memory, psychomotor slowing and word-finding even at very low dosages (25–50 mg/day). This impairment is reversible after discontinuation of the drug (Goldberg 2008; Salinsky et al. 2005).

Neuroleptics have been associated with sustained attention and visuomotor speed deficits (King 1994). Current antipsychotic treatment in BD patients is reported to relate to worse performance across all executive function tests as well as in semantic fluency, verbal learning and recognition memory, even when clinical features were controlled for (Frangou et al. 2005a; Jamrozinski et al. 2009; Altshuler et al. 2004). One study reported no adverse effect concerning risperidone (Reinares et al. 2000). One study found that the executive function deficit was correlated with years of exposure to antipsychotic drugs (Zubieta et al. 2001). In general, it is unclear whether this deficit constitutes a true medication adverse effect or the consequence of the manifestation of psychotic symptoms, for the treatment of whom, antipsychotics were prescribed.

Overall, the literature suggests that medications have a limited adverse effect on cognitive function (Maalouf et al. 2010) if any at all (Goswami et al. 2009; Roiser et al. 2009; Lopez-Jaramillo et al. 2010). On the contrary, there seems to be a close relationship between poor treatment adherence and neurocognitive impairment, but the causal inferences of these findings are uncertain. It is unclear whether it is the poor treatment adherence which leads to a worse neurocognitive performance through worsening of the overall course of BD or, on the contrary, it is the neurocognitive impairment which causes poor treatment adherence and reflects more severe illness (Martinez-Aran et al. 2009).

BD patients are often treated with benzodiazepines which are known to interfere with memory (Stein and Strickland 1998). It is also important to note that they are often treated with complex combinations of lithium, antipsychotics, antiepilectics, antidepressants and benzodiazepines and the combinatorial effects of these drugs on neurocognition is a matter of speculation rather than research.

It is evident that medication probably causes some degree of neurocognitive impairment especially in psychomotor speed and sustained attention (Bora et al. 2009a). This impairment is difficult to distinguish from the impairment caused by the illness. Studies comparing euthymic patients on or off medication have found little effects of medication on neurocognitive test performance (Strakowski et al. 2004; Joffe et al. 1988). Additionally, patients assessed during their first episode, and thus before any exposure to medications, also show evidence of neurocognitive deficits that are more or less similar to those observed in chronically medicated patients (Nehra et al. 2006). However, a study that compared unmedicated vs. medicated depressed BD-II patients found that medicated patients performed poorer in sustained attention (Holmes et al. 2008).

In those individuals with full inter-episode remission doing well off medication, this adverse effect might be obvious; however, it is also well known that staying off medication will adversely affect the overall course of the illness. It is unfortunate that no currently known pharmacotherapy improves substantially the neurocognition in BD. Preliminary findings suggest some potential value for adjunctive stimulants such as modafinil and novel experimental agents (Goldberg and Chengappa 2009).

4.9.2 The Effect of Psychotic Symptoms

Albus et al. (1996) hypothesized that neuropsychological dysfunction is a product of psychosis, rather than affective illness per se. This hypothesis was partially confirmed by other researchers since the presence of psychotic symptoms is strongly related to a worse overall neurocognitive performance (Zubieta et al. 2001; Bora et al. 2007; Levy and Weiss 2010; Sheffield et al. 2012; Liu et al. 2002; Glahn et al. 2006a, c, 2007; Lahera et al. 2008; Martinez-Aran et al. 2008; Selva et al. 2007; Savitz et al. 2009; Simonsen et al. 2011; Szoke et al. 2008; Daban et al. 2006). In psychotic BD patients several aspects of the neurocognitive deficit are reported to be similar in magnitude to those observed in patients with schizophrenia (Hill et al. 2009; McGrath et al. 2001; Daban et al. 2006). There is a strong consensus on this effect, in spite of some negative data (Basso et al. 2009; Lahera et al. 2008; Selva et al. 2007; Bora et al. 2010a). Negative studies suggest that the deficit in BD is overall less pronounced than in schizophrenia; however, it is similar with schizophrenia in working memory and executive function and as a general profile similar to unipolar psychotic depression (Bora et al. 2010a).

A meta-analyses suggested that BD patients generally perform better than patients with schizophrenia, and the effect sizes of the difference varied between 0.26 and 0.63 for IQ, mental speed, verbal working memory, immediate visual memory, verbal fluency (with the largest effect size of 0.63), executive control and concept formation, but without any difference concerning the rest of the domains (Krabbendam et al. 2005). It is important that there were only quantitative, and not qualitative, differences. Significant heterogeneity in effect sizes was present between studies, partially because of methodological issues and the size and clinical characteristics of the study samples (Daban et al. 2006).

In the absence of current psychotic symptoms, a history of psychotic features is also strongly related to worse neurocognitive function (Simonsen et al. 2011; de Almeida Rocca et al. 2008) especially concerning measures of executive functioning and verbal and spatial working memory (Glahn et al. 2007; Martinez-Aran et al. 2008). However, this effect is modest, and there does not seem to exist a complete categorical distinction between psychotic and nonpsychotic BD (Bora et al. 2010b). The presence of family history is correlated with worse visuomotor attention in psychotic BD patients (Tabares-Seisdedos et al. 2003); however, this load is less severe in comparison with schizophrenia since it has been reported that the offspring of mothers with BD have less neurocognitive impairment in comparison to offspring of mothers with schizophrenia (Schubert and McNeil 2005). Probably depending on the study sample (proportion of BD-I and BD-II patients) and the definition of psychosis, results vary and are suggestive of a nosological continuum between psychotic and nonpsychotic cases. It is interesting that such a history of psychotic symptoms is inversely related to the cognitive function in the patients' relatives (Jabben et al. 2009).

Meta-analysis suggests that between patients with and without history of psychotic symptoms, there are no differences concerning attention and visual memory. The observed differences in global IQ, mental speed, working memory, planning and reasoning and executive functions are small, and only after excluding one outlier study (Lahera et al. 2008), the effect size concerning the executive functions increases to 0.55 (Bora et al. 2010b).

One cannot exclude the possibility that cognitive differences between psychotic and nonpsychotic BD patients are in fact the result of an earlier onset of illness or medication use rather than a result of psychosis per se. In accord with this, the meta-analysis of cases suggested that psychotic BD patients in the above studies had a younger age of illness onset and more hospital admissions and a larger proportion of them were using antipsychotics. Also they had lower education (Bora et al. 2010b) and it has been reported that education plays a significant moderator role (Kurtz and Gerraty 2009).

Schizoaffective patients perform poorer in a global way, maybe because current psychotic symptoms or history of psychosis is correlated to more severe neurocognitive impairment no matter the specific diagnosis (Simonsen et al. 2011; Szoke et al. 2008; Torrent et al. 2007). Euthymic and stabilized schizoaffective patients are reported to perform worse than BD patients in attention, concentration, declarative memory, executive function and perceptuomotor function (Studentkowski et al. 2010; Torrent et al. 2007)

4.9.3 The Effect of Mood Symptoms

Very severely manic or depressed patients cannot be tested and thus data are not available. Extrapolating conclusions on these patients from the study of less severe cases is problematic.

For patients whose neurocognitive functions can be assessed, the overall severity of mood symptoms might not affect memory performance (Bearden et al. 2006a). Acute mania is reported to adversely affect impulse control (Ryan et al. 2012) and executive function (Dixon et al. 2004). Acute bipolar depression is associated with an attentional bias (Holmes et al. 2008) with lowering of mental speed, impaired attention in general (van der Werf-Eldering et al. 2010; Liu et al. 2002) and verbal fluency (Chaves et al. 2011), verbal recall and fine motor skills impairment (Malhi et al. 2007a). In both acutely depressed and manic patients, impaired performance on theory of mind tests was found, even when memory was controlled for (Kerr et al. 2003). Of course there are also studies suggesting there is no effect of either acute phase on the neurocognitive function of BD patients (Burdick et al. 2005). No effect specifically for acute mania has also been reported (Chaves et al. 2011). Fluctuations in both manic and depressive symptoms have an appreciable impact on cognitive functioning (Kurtz and Gerraty 2009). Additionally, moderate changes in affective symptoms did not covary with cognitive ability (Depp et al. 2012); however, when changes are more severe or when rapid cycling emerges, this is reported to adversely affect the neurocognitive function (McKay et al. 1995).

A number of research studies and meta-analyses suggest that significant neurocognitive impairment is present during remission in many domains (Daban et al. 2006; Bora et al. 2009a, 2010a; Arts et al. 2008; Jamrozinski 2010), in spite of some reservations (Gruber et al. 2007; Kerr et al. 2003). A meta-analysis reported that the illness phase had no effect on the short-term memory impairment (Goodwin and Jamison 2007), but some authors suggest that the impairment observed during the euthymic phase might be a consequence of antipsychotic medication alone (Jamrozinski et al. 2009).

The impairment in executive functions is reported to be independent from illness phase; however, there are reports suggesting aspects of it are related to affective lability (Aminoff et al. 2012), duration of illness, residual mood symptoms and current antipsychotic treatment (Frangou et al. 2005a) and history of psychosis (Glahn et al. 2007). One study related impairment in executive function to the severity of general psychopathology as it is measured by the PANSS (Martinez-Aran et al. 2002). It has also been reported that impaired insight is related to impaired executive functions (Dias et al. 2008). Finally, differences in somatic comorbidity (and comedication) between BD patients and normal controls could contribute to differences in cognitive performance (Newcomer 2006).

An important methodological problem is that the definition criteria for euthymia differ considerably between studies in respect of duration and parameter values, thus making conclusions suspect. Even subsyndromal conditions might affect verbal memory (Goswami et al. 2006). The presence of residual mood symptoms, regardless of polarity, might have a negative impact, primarily on measures of attentional interference (Frangou et al. 2005a). Residual mania, but not depression, impairs ideational fluency (Jaeger et al. 2007). It is possible that controlling for residual symptoms in stabilized euthymic patients might change our picture concerning the presence of neurocognitive impairment during euthymia (Clark et al. 2002; Ferrier et al. 1999; Thompson et al. 2005).

Apart from current symptomatology, it has been reported that the memory deficit in BD patients might depend on the number of previous hospitalizations and family history of mood disorder (Bearden et al. 2006b). Especially the impairment of verbal memory might relate to the presence of subsyndromal mood symptoms, the duration of illness and the numbers of previous manic episodes, hospitalizations and suicide attempts (Martinez-Aran et al. 2004; Cavanagh et al. 2002; Goswami et al. 2006).

The first follow-up study suggested that from patients without any neurocognitive impairment at first episode, one-third had significant deficits after 5–7 years (Dhingra and Rabins 1991). However, in adult patients, the picture is more complex. During the first episode of the illness, there might be no impairment at all in nonpsychotic patients, while those with psychotic features manifest a deficit comparable to that seen in patients with schizophrenia (Albus et al. 1996). After the first episode, the time to recover was associated with executive function and possibly with verbal fluency (Gruber et al. 2008).

A meta-analysis suggested neurocognitive impairment is present during all phases of BD and calculated the respected effect sizes for specific neurocognitive domains separately for each phase. During the acute manic/mixed states, the effect sizes showed a clear impairment in attention (0.79–0.90), impairment in verbal learning (1.43), delayed free verbal recall (1.05), delayed letter fluency (0.51), delayed semantic fluency (0.59), impairment in general executive function (0.72) and impairment in speeded set-shifting (0.64). During acute bipolar depression, the effect sizes revealed an impairment concerning attention (0.80), verbal memory (1.20), phonemic fluency (0.93) and executive function in speeded set-shifting (0.64). During the euthymic phase, the effect sizes showed a clear impairment in auditory (0.41) and sustained visual vigilance (0.69) and speeded visual scanning (0.65); working memory (0.65), verbal learning (0.81) and long-delay verbal free recall (0.78); executive functions concerning problem-solving tasks (0.54), verbal interference (0.75) and set-switching tasks (0.73) and immediate nonverbal memory (0.73), delayed nonverbal recall (0.80), visuospatial function (0.55), phonemic (0.51) and semantic (0.75) verbal fluency and psychomotor speed (0.66) (Kurtz and Gerraty 2009). Overall, these results suggested that patients in a manic or depressed state had significantly greater effect-size impairment in verbal learning than patients in an euthymic state.

Although the relationship between mood symptoms and neurocognitive decline seems to be strong, the overall evidence suggests that the observed neurocognitive deficit in BD patients is not merely the product of mood symptomatology or exposure to medication, but reflects deeper neurobiological dysfunction probably including the presence of premorbid developmental abnormalities (Savitz et al. 2005).

4.9.4 The Effect of Age and Age at Onset and Personal Psychiatric History

There is a line of research with sufficient data support, suggesting that the overall progression of the illness causes neurocognitive deterioration. The progression is a concept difficult to define and operationalize; however, a number of factors and indices can be utilized to reflect it, e.g. age of onset, duration of illness, number of previous episodes, etc. This concept is discussed in detail in Chap. 20 of this book (Staging). Overall, the severity of the disease is strongly related to neurocognitive function (Yates et al. 2011).

Onset in childhood or adolescence is related to more severe impairment (Jamrozinski 2010). In paediatric BD patients, a neurocognitive impairment is observed which is similar to adult patients (Dickstein et al. 2004). In more general terms, age at onset correlates with the severity of the neurocognitive impairment (Bora et al. 2007; Osuji and Cullum 2005), especially in verbal memory and psychomotor speed (Bora et al. 2009a).

In the course of BD, the number of episodes (Denicoff et al. 1999), number of prior hospitalizations (Tham et al. 1997; Denicoff et al. 1999; Bearden et al. 2006b; de Almeida Rocca et al. 2008) and longer duration (Denicoff et al. 1999) were associated with worse neurocognitive function. The duration of illness was reported to be related with the loss of inhibitory control (Frangou et al. 2005a) and with impairment of general memory (Bearden et al. 2006a) and of verbal memory (Martinez-Aran et al. 2004). Two studies reported that the number of episodes but not duration of the illness were associated with worse neurocognitive function (Kessing 1998; de

Almeida Rocca et al. 2008). The magnitude of the attentional deficit is correlated with the duration of the illness, the age of onset and the age of first hospitalization (Ancin et al. 2010).

Any history of mood disorder has an adverse effect especially on memory (Bearden et al. 2006a, b). The number of past manic episodes, hospitalizations and suicide attempts was correlated with worse neurocognitive performance (Martinez-Aran et al. 2004). Manic episodes was correlated with the deficit in verbal learning and memory (Cavanagh et al. 2002) and in attention and executive function (Lopez-Jaramillo et al. 2010), while the number of past depressive episodes was reported to have a negative influence on verbal memory (Fossati et al. 2004) and reaction times (MacQueen et al. 2004).

In the assessment of neurocognitive functioning, the age of the study sample was also proven to be important, since young BD patients perform better in comparison to young unipolar patients, but the reverse is true in the elderly (Burt et al. 2000). Overall, age seems to play a complex role. One meta-analysis reported a significant deterioration of neurocognitive function with age (Arts et al. 2008), while a second one suggested that the difference between BD patients and controls attenuates with age, probably because the neurocognitive performance of healthy people deteriorates with age at a rate which seems to be faster in comparison to what is observed in BD patients (Mann-Wrobel et al. 2011). A similar phenomenon has been reported concerning schizophrenia (Fountoulakis et al. 2008a, 2011a, b). A third meta-analysis is suggested no effect for age (Bora et al. 2010a).

Of course, again, a reverse explanation could be proposed, with the neurocognitive impairment being the cause rather than the effect of worse course and outcome (Martino et al. 2012). One cannot exclude the possibility that cognitive differences between psychotic and nonpsychotic BD patients are in fact the result of an earlier onset of illness or medication use rather than a result of psychosis per se. In accord with this, the meta-analysis of cases suggested that psychotic BD patients had a younger age of illness onset and more hospital admissions and a larger proportion of them were using antipsychotics. Also they had lower education (Bora et al. 2010b), and this should be taken into consideration having also in mind that it has been reported that education plays a significant moderator role (Kurtz and Gerraty 2009). Finally, there are two meta-analyses which report no significant effect for age at onset, duration or severity of illness, as defined by the number of episodes (Bora et al. 2009a, 2010a).

4.9.5 The Role of Other Clinical Factors

A variety of other clinical factors have also been studied concerning their effect on the neurocognitive performance of BD patients. These include the possible adverse effect of brain white matter lesions that are sometimes found in remitted BD patients and in patients with schizophrenia but apparently do not underlie cognitive deficits per se (Krabbendam et al. 2000). Similarly, a lifetime comorbid alcohol use disorder, also does not seem to correlate with neurocognitive performance (van der Werf-Eldering et al. 2010).

Education could constitute an additional confounding variable, since BD patients have less educational attainment despite comparable IQ levels in comparison to normal controls. Thus, controlling for it might attenuate the magnitude of the observed neurocognitive impairment (Glahn et al. 2006b). In general the neurocognitive impairment effect sizes seem to decrease as a function of education (Mann-Wrobel et al. 2011; Arts et al. 2008) and it has been reported that shorter duration of education is related to a more pronounced deficit in letter fluency, WCST categories and the Stroop test (Bora et al. 2010a). The explanation might include both the possibility that education is a marker related to the onset and severity of illness, since early and severe illness interferes with educational attainment, but also the possibility that education constitutes a protective factor.

Finally, overweight and obese BD patients might perform worse on verbal fluency testing (Yim et al. 2012).

4.10 BD-II

In spite of research efforts during the last few years, no specific neurocognitive profile has been clearly delineated for the different bipolar subtypes (Sole et al. 2012). This is partially due to the fact that research on BD-II patients is rare, with large differences between studies in terms of methodology and the results are largely inconclusive. Research on other subtypes of the bipolar spectrum is literally non-existent, with only one paper reporting data on 'bipolar spectrum' patients. That paper reported the presence of a widespread neurocognitive deficit, especially affecting the executive functions and verbal memory (Smith et al. 2006).

In this frame, all possible combinations of results have been reported. Thus, BD-II patients have been reported to perform similar to healthy controls (Savitz et al. 2008; Taylor Tavares et al. 2007; Derntl et al. 2009); to perform in-between healthy controls and BD-I patients (Dittmann et al. 2008a; Martino et al. 2011a; Simonsen et al. 2008; Andersson et al. 2008; Torrent et al. 2006; Derntl et al. 2009; Xu et al. 2012; Hsiao et al. 2009), specifically in verbal memory (Martinez-Aran et al. 2004; Torrent et al. 2006) and executive functions (Torrent et al. 2006); to perform similar to BD-I patients (Chang et al. 2011; Ha et al. 2012; Dittmann et al. 2008a; Martino et al. 2011a); or even to perform worse than BD-I, at least in some specific neurocognitive domains, that is, aspects of reaction time and inhibition (Summers et al. 2006; Harkavy-Friedman et al. 2006).

The above confusing picture does not permit any answer to the question whether there is any qualitative difference between bipolar subtypes, that is, a different pattern of neurocognitive deficit between BD-I and BD-II. Such a difference would suggest (although that would not be mandatory) that possibly, different neurobiological mechanisms underlie the two types. However, both questions (concerning a quantitative and a qualitative difference) remain unanswered. There are data in both in favour and against.

A global neurocognitive impairment has been reported, with only phonemic verbal fluency being preserved and with moderate to strong effect sizes ranging from 0.62 to 1.34 (Andersson et al. 2008). Concerning premorbid IQ, there is only one study and it reports no difference between BD-I and BD-II patients, with both groups performing significantly worse in comparison to healthy controls (Dittmann et al. 2008a). Two other studies found that the intellectual decline was less pronounced in BD-II in comparison to BD-I patients (Summers et al. 2006; Bruno et al. 2006). There are several studies indicating an impairment in attention and psychomotor speed (Torrent et al. 2006; Andersson et al. 2008; Dittmann et al. 2008a; Hsiao et al. 2009; Harkavy-Friedman et al. 2006; Holmes et al. 2008), but other studies disagree (Simonsen et al. 2008; Savitz et al. 2008). Reaction time was reported to be similar to that of controls (Berns et al. 2002). One study reported intact attention but impaired psychomotor speed (Xu et al. 2012). Concerning memory, some studies report an impairment in verbal memory and verbal learning (Xu et al. 2012; Martinez-Aran et al. 2004; Summers et al. 2006; Torrent et al. 2006; Andersson et al. 2008), but others do not support such an assumption (Dittmann et al. 2008a; Harkavy-Friedman et al. 2006; Hsiao et al. 2009; Simonsen et al. 2008; Savitz et al. 2008). Some data suggest the presence of a less disorganized semantic structure in BD-II in comparison to BD-I (Chang et al. 2011; Ha et al. 2012). Delayed memory is reported to be intact (Dittmann et al. 2008a). An impairment in the visual memory is reported by some authors (Summers et al. 2006; Andersson et al. 2008; Dittmann et al. 2008a), but this is disputed by others (Harkavy-Friedman et al. 2006; Hsiao et al. 2009; Savitz et al. 2008; Taylor Tavares et al. 2007; Holmes et al. 2008). Similarly, some authors have found a deficit in working memory and executive functions (Martinez-Aran et al. 2004; Summers et al. 2006; Andersson et al. 2008; Dittmann et al. 2008a; Torrent et al. 2006; Simonsen et al. 2008; Harkavy-Friedman et al. 2006; Xu et al. 2012), while others did not (Savitz et al. 2008; Taylor Tavares et al. 2007). Another study suggested BD-II patients were impaired only in working memory but not in executive functions (Hsiao et al. 2009). Interestingly, all the studies using the Stroop Colour–Word Test, which assesses interference, reported impaired inhibitory control in BD-II patients (Simonsen et al. 2008; Torrent et al. 2006; Andersson et al. 2008; Summers et al. 2006). The emotional processing might suffer from a deficit (Summers et al. 2006; Holmes et al. 2008); however, the emotion recognition seems to be intact (Derntl et al. 2009). One study on a small sample of unmedicated depressed BD-II patients reported intact decision-making performance (Taylor Tavares et al. 2007).

An interesting study which compared depressed unmedicated vs. medicated BD-II patients found that the latter group performed poorer than the former in sustained attention (Holmes et al. 2008).

A number of reviews and meta-analyses have already been conducted. With regard to general intellectual function, these meta-analyses report that there is no difference between BD-II and healthy subjects neither in the estimated current intelligence quotient (IQ) nor the premorbid IQ (Sole et al. 2011, 2012). Concerning specific neurocognitive functions, one meta-analysis reported that with the exception of memory and semantic fluency, cognitive impairment in BD-II patients is as severe as in BD-I patients (Bora et al. 2011). Another meta-analysis reported that the data concerning psychomotor speed and verbal and visual memory are contradictory and the impairment probably small in magnitude, while on the contrary the data are relatively robust concerning the presence of a working memory deficit and a decrease of cognitive flexibility and impaired inhibitory control in BD-II. Also BD-II patients were impaired in recognizing emotions (Sole et al. 2011). Overall, the literature supports that in quantitative terms, BD-II does not differ much from BD-I (Arts et al. 2011) although it seems that the prevailing opinion is that BD-II patients perform better than BD-I but worse than healthy controls and are positioned in between these two groups.

4.11 Long-Term Development of the Neurocognitive Deficit

BD is a complex illness with different phases and clinical characters. Two BD patients might differ from each other not only in the polarity and the number of episodes but also in the degree of remission between episodes, the presence or not of psychotic symptoms, the overall psychiatric and somatic comorbidity and other issues. Thus, it is difficult to chart the long-term course of the illness and so far, in spite of efforts to stage BD, there are no reliable indices to describe the course in a global way. In this frame, it is also difficult to study whether the progression of the illness causes further impairment in the neurocognitive function.

It is important to note that the direction of causality is unclear. One possibility is that the accumulation of mood episodes adversely affects the neurocognitive function; however, the reverse is equally possible. A third possibility is that both the mood symptoms and the neurocognitive impairment independently reflect a specific pattern of clinical course and disease phenotype without any direct relationship to each other.

Overall, it is believed that in contrast to schizophrenia patients, BD patients exhibit a relatively intact cognitive functioning throughout childhood and adolescence and the neurocognitive deterioration is observed only after the overt symptom onset (Lewandowski et al. 2011). A graphic illustration of this difference is shown in Fig. 4.1. In line with this, the retrospective investigations and record reviews suggest that children who later develop BD exhibit good academic functioning prior to illness onset (Quackenbush et al. 1996; Kutcher et al. 1998; Uzelac et al. 2006; Reichenberg et al. 2002; Toulopoulou et al. 2006).

However, there are some data suggesting the opposite. A prospective investigation of executive functioning in at-risk adolescents found executive function deficits in those who later developed BD (Meyer et al. 2004). Another study reported an increased prevalence of abnormal developmental history with retarded language and social and motor development in a group of adolescents with BD (Sigurdsson et al. 1999). A large Finnish cohort study examining verbal, arithmetic and visuospatial reasoning in healthy male conscripts (mean age 19.9 years) found that the premorbid visuospatial deficits were associated with later development of both BD and schizophrenia (Tiihonen et al. 2005). Another prospective study from Sweden

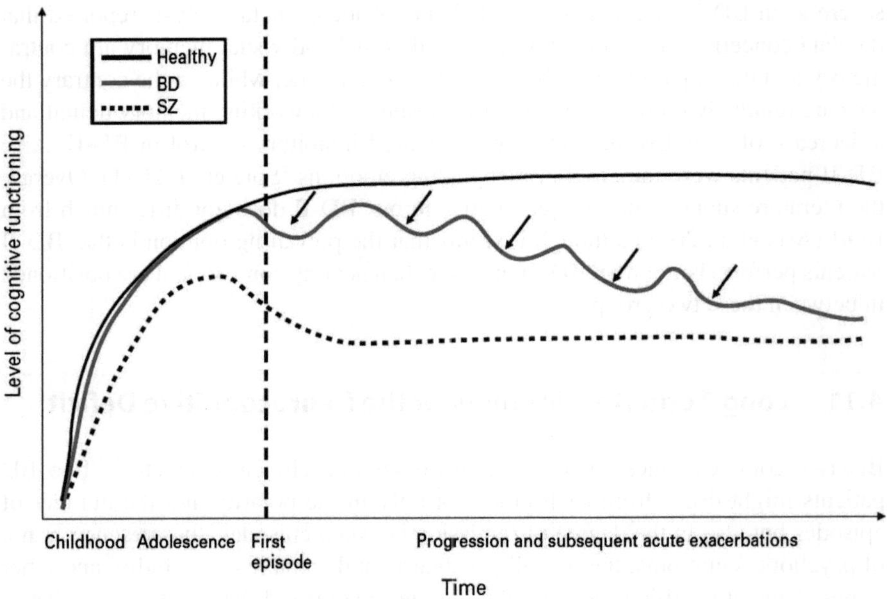

Fig. 4.1 Long-term evolution of the neurocognitive deficit in BD patients, in comparison to patients with schizophrenia and normal subjects. Overall, in contrast to schizophrenia patients, BD patients exhibit a relatively intact cognitive functioning throughout childhood and adolescence, and the neurocognitive deterioration is observed only after the overt symptom onset (Reproduced after permission from Lewandowski et al. (2011))

followed 56 Swedish adolescents with developmental deficits at the age of 6 years and reported that 7 % of them went on to develop BD, compared with none from the control group (Hellgren et al. 1994).

When BD develops during childhood, then it adversely affects the neurocognitive maturation and development of the child (Pavuluri et al. 2009). The overall neuropsychological deficit has been associated with earlier age at onset (Osuji and Cullum 2005). Immediately following illness onset, adolescents with BD exhibit significant deterioration in cognitive and social domains (Quackenbush et al. 1996). Similarly, in adults, it has been reported that the deficit is present already during the first mood episode (Nehra et al. 2006). At illness onset, sustained attention (Clark et al. 2002), learning and recall, spatial/nonverbal reasoning and several aspects of executive function (Torres et al. 2010) as well as memory, verbal fluency and executive function (Barrett et al. 2009) are reported to be impaired.

Patients with two or more illness episodes performed significantly worse than patients with just one episode (Kessing 1998) and it is reported that as soon as within 1–3 years, significant further deterioration might be observed in the executive function (Torrent et al. 2012), which along with processing speed are considered to be the main long-term neurocognitive deficits in BD (Mur et al. 2008). The rest neurocognitive functions seem to be stable at 1–3-year follow-up (Balanza-Martinez et al. 2005; Torrent et al. 2012). However, the complete picture of the results in the literature is controversial concerning the short-term deterioration (van Gorp et al. 1998; Tham et al. 1997; Ferrier et al. 1999; Atre-Vaidya et al. 1998; Hoff et al. 1990; Verdoux and Liraud 2000).

Later in the course of the illness, the neurocognitive functioning worsens with repeated acute episodes (Lewandowski et al. 2011), and it is reported to correlate with both the number of affective episodes and the overall duration of illness (Clark et al. 2002; Cavanagh et al. 2002; Lebowitz et al. 2001; Zubieta et al. 2001; Denicoff et al. 1999; El-Badri et al. 2001). Duration of illness and disease course are reported to correlate with executive function, verbal memory and visual memory (Sanchez-Morla et al. 2009; Robinson and Ferrier 2006; Zubieta et al. 2001). The comparison of young, elderly and chronic BD patients reported that a greater number of chronic patients scored in the severely impaired range on a memory and executive battery than their counterparts with fewer past episodes (McKay et al. 1995). Thus, it is possible that, instead of reflecting long-term damage to the brain because of repeated acute episodes, poor cognitive performance in multi-episode patients may be the result of the presence of chronic residual mood symptoms. It is known that BD patients experience mood lability (Kruger et al. 2003; Tsuang et al. 1979) and residual symptoms, usually depressive, during periods of euthymia in spite of the fact that they were rated as euthymic by clinicians (Scott et al. 2000).

The presence of complex comorbidity in chronic patients with incomplete remission is an additional issue. Indeed, it has been reported that the length of illness was predictive of greater cognitive impairment in a group of BD patients with alcohol dependence in comparison to a non-alcoholic group (van Gorp et al. 1998). And although, in many cases, the acute effects of alcohol or drug intoxication have been ruled out (van Gorp et al. 1999; Krabbendam et al. 2000; Atre-Vaidya et al. 1998), the effects of past exposures have not been taken into account, and this remains a weak point in the literature.

Continuous medication could also play an important confounding role. Although in patients under long-term lithium treatment, no further decline of neurocognitive function was observed (Engelsmann et al. 1988); in another study (as already mentioned above), it was found that the executive function deficit was negatively correlated with years of exposure to antipsychotic drugs (Zubieta et al. 2001). This latter finding could reflect either the toxic effect of chronic psychosis, the toxic effect of long-term medication or both.

In the long term, the neurocognitive deficit seems to be associated with the functional outcome. This relationship is particularly true for attention, processing speed and memory (Bearden et al. 2010) as well as the visual/motor processing domain (Tabares-Seisdedos et al. 2008). One study used cross-sectional data from a large case-register study of 14,000 people hospitalized with a mood disorder, 81,380 patients with osteoarthritis and 69,149 patients with diabetes. The results suggested that BD patients have a 6 % increase in the risk of dementia with every episode leading to admission and this risk was increased in comparison to the two control groups (Kessing and Andersen 2004; Kessing and Nilsson 2003). Although these data are in favour of a neurodegenerative process, it is also possible that the findings reflect different courses of the illness plus a different probability of long-term medication treatment and electroconvulsive therapy (ECT) with unknown long-term effects (Paradiso et al. 1997).

The specific clinical course of the illness seems to play an important role, with a course characterized by chronicity and residual symptoms with lack of remission between episodes being related to a progressive neurocognitive deficit (McKay et al. 1995; Denicoff et al. 1999). Of prime importance is the deleterious effect of psychotic symptoms (Lewandowski et al. 2011). In accord with the latter, antipsychotic medication is associated with poorer performance on IQ, memory and working memory assessments (Donaldson et al. 2003). Also, patients with more severe and frequent affective episodes perform more poorly on cognitive testing (Denicoff et al. 1999).

According to one systematic review, the most robust finding was a relationship between the number of manic episodes and the impairment in delayed verbal memory, sustained attention and executive function. The correlation of the number of depressive episodes to neurocognitive impairment was lower in comparison to that of manic episodes and concerned executive function, verbal learning, visual memory and spatial working memory (Robinson and Ferrier 2006). According to a meta-analysis, first episode BD patients were impaired in comparison to controls; however, the magnitude of this deficit was significantly smaller in comparison to multi-episode patients (Bora et al. 2010a).

The overall longitudinal course suggests that neurodevelopmental factors play, at most, a minor role in the emergence of neuropsychological dysfunction in BD (Savitz et al. 2005; Lewandowski et al. 2011). Psychopathological factors during the course of the disorder itself are associated with the neurocognitive deficit, but the nature of this association is unknown.

4.12 Awareness of the Neurocognitive Deficit

BD patients frequently report neurocognitive problems especially concerning attention, concentration and memory. However, there is little research on the relationship of subjective cognitive complaints relative to objective neuropsychological deficits.

The limited literature suggests that in general, the patients' self-reports of impairment do not correlate or predict objective neuropsychological deficits (Burdick et al. 2005; Chan et al. 2012; van der Werf-Eldering et al. 2011). Maybe there is some weak correlation between subjective complains and deficits in attention, memory and execute function (Martinez-Aran et al. 2005). Mood symptoms and severity of mania and depression do not correlate with self-report (Burdick et al. 2005) although it is possible that patients with a higher number of episodes, especially with a higher number of mixed episodes, longer duration of the illness and the onset of the illness at an earlier age might show more subjective complaints (Martinez-Aran et al. 2005). In this frame and since with the progression of the illness, depression seem to predominate in the majority of patients, there seems to be some association between depressive symptoms with cognitive complaints; however, the association between cognitive complaints and objective cognitive functioning is not moderated by mood symptoms (van der Werf-Eldering et al. 2011).

4.13 Gender and the Neurocognitive Deficit

There are limited data concerning a possible role gender plays, and no conclusions can be derived yet. There are studies suggesting that male BD patients manifest a more severe deficit in immediate memory (Carrus et al. 2010) and executive function (Barrett et al. 2008), while one study reported no gender effect on emotion recognition (Derntl et al. 2009). However, one study suggested that female gender, instead of impairment, is related to a better memory performance (Bearden et al. 2006a). It has been suggested that the verbal memory deficit as endophenotype might relate to female gender (Kieseppa et al. 2005). Three recent meta-analyses report conflicting results, one in favour (Arts et al. 2008) and two against the presence of a gender effect (Mann-Wrobel et al. 2011; Bora et al. 2010a).

4.14 The Neurocognitive Deficit as an Endophenotype for BD

Endophenotype refers to a stable pattern of behavioural symptoms with a clear genetic connection. It can be used to bridge the gap between high-level symptom presentation and low-level genetic variability. Ideally, an endophenotype might be useful in the differential diagnosis between disorders when they present with similar symptoms.

An endophenotype should be associated with the specific disorder in the population and also be heritable and state-independent. It is expected that within families, endophenotype and the specific diagnosis co-segregate and the endophenotype is found in non-affected family members at a higher rate than in the general population. Concerning the prevalence of BD in families, it is well known that the offspring of BD parents are at a four times higher risk (Chang et al. 2003), while first-degree relative are at a 10-to-20-fold higher risk to develop BD (Glahn et al. 2004; Smoller and Finn 2003).

As shown previously, the neurocognitive deficit of BD patients is at least partially different in comparison to the deficit seen in patients with schizophrenia. It is also at least partially state-independent and definitely present during periods of complete recovery and euthymia. However, the data so far do not support the use of global measures of cognition as endophenotypes (Burdick et al. 2009; Jabben et al. 2010; Kremen et al. 1998). On the other hand, specific neurocognitive impairments might be relevant, although further research is needed. There is strong evidence that unaffective relatives of patients occupy an intermediate position between patients and healthy controls concerning specific neurocognitive functions (Frantom et al. 2008).

4.14.1 Twin Studies

There are only a limited number of studies on discordant monozygotic or dizygotic twins. Healthy co-twins perform worse than controls in aspects of concentration, verbal and visual memory and verbal recognition and executive function (Gourovitch et al. 1999). However, a population-based study suggested that the verbal memory deficit as an endophenotype might relate to female gender alone (Kieseppa et al. 2005). A study with significant overlapping of study sample with the previous one suggested that neither BD patients nor their unaffected co-twins differed from control subjects in spatial working memory (Pirkola et al. 2005). Another population-based study on healthy monozygotic and dizygotic twins showed that monozygotic high-risk twins manifested significant impairment on selective and sustained attention, executive function, language processing and working and declarative memory, while the dizygotic high-risk twins manifested lower scores only on language processing and episodic memory (Christensen et al. 2006). A more recent study on response inhibition found no impairment in discordant twins of BD patients (event with a psychotic and familial form). The presence of depressive symptoms in twins explained lower performance in the testing (Kravariti et al. 2009). In most of these studies, unaffected co-twins suffered from minor or subthreshold mental disorders and dysthymia. Overall, twin studies provide some but not strong support for the presence of an endophenotype based on neurocognitive impairment.

4.14.2 Studies on First-Degree Relatives

The studies on children of parents suffering from BD are also very few. These high-risk children were reported to differ from controls in reaction time; however, the quality of that study was low (Winters et al. 1981). The same research group published a second study (with overlapping study samples) and reported that high-risk children were similar to controls in speech competence (Harvey et al. 1982). In two other studies, high-risk children were impaired in PIQ but not in VIQ; however, half of them were suffering from depression (Kron et al. 1982; Decina et al. 1983). On the contrary, IQ was similar in high-risk children and controls although controls performed better in some reading and arithmetic cognitive tasks and there was an increased rate of VIQ–PIQ discrepancy (McDonough-Ryan et al. 2002). A study on visual backward masking was also negative (MacQueen et al. 2004). High-risk relatives were reported to manifest slower reaction time on a sustained auditory attention task (Pierson et al. 2000). A small recent study suggested that specific executive functions which are supposedly located in the ventral frontal cortex might be impaired in high-risk children in comparison to controls (Frangou et al. 2005b). The most recent study was very well designed and executed and suggested the presence of impairment in healthy high-risk children in spatial memory and attention as well as in executive functions, even after correction for multiple confounding factors (Klimes-Dougan et al. 2006). Overall, these studies provide evidence for the usefulness of executive function impairment as an endophenotype for BD.

4.14.3 Studies on Mixed Samples of Relatives

The literature is significantly greater concerning families of BD patients. These studies utilized mixed samples of first- and second-degree patients.

The first of them utilized only female relatives of patients (most of them psychotic) and suggested their IQ was superior to the IQ of controls and provided some support for the usefulness of executive function and visual memory as endophenotypes (Kremen et al. 1998). Another study suggested an IQ similar to controls (Gilvarry et al. 2000), while on the contrary, another one reported the presence of a general and non-specific IQ impairment with some pronounced effect on verbal fluency (McIntosh et al. 2005). A more recent study reported the presence of a higher discrepancy between VIQ and PIQ in families of BD patients in comparison to controls; however, these results were inconsistent with previous findings of higher VIQ in comparison to PIQ (Toulopoulou et al. 2006).

Impairment in psychomotor speed has been reported (Antila et al. 2007a, b, 2009; Zalla et al. 2004), and while studies revealed a deficit in concentration (Ferrier et al. 2004), others suggested there is an impairment in shifting, but not in sustaining attention (concentration) (Schulze et al. 2011; Clark et al. 2005a, b). One study reported that well-educated siblings with high IQ manifested impairment in delayed recall (Keri et al. 2001). Other studies reported the presence of a deficit in concentration and in the visuospatial declarative memory (Ferrier et al. 2004); verbal working memory (Bora et al. 2008); verbal (Christodoulou et al. 2012; Antila et al. 2007a, b, 2009), visual (Frantom et al. 2008) and auditory verbal learning (Kulkarni et al. 2010) and working memory (Glahn et al. 2010). Other research groups reported an impairment executive function domain (Antila et al. 2007a, b, 2009; Bora et al. 2008; Szoke et al. 2006; Zalla et al. 2004).

There is one report on increased emotional interference with a bias towards mood-related information (Besnier et al. 2009). At-risk youths were reported to make more errors when identifying facial emotions, and the magnitude of impairment was similar to that seen in BD patients (Brotman et al. 2008); however, another study reported no impairment either in BD patients or in their first-degree relatives (Surguladze et al. 2010).

It is interesting that even subtle impairment might be present in first-degree relatives of BD patients with otherwise normal neurocognitive testing. A study which utilized L-tryptophan challenge showed that under challenge, memory, focused and divided attention and psychomotor performance were impaired in relatives of BD patients in comparison to controls. Relatives of BD-I patients showed more pronounced cognitive impairments than relatives of BD-II patients (Sobczak et al. 2002, 2003).

4.14.4 Reviews and Meta-analyses

Overall, the literature suggests that executive function impairment could serve as an endophenotype for BD, especially concerning psychotic cases. There are some data, however, which dispute the usefulness of specific executive functions, including cognitive control during episodic memory retrieval (Christodoulou et al. 2012), response inhibition (Kravariti et al. 2009) and cognitive set-shifting (Schulze et al. 2011). The data also suggest that although a widespread attention and memory deficit might be present in families of BD, there are some negative data concerning concentration (Clark et al. 2005a), psychomotor performance (Bora et al. 2008; Szoke et al. 2006), working memory (Schulze et al. 2011), spatial working memory (Pirkola et al. 2005), verbal learning (Antila et al. 2007b), verbal memory (Bora et al. 2008) and executive functions (Szoke et al. 2006). It is almost certain that IQ cannot serve as an endophenotype.

Reviews and meta-analyses support that the executive function and the verbal memory deficit could constitute central endophenotypes for BD (Balanza-Martinez et al. 2008; Arts et al. 2008; Robinson and Ferrier 2006), but conclusions are premature. The effect sizes reported are 0.49 with the Stroop test and 0.37 with the TMT-B, and concerning immediate verbal memory, the effect size is 0.42. Thus, in first-degree relatives, effect sizes were small ($d<0.5$), but significantly different from healthy controls for executive function and verbal memory in particular (Arts et al. 2008).

In accord with the above, another meta-analysis reported small effect sizes, that is, 0.20 for current IQ, 0.18–0.36 for attention and 0.17–0.22 for mental speed, 0.13–0.33 for various aspects of memory, 0.27 for verbal fluency and 0.24–0.51 for executive functions with the effect for the Stroop test being the highest (0.51). This meta-analytic study demonstrated that impaired response inhibition might be the most prominent cognitive endophenotype of BD. Another executive measure, set-shifting (TMT-B, 0.38; WCST perseveration, 0.36), and two other cognitive domains, verbal memory (0.27–0.33) and sustained attention (0.36), also met the criteria as potential endophenotypes of BD. These results suggest that the response inhibition deficit, a potential marker of ventral prefrontal dysfunction, seems to be the most prominent endophenotype of BD (Bora et al. 2009a).

In Table 4.2, the effect sizes of neurocognitive impairment in relatives of BD patients are shown. These effect sizes determine whether a specific impairment is of sufficient magnitude to be considered as an endophenotype.

Conclusion

As already mentioned, the neurocognitive function of BD patients has been the focus of debate for decades, and still many areas remain uncharted. It seems that a little less than half of BD patients suffer from significant neurocognitive impairment. While the majority of patients might not differ from normal subjects even in the eyes of the experienced clinician, it is also true that some others do not differ from patients with schizophrenia.

BD is a complex disease and this complexity reflects also in the patients' neurocognitive function and its assessment. The core deficit, which is the direct consequence of the disease itself, seems to be independent from the other components of the disease and more specifically seems to be independent of mood symptoms. This is important to note, because not long ago, the neurocognitive deficit was considered to be a 'functional' state and not trait, a direct consequence of mood symptoms. This core deficit is confounded (either increased or attenuated) by the disease phase, specific personal characteristics of the patients (age, gender, education etc.), current symptomatology and its treatment and long-term course and long term exposure to medication, psychiatric and somatic comorbidity and alcohol and/or substance abuse.

The origin of the core neurocognitive deficit is also unclear. Probably the neurodevelopmental component is either absent or very weak, while the neurodegenerative component as a consequence of repeated mood episodes and psychotic features as well as of chronicity is quite strong. This probably differentiates BD from schizophrenia, in which the neurodevelopmental component is strong.

The general picture from the individual studies and meta-analyses is that the neurocognitive deficit concerns almost all domains with only a few exceptions. Its magnitude is at the severe range during the acute episodes and at the medium range during euthymia. A summary of effect sizes by neurocognitive domain and illness phase is shown in Table 4.2.

While premorbid IQ and general neurocognitive function seems to be intact, there seems to be a small to moderate reduction in current IQ and general neurocognitive function during all phases of the illness. Psychomotor speed, attention, working memory and most of the verbal and some nonverbal components of memory as well as verbal fluency, executive functions and social cognition are also impaired. Impairment is typically severe during the acute phases and moderate during euthymia. The studies on memory suggest that overall BD is characterized by a significant impairment in the acquisition of new information, but not in retention, irrespective of illness phase probably because of a disruption in the engagement of effortful processes. An important exception is visuospatial impairment which is present only during the acute phases and not during euthymia, like the deficit in the other domains.

There is an ongoing debate concerning euthymia, mainly because different studies utilize different definitions of euthymia. Thus, it is unclear whether subthreshold residual symptoms are present or not, what their polarity is and whether they are responsible for the deficit observed during remission.

The overall adverse influence of medication is small and is confounded by the specific clinical symptoms, for which medication is used for their treatment. This is especially true concerning antipsychotics and psychotic symptoms.

Overall, the literature supports that in quantitative terms, BD-II does not differ much from BD-I although it seems that the prevailing opinion is that BD-II patients perform better than BD-I but worse than healthy controls and are positioned in between these two groups.

The specific clinical course of the illness seems to play an important role, with a course characterized by chronicity and residual symptoms with lack of remission between episodes being related to a progressive neurocognitive deficit. Of prime importance is the deleterious effect of psychotic symptoms, while manic episodes seem to affect neurocognitive function more than depressive episodes do. Age, age at onset, duration of the illness and number of episodes all reflect distinct but overlapping aspects of the overall disease burden and are related to the neurocognitive impairment and its progression. However, the data are inconclusive concerning the magnitude and the true nature of this relationship.

Reviews and meta-analyses support that the executive function and the verbal memory deficit could constitute central endophenotypes for BD. The response inhibition deficit seems to be the most prominent endophenotype of BD. It is interesting to note that in most family studies, unaffected at-risk family members do not suffer from BD, but they do manifest dysthymic or other, often subthreshold mood states, often in the form of temperament. The effect sizes concerning endophenotypes are shown in Table 4.2.

References

Addington J, Addington D (1997) Attentional vulnerability indicators in schizophrenia and bipolar disorder. Schizophr Res 23(3):197–204. doi:S0920996496001053 [pii]

Addington J, Addington D (1998) Facial affect recognition and information processing in schizophrenia and bipolar disorder. Schizophr Res 32(3):171–181. doi:S0920996498000425 [pii]

Adida M, Jollant F, Clark L, Besnier N, Guillaume S, Kaladjian A, Mazzola-Pomietto P, Jeanningros R, Goodwin GM, Azorin JM, Courtet P (2011) Trait-related decision-making impairment in the three phases of bipolar disorder. Biol Psychiatry 70(4):357–365. doi:10.1016/j.biopsych.2011.01.018, S0006-3223(11)00075-8 [pii]

Albus M, Hubmann W, Wahlheim C, Sobizack N, Franz U, Mohr F (1996) Contrasts in neuropsychological test profile between patients with first-episode schizophrenia and first-episode affective disorders. Acta Psychiatr Scand 94(2):87–93

Ali SO, Denicoff KD, Altshuler LL, Hauser P, Li X, Conrad AJ, Mirsky AF, Smith-Jackson EE, Post RM (2000) A preliminary study of the relation of neuropsychological performance to neuroanatomic structures in bipolar disorder. Neuropsychiatry Neuropsychol Behav Neurol 13(1):20–28

Almeida JR, Versace A, Hassel S, Kupfer DJ, Phillips ML (2010) Elevated amygdala activity to sad facial expressions: a state marker of bipolar but not unipolar depression. Biol Psychiatry 67(5):414–421. doi:10.1016/j.biopsych.2009.09.027, S0006-3223(09)01154-8 [pii]

Altshuler LL, Ventura J, van Gorp WG, Green MF, Theberge DC, Mintz J (2004) Neurocognitive function in clinically stable men with bipolar I disorder or schizophrenia and normal control subjects. Biol Psychiatry 56(8):560–569. doi:10.1016/j.biopsych.2004.08.002, S0006-3223(04)00853-4 [pii]

Aminoff SR, Jensen J, Lagerberg TV, Hellvin T, Sundet K, Andreassen OA, Melle I (2012) An association between affective lability and executive functioning in bipolar disorder. Psychiatry Res 198(1):58–61. doi:10.1016/j.psychres.2011.12.044, S0165-1781(12)00002-9 [pii]

Amodio DM, Frith CD (2006) Meeting of minds: the medial frontal cortex and social cognition. Nat Rev Neurosci 7(4):268–277. doi:10.1038/nrn1884, nrn1884 [pii]

Ancin I, Santos JL, Teijeira C, Sanchez-Morla EM, Bescos MJ, Argudo I, Torrijos S, Vazquez-Alvarez B, De La Vega I, Lopez-Ibor JJ, Barabash A, Cabranes-Diaz JA (2010) Sustained attention as a potential endophenotype for bipolar disorder. Acta Psychiatr Scand 122(3):235–245. doi:10.1111/j.1600-0447.2009.01532.x, ACP1532 [pii]

Andersson S, Barder HE, Hellvin T, Lovdahl H, Malt UF (2008) Neuropsychological and electrophysiological indices of neurocognitive dysfunction in bipolar II disorder. Bipolar Disord 10(8):888–899. doi:10.1111/j.1399-5618.2008.00638.x, BDI638 [pii]

Andreasen NC (1987) Creativity and mental illness: prevalence rates in writers and their first-degree relatives. Am J Psychiatry 144(10):1288–1292

Andreasen NC (2008) The relationship between creativity and mood disorders. Dialogues Clin Neurosci 10(2):251–255

Andreasen NC, Glick ID (1988) Bipolar affective disorder and creativity: implications and clinical management. Compr Psychiatry 29(3):207–217. doi:0010-440X(88)90044-2 [pii]

Antila M, Tuulio-Henriksson A, Kieseppa T, Eerola M, Partonen T, Lonnqvist J (2007a) Cognitive functioning in patients with familial bipolar I disorder and their unaffected relatives. Psychol Med 37(5):679–687. doi:10.1017/S0033291706009627, S0033291706009627 [pii]

Antila M, Tuulio-Henriksson A, Kieseppa T, Soronen P, Palo OM, Paunio T, Haukka J, Partonen T, Lonnqvist J (2007b) Heritability of cognitive functions in families with bipolar disorder. Am J Med Genet B Neuropsychiatr Genet 144B(6):802–808. doi:10.1002/ajmg.b.30538

Antila M, Partonen T, Kieseppa T, Suvisaari J, Eerola M, Lonnqvist J, Tuulio-Henriksson A (2009) Cognitive functioning of bipolar I patients and relatives from families with or without schizophrenia or schizoaffective disorder. J Affect Disord 116(1–2):70–79. doi:10.1016/j.jad.2008.11.006, S0165-0327(08)00462-X [pii]

Antila M, Kieseppa T, Partonen T, Lonnqvist J, Tuulio-Henriksson A (2011) The effect of processing speed on cognitive functioning in patients with familial bipolar I disorder and their unaffected relatives. Psychopathology 44(1):40–45. doi:10.1159/000317577, 000317577 [pii]

Arduini L, Kalyvoka A, Stratta P, Rinaldi O, Daneluzzo E, Rossi A (2003) Insight and neuropsychological function in patients with schizophrenia and bipolar disorder with psychotic features. Can J Psychiatry 48(5):338–341

Arts B, Jabben N, Krabbendam L, van Os J (2008) Meta-analyses of cognitive functioning in euthymic bipolar patients and their first-degree relatives. Psychol Med 38(6):771–785. doi:10.1017/S0033291707001675, S0033291707001675 [pii]

Arts B, Jabben N, Krabbendam L, van Os J (2011) A 2-year naturalistic study on cognitive functioning in bipolar disorder. Acta Psychiatr Scand 123(3):190–205. doi:10.1111/j.1600-0447.2010.01601.x

Asarnow RF, MacCrimmon DJ (1981) Span of apprehension deficits during the postpsychotic stages of schizophrenia. A replication and extension. Arch Gen Psychiatry 38(9): 1006–1011

Atre-Vaidya N, Taylor MA, Seidenberg M, Reed R, Perrine A, Glick-Oberwise F (1998) Cognitive deficits, psychopathology, and psychosocial functioning in bipolar mood disorder. Neuropsychiatry Neuropsychol Behav Neurol 11(3):120–126

Ayres AM, Busatto GF, Menezes PR, Schaufelberger MS, Coutinho L, Murray RM, McGuire PK, Rushe T, Scazufca M (2007) Cognitive deficits in first-episode psychosis: a population-based study in Sao Paulo, Brazil. Schizophr Res 90(1–3):338–343. doi:10.1016/j.schres.2006.09.026, S0920-9964(06)00425-7 [pii]

Badcock JC, Michiel PT, Rock D (2005) Spatial working memory and planning ability: contrasts between schizophrenia and bipolar I disorder. Cortex 41(6):753–763

Balanza-Martinez V, Tabares-Seisdedos R, Selva-Vera G, Martinez-Aran A, Torrent C, Salazar-Fraile J, Leal-Cercos C, Vieta E, Gomez-Beneyto M (2005) Persistent cognitive dysfunctions in bipolar I disorder and schizophrenic patients: a 3-year follow-up study. Psychother Psychosom 74(2):113–119. doi:10.1159/000083170, 83170 [pii]

Balanza-Martinez V, Rubio C, Selva-Vera G, Martinez-Aran A, Sanchez-Moreno J, Salazar-Fraile J, Vieta E, Tabares-Seisdedos R (2008) Neurocognitive endophenotypes (endophenocognitypes) from studies of relatives of bipolar disorder subjects: a systematic review. Neurosci Biobehav Rev 32(8):1426–1438. doi:10.1016/j.neubiorev.2008.05.019, S0149-7634(08)00089-4 [pii]

Barbosa IG, Rocha NP, Huguet RB, Ferreira RA, Salgado JV, Carvalho LA, Pariante CM, Teixeira AL (2012) Executive dysfunction in euthymic bipolar disorder patients and its association with plasma biomarkers. J Affect Disord 137(1–3):151–155. doi:10.1016/j.jad.2011.12.034, S0165-0327(11)00797-X [pii]

Barrera A, Vazquez G, Tannenhaus L, Lolich M, Herbst L (2012) Theory of mind and functionality in bipolar patients with symptomatic remission. Rev Psiquiatr Salud Ment. doi:10.1016/j.rpsm.2012.07.004, S1888-9891(12)00151-6 [pii]

Barrett SL, Kelly C, Bell R, King DJ (2008) Gender influences the detection of spatial working memory deficits in bipolar disorder. Bipolar Disord 10(5):647–654. doi:10.1111/j.13995618.2008.00592.x, BDI592 [pii]

Barrett SL, Mulholland CC, Cooper SJ, Rushe TM (2009) Patterns of neurocognitive impairment in first-episode bipolar disorder and schizophrenia. Br J Psychiatry 195(1):67–72. doi:10.1192/bjp.bp.108.054874, 195/1/67 [pii]

Basso MR, Lowery N, Ghormley C, Ward T, Purdie R, Neel J, Combs DR, Bornstein RA (2009) Neuropsychological impairment and psychosis in mania. J Clin Exp Neuropsychol 31(5):523–532. doi:10.1080/13803390802304516, 901726272 [pii]

Bearden CE, Hoffman KM, Cannon TD (2001) The neuropsychology and neuroanatomy of bipolar affective disorder: a critical review. Bipolar Disord 3(3):106–150; discussion 151–153

Bearden CE, Glahn DC, Monkul ES, Barrett J, Najt P, Kaur S, Sanches M, Villarreal V, Bowden C, Soares JC (2006a) Sources of declarative memory impairment in bipolar disorder: mnemonic processes and clinical features. J Psychiatr Res 40(1):47–58. doi:10.1016/j.jpsychires.2005.08.006, S0022-3956(05)00101-9 [pii]

Bearden CE, Glahn DC, Monkul ES, Barrett J, Najt P, Villarreal V, Soares JC (2006b) Patterns of memory impairment in bipolar disorder and unipolar major depression. Psychiatry Res 142(2–3): 139–150. doi:10.1016/j.psychres.2005.08.010, S0165-1781(05)00260-X [pii]

Bearden CE, Woogen M, Glahn DC (2010) Neurocognitive and neuroimaging predictors of clinical outcome in bipolar disorder. Curr Psychiatry Rep 12(6):499–504. doi:10.1007/s11920-010-0151-5

Bellack AS, Blanchard JJ, Mueser KT (1996) Cue availability and affect perception in schizophrenia. Schizophr Bull 22(3):535–544

Berns GS, Martin M, Proper SM (2002) Limbic hyperreactivity in bipolar II disorder. Am J Psychiatry 159(2):304–306

Besnier N, Richard F, Zendjidjian X, Kaladjian A, Mazzola-Pomietto P, Adida M, Azorin JM (2009) Stroop and emotional Stroop interference in unaffected relatives of patients with schizophrenic and bipolar disorders: distinct markers of vulnerability? World J Biol Psychiatry 10(4 Pt 3):809–818. doi:10.1080/15622970903131589, 914182822 [pii]

Blackburn IM (1975) Mental and psychomotor speed in depression and mania. Br J Psychiatry 126:329–335

Blumberg HP, Leung HC, Skudlarski P, Lacadie CM, Fredericks CA, Harris BC, Charney DS, Gore JC, Krystal JH, Peterson BS (2003) A functional magnetic resonance imaging study of bipolar disorder: state- and trait-related dysfunction in ventral prefrontal cortices. Arch Gen Psychiatry 60(6):601–609. doi:10.1001/archpsyc.60.6.601, 60/6/601 [pii]

Bonnin CM, Sanchez-Moreno J, Martinez-Aran A, Sole B, Reinares M, Rosa AR, Goikolea JM, Benabarre A, Ayuso-Mateos JL, Ferrer M, Vieta E, Torrent C (2012) Subthreshold symptoms in bipolar disorder: impact on neurocognition, quality of life and disability. J Affect Disord 136(3):650–659. doi:10.1016/j.jad.2011.10.012, S0165-0327(11)00656-2 [pii]

Bonshtein U, Leiser D, Levine J (2006) Naive theory impairment in schizophrenia: is it domain-specific? J Nerv Ment Dis 194(10):753–759. doi:10.1097/01.nmd.0000243083.75008.ae, 00005053-200610000-00005 [pii]

Bora E, Vahip S, Gonul AS, Akdeniz F, Alkan M, Ogut M, Eryavuz A (2005) Evidence for theory of mind deficits in euthymic patients with bipolar disorder. Acta Psychiatr Scand 112(2):110–116. doi:10.1111/j.1600-0447.2005.00570.x, ACP570[pii]

Bora E, Vahip S, Akdeniz F, Gonul AS, Eryavuz A, Ogut M, Alkan M (2007) The effect of previous psychotic mood episodes on cognitive impairment in euthymic bipolar patients. Bipolar Disord 9(5):468–477. doi:10.1111/j.1399-5618.2007.00469.x, BDI469 [pii]

Bora E, Vahip S, Akdeniz F, Ilerisoy H, Aldemir E, Alkan M (2008) Executive and verbal working memory dysfunction in first-degree relatives of patients with bipolar disorder. Psychiatry Res 161(3):318–324. doi:10.1016/j.psychres.2007.09.002, S0165-1781(07)00327-7 [pii]

Bora E, Yucel M, Pantelis C (2009a) Cognitive endophenotypes of bipolar disorder: a meta-analysis of neuropsychological deficits in euthymic patients and their first-degree relatives. J Affect Disord 113(1–2):1–20. doi:10.1016/j.jad.2008.06.009, S0165-0327(08)00246-2 [pii]

Bora E, Yucel M, Pantelis C (2009b) Theory of mind impairment: a distinct trait-marker for schizophrenia spectrum disorders and bipolar disorder? Acta Psychiatr Scand 120(4):253–264. doi:10.1111/j.1600-0447.2009.01414.x, ACP1414 [pii]

Bora E, Yucel M, Pantelis C (2010a) Cognitive impairment in affective psychoses: a meta-analysis. Schizophr Bull 36(1):112–125. doi:10.1093/schbul/sbp093, sbp093 [pii]

Bora E, Yucel M, Pantelis C (2010b) Neurocognitive markers of psychosis in bipolar disorder: a meta-analytic study. J Affect Disord 127(1–3):1–9. doi:10.1016/j.jad.2010.02.117, S0165-0327(10)00238-7 [pii]

Bora E, Yucel M, Pantelis C, Berk M (2011) Meta-analytic review of neurocognition in bipolar II disorder. Acta Psychiatr Scand 123(3):165–174. doi:10.1111/j.1600-0447.2010.01638.x

Borkowska A, Rybakowski JK (2001) Neuropsychological frontal lobe tests indicate that bipolar depressed patients are more impaired than unipolar. Bipolar Disord 3(2):88–94

Bozikas VP, Tonia T, Fokas K, Karavatos A, Kosmidis MH (2006) Impaired emotion processing in remitted patients with bipolar disorder. J Affect Disord 91(1):53–56. doi:10.1016/j.jad.2005.11.013, S0165-0327(05)00349-6 [pii]

Brambilla P, Macdonald AW 3rd, Sassi RB, Johnson MK, Mallinger AG, Carter CS, Soares JC (2007) Context processing performance in bipolar disorder patients. Bipolar Disord 9(3):230–237. doi:10.1111/j.1399-5618.2007.00398.x, BDI398 [pii]

Brambilla P, Cerruti S, Bellani M, Perlini C, Ferro A, Marinelli V, Giusto D, Tomelleri L, Rambaldelli G, Tansella M, Diwadkar VA (2011) Shared impairment in associative learning in schizophrenia and bipolar disorder. Prog Neuropsychopharmacol Biol Psychiatry 35(4):1093–1099. doi:10.1016/j.pnpbp.2011.03.007, S0278-5846(11)00088-1 [pii]

Brotman MA, Guyer AE, Lawson ES, Horsey SE, Rich BA, Dickstein DP, Pine DS, Leibenluft E (2008) Facial emotion labeling deficits in children and adolescents at risk for bipolar disorder. Am J Psychiatry 165(3):385–389. doi:10.1176/appi.ajp.2007.06122050, appi.ajp.2007.06122050 [pii]

Brown GG, Lohr J, Notestine R, Turner T, Gamst A, Eyler LT (2007) Performance of schizophrenia and bipolar patients on verbal and figural working memory tasks. J Abnorm Psychol 116(4):741–753. doi:10.1037/0021-843X.116.4.741, 2007-17062-007 [pii]

Bruno SD, Papadopoulou K, Cercignani M, Cipolotti L, Ron MA (2006) Structural brain correlates of IQ changes in bipolar disorder. Psychol Med 36(5):609–618. doi:10.1017/S0033291706007112, S0033291706007112 [pii]

Burdick KE, Endick CJ, Goldberg JF (2005) Assessing cognitive deficits in bipolar disorder: are self-reports valid? Psychiatry Res 136(1):43–50. doi:10.1016/j.psychres.2004.12.009, S0165-1781(05)00153-8 [pii]

Burdick KE, Gunawardane N, Woodberry K, Malhotra AK (2009) The role of general intelligence as an intermediate phenotype for neuropsychiatric disorders. Cogn Neuropsychiatry 14(4–5):299–311. doi:10.1080/13546800902805347, 913383382 [pii]

Burdick KE, Goldberg JF, Harrow M (2010) Neurocognitive dysfunction and psychosocial outcome in patients with bipolar I disorder at 15-year follow-up. Acta Psychiatr Scand 122(6):499–506. doi:10.1111/j.1600-0447.2010.01590.x, ACP1590 [pii]

Burt T, Prudic J, Peyser S, Clark J, Sackeim HA (2000) Learning and memory in bipolar and unipolar major depression: effects of aging. Neuropsychiatry Neuropsychol Behav Neurol 13(4):246–253

Carrus D, Christodoulou T, Hadjulis M, Haldane M, Galea A, Koukopoulos A, Kumari V, Frangou S (2010) Gender differences in immediate memory in bipolar disorder. Psychol Med 40(8):1349–1355. doi:10.1017/S0033291709991644, S0033291709991644 [pii]

Cavanagh JT, Van Beck M, Muir W, Blackwood DH (2002) Case-control study of neurocognitive function in euthymic patients with bipolar disorder: an association with mania. Br J Psychiatry 180:320–326

Chan RC, Lui SS, Wang Y, Liu AC, Chui WW, Shum DH, Cheung EF (2012) Patients with bipolar disorders share similar but attenuated prospective memory impairments with patients with schizophrenia. Psychol Med 43(8):1639–1649. doi:10.1017/S003329171200236X, S003329171200236X [pii]

Chandler RA, Wakeley J, Goodwin GM, Rogers RD (2009) Altered risk-aversion and risk-seeking behavior in bipolar disorder. Biol Psychiatry 66(9):840–846. doi:10.1016/j.biopsych.2009.05.011, S0006-3223(09)00635-0 [pii]

Chang K, Steiner H, Ketter T (2003) Studies of offspring of parents with bipolar disorder. Am J Med Genet C Semin Med Genet 123C(1):26–35. doi:10.1002/ajmg.c.20011

Chang JS, Choi S, Ha K, Ha TH, Cho HS, Choi JE, Cha B, Moon E (2011) Differential pattern of semantic memory organization between bipolar I and II disorders. Prog Neuropsychopharmacol Biol Psychiatry 35(4):1053–1058. doi:10.1016/j.pnpbp.2011.02.020, S0278-5846(11)00076-5 [pii]

Chaves OC, Lombardo LE, Bearden CE, Woolsey MD, Martinez DM, Barrett JA, Miller AL, Velligan DI, Glahn DC (2011) Association of clinical symptoms and neurocognitive performance in bipolar disorder: a longitudinal study. Bipolar Disord 13(1):118–123. doi:10.1111/j.1399-5618.2011.00888.x

Chen Y, Bidwell LC, Holzman PS (2005) Visual motion integration in schizophrenia patients, their first-degree relatives, and patients with bipolar disorder. Schizophr Res 74(2–3):271–281. doi:10.1016/j.schres.2004.04.002, S0920996404001331 [pii]

Christensen H, Griffiths K, Mackinnon A, Jacomb P (1997) A quantitative review of cognitive deficits in depression and Alzheimer-type dementia. J Int Neuropsychol Soc 3(6):631–651

Christensen MV, Kyvik KO, Kessing LV (2006) Cognitive function in unaffected twins discordant for affective disorder. Psychol Med 36(8):1119–1129. doi:10.1017/S0033291706007896, S0033291706007896 [pii]

Christodoulou T, Messinis L, Papathanasopoulos P, Frangou S (2012) The impact of familial risk for schizophrenia or bipolar disorder on cognitive control during episodic memory retrieval. Psychiatry Res 197(3):212–216. doi:10.1016/j.psychres.2011.12.028, S0165-1781(11)00812-2 [pii]

Clark L, Goodwin GM (2004) State- and trait-related deficits in sustained attention in bipolar disorder. Eur Arch Psychiatry Clin Neurosci 254(2):61–68. doi:10.1007/s00406-004-0460-y

Clark L, Iversen SD, Goodwin GM (2002) Sustained attention deficit in bipolar disorder. Br J Psychiatry 180:313–319

Clark L, Kempton MJ, Scarna A, Grasby PM, Goodwin GM (2005a) Sustained attention-deficit confirmed in euthymic bipolar disorder but not in first-degree relatives of bipolar patients or euthymic unipolar depression. Biol Psychiatry 57(2):183–187. doi:10.1016/j.biopsych.2004.11.007, S0006-3223(04)01165-5 [pii]

Clark L, Sarna A, Goodwin GM (2005b) Impairment of executive function but not memory in first-degree relatives of patients with bipolar I disorder and in euthymic patients with unipolar depression. Am J Psychiatry 162(10):1980–1982. doi:10.1176/appi.ajp.162.10.1980, 162/10/1980 [pii]

Coffman JA, Bornstein RA, Olson SC, Schwarzkopf SB, Nasrallah HA (1990) Cognitive impairment and cerebral structure by MRI in bipolar disorder. Biol Psychiatry 27(11):1188–1196. doi:0006-3223(90)90416-Y [pii]

Connelly CE, Davenport YB, Nurnberger JI Jr (1982) Adherence to treatment regimen in a lithium carbonate clinic. Arch Gen Psychiatry 39(5):585–588

Coryell W, Endicott J, Keller M, Andreasen N, Grove W, Hirschfeld RM, Scheftner W (1989) Bipolar affective disorder and high achievement: a familial association. Am J Psychiatry 146(8):983–988

Cusi A, Macqueen GM, McKinnon MC (2010) Altered self-report of empathic responding in patients with bipolar disorder. Psychiatry Res 178(2):354–358. doi:10.1016/j.psychres.2009.07.009, S0165-1781(09)00275-3 [pii]

Cusi AM, Macqueen GM, McKinnon MC (2012) Patients with bipolar disorder show impaired performance on complex tests of social cognition. Psychiatry Res 200(2–3):258–264. doi:10.1016/j.psychres.2012.06.021, S0165-1781(12)00332-0 [pii]

Czobor P, Jaeger J, Berns SM, Gonzalez C, Loftus S (2007) Neuropsychological symptom dimensions in bipolar disorder and schizophrenia. Bipolar Disord 9(1–2):71–92. doi:10.1111/j.1399-5618.2007.00428.x, BDI428 [pii]

Daban C, Martinez-Aran A, Torrent C, Tabares-Seisdedos R, Balanza-Martinez V, Salazar-Fraile J, Selva-Vera G, Vieta E (2006) Specificity of cognitive deficits in bipolar disorder versus schizophrenia. A systematic review. Psychother Psychosom 75(2):72–84. doi:10.1159/000090891, 90891 [pii]

Dalby JT, Williams R (1986) Preserved reading and spelling ability in psychotic disorders. Psychol Med 16(1):171–175

David AS, Cutting JC (1990) Affect, affective disorder and schizophrenia. A neuropsychological investigation of right hemisphere function. Br J Psychiatry 156:491–495

de Almeida Rocca CC, de Macedo-Soares MB, Gorenstein C, Tamada RS, Isller CK, Dias RS, de Almeida KM, Schwartzmann AM, Amaral JA, Lafer B (2008) Verbal fluency dysfunction in euthymic bipolar patients: a controlled study. J Affect Disord 107(1–3):187–192. doi:10.1016/j.jad.2007.07.013, S0165-0327(07)00266-2 [pii]

Decina P, Kestenbaum CJ, Farber S, Kron L, Gargan M, Sackeim HA, Fieve RR (1983) Clinical and psychological assessment of children of bipolar probands. Am J Psychiatry 140(5):548–553

Deckersbach T, McMurrich S, Ogutha J, Savage CR, Sachs G, Rauch SL (2004a) Characteristics of non-verbal memory impairment in bipolar disorder: the role of encoding strategies. Psychol Med 34(5):823–832

Deckersbach T, Savage CR, Reilly-Harrington N, Clark L, Sachs G, Rauch SL (2004b) Episodic memory impairment in bipolar disorder and obsessive-compulsive disorder: the role of memory strategies. Bipolar Disord 6(3):233–244. doi:10.1111/j.1399-5618.2004.00118.x, BDI118 [pii]

Den Hartog HM, Derix MM, Van Bemmel AL, Kremer B, Jolles J (2003) Cognitive functioning in young and middle-aged unmedicated out-patients with major depression: testing the effort and cognitive speed hypotheses. Psychol Med 33(8):1443–1451

Denicoff KD, Ali SO, Mirsky AF, Smith-Jackson EE, Leverich GS, Duncan CC, Connell EG, Post RM (1999) Relationship between prior course of illness and neuropsychological functioning in patients with bipolar disorder. J Affect Disord 56(1):67–73. doi:S0165-0327(99)00028-2 [pii]

Depp CA, Savla GN, de Dios LA, Mausbach BT, Palmer BW (2012) Affective symptoms and intra-individual variability in the short-term course of cognitive functioning in bipolar disorder. Psychol Med 42(7):1409–1416. doi:10.1017/S0033291711002662, S0033291711002662 [pii]

Derntl B, Seidel EM, Kryspin-Exner I, Hasmann A, Dobmeier M (2009) Facial emotion recognition in patients with bipolar I and bipolar II disorder. Br J Clin Psychol 48(Pt 4):363–375. doi: 10.1348/014466509X404845, bjcp682 [pii]

Dhingra U, Rabins PV (1991) Mania in the elderly: a 5–7 year follow-up. J Am Geriatr Soc 39(6):581–583

Dias VV, Brissos S, Carita AI (2008) Clinical and neurocognitive correlates of insight in patients with bipolar I disorder in remission. Acta Psychiatr Scand 117(1):28–34. doi:10.1111/j.1600-0447.2007.01110.x, ACP1110 [pii]

Dickerson FB, Sommerville J, Origoni AE, Ringel NB, Parente F (2001) Outpatients with schizophrenia and bipolar I disorder: Do they differ in their cognitive and social functioning? Psychiatry Res 102(1):21–27. doi:S0165-1781(01)00247-5 [pii]

Dickerson F, Boronow JJ, Stallings C, Origoni AE, Cole SK, Yolken RH (2004) Cognitive functioning in schizophrenia and bipolar disorder: comparison of performance on the Repeatable Battery for the Assessment of Neuropsychological Status. Psychiatry Res 129(1):45–53. doi:10.1016/j.psychres.2004.07.002, S0165-1781(04)00176-3 [pii]

Dickstein DP, Treland JE, Snow J, McClure EB, Mehta MS, Towbin KE, Pine DS, Leibenluft E (2004) Neuropsychological performance in pediatric bipolar disorder. Biol Psychiatry 55(1):32–39. doi:S0006322303007017 [pii]

Dittmann S, Hennig-Fast K, Gerber S, Seemuller F, Riedel M, Emanuel Severus W, Langosch J, Engel RR, Moller HJ, Grunze HC (2008a) Cognitive functioning in euthymic bipolar I and bipolar II patients. Bipolar Disord 10(8):877–887. doi:10.1111/j.1399-5618.2008.00640.x, BDI640 [pii]

Dittmann S, Seemuller F, Grunze HC, Schwarz MJ, Zach J, Fast K, Born C, Dargel S, Engel RR, Bernhard B, Moller HJ, Riedel M, Severus WE (2008b) The impact of homocysteine levels on cognition in euthymic bipolar patients: a cross-sectional study. J Clin Psychiatry 69(6):899–906. doi:ej07m03446 [pii]

Dixon T, Kravariti E, Frith C, Murray RM, McGuire PK (2004) Effect of symptoms on executive function in bipolar illness. Psychol Med 34(5):811–821

Docherty NM, Hawkins KA, Hoffman RE, Quinlan DM, Rakfeldt J, Sledge WH (1996) Working memory, attention, and communication disturbances in schizophrenia. J Abnorm Psychol 105(2):212–219

Donaldson S, Goldstein LH, Landau S, Raymont V, Frangou S (2003) The Maudsley Bipolar Disorder Project: the effect of medication, family history, and duration of illness on IQ and memory in bipolar I disorder. J Clin Psychiatry 64(1):86–93

Donohoe G, Duignan A, Hargreaves A, Morris DW, Rose E, Robertson D, Cummings E, Moore S, Gill M, Corvin A (2012) Social cognition in bipolar disorder versus schizophrenia: comparability in mental state decoding deficits. Bipolar Disord 14(7):743–748. doi:10.1111/bdi.12011 el Massioui F, Lesevre N (1988) Attention impairment and psychomotor retardation in depressed patients: an event-related potential study. Electroencephalogr Clin Neurophysiol 70(1):46–55

El-Badri SM, Ashton CH, Moore PB, Marsh VR, Ferrier IN (2001) Electrophysiological and cognitive function in young euthymic patients with bipolar affective disorder. Bipolar Disord 3(2):79–87

Elshahawi HH, Essawi H, Rabie MA, Mansour M, Beshry ZA, Mansour AN (2011) Cognitive functions among euthymic bipolar I patients after a single manic episode versus recurrent episodes. J Affect Disord 130(1–2):180–191. doi:10.1016/j.jad.2010.10.027, S0165-0327(10)00641-5 [pii]

Engelsmann F, Katz J, Ghadirian AM, Schachter D (1988) Lithium and memory: a long-term follow-up study. J Clin Psychopharmacol 8(3):207–212

Ferrier IN, Stanton BR, Kelly TP, Scott J (1999) Neuropsychological function in euthymic patients with bipolar disorder. Br J Psychiatry 175:246–251

Ferrier IN, Chowdhury R, Thompson JM, Watson S, Young AH (2004) Neurocognitive function in unaffected first-degree relatives of patients with bipolar disorder: a preliminary report. Bipolar Disord 6(4):319–322. doi:10.1111/j.1399-5618.2004.00122.x, BDI122 [pii]

Fitzgerald D, Lucas S, Redoblado MA, Winter V, Brennan J, Anderson J, Harris A (2004) Cognitive functioning in young people with first episode psychosis: relationship to diagnosis and clinical characteristics. Aust N Z J Psychiatry 38(7):501–510. doi:10.1111/j.1440-1614.2004.01403.x, ANP1403 [pii]

Fleck DE, Shear PK, Zimmerman ME, Getz GE, Corey KB, Jak A, Lebowitz BK, Strakowski SM (2003) Verbal memory in mania: effects of clinical state and task requirements. Bipolar Disord 5(5):375–380. doi:055 [pii]

Fleck DE, Shear PK, Strakowski SM (2005) Processing efficiency and directed forgetting in bipolar disorder. J Int Neuropsychol Soc 11(7):871–880

Fleck DE, Shear PK, Madore M, Strakowski SM (2008) Wisconsin Card Sorting Test performance in bipolar disorder: effects of mood state and early course. Bipolar Disord 10(4):539–545. doi:10.1111/j.1399-5618.2008.00582.x, BDI582 [pii]

Fossati P, Harvey PO, Le Bastard G, Ergis AM, Jouvent R, Allilaire JF (2004) Verbal memory performance of patients with a first depressive episode and patients with unipolar and bipolar recurrent depression. J Psychiatr Res 38(2):137–144. doi:S0022395603001110 [pii]

Fountoulakis KN, Panagiotidis PT, Siamouli M, Magiria S, Sokolaki S, Kantartzis S, Rova K, Papastergiou N, Shoretstanitis G, Oral T, Mavridis T, Iacovides A, Kaprinis G (2008a) Development of a standardized scoring method for the Graphic Sequence Test suitable for use in psychiatric populations. Cogn Behav Neurol 21(1):18–27. doi:10.1097/WNN.0b013e318165b120, 00146965-200803000-00005 [pii]

Fountoulakis KN, Vieta E, Bouras C, Notaridis G, Giannakopoulos P, Kaprinis G, Akiskal H (2008b) A systematic review of existing data on long-term lithium therapy: neuroprotective or neurotoxic? Int J Neuropsychopharmacol 11(2):269–287. doi:10.1017/S1461145707007821, S1461145707007821 [pii]

Fountoulakis KN, Siamouli M, Magiria S, Panagiotidis PT, Kantartzis S, Terzoglou VA, Oral T (2011a) A standardized scoring method for the copy of cube test, developed to be suitable for use in psychiatric populations. Ann Gen Psychiatry 10(1):19. doi:10.1186/1744-859X-10-19, 1744-859X-10-19 [pii]

Fountoulakis KN, Siamouli M, Panagiotidis PT, Magiria S, Kantartzis S, Terzoglou VA, Oral T (2011b) The standardised copy of pentagons test. Ann Gen Psychiatry 10(1):13. doi:10.1186/1744-859X-10-13, 1744-859X-10-13 [pii]

Frangou S, Donaldson S, Hadjulis M, Landau S, Goldstein LH (2005a) The Maudsley Bipolar Disorder Project: executive dysfunction in bipolar disorder I and its clinical correlates. Biol Psychiatry 58(11):859–864. doi:10.1016/j.biopsych.2005.04.056, S0006-3223(05)00579-2 [pii]

Frangou S, Haldane M, Roddy D, Kumari V (2005b) Evidence for deficit in tasks of ventral, but not dorsal, prefrontal executive function as an endophenotypic marker for bipolar disorder. Biol Psychiatry 58(10):838–839. doi:10.1016/j.biopsych.2005.05.020, S0006-3223(05)00616-5 [pii]

Frantom LV, Allen DN, Cross CL (2008) Neurocognitive endophenotypes for bipolar disorder. Bipolar Disord 10(3):387–399. doi:10.1111/j.1399-5618.2007.00529.x, BDI529 [pii]

Friedman MJ, Culver CM, Ferrell RB (1977) On the safety of long-term treatment with lithium. Am J Psychiatry 134(10):1123–1126

Gale CR, Batty GD, McIntosh AM, Porteous DJ, Deary IJ, Rasmussen F (2012) Is bipolar disorder more common in highly intelligent people? A cohort study of a million men. Mol Psychiatry. doi:10.1038/mp.2012.26, mp201226 [pii]

Gard D, Harrell EH, Poreh A (1999) Cognitive deficits in schizophrenia on the WAIS-R NI Sentence Arrangement Subtest. Wechsler Adult Intelligence Scale-Revised Neuropsychological Inventory. J Clin Psychol 55(9):1085–1094. doi:10.1002/(SICI)1097-4679(199909)55:9<1085::AID-JCLP6>3.0.CO;2-G [pii]

Getz GE, Shear PK, Strakowski SM (2003) Facial affect recognition deficits in bipolar disorder. J Int Neuropsychol Soc 9(4):623–632. doi:10.1017/S1355617703940021, S1355617703940021 [pii]

Gilvarry C, Takei N, Russell A, Rushe T, Hemsley D, Murray RM (2000) Premorbid IQ in patients with functional psychosis and their first-degree relatives. Schizophr Res 41(3):417–429. doi:S0920-9964(99)00092-4 [pii]

Glahn DC, Bearden CE, Niendam TA, Escamilla MA (2004) The feasibility of neuropsychological endophenotypes in the search for genes associated with bipolar affective disorder. Bipolar Disord 6(3):171–182. doi:10.1111/j.1399-5618.2004.00113.x, BDI113 [pii]

Glahn DC, Barrett J, Bearden CE, Mintz J, Green MF, Serap Monkul E, Najt P, Soares JC, Velligan DI (2006a) Dissociable mechanisms for memory impairment in bipolar disorder and schizophrenia. Psychol Med 36(8):1085–1095. doi:10.1017/S0033291706007902, S0033291706007902 [pii]

Glahn DC, Bearden CE, Bowden CL, Soares JC (2006b) Reduced educational attainment in bipolar disorder. J Affect Disord 92(2–3):309–312. doi:10.1016/j.jad.2006.01.025, S0165-0327(06)00046-2 [pii]

Glahn DC, Bearden CE, Cakir S, Barrett JA, Najt P, Serap Monkul E, Maples N, Velligan DI, Soares JC (2006c) Differential working memory impairment in bipolar disorder and schizophrenia: effects of lifetime history of psychosis. Bipolar Disord 8(2):117–123. doi:10.1111/j.1399-5618.2006.00296.x, BDI296 [pii]

Glahn DC, Bearden CE, Barguil M, Barrett J, Reichenberg A, Bowden CL, Soares JC, Velligan DI (2007) The neurocognitive signature of psychotic bipolar disorder. Biol Psychiatry 62(8):910–916. doi:10.1016/j.biopsych.2007.02.001, S0006-3223(07)00102-3 [pii]

Glahn DC, Almasy L, Barguil M, Hare E, Peralta JM, Kent JW Jr, Dassori A, Contreras J, Pacheco A, Lanzagorta N, Nicolini H, Raventos H, Escamilla MA (2010) Neurocognitive endophenotypes for bipolar disorder identified in multiplex multigenerational families. Arch Gen Psychiatry 67(2):168–177. doi:10.1001/archgenpsychiatry.2009.184, 67/2/168 [pii]

Goldberg J (2008) Adverse cognitive effects of psychotropic medications. In: Goldberg J, Burdick K (eds) Cognitive dysfunction in bipolar disorder: a guide for clinicians. American Psychiatric Press, Washington, DC, pp 137–158

Goldberg JF, Chengappa KN (2009) Identifying and treating cognitive impairment in bipolar disorder. Bipolar Disord 11(Suppl 2):123–137. doi:10.1111/j.1399-5618.2009.00716.x, BDI716 [pii]

Goldberg TE, Gold JM, Greenberg R, Griffin S, Schulz SC, Pickar D, Kleinman JE, Weinberger DR (1993) Contrasts between patients with affective disorders and patients with schizophrenia on a neuropsychological test battery. Am J Psychiatry 150(9):1355–1362

Gooding DC, Tallent KA (2001) The association between antisaccade task and working memory task performance in schizophrenia and bipolar disorder. J Nerv Ment Dis 189(1):8–16

Goodwin F, Jamison K (2007) Manic-depressive illness, 2nd edn. Oxford University Press, New York

Gorlyn M, Keilp JG, Oquendo MA, Burke AK, Sackeim HA, John Mann J (2006) The WAIS-III and major depression: absence of VIQ/PIQ differences. J Clin Exp Neuropsychol 28(7):1145–1157. doi:10.1080/13803390500246944, H44344LVQ511N361 [pii]

Goswami U, Sharma A, Khastigir U, Ferrier IN, Young AH, Gallagher P, Thompson JM, Moore PB (2006) Neuropsychological dysfunction, soft neurological signs and social disability in euthymic patients with bipolar disorder. Br J Psychiatry 188:366–373. doi:10.1192/bjp.188.4.366, 188/4/366 [pii]

Goswami U, Sharma A, Varma A, Gulrajani C, Ferrier IN, Young AH, Gallagher P, Thompson JM, Moore PB (2009) The neurocognitive performance of drug-free and medicated euthymic bipolar patients do not differ. Acta Psychiatr Scand 120(6):456–463. doi:10.1111/j.1600-0447.2009.01390.x, ACP1390 [pii]

Gourovitch ML, Torrey EF, Gold JM, Randolph C, Weinberger DR, Goldberg TE (1999) Neuropsychological performance of monozygotic twins discordant for bipolar disorder. Biol Psychiatry 45(5):639–646. doi:S0006-3223(98)00148-6 [pii]

Green MF, Nuechterlein KH, Mintz J (1994a) Backward masking in schizophrenia and mania. I. Specifying a mechanism. Arch Gen Psychiatry 51(12):939–944

Green MF, Nuechterlein KH, Mintz J (1994b) Backward masking in schizophrenia and mania. II. Specifying the visual channels. Arch Gen Psychiatry 51(12):945–951

Gruber S, Rathgeber K, Braunig P, Gauggel S (2007) Stability and course of neuropsychological deficits in manic and depressed bipolar patients compared to patients with major depression. J Affect Disord 104(1–3):61–71. doi:10.1016/j.jad.2007.02.011, S0165-0327(07)00083-3 [pii]

Gruber SA, Rosso IM, Yurgelun-Todd D (2008) Neuropsychological performance predicts clinical recovery in bipolar patients. J Affect Disord 105(1–3):253–260. doi:10.1016/j.jad.2007.04.014, S0165-0327(07)00138-3 [pii]

Gruzelier J, Seymour K, Wilson L, Jolley A, Hirsch S (1988) Impairments on neuropsychologic tests of temporohippocampal and frontohippocampal functions and word fluency in remitting schizophrenia and affective disorders. Arch Gen Psychiatry 45(7):623–629

Gualtieri CT, Morgan DW (2008) The frequency of cognitive impairment in patients with anxiety, depression, and bipolar disorder: an unaccounted source of variance in clinical trials. J Clin Psychiatry 69(7):1122–1130. doi:ej07m03786 [pii]

Ha TH, Kim JS, Chang JS, Oh SH, Her JY, Cho HS, Park TS, Shin SY, Ha K (2012) Verbal and visual memory impairments in bipolar I and II disorder. Psychiatry Investig 9(4):339–346. doi:10.4306/pi.2012.9.4.339

Hammar A (2003) Automatic and effortful information processing in unipolar major depression. Scand J Psychol 44(5):409–413

Hammar A, Lund A, Hugdahl K (2003a) Long-lasting cognitive impairment in unipolar major depression: a 6-month follow-up study. Psychiatry Res 118(2):189–196. doi:S0165178103000751 [pii]

Hammar A, Lund A, Hugdahl K (2003b) Selective impairment in effortful information processing in major depression. J Int Neuropsychol Soc 9(6):954–959. doi:10.1017/S1355617703960152, S1355617703960152 [pii]

Harkavy-Friedman JM, Keilp JG, Grunebaum MF, Sher L, Printz D, Burke AK, Mann JJ, Oquendo M (2006) Are BPI and BPII suicide attempters distinct neuropsychologically? J Affect Disord 94(1–3):255–259. doi:10.1016/j.jad.2006.04.010, S0165-0327(06)00182-0 [pii]

Harmer CJ, Clark L, Grayson L, Goodwin GM (2002a) Sustained attention deficit in bipolar disorder is not a working memory impairment in disguise. Neuropsychologia 40(9):1586–1590. doi:S0028393202000192 [pii]

Harmer CJ, Grayson L, Goodwin GM (2002b) Enhanced recognition of disgust in bipolar illness. Biol Psychiatry 51(4):298–304. doi:S0006322301012495 [pii]

Hartlage S, Alloy LB, Vazquez C, Dykman B (1993) Automatic and effortful processing in depression. Psychol Bull 113(2):247–278

Harvey PD, Weintraub S, Neale JM (1982) Speech competence of children vulnerable to psychopathology. J Abnorm Child Psychol 10(3):373–387

Hawkins KA, Hoffman RE, Quinlan DM, Rakfeldt J, Docherty NM, Sledge WH (1997) Cognition, negative symptoms, and diagnosis: a comparison of schizophrenic, bipolar, and control samples. J Neuropsychiatry Clin Neurosci 9(1):81–89

Hellgren L, Gillberg IC, Bagenholm A, Gillberg C (1994) Children with deficits in attention, motor control and perception (DAMP) almost grown up: psychiatric and personality disorders at age 16 years. J Child Psychol Psychiatry 35(7):1255–1271

Hill SK, Reilly JL, Harris MS, Rosen C, Marvin RW, Deleon O, Sweeney JA (2009) A comparison of neuropsychological dysfunction in first-episode psychosis patients with unipolar depression, bipolar disorder, and schizophrenia. Schizophr Res 113(2–3):167–175. doi:10.1016/j.schres.2009.04.020, S0920-9964(09)00177-7 [pii]

Hobart MP, Goldberg R, Bartko JJ, Gold JM (1999) Repeatable battery for the assessment of neuropsychological status as a screening test in schizophrenia, II: convergent/discriminant validity and diagnostic group comparisons. Am J Psychiatry 156(12):1951–1957

Hoff AL, Shukla S, Aronson T, Cook B, Ollo C, Baruch S, Jandorf L, Schwartz J (1990) Failure to differentiate bipolar disorder from schizophrenia on measures of neuropsychological function. Schizophr Res 3(4):253–260. doi:0920-9964(90)90006-S [pii]

Holmes MK, Erickson K, Luckenbaugh DA, Drevets WC, Bain EE, Cannon DM, Snow J, Sahakian BJ, Manji HK, Zarate CA Jr (2008) A comparison of cognitive functioning in medicated and unmedicated subjects with bipolar depression. Bipolar Disord 10(7):806–815. doi:10.1111/j.1399-5618.2008.00628.x, BDI628 [pii]

Honig A, Arts BM, Ponds RW, Riedel WJ (1999) Lithium induced cognitive side-effects in bipolar disorder: a qualitative analysis and implications for daily practice. Int Clin Psychopharmacol 14(3):167–171

Hsiao YL, Wu YS, Wu JY, Hsu MH, Chen HC, Lee SY, Lee IH, Yeh TL, Yang YK, Ko HC, Lu RB (2009) Neuropsychological functions in patients with bipolar I and bipolar II disorder. Bipolar Disord 11(5):547–554. doi:10.1111/j.1399-5618.2009.00723.x, BDI723 [pii]

Inoue Y, Tonooka Y, Yamada K, Kanba S (2004) Deficiency of theory of mind in patients with remitted mood disorder. J Affect Disord 82(3):403–409. doi:10.1016/j.jad.2004.04.004, S016503270400148X [pii]

Jabben N, Arts B, Krabbendam L, van Os J (2009) Investigating the association between neurocognition and psychosis in bipolar disorder: further evidence for the overlap with schizophrenia. Bipolar Disord 11(2):166–177. doi:10.1111/j.1399-5618.2009.00663.x, BDI663 [pii]

Jabben N, Arts B, van Os J, Krabbendam L (2010) Neurocognitive functioning as intermediary phenotype and predictor of psychosocial functioning across the psychosis continuum: studies in schizophrenia and bipolar disorder. J Clin Psychiatry 71(6):764–774. doi:10.4088/JCP.08m04837yel

Jaeger J, Berns S, Loftus S, Gonzalez C, Czobor P (2007) Neurocognitive test performance predicts functional recovery from acute exacerbation leading to hospitalization in bipolar disorder. Bipolar Disord 9(1–2):93–102. doi:10.1111/j.1399-5618.2007.00427.x, BDI427 [pii]

Jamison KR (1989) Mood disorders and patterns of creativity in British writers and artists. Psychiatry 52(2):125–134

Jamison KR (1995) Manic-depressive illness and creativity. Sci Am 272(2):62–67

Jamrozinski K (2010) Do euthymic bipolar patients have normal cognitive functioning? Curr Opin Psychiatry 23(3):255–260. doi:10.1097/YCO.0b013e328338620a

Jamrozinski K, Gruber O, Kemmer C, Falkai P, Scherk H (2009) Neurocognitive functions in euthymic bipolar patients. Acta Psychiatr Scand 119(5):365–374. doi:10.1111/j.1600-0447.2008.01320.x, ACP1320 [pii]

Joffe RT, MacDonald C, Kutcher SP (1988) Lack of differential cognitive effects of lithium and carbamazepine in bipolar affective disorder. J Clin Psychopharmacol 8(6):425–428

Jones PB, Bebbington P, Foerster A, Lewis SW, Murray RM, Russell A, Sham PC, Toone BK, Wilkins S (1993) Premorbid social underachievement in schizophrenia. Results from the Camberwell Collaborative Psychosis Study. Br J Psychiatry 162:65–71

Karniol IG, Dalton J, Lader MH (1978) Acute and chronic effects of lithium chloride on physiological and psychological measures in normals. Psychopharmacology (Berl) 57(3):289–294

Kathleen Holmes M, Bearden CE, Barguil M, Fonseca M, Serap Monkul E, Nery FG, Soares JC, Mintz J, Glahn DC (2009) Conceptualizing impulsivity and risk taking in bipolar disorder: importance of history of alcohol abuse. Bipolar Disord 11(1):33–40. doi:10.1111/j.1399-5618.2008.00657.x, BDI657 [pii]

Kaya E, Aydemir O, Selcuki D (2007) Residual symptoms in bipolar disorder: the effect of the last episode after remission. Prog Neuropsychopharmacol Biol Psychiatry 31(7):1387–1392. doi:10.1016/j.pnpbp.2007.06.003, S0278-5846(07)00194-7 [pii]

Keri S, Kelemen O, Benedek G, Janka Z (2001) Different trait markers for schizophrenia and bipolar disorder: a neurocognitive approach. Psychol Med 31(5):915–922

Kerr N, Dunbar RI, Bentall RP (2003) Theory of mind deficits in bipolar affective disorder. J Affect Disord 73(3):253–259. doi:S0165032702000083 [pii]

Kerr N, Scott J, Phillips ML (2005) Patterns of attentional deficits and emotional bias in bipolar and major depressive disorder. Br J Clin Psychol 44(Pt3):343–356. doi:10.1348/014466505X57755

Kerry RJ, McDermott CM, Orme JE (1983) Affective disorders and cognitive performance. A clinical report. J Affect Disord 5(4):349–352

Kessing LV (1998) Cognitive impairment in the euthymic phase of affective disorder. Psychol Med 28(5):1027–1038

Kessing LV, Andersen PK (2004) Does the risk of developing dementia increase with the number of episodes in patients with depressive disorder and in patients with bipolar disorder? J Neurol Neurosurg Psychiatry 75(12):1662–1666. doi:10.1136/jnnp.2003.031773, 75/12/1662 [pii]

Kessing LV, Nilsson FM (2003) Increased risk of developing dementia in patients with major affective disorders compared to patients with other medical illnesses. J Affect Disord 73(3): 261–269. doi:S0165032702000046 [pii]

Kieseppa T, Tuulio-Henriksson A, Haukka J, Van Erp T, Glahn D, Cannon TD, Partonen T, Kaprio J, Lonnqvist J (2005) Memory and verbal learning functions in twins with bipolar-I disorder, and the role of information-processing speed. Psychol Med 35(2):205–215

Kim E, Jung YC, Ku J, Kim JJ, Lee H, Kim SY, Kim SI, Cho HS (2009) Reduced activation in the mirror neuron system during a virtual social cognition task in euthymic bipolar disorder. Prog Neuropsychopharmacol Biol Psychiatry 33(8):1409–1416. doi:10.1016/j.pnpbp.2009.07.019, S0278-5846(09)00247-4 [pii]

King DJ (1994) Psychomotor impairment and cognitive disturbances induced by neuroleptics. Acta Psychiatr Scand Suppl 380:53–58

Klimes-Dougan B, Ronsaville D, Wiggs EA, Martinez PE (2006) Neuropsychological functioning in adolescent children of mothers with a history of bipolar or major depressive disorders. Biol Psychiatry 60(9):957–965. doi:10.1016/j.biopsych.2006.03.031, S0006-3223(06)00460-4 [pii]

Kluger A, Goldberg E (1990) IQ patterns in affective disorder, lateralized and diffuse brain damage. J Clin Exp Neuropsychol 12(2):182–194. doi:10.1080/01688639008400966

Kocsis JH, Shaw ED, Stokes PE, Wilner P, Elliot AS, Sikes C, Myers B, Manevitz A, Parides M (1993) Neuropsychologic effects of lithium discontinuation. J Clin Psychopharmacol 13(4):268–275

Koenen KC, Moffitt TE, Roberts AL, Martin LT, Kubzansky L, Harrington H, Poulton R, Caspi A (2009) Childhood IQ and adult mental disorders: a test of the cognitive reserve hypothesis. Am J Psychiatry 166(1):50–57. doi:10.1176/appi.ajp.2008.08030343, appi.ajp.2008.08030343 [pii]

Kolur US, Reddy YC, John JP, Kandavel T, Jain S (2006) Sustained attention and executive functions in euthymic young people with bipolar disorder. Br J Psychiatry 189:453–458. doi:10.1192/bjp.bp.106.022921, 189/5/453 [pii]

Krabbendam L, Honig A, Wiersma J, Vuurman EF, Hofman PA, Derix MM, Nolen WA, Jolles J (2000) Cognitive dysfunctions and white matter lesions in patients with bipolar disorder in remission. Acta Psychiatr Scand 101(4):274–280

Krabbendam L, Arts B, van Os J, Aleman A (2005) Cognitive functioning in patients with schizophrenia and bipolar disorder: a quantitative review. Schizophr Res 80(2–3):137–149. doi:10.1016/j.schres.2005.08.004, S0920-9964(05)00360-9 [pii]

Kravariti E, Schulze K, Kane F, Kalidindi S, Bramon E, Walshe M, Marshall N, Hall MH, Georgiades A, McDonald C, Murray RM (2009) Stroop-test interference in bipolar disorder. Br J Psychiatry 194(3):285–286. doi:10.1192/bjp.bp.108.052639, 194/3/285 [pii]

Kremen WS, Faraone SV, Seidman LJ, Pepple JR, Tsuang MT (1998) Neuropsychological risk indicators for schizophrenia: a preliminary study of female relatives of schizophrenic and bipolar probands. Psychiatry Res 79(3):227–240. doi:S0165-1781(98)00042-0 [pii]

Kremen WS, Seidman LJ, Faraone SV, Tsuang MT (2003) Is there disproportionate impairment in semantic or phonemic fluency in schizophrenia? J Int Neuropsychol Soc 9(1):79–88

Kron L, Decina P, Kestenbaum CJ, Farber S, Gargan M, Fieve R (1982) The offspring of bipolar manic-depressives: clinical features. Adolesc Psychiatry 10:273–291

Kropf D, Muller-Oerlinghausen B (1979) Changes in learning, memory, and mood during lithium treatment. Approach to a research strategy. Acta Psychiatr Scand 59(1):97–124
Kruger S, Seminowicz D, Goldapple K, Kennedy SH, Mayberg HS (2003) State and trait influences on mood regulation in bipolar disorder: blood flow differences with an acute mood challenge. Biol Psychiatry 54(11):1274–1283. doi:S0006322303006917 [pii]
Kucharska-Pietura K, David AS (2003) The perception of emotional chimeric faces in patients with depression, mania and unilateral brain damage. Psychol Med 33(4):739–745
Kulkarni S, Jain S, Janardhan Reddy YC, Kumar KJ, Kandavel T (2010) Impairment of verbal learning and memory and executive function in unaffected siblings of probands with bipolar disorder. Bipolar Disord 12(6):647–656. doi:10.1111/j.1399-5618.2010.00857.x
Kurtz MM, Gerraty RT (2009) A meta-analytic investigation of neurocognitive deficits in bipolar illness: profile and effects of clinical state. Neuropsychology 23(5):551–562. doi:10.1037/a0016277, 2009-12548-002 [pii]
Kutcher S, Robertson HA, Bird D (1998) Premorbid functioning in adolescent onset bipolar I disorder: a preliminary report from an ongoing study. J Affect Disord 51(2):137–144. doi:S0165032798002122 [pii]
Lahera G, Montes JM, Benito A, Valdivia M, Medina E, Mirapeix I, Saiz-Ruiz J (2008) Theory of mind deficit in bipolar disorder: is it related to a previous history of psychotic symptoms? Psychiatry Res 161(3):309–317. doi:10.1016/j.psychres.2007.08.009, S0165-1781(07)00293-4 [pii]
Lahera G, Ruiz-Murugarren S, Iglesias P, Ruiz-Bennasar C, Herreria E, Montes JM, Fernandez-Liria A (2012) Social cognition and global functioning in bipolar disorder. J Nerv Ment Dis 200(2):135–141. doi:10.1097/NMD.0b013e3182438eae, 00005053-201202000-00004 [pii]
Landro NI, Orbeck AL, Rund BR (1993) Memory functioning in chronic and non-chronic schizophrenics, affectively disturbed patients and normal controls. Schizophr Res 10(1):85–92
Langenecker SA, Saunders EF, Kade AM, Ransom MT, McInnis MG (2010) Intermediate: cognitive phenotypes in bipolar disorder. J Affect Disord 122(3):285–293. doi:10.1016/j.jad.2009.08.018, S0165-0327(09)00399-1 [pii]
Larson ER, Shear PK, Krikorian R, Welge J, Strakowski SM (2005) Working memory and inhibitory control among manic and euthymic patients with bipolar disorder. J Int Neuropsychol Soc 11(2):163–172
Lebowitz BK, Shear PK, Steed MA, Strakowski SM (2001) Verbal fluency in mania: relationship to number of manic episodes. Neuropsychiatry Neuropsychol Behav Neurol 14(3):177–182
Lembke A, Ketter TA (2002) Impaired recognition of facial emotion in mania. Am J Psychiatry 159(2):302–304
Lennox BR, Jacob R, Calder AJ, Lupson V, Bullmore ET (2004) Behavioural and neurocognitive responses to sad facial affect are attenuated in patients with mania. Psychol Med 34(5):795–802
Levy B, Weiss RD (2010) Neurocognitive impairment and psychosis in bipolar I disorder during early remission from an acute episode of mood disturbance. J Clin Psychiatry 71(2):201–206. doi:10.4088/JCP.08m04663yel
Lewandowski KE, Cohen BM, Ongur D (2011) Evolution of neuropsychological dysfunction during the course of schizophrenia and bipolar disorder. Psychol Med 41(2):225–241. doi:10.1017/S0033291710001042, S0033291710001042 [pii]
Lior R, Nachson I (1999) Impairments in judgment of chimeric faces by schizophrenic and affective patients. Int J Neurosci 97(3–4):185–209
Liu SK, Chiu CH, Chang CJ, Hwang TJ, Hwu HG, Chen WJ (2002) Deficits in sustained attention in schizophrenia and affective disorders: stable versus state-dependent markers. Am J Psychiatry 159(6):975–982
Lopez-Jaramillo C, Lopera-Vasquez J, Gallo A, Ospina-Duque J, Bell V, Torrent C, Martinez-Aran A, Vieta E (2010) Effects of recurrence on the cognitive performance of patients with bipolar I disorder: implications for relapse prevention and treatment adherence. Bipolar Disord 12(5):557–567. doi:10.1111/j.1399-5618.2010.00835.x, BDI835 [pii]
Loughland CM, Williams LM, Gordon E (2002) Schizophrenia and affective disorder show different visual scanning behavior for faces: a trait versus state-based distinction? Biol Psychiatry 52(4):338–348. doi:S0006322302013562 [pii]

Lund Y, Nissen M, Rafaelsen OJ (1982) Long-term lithium treatment and psychological functions. Acta Psychiatr Scand 65(3):233–244

Maalouf FT, Klein C, Clark L, Sahakian BJ, Labarbara EJ, Versace A, Hassel S, Almeida JR, Phillips ML (2010) Impaired sustained attention and executive dysfunction: bipolar disorder versus depression-specific markers of affective disorders. Neuropsychologia 48(6):1862–1868. doi:10.1016/j.neuropsychologia.2010.02.015, S0028-3932(10)00069-2 [pii]

Maarbjerg K, Aagaard J, Vestergaard P (1988) Adherence to lithium prophylaxis: I. Clinical predictors and patient's reasons for nonadherence. Pharmacopsychiatry 21(3):121–125. doi:10.1055/s-2007-1014662

MacQueen GM, Grof P, Alda M, Marriott M, Young LT, Duffy A (2004) A pilot study of visual backward masking performance among affected versus unaffected offspring of parents with bipolar disorder. Bipolar Disord 6(5):374–378. doi:10.1111/j.1399-5618.2004.00133.x, BDI133 [pii]

Malhi GS, Ivanovski B, Szekeres V, Olley A (2004) Bipolar disorder: it's all in your mind? The neuropsychological profile of a biological disorder. Can J Psychiatry 49(12):813–819

Malhi GS, Ivanovski B, Hadzi-Pavlovic D, Mitchell PB, Vieta E, Sachdev P (2007a) Neuropsychological deficits and functional impairment in bipolar depression, hypomania and euthymia. Bipolar Disord 9(1–2):114–125. doi:10.1111/j.1399-5618.2007.00324.x, BDI324 [pii]

Malhi GS, Lagopoulos J, Sachdev PS, Ivanovski B, Shnier R, Ketter T (2007b) Is a lack of disgust something to fear? A functional magnetic resonance imaging facial emotion recognition study in euthymic bipolar disorder patients. Bipolar Disord 9(4):345–357. doi:10.1111/j.1399-5618.2007.00485.x, BDI485 [pii]

Malloy-Diniz LF, Neves FS, Abrantes SS, Fuentes D, Correa H (2009) Suicide behavior and neuropsychological assessment of type I bipolar patients. J Affect Disord 112(1–3):231–236. doi:10.1016/j.jad.2008.03.019, S0165-0327(08)00143-2 [pii]

Mann-Wrobel MC, Carreno JT, Dickinson D (2011) Meta-analysis of neuropsychological functioning in euthymic bipolar disorder: an update and investigation of moderator variables. Bipolar Disord 13(4):334–342. doi:10.1111/j.1399-5618.2011.00935.x

Martinez-Aran A, Penades R, Vieta E, Colom F, Reinares M, Benabarre A, Salamero M, Gasto C (2002) Executive function in patients with remitted bipolar disorder and schizophrenia and its relationship with functional outcome. Psychother Psychosom 71(1):39–46. doi:pps71039 [pii]

Martinez-Aran A, Vieta E, Reinares M, Colom F, Torrent C, Sanchez-Moreno J, Benabarre A, Goikolea JM, Comes M, Salamero M (2004) Cognitive function across manic or hypomanic, depressed, and euthymic states in bipolar disorder. Am J Psychiatry 161(2):262–270

Martinez-Aran A, Vieta E, Colom F, Torrent C, Reinares M, Goikolea JM, Benabarre A, Comes M, Sanchez-Moreno J (2005) Do cognitive complaints in euthymic bipolar patients reflect objective cognitive impairment? Psychother Psychosom 74(5):295–302. doi:10.1159/000086320, 86320 [pii]

Martinez-Aran A, Vieta E, Torrent C, Sanchez-Moreno J, Goikolea JM, Salamero M, Malhi GS, Gonzalez-Pinto A, Daban C, Alvarez-Grandi S, Fountoulakis K, Kaprinis G, Tabares-Seisdedos R, Ayuso-Mateos JL (2007) Functional outcome in bipolar disorder: the role of clinical and cognitive factors. Bipolar Disord 9(1–2):103–113. doi:10.1111/j.1399-5618.2007.00327.x, BDI327 [pii]

Martinez-Aran A, Torrent C, Tabares-Seisdedos R, Salamero M, Daban C, Balanza-Martinez V, Sanchez-Moreno J, Manuel Goikolea J, Benabarre A, Colom F, Vieta E (2008) Neurocognitive impairment in bipolar patients with and without history of psychosis. J Clin Psychiatry 69(2):233–239. doi:ej06m02909 [pii]

Martinez-Aran A, Scott J, Colom F, Torrent C, Tabares-Seisdedos R, Daban C, Leboyer M, Henry C, Goodwin GM, Gonzalez-Pinto A, Cruz N, Sanchez-Moreno J, Vieta E (2009) Treatment nonadherence and neurocognitive impairment in bipolar disorder. J Clin Psychiatry 70(7):1017–1023. doi:10.4088/JCP.08m04408

Martino DJ, Strejilevich SA, Scapola M, Igoa A, Marengo E, Ais ED, Perinot L (2008) Heterogeneity in cognitive functioning among patients with bipolar disorder. J Affect Disord 109(1–2):149–156. doi:10.1016/j.jad.2007.12.232, S0165-0327(07)00656-8 [pii]

Martino DJ, Igoa A, Marengo E, Scapola M, Strejilevich SA (2011a) Neurocognitive impairments and their relationship with psychosocial functioning in euthymic bipolar II disorder. J Nerv Ment Dis 199(7):459–464. doi:10.1097/NMD.0b013e3182214190, 00005053-201107000-00007 [pii]

Martino DJ, Strejilevich SA, Fassi G, Marengo E, Igoa A (2011b) Theory of mind and facial emotion recognition in euthymic bipolar I and bipolar II disorders. Psychiatry Res 189(3):379–384. doi:10.1016/j.psychres.2011.04.033, S0165-1781(11)00364-7 [pii]

Martino DJ, Strejilevich SA, Marengo E, Igoa A, Fassi G, Teitelbaum J, Caravotta P (2012) Relationship between neurocognitive functioning and episode recurrences in bipolar disorder. J Affect Disord. doi:10.1016/j.jad.2012.11.037, S0165-0327(12)00804-X [pii]

Marvel CL, Paradiso S (2004) Cognitive and neurological impairment in mood disorders. Psychiatr Clin North Am 27(1):19–36, vii–viii. doi:10.1016/S0193-953X(03)00106-0, S0193953X03001060 [pii]

Mason CF (1956) Pre-illness intelligence of mental hospital patients. J Consult Psychol 20(4): 297–300

McDonough-Ryan P, DelBello M, Shear PK, Ris DM, Soutullo C, Strakowski SM (2002) Academic and cognitive abilities in children of parents with bipolar disorder: a test of the nonverbal learning disability model. J Clin Exp Neuropsychol 24(3):280–285. doi:10.1076/jcen.24.3.280.980

McGrath J, Scheldt S, Welham J, Clair A (1997) Performance on tests sensitive to impaired executive ability in schizophrenia, mania and well controls: acute and subacute phases. Schizophr Res 26(2–3):127–137. doi:S0920-9964(97)00070-4 [pii]

McGrath J, Chapple B, Wright M (2001) Working memory in schizophrenia and mania: correlation with symptoms during the acute and subacute phases. Acta Psychiatr Scand 103(3):181–188. doi:acp114 [pii]

McIntosh AM, Harrison LK, Forrester K, Lawrie SM, Johnstone EC (2005) Neuropsychological impairments in people with schizophrenia or bipolar disorder and their unaffected relatives. Br J Psychiatry 186:378–385. doi:10.1192/bjp.186.5.378, 186/5/378 [pii]

McKay AP, Tarbuck AF, Shapleske J, McKenna PJ (1995) Neuropsychological function in manic-depressive psychosis. Evidence for persistent deficits in patients with chronic, severe illness. Br J Psychiatry 167(1):51–57

Meyer SE, Carlson GA, Wiggs EA, Martinez PE, Ronsaville DS, Klimes-Dougan B, Gold PW, Radke-Yarrow M (2004) A prospective study of the association among impaired executive functioning, childhood attentional problems, and the development of bipolar disorder. Dev Psychopathol 16(2):461–476

Mojtabai R, Bromet EJ, Harvey PD, Carlson GA, Craig TJ, Fennig S (2000) Neuropsychological differences between first-admission schizophrenia and psychotic affective disorders. Am J Psychiatry 157(9):1453–1460

Montag C, Ehrlich A, Neuhaus K, Dziobek I, Heekeren HR, Heinz A, Gallinat J (2010) Theory of mind impairments in euthymic bipolar patients. J Affect Disord 123(1–3):264–269. doi:10.1016/j.jad.2009.08.017, S0165-0327(09)00390-5 [pii]

Morice R (1990) Cognitive inflexibility and pre-frontal dysfunction in schizophrenia and mania. Br J Psychiatry 157:50–54

Mur M, Portella MJ, Martinez-Aran A, Pifarre J, Vieta E (2007) Persistent neuropsychological deficit in euthymic bipolar patients: executive function as a core deficit. J Clin Psychiatry 68(7):1078–1086

Mur M, Portella MJ, Martinez-Aran A, Pifarre J, Vieta E (2008) Long-term stability of cognitive impairment in bipolar disorder: a 2-year follow-up study of lithium-treated euthymic bipolar patients. J Clin Psychiatry 69(5):712–719. doi:ej07m03354 [pii]

Nehra R, Chakrabarti S, Pradhan BK, Khehra N (2006) Comparison of cognitive functions between first- and multi-episode bipolar affective disorders. J Affect Disord 93(1–3):185–192. doi:10.1016/j.jad.2006.03.013, S0165-0327(06)00139-X [pii]

Newcomer JW (2006) Medical risk in patients with bipolar disorder and schizophrenia. J Clin Psychiatry 67(11):e16

Olley AL, Malhi GS, Bachelor J, Cahill CM, Mitchell PB, Berk M (2005) Executive functioning and theory of mind in euthymic bipolar disorder. Bipolar Disord 7(Suppl 5):43–52. doi:10.1111/j.1399-5618.2005.00254.x, BDI254 [pii]

Osuji IJ, Cullum CM (2005) Cognition in bipolar disorder. Psychiatr Clin North Am 28(2): 427–441. doi:10.1016/j.psc.2005.02.005, S0193-953X(05)00027-4 [pii]

Pan YJ, Hsieh MH, Liu SK (2011) Visuospatial working memory deficits in remitted patients with bipolar disorder: susceptibility to the effects of GABAergic agonists. Bipolar Disord 13(4):365–376. doi:10.1111/j.1399-5618.2011.00931.x

Paradiso S, Lamberty GJ, Garvey MJ, Robinson RG (1997) Cognitive impairment in the euthymic phase of chronic unipolar depression. J Nerv Ment Dis 185(12):748–754

Park S (1997) Association of an oculomotor delayed response task and the Wisconsin Card Sort Test in schizophrenic patients. Int J Psychophysiol 27(2):147–151. doi:S0167876097000457 [pii]

Park S, Holzman PS (1992) Schizophrenics show spatial working memory deficits. Arch Gen Psychiatry 49(12):975–982

Pavuluri MN, West A, Hill SK, Jindal K, Sweeney JA (2009) Neurocognitive function in pediatric bipolar disorder: 3-year follow-up shows cognitive development lagging behind healthy youths. J Am Acad Child Adolesc Psychiatry 48(3):299–307. doi:10.1097/CHI.0b013e318196b907, S0890-8567(09)60030-7 [pii]

Petterson U (1977) Manic-depressive illness. A clinical, social and genetic study. Acta Psychiatr Scand Suppl 269:1–93

Pierson A, Jouvent R, Quintin P, Perez-Diaz F, Leboyer M (2000) Information processing deficits in relatives of manic depressive patients. Psychol Med 30(3):545–555

Pirkola T, Tuulio-Henriksson A, Glahn D, Kieseppa T, Haukka J, Kaprio J, Lonnqvist J, Cannon TD (2005) Spatial working memory function in twins with schizophrenia and bipolar disorder. Biol Psychiatry 58(12):930–936. doi:10.1016/j.biopsych.2005.05.041, S0006-3223(05)00694-3 [pii]

Quackenbush D, Kutcher S, Robertson HA, Boulos C, Chaban P (1996) Premorbid and postmorbid school functioning in bipolar adolescents: description and suggested academic interventions. Can J Psychiatry 41(1):16–22

Quraishi S, Frangou S (2002) Neuropsychology of bipolar disorder: a review. J Affect Disord 72(3):209–226. doi:S0165032702000915 [pii]

Reichenberg A, Weiser M, Rabinowitz J, Caspi A, Schmeidler J, Mark M, Kaplan Z, Davidson M (2002) A population-based cohort study of premorbid intellectual, language, and behavioral functioning in patients with schizophrenia, schizoaffective disorder, and nonpsychotic bipolar disorder. Am J Psychiatry 159(12):2027–2035

Reichenberg A, Harvey PD, Bowie CR, Mojtabai R, Rabinowitz J, Heaton RK, Bromet E (2009) Neuropsychological function and dysfunction in schizophrenia and psychotic affective disorders. Schizophr Bull 35(5):1022–1029. doi:10.1093/schbul/sbn044, sbn044 [pii]

Reinares M, Martinez-Aran A, Colom F, Benabarre A, Salamero M, Vieta E (2000) Long-term effects of the treatment with risperidone versus conventional neuroleptics on the neuropsychological performance of euthymic bipolar patients. Actas Esp Psiquiatr 28(4):231–238

Reus VI, Targum SD, Weingarter H, Post RM (1979) Effect of lithium carbonate on memory processes of bipolar affectively ill patients. Psychopharmacology (Berl) 63(1):39–42

Robinson LJ, Ferrier IN (2006) Evolution of cognitive impairment in bipolar disorder: a systematic review of cross-sectional evidence. Bipolar Disord 8(2):103–116. doi:10.1111/j.1399-5618.2006.00277.x, BDI277 [pii]

Robinson LJ, Thompson JM, Gallagher P, Goswami U, Young AH, Ferrier IN, Moore PB (2006) A meta-analysis of cognitive deficits in euthymic patients with bipolar disorder. J Affect Disord 93(1–3):105–115. doi:10.1016/j.jad.2006.02.016, S0165-0327(06)00093-0 [pii]

Robinson JL, Monkul ES, Tordesillas-Gutierrez D, Franklin C, Bearden CE, Fox PT, Glahn DC (2008) Fronto-limbic circuitry in euthymic bipolar disorder: evidence for prefrontal hyperactivation. Psychiatry Res 164(2):106–113. doi:10.1016/j.pscychresns.2007.12.004, S0925-4927(07)00250-8 [pii]

Rocca CC, Heuvel E, Caetano SC, Lafer B (2009) Facial emotion recognition in bipolar disorder: a critical review. Rev Bras Psiquiatr 31(2):171–180. doi:S1516-44462009000200015 [pii]

Roiser JP, Cannon DM, Gandhi SK, Taylor Tavares J, Erickson K, Wood S, Klaver JM, Clark L, Zarate CA Jr, Sahakian BJ, Drevets WC (2009) Hot and cold cognition in unmedicated depressed subjects with bipolar disorder. Bipolar Disord 11(2):178–189. doi:10.1111/j.1399-5618.2009.00669.x, BDI669 [pii]

Rossi A, Arduini L, Daneluzzo E, Bustini M, Prosperini P, Stratta P (2000) Cognitive function in euthymic bipolar patients, stabilized schizophrenic patients, and healthy controls. J Psychiatr Res 34(4–5):333–339. doi:S0022-3956(00)00025-X [pii]

Roy-Byrne PP, Weingartner H, Bierer LM, Thompson K, Post RM (1986) Effortful and automatic cognitive processes in depression. Arch Gen Psychiatry 43(3):265–267
Rubinow DR, Post RM (1992) Impaired recognition of affect in facial expression in depressed patients. Biol Psychiatry 31(9):947–953
Rubinsztein JS, Michael A, Paykel ES, Sahakian BJ (2000) Cognitive impairment in remission in bipolar affective disorder. Psychol Med 30(5):1025–1036
Rund BR, Orbeck AL, Landro NI (1992) Vigilance deficits in schizophrenics and affectively disturbed patients. Acta Psychiatr Scand 86(3):207–212
Ryan KA, Vederman AC, McFadden EM, Weldon AL, Kamali M, Langenecker SA, McInnis MG (2012) Differential executive functioning performance by phase of bipolar disorder. Bipolar Disord 14(5):527–536. doi:10.1111/j.1399-5618.2012.01032.x
Sackeim HA, Freeman J, McElhiney M, Coleman E, Prudic J, Devanand DP (1992) Effects of major depression on estimates of intelligence. J Clin Exp Neuropsychol 14(2):268–288. doi:10.1080/01688639208402828
Salinsky MC, Storzbach D, Spencer DC, Oken BS, Landry T, Dodrill CB (2005) Effects of topiramate and gabapentin on cognitive abilities in healthy volunteers. Neurology 64(5):792–798. doi:10.1212/01.WNL.0000152877.08088.87, 64/5/792 [pii]
Samame C, Martino DJ, Strejilevich SA (2012) Social cognition in euthymic bipolar disorder: systematic review and meta-analytic approach. Acta Psychiatr Scand 125(4):266–280. doi:10.1111/j.1600-0447.2011.01808.x
Sanchez-Morla EM, Barabash A, Martinez-Vizcaino V, Tabares-Seisdedos R, Balanza-Martinez V, Cabranes-Diaz JA, Baca-Baldomero E, Gomez JL (2009) Comparative study of neurocognitive function in euthymic bipolar patients and stabilized schizophrenic patients. Psychiatry Res 169(3):220–228. doi:10.1016/j.psychres.2008.06.032, S0165-1781(08)00200-X [pii]
Sapin LR, Berrettini WH, Nurnberger JI Jr, Rothblat LA (1987) Mediational factors underlying cognitive changes and laterality in affective illness. Biol Psychiatry 22(8):979–986
Sarfati Y, Hardy-Bayle MC (1999) How do people with schizophrenia explain the behaviour of others? A study of theory of mind and its relationship to thought and speech disorganization in schizophrenia. Psychol Med 29(3):613–620
Savard RJ, Rey AC, Post RM (1980) Halstead-Reitan Category Test in bipolar and unipolar affective disorders. Relationship to age and phase of illness. J Nerv Ment Dis 168(5):297–304
Savitz J, Solms M, Ramesar R (2005) Neuropsychological dysfunction in bipolar affective disorder: a critical opinion. Bipolar Disord 7(3):216–235. doi:10.1111/j.1399-5618.2005.00203.x, BDI203 [pii]
Savitz JB, van der Merwe L, Stein DJ, Solms M, Ramesar RS (2008) Neuropsychological task performance in bipolar spectrum illness: genetics, alcohol abuse, medication and childhood trauma. Bipolar Disord 10(4):479–494. doi:10.1111/j.1399-5618.2008.00591.x, BDI591 [pii]
Savitz J, van der Merwe L, Stein DJ, Solms M, Ramesar R (2009) Neuropsychological status of bipolar I disorder: impact of psychosis. Br J Psychiatry 194(3):243–251. doi:10.1192/bjp.bp.108.052001, 194/3/243 [pii]
Schretlen DJ, Cascella NG, Meyer SM, Kingery LR, Testa SM, Munro CA, Pulver AE, Rivkin P, Rao VA, Diaz-Asper CM, Dickerson FB, Yolken RH, Pearlson GD (2007) Neuropsychological functioning in bipolar disorder and schizophrenia. Biol Psychiatry 62(2):179–186. doi:10.1016/j.biopsych.2006.09.025, S0006-3223(06)01198-X [pii]
Schubert EW, McNeil TF (2005) Neuropsychological impairment and its neurological correlates in adult offspring with heightened risk for schizophrenia and affective psychosis. Am J Psychiatry 162(4):758–766. doi:10.1176/appi.ajp.162.4.758, 162/4/758 [pii]
Schulze KK, Walshe M, Stahl D, Hall MH, Kravariti E, Morris R, Marshall N, McDonald C, Murray RM, Bramon E (2011) Executive functioning in familial bipolar I disorder patients and their unaffected relatives. Bipolar Disord 13(2):208–216. doi:10.1111/j.1399-5618.2011.00901.x
Scott J, Stanton B, Garland A, Ferrier IN (2000) Cognitive vulnerability in patients with bipolar disorder. Psychol Med 30(2):467–472
Seidman LJ, Kremen WS, Koren D, Faraone SV, Goldstein JM, Tsuang MT (2002) A comparative profile analysis of neuropsychological functioning in patients with schizophrenia and bipolar psychoses. Schizophr Res 53(1–2):31–44. doi:S0920996401001621 [pii]

Seidman LJ, Lanca M, Kremen WS, Faraone SV, Tsuang MT (2003) Organizational and visual memory deficits in schizophrenia and bipolar psychoses using the Rey-Osterrieth complex figure: effects of duration of illness. J Clin Exp Neuropsychol 25(7):949–964. doi:10.1076/jcen.25.7.949.16482

Selva G, Salazar J, Balanza-Martinez V, Martinez-Aran A, Rubio C, Daban C, Sanchez-Moreno J, Vieta E, Tabares-Seisdedos R (2007) Bipolar I patients with and without a history of psychotic symptoms: do they differ in their cognitive functioning? J Psychiatr Res 41(3–4):265–272. doi:10.1016/j.jpsychires.2006.03.007, S0022-3956(06)00062-8 [pii]

Senturk V, Goker C, Bilgic A, Olmez S, Tugcu H, Oncu B, Atbasoglu EC (2007) Impaired verbal memory and otherwise spared cognition in remitted bipolar patients on monotherapy with lithium or valproate. Bipolar Disord 9(Suppl 1):136–144. doi:10.1111/j.1399-5618.2007.00481.x, BDI481 [pii]

Shamay-Tsoory S, Harari H, Szepsenwol O, Levkovitz Y (2009) Neuropsychological evidence of impaired cognitive empathy in euthymic bipolar disorder. J Neuropsychiatry Clin Neurosci 21(1):59–67. doi:10.1176/appi.neuropsych.21.1.59, 21/1/59 [pii]

Shaw ED, Mann JJ, Stokes PE, Manevitz AZ (1986) Effects of lithium carbonate on associative productivity and idiosyncrasy in bipolar outpatients. Am J Psychiatry 143(9):1166–1169

Shaw ED, Stokes PE, Mann JJ, Manevitz AZ (1987) Effects of lithium carbonate on the memory and motor speed of bipolar outpatients. J Abnorm Psychol 96(1):64–69

Sheffield JM, Williams LE, Cohen N, Heckers S (2012) Relational memory in psychotic bipolar disorder. Bipolar Disord 14(5):537–546. doi:10.1111/j.1399-5618.2012.01036.x

Sigurdsson E, Fombonne E, Sayal K, Checkley S (1999) Neurodevelopmental antecedents of early-onset bipolar affective disorder. Br J Psychiatry 174:121–127

Silverstein ML, McDonald C, Fogg L (1990) Intelligence and neuropsychological functioning in psychiatric disorders. Arch Clin Neuropsychol 5(3):317–323. doi:0887-6177(90)90030-S [pii]

Simonsen C, Sundet K, Vaskinn A, Birkenaes AB, Engh JA, Hansen CF, Jonsdottir H, Ringen PA, Opjordsmoen S, Friis S, Andreassen OA (2008) Neurocognitive profiles in bipolar I and bipolar II disorder: differences in pattern and magnitude of dysfunction. Bipolar Disord 10(2):245–255. doi:10.1111/j.1399-5618.2007.00492.x, BDI492 [pii]

Simonsen C, Sundet K, Vaskinn A, Birkenaes AB, Engh JA, Faerden A, Jonsdottir H, Ringen PA, Opjordsmoen S, Melle I, Friis S, Andreassen OA (2011) Neurocognitive dysfunction in bipolar and schizophrenia spectrum disorders depends on history of psychosis rather than diagnostic group. Schizophr Bull 37(1):73–83. doi:10.1093/schbul/sbp034, sbp034 [pii]

Smith DJ, Muir WJ, Blackwood DH (2006) Neurocognitive impairment in euthymic young adults with bipolar spectrum disorder and recurrent major depressive disorder. Bipolar Disord 8(1):40–46. doi:10.1111/j.1399-5618.2006.00275.x, BDI275 [pii]

Smoller JW, Finn CT (2003) Family, twin, and adoption studies of bipolar disorder. Am J Med Genet C Semin Med Genet 123C(1):48–58. doi:10.1002/ajmg.c.20013

Sobczak S, Riedel WJ, Booij I, Aan Het Rot M, Deutz NE, Honig A (2002) Cognition following acute tryptophan depletion: difference between first-degree relatives of bipolar disorder patients and matched healthy control volunteers. Psychol Med 32(3):503–515

Sobczak S, Honig A, Schmitt JA, Riedel WJ (2003) Pronounced cognitive deficits following an intravenous L-tryptophan challenge in first-degree relatives of bipolar patients compared to healthy controls. Neuropsychopharmacology 28(4):711–719. doi:10.1038/sj.npp.1300055, 1300055 [pii]

Sole B, Martinez-Aran A, Torrent C, Bonnin CM, Reinares M, Popovic D, Sanchez-Moreno J, Vieta E (2011) Are bipolar II patients cognitively impaired? A systematic review. Psychol Med 41(9):1791–1803. doi:10.1017/S0033291711000018, S0033291711000018 [pii]

Sole B, Bonnin CM, Torrent C, Martinez-Aran A, Popovic D, Tabares-Seisdedos R, Vieta E (2012) Neurocognitive impairment across the bipolar spectrum. CNS Neurosci Ther 18(3):194–200. doi:10.1111/j.1755-5949.2011.00262.x

Sorensen HJ, Saebye D, Urfer-Parnas A, Mortensen EL, Parnas J (2012) Premorbid intelligence and educational level in bipolar and unipolar disorders: a Danish draft board study. J Affect Disord 136(3):1188–1191. doi:10.1016/j.jad.2011.12.007, S0165-0327(11)00767-1 [pii]

Souza VB, Muir WJ, Walker MT, Glabus MF, Roxborough HM, Sharp CW, Dunan JR, Blackwood DH (1995) Auditory P300 event-related potentials and neuropsychological performance in schizophrenia and bipolar affective disorder. Biol Psychiatry 37(5):300–310. doi:10.1016/0006-3223(94)00131-L, 0006-3223(94)00131-L [pii]

Squire LR, Judd LL, Janowsky DS, Huey LY (1980) Effects of lithium carbonate on memory and other cognitive functions. Am J Psychiatry 137(9):1042–1046

Stein RA, Strickland TL (1998) A review of the neuropsychological effects of commonly used prescription medications. Arch Clin Neuropsychol 13(3):259–284. doi:S0887-6177(97)00027-9 [pii]

Stern Y, Sackeim HA (2002) The neuropsychology of memory and amnesia. In: Yudofsky SC, Hales RE (eds) The American psychiatric press textbook of neuropsychiatry and clinical neurosciences, 4th edn. American Psychiatric Press, Washington, DC, pp 597–622

Stoddart SD, Craddock NJ, Jones LA (2007) Differentiation of executive and attention impairments in affective illness. Psychol Med 37(11):1613–1623. doi:10.1017/S0033291707000712, S0033291707000712 [pii]

Stoll AL, Locke CA, Vuckovic A, Mayer PV (1996) Lithium-associated cognitive and functional deficits reduced by a switch to divalproex sodium: a case series. J Clin Psychiatry 57(8): 356–359

Strakowski SM, Adler CM, Holland SK, Mills N, DelBello MP (2004) A preliminary FMRI study of sustained attention in euthymic, unmedicated bipolar disorder. Neuropsychopharmacology 29(9):1734–1740. doi:10.1038/sj.npp.1300492, 1300492 [pii]

Studentkowski G, Scheele D, Calabrese P, Balkau F, Hoffler J, Aubel T, Edel MA, Juckel G, Assion HJ (2010) Cognitive impairment in patients with a schizoaffective disorder: a comparison with bipolar patients in euthymia. Eur J Med Res 15(2):70–78

Summers M, Papadopoulou K, Bruno S, Cipolotti L, Ron MA (2006) Bipolar I and bipolar II disorder: cognition and emotion processing. Psychol Med 36(12):1799–1809. doi:10.1017/S0033291706008804, S0033291706008804 [pii]

Surguladze SA, Marshall N, Schulze K, Hall MH, Walshe M, Bramon E, Phillips ML, Murray RM, McDonald C (2010) Exaggerated neural response to emotional faces in patients with bipolar disorder and their first-degree relatives. Neuroimage 53(1):58–64. doi:10.1016/j.neuroimage.2010.05.069, S1053-8119(10)00821-9 [pii]

Swann AC, Pazzaglia P, Nicholls A, Dougherty DM, Moeller FG (2003) Impulsivity and phase of illness in bipolar disorder. J Affect Disord 73(1–2):105–111. doi:S0165032702003282 [pii]

Szoke A, Schurhoff F, Golmard JL, Alter C, Roy I, Meary A, Etain B, Bellivier F, Leboyer M (2006) Familial resemblance for executive functions in families of schizophrenic and bipolar patients. Psychiatry Res 144(2–3):131–138. doi:10.1016/j.psychres.2005.11.013, S0165-1781(05)00418-X [pii]

Szoke A, Meary A, Trandafir A, Bellivier F, Roy I, Schurhoff F, Leboyer M (2008) Executive deficits in psychotic and bipolar disorders – implications for our understanding of schizoaffective disorder. Eur Psychiatry 23(1):20–25. doi:10.1016/j.eurpsy.2007.10.006, S0924-9338(07)01422-8 [pii]

Tabares-Seisdedos R, Balanza-Martinez V, Salazar-Fraile J, Selva-Vera G, Leal-Cercos C, Gomez-Beneyto M (2003) Specific executive/attentional deficits in patients with schizophrenia or bipolar disorder who have a positive family history of psychosis. J Psychiatr Res 37(6):479–486. doi:S0022395603000712 [pii]

Tabares-Seisdedos R, Balanza-Martinez V, Sanchez-Moreno J, Martinez-Aran A, Salazar-Fraile J, Selva-Vera G, Rubio C, Mata I, Gomez-Beneyto M, Vieta E (2008) Neurocognitive and clinical predictors of functional outcome in patients with schizophrenia and bipolar I disorder at one-year follow-up. J Affect Disord 109(3):286–299. doi:10.1016/j.jad.2007.12.234, S0165-0327(08)00015-3 [pii]

Tam WC, Liu Z (2004) Comparison of neurocognition between drug-free patients with schizophrenia and bipolar disorder. J Nerv Ment Dis 192(7):464–470. doi:00005053-200407000-00003 [pii]

Tam WC, Sewell KW, Deng HC (1998) Information processing in schizophrenia and bipolar disorder: a discriminant analysis. J Nerv Ment Dis 186(10):597–603

Taylor Tavares JV, Clark L, Cannon DM, Erickson K, Drevets WC, Sahakian BJ (2007) Distinct profiles of neurocognitive function in unmedicated unipolar depression and bipolar II depression. Biol Psychiatry 62(8):917–924. doi:10.1016/j.biopsych.2007.05.034, S0006-3223(07)00612-9 [pii]

Tham A, Engelbrektson K, Mathe AA, Johnson L, Olsson E, Aberg-Wistedt A (1997) Impaired neuropsychological performance in euthymic patients with recurring mood disorders. J Clin Psychiatry 58(1):26–29

Thomas P, Kearney G, Napier E, Ellis E, Leuder I, Johnson M (1996) Speech and language in first onset psychosis differences between people with schizophrenia, mania, and controls. Br J Psychiatry 168(3):337–343

Thompson PJ, Trimble MR (1982) Anticonvulsant drugs and cognitive functions. Epilepsia 23(5):531–544

Thompson JM, Gallagher P, Hughes JH, Watson S, Gray JM, Ferrier IN, Young AH (2005) Neurocognitive impairment in euthymic patients with bipolar affective disorder. Br J Psychiatry 186:32–40. doi:10.1192/bjp.186.1.32, 186/1/32 [pii]

Thompson JM, Hamilton CJ, Gray JM, Quinn JG, Mackin P, Young AH, Ferrier IN (2006) Executive and visuospatial sketchpad resources in euthymic bipolar disorder: Implications for visuospatial working memory architecture. Memory 14(4):437–451. doi:10.1080/09658210500464293, JJ45X74532377351 [pii]

Thompson JM, Gray JM, Hughes JH, Watson S, Young AH, Ferrier IN (2007) Impaired working memory monitoring in euthymic bipolar patients. Bipolar Disord 9(5):478–489. doi:10.1111/j.1399-5618.2007.00470.x, BDI470 [pii]

Tien AY, Ross DE, Pearlson G, Strauss ME (1996) Eye movements and psychopathology in schizophrenia and bipolar disorder. J Nerv Ment Dis 184(6):331–338

Tiihonen J, Haukka J, Henriksson M, Cannon M, Kieseppa T, Laaksonen I, Sinivuo J, Lonnqvist J (2005) Premorbid intellectual functioning in bipolar disorder and schizophrenia: results from a cohort study of male conscripts. Am J Psychiatry 162(10):1904–1910. doi:10.1176/appi.ajp.162.10.1904, 162/10/1904 [pii]

Torralva T, Strejilevich S, Gleichgerrcht E, Roca M, Martino D, Cetkovich M, Manes F (2012) Deficits in tasks of executive functioning that mimic real-life scenarios in bipolar disorder. Bipolar Disord 14(1):118–125. doi:10.1111/j.1399-5618.2012.00987.x

Torrent C, Martinez-Aran A, Daban C, Sanchez-Moreno J, Comes M, Goikolea JM, Salamero M, Vieta E (2006) Cognitive impairment in bipolar II disorder. Br J Psychiatry 189:254–259. doi:10.1192/bjp.bp.105.017269, 189/3/254 [pii]

Torrent C, Martinez-Aran A, Amann B, Daban C, Tabares-Seisdedos R, Gonzalez-Pinto A, Reinares M, Benabarre A, Salamero M, McKenna P, Vieta E (2007) Cognitive impairment in schizoaffective disorder: a comparison with non-psychotic bipolar and healthy subjects. Acta Psychiatr Scand 116(6):453–460. doi:10.1111/j.1600-0447.2007.01072.x, ACP1072 [pii]

Torrent C, Martinez-Aran A, del Mar BC, Reinares M, Daban C, Sole B, Rosa AR, Tabares-Seisdedos R, Popovic D, Salamero M, Vieta E (2012) Long-term outcome of cognitive impairment in bipolar disorder. J Clin Psychiatry 73(7):e899–e905. doi:10.4088/JCP.11m07471

Torres IJ, Boudreau VG, Yatham LN (2007) Neuropsychological functioning in euthymic bipolar disorder:ameta-analysis.ActaPsychiatrScandSuppl434:17–26.doi:10.1111/j.1600-0447.2007.01055.x, ACP1055 [pii]

Torres IJ, DeFreitas VG, DeFreitas CM, Kauer-Sant'Anna M, Bond DJ, Honer WG, Lam RW, Yatham LN (2010) Neurocognitive functioning in patients with bipolar I disorder recently recovered from a first manic episode. J Clin Psychiatry 71(9):1234–1242. doi:10.4088/JCP.08m04997yel

Toulopoulou T, Quraishi S, McDonald C, Murray RM (2006) The Maudsley Family Study: premorbid and current general intellectual function levels in familial bipolar I disorder and schizophrenia. J Clin Exp Neuropsychol 28(2):243–259. doi:10.1080/13803390500360513, K811333911PM55L1 [pii]

Tsuang MT, Woolson RF, Fleming JA (1979) Long-term outcome of major psychoses. I. Schizophrenia and affective disorders compared with psychiatrically symptom-free surgical conditions. Arch Gen Psychiatry 36(12):1295–1301

Uzelac S, Jaeger J, Berns S, Gonzales C (2006) Premorbid adjustment in bipolar disorder: comparison with schizophrenia. J Nerv Ment Dis 194(9):654–658. doi:10.1097/01.nmd.0000235767.00901.e2, 00005053-200609000-00004 [pii]

van der Werf-Eldering MJ, Burger H, Holthausen EA, Aleman A, Nolen WA (2010) Cognitive functioning in patients with bipolar disorder: association with depressive symptoms and alcohol use. PLoS One 5(9) doi:10.1371/journal.pone.0013032 e13032 [pii]

van der Werf-Eldering MJ, Burger H, Jabben N, Holthausen EA, Aleman A, Nolen WA (2011) Is the lack of association between cognitive complaints and objective cognitive functioning in patients with bipolar disorder moderated by depressive symptoms? J Affect Disord 130(1–2):306–311. doi:10.1016/j.jad.2010.10.005, S0165-0327(10)00619-1 [pii]

van Gorp WG, Altshuler L, Theberge DC, Wilkins J, Dixon W (1998) Cognitive impairment in euthymic bipolar patients with and without prior alcohol dependence. A preliminary study. Arch Gen Psychiatry 55(1):41–46

van Gorp WG, Altshuler L, Theberge DC, Mintz J (1999) Declarative and procedural memory in bipolar disorder. Biol Psychiatry 46(4):525–531. doi:S0006-3223(98)00336-9 [pii]

Varga M, Magnusson A, Flekkoy K, Ronneberg U, Opjordsmoen S (2006) Insight, symptoms and neurocognition in bipolar I patients. J Affect Disord 91(1):1–9. doi:10.1016/j.jad.2005.09.002, S0165-0327(05)00285-5 [pii]

Vaskinn A, Sundet K, Friis S, Simonsen C, Birkenaes AB, Engh JA, Jonsdottir H, Ringen PA, Opjordsmoen S, Andreassen OA (2007) The effect of gender on emotion perception in schizophrenia and bipolar disorder. Acta Psychiatr Scand 116(4):263–270. doi:10.1111/j.1600-0447.2007.00991.x, ACP991 [pii]

Venn HR, Gray JM, Montagne B, Murray LK, Michael Burt D, Frigerio E, Perrett DI, Young AH (2004) Perception of facial expressions of emotion in bipolar disorder. Bipolar Disord 6(4):286–293. doi:10.1111/j.1399-5618.2004.00121.x, BDI121 [pii]

Verdoux H, Liraud F (2000) Neuropsychological function in subjects with psychotic and affective disorders. Relationship to diagnostic category and duration of illness. Eur Psychiatry 15(4):236–243. doi:S0924-9338(00)00238-8 [pii]

Waddington JL, Brown K, O'Neill J, McKeon P, Kinsella A (1989) Cognitive impairment, clinical course and treatment history in out-patients with bipolar affective disorder: relationship to tardive dyskinesia. Psychol Med 19(4):897–902

Waters BG, Marchenko-Bouer I, Smiley D (1981) Educational achievement, IQ and affective disorder in the adult offspring of bipolar manic-depressives. Br J Psychiatry 139:457–462

Weingartner H, Miller H, Murphy DL (1977) Mood-state-dependent retrieval of verbal associations. J Abnorm Psychol 86(3):276–284

Weingartner H, Cohen RM, Murphy DL, Martello J, Gerdt C (1981) Cognitive processes in depression. Arch Gen Psychiatry 38(1):42–47

Wiegand LC, Warfield SK, Levitt JJ, Hirayasu Y, Salisbury DF, Heckers S, Dickey CC, Kikinis R, Jolesz FA, McCarley RW, Shenton ME (2004) Prefrontal cortical thickness in first-episode psychosis: a magnetic resonance imaging study. Biol Psychiatry 55(2):131–140. doi:S0006322303008552 [pii]

Wilder-Willis KE, Sax KW, Rosenberg HL, Fleck DE, Shear PK, Strakowski SM (2001) Persistent attentional dysfunction in remitted bipolar disorder. Bipolar Disord 3(2):58–62

Wingo AP, Wingo TS, Harvey PD, Baldessarini RJ (2009) Effects of lithium on cognitive performance: a meta-analysis. J Clin Psychiatry 70(11):1588–1597. doi:10.4088/JCP.08r04972

Winters KC, Stone AA, Weintraub S, Neale JM (1981) Cognitive and attentional deficits in children vulnerable to psychopathology. J Abnorm Child Psychol 9(4):435–453

Wolf F, Brune M, Assion HJ (2010) Theory of mind and neurocognitive functioning in patients with bipolar disorder. Bipolar Disord 12(6):657–666

Woodruff RA Jr, Robins LN, Winokur G, Walbran B (1968) Educational and occupational achievement in primary affective disorder. Am J Psychiatry 124(11):57–64, Suppl

Woodruff RA Jr, Robins LN, Winokur G, Reich T (1971) Manic depressive illness and social achievement. Acta Psychiatr Scand 47(3):237–249

Xu G, Lin K, Rao D, Dang Y, Ouyang H, Guo Y, Ma J, Chen J (2012) Neuropsychological performance in bipolar I, bipolar II and unipolar depression patients: a longitudinal, naturalistic study. J Affect Disord 136(3):328–339. doi:10.1016/j.jad.2011.11.029, S0165-0327(11)00746-4 [pii]

Yates DB, Dittmann S, Kapczinski F, Trentini CM (2011) Cognitive abilities and clinical variables in bipolar I depressed and euthymic patients and controls. J Psychiatr Res 45(4):495–504. doi:10.1016/j.jpsychires.2010.09.006, S0022-3956(10)00273-6 [pii]

Yechiam E, Hayden EP, Bodkins M, O'Donnell BF, Hetrick WP (2008) Decision making in bipolar disorder: a cognitive modeling approach. Psychiatry Res 161(2):142–152. doi:10.1016/j.psychres.2007.07.001, S0165-1781(07)00209-0 [pii]

Yim CY, Soczynska JK, Kennedy SH, Woldeyohannes HO, Brietzke E, McIntyre RS (2012) The effect of overweight/obesity on cognitive function in euthymic individuals with bipolar disorder. Eur Psychiatry 27(3):223–228. doi:10.1016/j.eurpsy.2011.02.004, S0924-9338(11)00029-0 [pii]

Young DA, Zakzanis KK, Bailey C, Davila R, Griese J, Sartory G, Thom A (1998) Further parameters of insight and neuropsychological deficit in schizophrenia and other chronic mental disease. J Nerv Ment Dis 186(1):44–50

Yurgelun-Todd DA, Gruber SA, Kanayama G, Killgore WD, Baird AA, Young AD (2000) fMRI during affect discrimination in bipolar affective disorder. Bipolar Disord 2(3 Pt 2):237–248

Zalla T, Joyce C, Szoke A, Schurhoff F, Pillon B, Komano O, Perez-Diaz F, Bellivier F, Alter C, Dubois B, Rouillon F, Houde O, Leboyer M (2004) Executive dysfunctions as potential markers of familial vulnerability to bipolar disorder and schizophrenia. Psychiatry Res 121(3):207–217. doi:S016517810300252X [pii]

Zammit S, Allebeck P, David AS, Dalman C, Hemmingsson T, Lundberg I, Lewis G (2004) A longitudinal study of premorbid IQ Score and risk of developing schizophrenia, bipolar disorder, severe depression, and other nonaffective psychoses. Arch Gen Psychiatry 61(4):354–360. doi:10.1001/archpsyc.61.4.354, 61/4/354 [pii]

Zubieta JK, Huguelet P, O'Neil RL, Giordani BJ (2001) Cognitive function in euthymic bipolar I disorder. Psychiatry Res 102(1):9–20. doi:S0165-1781(01)00242-6 [pii]

The Role of Temperament

5

5.1 Historical Perspective

While early versions of the concept of temperament might had existed in ancient Egypt and Mesopotamia, essentially this approach was developed by the school of Cos and specifically by Polybus who was a pupil and son-in-law to Hippocrates (fourth century BC) and author of the book 'Peri physeos anthropou' ('On the Nature of Man'). This theory is in fact a microcosmic form of the macrocosmic theory of the four elements (earth, water, air, fire) and the four qualities (dry, wet, cold, hot) as first proposed by Empedocles (fifth century BC). According to this ancient approach, temperament (in Greek *crasis* or *idiosyncrasia*), health and disease are the products of the balance four body humours (in Greek *choli*). According to the predominance of a given humour, four temperamental types were described: the choleric (yellow bile from the liver; cyclothymic), the sanguine (blood from the heart; hyperthymic), the melancholic (black bile from the kidneys; depressive) and the phlegmatic (phlegm from the lungs; self-content). The theory was further elaborated by Erasistratos, Asclepiades (first century BC) and eventually by Galen (second century AD) with his treatise 'Peri crasaion' ('De temperamentis'). This approach was the standard until the sixteenth century and in the India and the Muslim world constituted the basis of Yunani or Unani medicine (after Yunan that is Iones-Greeks in Eastern languages). In 'The Canon of Medicine', Avicenna (980–1037 AD) extended the theory of temperaments to include 'emotion, mental ability, moral attitudes, self-awareness, movement and dreams'. In English texts, temperament is mentioned in Wycliff's sermons (1380), in the writings of Shakespeare and in Robert Burton's Anatomy of Melancholy (Table 5.1).

The word 'temperament' itself comes from the Latin word 'temperare', which means 'to mix', while the Greek original word is 'crasis' or 'idiosyncrasia', standing for 'mixture' and 'unique admixture', respectively.

Temperament theory influenced philosophical thinking and played a predominant role in the shaping of the anthropological and humanitarian sciences. Prominent scholars like Ernst Platner (1744–1818), Immanuel Kant (1724–1804),

K.N. Fountoulakis, *Bipolar Disorder: An Evidence-Based Guide to Manic Depression*, DOI 10.1007/978-3-642-37216-2_5

Table 5.1 Chronological chart of theoretical elaboration on temperament

Theorist	Time period	Contribution
Polybus (school of Cos)	Fourth century BC	'Peri physeos anthropou' ('On the Nature of Man'). Theory of the four humours
Eristratos, Asclepiades	First century BC	Further elaboration on Polybus' theory
Galen	Second century AD	'Peri crasaion' ('De temperamentis')
Avicenna	980–1037 AD	Canon of medicine (includes emotion, mental ability, moral attitudes, self-awareness, movement and dreams)
Nicholas Culpeper	1616–1654	The first to disregard the idea of fluids as defining human behaviour
Georg Ernst Stahl	1660–1734	Animism/vitalism
Friedrich Hoffmann	1660–1742	Iatromechanism (hydraulic based theory)
Immanuel Kant	1724–1804	Anthropologie
Ernst Platner	1744–1818	Philosophische Aphorismen
Friedrich Schiller	1759–1805	Human types: idealist and realist
Franz Joseph Gall	1758–1828	Phrenologistic teachings; considered the study of temperaments as the first step in phrenology
Johann Spurzheim	1776–1832	
Friedrich Schelling	1775–1854	'Naturphilosophie'
Jacob Henle	1809–1885	The first to base a theory of temperaments on the tone of the nervous system
William James	1842–1910	Tough-minded and tender-minded temperaments
Friedrich Wilhelm Nietzsche	1844–1900	The Apollonian, or rational, and the Dionysian, or passionate, element of human nature (the birth of tragedy)
Carl Spitteler	1845–1924	Prometheus (forethinker, introvert) and Epimetheus (after-thinker, extrovert)
Rudolf Steiner	1861–1925	Suggested that temperament is under the persons' partial control, changes and matures; persons are a mixture of different temperaments which are characterized by different levels of maturity
Erich Adickes	1866–1928	'Four world views' in 1907: 'dogmatic', 'agnostic', 'traditional' and 'innovative'
Carl Gustav Jung	1875–1961	Interplay between an outer public self and a secret inner self as determining the direction of the libido (extroversion vs. introversion)
Alfred Adler	1879–1937	Four mistaken goals: 'recognition', 'power', 'service' and 'revenge'
Eduard Spränger	1882–1963	Four human values: 'religious', 'theoretic', 'economic' and 'artistic'

Table 5.1 (continued)

Theorist	Time period	Contribution
Ernst Kretschmer	1888–1964	Three body types (asthenic/leptosomic, athletic and pyknic/extrovert) and two temperaments ('schizothymic' with the hyperaesthetic–sensitive and anaesthetic–cold characters and the 'cyclothymic' with depressive–melancholic and the hypomanic characters)
William Sheldon	1898–1977	Three body types (endomorphic, mesomorphic and ectomorphic) and three related groups of temperament traits: 'viscerotonia' (relaxation, comfort, sociability, gluttony for food, for people and for affection), 'somatotonia' (muscular activity and of bodily assertiveness) and 'cerebrotonia' (restraint, inhibition, concealment)
Erich Fromm	1900–1980	Eight basic needs (relatedness, transcendence, creativity, rootedness, sense of identity, frame of orientation, excitation and stimulation, unity, effectiveness) and two factors (acquiring and assimilating things (assimilation) and reacting to people (socialization)) forming five types of malignant character (receptive, exploitative, hoarding, necrophilous and marketing) and one positive character (productive)
Hans Eysenck	1916–1997	The first psychologist to analyse personality differences using an empirical/statistical method
		He suggested that temperament is biologically based. Three dimensions of personality: neuroticism (tendency to experience negative emotions), extraversion (tendency to enjoy positive events) and psychoticism (cognitive style)
		His theory and the theories that derived from it, all concern approach/reward, inhibition/punishment and aggression/flight
Solomon Diamond	1957	In order to distinguish between 'the essential foundations of individuality and its cultural elaboration', one has to look at the animal world
		Four temperament traits in primates: fearfulness, aggressiveness, affiliativeness and impulsiveness
David Keirsey	1921–	Four temperament patterns (sensing perceiver, sensing judger, intuitive thinker and intuitive feeler) and 16 characters
Jeffrey Gray	1934–2004	Neural theory of the Behavioural Inhibition System (BIS) and Behavioural Approach System (BAS)

(continued)

Table 5.1 (continued)

Theorist	Time period	Contribution
Alexander Thomas, Stella Chess, Herbert G. Birch	1956	The 'New York Longitudinal Study' began in 1956
		Nine dimensions of temperament (activity level, rhythmicity of biological functions, approach/withdrawal, adaptability, threshold of responsiveness, intensity of responses, quality of mood, distractibility and persistence) and three distinct temperaments: the 'easy children' (40 % of sample, characterized by regularity, ease of approach, adaptability, mild to moderate mood intensity and a generally positive mood), the 'difficult children' (10 % of the sample with opposite qualities to the 'easy' type) and the 'slow-to-adapt children' (50 %)
		They put the emphasis on 'goodness of fit'
Buss and Plomin	1973	Temperament traits show early appearance in ontogenesis (infancy), are heritable and are predictive of later development
		Four temperament traits (emotionality, activity, sociability and impulsivity)
Robert Cloninger	1944–	He developed a theory of hierarchical temperament and character traits and dimensions; he attempted to intimately connect temperamental characteristics and neurotransmitter systems
		His theory suggests a link between novelty seeking and dopamine, harm avoidance and serotonin and reward dependence and noradrenaline
H. Hill Goldsmith and Joseph Campos	1990	Temperaments are individual differences in the primary emotions. Emphasis on the basic/primary emotions (anger, fear and pleasure) and also the way of regulating them. Central to this notion are three characteristics of response: threshold, latency and intensity
Hagop Akiskal	1945–	He focused on the affective components of temperament and their relationship to mood disorders and creativity
Mary Rothbart	1940–	She emphasized reactivity (meaning biological arousability), self-regulation (increase, decrease, maintain and restructure the patterning of reactivity) and cognitive processes (focus of attention)
		She identified three broad dimensions of temperament: surgency–extraversion (positive anticipation, activity level and sensation seeking), negative affectivity (fear, anger/frustration and social discomfort) and effortful control (inhibitory control, attentional focusing and perceptual sensitivity)
Jerome Kagan	1929–	Described two types of children: the 'inhibited' (cling to their mothers, cry and hesitate with unfamiliar persons or events, are timid and shy and represent about 20 %) and the 'uninhibited' (or exuberant)
		Inhibition can be better understood as intolerance of uncertainty and not as a proneness to fear

Friedrich Schiller (1759–1805) and Friedrich Wilhelm Nietzsche (1844–1900) included concepts similar to temperament in their writings. Gradually physiology and medicine returned to the field and eventually, on the borderline and interface between philosophy, sociology, psychology, anthropology and medicine, Rudolf Steiner (1861–1925), Ernst Kretschmer (1888–1964) and Erich Fromm (1900–1980) described human types and temperaments. Ernst Kretschmer (1888–1964) described the asthenic/leptosomic, athletic and pyknic body types with the pyknic body type being extrovert and related to manic depression. He also divided personality into two temperaments: The 'schizothymic' (with the hyperaesthetic–sensitive and anaesthetic–cold characters) and the 'cyclothymic' (with depressive-melancholic and the hypomanic characters). Hans Eysenck (1916–1997) was the first to analyse personality differences using an empirical/statistical method. He proposed that the basic factors were neuroticism (tendency to experience negative emotions), extraversion (tendency to enjoy positive events) and psychoticism (cognitive style). Eysenck's theory and all the theories that derived from it concern approach/reward, inhibition/punishment and aggression/flight (Eysenck and Eysenck 1962, 1964, 1967, 1968, 1969, 1972, 1977; Eysenck et al. 1974, 1976, 1977).

McCrae and Costa proposed the five-factor model (Big Five) (McCrae and Costa 1987) which includes neuroticism, extroversion agreeableness, openness and conscientiousness and constitutes a further development of Eysenck's theory. The older concept of 'psychoticism' was substituted by agreeableness and conscientiousness, while openness has some degree of overlap with extroversion (Markon et al. 2005).

The work of Robert Cloninger is characterized by an attempt to intimately connect temperamental characteristics with individual differences in genetics, neurotransmitter systems and behavioural conditioning. He described novelty seeking (anger), harm avoidance (fear), reward dependence (attachment) and persistence (ambition) (Cloninger 1987; Cloninger et al. 1993). His research suggests that temperament components can be assessed as early as preschool age (Constantino et al. 2002) and remain moderately stable throughout a person's lifespan except for changes from behavioural conditioning (Josefsson et al. 2012).

Hagop Akiskal has conceived temperament as the affective predisposition or reactivity, based on the original descriptions by Kraepelin (1921) of fundamental states (manic or hyperthymic, irritable, cyclothymic, anxious and depressive). Empirical research has confirmed the hypothesized four-dimensional factor structure and is in agreement with those previously proposed on clinical populations. In an additional exploratory analysis, a depressive type constituted the antipode of hyperthymia and was distinguished from cyclothymia; the irritable temperament appeared somewhat independent. These are close to the classic descriptions of Kraepelin, Kretschmer and Schneider (Akiskal et al. 1998b) (Table 5.2).

While personality refers to goals, coping styles, defensive styles, motives, self-views, life stories and identities (McAdams and Pals 2006), basic personality traits (e.g. extraversion or neuroticism) are essentially parts of temperament (Rothbart et al. 2000). The major theories taken together suggest that four-temperament model of Akiskal (Akiskal and Akiskal 2005), the cube model of Cloninger (Cloninger et al. 1999), the five-factor model represented by the NEO-PI (Costa and McCrae 1990), the seven-factor model of Tellegen (Tellegen et al. 1991) and Cattell's 16-factor

Table 5.2 Summary of the results of empirical studies on temperament

Researcher	Time period	Results
Alexander Thomas, Stella Chess, Herbert G. Birch	1956	Nine dimensions of temperament (activity level, rhythmicity of biological functions, approach/withdrawal, adaptability, threshold of responsiveness, intensity of responses, quality of mood, distractibility and persistence) and three distinct temperaments: the easy, the difficult and the slow-to-adapt children. Emphasis on 'goodness of fit'
Solomon Diamond	1957	Fearfulness, aggressiveness, affiliativeness and impulsiveness
Hans Eysenck	1964	Neuroticism (tendency to experience negative emotions), extraversion (tendency to enjoy positive events) and psychoticism (cognitive style)
Buss and Plomin	1973	Emotionality, activity, sociability and impulsivity
Robert Cloninger	1987	Four temperaments (novelty seeking, harm avoidance, reward dependence and persistence), 3 characters (self-directedness, cooperativeness, self-transcendence) and 25 facets
Mary Rothbart	1988	Reactivity, self-regulation and cognitive processes
		Three dimensions of temperament: surgency–extraversion, negative affectivity and effortful control
Jerome Kagan	1989	The inhibited and the uninhibited children
H. Hill Goldsmith and Joseph Campos	1990	Anger, fear and pleasure and the way of regulating them (threshold, latency and intensity)
Jeffrey Gray	1991	Behavioural Inhibition System (BIS) and Behavioural Approach System (BAS)
Hagop Akiskal	1998	Hyperthymic, cyclothymic, depressive, irritable and anxious
Diogo Lara and Hagop Akiskal	2006	The fear and anger model

model (Cattel et al. 1970) may in fact represent different levels of an hierarchical structure of normal and pathological personality with a two-superfactor solution at the top largely reflecting ego control and ego resiliency (Akiskal et al. 2005a; Cohen 1999), a limited number of temperaments in the middle (named under many labels, but significantly overlapping) (Maremmani et al. 2005) and many characters (15 or more) at the bottom. 'Temperament' corresponds to the 'higher' levels, while 'personality' and 'character' to the 'lower' (Cloninger et al. 2011).

The relationship of temperament to health suggests a strong link to general health and mortality (Friedman et al. 1993) to future mental health (Conley 1985) and to anxiety (Rosenbaum et al. 1988, 1991; Biederman et al. 1990, 2001; Kagan and Zentner 1996; Kagan et al. 1999, 2001; Smoller et al. 2005). It is established that premorbid temperamental predispositions are often present in mood patients and their relatives. These temperamental traits have a disorder-specific pattern of distribution (Evans et al. 2005; Kesebir et al. 2005; Akiskal et al. 2005a, b, c).

The anxious temperament seems to constitute a generic vulnerability factor and was shown to be a robust predictor of most mental disorders. On the contrary, the hyperthymic temperament has shown a uniquely protective effect on most mental disorders (with few exceptions including bipolar disorder) (Karam et al. 2010; Pompili et al. 2008). The dysthymic, cyclothymic and anxious temperaments are related to hopelessness and the irritable temperament to suicidality (Pompili et al. 2008).

Temperament assessment might help in differentiating between unipolar and bipolar depression. This is very important since in many patients the manifestation of a manic or mixed episode comes after several years of suffering and failed or false treatment efforts. The problem is that this 'temperament assessment' might reflect subclinical residual features of bipolar disorder (state) rather than true 'temperament' (i.e. basic long-standing characteristics of the patients or traits). To further complicate the picture, the assessment of temperament changes the definition of bipolarity itself and contributes to the concept of the 'bipolar spectrum'. In this frame it is one of the crucial factors in the increasing prevalence of bipolar cases (especially bipolar II) at the expense of unipolar ones. Although these above-mentioned thoughts constitute significant limitations, the presence of an affective temperament contributes additional affirmation of the early occurrence of mood symptoms in early-onset forms of both unipolar and bipolar depressions (Oedegaard et al. 2009).

The literature suggests that the clinical constellation of 'euphoric–grandiose', 'paranoid–anxious' and 'accelerated–sleepless' symptoms is related to the hyperthymic temperament, while the 'depressive' constellation is related to the depressive temperament and the cluster of 'irritable–agitated' symptoms is related to both temperaments (Perugi et al. 2001). Thus, 'hyperthymic' temperament characterizes manic patients with or without psychotic features (Perugi et al. 1997, 1998b; Dell'Osso et al. 1993) and its assessment reveals that one-third of depressed patients belong to the bipolar spectrum (Cassano et al. 1989).

The subgroup of 'unipolar' patients with hyperthymic temperament (12.4 % of unipolar cases) is similar to BD-II patients in terms of gender and bipolar family history (Cassano et al. 1992b). BD-II patients (40 % of depressed patients after systematic evaluation) manifest high scores on hypomania scales and cyclothymic and irritable temperaments. On the other hand, 88 % of cases, for which a cyclothymic temperament is recognized by clinicians, are diagnosed as BP-II. Cyclothymic temperament is significantly elevated in the bipolar vs. the unipolar depressive group (Mendlowicz et al. 2005a), but it seems that it is a robust clinical marker specifically for BP-II disorder (Hantouche et al. 1998) and is also higher in patients with a family history of bipolarity (Akiskal et al. 2005b).

BD-II patients with cyclothymia differ from those without as having younger age at onset and age at seeking help, higher depressive scores, more atypical features, longer delay between onset of illness and recognition of bipolarity, higher rate of psychiatric comorbidity and different personality disorders profiles (i.e. more histrionic, passive–aggressive and less obsessive–compulsive). Also, cyclothymic BP-II scored significantly much higher on irritable–risk-taking than 'classic' driven–euphoric items of hypomania (Akiskal et al. 2003). In comparison to hyperthymic patients, they might be more frequently females with more depressive and hypomanic episodes and suicide attempts and more comorbidities (most often panic disorder/agoraphobia and social anxiety disorder); they meet more borderline personality disorder criteria and have higher rates of first-degree family history for both mood and anxiety disorders. On the other hand, hyperthymic patients might have more frequent manic episodes and hospitalizations and more antisocial personality disorder features (Perugi et al. 2010).

Marked irritable–explosive traits (occurring in 2–3 % of young persons and tending to attenuate by middle age) often coexist with the mood-labile cyclothymic type, representing the dark 'borderline' side of this cyclothymic temperament (Akiskal et al. 2003; Merikangas et al. 2007, 2011). The type BP-II ½ manifests early onset, complex temperament structure and high mood instability, rapid switching, irritable ('dark') hypomania and suicidality and seems to be the most prevalent and severe expression of the bipolar spectrum, accounting for 33 % of all depressions (Akiskal et al. 2006a). BP-III which is associated with antidepressant treatment is reported to arise from depressive temperament and bipolar family history (Akiskal et al. 2006b).

More than half of depressed patients with atypical features are reported to have antecedent cyclothymic or hyperthymic temperaments and often family history for bipolar disorder (Perugi et al. 1998a). Most of them (78 %) could meet the criteria for bipolar spectrum (mainly BD-II). Atypical patients with cyclothymic temperament manifest higher reactivity of mood, interpersonal sensitivity, functional impairment, avoidance of relationships, other rejection avoidance and, on the interpersonal sensitivity, phobic anxiety, paranoid ideation and psychoticism (Perugi et al. 2003). Reversely, as mentioned before, cyclothymic BD-II patients are reported to manifest more atypical features (Akiskal et al. 2003).

The psychotic mixed patients seem to be closer to the BD-I and are characterized by a hyperthymic temperament with a familial background of psychotic mood disorders, while the nonpsychotic mixed patients are closer to the BD-II and more often have a cyclothymic temperament and a family background of nonpsychotic disorders and substance abuse (Dell'Osso et al. 1993). The EPIMAN study in France suggests that the higher prevalence of hyperthymic temperament in males is responsible for the higher frequency of pure mania in men and the higher prevalence of depressive temperament in females is responsible for the more frequent mixed episodes in women (Akiskal et al. 1998a). Mixed episodes in BD-I women are related to both hyperthymic and depressive temperaments and familial depressive (rather than bipolar) disorders (Dell'Osso et al. 1991; Perugi et al. 1997).

Suicide is related to hopelessness and in turn the dysthymic, cyclothymic and anxious temperaments are related to hopelessness with the irritable temperament relating specifically to suicidality (Pompili et al. 2008). Lifetime suicide is related (among others) to depressive or mixed polarity of first episode and cyclothymic temperament (Azorin et al. 2009).

Patients with non-violent suicide attempts in the past have higher depressive, cyclothymic, irritable and anxious temperaments, but they do not differ from the general population in terms of hyperthymic temperament (Rihmer et al. 2009; Azorin et al. 2010).

Patients with high depressive and low hyperthymic temperament seem to be more likely to have higher hopelessness scores, more white matter hyperintensities, higher suicidal risk and more recent suicide attempts than the rest (Serafini et al. 2010). Late-onset mood disorder is characterized by hyperthymic, cyclothymic and irritable temperaments (Ng et al. 2008).

In summary, the hyperthymic temperament is related to euphoria, grandiose and paranoid thinking, antisocial behaviour, psychomotor acceleration and reduced sleep, as well as to higher frequency of manic episodes and hospitalizations. The cyclothymic temperament is related to the BD-II bipolar type, the presence of panic disorder, agoraphobia and social anxiety disorder, nonpsychotic mixed episodes and suicidality. The depressive temperament is related to depressive symptoms and the irritable to suicidality.

A summary of the relationship of various temperaments and the clinical manifestations of bipolar illness is shown in Table 5.3.

The differences between genders concerning the manifestation of mood disorders can be explained at least partially through differences in temperament. Women are much higher in need for approval (reward dependence) and cooperativeness than men (Cloninger et al. 1994). Females manifest less hypomanic, and more depressive, episodes and more anxiety and somatization. Gender differences in temperament (higher prevalence of the depressive temperament in women vs. higher hyperthymic temperament in men) might account for the differences in rates between genders (Perugi et al. 1990). It has also been proposed that sexes are distinguished by the 'ruminative' and the 'active' cognitive response styles. It seems also possible that women are more vulnerable to childhood adversities and to adult stressors especially related to bonding with men and child rearing (Nolen-Hoeksema and Girgus 1994; Nolen-Hoeksema et al. 1999; Nolen-Hoeksema 2011), which is consistent with gender differences in personality being closely related to traits important for attachment.

Mixed episodes in BD-I women are related to lower hyperthymic temperament and familial depressive, rather than bipolar, disorders (Dell'Osso et al. 1991). These temperamental dysregulations seem to constitute the intermediate step between predisposing familial-genetic factors in affective illness and gender-related clinical expressions of mood disorders (Cassano et al. 1992a). Differences in clinical manifestations might also include more anxiety–depressive features in females (which is in line with female overrepresentation in mixed mania) vs. more social disinhibition in males (Hantouche et al. 2001).

Unipolar and bipolar depressive patients with hyperthymic temperament are reported to have high rates of bipolar family history (Kendler 1997; Kendler and Karkowski-Shuman 1997). In comparison, patients with depressive temperament are reported to have a higher familial loading for mood disorders in general (Cassano et al. 1992a). Cyclothymic patients have also bipolar family history (Akiskal et al. 2005b; Hantouche and Akiskal 2006). Many monozygotic twins discordant for full-blown mood disorders manifest temperamental features strongly suggesting the presence of a genetic component (Bertelsen 1978; Bertelsen et al. 1977).

Table 5.3 Summary of the relationship of bipolar clinical features with various temperaments

Bipolar clinical feature	Temperament
Classic bipolar disorder	
Euphoric–grandiose	Hyperthymic
Paranoid–anxious	Hyperthymic
Accelerated–sleepless	Hyperthymic
Manic patients with or without psychotic features	Hyperthymic
More frequent manic episodes and hospitalizations and more antisocial personality disorder features	Hyperthymic
Depressive' constellation	Depressive
Mixed episodes	
'Irritable–agitated' symptoms	Hyperthymic, depressive
Psychotic mixed patients	Hyperthymic
Nonpsychotic mixed patients	Cyclothymic
Mixed episodes in females	Hyperthymic, depressive
Comorbidity	
Panic disorder, agoraphobia and social anxiety disorder	Cyclothymic, anxious
Suicidality	
Hopelessness	Dysthymic, cyclothymic and anxious
Suicidality	Irritable
Lifetime suicidality	Cyclothymic
Non-violent lifetime suicidality	Depressive, cyclothymic, irritable, anxious
Bipolar spectrum types	
BD-II	Cyclothymic
BD-II ½	Cyclothymic, irritable
BD-III	Depressive
Atypical depression	Cyclothymic, hyperthymic
Late-onset mood disorder (BD-VI)	Hyperthymic, cyclothymic and irritable

In terms of relatives of patients, the cyclothymic temperament is more frequently present in first-degree relatives of patients with BD-I, followed by persons with family history of mood disorders. This loading was more pronounced in females. In the frame of a spectrum concept of bipolar disorder, cyclothymic temperament is distributed in ascending order in the well-relatives of patients from unipolar depression to bipolar disorders, thus possibly constituting a link between molecular and behavioural genetics (Chiaroni et al. 2005). Although peculiar, it is reported that controls have higher hyperthymic temperament in comparison to relatives of bipolar patients (Evans et al. 2005; Mendlowicz et al. 2005b). This is in accord with the above, but in contrast to the results of another study which suggests that BD-I patients and their relatives had significantly higher frequency of hyperthymic temperament than the controls (Kesebir et al. 2005). Relatives of bipolar probands showed lower cyclothymic temperament scores than bipolar patients but higher scores than controls. Patients and their relatives showed higher anxious temperament scores than controls (Mendlowicz et al. 2005b). It seems that the composition of the sample in terms of diagnosis might determine the outcome, by giving weight to depressive, anxious, irritable or cyclothymic temperament, but not hyperthymic which might be higher in controls. The presence of these temperaments might impact on the quality of life of relatives of mood patients (Vazquez et al. 2008). Finally it has been shown that personality traits of high harm avoidance and low self-directedness are heritable risk factors for major depression in the never depressed sibs of depressives (Farmer et al. 2003).

It is often very difficult to distinguish between 'personality' from one hand and 'bipolar disorder' on the other, especially if bipolar disorder has a very early onset with complex residual symptoms between episodes.

Many of subthreshold mood conditions that constitute subeffective disorders were previously subsumed under such rubrics as 'neurotic', 'characterological' and 'existential' depressions and more recently personality disorders. It is relevant that measures of Beck's dysfunctional attitudes are strongly correlated with low self-directedness but not with temperament. Any temperament profile as measured by Cloninger may occur in people who are well adjusted and clinically normal – it is individual differences in character that determine whether a person can self-regulate their emotional drives (temperament) and thereby function in a healthy adaptive manner regardless of stress (Cloninger and Zohar 2011; Cloninger et al. 2010).

Cluster B personality disorders are closer to mood disorders in terms of clinical manifestations. Depending on the population studied, anywhere from half to two-thirds of DSM-III borderline disorders seem to represent subaffective expressions, principally on the border of bipolar disorder, characterized by dysthymic, irritable and cyclothymic temperaments or anxious-sensitive temperament in continuum with hysteroid dysphoric and atypical depressive disorders (Akiskal 1994). This is particularly true for cyclothymic BD-II patients, who are often misclassified as borderline personality disorder because of their extreme mood instability (Perugi and Akiskal 2002).

Cyclothymic BP-II patients were more histrionic, passive–aggressive and less obsessive–compulsive in terms of personality disorders (Akiskal et al. 2003).

The concept of temperament has been developed since antiquity to serve the comprehensive understanding of how the human body works and more important what determines human behaviour. The many theories on temperament included biological interpretations, philosophical and ethical approaches as well as psychological and sociocultural elements. Therefore, a large amount of information concerning the patient is gathered under the umbrella of temperament, and thus it is reasonable to assume that by utilizing temperament and related concepts, one can understand mental illness in a more comprehensive way. This has been studied especially for mood disorders with fruitful results, although many areas remain to be further clarified.

Within the area of mood disorders, specific affective temperaments might constitute vulnerability factors, clinical picture and illness course modifiers, residual syndromes or genetically determined variations of mood disorders, or even the source of creativity. Considering the temperament issue in a wider sense, temperaments could constitute all the above in different proportions, but even in the same patient (Akiskal et al. 1989, 1997; Akiskal 1998, 2000, 2001; von Zerssen and Akiskal 1998; Kendler et al. 1992; Maier et al. 1992; Remick et al. 1996; Akiskal and Akiskal 2007). Affective temperaments seem to relate also to mood disorder family history, thus constituting an endophenotype bridge between genes and mood disorders (Cassano et al. 1992a; Akiskal et al. 2005b; Hantouche and Akiskal 2006; Chiaroni et al. 2005; Mendlowicz et al. 2005b). Viewing mood disorders under this prism gives birth to the concept of the bipolar spectrum with major implications for all aspects of mental health research and providing of care (Akiskal 2007).

Research so far indicates that the hyperthymic and the depressive temperaments are related to the more 'classic' bipolar picture (i.e. euphoria, grandiose and paranoid thinking, antisocial behaviour, psychomotor acceleration and reduced sleep and depressive episodes, respectively). On the contrary, cyclothymic, anxious and irritable temperaments are related to more complex pictures and might predict poor response to treatment, violent or suicidal behaviour and high comorbidity. Coexistence of temperaments or intrusion of a mood episode on a temperament of the opposite polarity also produces complex clinical manifestations and might lead to poor outcome. Often this poor outcome does not reflect inherent properties of the illness, but instead reflects the inability of the therapist to understand the illness and adequately plan treatment (Pompili et al. 2008; Oedegaard et al. 2009; Perugi et al. 1997, 1998b, 2001; Dell'Osso et al. 1993; Cassano et al. 1989, 1992b; Akiskal et al. 2005b, 2006a, b; Azorin et al. 2009, 2010; Rihmer et al. 2009; Ng et al. 2008). Temperament assessment could be especially helpful in understanding gender differences and plan treatment accordingly (Perugi et al. 1990; Dell'Osso et al. 1991; Cassano et al. 1992a; Hantouche et al. 2001).

Finally, the widening of our view concerning the information that could be useful for the diagnosis and treatment of bipolar disorder not only radically changes our understanding of the disease but also leads to better treatment and outcome of patients and probably can also lead to saving and better allocation of resources. Incorporating the concept of temperament and the bipolar spectrum in the standard training of psychiatric residents emerges as a pressing issue, but the way this can be achieved remains a challenge.

References

Akiskal HS (1994) The temperamental borders of affective disorders. Acta Psychiatr Scand Suppl 379:32–37

Akiskal HS (1998) The childhood roots of bipolar disorder. J Affect Disord 51(2):75–76. doi:S0165032798001736 [pii]

Akiskal HS (2000) Temperament and mood disorders. Harv Ment Health Lett 16(8):5–6. doi:M0100b [pii]

Akiskal HS (2001) Dysthymia and cyclothymia in psychiatric practice a century after Kraepelin. J Affect Disord 62(1–2):17–31. doi:S0165-0327(00)00347-5 [pii]

Akiskal HS (2007) The emergence of the bipolar spectrum: validation along clinical-epidemiologic and familial-genetic lines. Psychopharmacol Bull 40(4):99–115

Akiskal H, Akiskal K (2005) Epilogue. The renaissance of the ancient concept of temperament (with a focus on affective temperaments). In: Mai M, Akiskal H, Mezzich J, Okasha A (eds) Personality disorders. Wiley, San Diego, pp 479–500

Akiskal HS, Akiskal KK (2007) In search of Aristotle: temperament, human nature, melancholia, creativity and eminence. J Affect Disord 100(1–3):1–6. doi:10.1016/j.jad.2007.04.013, S0165-0327(07)00139-5 [pii]

Akiskal HS, Cassano GB, Musetti L, Perugi G, Tundo A, Mignani V (1989) Psychopathology, temperament, and past course in primary major depressions. 1. Review of evidence for a bipolar spectrum. Psychopathology 22(5):268–277

Akiskal HS, Judd LL, Gillin JC, Lemmi H (1997) Subthreshold depressions: clinical and polysomnographic validation of dysthymic, residual and masked forms. J Affect Disord 45(1–2):53–63. doi:S0165-0327(97)00059-1 [pii]

Akiskal HS, Hantouche EG, Bourgeois ML, Azorin JM, Sechter D, Allilaire JF, Lancrenon S, Fraud JP, Chatenet-Duchene L (1998a) Gender, temperament, and the clinical picture in dysphoric mixed mania: findings from a French national study (EPIMAN). J Affect Disord 50(2–3):175–186

Akiskal HS, Placidi GF, Maremmani I, Signoretta S, Liguori A, Gervasi R, Mallya G, Puzantian VR (1998b) TEMPS-I: delineating the most discriminant traits of the cyclothymic, depressive, hyperthymic and irritable temperaments in a nonpatient population. J Affect Disord 51(1): 7–19. doi:S0165-0327(98)00152-9 [pii]

Akiskal HS, Hantouche EG, Allilaire JF (2003) Bipolar II with and without cyclothymic temperament: "dark" and "sunny" expressions of soft bipolarity. J Affect Disord 73(1–2):49–57. doi:S0165032702003208 [pii]

Akiskal H, Akiskal K, Haykal R, Manning J, Connor PD (2005a) TEMPS-A: progress towards validation of a self-rated clinical version of the temperament evaluation of the Memphis, Pisa, Paris, and San Diego autoquestionnaire. J Affect Disord 85(1–2):3–16

Akiskal HS, Akiskal K, Allilaire JF, Azorin JM, Bourgeois ML, Sechter D, Fraud JP, Chatenet-Duchene L, Lancrenon S, Perugi G, Hantouche EG (2005b) Validating affective temperaments in their subaffective and socially positive attributes: psychometric, clinical and familial data from a French national study. J Affect Disord 85(1–2):29–36. doi:10.1016/j.jad.2003.12.009, S0165032704000242 [pii]

Akiskal HS, Mendlowicz MV, Jean-Louis G, Rapaport MH, Kelsoe JR, Gillin JC, Smith TL (2005c) TEMPS-A: validation of a short version of a self-rated instrument designed to measure variations in temperament. J Affect Disord 85(1–2):45–52. doi:10.1016/j.jad.2003.10.012, S0165032703003215 [pii]

Akiskal HS, Akiskal KK, Lancrenon S, Hantouche E (2006a) Validating the soft bipolar spectrum in the French National EPIDEP Study: the prominence of BP-II 1/2. J Affect Disord 96(3): 207–213. doi:10.1016/j.jad.2006.03.011, S0165-0327(06)00131-5 [pii]

Akiskal HS, Akiskal KK, Lancrenon S, Hantouche EG, Fraud JP, Gury C, Allilaire JF (2006b) Validating the bipolar spectrum in the French National EPIDEP Study: overview of the phenomenology and relative prevalence of its clinical prototypes. J Affect Disord 96(3):197–205. doi:10.1016/j.jad.2006.05.015, S0165-0327(06)00248-5 [pii]

Azorin JM, Kaladjian A, Adida M, Hantouche E, Hameg A, Lancrenon S, Akiskal HS (2009) Risk factors associated with lifetime suicide attempts in bipolar I patients: findings from a French National Cohort. Compr Psychiatry 50(2):115–120. doi:10.1016/j.comppsych.2008.07.004, S0010-440X(08)00105-3 [pii]

Azorin JM, Kaladjian A, Besnier N, Adida M, Hantouche E, Lancrenon S, Akiskal H (2010) Suicidal behaviour in a French Cohort of major depressive patients: characteristics of attempters and nonattempters. J Affect Disord 123(1–3):87–94. doi:10.1016/j.jad.2009.09.004, S0165-0327(09)00422-4 [pii]

Bertelsen A (1978) A Danish twin study of manic-depressive disorders. Prog Clin Biol Res 24A:119–124

Bertelsen A, Harvald B, Hauge M (1977) A Danish twin study of manic-depressive disorders. Br J Psychiatry 130:330–351

Biederman J, Rosenbaum JF, Hirshfeld DR, Faraone SV, Bolduc EA, Gersten M, Meminger SR, Kagan J, Snidman N, Reznick JS (1990) Psychiatric correlates of behavioral inhibition in young children of parents with and without psychiatric disorders. Arch Gen Psychiatry 47(1):21–26
Biederman J, Hirshfeld-Becker DR, Rosenbaum JF, Herot C, Friedman D, Snidman N, Kagan J, Faraone SV (2001) Further evidence of association between behavioral inhibition and social anxiety in children. Am J Psychiatry 158(10):1673–1679
Cassano GB, Akiskal HS, Musetti L, Perugi G, Soriani A, Mignani V (1989) Psychopathology, temperament, and past course in primary major depressions. 2. Toward a redefinition of bipolarity with a new semistructured interview for depression. Psychopathology 22(5):278–288
Cassano GB, Akiskal HS, Perugi G, Musetti L, Savino M (1992a) The importance of measures of affective temperaments in genetic studies of mood disorders. J Psychiatr Res 26(4):257–268
Cassano GB, Akiskal HS, Savino M, Musetti L, Perugi G (1992b) Proposed subtypes of bipolar II and related disorders: with hypomanic episodes (or cyclothymia) and with hyperthymic temperament. J Affect Disord 26(2):127–140
Cattel R, Eber H, Tatsuoka M (1970) The handbook for the sixteen personality factor questionnaire. Institute for Personality and Ability Testing, Champain
Chiaroni P, Hantouche EG, Gouvernet J, Azorin JM, Akiskal HS (2005) The cyclothymic temperament in healthy controls and familially at risk individuals for mood disorder: endophenotype for genetic studies? J Affect Disord 85(1–2):135–145. doi:10.1016/j.jad.2003.12.010, S0165032704000254 [pii]
Cloninger CR (1987) A systematic method for clinical description and classification of personality variants. A proposal. Arch Gen Psychiatry 44(6):573–588
Cloninger CR, Zohar AH (2011) Personality and the perception of health and happiness. J Affect Disord 128(1–2):24–32. doi:10.1016/j.jad.2010.06.012, S0165-0327(10)00425-8 [pii]
Cloninger CR, Svrakic DM, Przybeck TR (1993) A psychobiological model of temperament and character. Arch Gen Psychiatry 50(12):975–990
Cloninger CR, Przybeck TR, Svrakic DM, Wetzel RD (1994) The Temperament and Character Inventory (TCI): a guide to its development and use. Washington University Center for Psychobiology of Personality, St. Louis
Cloninger C, Svrakic D, Bayon C, Przybeck T (1999) Measurement of psychopathology as variants of personality. In: Cloninger C (ed) Personality and psychopathology. American Psychiatric Press Inc., Washington, DC, pp 33–65
Cloninger CR, Zohar AH, Cloninger KM (2010) Promotion of well-being in person-centered mental health care. Focus 8(2):165–179
Cloninger CR, Abou-Saleh MT, Mrazek DA, Moller H-J (2011) Biological perspective on psychiatry for the person. Int J Person Cent Med 1 (1) (in press)
Cohen P (1999) Personality development in childhood: old and new findings. In: Cloninger C (ed) Personality and psychopathology. American Psychiatric Press Inc, Washington, DC, pp 101–127
Conley JJ (1985) Longitudinal stability of personality traits: a multitrait-multimethod-multioccasion analysis. J Pers Soc Psychol 49(5):1266–1282
Constantino JN, Cloninger CR, Clarke AR, Hashemi B, Przybeck T (2002) Application of the seven-factor model of personality to early childhood. Psychiatry Res 109(3):229–243. doi:S0165178102000082 [pii]
Costa P, McCrae R (1990) Personality disorders and the five-factor model of personality. J Personal Disord 4:362–371
Dell'Osso L, Placidi GF, Nassi R, Freer P, Cassano GB, Akiskal HS (1991) The manic-depressive mixed state: familial, temperamental and psychopathologic characteristics in 108 female inpatients. Eur Arch Psychiatry Clin Neurosci 240(4–5):234–239
Dell'Osso L, Akiskal HS, Freer P, Barberi M, Placidi GF, Cassano GB (1993) Psychotic and non-psychotic bipolar mixed states: comparisons with manic and schizoaffective disorders. Eur Arch Psychiatry Clin Neurosci 243(2):75–81
Evans L, Akiskal HS, Keck PE Jr, McElroy SL, Sadovnick AD, Remick RA, Kelsoe JR (2005) Familiality of temperament in bipolar disorder: support for a genetic spectrum. J Affect Disord 85(1–2):153–168. doi:10.1016/j.jad.2003.10.015, S0165032703003252 [pii]

Eysenck HJ, Eysenck SB (1962) A factorial study of an interview-questionnaire. J Clin Psychol 18:286–290
Eysenck SB, Eysenck HJ (1964) An improved short questionnaire for the measurement of extraversion and neuroticism. Life Sci 3:1103–1109
Eysenck SB, Eysenck HJ (1967) Physiological reactivity to sensory stimulation as a measure of personality. Psychol Rep 20(1):45–46
Eysenck SB, Eysenck HJ (1968) The measurement of psychoticism: a study of factor stability and reliability. Br J Soc Clin Psychol 7(4):286–294
Eysenck SB, Eysenck HJ (1969) Scores on three personality variables as a function of age, sex and social class. Br J Soc Clin Psychol 8(1):69–76
Eysenck SB, Eysenck HJ (1972) The questionnaire measurement of psychoticism. Psychol Med 2(1):50–55
Eysenck SB, Eysenck HJ (1977) The place of impulsiveness in a dimensional system of personality description. Br J Soc Clin Psychol 16(1):57–68
Eysenck SB, Eysenck HJ, Shaw L (1974) The modification of personality and lie scale scores by special 'honesty' instructions. Br J Soc Clin Psychol 13(1):41–50
Eysenck SB, White O, Eysenck HJ (1976) Personality and mental illness. Psychol Rep 39(3):1011–1022
Eysenck SB, Adelaja O, Eysenck HJ (1977) A comparative study of personality in Nigerian and English subjects. J Soc Psychol 102(Second Half):171–178
Farmer A, Mahmood A, Redman K, Harris T, Sadler S, McGuffin P (2003) A sib-pair study of the temperament and character inventory scales in major depression. Arch Gen Psychiatry 60(5):490–496. doi:10.1001/archpsyc.60.5.490, 60/5/490 [pii]
Friedman HS, Tucker JS, Tomlinson-Keasey C, Schwartz JE, Wingard DL, Criqui MH (1993) Does childhood personality predict longevity? J Pers Soc Psychol 65(1):176–185
Hantouche EG, Akiskal HS (2006) Toward a definition of a cyclothymic behavioral endophenotype: which traits tap the familial diathesis for bipolar II disorder? J Affect Disord 96(3):233–237. doi:10.1016/j.jad.2004.08.013, S0165-0327(04)00279-4 [pii]
Hantouche EG, Akiskal HS, Lancrenon S, Allilaire JF, Sechter D, Azorin JM, Bourgeois M, Fraud JP, Chatenet-Duchene L (1998) Systematic clinical methodology for validating bipolar-II disorder: data in mid-stream from a French national multi-site study (EPIDEP). J Affect Disord 50(2–3):163–173
Hantouche EG, Allilaire JP, Bourgeois ML, Azorin JM, Sechter D, Chatenet-Duchene L, Lancrenon S, Akiskal HS (2001) The feasibility of self-assessment of dysphoric mania in the French national EPIMAN study. J Affect Disord 67(1–3):97–103. doi:S0165032701004426 [pii]
Josefsson K, Jokela M, Cloninger CR, Hintsanen M, Salo J, Hintsa T, Pulkki-Raback L, Keltikangas-Jarvinen L (2012) Maturity and change in personality: developmental trends of temperament and character in adulthood. Development and Psychopathology (in press)
Kagan J, Zentner M (1996) Early childhood predictors of adult psychopathology. Harv Rev Psychiatry 3(6):341–350
Kagan J, Snidman N, Zentner M, Peterson E (1999) Infant temperament and anxious symptoms in school age children. Dev Psychopathol 11(2):209–224
Kagan J, Snidman N, McManis M, Woodward S (2001) Temperamental contributions to the affect family of anxiety. Psychiatr Clin North Am 24(4):677–688
Karam EG, Salamoun MM, Yeretzian JS, Mneimneh ZN, Karam AN, Fayyad J, Hantouche E, Akiskal K, Akiskal HS (2010) The role of anxious and hyperthymic temperaments in mental disorders: a national epidemiologic study. World Psychiatry 9(2):103–110
Kendler KS (1997) Social support: a genetic-epidemiologic analysis. Am J Psychiatry 154(10):1398–1404
Kendler KS, Karkowski-Shuman L (1997) Stressful life events and genetic liability to major depression: genetic control of exposure to the environment? Psychol Med 27(3):539–547
Kendler KS, Neale MC, Kessler RC, Heath AC, Eaves LJ (1992) A population-based twin study of major depression in women. The impact of varying definitions of illness. Arch Gen Psychiatry 49(4):257–266

Kesebir S, Vahip S, Akdeniz F, Yuncu Z, Alkan M, Akiskal H (2005) Affective temperaments as measured by TEMPS-A in patients with bipolar I disorder and their first-degree relatives: a controlled study. J Affect Disord 85(1–2):127–133. doi:10.1016/j.jad.2003.10.013, S0165032703003227 [pii]

Kraepelin E (1921) Manic-Depressive Insanity and Paranoia. Edinburgh: Livingstone

Maier W, Lichtermann D, Minges J, Heun R, Hallmayer J (1992) The risk of minor depression in families of probands with major depression: sex differences and familiality. Eur Arch Psychiatry Clin Neurosci 242(2–3):89–92

Maremmani I, Akiskal H, Signoretta S, Liguori A, Perugi G, Cloninger C (2005) The relationship of Kraepelian affective temperaments (as measured by TEMPS-I) to the tridimensional personality questionnaire (TPQ). J Affect Disord 85:17–27

Markon KE, Krueger RF, Watson D (2005) Delineating the structure of normal and abnormal personality: an integrative hierarchical approach. J Pers Soc Psychol 88(1):139–157. doi:10.1037/0022-3514.88.1.139, 2004-22407-010 [pii]

McAdams DP, Pals JL (2006) A new Big Five: fundamental principles for an integrative science of personality. Am Psychol 61(3):204–217. doi:10.1037/0003-066X.61.3.204, 2006-03947-002 [pii]

McCrae RR, Costa PT Jr (1987) Validation of the five-factor model of personality across instruments and observers. J Pers Soc Psychol 52(1):81–90

Mendlowicz MV, Akiskal HS, Kelsoe JR, Rapaport MH, Jean-Louis G, Gillin JC (2005a) Temperament in the clinical differentiation of depressed bipolar and unipolar major depressive patients. J Affect Disord 84(2–3):219–223. doi:10.1016/j.jad.2004.01.013, S0165032704000849 [pii]

Mendlowicz MV, Jean-Louis G, Kelsoe JR, Akiskal HS (2005b) A comparison of recovered bipolar patients, healthy relatives of bipolar probands, and normal controls using the short TEMPS-A. J Affect Disord 85(1–2):147–151. doi:10.1016/j.jad.2004.01.012, S0165032704000825 [pii]

Merikangas KR, Akiskal HS, Angst J, Greenberg PE, Hirschfeld RM, Petukhova M, Kessler RC (2007) Lifetime and 12-month prevalence of bipolar spectrum disorder in the National Comorbidity Survey replication. Arch Gen Psychiatry 64(5):543–552. doi:10.1001/archpsyc.64.5.543, 64/5/543 [pii]

Merikangas KR, Jin R, He JP, Kessler RC, Lee S, Sampson NA, Viana MC, Andrade LH, Hu C, Karam EG, Ladea M, Medina-Mora ME, Ono Y, Posada-Villa J, Sagar R, Wells JE, Zarkov Z (2011) Prevalence and correlates of bipolar spectrum disorder in the world mental health survey initiative. Arch Gen Psychiatry 68(3):241–251. doi:10.1001/archgenpsychiatry.2011.12, 68/3/241 [pii]

Ng B, Camacho A, Lara DR, Brunstein MG, Pinto OC, Akiskal HS (2008) A case series on the hypothesized connection between dementia and bipolar spectrum disorders: bipolar type VI? J Affect Disord 107(1–3):307–315

Nolen-Hoeksema S (2011) Emotion regulation and psychopathology: the role of gender. Annu Rev Clin Psychol 8:161–187. doi:10.1146/annurev-clinpsy-032511-143109

Nolen-Hoeksema S, Girgus JS (1994) The emergence of gender differences in depression during adolescence. Psychol Bull 115(3):424–443

Nolen-Hoeksema S, Larson J, Grayson C (1999) Explaining the gender difference in depressive symptoms. J Pers Soc Psychol 77(5):1061–1072

Oedegaard KJ, Syrstad VE, Morken G, Akiskal HS, Fasmer OB (2009) A study of age at onset and affective temperaments in a Norwegian sample of patients with mood disorders. J Affect Disord 118(1–3):229–233. doi:10.1016/j.jad.2009.01.030, S0165-0327(09)00047-0 [pii]

Perugi G, Akiskal HS (2002) The soft bipolar spectrum redefined: focus on the cyclothymic, anxious-sensitive, impulse-dyscontrol, and binge-eating connection in bipolar II and related conditions. Psychiatr Clin North Am 25(4):713–737

Perugi G, Musetti L, Simonini E, Piagentini F, Cassano GB, Akiskal HS (1990) Gender-mediated clinical features of depressive illness. The importance of temperamental differences. Br J Psychiatry 157:835–841

Perugi G, Akiskal HS, Micheli C, Musetti L, Paiano A, Quilici C, Rossi L, Cassano GB (1997) Clinical subtypes of bipolar mixed states: validating a broader European definition in 143 cases. J Affect Disord 43(3):169–180. doi:S0165-0327(97)01446-8 [pii]

Perugi G, Akiskal HS, Lattanzi L, Cecconi D, Mastrocinque C, Patronelli A, Vignoli S, Bemi E (1998a) The high prevalence of "soft" bipolar (II) features in atypical depression. Compr Psychiatry 39(2):63–71. doi:S0010-440X(98)90080-3 [pii]

Perugi G, Akiskal HS, Rossi L, Paiano A, Quilici C, Madaro D, Musetti L, Cassano GB (1998b) Chronic mania. Family history, prior course, clinical picture and social consequences. Br J Psychiatry 173:514–518

Perugi G, Maremmani I, Toni C, Madaro D, Mata B, Akiskal HS (2001) The contrasting influence of depressive and hyperthymic temperaments on psychometrically derived manic subtypes. Psychiatry Res 101(3):249–258. doi:S0165-1781(01)00232-3 [pii]

Perugi G, Toni C, Travierso MC, Akiskal HS (2003) The role of cyclothymia in atypical depression: toward a data-based reconceptualization of the borderline-bipolar II connection. J Affect Disord 73(1–2):87–98. doi:S0165032702003294 [pii]

Perugi G, Toni C, Maremmani I, Tusini G, Ramacciotti S, Madia A, Fornaro M, Akiskal HS (2010) The influence of affective temperaments and psychopathological traits on the definition of bipolar disorder subtypes: a study on bipolar I Italian National sample. J Affect Disord. doi:10.1016/j.jad.2009.12.027, S0165-0327(10)00006-6 [pii]

Pompili M, Rihmer Z, Akiskal HS, Innamorati M, Iliceto P, Akiskal KK, Lester D, Narciso V, Ferracuti S, Tatarelli R, De Pisa E, Girardi P (2008) Temperament and personality dimensions in suicidal and nonsuicidal psychiatric inpatients. Psychopathology 41(5):313–321. doi:10.1159/000146069, 000146069 [pii]

Remick RA, Sadovnick AD, Lam RW, Zis AP, Yee IM (1996) Major depression, minor depression, and double depression: are they distinct clinical entities? Am J Med Genet 67(4):347–353. doi:10.1002/(SICI)1096-8628(19960726)67:4<347::AID-AJMG6>3.0.CO;2-J [pii]

Rihmer A, Rozsa S, Rihmer Z, Gonda X, Akiskal KK, Akiskal HS (2009) Affective temperaments, as measured by TEMPS-A, among nonviolent suicide attempters. J Affect Disord 116 (1–2):18–22. doi:10.1016/j.jad.2008.10.024, S0165-0327(08)00438-2 [pii]

Rosenbaum JF, Biederman J, Gersten M, Hirshfeld DR, Meminger SR, Herman JB, Kagan J, Reznick JS, Snidman N (1988) Behavioral inhibition in children of parents with panic disorder and agoraphobia. A controlled study. Arch Gen Psychiatry 45(5):463–470

Rosenbaum JF, Biederman J, Hirshfeld DR, Bolduc EA, Faraone SV, Kagan J, Snidman N, Reznick JS (1991) Further evidence of an association between behavioral inhibition and anxiety disorders: results from a family study of children from a non-clinical sample. J Psychiatr Res 25(1–2):49–65

Rothbart MK, Ahadi SA, Evans DE (2000) Temperament and personality: origins and outcomes. J Pers Soc Psychol 78(1):122–135

Serafini G, Pompili M, Innamorati M, Fusar-Poli P, Akiskal HS, Rihmer Z, Lester D, Romano A, de Oliveira IR, Strusi L, Ferracuti S, Girardi P, Tatarelli R (2010) Affective temperamental profiles are associated with white matter hyperintensity and suicidal risk in patients with mood disorders. J Affect Disord. doi:10.1016/j.jad.2010.07.020, S0165-0327(10)00501-X [pii]

Smoller JW, Yamaki LH, Fagerness JA, Biederman J, Racette S, Laird NM, Kagan J, Snidman N, Faraone SV, Hirshfeld-Becker D, Tsuang MT, Slaugenhaupt SA, Rosenbaum JF, Sklar PB (2005) The corticotropin-releasing hormone gene and behavioral inhibition in children at risk for panic disorder. Biol Psychiatry 57(12):1485–1492. doi:10.1016/j.biopsych.2005.02.018, S0006-3223(05)00183-6 [pii]

Tellegen A, Grove W, Waller N (1991) Inventory of personality characteristics #7 (IPC7). University of Minnesota Department of Psychology, Minneapolis

Vazquez GH, Kahn C, Schiavo CE, Goldchluk A, Herbst L, Piccione M, Saidman N, Ruggeri H, Silva A, Leal J, Bonetto GG, Zaratiegui R, Padilla E, Vilaprino JJ, Calvo M, Guerrero G, Strejilevich SA, Cetkovich-Bakmas MG, Akiskal KK, Akiskal HS (2008) Bipolar disorders and affective temperaments: a national family study testing the "endophenotype" and "subaffective" theses using the TEMPS-A Buenos Aires. J Affect Disord 108(1–2):25–32. doi:10.1016/j.jad.2007.09.011, S0165-0327(07)00340-0 [pii]

von Zerssen D, Akiskal HS (1998) Personality factors in affective disorders: historical developments and current issues with special reference to the concepts of temperament and character. J Affect Disord 51(1):1–5. doi:S0165032798001517 [pii]

6 The Bipolar Spectrum

As mentioned above, a significant number of patients are initially diagnosed as suffering from unipolar depression, and latter, when mania or hypomania emerges, the diagnosis is changed to bipolar disorder. This essentially poses another question, concerning the diagnosis of cases with subthreshold manic symptoms or long-lasting hyperthymia. These patients are reported to be refractory to standard therapeutic approaches. While the traditional bipolar vs. unipolar distinction is widely used and adopted by classification systems, it is doubtful whether it can capture the essence of the huge heterogeneity observed in mood disorders and their dynamic nature with frequent switches and changes in the clinical profile. The greatest disadvantage of both classification systems is that they perform better (and focus) when interepisodic remission is present; instead, the everyday real-life patients is more likely to suffer from a chronic disorder with residual and mixed symptoms. A dimensional concept (from normal to pathological) was proposed by Kretschmer in 1921 for schizophrenia (schizothymic–schizoid–schizophrenic) and for affective disorders (cyclothymic temperament–cycloid 'psychopathy'–manic–depressive disorder) as well as by Bleuler in 1922. The term 'spectrum' was first used in psychiatry in 1968 for the schizophrenia spectrum (Kety et al. 1968). However, the mood spectrum is solidly embedded in the spectrum of functional psychoses, including schizophrenia and schizoaffective and affective disorders. There is growing clinical evidence that the spectrum approach, with its dimensional nature, offers a real alternative to the traditional Kraepelinian dichotomy of schizophrenia v. manic–depressive insanity (Marneros 2006) and the unipolar–bipolar dichotomy.

The proposed mood spectrum models unify categorical classification, which is essential, with a dimensional view, which is true to nature; both are needed and both are empirically testable. Today the term 'bipolar spectrum' is mainly used in two complementary senses: (a) a spectrum of severity, which embraces psychotic and nonpsychotic major and minor bipolar disorders (including bipolar dysthymia, recurrent brief and minor depressions), cyclothymic disorders, hypomania and, at its broadest, even borderline disorders and cyclothymic temperament; (b) a proportional mood spectrum, which considers the two components mania and depression,

K.N. Fountoulakis, *Bipolar Disorder: An Evidence-Based Guide to Manic Depression*, DOI 10.1007/978-3-642-37216-2_6

on the level of major and minor mood disorders. This proportional model is an extension of Kleist's concept of bipolar disorder as a combination of the two monopolar disorders depression and mania (Kleist 1937). Thus, these two approaches to spectrum reflect two distinct continua: from normal to pathological and from unipolar to bipolar.

Clinical and epidemiological studies in the USA and Europe have revealed a richer range of hypomanic manifestations than those listed in the classification systems (cheerfulness and jocularity; gregariousness and people seeking; greater interest in sex; talkativeness, self-confidence, and optimism; and decreased inhibitions and sleep need). The use of stimulant and alcohol as well as chronic caffeine use and smoking might perplex the picture and make a reliable diagnosis difficult.

The everyday real-life patients most probably manifest depression with anxiety, atypical depressive features and reactivity of mood are frequent, hypomania tends to be dysphoric or irritable rather than euphoric and benzodiazepine abuse is frequent. If hypomania is euphoric, often it is perceived as a 'bright' depression-free period and is not mentioned either by the patient or by family. Mood swings start during adolescence and might last for lifetime. They are unpredictable in terms of polarity, severity and duration as well as additional symptomatology (e.g. anxiety or psychotic features). Sometimes they are related to the season of the year or to the menstrual cycle of females. It appears that multipolar mood disorder might be a more accurate designation for the soft bipolar spectrum.

Since many patients manifest symptoms of both poles, but the severity or duration of those in either pole (or both) is subthreshold (minor), a group of disorders can be proposed on the basis of 'subthreshold' bipolarity in cases where otherwise a 'unipolar' diagnosis would be more appropriate according to either classification system. Often these patients show episodic dysphoric hypomania associated with mood instability, irritability, impulsiveness, temper dyscontrol, impaired judgement, interpersonal difficulties and disability. Paranoid ideation is also frequent. This makes the concept of temperament highly important and useful.

Essentially, this line of thought is based on a 'dimensional' rather than a 'categorical' approach to psychopathology and diagnosis. Subsequently, this raises the question of the correct cut-off levels for caseness (Wing et al. 1978). Since the official standards concerning duration and severity no longer apply, the boundaries between health and disease, normality and illness become vague. Empirically validated, sensitive and operational definitions of hypomania and minor depression are essential and these definitions will allow early recognition of major and minor bipolar disorders. However, almost by definition, duration, severity and impairment cannot be used cross-sectionally as markers for the differentiation between normal psychological reactions and subthreshold mood disorders. Additionally, in chronic conditions, neither the patient nor his family can clearly describe a change in behaviour or in personality. It is expected that in the long term, patients manifest a significant degree of impairment, which often appears very early in the course and is disproportional to the acute symptomatology. These patients do not seem to benefit from taking leisure time. The personal history as well as the family history of past mood episodes could be of prime importance. Especially the family history can be used as an external validator particularly for those cases with a large number of family members being afflicted with mood disorder. Hypomanias with short duration (less than 4 days) are familially similar to those with longer duration (more than 4 days).

An important part of the 'bipolar spectrum' is cyclothymic disorder which is considered to be an attenuated form of BD. It typically starts before the age of 21 and is characterized by frequent short cycles of subsyndromal depression and hypomania. The course is continuous or intermittent, with infrequent periods of euthymia. Endogenous overreactivity seems to determine the sudden shifts in mood and behaviour. Mood swings in these ambulatory patients are overshadowed by the chaos that the swings produce in their personal lives. These patients are dilettantes; they show great promise in many areas, but rarely bring any of their efforts to fruition. As a result, their lives are often a string of improvident activities. Geographical instability is a characteristic feature; easily attracted to a new locale job or love partner, they soon lose interest and leave in dissatisfaction. Their behaviour is characterized by the alternation of extremes: introverted self-absorption vs. uninhibited people seeking, taciturn vs. talkative, unexplained tearfulness vs. buoyant jocularity, psychomotor inertia vs. restless pursuit of activities, lethargy and somatic discomfort vs. eutonia, dulling of senses vs. keen perceptions, slow-witted thinking vs. sharpened thinking, shaky self-esteem alternating between low self-confidence and overconfidence and pessimistic brooding vs. optimism and carefree attitudes (Akiskal et al. 1977). Polysubstance abuse which occurs in as many as 50 % of such persons is often an attempt at self-treatment. Depending on the threshold of traits used in determining the presence of hyperthymia, cyclothymic patients may constitute 10–20 % of those with major depressive disorder. Also, cyclothymia is often a prodromal of bipolar disorder (Akiskal et al. 1979).

Another important part of the bipolar spectrum is those patients who experience an antidepressant-induced switch. Although antidepressant-induced switch is still not proven beyond reasonable doubt and many authors suggest it might not exist at all (Grunze 2008), the prevailing opinion among researchers and clinicians is that at least some antidepressants (and especially double acting ones) pose the patient at a significant risk to switch to the opposite pole or to slip into a mixed episode. These patients are reported to have family history of bipolarity and often their depression is superimposed on a hyperthymic temperament. Thus, many patients with so-called unipolar depression are actually 'pseudounipolar'. The presence of marked narcissistic traits is a helpful clinical clue that a clinically depressed patient might belong to the group of those with hyperthymic depressions.

An important issue in the bipolar spectrum research is the nature of the concepts and tools used to assess mood patients. The standard methodology restricts itself to the current DSM diagnostic concepts, and no additional data are collected. On the other hand, when too broad definitions and concepts and tools are used, the data might be contaminated by some kind of 'noise' which might obscure diagnostic boundaries, leading to uncritical generalizations and over-inclusiveness. This is especially true, since most of anxiety and dysphoric symptoms can be considered 'transnosological' and non-specific (i.e. they can be observed in most 'primary' diagnoses, from schizophrenia to personality disorders). This is of course a consequence of the fact that psychiatric diagnosis is based on phenomenology and diagnostic biological markers are missing. This is an important problem since in the rest of medicine, it is known that similar symptoms may arise from different underlying pathologies and require different therapeutic interventions. Polythetic criteria in classification systems, huge comorbidity, the great overlapping of genetic and other biological data and the non-specificity of overall outcome obscure the picture. Also diagnostic tendencies are influenced by available treatment options (mostly pharmacotherapy). It is well known that in the past, borderline behaviour was considered to be a variant of psychosis, depression or posttraumatic stress disorder (Paris 2004).

There are a number of studies suggesting that 'phenomenological similarity' does not necessarily imply 'nosological similarity' in psychiatry. For example, subthreshold hypomania during adolescence does not predict hypomania during adulthood and thus treatment might not be necessary (Aivar et al. 2012). Different phenomenology, family history, course and response to treatment have been reported for bipolar spectrum disorders in comparison to the classical BD (Paris 2009). Some authors suggest that a significant part of the literature consists mostly of expert opinion overemphasizing various links between bipolar and unipolar mood disorders and personality disorders (Patten and Paris 2008; Paris et al. 2007). For some authors, it is simply a matter of 'bipolar imperialism'.

However, in modern medicine and psychiatry, data and not arguments prevail and determine (or should prevail and should determine) the conclusions.

During the last 10 years, several studies reported epidemiological and clinical data in support for a continuous distribution of depressive and hypomanic/manic symptomatology from normal to pathological (Judd and Akiskal 2003; Judd et al. 2003; Merikangas et al. 2007, 2011). It is interesting that these studies suggest that only a small minority (around 15 %) of the general population reports no such symptoms ever in lifetime. These persons might be considered to be 'supernormal', with high ego resiliency and strength. It has also been reported that brief episodes of hypomania (1–3 days) are more common than those with longer duration (4 days to 1 week) (Angst 2007). Recently the first solid international epidemiological data in support of the bipolar spectrum have been published (Merikangas et al. 2007, 2011; Angst et al. 2010). According to these authors there is a direct association between increasingly restrictive definitions of BD and indicators of clinical severity including symptom severity, role impairment, comorbidity, suicidality and treatment. For example, the proportion of mood episodes rated as clinically severe increased from 42.5 % for subthreshold BD to 68.8 % for BD-II to 74.5 % for BD-I. However, since clinical diagnosis and severity share confounding factors and definitions overlap, it is also important to note that these studies also showed that the proportion of cases reporting severe role impairment ranged from 46.3 % for subthreshold BD to 57.1 % for BD-I (Merikangas et al. 2011).

High comorbidity of BD with other mental disorders is reported (Merikangas et al. 2011) and particularly there seems to be a strong link between BD and anxiety. Prospective studies in adolescents (Lewinsohn et al. 2000, 2002) and children of parents with BD suggest that anxiety may constitute an early step in the developmental pathway of bipolarity (Duffy et al. 2007; Henin et al. 2005).

On the basis of both epidemiological data and clinical wisdom, a limited number of models reflecting the structure of the bipolar spectrum have been proposed. The first effort was a dimensional concept (from normal to pathological) proposed by Kretschmer in 1921 for schizophrenia (schizothymic–schizoid–schizophrenic) and for affective disorders (cyclothymic temperament–cycloid 'psychopathy'–manic–depressive disorder). Bleuler suggested a similar concept in 1922.

Emil Kraepelin conceptualized a continuum that included today's DSM-IV subtypes, mixed and rapid cycling states, many of the soft bipolar variations and also episodic depressions. This view prevailed until the 1960s, at which time the creators of DSM-I proposed a differentiation between major depression and manic–depressive illness. In later DSM editions, this evolved to the unipolar–bipolar dichotomy. In the 1970s Fieve et al. (1976a, b) discriminated bipolar I from bipolar II disorder, a seminal event in the evolution of the soft bipolar spectrum.

In 1977 Akiskal proposed a cyclothymic–bipolar spectrum (Akiskal et al. 1977).

A simple model system was introduced in 1978 by Jules Angst (Angst 1978; Angst et al. 1978), who used the following codes: M for severe mania, D for severe depression (unipolar depression), m for less severe mania (hypomania) and d for less severe depression. The combination of these codes describes the different entities which are supposed to comprise the bipolar spectrum. For example, according to this, mD stands for hypomania and major depression. Also the order of the code letters denotes the order of the episodes at the onset of the disorder. Thus, MD stands for a first episode of mania followed by depression while DM stands for the opposite.

In 1981 Gerald Klerman suggested a mania spectrum (Klerman 1981). His classification of primary bipolar subtypes is summarized as follows (Klerman 1987):

Bipolar I: Mania and depression
Bipolar II: Hypomania and depression
Bipolar III: Cyclothymic disorder
Bipolar IV: Hypomania or mania precipitated by antidepressant drugs
Bipolar V: Depressed patients with a family history of bipolar illness
Bipolar VI: Mania without depression [unipolar mania]

Today's leading conceptual thinker in the area of bipolar subtyping is Hagop Akiskal. Akiskal's description of the bipolar subtypes differs from that of Klerman. He proposes six subtypes, some of which are further subdivided according to their unique clinical features. A summary of his proposed subtype schema is as follows (Akiskal and Pinto 1999; Ng et al. 2007; Akiskal and Benazzi 2005; Fountoulakis 2008).

BD type	Description
BD-0	Schizophrenia
BD-1/2	Schizobipolar disorder
BD-I	Bipolar disorder with full blown mania
BD-I1/2	Depression with protracted hypomania
BD-II	Hypomania plus major depression
BD-II1/2	Depression superimposed on cyclothymic temperament
BD-III	Recurrent depression, plus hypomania occurring solely in association with antidepressant or other somatotherapy
BD-III1/2	Mood swings associated with substance and/or alcohol abuse
BD-IV	Depression superimposed on a hyperthymic temperament
BD-V	Recurrent depressions without discrete hypomania, but mixed hypomanic episodes (irritability/agitation/racing thoughts) during depression
BD-VI	Bipolarity in the frame of dementia

At present, we have no solid evidence that persons who belong to the 'bipolar spectrum' respond to treatments with proven efficacy against more classical forms of BD. Critics suggest that it is possible the broadening of the label of bipolar disorder to include the bipolar spectrum might lead to psychotropic drug overuse, especially of antipsychotics, antiepileptics and lithium.

References

Aivar P, Anne-Liis VK, Gunilla O, Lars VK, Hannes B, Ulf J (2012) Hypomania spectrum disorders from adolescence to adulthood: a 15-year follow-up of a community sample. J Affect Disord. doi:10.1016/j.jad.2012.07.031, S0165-0327(12)00562-9 [pii]

Akiskal HS, Benazzi F (2005) Atypical depression: a variant of bipolar II or a bridge between unipolar and bipolar II? J Affect Disord 84(2–3):209–217

Akiskal HS, Pinto O (1999) The evolving bipolar spectrum. Prototypes I, II, III, and IV. Psychiatr Clin N Am 22(3):517–534, vii

Akiskal HS, Djenderedjian AM, Rosenthal RH, Khani MK (1977) Cyclothymic disorder: validating criteria for inclusion in the bipolar affective group. Am J Psychiatry 134(11):1227–1233

Akiskal HS, Rosenthal RH, Rosenthal TL, Kashgarian M, Khani MK, Puzantian VR (1979) Differentiation of primary affective illness from situational, symptomatic, and secondary depressions. Arch Gen Psychiatry 36(6):635–643

Angst J (1978) The course of affective disorders. II Typology of bipolar manic-depressive illness. Arch Psychiatr Nervenkr 226(1):65–73

Angst J (2007) The bipolar spectrum. Br J Psychiatry 190:189–191. doi:10.1192/bjp.bp.106.030957, 190/3/189 [pii]

Angst J, Felder W, Frey R, Stassen HH (1978) The course of affective disorders. I. Change of diagnosis of monopolar, unipolar, and bipolar illness. Arch Psychiatr Nervenkr 226(1):57–64

Angst J, Cui L, Swendsen J, Rothen S, Cravchik A, Kessler RC, Merikangas KR (2010) Major depressive disorder with subthreshold bipolarity in the National Comorbidity Survey Replication. Am J Psychiatry 167(10):1194–1201. doi:10.1176/appi.ajp.2010.09071011, appi.ajp.2010.09071011 [pii]

Duffy A, Alda M, Crawford L, Milin R, Grof P (2007) The early manifestations of bipolar disorder: a longitudinal prospective study of the offspring of bipolar parents. Bipolar Disord 9(8):828–838. doi:10.1111/j.1399-5618.2007.00421.x, BDI421 [pii]

Fieve RR, Dunner DL, Kumbaraci T, Stallone F (1976a) Lithium carbonate prophylaxis of depression in three subtypes in primary affective disorder. Pharmakopsychiatr Neuropsychopharmakol 9(3):100–107. doi:10.1055/s-0028-1094484

Fieve RR, Kumbaraci T, Dunner DL (1976b) Lithium prophylaxis of depression in bipolar I, bipolar II, and unipolar patients. Am J Psychiatry 133(8):925–929

Fountoulakis KN (2008) The contemporary face of bipolar illness: complex diagnostic and therapeutic challenges. CNS Spectr 13(9):763–774, 777–779

Grunze HC (2008) Switching, induction of rapid cycling, and increased suicidality with antidepressants in bipolar patients: fact or overinterpretation? CNS Spectr 13(9):790–795

Henin A, Biederman J, Mick E, Sachs GS, Hirshfeld-Becker DR, Siegel RS, McMurrich S, Grandin L, Nierenberg AA (2005) Psychopathology in the offspring of parents with bipolar disorder: a controlled study. Biol Psychiatry 58(7):554–561. doi:10.1016/j.biopsych.2005.06.010, S0006-3223(05)00716-X [pii]

Judd LL, Akiskal HS (2003) The prevalence and disability of bipolar spectrum disorders in the US population: re-analysis of the ECA database taking into account subthreshold cases. J Affect Disord 73(1–2):123–131

Judd LL, Akiskal HS, Schettler PJ, Coryell W, Endicott J, Maser JD, Solomon DA, Leon AC, Keller MB (2003) A prospective investigation of the natural history of the long-term weekly symptomatic status of bipolar II disorder. Arch Gen Psychiatry 60(3):261–269, doi:yoa20225 [pii]

Kety S, Rosenthal D, Wender P, Schulschinger F (1968) The types and prevalence of mental illness in the biological and adoptive families of adopted schizophrenics. J Psychiatr Res 6:345–362

Kleist K (1937) Zustandsbilder und Krankheitsarten im Lichte der Gehirnpathologie. Psychiatrischneurologische Wochenschrift 39:420–422

Klerman GL (1981) The spectrum of mania. Compr Psychiatry 22(1):11–20

Klerman GL (1987) The classification of bipolar disorders. Psychiatr Ann 17(1):13–17

Lewinsohn PM, Klein DN, Seeley JR (2000) Bipolar disorder during adolescence and young adulthood in a community sample. Bipolar Disord 2(3 Pt 2):281–293

Lewinsohn PM, Seeley JR, Buckley ME, Klein DN (2002) Bipolar disorder in adolescence and young adulthood. Child Adolesc Psychiatr Clin N Am 11(3):461–475, vii

Marneros A (2006) Beyond the Kraepelinian dichotomy: acute and transient psychotic disorders and the necessity for clinical differentiation. Br J Psychiatry 189:1–2. doi:10.1192/bjp.bp.106.024257, 189/1/1 [pii]

Merikangas KR, Akiskal HS, Angst J, Greenberg PE, Hirschfeld RM, Petukhova M, Kessler RC (2007) Lifetime and 12-month prevalence of bipolar spectrum disorder in the National Comorbidity Survey replication. Arch Gen Psychiatry 64(5):543–552. doi:10.1001/archpsyc.64.5.543, 64/5/543 [pii]

Merikangas KR, Jin R, He JP, Kessler RC, Lee S, Sampson NA, Viana MC, Andrade LH, Hu C, Karam EG, Ladea M, Medina-Mora ME, Ono Y, Posada-Villa J, Sagar R, Wells JE, Zarkov Z (2011) Prevalence and correlates of bipolar spectrum disorder in the world mental health survey initiative. Arch Gen Psychiatry 68(3):241–251. doi:10.1001/archgenpsychiatry.2011.12, 68/3/241 [pii]

Ng B, Camacho A, Lara DR, Brunstein MG, Pinto OC, Akiskal HS (2007) A case series on the hypothesized connection between dementia and bipolar spectrum disorders: bipolar type VI? J Affect Disord 107(1–3):307–315

Paris J (2004) Borderline or bipolar? Distinguishing borderline personality disorder from bipolar spectrum disorders. Harv Rev Psychiatry 12(3):140–145. doi:10.1080/10673220490472373, 6RNMQUVU66LH5YJK [pii]

Paris J (2009) The bipolar spectrum: a critical perspective. Harv Rev Psychiatry 17(3):206–213. doi:10.1080/10673220902979888, 912030914 [pii]

Paris J, Gunderson J, Weinberg I (2007) The interface between borderline personality disorder and bipolar spectrum disorders. Compr Psychiatry 48(2):145–154. doi:10.1016/j.comppsych.2006.10.001, S0010-440X(06)00107-6 [pii]

Patten SB, Paris J (2008) The bipolar spectrum – a bridge too far? Can J Psychiatry 53(11):762–768

Wing JK, Mann SA, Leff JP, Nixon JM (1978) The concept of a 'case' in psychiatric population surveys. Psychol Med 8(2):203–217

Schizoaffective Disorder

7

It is well known that Kraepelin divided the psychoses into dementia praecox and manic–depressive illness on the basis of a supposed progressive deterioration for the first and a better long-term outcome for the latter. However, even Kraepelin himself reported that his clinical experience included many patients with features of both disorders. These patients were so many that he characterized their frequency as 'displeasing' (Angst 1986b). These cases have attracted the interest of researchers in the last few decades, but their diagnostic status is still uncertain.

In the early twentieth century, several authors also described forms of dementia praecox with an intermittent course and periods of excitement or depression. Lange described even catatonic syndromes in 14 % of those called 'circular disorders'. Bleuler suggested that the existence of mood and schizophrenic symptoms during the same episode should not change the diagnosis of schizophrenia (Angst 1986b). He also pointed out the need for prolonged observation to correctly differentiate schizophrenia from manic–depressive psychosis. In this frame he considered mixed cases to be isolated exceptions.

In 1878, Shulle regarded these cases as a transitional phase from manic depression to paranoia, while Hoffman in 1925 and Mayer-Gross in 1932 described the longitudinal course as beginning with mood symptoms and ending as schizophrenia and vice versa (Angst 1986b). But it was Jacob Kasanin (1897–1946) who first coined the term schizoaffective psychosis in 1933 (Kasanin 1933, 1994). Kasanin reported the course of nine young patients with good premorbid functioning, a sudden onset of both schizophrenic and mood symptoms and a good outcome. However, a review of these case histories might suggest they were essentially patients suffering from a mood disorder with psychotic features, according to contemporary classification systems. In 1937, Langfeldt described the so-called schizophreniform psychoses with many affective clinical elements and favourable outcome (Langfeldt 1937), while Kant in 1940 described 'recovered schizophrenics' as having more affective psychosis among their relatives in comparison to schizophrenic patients (Kant 1940). Valuable contributions in the nosology were made by Kurt Schneider (1887–1967) who described the so-called 'cases in between' (zwischen-fälle)

K.N. Fountoulakis, *Bipolar Disorder: An Evidence-Based Guide to Manic Depression*, DOI 10.1007/978-3-642-37216-2_7

schizophrenia and affective psychosis. In his view, no differential diagnosis between these two diseases could be made concerning the 'in-between cases'. Schneider also described for the first time a 'concurrent' and a 'sequential' form concerning these cases (Schneider 1973; Marneros 1983, 2003). In 1957 Karl Leonhard coined the term 'cycloid psychoses' (Leonhard 1957a, b).

After these studies which were based almost exclusively on clinical description and following Kant's report (in 1940) concerning the family history of 'recovered schizophrenics', George Vaillant also reported in 1962 that these patients were loaded with a family history of unipolar mood disorder and were depressed themselves (Vaillant 1962). In 1966 this was confirmed by the work of Astrup and Noreik. These authors suggested that the presence of mood symptoms and excitational confusion vs. blunted affect was predictive of a favourable course and outcome (Holmboe et al. 1968; Noreik et al. 1967; Astrup and Noreik 1966). Furthermore, in the late 1970s, a review of all available evidence at the time suggested that mood symptoms were predictive of better outcome, but on the contrary, 'schizophrenic' symptoms were not predictive of a worse outcome (Pope and Lipinski 1978). It is important to note, however, that a number of latter studies disputed the predictive value of mood symptoms as well (Croughan and Robins 1974; Welner et al. 1977a, b; Gift et al. 1980; Moller et al. 1982).

More recently it has been argued that schizoaffective disorder is simply the result of a number of weaknesses in contemporal classification systems (Malhi et al. 2008). However, while a psychiatrist with a broad concept of schizophrenia and bipolar disorder might be able to classify any patient (however, with a certain loss of reliability and validity), when a narrow concept is used, many patients do not fall into either diagnostic category. It is obvious that with strict application of the operationalized criteria, the diagnosis of schizoaffective disorder is limited to a small group of individuals, which might more probably be chronically ill and relatively treatment resistant (Averill et al. 2004). These in-between patients can be conceptualized as schizophrenics with mood symptoms, as mood patients with psychotic symptoms, as suffering from both schizophrenia and mood disorder, as suffering from an independent type of psychotic disorder or as 'interforms' that is as patients which an admixture of the aetiological factors causing schizophrenia and mood disorders. Since schizoaffective patients have better prognosis in comparison to patients with schizophrenia, this fact precludes the possibility of suffering from both schizophrenia and mood disorders. Additionally, the family history data with heavy loading of either schizophrenic or mood disorder cases is also against the idea of a distinct third kind of psychosis. No data in favour of an independent transmission of psychotic symptoms has been reported (Winokur et al. 1985), although the research efforts concerning this question are old and inadequate and the issue needs further study. The failure of a number of studies to recognize two clearly separate populations is in support of the last suggestion, that is, of the admixture of schizophrenic and mood aetiopathological factors (Kendell 1986). The existence of these cases can be conceived as a strong argument in favour of the 'unitary psychosis theory' (einheitspsychose), as conceived in the works of Joseph Guislain (1797–1860), Ernst Albrecht von Zeller (1804–1877), Wilhelm Griesinger (1817–1868) and

Heinrich Neumann (1814–1888) (Angst 2002; Berrios and Beer 1994; Moller 2008; Lake and Hurwitz 2006). Also at least to some extent, the concept of schizoaffective patients as cases in between disputes Jasper's hierarchical principle which is largely adopted by contemporary classification systems (Berner and Lenz 1986; Jaspers 1973). Probably with an attitude to compromise and synthesize the conflicting data, some authors suggest that schizoaffective disorder is a heterogenous group which includes both patients with schizophrenia and mood disorders as well as intermediate cases (Cheniaux et al. 2008; Laursen et al. 2005).

Nomenclature and classification of these cases has always been a problem. In most of the literature, the terms 'cycloid psychosis', 'psychogenic', 'reactive psychosis' and 'bouffee delirante' were used as synonyms of what today is called schizoaffective disorder. Several operationalized criteria sets were developed, and all of them required the presence of both affective and schizophrenic symptoms in some kind of combination and with a minimum duration (Kendell and Gourlay 1970; Welner et al. 1979, 1977b; Angst et al. 1979; Mendlewicz et al. 1980; Perris 1966; Tsuang et al. 1976). The best known are the Research Diagnostic Criteria developed by Spitzer et al. in 1978 (Spitzer et al. 1978a, b; Endicott et al. 1978). These criteria defined schizoaffective disorder as the acute co-occurrence of a full mood syndrome and one of a set of 'core schizophrenic' symptoms (e.g. bizarre delusions, first-rank symptoms or hallucinations). They further defined a depressed and a manic subtypes, as well as chronic and nonchronic subtypes. According to overall outcome, RDC defined a 'mainly schizophrenic subtype' and a 'mainly affective subtype'.

DSM-I proposed a schizoaffective type of schizophrenia reaction for patients with 'significant admixtures of schizophrenic and affective reactions'. However, the whole concept suggested that these patients are schizophrenics in nature. DSM-II introduced the excited and the depressed subtypes. It is to be noted that in line with the earlier editions of the DSM, most pharmaceutical trials of schizophrenia include also schizoaffective patients. DSM-III classified most 'in-between' cases as suffering from a mood disorder (e.g. with mood-incongruent psychotic symptoms) and grouped schizoaffective disorder under the category psychotic disorders not elsewhere classified. Essentially this constituted a residual category, although a description was available. DSM-III-R, DSM-IV and the DSM-IV-TR focused on defining better the duration and the relationship between 'schizophrenic' and mood symptoms. The ICD-10 follows a different approach and requires that both mood and psychotic symptoms constitute a prominent part of the clinical picture with a balance between their number, severity and duration. A problem still unsolved is that since all diagnostic approaches require the utilization of long-term data and the past history of the patient, the diagnosis might change over the course of such a lengthy illness, with patients and their families often being unable to provide with reliable descriptions of past episodes (Marneros et al. 1988a). As a result, schizoaffective disorder has a polymorphic course and low levels of diagnostic stability as compared to schizophrenia or mood disorders. Thus, prognosis and outcomes may fluctuate with changes in diagnosis and success of treatment (Astrup et al. 1959; Avery and Winokur 1976; Tsuang and Dempsey 1979; Tsuang et al. 1979; Clark and Mallett 1963; Marneros et al. 1988b, 1991).

Until today, most of studies on schizoaffective disorder focus on outcome, since outcome was the specific validator defined by Kraepelin in order to separate schizophrenia from manic–depressive illness. Earlier studies suggested a more favourable outcome for schizoaffective disorder in comparison to schizophrenia (Coryell et al. 1984; Holmboe and Astrup 1957; Clayton 1982; Cutting et al. 1978; Post 1971; Clark and Mallett 1963; Angst et al. 1980; Grossman et al. 1984; Brockington et al. 1980, 1982; Tsuang et al. 1977, 1979; Pope et al. 1980; Tsuang and Dempsey 1979; Armbruster et al. 1983; Koehler 1983) and in fact they were suggesting that the outcome lays on a continuum with nonpsychotic mood disorders at the one end and psychotic disorders with noncongruent psychotic features at the opposite one (Coryell and Tsuang 1982). Although the course and prognosis of schizoaffective disorder may vary, it is solidly established that the outcome is generally poorer than for patients with mood disorder but somewhat better than for patients with schizophrenia (Marneros et al. 1988b).

However, it has been shown that during inter-episode intervals, schizoaffective patients often manifest residual mood symptoms and mood liability (Astrup et al. 1959). They may also manifest neurocognitive impairment and deficits in social and occupational functioning. This impairment is greater than that of bipolar patients. Recent studies suggested that the neuropsychological deficit observed in schizoaffective patients is quantitatively but not qualitatively different from those with schizophrenia (Reichenberg et al. 2009) which is partially in accord with the above. Schizoaffective patients perform poorer in a global way probably because current psychotic symptoms or history of psychosis is correlated to more severe neurocognitive impairment no matter the specific diagnosis (Simonsen et al. 2011; Szoke et al. 2008; Torrent et al. 2007). Euthymic and stabilized schizoaffective patients are reported to perform worse than BD patients in attention, concentration, declarative memory, executive function and perceptuomotor function (Studentkowski et al. 2010; Torrent et al. 2007).

Also a progress in the understanding of the clinical picture has been done recently. The age of onset of schizoaffective disorder is reported to be in the mid-1920s and is lower than that of mood disorder but higher than that of schizophrenia (Angst 1980; Angst et al. 1980; Joyce 1984; Himmelhoch et al. 1981; Ballenger et al. 1982; Carlson and Strober 1978; Tsuang et al. 1976, 1977; Coryell et al. 1984; Angst 1986a). In terms of the quality of mood episodes, it has been documented that mixed mood episodes are not uncommon (Marneros et al. 2004). A seasonal pattern is less common in comparison to mood disorders. The average length of episodes is shorter than that of pure mood episodes and around 4–4.5 months. It has been reported that the length of circles decreases with increasing number of cycles and this decrease seems to correlate with age at onset (Angst 1986b; Marneros et al. 1988b). It is interesting to note that it is widely believed that the male-to-female ratio seems to depend on the subtype, with the depressive subtype having similar ratio to unipolar depression and the bipolar type similar to bipolar disorder. This has not been adequately confirmed however. Genetic studies have shown that relatives of probands with schizoaffective disorder have higher rates of mood disorder than relatives of probands with schizophrenia and higher rates of schizophrenia than relatives of probands with mood disorder (Baron et al. 1982; Scharfetter and Nusperli 1980) and that schizophrenia, schizoaffective disorder and bipolar disorder might share common disrupted genes (Jabs et al. 2002; Barnett and Smoller 2009; Craddock et al. 2009; Hamshere et al. 2011), although research in this field is problematic among other reasons because it is not unusual for schizoaffective patients to be included along with schizophrenics in many genetic studies.

Taken all the above together, it seems that the question whether schizoaffective disorder is similar to schizophrenia or to mood disorders still remains unanswered. It seems reasonable to assume that since both schizophrenia and mood disorders develop out of multiple causality factors and also share some of them, schizoaffective disorder does not merely constitute the admixture of their clinical pictures but maybe also of their causalities. Thus, the probable answer is that schizoaffective disorder is a highly heterogenous disorder which bridges the two major groups of mental disorders.

References

Angst J (1980) Course of unipolar depressive, bipolar manic-depressive, and schizoaffective disorders. Results of a prospective longitudinal study (author's transl). Fortschr Neurol Psychiatr Grenzgeb 48(1):3–30. doi:10.1055/s-2007-1002365

Angst J (1986a) The course of affective disorders. Psychopathology 19(Suppl 2):47–52

Angst J (1986b) The course of schizoaffective disorders. In: Marneros A, Tsuang MT (eds) Schizoaffective psychoses. Springer, Berlin, pp 18–30

Angst J (2002) Historical aspects of the dichotomy between manic-depressive disorders and schizophrenia. Schizophr Res 57(1):5–13. doi:S0920996402003286 [pii]

Angst J, Felder W, Lohmeyer B (1979) Schizoaffective disorders. Results of a genetic investigation, I. J Affect Disord 1(2):139–153. doi:0165-0327(79)90033-8 [pii]

Angst J, Felder W, Lohmeyer B (1980) Course of schizoaffective psychoses: results of a followup study. Schizophr Bull 6(4):579–585

Armbruster B, Gross G, Huber G (1983) Long-term prognosis and course of schizo-affective, schizophreniform, and cycloid psychoses. Psychiatr Clin (Basel) 16(2–4):156–168

Astrup C, Noreik K (1966) Functional psychoses: diagnostic and prognostic models. Charles C Thomas, Springfield

Astrup C, Fossum A, Holmboe R (1959) A follow-up of 270 patients with acute affective psychoses. Acta Psychiatr Scand Suppl 34(135):1–65

Averill PM, Reas DL, Shack A, Shah NN, Cowan K, Krajewski K, Kopecky C, Guynn RW (2004) Is schizoaffective disorder a stable diagnostic category: a retrospective examination. Psychiatr Q 75(3):215–227

Avery D, Winokur G (1976) Mortality in depressed patients treated with electroconvulsive therapy and antidepressants. Arch Gen Psychiatry 33(9):1029–1037

Ballenger JC, Reus VI, Post RM (1982) The "atypical" clinical picture of adolescent mania. Am J Psychiatry 139(5):602–606

Barnett JH, Smoller JW (2009) The genetics of bipolar disorder. Neuroscience 164(1):331–343. doi:10.1016/j.neuroscience.2009.03.080, S0306-4522(09)00576-4 [pii]

Baron M, Gruen R, Asnis L, Kane J (1982) Schizoaffective illness, schizophrenia and affective disorders: morbidity risk and genetic transmission. Acta Psychiatr Scand 65(4):253–262

Berner P, Lenz G (1986) Definitions of schizoaffective psychosis: mutual concordance and relationship to schizophrenia and affective disorder. In: Marneros A, Tsuang MT (eds) Schizoaffective psychoses. Springer, Berlin, pp 18–30

Berrios GE, Beer D (1994) The notion of a unitary psychosis: a conceptual history. Hist Psychiatry 5(17 Pt 1):13–36

Brockington IF, Kendell RE, Wainwright S (1980) Depressed patients with schizophrenic or paranoid symptoms. Psychol Med 10(4):665–675

Brockington IF, Helzer JE, Hillier VF, Francis AF (1982) Definitions of depression: concordance and prediction of outcome. Am J Psychiatry 139(8):1022–1027

Carlson GA, Strober M (1978) Affective disorder in adolescence: issues in misdiagnosis. J Clin Psychiatry 39(1):59–66

Cheniaux E, Landeira-Fernandez J, Lessa Telles L, Lessa JL, Dias A, Duncan T, Versiani M (2008) Does schizoaffective disorder really exist? A systematic review of the studies that compared schizoaffective disorder with schizophrenia or mood disorders. J Affect Disord 106(3):209–217. doi:10.1016/j.jad.2007.07.009, S0165-0327(07)00262-5 [pii]

Clark JA, Mallett BL (1963) A follow up study of schizophrenia and depression in young adults. Br J Psychiatry 109:491–499

Clayton PJ (1982) Schizoaffective disorders. J Nerv Ment Dis 170(11):646–650

Coryell W, Tsuang MT (1982) Primary unipolar depression and the prognostic importance of delusions. Arch Gen Psychiatry 39(10):1181–1184

Coryell W, Lavori P, Endicott J, Keller M, VanEerdewegh M (1984) Outcome in schizoaffective, psychotic, and nonpsychotic depression. Course during a six- to 24-month follow-up. Arch Gen Psychiatry 41(8):787–791

Craddock N, O'Donovan MC, Owen MJ (2009) Psychosis genetics: modeling the relationship between schizophrenia, bipolar disorder, and mixed (or "schizoaffective") psychoses. Schizophr Bull 35(3):482–490. doi:10.1093/schbul/sbp020, sbp020 [pii]

Croughan JL, Robins E (1974) The group of schizoaffective and related psychoses–critique, record, follow-up and family studies. II Record studies. Arch Gen Psychiatry 31(5):632–637

Cutting JC, Clare AW, Mann AH (1978) Cycloid psychosis: an investigation of the diagnostic concept. Psychol Med 8(4):637–648

Endicott J, Forman JB, Spitzer RL (1978) Research approaches to diagnostic classification in schizophrenia. Birth Defects Orig Artic Ser 14(5):41–57

Gift TE, Strauss JS, Kokes RF, Harder DW, Ritzler BA (1980) Schizophrenia: affect and outcome. Am J Psychiatry 137(5):580–585

Grossman LS, Harrow M, Fudala JL, Meltzer HY (1984) The longitudinal course of schizoaffective disorders. A prospective follow-up study. J Nerv Ment Dis 172(3):140–149

Hamshere ML, O'Donovan MC, Jones IR, Jones L, Kirov G, Green EK, Moskvina V, Grozeva D, Bass N, McQuillin A, Gurling H, St Clair D, Young AH, Ferrier IN, Farmer A, McGuffin P, Sklar P, Purcell S, Holmans PA, Owen MJ, Craddock N (2011) Polygenic dissection of the bipolar phenotype. Br J Psychiatry 198(4):284–288. doi:10.1192/bjp.bp.110.087866, 198/4/284 [pii]

Himmelhoch JM, Fuchs CZ, May SJ, Symons BJ, Neil JF (1981) When a schizoaffective diagnosis has meaning. J Nerv Ment Dis 169(5):277–282

Holmboe R, Astrup C (1957) A follow-up study of 255 patients with acute schizophrenia and schizophreniform psychoses. Acta Psychiatr Neurol Scand Suppl 115:9–61

Holmboe R, Noreik K, Astrup C (1968) Follow-up of functional psychoses at two Norwegian mental hospitals. Acta Psychiatr Scand 44(3):298–310

Jabs BE, Pfuhlmann B, Bartsch AJ, Cetkovich-Bakmas MG, Stober G (2002) Cycloid psychoses – from clinical concepts to biological foundations. J Neural Transm 109(5–6):907–919. doi:10.1007/s007020200074

Jaspers K (1973) Allgemeine psychopathologie, 9th edn. Springer, Berlin

Joyce PR (1984) Age of onset in bipolar affective disorder and misdiagnosis as schizophrenia. Psychol Med 14(1):145–149

Kant O (1940) Types and analyses of the clinical pictures of recovered schizophrenics. Psychiat Q 14:676–700

Kasanin J (1933) The acute schizoaffective psychoses. Am J Psychiatry 13:97–126

Kasanin J (1994) The acute schizoaffective psychoses. 1933. Am J Psychiatry 151(6 Suppl): 144–154

Kendell RE (1986) The relationship of schizoaffective illnesses to schizophrenic and affective disorders. In: Marneros A, Tsuang MT (eds) Schizoaffective psychoses. Springer, Berlin, pp 18–30
Kendell RE, Gourlay J (1970) The clinical distinction between the affective psychoses and schizophrenia. Br J Psychiatry 117(538):261–266
Koehler K (1983) Prognostic prediction in RDC schizo-affective disorder on the basis of first-rank symptoms weighted in terms of outcome. Psychiatr Clin (Basel) 16(2–4):186–197
Lake CR, Hurwitz N (2006) Schizoaffective disorders are psychotic mood disorders; there are no schizoaffective disorders. Psychiatry Res 143(2–3):255–287. doi:10.1016/j.psychres.2005.08.012, S0165-1781(05)00264-7 [pii]
Langfeldt G (1937) The prognosis of schizophrenia and the factors influencing the course of the disease. Acta Psychiatr Neurol Scand Suppl 13:1–128
Laursen TM, Labouriau R, Licht RW, Bertelsen A, Munk-Olsen T, Mortensen PB (2005) Family history of psychiatric illness as a risk factor for schizoaffective disorder: a Danish register-based cohort study. Arch Gen Psychiatry 62(8):841–848. doi:10.1001/archpsyc.62.8.841, 62/8/841 [pii]
Leonhard K (1957a) Cycloid psychoses, often erroneously considered as schizophrenia. Psychiatr Neurol Med Psychol (Leipz) 9(12):359–365
Leonhard K (1957b) Pathogenesis of manic-depressive disease. Nervenarzt 28(6):271–272
Malhi GS, Green M, Fagiolini A, Peselow ED, Kumari V (2008) Schizoaffective disorder: diagnostic issues and future recommendations. Bipolar Disord 10(1 Pt 2):215–230. doi:10.1111/j.1399-5618.2007.00564.x, BDI564 [pii]
Marneros A (1983) Kurt Schneider's 'Zwischen-Falle', 'mid-cases' or 'cases in between'. Psychiatr Clin (Basel) 16(2–4):87–102
Marneros A (2003) The schizoaffective phenomenon: the state of the art. Acta Psychiatr Scand Suppl 418:29–33. doi:177 [pii]
Marneros A, Deister A, Rohde A (1988a) Syndrome shift in the long-term course of schizoaffective disorders. Eur Arch Psychiatry Neurol Sci 238(2):97–104
Marneros A, Rohde A, Deister A, Fimmers R, Junemann H (1988b) Long-term course of schizoaffective disorders. Part III: onset, type of episodes and syndrome shift, precipitating factors, suicidality, seasonality, inactivity of illness, and outcome. Eur Arch Psychiatry Neurol Sci 237(5):283–290
Marneros A, Deister A, Rohde A (1991) Stability of diagnoses in affective, schizoaffective and schizophrenic disorders. Cross-sectional versus longitudinal diagnosis. Eur Arch Psychiatry Clin Neurosci 241(3):187–192
Marneros A, Rottig S, Wenzel A, Bloink R, Brieger P (2004) Affective and schizoaffective mixed states. Eur Arch Psychiatry Clin Neurosci 254(2):76–81. doi:10.1007/s00406-004-0462-9
Mendlewicz J, Linkowski P, Wilmotte J (1980) Relationship between schizoaffective illness and affective disorders or schizophrenia. Morbidity risk and genetic transmission. J Affect Disord 2(4):289–302
Moller HJ (2008) Systematic of psychiatric disorders between categorical and dimensional approaches: Kraepelin's dichotomy and beyond. Eur Arch Psychiatry Clin Neurosci 258(Suppl 2):48–73. doi:10.1007/s00406-008-2004-3
Moller HJ, Werner-Eilert K, Wuschner-Stockheim M, von Zerssen D (1982) Relevant predictors of the 5 year outcome of patients with schizophrenic or similar paranoid psychoses (author's transl). Arch Psychiatr Nervenkr 231(4):305–322
Noreik K, Astrup C, Dalgard OS, Holmboe R (1967) A prolonged follow-up of acute schizophrenic and schizophreniform psychoses. Acta Psychiatr Scand 43(4):432–443
Perris C (1966) A study of bipolar (manic-depressive) and unipolar recurrent depressive psychoses. Introduction. Acta Psychiatr Scand Suppl 194:9–14
Pope HG Jr, Lipinski JF Jr (1978) Diagnosis in schizophrenia and manic-depressive illness: a reassessment of the specificity of 'schizophrenic' symptoms in the light of current research. Arch Gen Psychiatry 35(7):811–828
Pope HG Jr, Lipinski JF, Cohen BM, Axelrod DT (1980) "Schizoaffective disorder": an invalid diagnosis? A comparison of schizoaffective disorder, schizophrenia, and affective disorder. Am J Psychiatry 137(8):921–927

Post F (1971) Schizo-affective symptomatology in late life. Br J Psychiatry 118(545):437–445
Reichenberg A, Harvey PD, Bowie CR, Mojtabai R, Rabinowitz J, Heaton RK, Bromet E (2009) Neuropsychological function and dysfunction in schizophrenia and psychotic affective disorders. Schizophr Bull 35(5):1022–1029. doi:10.1093/schbul/sbn044, sbn044 [pii]
Scharfetter C, Nusperli M (1980) The group of schizophrenias, schizoaffective psychoses, and affective disorders. Schizophr Bull 6(4):586–591
Schneider K (1973) Klinische psychopathologie, 10th edn. Thieme, Stuttgart
Simonsen C, Sundet K, Vaskinn A, Birkenaes AB, Engh JA, Faerden A, Jonsdottir H, Ringen PA, Opjordsmoen S, Melle I, Friis S, Andreassen OA (2011) Neurocognitive dysfunction in bipolar and schizophrenia spectrum disorders depends on history of psychosis rather than diagnostic group. Schizophr Bull 37(1):73–83. doi:10.1093/schbul/sbp034 sbp034
Spitzer RL, Andreasen NC, Endicott J (1978a) Schizophrenia and other psychotic disorders in DSM-III. Schizophr Bull 4(4):489–510
Spitzer RL, Endicott J, Robins E (1978b) Research diagnostic criteria: rationale and reliability. Arch Gen Psychiatry 35(6):773–782
Studentkowski G, Scheele D, Calabrese P, Balkau F, Hoffler J, Aubel T, Edel MA, Juckel G, Assion HJ (2010) Cognitive impairment in patients with a schizoaffective disorder: a comparison with bipolar patients in euthymia. Eur J Med Res 15(2):70–78
Szoke A, Meary A, Trandafir A, Bellivier F, Roy I, Schurhoff F, Leboyer M (2008) Executive deficits in psychotic and bipolar disorders – implications for our understanding of schizoaffective disorder. Eur Psychiatry 23(1):20–25. doi:10.1016/j.eurpsy.2007.10.006, S0924-9338(07)01422-8 [pii]
Torrent C, Martinez-Aran A, Amann B, Daban C, Tabares-Seisdedos R, Gonzalez-Pinto A, Reinares M, Benabarre A, Salamero M, McKenna P, Vieta E (2007) Cognitive impairment in schizoaffective disorder: a comparison with non-psychotic bipolar and healthy subjects. Acta Psychiatr Scand 116(6):453–460. doi:10.1111/j.1600-0447.2007.01072.x, ACP1072 [pii]
Tsuang MT, Dempsey GM (1979) Long-term outcome of major psychoses. II. Schizoaffective disorder compared with schizophrenia, affective disorders, and a surgical control group. Arch Gen Psychiatry 36(12):1302–1304
Tsuang MT, Dempsey M, Rauscher F (1976) A study of "atypical schizophrenia". Comparison with schizophrenia and affective disorder by sex, age of admission, precipitant, outcome, and family history. Arch Gen Psychiatry 33(10):11157–11160
Tsuang MT, Dempsey GM, Dvoredsky A, Struss A (1977) A family history study of schizoaffective disorder. Biol Psychiatry 12(3):331–338
Tsuang MT, Woolson RF, Fleming JA (1979) Long-term outcome of major psychoses. I Schizophrenia and affective disorders compared with psychiatrically symptom-free surgical conditions. Arch Gen Psychiatry 36(12):1295–1301
Vaillant GE (1962) The prediction of recovery in schizophrenia. J Nerv Ment Dis 135:534–543
Welner A, Croughan J, Fishman R, Robins E (1977a) The group of schizoaffective and related psychoses: a follow-up study. Compr Psychiatry 18(5):413–422. doi:0010-440X(77)90039-6 [pii]
Welner A, Welner Z, Leonard MA (1977b) Bipolar manic-depressive disorder: a reassessment of course and outcome. Compr Psychiatry 18(4):327–332. doi:0010-440X(77)90003-7 [pii]
Welner A, Welner Z, Fishman R (1979) The group of schizoaffective and related psychoses: IV. A family study. Compr Psychiatry 20(1):21–26. doi:0010-440X(79)90056-7 [pii]
Winokur G, Scharfetter C, Angst J (1985) A family study of psychotic symptomatology in schizophrenia, schizoaffective disorder, unipolar depression, and bipolar disorder. Eur Arch Psychiatry Neurol Sci 234(5):295–298

Personality Disorders (Narcissistic, Antisocial, Borderline)

8

The concept of personality and of PDs is both essential and controversial for psychiatry. Most definitions of personality focus on motivation and mental adaptation. Personality refers to the way a person shapes and adapts to an ever-changing internal and external environment. Its basic functions are to feel (emotional responses), to think and perceive (cognitive interpretation of self, the others and the environment) and to incorporate these into purposeful behaviours (interpersonal functioning, impulse control).

Different persons differ greatly in many aspects of their behaviour, but on the other hand, they share the ability to expresses many potentially different lifestyles. One of the core characteristics of personality is 'free will' which refers mostly to the ability people have to be self-aware and to modify behaviour in a way not predictable or predetermined and to be responsible for their choices. Personality is usually conceptualized as a complex interaction among temperament, character (rational concepts about self and interpersonal relations) and psyche (intuitive self-awareness and fluid intelligence). Personality is by definition stable, of long duration and already shaped during adolescence or early adulthood.

Personality disorders (PDs) are inflexible dysfunctional patterns of personality. Frequently they coexist with other mental disorders and conditions. They tend to cause chronic impairments in work, interpersonal relationships and marriage. People with PDs tend to be less educated, single and unemployed and manifest more often drug or alcohol abuse or dependence. PDs are reported to occur in 10–20 % of the general population and in more than half of psychiatric patients (Cloninger and Svrakic 2009). Persons with a PD are generally considered to have poor prognosis and often challenge the limits of the therapist's knowledge, skills and even personal maturity. Characteristically they are externalizing responsibility by blaming other people or unfavourable circumstances for their problems. This is because their symptoms and behaviours are ego-syntonic and they are alloplastic, that is, they aim to change others, not themselves. Of course there are some exceptions to the above rules.

K.N. Fountoulakis, *Bipolar Disorder: An Evidence-Based Guide to Manic Depression*, DOI 10.1007/978-3-642-37216-2_8

The separation between 'personality disorders' and 'clinical syndromes' which was the product of the separation between Axis I vs. Axis II in DSM-III reflects a number of concepts and approaches which remain controversial in contemporary psychiatry, including the biomedical–pharmacological (Axis II) vs. the social–psychological (Axis II) (Fountoulakis and Kaprinis 2006). Characteristically, much of the literature and research on personality is based directly or indirectly on the classical psycholexical study by Gordon Allport and Henry Odbert (Allport and Odbert 1936; Waller 1999). In spite of the fact that traditionally 'clinical syndromes' were considered to be the product of 'personality' both according to psychodynamic and psychobiological theories, the new multiaxial approach broke that link and separated them at a number of levels. It can be argued that Axis II disorders are determined more on the basis of social norms and they reflect developmental conditions with early onset and chronic and stable course without major fluctuations (apart from comorbidity with Axis I disorders). On the contrary, Axis I disorders are more consistent with the biomedical model and are frequently episodic with remission and relapse of symptoms. However, there are studies reporting that PDs may have a late onset (Bolton and Gunderson 1996; Parnas et al. 2005), attenuate or even diminish after several years (Stone 1993; Grilo et al. 2004, 2005; McGlashan 1986; McGlashan et al. 2005; Zanarini et al. 2004) and this is even accepted by the DSM-5 which accepts that borderline personality may remit within 1 year and within 10 years as many as half of patients do not manifest any more a pattern indicative of the existence of a borderline personality (American Psychiatric Association 2013). Coexistence of these two groups of disorders often makes differential diagnosis difficult and suggests a close relationship between them.

An existential component is often present in PDs and constitutes an intensified extension of normal existential thoughts. Often patients struggle with questions of purpose; they are ambivalent and feel empty. Frequently, they cannot precisely describe their problems. Guilt, anxiety and depression might not dominate the clinical picture. Their core problem is often an unusual inability to learn from adverse and painful experience and because of this they tend to repeat problematic behaviours.

According to DSM-5 (American Psychiatric Association 2013), PDs are classified into three clusters: cluster A (paranoid, schizoid and schizotypal PDs that is odd or eccentric), cluster B (borderline, antisocial, narcissistic and histrionic PDs that is emotionally unstable and impulsive) and cluster C (avoidant, dependent and obsessive–compulsive PDs that are anxious). Theoretically there are three dimensions underlying these clusters, that is, detachment, impulsivity and fearfulness. The latter two constitute also components of mood disorders and especially BD.

Since it is considered that at least some PDs constitute attenuated forms of mood and psychotic disorders and essentially belong to the respected spectrums, concerning BD it is important to start by exploring comorbidity. In this frame, it has been reported that 20–41 % of BD patients meet DSM criteria for a PD (Brieger et al. 2003; George et al. 2003; Kay et al. 2002; Mantere et al. 2006; Weber et al. 2011) with dramatic/emotionally erratic and fearful/avoidant PDs being more common than odd/eccentric (Mantere et al. 2006). More specifically 17 % of patients might suffer also from borderline (BPD), 6 % from antisocial (ASPD), 5 % from histrionic

(HPD) and 8 % from narcissistic (NPD) (Garno et al. 2005). Another study reported higher percentages with 62 % of BD patients suffering from a PD, usually HPD, BPD, passive–aggressive and ASPD (Pica et al. 1990). However, when the sample includes only inpatients, it is reported that up to 71.8 % of BD inpatients suffer from a PD and most frequently BPD (41 %), NPD (20.5 %), dependent (12.8 %) and HPD (10.3 %) (Schiavone et al. 2004). The literature generally suggests that depending on the study sample quality, 14–71.8 % of BD patients suffer from a PD most usually BPD, NPD and ASPD (Joyce et al. 2004; Turley et al. 1992; Brieger et al. 2003; Gunderson et al. 2006; Perugi et al. 2012; Weber et al. 2011). Recent reviews confirmed the above but also suggested that the true magnitude of comorbidity is inconclusive because of a variety of factors including the phase of the illness the patients are in and the effect mood symptoms have on the assessment of personality (Fan and Hassell 2008; Krishnan 2005). For example, in hospitalized BD patients the prevalence of PDs is reported to be as low as 6 % (Sorvaniemi and Hintikka 2005). The presence of a PD is reported to be associated with poor outcome (Bieling et al. 2003; Kay et al. 2002; Preston et al. 2004) and with significantly more lifetime suicide attempts and current depression (Garno et al. 2005), which in turn points to a vicious logical diagnostic circle.

ASPD is characterized by a pervasive disregard and violation of the rights of others and these patients do not conform to social norms. This kind of behaviour starts before the age of 15 and continues into adult life. Deceitfulness, impulsivity, irritability and physical aggressiveness, recklessness and promiscuity constitute the hallmarks of this disorder. Lack of remorse and irresponsibility, as well as inflated and arrogant self-appraisal, are also present. They are often arrested and have problems with the law. Their inner experience includes severe dysphoria, tension and painful boredom but rarely true depression. It is present in 0.2–3.3 % of persons in the general population with males being the majority. The prevalence is much higher in clinical populations, forensic samples and substance abusers (American Psychiatric Association 2013).

ASPD and BD share many common features, including impulsivity, increased incarceration or arrest, substance and behavioural addictions and suicidality. In cases these disorders coexist, these features are even more pronounced (Swann et al. 2010, 2011). BD patients with comorbid ASPD have earlier onset and manic predominant polarity. It has been suggested that this pattern of features suggests a distinct underlying neurobiological dysfunction for each of these disorders (Swann 2011; Swann et al. 2011). Coexistence of ASPD seems to worsen the long-term course of BD, but does not alter the nature of episodic affective symptoms (Swann et al. 2012).

NPD is characterized by a pervasive sense of grandiosity (in fantasy, behaviour or both). Narcissistic patients have an intense need for admiration and are preoccupated with fantasies of unlimited success, power, brilliance, beauty or ideal love. They lack empathy, have a sense of entitlement, are exploitative and arrogant towards others and manifest a haughty attitude. They often experience chronic intense envy. They are hypersensitive to criticism, and although often they are high achievers, the combination of strong feelings of shame and humiliation with exhibitionism frequently leads them to social withdrawal, depression and high levels of dysphoria, with pessimism developing and predominating after the age of 40 (Cloninger and Svrakic 2009).

The prevalence of NPD in the general population is not known since estimations vary from 0 to 6.2 %. It is clearly more often seen in clinical samples, and it is more often diagnosed in males (2–3:1) (American Psychiatric Association 2013). Higher rates in the general population (up to 8 %) have been reported and after controlling for additional comorbidity controlled for, associations with bipolar I disorder, remained significant (Stinson et al. 2008).

Excessive self-dramatization, emotionality and attention seeking constitute the hallmarks of HPD. Also core characteristics are inappropriate sexual seductiveness or provocativeness, excessive need to be at the centre of attention, rapidly shifting and shallow expression of emotions, impressionistic speech lacking detail, self-dramatization, theatricality, exaggerated expression of emotions and relationships considered more intimate than they really are, crave for excitement and stimulation and often sexual indiscreteness with low tolerance for delayed gratification (Cloninger and Svrakic 2009). The prevalence for HDP is approximately 2 % in the general population and higher in clinical samples. Males and females manifest similar rates (American Psychiatric Association 2013).

It is interesting to mention that NPD, ASPD and HPD can be considered to belong to a spectrum of disorders, since they aggregate in families and coexist in the same patients. This spectrum approach is based on the presence of a common antisocial trait which is present in all three PDs and increases in severity from HPD (manipulation) via NPD (exploitation) to ASPD (violence and property crime) (Cloninger and Svrakic 2009).

BPD is characterized by pervasive and excessive instability of affects, self-image, sense of self and interpersonal relationships. Significant impulsivity is also present. The constellation of symptoms and behaviours includes frantic efforts to avoid real or imagined abandonment, alternation between idealization and devaluation, impulsivity, marked reactivity of mood, chronic feelings of emptiness, anger, suicidal or self-mutilating behaviour and stress-related, transient paranoid ideation or dissociative symptoms. Maybe one of the best-ever-said phrases to describe the riddle of borderline personality is 'borderline an adjective in search of a noun' (Akiskal et al. 1985). BPD is reported to afflict 1.6 % of the general population, 6 % in primary care settings, 10 % for psychiatric outpatients and 20 % of psychiatric inpatients and constitutes 30–60 % of PD patients. The male-to-female ratio is 3:1 (American Psychiatric Association 2013).

Recent systematic reviews suggested that BPD and BD are separate entities but share some common elements, especially genetic (Bassett 2012; Coulston et al. 2012; Paris et al. 2007). More than half borderline patients seem to belong to the bipolar spectrum (Deltito et al. 2001; Perugi and Akiskal 2002). Often BPD manifests a long-term course resembling that of an Axis I clinical syndrome. It has been reported that of the subjects with BPD, 34.5 % met the criteria for remission at 2 years, 49.4 % at 4 years, 68.6 % at 6 years and 73.5 % over the entire follow-up. Only 5.9 % of those with remissions experienced recurrences (Zanarini et al. 2003).

The spectrum hypothesis suggests that specific PDs may be an attenuated form of mood disorders. A line of research suggests PD symptoms appear to be dimensional, trait-like characteristics of BD (Perugi et al. 2003). ASPD and BPD symptoms are differentially related to impulsivity and course of illness (Swann et al. 2012). An aetiopathogenetic nature of this Axis I–Axis II relationship has not been established, and the spectrum hypothesis is based on the obvious symptomatic similarity and some family data. In this frame, PDs might be predisposing factors, premorbid conditions or attenuated forms of major mood disorders.

According to both the psychodynamic model and the psychobiological model, the borderline personality organization (Kernberg 1975), which includes chronic free-floating anxiety, polysymptomatic neurosis, polymorphous perverse sexual trends, poor impulse control and addictions, shift towards primary process thinking and partially impaired reality testing, constitutes 'the core feature', which extends across discrete subtypes of personality syndromes (Reich and Frances 1984). Both models suggest that excessive negative emotionality (fear and anger or high harm avoidance and high novelty seeking) influences the developmental processes and leads to the formation of a PD. This understanding can bridge the lack of knowledge on the differences and similarities between PDs and BD.

However, the standard approach is that BPD is distinguished from mood disorders on the basis of behaviours like efforts to avoid abandonment, unstable relationships with alternation between idealization and devaluation, identity disturbance, impulsivity in potentially self-damaging areas, chronic feelings of emptiness and inappropriately intensive anger or difficulty in controlling anger. Some of these features are not typically considered to be part of a mood disorder, although one can argue against such an assumption, especially when the bipolar spectrum is taken into consideration. ASPD and NPD are distinguished from BD on the basis of the episodic nature of the latter and the greater intensity of symptomatology. Euphoric mood is not present in PDs; however, less typical forms of BD might pose a diagnostic challenge.

The pharmacological treatment of PDs and especially for BPD is generally similar to BD, although less well documented (Abraham and Calabrese 2008; Bellino et al. 2008, 2011; Binks et al. 2006; Feurino and Silk 2011; Herpertz et al. 2007; Ingenhoven and Duivenvoorden 2011; Lieb et al. 2010; Mercer et al. 2009; Stoffers et al. 2010; Vita et al. 2011; Frankenburg and Zanarini 2002; Preston et al. 2004). A problem is that this pharmacological approach is rather generic for all PDs (Ingenhoven et al. 2010).

Conclusively, it can be said that a significant percentage of PD patients are in fact mood patients and belong to the bipolar spectrum. However, this cannot be assumed for all PD patients by definition, but mainly for those with a predominant affective component in their symptomatology. Impulsivity, although prevalent both in PDs and BD, seems to differ in terms of quality between these groups of patients. Existential dilemata and interpersonal difficulties are more characteristic of 'personality pathology' rather than of 'mood disorder' although they are not uncommon in BD patients.

References

Abraham PF, Calabrese JR (2008) Evidenced-based pharmacologic treatment of borderline personality disorder: a shift from SSRIs to anticonvulsants and atypical antipsychotics? J Affect Disord 111(1):21–30. doi:10.1016/j.jad.2008.01.024, S0165-0327(08)00063-3 [pii]

Akiskal HS, Chen SE, Davis GC, Puzantian VR, Kashgarian M, Bolinger JM (1985) Borderline: an adjective in search of a noun. J Clin Psychiatry 46(2):41–48

Allport G, Odbert H (1936) Trait-names: a psycho-lexical study. Psychol Monogr 47(1):1–177

American Psychiatric Association (2013) Diagnostic and statistical manual of mental disorders, 5th edn, DSM-5. American Psychiatric Publishing, Washington, DC

Bassett D (2012) Borderline personality disorder and bipolar affective disorder. Spectra or spectre? A review. Aust N Z J Psychiatry 46(4):327–339. doi:10.1177/0004867411435289, 0004867411435289 [pii]

Bellino S, Paradiso E, Bogetto F (2008) Efficacy and tolerability of pharmacotherapies for borderline personality disorder. CNS Drugs 22(8):671–692. doi:2285 [pii]

Bellino S, Rinaldi C, Bozzatello P, Bogetto F (2011) Pharmacotherapy of borderline personality disorder: a systematic review for publication purpose. Curr Med Chem 18(22):3322–3329. doi:BSP/CMC/E-Pub/2011/ 239 [pii]

Bieling PJ, MacQueen GM, Marriot MJ, Robb JC, Begin H, Joffe RT, Young LT (2003) Longitudinal outcome in patients with bipolar disorder assessed by life-charting is influenced by DSM-IV personality disorder symptoms. Bipolar Disord 5(1):14–21. doi:014 [pii]

Binks CA, Fenton M, McCarthy L, Lee T, Adams CE, Duggan C (2006) Pharmacological interventions for people with borderline personality disorder. Cochrane Database Syst Rev (1):CD005653. doi:10.1002/14651858.CD005653

Bolton S, Gunderson J (1996) Distinguishing borderline personality disorder from bipolar disorder: differential diagnosis and implications. Am J Psychiatry 153:1202–1207

Brieger P, Ehrt U, Marneros A (2003) Frequency of comorbid personality disorders in bipolar and unipolar affective disorders. Compr Psychiatry 44(1):28–34. doi:10.1053/comp.2003.50009, S0010440X03000294 [pii]

Cloninger C, Svrakic D (2009) Personality disorders. In: Sadock B, Sadock V, Ruiz P (eds) Kaplan & Sadock's comprehensive textbook of psychiatry, vol 2, 9th edn. Lippincott Williams & Wilkins, Philadelphia, pp 2198–2240

Coulston CM, Tanious M, Mulder RT, Porter RJ, Malhi GS (2012) Bordering on bipolar: the overlap between borderline personality and bipolarity. Aust N Z J Psychiatry 46(6):506–521. doi:10.1177/0004867412445528, 0004867412445528 [pii]

Deltito J, Martin L, Riefkohl J, Austria B, Kissilenko A, Corless CMP (2001) Do patients with borderline personality disorder belong to the bipolar spectrum? J Affect Disord 67(1-3):221–228. doi:S0165032701004360 [pii]

Fan AH, Hassell J (2008) Bipolar disorder and comorbid personality psychopathology: a review of the literature. J Clin Psychiatry 69(11):1794–1803. doi:ej08r04175 [pii]

Feurino L 3rd, Silk KR (2011) State of the art in the pharmacologic treatment of borderline personality disorder. Curr Psychiatry Rep 13(1):69–75. doi:10.1007/s11920-010-0168-9

Fountoulakis KN, Kaprinis GS (2006) Personality disorders: new data versus old concepts. Curr Opin Psychiatry 19(1):90–94. doi:10.1097/01.yco.0000196158.98540.b6, 00001504-200601000-00017 [pii]

Frankenburg FR, Zanarini MC (2002) Divalproex sodium treatment of women with borderline personality disorder and bipolar II disorder: a double-blind placebo-controlled pilot study. J Clin Psychiatry 63(5):442–446

Garno JL, Goldberg JF, Ramirez PM, Ritzler BA (2005) Bipolar disorder with comorbid cluster B personality disorder features: impact on suicidality. J Clin Psychiatry 66(3):339–345

George EL, Miklowitz DJ, Richards JA, Simoneau TL, Taylor DO (2003) The comorbidity of bipolar disorder and axis II personality disorders: prevalence and clinical correlates. Bipolar Disord 5(2):115–122. doi:028 [pii]

Grilo C, Sanislow C, Gunderson J, Pagano M, Yen S, Zanarini M, Shea M, Skodol A, Stout R, Morey L, McClashan T (2004) Two-year stability and change of schizotypal, borderline, avoidant and obsessive-compulsive personality disorders. J Consult Clin Psychol 72(5):767–775

Grilo C, Skodol A, Gunderson J, Sanislow C, Stout R, Shea M, Morey L, Zanarini M, Bender D, Yen S, McClashan T (2005) Longitudinal diagnostic efficiency of DSM-IV criteria for obsessive-compulsive personality disorder: a 2-year prospective study. Acta Psychiatr Scand 110:64–68

Gunderson JG, Weinberg I, Daversa MT, Kueppenbender KD, Zanarini MC, Shea MT, Skodol AE, Sanislow CA, Yen S, Morey LC, Grilo CM, McGlashan TH, Stout RL, Dyck I (2006) Descriptive and longitudinal observations on the relationship of borderline personality disorder and bipolar disorder. Am J Psychiatry 163(7):1173–1178. doi:10.1176/appi.ajp.163.7.1173, 163/7/1173 [pii]

Herpertz SC, Zanarini M, Schulz CS, Siever L, Lieb K, Moller HJ (2007) World Federation of Societies of Biological Psychiatry (WFSBP) guidelines for biological treatment of personality disorders. World J Biol Psychiatry 8(4):212–244. doi:10.1080/15622970701685224, 783497647 [pii]

Ingenhoven TJ, Duivenvoorden HJ (2011) Differential effectiveness of antipsychotics in borderline personality disorder: meta-analyses of placebo-controlled, randomized clinical trials on symptomatic outcome domains. J Clin Psychopharmacol 31(4):489–496. doi:10.1097/JCP.0b013e3182217a69

Ingenhoven T, Lafay P, Rinne T, Passchier J, Duivenvoorden H (2010) Effectiveness of pharmacotherapy for severe personality disorders: meta-analyses of randomized controlled trials. J Clin Psychiatry 71(1):14–25. doi:10.4088/JCP.08r04526gre

Joyce PR, Luty SE, McKenzie JM, Mulder RT, McIntosh VV, Carter FA, Bulik CM, Sullivan PF (2004) Bipolar II disorder: personality and outcome in two clinical samples. Aust N Z J Psychiatry 38(6):433–438. doi:10.1111/j.1440-1614.2004.01380.x, ANP1380 [pii]

Kay JH, Altshuler LL, Ventura J, Mintz J (2002) Impact of axis II comorbidity on the course of bipolar illness in men: a retrospective chart review. Bipolar Disord 4(4):237–242

Kernberg O (1975) Borderline conditions and pathological narcissism. Jason Aronson, New York

Krishnan KR (2005) Psychiatric and medical comorbidities of bipolar disorder. Psychosom Med 67(1):1–8. doi:10.1097/01.psy.0000151489.36347.18, 67/1/1 [pii]

Lieb K, Vollm B, Rucker G, Timmer A, Stoffers JM (2010) Pharmacotherapy for borderline personality disorder: cochrane systematic review of randomised trials. Br J Psychiatry 196(1):4–12. doi:10.1192/bjp.bp.108.062984, 196/1/4 [pii]

Mantere O, Melartin TK, Suominen K, Rytsala HJ, Valtonen HM, Arvilommi P, Leppamaki S, Isometsa ET (2006) Differences in axis I and II comorbidity between bipolar I and II disorders and major depressive disorder. J Clin Psychiatry 67(4):584–593

McGlashan T (1986) The chestnut lodge follow-up study III. Long-term outcome of borderline personalities. Arch Gen Psychiatry 43:20–30

McGlashan T, Grilo C, Sanislow C, Ralevski E, Morey L, Gunderson J, Skodol A, Tracie Shea M, Zanarini M, Bender D, Stout R, Yen S, Pagano M (2005) Two-year prevalence and stability of individual DSM-IV criteria for schizotypal, borderline, avoidant, and obsessive-compulsive personality disorders: toward a hybrid model of axis II disorders. Am J Psychiatry 162:883–889

Mercer D, Douglass AB, Links PS (2009) Meta-analyses of mood stabilizers, antidepressants and antipsychotics in the treatment of borderline personality disorder: effectiveness for depression and anger symptoms. J Pers Disord 23(2):156–174. doi:10.1521/pedi.2009.23.2.156 [pii]

Paris J, Gunderson J, Weinberg I (2007) The interface between borderline personality disorder and bipolar spectrum disorders. Compr Psychiatry 48(2):145–154. doi:10.1016/j.comppsych.2006.10.001, S0010-440X(06)00107-6 [pii]

Parnas J, Licht D, Bovet P (2005) Cluster A personality disorders: a review. In: Mai M, Akiskal H, JE M, Okasha A (eds) Personality disorders. Wiley, New York, pp 1–74

Perugi G, Akiskal HS (2002) The soft bipolar spectrum redefined: focus on the cyclothymic, anxious-sensitive, impulse-dyscontrol, and binge-eating connection in bipolar II and related conditions. Psychiatr Clin North Am 25(4):713–737

Perugi G, Toni C, Travierso MC, Akiskal HS (2003) The role of cyclothymia in atypical depression: toward a data-based reconceptualization of the borderline-bipolar II connection. J Affect Disord 73(1–2):87–98. doi:S0165032702003294 [pii]

Perugi G, Angst J, Azorin JM, Bowden C, Vieta E, Young AH (2012) Is comorbid borderline personality disorder in patients with major depressive episode and bipolarity a developmental subtype? Findings from the international BRIDGE study. J Affect Disord 144:72–78. doi:10.1016/j.jad.2012.06.008, S0165-0327(12)00452-1 [pii]

Pica S, Edwards J, Jackson HJ, Bell RC, Bates GW, Rudd RP (1990) Personality disorders in recent-onset bipolar disorder. Compr Psychiatry 31(6):499–510

Preston GA, Marchant BK, Reimherr FW, Strong RE, Hedges DW (2004) Borderline personality disorder in patients with bipolar disorder and response to lamotrigine. J Affect Disord 79(1-3):297–303. doi:10.1016/S0165-0327(02)00358-0, S0165032702003580 [pii]

Reich J, Frances A (1984) The structural interview method for diagnosing borderline disorders: a critique. Psychiatry Q 56(3):229–235

Schiavone P, Dorz S, Conforti D, Scarso C, Borgherini G (2004) Comorbidity of DSM-IV personality disorders in unipolar and bipolar affective disorders: a comparative study. Psychol Rep 95(1):121–128

Sorvaniemi M, Hintikka J (2005) Recorded psychiatric comorbidity with bipolar disorder–a Finnish hospital discharge register study. Nord J Psychiatry 59(6):531–533. doi:10.1080/08039480500360773, VL0375G732718418 [pii]

Stinson FS, Dawson DA, Goldstein RB, Chou SP, Huang B, Smith SM, Ruan WJ, Pulay AJ, Saha TD, Pickering RP, Grant BF (2008) Prevalence, correlates, disability, and comorbidity of DSM-IV narcissistic personality disorder: results from the wave 2 national epidemiologic survey on alcohol and related conditions. J Clin Psychiatry 69(7):1033–1045. doi:ej08m04183 [pii]

Stoffers J, Vollm BA, Rucker G, Timmer A, Huband N, Lieb K (2010) Pharmacological interventions for borderline personality disorder. Cochrane Database Syst Rev (6):CD005653. doi:10.1002/14651858.CD005653.pub2

Stone M (1993) Long-term outcome in personality disorders. Br J Psychiatry 162:229–313

Swann AC (2011) Antisocial personality and bipolar disorder: interactions in impulsivity and course of illness. Neuropsychiatry (Lond) 1(6):599–610. doi:10.2217/NPY.11.69

Swann AC, Lijffijt M, Lane SD, Steinberg JL, Moeller FG (2010) Interactions between bipolar disorder and antisocial personality disorder in trait impulsivity and severity of illness. Acta Psychiatr Scand 121(6):453–461. doi:10.1111/j.1600-0447.2009.01528.x, ACP1528 [pii]

Swann AC, Lijffijt M, Lane SD, Steinberg JL, Moeller FG (2011) Interacting mechanisms of impulsivity in bipolar disorder and antisocial personality disorder. J Psychiatr Res 45(11):1477–1482. doi:10.1016/j.jpsychires.2011.06.009, S0022-3956(11)00125-7 [pii]

Swann AC, Lijffijt M, Lane SD, Steinberg JL, Moeller FG (2012) Antisocial personality disorder and borderline symptoms are differentially related to impulsivity and course of illness in bipolar disorder. J Affect Disord. doi:10.1016/j.jad.2012.06.027, S0165-0327(12)00490-9 [pii]

Turley B, Bates GW, Edwards J, Jackson HJ (1992) MCMI-II personality disorders in recent-onset bipolar disorders. J Clin Psychol 48(3):320–329

Vita A, De Peri L, Sacchetti E (2011) Antipsychotics, antidepressants, anticonvulsants, and placebo on the symptom dimensions of borderline personality disorder: a meta-analysis of randomized controlled and open-label trials. J Clin Psychopharmacol 31(5):613–624. doi:10.1097/JCP.0b013e31822c1636

Waller N (1999) Evaluating the structure of personality. In: Cloninger C (ed) Personality and psychopathology. American Psychiatric Press, Washington, DC, pp 155–197

Weber NS, Fisher JA, Cowan DN, Niebuhr DW (2011) Psychiatric and general medical conditions comorbid with bipolar disorder in the National Hospital Discharge Survey. Psychiatr Serv 62(10):1152–1158. doi:10.1176/appi.ps.62.10.1152, 62/10/1152 [pii]

Zanarini MC, Frankenburg FR, Hennen J, Silk KR (2003) The longitudinal course of borderline psychopathology: 6-year prospective follow-up of the phenomenology of borderline personality disorder. Am J Psychiatry 160(2):274–283

Zanarini M, Frankenburg F, Vujanovic A, Hennen J, Reich D, Silk K (2004) Axis II comorbidity of borderline personality disorder: description of 6-year course and prediction to time-to-remission. Acta Psychiatr Scand 110:416–420

Alcohol and Substance Use in BD Patients

9

It is common knowledge among clinicians that BD and substance use disorders (SUD) often co-occur in the same patient. However a number of methodological problems and limitations made research difficult on this specific topic. Additionally, clinicians are often unwilling to invest the time and effort needed to elicit the key features of the personal and psychiatric history which will reveal the presence of a SUD and elucidate its relationship with the development of BD and its role in the shaping of the patient's clinical picture.

Both for research as well as for clinical practice, a core issue is the direction of cause and effect in the relationship between BD and SUD. BD has a higher prevalence of SUD than that observed in any other mental disorder, and patients with both disorders have a more severe course of BD and worse outcome. They usually manifest an earlier age at onset, more frequent episodes, and more comorbid conditions. They more often face problems with the law and exhibit higher suicidality (Swann 2010). Some patients manifest BD first and SUD follows, while in others the sequence is the opposite. Obtaining a detailed chronology of the clinical history of the patient as well as a careful family history will be essential for the correct assessment and diagnosis.

9.1 Epidemiology

The data from the Epidemiological Catchment Area (ECA) suggest that drug abuse is present in 13 % of BD-I and in 9 % of BD-II patients and drug dependence is present in 28 and 12 % respectively. These rates suggest that BD-II patients had similar SUD rates in comparison to unipolar depressive patients but BD-I had double rates. All patient groups had much higher frequency of SUD (three to seven times) in comparison to the general population (Regier et al. 1990).

The most recent literature supports the high prevalence of alcohol and substance abuse comorbidity in BD, and this seems more pronounced in BD-I males which are

K.N. Fountoulakis, *Bipolar Disorder: An Evidence-Based Guide to Manic Depression*, DOI 10.1007/978-3-642-37216-2_9

single, with low education and with interepisodic cyclothymia and hyperthymia (Azorin et al. 2013; Lagerberg et al. 2010b). However, there are some data which relate SUD more with BD-II than with BD-I (Mazza et al. 2009). This high prevalence includes also the bipolar spectrum and extends to include the use of social drugs such as tobacco and coffee (Maremmani et al. 2011). The comorbidity is especially high in teenagers and young adults, and in these age groups, it often represents self-treatment of mood instability. It has been reported that the lifetime prevalence of any SUD among adolescents with BD was 16 % (Goldstein et al. 2008b). SUD usually arises during the early course of BD, even before the first mood episode. The peak hazard is between 14 and 20 years of age, and it constitutes a risk factor or alternatively a prognostic sign for the development of BD with psychotic features (Hazard Ratio HR=3) (Duffy et al. 2012).

In adults, the lifetime prevalence of SUDs is at least 40 % in BD-I patients, with alcohol and cannabis being those most often abused, followed by cocaine and opioids (Cerullo and Strakowski 2007; Lagerberg et al. 2010a). In comparison to the general population, BD is associated with a significant age-adjusted risk for any substance use disorder (HR=8.68) including alcohol abuse (HR=7.66), drug abuse (HR=18.5) and dependence (HR=12.1) and cigarette smoking (HR=12.3), and this relationship is independent of a comorbid attention deficit/hyperactivity disorder, multiple anxiety, and conduct disorder (Wilens et al. 2008).

SUD is higher among patients with BD-I, followed by BD-II, and unipolar depression (Moreno et al. 2012). In terms of specific substance use, it seems that BD patients have higher rates of alcohol consumption and cannabis use, while schizophrenia patients more often use stimulants and other substances except alcohol (Ringen et al. 2008).

9.1.1 Epidemiology of Alcohol Use Disorder

BD and alcohol use disorder represent a significant comorbid population (Farren et al. 2012; Bernadt and Murray 1986). From all mental patients, BD patients might be at a particularly higher risk to develop alcoholism during lifetime, especially during periods of acute mania (Helzer and Pryzbeck 1988).

In clinical samples, alcohol use disorder is reported to affect more than one-third and up to 75 % of BD patients. However, the reports vary significantly by geographical location, gender (with males having double rates in comparison to females) and specific clinical characteristics of the study sample (Di Florio et al. 2013; Lai et al. 2012; Farren et al. 2012; Freed 1969; Morrison 1974; Estroff et al. 1985). This specific comorbidity is reported to be higher for BD-I males which are single and with interepisodic cyclothymia and hyperthymia (Azorin et al. 2013). The data of the ECA suggest that alcohol abuse is present in 15 % of BD-I and in 18 % of BD-II patients and alcohol dependence in 31 and 21 %, respectively. These rates are two to three times higher than those observed in unipolar depressive patients and four times higher in comparison to the general population (Regier et al. 1990).

9.1.2 Epidemiology of Cannabis Use Disorder

The cannabis use disorder rate is reported to be 5.7 % in patients with BD (Lai and Sitharthan 2012) but probably this is not higher in comparison to the rate observed in the general population. Other studies report much higher rates (15–65 %) especially during acute mania (Goodwin and Jamison 2007), but they were presented as posters or chapters in books and thus the methodology is of unknown quality.

9.1.3 Epidemiology of Gambling

The large Canadian Community Health Survey on Mental Health and Well-Being (CCHS 1.2), which included 36,984 individuals (aged 15 years or older), reported that the weighted prevalence of problem gambling was significantly higher for BD patients in comparison to the general population (6.3 % vs. 2.0 %; $p<0.001$) with an odds ratio (OR) equal to 2.3 even after controlling for potential confounders. Being male, single and with low education were factors that were increasing the risk. The risk was also increased in the presence of alcohol and illicit drug dependence and decreased with moderate to active physical activity level (McIntyre et al. 2007b). This strong relationship of problematic gambling to mood disorders and BD in particular is observed even after adjustment for medical conditions, health-related quality of life and recent stressful life events (Chou and Afifi 2011). In clinical samples the prevalence might be even higher. One study reported a rate of 12.5 % of problem gambling in BD and a similar rate in unipolar depression with males having more than double rates in comparison to females in the BD group (19.5 % vs. 7.8 %). Mood disorder appeared before gambling in the majority of patients (71 %) and was associated with a comorbid anxiety disorder and lower quality of life (Kennedy et al. 2010).

9.1.4 Epidemiology of Methadone

One study in BD-I and BD-II patients or patients with cyclothymia both HIV-infected and HIV-noninfected reported that 6.4 % were receiving methadone maintenance therapy (Applebaum et al. 2010).

9.1.5 Epidemiology of Cocaine

In a clinical sample of BD patients, 3.4 % were found to suffer from cocaine abuse and 6.7 % from cocaine dependence (Chengappa et al. 2000). The literature suggests that cocaine use is mostly related with periods of acute mania (Estroff et al. 1985; Weiss and Mirin 1986; Weiss et al. 1986).

9.1.6 Epidemiology of Opioids

It has been reported that 5.4 % of opiate users were suffering from BD (Kosten and Rounsaville 1986; Rounsaville et al. 1986), while up to 5–25 % of BD patients might suffer from heroin abuse especially during periods of acute mania (Estroff et al. 1985; Miller et al. 1989).

9.1.7 Epidemiology of Smoking

A study which covered the period 1999–2011 reported that 44 % of BD patients in comparison to 64 % of patients with schizophrenia and to 19 % of controls were smoking. It also reported that these rates were relatively stable without any detectable time trends. These authors reported that in psychiatric patients smoking was correlated with less education, a history of substance abuse, longer illness duration and Caucasian race, but not with psychiatric symptom severity (Dickerson et al. 2013). Somewhat lower rates were reported by another study which however utilized a different research approach and studied 80 adolescents between 13 and 22 years of age with co-occurring BD-I and cannabis abuse or dependence who reported ever trying a cigarette. These authors reported that 49 % of these participants were current heavy smokers and 70 % of these met DSM-IV-TR lifetime criteria for nicotine dependence (Heffner et al. 2013). A similar prevalence for smoking (45.5 %) has been reported concerning the time of first hospitalization. Also, it has been reported that cigarette smokers were significantly more likely in comparison to non-smokers to report recent use of marijuana (55.7 % vs. 18.1 %) and alcohol (67.2 % vs. 25.4 %) (Heffner et al. 2008).

A similar prevalence of smoking (53.9 %) was reported in BD-I patients from Israel and this rate that was 2.36 times higher in comparison to that of the general population in Israel (22.8 %) (Kreinin et al. 2012). This higher risk is comparable to that reported in the US population (2.4 times) and might correlate with specific genes (COMT, SLC6A3 and SLC6A4) (McEachin et al. 2010).

Overall, the epidemiological data suggest that in comparison to the general population, half of BD patients are current smokers in comparison to approximately one-fifth of the general population (2.5 higher percentage), one-third regularly use alcohol and more than 6 % marijuana and methadone and manifest problematic gambling behaviours (three times higher in comparison to general population).

9.2 Etiopathogenesis of SUD in BD

9.2.1 General Causative Factors and Mechanisms

The high comorbidity of alcohol and substance use disorders with mood disorders cannot be explained as merely the chance occurrence of two prevalent disorders (Farren et al. 2012). Although the classical interpretation for the increased prevalence of SUD in mood disorders is that of self-treatment, this might not be the sole valid approach concerning BD. In the case of this specific disorder, it might also concern the augmentation or the triggering of desired or pleasurable states (e.g. use of stimulants to trigger hypomania or mania) (Bizzarri et al. 2007). Alcohol is usually used for both reasons, both because it exerts a disinhibiting effect but also because it possesses sedative and anxiolytic properties (McDonald and Meyer 2011) and thus alcohol use is related in a differential way to different phases of BD (Meyer et al. 2012).

The research on the causative relationship of BD with SUDs is limited in contrast to the significant amount of data which exist concerning schizophrenia. Recent research suggests that a subgroup of BD patients might develop a relatively milder form of the disorder only after extended exposure to alcohol or substance abuse (Cerullo and Strakowski 2007; Winokur et al. 1995; Feinman and Dunner 1996) and at a relatively later age at onset (Goldstein and Levitt 2006a, b).

The reverse, that is, how many BD patients develop alcohol and SUD secondary to an underlying bipolar diathesis, remains to be determined. Adolescents with BD are more likely than SUD patients without a mood disorder to report that they had started using the specific substance for its mood-altering effects. After the development of the SUD, there was no difference between mood disorder and non-mood disorder SUD patients concerning the reason why they continue using the substance (Lorberg et al. 2010). Early-onset and especially adolescent-onset BD especially in males was reported to predict the development of SUD but this was not the case concerning BD type or family history of BD (Kenneson et al. 2013; Feinman and Dunner 1996).

9.2.2 Neurobiology

The evidence suggests that intermittent stressors, mood episodes and bouts of cocaine use not only show sensitization to themselves but cross-sensitization to the others, and thus a vicious cycle is set to action (Post and Kalivas 2013). In addition, specific vulnerabilities seem to exist. There are some data suggesting that specific genes (COMT, SLC6A3 and SLC6A4) might predispose to the development both of BD and SUD; however the evidence is rare and sparse (McEachin et al. 2010). One study reported that patients with both BD and alcohol use disorders have smaller grey matter volume in the left medial frontal and the right anterior cingulate gyri in comparison to BD patients without alcohol use which had grey matter volumes similar to healthy controls. However it is unclear what is the cause and what is the effect (Nery et al. 2011). In line with this, in young persons with emerging BD who drink at risky levels, there is evidence suggesting there are reduced levels of glutathione which is the main brain antioxidant factor, in the anterior cingulate cortex (Chitty et al. 2013).

9.2.2.1 Endophenotypes

There are family data suggesting that BD and SUD do not share familial risk factors, since they correlate with different family histories. BD patients have mainly psychiatric family history, while SUD patients mainly have a family history of alcohol abuse (Sbrana et al. 2007). However there are data suggesting a more complex relationship with relatives of patients with BD being at a higher risk to develop SUD no matter whether SUD is present in BD patients themselves (Wilens et al. 2007). Also, SUD in parents predicts BD in the offspring (Duffy et al. 2012).

9.3 Clinical Issues

A major clinical problem is the fact that many patients with active SUD living in the community present with a pattern of mood instability which does not fit into contemporary classification systems (Goldberg et al. 2008). The task to identify and diagnose a SUD in BD patients, and especially in adolescents, might prove to be very difficult since repeated and targeted interviews might be necessary to elicit relevant, accurate and reliable information (Black et al. 2012).

It is important to recognize both the specific SUD as well as BD so that competent treatment is provided to both. Unfortunately in most programmes which aim SUD, the diagnosis of BD is often neglected even when properly put. Since BD is a treatable mental disorder, missing the opportunity to properly treat it is unacceptable, and this concerns also the whole bipolar spectrum (Maremmani et al. 2008), which appears particularly likely to invite self-medication.

There are several reports which link specific clinical features of BD with the presence of SUD. In many cases, substance use and abuse is associated with mood states (Baethge et al. 2008). It has been reported that during an acute depressive episode, SUD patients were using more often non-prescribed anxiolytic hypnotics, while during a hypomanic episode, they were using cocaine and amphetamines. During a full-blown acute manic episode, they were using more frequently cannabis and cocaine amphetamines, while during mixed episodes, the pattern of use included alcohol, cocaine amphetamines and cannabinoids. According to these data, the use of stimulants is more prevalent during the 'up' rather than the 'down' phase of the illness (Maremmani et al. 2012). It is possible that SUD alters the clinical presentation of BD and induces a kind of 'mixed' states (Winokur et al. 1969; Himmelhoch et al. 1976) and it might also increase the risk of switching during treatment with antidepressants (Goldberg and Whiteside 2002). According to one study, current psychomotor agitation and lifetime BD each were associated with increased prevalence of lifetime nicotine, alcohol and drug dependence (Leventhal and Zimmerman 2010). Concerning the bipolar type, the literature is inconclusive with some authors suggesting that SUD is related more with BD-I (Azorin et al. 2013; Lagerberg et al. 2010b), while others suggest it is related more with BD-II (Mazza et al. 2009). In patients with both BD and SUD, often there is also a comorbid personality disorder and the impairment is more severe (Mazza et al. 2009; Merikangas et al. 2008). An important psychological characteristic linking BD with SUD seems to be increased trait impulsivity (Powers et al. 2013).

BD preceded by substance misuse may represent a clinically milder subtype of bipolar illness. This subtype would be less 'primary' and might be more early targeted by primary prevention with programmes focused on substance misuse (Pacchiarotti et al. 2009). Overall, it seems that patients with a manic predominant polarity have a better prognosis concerning their substance use (Gonzalez-Pinto et al. 2010). However, even if remitted, substance use is related to a poorer acute treatment response, longer time to remission and more time with subthreshold symptoms, more often depressive. There is also a relationship of rapid cycling with SUD but the direction of causality is unknown (Schneck et al. 2004). This poor outcome does not seem to correlate with sporadic subsequent substance abuse during follow-up (Gaudiano et al. 2008). It is reflected also in the rates of hospitalization. It is reported that practically all BD patients with substance abuse will be rehospitalized within a year in comparison to only one-fifth of the rest. This is especially true for polysubstance abuse in combination with separation from their spouse or partner. For those patients who were not separated, only half will be rehospitalized, and in comparison only one in ten patients without substance abuse and without being separated from spouse or partner would be rehospitalized within a year (Hoblyn et al. 2009). In contrast to these, there are some studies which report that the overall long-term outcome of BD is not necessarily worse in SUD patients (Mandelli et al. 2012; Lagerberg et al. 2010a).

A significant issue is that the presence of SUD is also related to higher medical comorbidity (Magalhaes et al. 2012) with the exception of obesity, since BD patients with SUD had a lower rate of overweight/obesity when compared with non-substance-dependent bipolar patients (39 % vs. 54 %, $p<0.01$) (McIntyre et al. 2007a). It is important to note that one of the most important medical comorbidities is HIV infection which is related with greater drug use severity (Meade et al. 2008). Another important fact is that SUD among bipolar adolescents is associated with a higher risk for suicide attempts and teenage pregnancy and abortion (Goldstein et al. 2008b; Goldstein and Levitt 2008).

As a result, the prevalence of comorbid SUD was reported to be higher among unipolar and BD deaths than that among all other deaths, and this was mainly because of suicide and other unnatural death in both men and women. Consequently, SUD is associated with a reduced mean age at death in comparison to the general population (11.7–33.8 years). In general, these effects were much stronger for drug use disorders than for alcohol use disorders (Yoon et al. 2011).

9.3.1 Clinical Issues Related to Alcohol Use

Overall, the literature suggests that the presence of mood symptoms is related to alcohol abuse and dependence. One consistent finding in BD patients is that alcohol use and abuse preceded or coincided with depression (Baethge et al. 2008; Reich et al. 1974), but it has also been reported that it increases only during periods of mania (Winokur et al. 1969). In the general population, the presence of hypomanic symptoms increases the likelihood of alcohol abuse and dependence (Do and Mezuk 2013). Some authors suggest that problems with alcohol in BD patients exist irrespective of phase of the illness (Hensel et al. 1979; Dunner et al. 1979; Bernadt and Murray 1986). There are some inconsistent data suggesting that BD disorder has a later onset when comorbid with alcohol abuse. This implies that alcohol probably does not trigger BD but instead it is used as a self-healing method (Lagerberg et al. 2011). However, on the contrary, another study suggested that alcohol use is related to an earlier age at onset (Cardoso et al. 2008).

From a reverse angle, the risk to develop hypomania was specifically related to an unstable drinking pattern and binge drinking, but not higher consumption or alcohol abuse in general (Meyer and Wolkenstein 2010). Generally, bipolar alcoholics might have a better outcome concerning their alcohol problem in comparison to unipolar depressives (Farren et al. 2013).

Alcohol abuse and dependence are associated with a number of sociodemographic factors, including male gender and lower education. They are also related to a number of clinical characteristics, including the presence of psychotic features during the first episode, depressive symptoms, generalized anxiety and worse overall functioning (Mitchell et al. 2007; Cardoso et al. 2008). In this frame it is important for the clinician to have in mind that the number of days of alcohol use as well as any increase in this number are strong predictors of the emergence of a depressive episode in the subsequent month (Jaffee et al. 2009).

Increased impulsivity might mediate some severe manifestations of this comorbidity (Nery et al. 2013) including the remarkably high rates of suicide attempt observed in patients with comorbid BD and alcohol use. This increased suicidality might also be caused at least in part because of the greater overall burden of the disease which is experienced by these patients (Cardoso et al. 2008).

A specific clinical feature of comorbid alcohol abuse and dependence concerns the worse neurocognitive function both in BD-I and BD-II patients (Chang et al. 2012). These patients might have severe impairment on tests of executive functioning, verbal and visual memory as well as performance IQ (Levy et al. 2008). Patients without concomitant alcohol abuse show a much better recovery of their neurocognitive function when in remission (Levy et al. 2012).

In spite of the worse overall clinical picture related with alcohol abuse and dependence in BD patients, the literature does not suggest that these patients suffer from prolonged mood episodes of any type in comparison to the rest of patients. Concerning whether high levels of alcohol intake increase the risk of a mood recurrence, increase the rates of rapid-cycling and worsen the overall course of BD, the data are contradictory and inconclusive (Rakofsky and Dunlop 2013; van Zaane et al. 2010).

9.3.2 Clinical Issues Related to Cannabis Use

Cannabis abuse is reported to be significantly and independently associated with earlier onset of BD probably in a dose-dependent way (Lev-Ran et al. 2013; Lagerberg et al. 2011, 2013; De Hert et al. 2011; Aas et al. 2013). This implies that cannabis might trigger BD in vulnerable individuals (Lagerberg et al. 2011). The literature suggests that very often cannabis use selectively and strongly preceded and coincided with mania/hypomania (Baethge et al. 2008), and it was reported to correlate with a greater number of mood episodes of any type, a more severe course of BD

(Lev-Ran et al. 2013) and with prolonged mood episodes (Strakowski et al. 2007). BD patients who suffer from a concomitant cannabis abuse are similar to patients with schizophrenia in terms of worse outcome (De Hert et al. 2011).

Cannabis use was also related with lifetime history of at least one suicide attempt (Aas et al. 2013) and a trend for rapid cycling (Aas et al. 2013; Strakowski et al. 2007).

9.3.3 Clinical Issues Related to Cocaine Use

It has been reported that BD patients with concomitant cocaine use manifest higher rates of post-traumatic stress disorder and antisocial personality traits and are more likely to present with a mixed episode. They were also more likely to suffer from BD-I instead of BD-II (Mitchell et al. 2007). It is interesting that greater cocaine use severity was an independent predictor of total HIV risk, risk-taking sexual behaviour and an increased risk of sex trading (Meade et al. 2008, 2011).

9.3.4 Clinical Issues Related to Opioid Use

The literature on opioid use in BD patients is rather limited and does not suggest any difference between those patients that use opioids and the rest in terms of any of the examined clinical and course indices (Shabani et al. 2010).

9.3.5 Clinical Issues Related to Nicotine Use and Smoking

According to a recent study, in most BD patients with lifetime nicotine dependence, BD appears first and smoking follows. In these patients the onset of BD occurred at an earlier age and was characterized by a higher number of manic episodes. In the minority of BD patients where nicotine dependence preceded the onset of BD, the age at onset of both BD and smoking was earlier and there was an increased coexistence of alcohol use disorder (Martinez-Ortega et al. 2013). On the other hand, it seems that in BD patients, smoking is related more with the concomitant use and abuse of other substances, rather than with the clinical characteristics of BD (Kreinin et al. 2012; Heffner et al. 2008), and it is specifically related with earlier age at onset of regular marijuana and alcohol use (Heffner et al. 2008).

In comparison to non-smokers, current smokers with BD showed greater episode severity (Baek et al. 2013), higher rate of history of conduct disorder (Goldstein et al. 2008a; Wilens et al. 2009), more frequent concomitant alcohol and drug use (Goldstein et al. 2008a; Baek et al. 2013) and poorer functional levels (Baek et al. 2013). Previous smokers displayed intermediate characteristics between current smokers and non-smokers. Current smoking status but not lifetime smoking history was related to a higher suicide risk but the data for lifetime history are controversial (Baek et al. 2013; Goldstein et al. 2008a).

There seems to be a dose–response relationship between smoking and worse overall clinical picture and long-term outcome in BD patients (Goldstein et al. 2008a). Probably the dose–response relationship and the complex pattern of smoking and nicotine use and dependence are responsible of a number of studies which report no relationship between the clinical characteristics of BD and smoking (Heffner et al. 2008; Kreinin et al. 2012).

9.3.6 Substance Use and Neurocognitive Disorder

There are only limited data concerning the neurocognitive deficit specifically in BD patients with concomitant SUD. BD patients with a history of alcohol abuse or dependence obtained lower scores in the interference task of the Stroop test compared to patients with BD alone. Both patient groups showed a poorer performance in some verbal memory and executive function measures than healthy controls. In those BD patients with history of alcohol misuse, greater difficulties of inhibitory control were found, and this could be attributed to higher impulsivity (Sanchez-Moreno et al. 2009). A rather consistent finding suggests that the history of alcohol abuse is not associated with the current neurocognitive deficit in BD patients (Sanchez-Moreno et al. 2009; van der Werf-Eldering et al. 2010).

It is interesting that one study reported a better than expected neurocognitive function in BD patients with concomitant cannabis use, which is in sharp contrast to the findings reported concerning patients with schizophrenia (Ringen et al. 2010).

9.3.7 Comorbidity

In comparison to controls, patients with BD and comorbid SUD seem to have an over fourfold increase in the relative risk for HCV and this increased risk can be attributed to both conditions (Matthews et al. 2008).

9.3.8 Disability

When SUD is present, the overall disability of BD patients is reported to be similar to that of patients with schizophrenia. Also, in the BD plus SUD group, a number of features, including suicide attempts, poor compliance, longer hospitalizations, shorter periods of remission and criminal activity, were also more frequently observed. It seems that the presence of SUD has a greater impact than the main diagnosis (schizophrenia vs. BD) in the prediction of worse social adjustment and poorer outcome (Jaworski et al. 2011).

9.3.9 Suicidality

It has been reported that SUD was associated with suicide attempts especially in BD patients (Harris and Barraclough 1997). This effect seems to be present in BD-I but not BD-II, and this was mostly explained by higher impulsivity, hostility and aggression scores and earlier age at BD onset (Elizabeth Sublette et al. 2009). A more recent study suggested that specifically comorbid alcohol use puts the BD patient at a greater risk for a suicide attempt (OR=2.25; 95 % CI, 1.61–3.14). In contrast, nicotine dependence and drug use disorders did not seem to increase the risk for suicidal behaviour. The data concerning the interaction between alcohol use and other SUDs in the emergence of an additional risk among BD patients are controversial (Oquendo et al. 2010; Elizabeth Sublette et al. 2009).

9.4 Legal Issues

Legal problems are consistently found to be more frequent in patients with both BD and SUD in comparison to BD alone (Goldstein et al. 2008b; Goldstein and Levitt 2008; McCabe et al. 2013). The odds of having a comorbid SUD diagnosis for arrested female BD patients was more than 38 times higher in comparison to community female BD patients (McDermott et al. 2007).

Women were more likely to have been arrested for violent and substance use charges, while men were more likely to have been arrested for theft and miscellaneous charges (McDermott et al. 2007). Apart from criminal activities, patients with BD and SUD are more likely to be involved in a variety of activities with potential legal implications, including teenage pregnancy and abortion (Goldstein et al. 2008b; Goldstein and Levitt 2008).

9.5 Treatment

Three open-label medication trials provide limited evidence that quetiapine, aripiprazole, and lamotrigine may be effective in treating affective and SUD symptoms in BD patients with cocaine dependence. Also, aripiprazole might be helpful in patients with alcohol use disorders (Cerullo and Strakowski 2007). There are two placebo controlled trials to date which suggest that valproate given as an adjunct to lithium in BD patients with co-occurring alcohol dependence improves both mood and alcohol use symptoms and that lithium treatment in BD adolescents improves mood and SUD symptoms (Cerullo and Strakowski 2007). It is important to note that there are data suggesting that substance use might increase the risk of switching during treatment with antidepressants (Goldberg and Whiteside 2002).

Overall the data are insufficient to support an informed design of pharmaceutical treatment strategy in BD patients with SUD. Some data are available for alcohol, cannabis and cocaine SUD comorbid with BD but the literature is poor concerning heroin, amphetamine, methamphetamine and polysubstance SUD comorbid with BD (Beaulieu et al. 2012).

Psychotherapeutically, it is important to investigate and recognize the patterns and reasons of substance use as well as the motivation for treatment. The reasons are usually idiosyncratic to the patient and evolve through personal experience (Healey et al. 2009). Further well-designed studies are needed in order to properly assess the potential usefulness of psychotherapeutic interventions in a specific and targeted manner in the treatment of specific SUDs comorbid with BD (Beaulieu et al. 2012).

The observed positive associations between GAD, later treatment with a mood stabilizer, and early childhood trauma and history of SUDs suggest that adequate treatment of comorbid anxiety, early treatment with a mood stabilizer and prevention of childhood trauma may reduce the risk for the development of SUDs in patients with BD (Gao et al. 2010a).

However the literature suggests not only that half of the patients might not receive correct treatment (Gao et al. 2010b) but also that the risk of long treatment delays is increased in patients with excessive substance use, and this puts the patients in vicious cycles and worsens the outcome (Lagerberg et al. 2010b).

An important implication of the comorbid SUDs in BD patients is the frequent manifestation of poor medication adherence and the presence of negative attitudes concerning medication management (Keck et al. 1997) which often leads to poorer outcome (Calabrese and Delucchi 1990). Helping patients with BD achieve remission from SUD may lead to a more successful course of BD treatment (Teter et al. 2011; Manwani et al. 2007).

References

Aas M, Etain B, Bellivier F, Henry C, Lagerberg T, Ringen A, Agartz I, Gard S, Kahn JP, Leboyer M, Andreassen OA, Melle I (2014) Additive effects of childhood abuse and cannabis abuse on clinical expressions of bipolar disorders. Psychol Med 44(8):1653–1662. doi:10.1017/S0033291713002316, S0033291713002316 [pii]

Applebaum AJ, Bullis JR, Traeger LN, O'Cleirigh C, Otto MW, Pollack MH, Safren SA (2010) Rates of mood and anxiety disorders and contributors to continued heroin use in methadone maintenance patients: a comparison by HIV status. J Neurobehav HIV Med 2010(2):49–57. doi:10.2147/NBHIV.S12371

Azorin JM, Belzeaux R, Kaladjian A, Adida M, Hantouche E, Lancrenon S, Fakra E (2013) Risks associated with gender differences in bipolar I disorder. J Affect Disord 151(3):1033–1040. doi:10.1016/j.jad.2013.08.031, S0165-0327(13)00665-4 [pii]

Baek JH, Eisner LR, Nierenberg AA (2013) Smoking and suicidality in subjects with bipolar disorder: results from the National Epidemiologic Survey on Alcohol and Related Conditions (NESARC). Depress Anxiety 30(10):982–990. doi:10.1002/da.22107

Baethge C, Hennen J, Khalsa HM, Salvatore P, Tohen M, Baldessarini RJ (2008) Sequencing of substance use and affective morbidity in 166 first-episode bipolar I disorder patients. Bipolar Disord 10(6):738–741. doi:10.1111/j.1399-5618.2007.00575.x, BDI575 [pii]

Beaulieu S, Saury S, Sareen J, Tremblay J, Schutz CG, McIntyre RS, Schaffer A (2012) The Canadian Network for Mood and Anxiety Treatments (CANMAT) task force recommendations for the management of patients with mood disorders and comorbid substance use disorders. Ann Clin Psychiatry 24(1):38–55, acp_2401e [pii]

Bernadt MW, Murray RM (1986) Psychiatric disorder, drinking and alcoholism: what are the links? Br J Psychiatry 148:393–400

Bizzarri JV, Sbrana A, Rucci P, Ravani L, Massei GJ, Gonnelli C, Spagnolli S, Doria MR, Raimondi F, Endicott J, Dell'Osso L, Cassano GB (2007) The spectrum of substance abuse in bipolar disorder: reasons for use, sensation seeking and substance sensitivity. Bipolar Disord 3:213–220. doi:10.1111/j.1399-5618.2007.00383.x, BDI383 [pii]

Black JJ, Heffner JL, Anthenelli RM, Beavers JN, Albertz A, Blom T, Adler C, Delbello MP (2012) Diagnosing alcohol and cannabis use disorders in adolescents with bipolar disorder: a preliminary investigation. J Dual Diagn 8(1):13–18. doi:10.1080/15504263.2012.647349

Calabrese JR, Delucchi GA (1990) Spectrum of efficacy of valproate in 55 patients with rapid-cycling bipolar disorder. Am J Psychiatry 147(4):431–434

Cardoso BM, Kauer Sant'Anna M, Dias VV, Andreazza AC, Cereser KM, Kapczinski F (2008) The impact of co-morbid alcohol use disorder in bipolar patients. Alcohol 42(6):451–457. doi:10.1016/j.alcohol.2008.05.003, S0741-8329(08)00248-6 [pii]

Cerullo MA, Strakowski SM (2007) The prevalence and significance of substance use disorders in bipolar type I and II disorder. Subst Abuse Treat Prev Policy 2:29. doi:10.1186/1747-597X-2-29, 1747-597X-2-29 [pii]

Chang YH, Chen SL, Lee SY, Hsu YW, Wu JY, Chen SH, Chu CH, Lee IH, Yeh TL, Tzeng NS, Huang SY, Yang YK, Lu RB (2012) Neuropsychological functions in bipolar disorders I and II with and without comorbid alcohol dependence. Prog Neuropsychopharmacol Biol Psychiatry 37(2):211–216. doi:10.1016/j.pnpbp.2012.01.015, S0278-5846(12)00019-X [pii]

Chengappa KN, Levine J, Gershon S, Kupfer DJ (2000) Lifetime prevalence of substance or alcohol abuse and dependence among subjects with bipolar I and II disorders in a voluntary registry. Bipolar Disord 2(3 Pt 1):191–195

Chitty KM, Lagopoulos J, Hickie IB, Hermens DF (2013) Risky alcohol use in young persons with emerging bipolar disorder is associated with increased oxidative stress. J Affect Disord 150(3):1238–1241. doi:10.1016/j.jad.2013.06.003, S0165-0327(13)00476-X [pii]

Chou KL, Afifi TO (2011) Disordered (pathologic or problem) gambling and axis I psychiatric disorders: results from the National Epidemiologic Survey on Alcohol and Related Conditions. Am J Epidemiol 173(11):1289–1297. doi:10.1093/aje/kwr017, kwr017 [pii]

De Hert M, Wampers M, Jendricko T, Franic T, Vidovic D, De Vriendt N, Sweers K, Peuskens J, van Winkel R (2011) Effects of cannabis use on age at onset in schizophrenia and bipolar disorder. Schizophr Res 126(1–3):270–276. doi:10.1016/j.schres.2010.07.003, S0920-9964(10)01418-0 [pii]

Di Florio A, Craddock N, van den Bree M (2013) Alcohol misuse in bipolar disorder. A systematic review and meta-analysis of comorbidity rates. Eur Psychiatry. doi:10.1016/j.eurpsy.2013.07.004, S0924-9338(13)00100-4 [pii]

Dickerson F, Stallings CR, Origoni AE, Vaughan C, Khushalani S, Schroeder J, Yolken RH (2013) Cigarette smoking among persons with schizophrenia or bipolar disorder in routine clinical settings, 1999–2011. Psychiatr Serv 64(1):44–50. doi:10.1176/appi.ps.201200143, 1487305 [pii]

Do EK, Mezuk B (2013) Comorbidity between hypomania and substance use disorders. J Affect Disord 150(3):974–980. doi:10.1016/j.jad.2013.05.023, S0165-0327(13)00382-0 [pii]

Duffy A, Horrocks J, Milin R, Doucette S, Persson G, Grof P (2012) Adolescent substance use disorder during the early stages of bipolar disorder: a prospective high-risk study. J Affect Disord 142(1–3):57–64. doi:10.1016/j.jad.2012.04.010, S0165-0327(12)00271-6 [pii]

Dunner DL, Hensel BM, Fieve RR (1979) Bipolar illness: factors in drinking behavior. Am J Psychiatry 136(4B):583–585

Elizabeth Sublette M, Carballo JJ, Moreno C, Galfalvy HC, Brent DA, Birmaher B, John Mann J, Oquendo MA (2009) Substance use disorders and suicide attempts in bipolar subtypes. J Psychiatr Res 43(3):230–238. doi:10.1016/j.jpsychires.2008.05.001, S0022-3956(08)00114-3 [pii]

Estroff TW, Dackis CA, Gold MS, Pottash AL (1985) Drug abuse and bipolar disorders. Int J Psychiatry Med 15(1):37–40

Farren CK, Hill KP, Weiss RD (2012) Bipolar disorder and alcohol use disorder: a review. Curr Psychiatry Rep 14(6):659–666. doi:10.1007/s11920-012-0320-9

Farren CK, Snee L, Daly P, McElroy S (2013) Prognostic factors of 2-year outcomes of patients with comorbid bipolar disorder or depression with alcohol dependence: importance of early abstinence. Alcohol Alcohol 48(1):93–98. doi:10.1093/alcalc/ags112, ags112 [pii]

Feinman JA, Dunner DL (1996) The effect of alcohol and substance abuse on the course of bipolar affective disorder. J Affect Disord 37(1):43–49

Freed EX (1969) Alcohol abuse by manic patients. Psychol Rep 25(1):280

Gao K, Chan PK, Verduin ML, Kemp DE, Tolliver BK, Ganocy SJ, Bilali S, Brady KT, Findling RL, Calabrese JR (2010a) Independent predictors for lifetime and recent substance use disorders in patients with rapid-cycling bipolar disorder: focus on anxiety disorders. Am J Addict 19(5):44–449. doi:10.1111/j.1521-0391.2010.00060.x, AJAD60 [pii]

Gao K, Kemp DE, Conroy C, Ganocy SJ, Findling RL, Calabrese JR (2010b) Comorbid anxiety and substance use disorders associated with a lower use of mood stabilisers in patients with rapid cycling bipolar disorder: a descriptive analysis of the cross-sectional data of 566 patients. Int J Clin Pract 64(3):336–344. doi:10.1111/j.1742-1241.2009.02284.x, IJCP2284 [pii]

Gaudiano BA, Uebelacker LA, Miller IW (2008) Impact of remitted substance use disorders on the future course of bipolar I disorder: findings from a clinical trial. Psychiatry Res 160(1):63–71. doi:10.1016/j.psychres.2007.05.014, S0165-1781(07)00163-1 [pii]

Goldberg JF, Whiteside JE (2002) The association between substance abuse and antidepressant-induced mania in bipolar disorder: a preliminary study. J Clin Psychiatry 63(9):791–795

Goldberg JF, Garno JL, Callahan AM, Kearns DL, Kerner B, Ackerman SH (2008) Overdiagnosis of bipolar disorder among substance use disorder inpatients with mood instability. J Clin Psychiatry 69(11):1751–1757, ej07m04020 [pii]

Goldstein BI, Levitt AJ (2006a) Factors associated with temporal priority in comorbid bipolar I disorder and alcohol use disorders: results from the national epidemiologic survey on alcohol and related conditions. J Clin Psychiatry 67(4):643–649

Goldstein BI, Levitt AJ (2006b) Further evidence for a developmental subtype of bipolar disorder defined by age at onset: results from the national epidemiologic survey on alcohol and related conditions. Am J Psychiatry 163(9):1633–1636. doi:10.1176/appi.ajp.163.9.1633

Goldstein BI, Levitt AJ (2008) The specific burden of comorbid anxiety disorders and of substance use disorders in bipolar I disorder. Bipolar Disord 10(1):67–78. doi:10.1111/j.1399-5618.2008.00461.x, BDI461 [pii]

Goldstein BI, Birmaher B, Axelson DA, Goldstein TR, Esposito-Smythers C, Strober MA, Hunt J, Leonard H, Gill MK, Iyengar S, Grimm C, Yang M, Ryan ND, Keller MB (2008a) Significance of cigarette smoking among youths with bipolar disorder. Am J Addict 17(5):364–371. doi:10.1080/10550490802266151, 902146255 [pii]

Goldstein BI, Strober MA, Birmaher B, Axelson DA, Esposito-Smythers C, Goldstein TR, Leonard H, Hunt J, Gill MK, Iyengar S, Grimm C, Yang M, Ryan ND, Keller MB (2008b) Substance use disorders among adolescents with bipolar spectrum disorders. Bipolar Disord 10(4):469–478. doi:10.1111/j.1399-5618.2008.00584.x, BDI584 [pii]

Gonzalez-Pinto A, Alberich S, Barbeito S, Alonso M, Vieta E, Martinez-Aran A, Saenz M, Lopez P (2010) Different profile of substance abuse in relation to predominant polarity in bipolar disorder: the Vitoria long-term follow-up study. J Affect Disord 124(3):250–255. doi:10.1016/j.jad.2009.11.005, S0165-0327(09)00498-4 [pii]

Goodwin F, Jamison K (2007) Manic-depressive illness, 2nd edn. Oxford University Press, New York

Harris EC, Barraclough B (1997) Suicide as an outcome for mental disorders. A meta-analysis. Br J Psychiatry 170:205–228

Healey C, Peters S, Kinderman P, McCracken C, Morriss R (2009) Reasons for substance use in dual diagnosis bipolar disorder and substance use disorders: a qualitative study. J Affect Disord 113(1–2):118–126. doi:10.1016/j.jad.2008.05.010, S0165-0327(08)00225-5 [pii]

Heffner JL, DelBello MP, Fleck DE, Anthenelli RM, Strakowski SM (2008) Cigarette smoking in the early course of bipolar disorder: association with ages-at-onset of alcohol and marijuana use. Bipolar Disord 10(7):838–845. doi:10.1111/j.1399-5618.2008.00630.x, BDI630 [pii]

Heffner JL, Anthenelli RM, Adler CM, Strakowski SM, Beavers J, Delbello MP (2013) Prevalence and correlates of heavy smoking and nicotine dependence in adolescents with bipolar and cannabis use disorders. Psychiatry Res 210(3):857–862. doi:10.1016/j.psychres.2013.04.010, S0165-1781(13)00198-4 [pii]

Helzer JE, Pryzbeck TR (1988) The co-occurrence of alcoholism with other psychiatric disorders in the general population and its impact on treatment. J Stud Alcohol 49(3):219–224

Hensel B, Dunner DL, Fieve RR (1979) The relationship of family history of alcoholism to primary affective disorder. J Affect Disord 1(2):105–113

Himmelhoch JM, Mulla D, Neil JF, Detre TP, Kupfer DJ (1976) Incidence and significance of mixed affective states in a bipolar population. Arch Gen Psychiatry 33(9):1062–1066

Hoblyn JC, Balt SL, Woodard SA, Brooks JO 3rd (2009) Substance use disorders as risk factors for psychiatric hospitalization in bipolar disorder. Psychiatr Serv 60(1):50–55. doi:10.1176/appi.ps.60.1.50, 60/1/50 [pii]

Jaffee WB, Griffin ML, Gallop R, Meade CS, Graff F, Bender RE, Weiss RD (2009) Depression precipitated by alcohol use in patients with co-occurring bipolar and substance use disorders. J Clin Psychiatry 70(2):171–176, ej07m04011 [pii]

Jaworski F, Dubertret C, Ades J, Gorwood P (2011) Presence of co-morbid substance use disorder in bipolar patients worsens their social functioning to the level observed in patients with schizophrenia. Psychiatry Res 185(1–2):129–134. doi:10.1016/j.psychres.2010.06.005, S0165-1781(10)00311-2 [pii]

Keck PE Jr, McElroy SL, Strakowski SM, Bourne ML, West SA (1997) Compliance with maintenance treatment in bipolar disorder. Psychopharmacol Bull 33(1):87–91

Kennedy SH, Welsh BR, Fulton K, Soczynska JK, McIntyre RS, O'Donovan C, Milev R, le Melledo JM, Bisserbe JC, Zimmerman M, Martin N (2010) Frequency and correlates of gambling problems in outpatients with major depressive disorder and bipolar disorder. Can J Psychiatry 55(9):568–576

Kenneson A, Funderburk JS, Maisto SA (2013) Risk factors for secondary substance use disorders in people with childhood and adolescent-onset bipolar disorder: opportunities for prevention. Compr Psychiatry 54(5):439–446. doi:10.1016/j.comppsych.2012.12.008, S0010-440X(12)00264-7 [pii]

Kosten TR, Rounsaville BJ (1986) Psychopathology in opioid addicts. Psychiatr Clin North Am 9(3):515–532

Kreinin A, Novitski D, Rabinowitz D, Weizman A, Grinshpoon A (2012) Association between tobacco smoking and bipolar affective disorder: clinical, epidemiological, cross-sectional, retrospective study in outpatients. Compr Psychiatry 53(3):269–274. doi:10.1016/j.comppsych.2011.04.063, S0010-440X(11)00109-X [pii]

Lagerberg TV, Andreassen OA, Ringen PA, Berg AO, Larsson S, Agartz I, Sundet K, Melle I (2010a) Excessive substance use in bipolar disorder is associated with impaired functioning rather than clinical characteristics, a descriptive study. BMC Psychiatry 10:9. doi:10.1186/1471-244X-10-9, 1471-244X-10-9 [pii]

Lagerberg TV, Larsson S, Sundet K, Hansen CB, Hellvin T, Andreassen OA, Melle I (2010b) Treatment delay and excessive substance use in bipolar disorder. J Nerv Ment Dis 198(9):628–633. doi:10.1097/NMD.0b013e3181ef3ef4, 00005053-201009000-00004 [pii]

Lagerberg TV, Sundet K, Aminoff SR, Berg AO, Ringen PA, Andreassen OA, Melle I (2011) Excessive cannabis use is associated with earlier age at onset in bipolar disorder. Eur Arch Psychiatry Clin Neurosci 261(6):397–405. doi:10.1007/s00406-011-0188-4

Lagerberg TV, Kvitland LR, Aminoff SR, Aas M, Ringen PA, Andreassen OA, Melle I (2013) Indications of a dose-response relationship between cannabis use and age at onset in bipolar disorder. Psychiatry Res. doi:10.1016/j.psychres.2013.10.029, S0165-1781(13)00680-X [pii]

Lai HM, Sitharthan T (2012) Exploration of the comorbidity of cannabis use disorders and mental health disorders among inpatients presenting to all hospitals in New South Wales, Australia. Am J Drug Alcohol Abuse 38(6):567–574. doi:10.3109/00952990.2012.694523

Lai HM, Sitharthan T, Huang QR (2012) Exploration of the comorbidity of alcohol use disorders and mental health disorders among inpatients presenting to all hospitals in New South Wales, Australia. Subst Abus 33(2):138–145. doi:10.1080/08897077.2011.634967

Leventhal AM, Zimmerman M (2010) The relative roles of bipolar disorder and psychomotor agitation in substance dependence. Psychol Addict Behav 24(2):360–365. doi:10.1037/a0019217, 2010-12599-020 [pii]

Lev-Ran S, Le Foll B, McKenzie K, George TP, Rehm J (2013) Bipolar disorder and co-occurring cannabis use disorders: characteristics, co-morbidities and clinical correlates. Psychiatry Res 209(3):459–465. doi:10.1016/j.psychres.2012.12.014, S0165-1781(12)00811-6 [pii]

Levy B, Monzani BA, Stephansky MR, Weiss RD (2008) Neurocognitive impairment in patients with co-occurring bipolar disorder and alcohol dependence upon discharge from inpatient care. Psychiatry Res 161(1):28–35. doi:10.1016/j.psychres.2007.09.009, S0165-1781(07)00334-4 [pii]

Levy B, Manove E, Weiss RD (2012) Recovery of cognitive functioning in patients with co-occurring bipolar disorder and alcohol dependence during early remission from an acute mood episode. Ann Clin Psychiatry 24(2):143–154, acp_2402e [pii]

Lorberg B, Wilens TE, Martelon M, Wong P, Parcell T (2010) Reasons for substance use among adolescentswithbipolardisorder.AmJAddict19(6):474–480.doi:10.1111/j.1521-0391.2010.00077.x

Magalhaes PV, Kapczinski F, Nierenberg AA, Deckersbach T, Weisinger D, Dodd S, Berk M (2012) Illness burden and medical comorbidity in the Systematic Treatment Enhancement Program for Bipolar Disorder. Acta Psychiatr Scand 125(4):303–308. doi:10.1111/j.1600-0447.2011.01794.x

Mandelli L, Mazza M, Di Nicola M, Zaninotto L, Harnic D, Catalano V, Tedeschi D, Martinotti G, Bria P, Janiri L, Serretti A (2012) Role of substance abuse comorbidity and personality on the outcome of depression in bipolar disorder: harm avoidance influences medium-term treatment outcome. Psychopathology 45(3):174–178. doi:10.1159/000330364, 000330364 [pii]

Manwani SG, Szilagyi KA, Zablotsky B, Hennen J, Griffin ML, Weiss RD (2007) Adherence to pharmacotherapy in bipolar disorder patients with and without co-occurring substance use disorders. J Clin Psychiatry 68(8):1172–1176

Maremmani I, Pacini M, Perugi G, Deltito J, Akiskal H (2008) Cocaine abuse and the bipolar spectrum in 1090 heroin addicts: clinical observations and a proposed pathophysiologic model. J Affect Disord 106(1–2):55–61. doi:10.1016/j.jad.2007.03.015

Maremmani I, Perugi G, Rovai L, Maremmani AG, Pacini M, Canonico PL, Carbonato P, Mencacci C, Muscettola G, Pani L, Torta R, Vampini C, Akiskal HS (2011) Are "social drugs" (tobacco, coffee and chocolate) related to the bipolar spectrum? J Affect Disord 133(1–2):227–233. doi:10.1016/j.jad.2011.04.019, S0165-0327(11)00186-8 [pii]

Maremmani I, Maremmani AG, Rugani F, Rovai L, Pacini M, Bacciardi S, Deltito J, Dell'osso L, Akiskal HS (2012) Clinical presentations of substance abuse in bipolar heroin addicts at time of treatment entry. Ann Gen Psychiatr 11(1):23. doi:10.1186/1744-859X-11-23, 1744-859X-11-23 [pii]

Martinez-Ortega JM, Goldstein BI, Gutierrez-Rojas L, Sala R, Wang S, Blanco C (2013) Temporal sequencing of nicotine dependence and bipolar disorder in the National Epidemiologic Survey on Alcohol and Related Conditions (NESARC). J Psychiatr Res 47(7):858–864. doi:10.1016/j.jpsychires.2013.03.012, S0022-3956(13)00095-2 [pii]

Matthews AM, Huckans MS, Blackwell AD, Hauser P (2008) Hepatitis C testing and infection rates in bipolar patients with and without comorbid substance use disorders. Bipolar Disord 10(2):266–270. doi:10.1111/j.1399-5618.2007.00472.x, BDI472 [pii]

Mazza M, Mandelli L, Di Nicola M, Harnic D, Catalano V, Tedeschi D, Martinotti G, Colombo R, Bria P, Serretti A, Janiri L (2009) Clinical features, response to treatment and functional outcome of bipolar disorder patients with and without co-occurring substance use disorder: 1-year follow-up. J Affect Disord 115(1–2):27–35. doi:10.1016/j.jad.2008.08.019, S0165-0327(08)00357-1 [pii]

McCabe PJ, Christopher PP, Pinals DA, Fisher WH (2013) Predictors of criminal justice involvement in severe mania. J Affect Disord 149(1–3):367–374. doi:10.1016/j.jad.2013.02.015, S0165-0327(13)00170-5 [pii]

McDermott BE, Quanbeck CD, Frye MA (2007) Comorbid substance use disorder in women with bipolar disorder associated with criminal arrest. Bipolar Disord 9(5):536–540. doi:10.1111/j.1399-5618.2007.00346.x, BDI346 [pii]

McDonald JL, Meyer TD (2011) Self-report reasons for alcohol use in bipolar disorders: why drink despite the potential risks? Clin Psychol Psychother 18(5):418–425. doi:10.1002/cpp.782

McEachin RC, Saccone NL, Saccone SF, Kleyman-Smith YD, Kar T, Kare RK, Ade AS, Sartor MA, Cavalcoli JD, McInnis MG (2010) Modeling complex genetic and environmental influences on comorbid bipolar disorder with tobacco use disorder. BMC Med Genet 11:14. doi:10.1186/1471-2350-11-14, 1471-2350-11-14 [pii]

McIntyre RS, McElroy SL, Konarski JZ, Soczynska JK, Bottas A, Castel S, Wilkins K, Kennedy SH (2007a) Substance use disorders and overweight/obesity in bipolar I disorder: preliminary evidence for competing addictions. J Clin Psychiatry 68(9):1352–1357

McIntyre RS, McElroy SL, Konarski JZ, Soczynska JK, Wilkins K, Kennedy SH (2007b) Problem gambling in bipolar disorder: results from the Canadian Community Health Survey. J Affect Disord 102(1–3):27–34. doi:10.1016/j.jad.2006.12.005, S0165-0327(06)00534-9 [pii]

Meade CS, Graff FS, Griffin ML, Weiss RD (2008) HIV risk behavior among patients with co-occurring bipolar and substance use disorders: associations with mania and drug abuse. Drug Alcohol Depend 92(1–3):296–300. doi:10.1016/j.drugalcdep.2007.07.013, S0376-8716(07)00285-2 [pii]

Meade CS, Fitzmaurice GM, Sanchez AK, Griffin ML, McDonald LJ, Weiss RD (2011) The relationship of manic episodes and drug abuse to sexual risk behavior in patients with co-occurring bipolar and substance use disorders: a 15-month prospective analysis. AIDS Behav 15(8):1829–1833. doi:10.1007/s10461-010-9814-9

Merikangas KR, Herrell R, Swendsen J, Rossler W, Ajdacic-Gross V, Angst J (2008) Specificity of bipolar spectrum conditions in the comorbidity of mood and substance use disorders: results from the Zurich cohort study. Arch Gen Psychiatry 65(1):47–52. doi:10.1001/archgenpsychiatry.2007.18, 65/1/47 [pii]

Meyer TD, Wolkenstein L (2010) Current alcohol use and risk for hypomania in male students: generally more or more binging? Compr Psychiatry 51(2):171–176. doi:10.1016/j.comppsych.2009.05.002, S0010-440X(09)00064-9 [pii]

Meyer TD, McDonald JL, Douglas JL, Scott J (2012) Do patients with bipolar disorder drink alcohol for different reasons when depressed, manic or euthymic? J Affect Disord 136(3):926–932. doi:10.1016/j.jad.2011.09.005, S0165-0327(11)00531-3 [pii]

Miller FT, Busch F, Tanenbaum JH (1989) Drug abuse in schizophrenia and bipolar disorder. Am J Drug Alcohol Abuse 15(3):291–295

Mitchell JD, Brown ES, Rush AJ (2007) Comorbid disorders in patients with bipolar disorder and concomitant substance dependence. J Affect Disord 102(1–3):281–287. doi:10.1016/j.jad.2007.01.005, S0165-0327(07)00005-5 [pii]

Moreno C, Hasin DS, Arango C, Oquendo MA, Vieta E, Liu S, Grant BF, Blanco C (2012) Depression in bipolar disorder versus major depressive disorder: results from the National Epidemiologic Survey on Alcohol and Related Conditions. Bipolar Disord 14(3):271–282. doi:10.1111/j.1399-5618.2012.01009.x

Morrison JR (1974) Bipolar affective disorder and alcoholism. Am J Psychiatry 131(10):1130–1133

Nery FG, Matsuo K, Nicoletti MA, Monkul ES, Zunta-Soares GB, Hatch JP, Lafer B, Soares JC (2011) Association between prior alcohol use disorders and decreased prefrontal gray matter volumes in bipolar I disorder patients. Neurosci Lett 503(2):136–140. doi:10.1016/j.neulet.2011.08.026, S0304-3940(11)01211-0 [pii]

Nery FG, Hatch JP, Monkul ES, Matsuo K, Zunta-Soares GB, Bowden CL, Soares JC (2013) Trait impulsivity is increased in bipolar disorder patients with comorbid alcohol use disorders. Psychopathology 46(3):145–152. doi:10.1159/000336730, 000336730 [pii]

Oquendo MA, Currier D, Liu SM, Hasin DS, Grant BF, Blanco C (2010) Increased risk for suicidal behavior in comorbid bipolar disorder and alcohol use disorders: results from the National Epidemiologic Survey on Alcohol and Related Conditions (NESARC). J Clin Psychiatry 71(7):902–909. doi:10.4088/JCP.09m05198gry

Pacchiarotti I, Di Marzo S, Colom F, Sanchez-Moreno J, Vieta E (2009) Bipolar disorder preceded by substance abuse: a different phenotype with not so poor outcome? World J Biol Psychiatry 10(3):209–216. doi:10.1080/15622970701558488, 781983075 [pii]

Post RM, Kalivas P (2013) Bipolar disorder and substance misuse: pathological and therapeutic implications of their comorbidity and cross-sensitisation. Br J Psychiatry 202(3):172–176. doi:10.1192/bjp.bp.112.116855, 202/3/172 [pii]

Powers RL, Russo M, Mahon K, Brand J, Braga RJ, Malhotra AK, Burdick KE (2013) Impulsivity in bipolar disorder: relationships with neurocognitive dysfunction and substance use history. Bipolar Disord. doi:10.1111/bdi.12124

Rakofsky JJ, Dunlop BW (2013) Do alcohol use disorders destabilize the course of bipolar disorder? J Affect Disord 145(1):1–10. doi:10.1016/j.jad.2012.06.012, S0165-0327(12)00461-2 [pii]

Regier DA, Farmer ME, Rae DS, Locke BZ, Keith SJ, Judd LL, Goodwin FK (1990) Comorbidity of mental disorders with alcohol and other drug abuse. Results from the Epidemiologic Catchment Area (ECA) Study. JAMA 264(19):2511–2518

Reich LH, Davies RK, Himmelhoch JM (1974) Excessive alcohol use in manic-depressive illness. Am J Psychiatry 131(1):83–86

Ringen PA, Lagerberg TV, Birkenaes AB, Engn J, Faerden A, Jonsdottir H, Nesvag R, Friis S, Opjordsmoen S, Larsen F, Melle I, Andreassen OA (2008) Differences in prevalence and patterns of substance use in schizophrenia and bipolar disorder. Psychol Med 38(9):1241–1249. doi:10.1017/S003329170700236X, S003329170700236X [pii]

Ringen PA, Vaskinn A, Sundet K, Engh JA, Jonsdottir H, Simonsen C, Friis S, Opjordsmoen S, Melle I, Andreassen OA (2010) Opposite relationships between cannabis use and neurocognitive functioning in bipolar disorder and schizophrenia. Psychol Med 40(8):1337–1347. doi:10.1017/S0033291709991620, S0033291709991620 [pii]

Rounsaville BJ, Kosten TR, Kleber HD (1986) Long-term changes in current psychiatric diagnoses of treated opiate addicts. Compr Psychiatry 27(5):480–498

Sanchez-Moreno J, Martinez-Aran A, Colom F, Scott J, Tabares-Seisdedos R, Sugranyes G, Torrent C, Daban C, Benabarre A, Goikolea JM, Franco C, Gonzalez-Pinto A, Ayuso-Mateos JL, Vieta E (2009) Neurocognitive dysfunctions in euthymic bipolar patients with and without prior history of alcohol use. J Clin Psychiatry 70(8):1120–1127. doi:10.4088/JCP.08m04302

Sbrana A, Bizzarri JV, Rucci P, Gonnelli C, Massei JG, Ravani L, Endicott J, Maser JD, Cassano GB (2007) Family history of psychiatric disorders and alcohol and substance misuse in patients with bipolar I disorder, substance use disorder, or both. Am J Addict 16(3):227–231. doi:10.1080/10550490701375699, 779832597 [pii]

Schneck CD, Miklowitz DJ, Calabrese JR, Allen MH, Thomas MR, Wisniewski SR, Miyahara S, Shelton MD, Ketter TA, Goldberg JF, Bowden CL, Sachs GS (2004) Phenomenology of rapid-cycling bipolar disorder: data from the first 500 participants in the Systematic Treatment Enhancement Program. Am J Psychiatry 161(10):1902–1908. doi:10.1176/appi.ajp.161.10.1902

Shabani A, Jolfaei AG, Vazmalaei HA, Ebrahimi AA, Naserbakht M (2010) Clinical and course indicators of bipolar disorder type I with and without opioid dependence. J Res Med Sci 15(1):20–26

Strakowski SM, DelBello MP, Fleck DE, Adler CM, Anthenelli RM, Keck PE Jr, Arnold LM, Amicone J (2007) Effects of co-occurring cannabis use disorders on the course of bipolar disorder after a first hospitalization for mania. Arch Gen Psychiatry 64(1):57–64. doi:10.1001/archpsyc.64.1.57, 64/1/57 [pii]

Swann AC (2010) The strong relationship between bipolar and substance-use disorder. Ann N Y Acad Sci 1187:276–293. doi:10.1111/j.1749-6632.2009.05146.x, NYAS5146 [pii]

Teter CJ, Falone AE, Bakaian AM, Tu C, Ongur D, Weiss RD (2011) Medication adherence and attitudes in patients with bipolar disorder and current versus past substance use disorder. Psychiatry Res 190(2–3):253–258. doi:10.1016/j.psychres.2011.05.042, S0165-1781(11)00439-2 [pii]

van der Werf-Eldering MJ, Burger H, Holthausen EA, Aleman A, Nolen WA (2010) Cognitive functioning in patients with bipolar disorder: association with depressive symptoms and alcohol use. PLoS One 5(9). doi:10.1371/journal.pone.0013032

van Zaane J, van den Brink W, Draisma S, Smit JH, Nolen WA (2010) The effect of moderate and excessive alcohol use on the course and outcome of patients with bipolar disorders: a prospective cohort study. J Clin Psychiatry 71(7):885–893. doi:10.4088/JCP.09m05079gry

Weiss RD, Mirin SM (1986) Subtypes of cocaine abusers. Psychiatr Clin North Am 9(3):491–501

Weiss RD, Mirin SM, Michael JL, Sollogub AC (1986) Psychopathology in chronic cocaine abusers. Am J Drug Alcohol Abuse 12(1–2):17–29

Wilens TE, Biederman J, Adamson J, Monuteaux M, Henin A, Sgambati S, Santry A, Faraone SV (2007) Association of bipolar and substance use disorders in parents of adolescents with bipolar disorder. Biol Psychiatry 62(2):129–134. doi:10.1016/j.biopsych.2006.11.022, S0006-3223(06)01511-3 [pii]

Wilens TE, Biederman J, Adamson JJ, Henin A, Sgambati S, Gignac M, Sawtelle R, Santry A, Monuteaux MC (2008) Further evidence of an association between adolescent bipolar disorder with smoking and substance use disorders: a controlled study. Drug Alcohol Depend 95(3):188–198. doi:10.1016/j.drugalcdep.2007.12.016, S0376-8716(08)00050-1 [pii]

Wilens TE, Martelon M, Kruesi MJ, Parcell T, Westerberg D, Schillinger M, Gignac M, Biederman J (2009) Does conduct disorder mediate the development of substance use disorders in adolescents with bipolar disorder? A case-control family study. J Clin Psychiatry 70(2):259–265, ej08m04438 [pii]

Winokur G, Clayton P, Reich T (1969) Manic depressive illness. CV Mosby, Saint Louis

Winokur G, Coryell W, Akiskal HS, Maser JD, Keller MB, Endicott J, Mueller T (1995) Alcoholism in manic-depressive (bipolar) illness: familial illness, course of illness, and the primary-secondary distinction. Am J Psychiatry 152(3):365–372

Yoon YH, Chen CM, Yi HY, Moss HB (2011) Effect of comorbid alcohol and drug use disorders on premature death among unipolar and bipolar disorder decedents in the United States, 1999 to 2006. Compr Psychiatry 52(5):453–464. doi:10.1016/j.comppsych.2010.10.005, S0010-440X(10)00172-0 [pii]

Comorbidity

10

'Comorbidity' is a term introduced by Feinstein to refer to the coexistence of two essentially independent and distinct disorders. According to this early concept, there exists an 'index' or 'primary' disorder and a comorbid separate second disorder which potentially affects the selection of treatment and the prognosis of the index one (Feinstein 1970). Comorbidity may be due to chance or to ascertainment bias (Berkson's bias); however, the consistent pattern of comorbidity concerning several disorders (e.g. comorbid anxiety and depression) makes unlikely the suggestion it is happening by chance (Kessler et al. 2007). According to some authors, the conceptual overlapping especially between mood and anxiety disorders and the overlapping of symptoms might produce an 'artefactual comorbidity' (Maj 2005).

Most authors and textbooks clearly suggest that comorbidity, both with mental as well as with somatic diseases, is the rule rather than the exception in BD. Many go even further and suggest that the clinical picture of BD is grossly complicated because of comorbidity. In terms of official classification systems, this complex picture is reflected by the finding that most BD patients suffer from more than two distinct 'comorbid' mental disorders.

The literature is conclusive concerning the overall high rate of comorbidity and its adverse effect on overall outcome of the patients; however, it is rather inconclusive concerning certain diseases and specific rates. This is because of differences in study samples (e.g. inpatients, outpatients, epidemiological samples, registered and insured which by definition might suffer from a less severe form, etc.) and assessment methods. General population epidemiological studies often use trained lay interviewers, while clinical studies often utilize only highly experienced researchers. Thus, there is an unsolved riddle in place: Clinical samples are more reliably evaluated, but they might include patients with more severe form of the illness and higher comorbidity, while general population samples have problematic assessment, almost always with the use of structured interviews and thus an artificial inflation of rates, because of false allocation or multiple allocation of the same symptom.

K.N. Fountoulakis, *Bipolar Disorder: An Evidence-Based Guide to Manic Depression*, DOI 10.1007/978-3-642-37216-2_10

This chapter will deal with mental and medical comorbidity in adult BD patients with the exception of personality disorders, alcohol and substance abuse as well as behavioural addictions (e.g. gambling, Internet addiction, etc.). Also, this chapter will not cover the issue of comorbidity in children, adolescents and the elderly. These topics will be covered in especially dedicated chapters of this book. Treatment of comorbid disorders will be covered in the chapters specifically dedicated to treatment options.

In general, with the exception of substance use disorders, medical and psychiatric comorbidity is more common in females than in males (Arnold 2003). It is interesting that while bipolar males and females have similar rates of migraine headache (Mahmood et al. 1999), migraine is more frequent among females than males in community samples. Also, bipolar males are less likely than females to develop hypothyroidism as a consequence of lithium treatment (Kupka et al. 2002).

This chapter will also include detailed tables with lists of published papers concerning the rates of comorbid conditions in BD patients. Where possible, these tables will also include an estimation of the probable rate of the specific comorbid disorder after pooling all study samples together. This does not constitute a meta-analysis, but it can give a rough approximation of the average reported rate weighted by sample size and should be considered only as indicative. It should be noted that study samples often overlap and while in many instances this is obvious, in other instances it is very difficult to clarify even when concerning the same group of authors or the same institution. In this weighted averaging, the data from the general population, from non-bipolar medical patients' registries and from other nonmental patients control groups will be pooled together in a group named 'general population' which of course is not representative of the general population in epidemiological terms. Since this was in no way a formal meta-analysis, the author kept the privilege to exclude from pooling a small number of studies which were clearly outliers or of unknown composition or quality. Therefore, in several cases, the numbers shown as results of the pooling process do not correspond to the sum of all studies.

10.1 Psychiatric Comorbidity

In spite of the large theoretical debate on the true rates of comorbid conditions in BD, the everyday clinical reality is that of gross under-recognition and under-treatment of comorbidities (Simon et al. 2004a). This is because in everyday clinical practice the average psychiatrist is inclined to utilize a single comprehensive primary diagnosis and neglect the 'residual' symptomatology. This might lead not only to residual untreated symptoms, but also there is a danger that treating the 'primary' condition might worsen 'comorbidities'.

General population surveys suggest that almost all BD patients manifested at least a second mental disorder and almost two-thirds of patients reported that the 'comorbid' condition appeared first and BD followed (Kessler et al. 1997). Studies on clinical samples reported lower comorbidity rates.

Several studies suggested that from one-half to two-thirds of BD patients were suffering from one comorbid condition during lifetime (Subramaniam et al. 2013; Krishnan 2005; Leverich et al. 2003; Vieta et al. 2001; Tohen et al. 2003; Sasson et al. 2003; McElroy et al. 2001; Mantere et al. 2006; Strakowski et al. 1992; Dell'Osso et al. 2011) although unusually low rates have also been reported (Szadoczky et al. 1998). Additionally, 42 % of them manifested two, and 25 % manifested three comorbid psychiatric conditions (McElroy et al. 2001).

However, the prevalence of current (cross-sectional) comorbidity is significantly lower with around one-third of BD patients suffering from any psychiatric comorbidity (Mantere et al. 2006; Oreski et al. 2012; Vieta et al. 2001). The age of the sample seems to play a role since younger patients seem to manifest higher rates of current psychiatric comorbidity (Dell'Osso et al. 2011). Rates as high as almost 80 % have been reported (Bellani et al. 2012). It is important to note that when the official records are used in a retrospective way, only 18 % of hospitalized BD patients are reported to suffer from some additional mental disorder, and only approximately 3.5 % from two with any anxiety disorder present in only 1 % (Sorvaniemi and Hintikka 2005). These very low rates might reflect mainly the usual practice of clinicians to stick to a single major diagnosis in everyday clinical practice.

Mental comorbidity seems to relate with a more overall complicated clinical picture for BD, with younger age at onset (Moor et al. 2012) and worse long-term outcome, including increased suicidality and self-harm (Vieta et al. 2001; Moor et al. 2012; McElroy et al. 2001; Leverich et al. 2003; Young et al. 1993), poor adherence to treatment (Vieta et al. 2001) and less favourable response to lithium (Sasson et al. 2003; Young et al. 1993). However, at least one study does not support the relationship between comorbidity and outcome (Strakowski et al. 1992).

During manic and hypo-manic episodes, the overall psychiatric comorbidity is lower in comparison to depressive and mixed episodes (56.8 % vs. 82.9 %) (Mantere et al. 2006). Community studies suggest that the 'comorbid' condition appears first and BD follows (Kessler et al. 1997; Johnson et al. 2000), but studies on clinical samples suggest the opposite (Kupka et al. 2001).

Probably the most frequent comorbid condition is any anxiety disorder with substance abuse/dependence, impulse control disorders, eating disorders and attention deficit hyperactivity disorder (ADHD) following (Singh and Zarate 2006).

The reported rates concerning the presence of any comorbid mental disorder in BD patients are shown in detail in Table 10.1. The pooled rate suggests that two-thirds of BD patients are suffering from at least one comorbid mental disorder and the rate is similar to the respected which is reported for unipolar depression.

In the same Table (10.1), the rate of comorbid BD on other mental disorders is also shown.

Table 10.1 Rates of any mental comorbidity in BD patients and of BD on top of other mental disorders

Study	*N*	Control population	*N*	Prevalence in BD *N*(%)	Prevalence in control *N*%	Comments
Any mental comorbidity in pts with BD						
Szadoczky et al. (1998)	149	MDD	443	57 (38.3 %)	315 (71.1 %)	Lifetime rate
Bellani et al. (2012)	205	MDD	105	161 (78.5 %)	47 (44.8 %)	Cross-sectional rate
Kessler et al. (1997)	29			29 (100 %)		BD-I patients, National Comorbidity Survey, lifetime rate
Pooled	383		548	247 (64.5 %)	362 (66.05 %)	

Study	Study population	*N*	*N*	Prevalence in study population	Comments
Prevalence of BD in PD with other mental disorders					
Bowen et al. (1994)	Panic disorder	108		BD depression 19.4 % BD hypomanic 3.7 %	Self-report questionnaires
Darby et al. (2011)	OCD			BD-I 5.3 % BD-II 10.7 %	
Goldstein and Levitt (2007)	Youth-onset anxiety disorder	1,571	41,522	BD-I 14.57 %	National Epidemiologic Study, lifetime
Judd et al. (1998)	GAD			BD 17 %	National Comorbidity Survey
Lensi et al. (1996)	OCD	263		BD-I 1.5 % BD-II 13 %	Lifetime rates, probably overlapping with Perugi et al. (1997)
MacKinnon et al. (1997)	Panic dis	41		BD 88 %	
Perugi et al. (1997)	OCD	315		BD-I 2 % BD-II 13.6 %	Lifetime rates, probably including Lensi et al. (1996)
Perugi et al. (1999)	Panic disorder	119		BD-I 0.8 % BD-II 5 %	

Perugi et al. (1999)	Social phobia	71		BD-I 0 % BD-II 21.1 %	
Perugi et al. (1999)	OCD	79		BD-I 3.8 % BD-II 17.7 %	Overlapping with previous studies
Perugi et al. (2001)	Social phobia	153		BD-II 9.1 %	Overlapping with previous studies
Savino et al. (1993)	Panic disorder	140		7.1 %	Lifetime rates
Schneier et al. (1992)	Social phobia	361			Epidemiological Catchment Area study, lifetime rates
Wittchen et al. (1994)	GAD	8,098		10.5 %	National Comorbidity Survey, lifetime rates

MDD major depressive disorder

10.1.1 Comorbid Anxiety

Anxiety is extremely common in psychiatric patients, either as isolated symptoms or as full-blown comorbid disorders. This 'comorbidity' is so frequent that symptoms of anxiety could be considered to be 'non-specific' and 'transnosological'. Kraepelin was the first to describe it as a core feature of BD, and he embedded it in the clinical subtypes he described. However, only during the last couple of decades, there was a huge increase in published papers on this specific topic (Provencher et al. 2012). Especially in the frame of mixed episodes or anxious and agitated depression, anxiety and psychic tension are core components of the clinical picture in almost half of acutely ill patients (Cassidy et al. 1998a, b). This is partially responsible for the varying prevalence rates among studies and the conflicting opinions between authors.

Any anxiety disorder is reported to be present in 42–93 % of patients during lifetime and in almost 11–70 % cross-sectionally (Young et al. 2013; Tamam and Ozpoyraz 2002; Altshuler et al. 2010; Zutshi et al. 2006; Simon et al. 2004b; Kawa et al. 2005; Kessler et al. 1997; Levander et al. 2007; Nakagawa et al. 2008; Goldstein and Levitt 2008; Schaffer et al. 2006; Otto et al. 2006; Nery-Fernandes et al. 2009; Mantere et al. 2006, 2010; Henry et al. 2003; Freeman et al. 2002; Dittmann et al. 2002; Das 2013; Cosoff and Hafner 1998; Ciapparelli et al. 2007; Bellani et al. 2012; McElroy et al. 2001; Boylan et al. 2004; Szadoczky et al. 1998; Weber et al. 2011; Azorin et al. 2009). Up to half of these BD patients with comorbid anxiety manifest at least two anxiety disorders (Henry et al. 2003).

Comorbid anxiety is probably related to predominant depressive polarity (Das 2013; Coryell et al. 2009), the presence of depressive symptoms during a manic episode (Post et al. 1989), the severity of manic symptoms and overall severity of the disease (Lee and Dunner 2008; Gonzalez-Pinto et al. 2012; Toniolo et al. 2009), worse outcome (Young et al. 1993; Lee and Dunner 2008; Keller 2006; Gaudiano and Miller 2005; Frank et al. 2002; Otto et al. 2006; Feske et al. 2000; Keck et al. 1998; Conus et al. 2006; El-Mallakh and Hollifield 2008; Tohen et al. 2007), longer recovery time from index mood episode and especially depression (Frank et al. 2002; Das 2013; Coryell et al. 2009; Otto et al. 2006), earlier relapse (Otto et al. 2006) and lower quality of life (Kauer-Sant'Anna et al. 2007). Generalized anxiety disorder (GAD) and social phobia have the worst impact, probably because they are chronic in nature and trait-like (Boylan et al. 2004). However, some authors suggest that no such a relationship exists (Henry et al. 2003). The relationship of comorbid anxiety with suicidality is questionable (Slama et al. 2004). Probably it is more frequent in BD-II than in BD-I patients (Dittmann et al. 2002), although rapid cycling and substance abuse might reverse this and dramatically increase anxiety rates in BD-I (Gao et al. 2008).

Concerning the rates of BD in anxiety patients, they vary from study to study depending mainly on the specific anxiety disorder and probably on the phase of the illness. It has been reported that up to 21 % of anxiety patients also suffer from BD (Yerevanian et al. 2001; Savino et al. 1993; Schneier et al. 1992; Wittchen et al. 1994; Lensi et al. 1996; Perugi et al. 1997, 1999; Bowen et al. 1994; Goldstein and Levitt 2007) and in these patients anxiety has a very early age at onset, often preceding the onset of BD itself (Goldstein and Levitt 2007). The phase of the disorder plays an important role; rates of anxiety are very low in purely and euphoric manic patients, while multiple anxiety disorders are present in the majority of mixed or depressive (Gaudiano and Miller 2005; Dilsaver and Chen 2003; McElroy et al. 1995; Himmelhoch and Garfinkel 1986) and seem to correlate with rapid cycling (Boylan et al. 2004; MacKinnon et al. 2002, 2003a). The literature suggest a strong connection between anxiety and impulsivity in BD patients, probably because increased arousal and reduced cognitive efficiency associated with anxiety could result in less rational and more impulsive thinking (Taylor et al. 2008; Bellani et al. 2012).

It is reported that anxiety is more common in BD in comparison to unipolar depression (Bellani et al. 2012; Szadoczky et al. 1998; Yerevanian et al. 2001; Chen and Dilsaver 1995); however, this does not accurately reflect the accumulated data (Table 10.2). At least one study found close to 80 % of BD patients to manifest any anxiety disorder, and it also reported that unipolar patients manifested even higher rates (>90 %) (Pini et al. 1997).

The reported rates concerning the presence of any anxiety disorder in BD patients are shown in detail in Table 10.2. The pooled rate suggests that cross-sectionally 14 % of BD patients suffer from any anxiety disorder. This rate is three times higher to that reported for the control population but three to four times or more lower in comparison to that reported for patients with schizophrenia or unipolar depression. The pooled lifetime rate for any anxiety disorder for BD patients is 42 % and still lower but very close to that reported for unipolar depressive patients and again almost three times higher in comparison to the control population. The great discrepancy of cross-sectional and lifetime rates suggest an episodic character in the presence of anxiety disorders in BD patients, while on the contrary it seems that in unipolar patients anxiety runs a more chronic course.

10.1.1.1 Comorbid Generalized Anxiety Disorder (GAD)

GAD tends to be chronic and thus lifetime and cross-sectional rates are almost identical; however, the prevalence varies widely from below 2 % up to above 40 % (Schaffer et al. 2006; Tamam and Ozpoyraz 2002; Zutshi et al. 2006; Simon et al. 2004b; Kessler et al. 1997; Nakagawa et al. 2008; Goldstein and Levitt 2008; Rihmer et al. 2001; Azorin et al. 2009; Otto et al. 2006; Slama et al. 2004; Dell'Osso et al. 2011; Cosoff and Hafner 1998; Pini et al. 1997; Mantere et al. 2006; McElroy et al. 2001; Bellani et al. 2012; Young et al. 1993; Boylan et al. 2004; Coryell et al. 2009) (Szadoczky et al. 1998). It is important to note that the overall prevalence of comorbid anxiety is lower in BD-I in comparison to BD-II, which is higher and similar to that observed in unipolar major depression (Mantere et al. 2006). Comorbid GAD might relate to increased suicidality (Neves et al. 2009).

From a reverse angle, it has been reported that 8.6–17 % of GAD patients also suffer from BD (Wittchen et al. 1994; Yerevanian et al. 2001; Judd et al. 1998).

The reported rates concerning the presence of GAD in BD patients are shown in detail in Table 10.3. The pooled rate suggests that cross-sectionally 11.2 % of BD patients suffer from GAD. This rate is twice as much as that reported for the control population but similar to that reported for patients with schizophrenia or unipolar depression. The pooled lifetime rate for GAD in BD patients is 17.6 %, and it is three

Table 10.2 Cross-sectional and lifetime rates of any anxiety disorder comorbidity in BD patients

Study	*N*	Control population	*N*	Prevalence in BD *N*(%)	Prevalence in control *N*%	Comments
Cross-sectional rates						
Bellani et al. (2012)	205	MDD	105	122 (59.5 %)	30 (28.6 %)	
Boylan et al. (2004)	138			77 (55.8 %)		
Cassidy et al. (1998b)	316			124 (39.2 %)		Acute mania, at least one anxiety symptom present at interview
Ciapparelli et al. (2007)	56	Schiz	98	23 (41.1 %)	72 (73.9 %)	BD with psychotic features
Cosoff and Hafner (1998)	20	Schiz	60	14 (70.0 %)	34 (56.7 %)	
Das (2013)	102			30 (29.4 %)		Acute mania
Mantere et al. (2006, 2010)	191	MDD	269	85 (44.5 %)	152 (56.5 %)	Acute phase BD, half pts depressed
McElroy et al. (2001)	288			86 (29.9 %)		STANLEY foundation data
Otto et al. (2006)	918			293 (31.9 %)		STEP-BD, >75 % BD-I, half in recovery, ~25 % depressed
Simon et al. (2004b)	360			123 (34.2 %)		BD-I
Simon et al. (2004b)	115			22 (19.1 %)		BD-II
Tamam and Ozpoyraz (2002)	70			36 (51.4 %)		BD-I
Weber et al. (2011)	27,054	All non-BD discharges	2,325,247	3,071 (11.4 %)	78,809 (3.4 %)	Hospital records
Zutshi et al. (2006)	80	Nonpsychiatric controls	50	40 (50.0 %)	7 (14.0 %)	Remitted BD pts
Pooled	*29,913*			*4,146 (13.9%)*		
		Schiz	*158*		*106 (67.1 %)*	
		MDD	*374*		*207 (55.4 %)*	
		Other controls	*2,325,297*		*78,816 (3.4 %)*	

Lifetime rates						
Altshuler et al. (2010)	711			277 (39.0 %)		STANLEY foundation data, >80 % BD-I
Azorin et al. (2009)	1,090			297 (27.2 %)		Acute mania, hospitalized pts
Das (2013)	102			72 (70.6 %)		Acute mania
Dittmann et al. (2002)	108			11 (10.4 %)		BD-I
Dittmann et al. (2002)	38			7 (18.4 %)		BD-II
Goldstein and Levitt (2008)	1,411			670 (47.5 %)		2001–2002 National Epidemiologic Survey
Henry et al. (2003)	318			75 (23.6 %)		75 % BD-I, half pts psychotic
Kawa et al. (2005)	211			90 (42.6 %)		
Kessler et al. (1994, 1997)	29			27 (93.1 %)		BD-I National Comorbidity Study, retrospective study, limited by recall bias
Levander et al. (2007)	350			163 (46.6 %)		STANLEY foundation data, 2/3 of patients with alcohol use lifetime
Mantere et al. (2006)	191	MDD	269	102 (53.40)	152 (56.5 %)	Acute phase BD
McElroy et al. (2001)	288			122 (42.0 %)		STANLEY foundation data
Nakagawa et al. (2008)	116			60 (51.7 %)		Depressed patients
Nery-Fernandes et al. (2009)	62			21 (33.7 %)		Euthymic patients
Pini et al. (1997)	24	MDD	38	19 (79.2 %)	35 (92.1 %)	Depressed patients
Schaffer et al. (2006)	852			441 (51.8 %)		Canadian Community Health Survey: mental health and well-being
Simon et al. (2004b)	360			190 (52.8 %)		BD-I
Simon et al. (2004b)	115			53 (46.1 %)		BD-II
Tamam and Ozpoyraz (2002)	70			43 (61.4 %)		BD-I

(continued)

Table 10.2 (continued)

Study	*N*	Control population	*N*	Prevalence in BD *N*(%)	Prevalence in control *N*%	Comments
Yerevanian et al. (2001)	35	MDD	98	13 (37.1 %)	47 (48.0 %)	Mostly BD-II
Young et al. (2013)	304			68 (22.4 %)		
Zutshi et al. (2006)	80	Nonpsychiatric controls	*50*	49 (61.3 %)	7 (14.0 %)	Remitted BD pts
Pooled	*6,865*			*2,870 (41.8 %)*		
		MDD	*405*		*234 (57.8 %)*	
		Nonpsychiatric controls	*50*		*7 (14.0 %)*	

MDD major depressive disorder, *Schiz* schizophrenia

Table 10.3 Cross-sectional and lifetime rates of generalized anxiety disorder comorbidity in BD patients

Study	*N*	Control population	*N*	Prevalence in BD *N*(%)	Prevalence in control *N*%	Comments
Cross-sectional						
Bellani et al. (2012)	205	MDD	105	28 (13.7 %)	4 (3.8 %)	
Boylan et al. (2004)	138			43 (31.2 %)		
Cosoff and Hafner (1998)	20	Schiz	60	2 (10.0 %)	7 (11.7 %)	
Dell'Osso et al. (2011)	508			7 (1.4 %)		
Mantere et al. (2006)	191	MDD	269	29 (15.18)	37 (13.75)	Acute phase BD
McElroy et al. (2001)	288			8 (2.78)		STANLEY foundation data
Otto et al. (2006)	918			122 (13.3 %)		STEP-BD. >75 % BD-I, half pts in recovery, ~25 % depressed
Simon et al. (2004b)	360			46 (12.8 %)		BD-I
Simon et al. (2004b)	115			12 (10.4 %)		BD-II
Tamam and Ozpoyraz (2002)	70			9 (12.9 %)		
Zutshi et al. (2006)	80	Controls	50	19 (23.8 %)	3 (6 %)	Remitted BD pts
Pooled	*2,893*	*Controls*	*50*	*325 (11.2 %)*	*3 (6 %)*	
		MDD	*374*		*41 (11.0 %)*	
		Schiz	*60*		*7 (11.7 %)*	
Lifetime						
Azorin et al. (2009)	1,090			217 (19.9 %)		Acutely manic hospitalized pts
Coryell et al. (2009)	427			20 (4.68 %)		
Goldstein and Levitt (2008)	1,411			346 (24.5 %)		2001–2002 National Epidemiologic Survey
Kessler et al. (1997)	29			12 (41.4 %)		BD-I, National Comorbidity Study

(continued)

Table 10.3 (continued)

Study	N	Control population	N	Prevalence in BD N(%)	Prevalence in control N%	Comments
McElroy et al. (2001)	288			8 (2.8 %)		STANLEY foundation data
Nakagawa et al. (2008)	116			2 (1.7 %)		Depressed pts
Pini et al. (1997)	24	MDD	38	8 (33.3 %)	14 (36.8 %)	Depressed pts
Rihmer et al. (2001)	95	MDD	443	10 (10.5 %)	62 (14.0 %)	BD-I, Hungarian epidemiological study
Rihmer et al. (2001)	24	MDD	443	5 (20.8 %)	62 (14.0 %)	BD-II, Hungarian epidemiological study
Simon et al. (2004b)	360			68 (18.9 %)		BD-I
Simon et al. (2004b)	115			19 (16.5 %)		BD-II
Slama et al. (2004)	180			7 (3.9 %)		Pts in remission
Szadoczky et al. (1998)	149	MDD	443	22 (14.4 %)	61 (13.7 %)	Epidemiological, rates weighted for sex
Tamam and Ozpoyraz (2002)	70			10 (14.3 %)		BD-I
Yerevanian et al. (2001)	35	MDD	98	3 (8.6 %)	22 (22.5 %)	Mostly BD-II
Young et al. (1993)	81			26 (32.1 %)		
Zutshi et al. (2006)	80	Controls	*50*	20 (25 %)	3 (6 %)	Remitted BD pts
Pooled	*4,574*			*803 (17.6 %)*		
		Controls	*50*		*3 (6 %)*	
		MDD	*1,022*		*159 (15.6 %)*	

MDD major depressive disorder, *Schiz* schizophrenia

times higher in comparison to that reported concerning the control population and similar to the rate reported for unipolar depressed patients. The small but obvious discrepancy of cross-sectional and lifetime rates suggests an admixture of an episodic and chronic character in the presence of GAD in BD and unipolar depressive patients.

10.1.1.2 Comorbid Panic Disorder

In BD patients, panic disorder is reported to have a cross-sectional prevalence of 2.3–62.5 % and a lifetime prevalence of 2.9–56.5 % (Vieta et al. 2001; Schaffer et al. 2006; Young et al. 1993, 2013; Tamam and Ozpoyraz 2002; Altshuler et al. 2010; Zutshi et al. 2006; Simon et al. 2004b; Kawa et al. 2005; Kessler et al. 1994, 1997; Levander et al. 2007; Nakagawa et al. 2008; Goldstein and Levitt 2008; Rihmer et al. 2001; Azorin et al. 2009; Pini et al. 1997, 2003; Otto et al. 2006; Okan Ibiloglu and Caykoylu 2011; Mula et al. 2008a; Henry et al. 2003; Dilsaver et al. 1997, 2008; Slama et al. 2004; Dell'Osso et al. 2011; Craig et al. 2002; Cosoff and Hafner 1998; Ciapparelli et al. 2007; Mantere et al. 2006; McElroy et al. 2001; Robins and Regier 1991; Chen and Dilsaver 1995; Bellani et al. 2012; Boylan et al. 2004; Coryell et al. 2009; Szadoczky et al. 1998). The phase of the disorder plays an important role; panic is virtually absent in purely manic patients and present in more than 80 % of mixed or depressive patients (Dilsaver and Chen 2003). Comorbid panic disorder is related to worse outcome of BD with younger age at onset (Schurhoff et al. 2000), more depressive episodes and possibly higher suicidality (Frank et al. 2002; Kilbane et al. 2009; Neves et al. 2009). Reversely, panic attacks constitute a risk factor for the future development of BD (Kinley et al. 2011; Goodwin and Hamilton 2002) and panic disorder when comorbid with BD has an earlier onset and greater severity (Goodwin and Hoven 2002).

Patients with panic disorder have rates of BD ranging from 6 to 88 % (Savino et al. 1993; Bowen et al. 1994; Perugi et al. 1997, 1999; MacKinnon et al. 1997; Yerevanian et al. 2001), and switching to mania or hypomania during treatment of panic disorder with antidepressants has been reported (Pecknold and Fleury 1986; Sholomskas 1990).

The reported rates concerning the presence of panic disorder in BD patients are shown in detail in Table 10.4. The pooled rate suggests that cross-sectionally 15.4 % of BD patients suffer from panic disorder. This rate is more than ten times the rate expected for the general population but similar to that reported for patients with schizophrenia or unipolar depression. The pooled lifetime rate for panic disorder in BD patients is 16.9 %, and it is again more than ten times higher in comparison to that reported concerning the control population and similar to that reported for unipolar depressive patients. The negligible difference between cross-sectional and lifetime prevalence suggests that panic disorder probably presents with a chronic rather than episodic course in BD and unipolar depressive patients.

10.1.1.3 Comorbid Simple (Specific) Phobia

Simple (specific) phobia is also comorbid with BD, and cross-sectional comorbid rates are reported to vary from 1.6 to 22.9 % (Boylan et al. 2004; Cosoff and Hafner 1998; Strakowski et al. 1992; Tamam and Ozpoyraz 2002; Vieta et al. 2001).

Table 10.4 Cross-sectional and lifetime rates of panic disorder comorbidity in BD patients

Study	*N*	Control population	*N*	Prevalence in BD *N*(%)	Prevalence in control *N*%	Comments
Cross-sectional rates						
Bellani et al. (2012)	205	MDD	105	60 (29.3 %)	10 (9.8 %)	
Boylan et al. (2004)	138			37 (26.8 %)		
Ciapparelli et al. (2007)	56	Schiz	98	13 (23.2 %)	24 (24.5 %)	BD with psychotic features
Coryell et al. (2009)	427			107 (25.5 %)		
Cosoff and Hafner (1998)	20	Schiz	60	3 (15.0 %)	3 (5.0 %)	
Dell'Osso et al. (2011)	508			32 (6.3 %)		
Dilsaver and Chen (2003)	25			1 (4.0 %)		Pure manic, >90 % of pts with psychotic features
Dilsaver and Chen (2003)	19			16 (84.2 %)		Depressive mania, >90 % of pts with psychotic features
Dilsaver et al. (1997)	53			33 (62.3 %)		Bipolar depression
Dilsaver et al. (1997)	32			1 (2.3 %)		Pure mania
Dilsaver et al. (1997)	44			20 (62.5 %)		Depressive mania
Mantere et al. (2006)	191	MDD	269	46 (24.1)	45 (16.7 %)	Acute phase BD pts
McElroy et al. (2001)	288			27 (9.4 %)		STANLEY foundation data
Okan Ibiloglu and Caykoylu (2011)	50			30 (60.0 %)		BD-I
Okan Ibiloglu and Caykoylu (2011)	46			22 (47.8 %)		BD-II
Otto et al. (2006)	918			78 (8.5 %)		STEP-BD, >75 % BD-I, half pts in recovery, ~25 % depressed
Pini et al. (2003)	151			35 (23.2 %)		
Simon et al. (2004b)	360			33 (9.2 %)		BD-I
Simon et al. (2004b)	115			5 (4.4 %)		BD-II
Strakowski et al. (1992)	41			2 (4.9 %)		First-episode manic/mixed inpatients
Tamam and Ozpoyraz (2002)	70			4 (5.7 %)		BD-I

Vieta et al. (2001)	129			3 (2.3 %)		BD-I, pts in remission
Zutshi et al. (2006)	80	Controls	50	4 (5.0 %)	0 (0 %)	Remitted BD
Pooled	*3,966*			*612 (15.4 %)*		
		MDD	*374*		*55 (14.7 %)*	
		Schiz	*158*		*27 (17.1 %)*	
		Controls	*50*		*0 (0.0 %)*	
Lifetime rates						
Altshuler et al. (2010)	711			122 (17.2 %)		>80 % BD-I, STANLEY foundation data
Azorin et al. (2009)	1,090			56 (5.1 %)		Acutely manic hospitalized pts
Chen and Dilsaver (1995; Robins and Regier (1991)	168	Gen pop	18,571	35 (20.8 %)	149 (0.8 %)	Epidemiological Catchment Area
Chen and Dilsaver (1995; Robins and Regier (1991)	168	MDD	557	35 (20.8 %)	56 (10.0 %)	Epidemiological Catchment Area
Coryell et al. (2009)	427			17 (4.0 %)		
Craig et al. (2002)	138	MDD with psychosis	87	4 (2.9 %)	7 (8.0 %)	BD with psychosis
Dilsaver et al. (2008)	69	MDD	118	39 (56.5 %)	27 (22.9 %)	Data from Latinos
Goldstein and Levitt (2008)	1,411			381 (27.0 %)		2001–2002 National Epidemiologic Survey on Alcohol and Related Conditions
Henry et al. (2003)	318			52 (16.4 %)		75 % BD-I, half psychotic, currently or lifetime
Kawa et al. (2005)	211			44 (20.8 %)		
Kessler et al. (1994)	130			43 (33.1 %)		BD-I Epidemiological Catchment Area
Kessler et al. (1997)	29			10 (34.5 %)		BD-I National Comorbidity Survey
Levander et al. (2007)	350			72 (20.6 %)		STANLEY foundation data, 2/3 with alcohol use
McElroy et al. (2001)	288			58 (20.1 %)		STANLEY foundation data
Mula et al. (2008a)	70	MDD	60	10 (14.3 %)	24 (40 %)	BD-I

(continued)

Table 10.4 (continued)

Study	*N*	Control population	*N*	Prevalence in BD *N*(%)	Prevalence in control *N*%	Comments
Mula et al. (2008a)	51	MDD	60	16 (31.4 %)	24 (40 %)	BD-II
Nakagawa et al. (2008)	116			37 (31.9 %)		BD depression
Pini et al. (1997)	24	MDD	38	9 (37.5 %)	12 (31.6 %)	BD depression
Rihmer et al. (2001)	95	MDD	443	7 (7.4 %)	55 (12.4 %)	BD-I pts, Hungarian epidemiological study
Rihmer et al. (2001)	24	MDD	443	3 (12.5 %)	55 (12.4 %)	BD-II pts, Hungarian epidemiological study
Schaffer et al. (2006)	852			164 (19.3 %)		Canadian Community Health Survey: mental health and well-being
Simon et al. (2004b)	360			66 (18.3 %)		BD-I
Simon et al. (2004b)	115			16 (13.9 %)		BD-II
Slama et al. (2004)	302			24 (7.9 %)		Pts in remission
Szadoczky et al. (1998)	149	MDD	443	16 (10.6 %)	55 (12.4 %)	Epidemiological study
Tamam and Ozpoyraz (2002)	70			7 (10.0 %)		BD-I
Yerevanian et al. (2001)	35	MDD	98	2 (5.7 %)	18 (18.4 %)	Most pts BD-II
Young et al. (1993)	81			26 (32.1 %)		
Young et al. (2013)	304			21 (6.9 %)		
Zutshi et al. (2006)	80	Controls	50	6 (7.5 %)	0 (0.0 %)	Remitted BD
Pooled	*8,068*			*1,363 (16.9 %)*		
		MDD	*1,401*		*199 (14.2 %)*	
		Controls	*18,621*		*149 (0.8 %)*	

MDD major depressive disorder, *Schiz* schizophrenia

Lifetime rates vary from 3 % to 65.5 % (Szadoczky et al. 1998; Yerevanian et al. 2001; Coryell et al. 2009; Pini et al. 1997; Kessler et al. 1997; Slama et al. 2004; Rihmer et al. 2001; Nakagawa et al. 2008; Kawa et al. 2005; Tamam and Ozpoyraz 2002; Levander et al. 2007; Altshuler et al. 2010).

The reported rates concerning the presence of simple (specific) phobia in BD patients are shown in detail in Table 10.5. The pooled rate suggests that cross-sectionally 9 % of BD patients suffer from simple phobia. This rate is double in comparison to that reported for patients with schizophrenia. The pooled lifetime rate for simple phobia in BD patients is 10.4 %, and thus it is similar to the cross-sectional rate, suggesting a chronic course for simple phobias in BD patients. The lifetime prevalence of simple phobia in unipolar depression is around 30 % higher in comparison to BD.

10.1.1.4 Comorbid Social Anxiety Disorder (Social Phobia)

Social phobia as comorbid condition in BD patients seems also to run a chronic course with cross-sectional rate ranging from 1.6 to 29 % and a lifetime ranging from 2.5 to 53.6 % (Vieta et al. 2001; Schaffer et al. 2006; Tamam and Ozpoyraz 2002; Altshuler et al. 2010; Zutshi et al. 2006; Simon et al. 2004b; Kawa et al. 2005; Levander et al. 2007; Nakagawa et al. 2008; Goldstein and Levitt 2008; Rihmer et al. 2001; Azorin et al. 2009; Pini et al. 2006; Otto et al. 2006; Okan Ibiloglu and Caykoylu 2011; Slama et al. 2004; Dilsaver et al. 2008; Kessler et al. 1994; Cosoff and Hafner 1998; Ciapparelli et al. 2007; McElroy et al. 2001; Bellani et al. 2012; Boylan et al. 2004; Szadoczky et al. 1998). In the ECA study, almost half of BD patients also had social anxiety disorder (Kessler et al. 1994), and in half of them, social phobia appeared more than a decade earlier than BD (Kessler et al. 1999). The phase of the disorder plays an important role; social phobia is virtually absent in purely manic patients and present in two-thirds of mixed or depressive (Dilsaver and Chen 2003). Peculiarly, one group of authors didn't find any such symptoms in depressed BD patients (Pini et al. 1997). In spite of the fact that social phobia is correlated to functional impairment, increased suicidality and overall severity and outcome, its presence is often neglected, and it is not adequately treated, even when not comorbid with major mood disorders (Olfson et al. 2000; Bisserbe et al. 1996; Weiller et al. 1996). However, when comorbid with BD, its treatment is problematic since the appropriate treatment is antidepressants, and it seems that almost 80 % of patients who respond also switch to hypomania (Himmelhoch 1998).

It is reported that on average, 9.1 % of patients with social phobia also manifest BD during lifetime (Perugi et al. 2001). Depending on the clinical state of the study sample, up to 20 % of social phobia patients suffer from BD-II, but BD-I seems to be rare or even absent (Perugi et al. 1999).

The reported rates concerning the presence of social phobia in BD patients are shown in detail in Table 10.6. The pooled rate suggests that cross-sectionally 13.9 % of BD patients suffer from social phobia. This rate is almost double in comparison to that reported in the control group and similar to that of unipolar depression but somewhat lower to that observed in patients with schizophrenia. The pooled lifetime rate for social phobia in BD patients is 18.8 %, and thus it is only marginally

Table 10.5 Cross-sectional and lifetime rates of simple (specific) phobia comorbidity in BD patients

Study	*N*	Control population	*N*	Prevalence in BD *N*(%)	Prevalence in control *N*%	Comments
Cross-sectional rates						
Boylan et al. (2004)	138			14 (10.1 %)		
Cosoff and Hafner (1998)	20	Schiz	60	2 (10 %)	3 (5 %)	
Strakowski et al. (1992)	41			2 (4.9 %)		First-episode manic/mixed inpatients
Tamam and Ozpoyraz (2002)	70			16 (22.9 %)		BD-I
Vieta et al. (2001)	129			2 (1.6 %)		BD-I pts in remission
Pooled	*398*			*36 (9.0 %)*		
		Schiz	*60*		*3 (5 %)*	
Lifetime rates						
Szadoczky et al. (1998)	149			19 (12.9 %)		Epidemiological study
Yerevanian et al. (2001)	35	MDD	98	6 (17.1 %)	25 (25.5 %)	Mostly BD-II pts
Coryell et al. (2009)	427			23 (5.38 %)		
Pini et al. (1997)	24	MDD	38	1 (5.3 %)	2 (5.7 %)	BD depression
Kessler et al. (1997)	29			19 (65.5 %)		BD-I pts National Comorbidity Study
Slama et al. (2004)	300			9 (3 %)		Pts in remission
Rihmer et al. (2001)	95	MDD	443	9 (9.5 %)	51 (11.5 %)	BD-I Hungarian epidemiological study
Rihmer et al. (2001)	24	MDD	443	4 (16.7 %)	51 (11.5 %)	BD-II Hungarian epidemiological study
Nakagawa et al. (2008)	116			12 (10.3 %)		BD depression
Kawa et al. (2005)	211			33 (15.6 %)		
Tamam and Ozpoyraz (2002)	70			18 (25.7 %)		BD-I pts
Levander et al. (2007)	350			47 (13.4 %)		STANLEY foundation data, 2/3 of pts with alcohol use
Altshuler et al. (2010)	711			63 (8,9 %)		>80 % BD-I pts, STANLEY foundation data
Pooled	*2,541*			*263 (10.4 %)*		
		MDD	*579*		*78 (13.5 %)*	

MDD major depressive disorder, *Schiz* schizophrenia

Table 10.6 Cross-sectional and lifetime rates of social phobia comorbidity in BD patients

Study	*N*	Control population	*N*	Prevalence in BD *N*(%)	Prevalence in control *N*%	Comments
Cross-sectional rates						
Bellani et al. (2012)	205	MDD	105	30 (14.6 %)	8 (7.6 %)	
Boylan et al. (2004)	138			24 (	17.4 %)	
Ciapparelli et al. (2007)	56	Schiz	98	6 (10.7 %)	19 (19.4 %)	BD with psychotic features
Cosoff and Hafner (1998)	20	Schiz	60	1 (5.0 %)	10 (16.7 %)	
Dilsaver and Chen (2003)	25			0 (0.0 %)		Pure manic, >90 % pts with psychotic features
Dilsaver and Chen (2003)	19			13 (68.4 %)		Depressive mania, >90 % pts with psychotic features
Mantere et al. (2006)	191	MDD	269	34 (17.8 %)	53 (19.7 %)	Acute BD pts
McElroy et al. (2001)	288			36 (12.5 %)		STANLEY foundation data
Okan Ibiloglu and Caykoylu (2011)	50			8 (16.0 %)		BD-I
Okan Ibiloglu and Caykoylu (2011)	46			7 (15.2 %)		BD-II
Otto et al. (2006)	918			122 (13.3 %)		STEP-BD, >75 % BD-I, half pts in recovery, ~25 % depressed
Simon et al. (2004b)	360			50 (13.9 %)		BD-I
Simon et al. (2004b)	115			10 (8.7 %)		BD-II
Tamam and Ozpoyraz (2002)	70			12 (17.1 %)		BD-I
Vieta et al. (2001)	129			2 (1.6 %)		BD-I patients in remission
Zutshi et al. (2006)	80	Controls	50	23 (28.8 %)	4 (8.0 %)	Remitted BD
Pooled	*2,710*			*378 (13.9 %)*		
		MDD	*374*		*61 (16.3 %)*	
		Schiz	*158*		*29 (18.4 %)*	
		Controls	*50*		*4 (8.0 %)*	

(continued)

Table 10.6 (continued)

Study	*N*	Control population	*N*	Prevalence in BD *N*(%)	Prevalence in control *N*%	Comments
Lifetime rates						
Altshuler et al. (2010)	711			80 (11.3 %)		>80 % BD-I pts, STANLEY foundation data
Azorin et al. (2009)	1,090			27 (2.5 %)		Acutely hospitalized manic pts
Dilsaver et al. (2008)	69	MDD	118	37 (53.6 %)	20 (16.9 %)	Latino pts
Goldstein and Levitt (2008)	1,411			320 (22.7 %)		2001–2002 National Epidemiologic Survey on Alcohol and Related Conditions
Kawa et al. (2005)	211			40 (18.9 %)		
Kessler et al. (1994)	130			61 (47.2 %)		BD-I Epidemiological Catchment Area
Kessler et al. (1997, 1999)	29	MDD	1,080	13 (44.8 %)	296 (26.5 %)	BD-I pts National Comorbidity Study
Levander et al. (2007)	350			65 (18.6 %)		STANLEY foundation data, 2/3 pts with alcohol use
McElroy et al. (2001)	288			47 (16.3 %)		STANLEY foundation data
Nakagawa et al. (2008)	116			13 (11.2 %)		Bipolar depression
Pini et al. (1997)	24	MDD	38	0 (0.0 %)	4 (10.5 %)	BD depression
Pini et al. (2006)	189			24 (12.7 %)		
Rihmer et al. (2001)	95	MDD	443	4 (4.2 %)	78 (17.6 %)	BD-I Hungarian epidemiological study
Rihmer et al. (2001)	24	MDD	443	3 (12.5 %)	78 (17.6 %)	BD-II Hungarian epidemiological study
Schaffer et al. (2006)	852			338 (39.7 %)		Canadian Community Health Survey: mental health and well-being
Simon et al. (2004b)	360			83 (23.1 %)		BD-I
Simon et al. (2004b)	115			21 (18.3 %)		BD-II
Slama et al. (2004)	302			24 (7.9 %)		Pts in remission

Szadoczky et al. (1998)	149	MDD	443	12 (7.8 %)	78 (17.6 %)	Epidemiological
Tamam and Ozpoyraz (2002)	70			14 (20.0 %)		BD-I
Zutshi et al. (2006)	80	Controls	50	24 (30.0 %)	4 (8.0 %)	Remitted BD pts
Pooled	*6,665*			*1,250 (18.8 %)*		
		MDD	*1,729*		*398 (23.0 %)*	
		Controls	*50*		*4 (8.0 %)*	

MDD major depressive disorder, *Schiz* schizophrenia

higher in comparison to the cross-sectional rate, suggesting a chronic course for social phobia in BD patients. It is more than double the rate observed in the control population. The lifetime prevalence of simple phobia in unipolar depression is around 23 %, and it is higher in comparison to BD.

10.1.1.5 Comorbid Post-traumatic Stress Disorder (PTSD)

PTSD is very frequent in BD patients with a cross-sectional rate between 0.9 and 21 % (Bellani et al. 2012; Boylan et al. 2004; Mantere et al. 2006; McElroy et al. 2001; Okan Ibiloglu and Caykoylu 2011; Otto et al. 2006; Simon et al. 2004b; Tamam and Ozpoyraz 2002; Keck et al. 1995; Neria et al. 2002; Strakowski et al. 1998) and a lifetime rate between 2 and 62.3 % (Freeman et al. 2002; Altshuler et al. 2010; Azorin et al. 2009; Dilsaver et al. 2008; Kessler et al. 1994, 1997; Levander et al. 2007; McElroy et al. 2001; Mueser et al. 2004; Nakagawa et al. 2008; Simon et al. 2004b; Tamam and Ozpoyraz 2002; Yerevanian et al. 2001).

The nature of this comorbidity is unknown; however, BD patients are vulnerable to develop PTSD both because they are at a higher risk to experience a traumatic situation mainly because of impulsivity and poor judgement but also because they are more likely to develop PTSD after experiencing a traumatic event. During periods of mania or hyperthymia, BD patients manifest a high resiliency to traumatic events, although during these specific periods most traumatic events are caused and experienced. This resiliency rapidly disappears after the resolution of the hyperthymic state. Especially during periods of depression, BD patients are extremely vulnerable to traumatic events. In turn, the presence of PTSD might worsen the overall course of BD since it disrupts sleep patterns and increases the overall stress. PTSD comorbidity is related to worse outcome, more substance abuse, low quality of life and more disability as well as higher suicidality (Simon et al. 2004b).

The reported rates concerning the presence of PTSD in BD patients are shown in detail in Table 10.7. The pooled rate suggests that cross-sectionally 7.8 % of BD patients suffer from PTSD. This rate is almost double in comparison to that reported in unipolar depression. The pooled lifetime rate for PTSD in BD patients is 11.7 %, and thus it is significantly higher in comparison to the cross-sectional rate, suggesting an episodic course for PTSD in BD patients. The lifetime prevalence of PTSD in unipolar depression is around 22 %, and it is double of that reported concerning BD.

Significantly lower in comparison to 16 % reported by an older meta-analysis on seven studies alone which did not distinguish between studies reporting cross-sectional and lifetime rates (Otto et al. 2004).

10.1.2 Comorbid Obsessive–Compulsive Disorder (OCD)

Comorbid OCD in BD patients is reported to have a prevalence ranging from 1.6 to 35 % cross-sectionally (Vieta et al. 2001; Pashinian et al. 2006; Krishnan 2005; Cosoff and Hafner 1998; Boylan et al. 2004; Kruger et al. 1995, 2000; Otto et al. 2006; Tamam and Ozpoyraz 2002; Dell'Osso et al. 2011; Ciapparelli et al. 2007;

Table 10.7 Cross-sectional and lifetime rates of PTSD comorbidity in BD patients

Study	*N*	Control population	*N*	Prevalence in BD *N*(%)	Prevalence in control *N*%	Comments
Cross-sectional rates						
Bellani et al. (2012)	205	MDD	105	37 (18.0 %)	11 (10.5 %)	
Boylan et al. (2004)	138			20 (14.5 %)		
Keck et al. (1995)	71			12 (16.9 %)		Manic/mixed inpatients
Mantere et al. (2006)	191	MDD	269	20 (10.5 %)	2 (0.7 %)	Acute BD pts
McElroy et al. (2001)	288			12 (4.2 %)		STANLEY foundation data
Neria et al. (2002)	102			11 (10.8 %)		First admission pts
Okan Ibiloglu and Caykoylu (2011)	50			5 (10.0 %)		BD-I pts
Okan Ibiloglu and Caykoylu (2011)	46			3 (6.5 %)		BD-II pts
Otto et al. (2006)	918			44 (4.8 %)		STEP-BD. >75 % BD-I, half pts in recovery, ~25 % depressed
Simon et al. (2004b)	360			23 (6.4 %)		BD-I pts
Simon et al. (2004b)	115			1 (0.9 %)		BD-II pts
Strakowski et al. (1998)	77			16 (20.8 %)		Manic/mixed first-episode inpatients
Tamam and Ozpoyraz (2002)	70			0 (0.0 %)		BD-I pts
Pooled	*2,631*			*204 (7.8 %)*		
		MDD	*374*		*13 (3.5 %)*	
Lifetime rates						
Altshuler et al. (2010)	711			56 (7.9 %)		>80 % BD-I STANLEY foundation data
Azorin et al. (2009)	1,090			22 (2.0 %)		Acutely manic hospitalized pts
Dilsaver et al. (2008)	69	MDD	118	43 (62.3 %)	28 (23.8 %)	Latinos
Kessler et al. (1994)	130			50 (38.8 %)		BD-I pts Epidemiological Catchment Area

(continued)

Table 10.7 (continued)

Study	*N*	Control population	*N*	Prevalence in BD *N*(%)	Prevalence in control *N*%	Comments
Kessler et al. (1997)	29			11 (37.9 %)		BD-I pts National Comorbidity Study
Levander et al. (2007)	350			36 (10.3 %)		STANLEY foundation data, 2/3 with alcohol use
McElroy et al. (2001)	288			19 (6.6 %)		STANLEY foundation data
Mueser et al. (2004)	141	MDD	78	55 (39.0 %)	35 (44.9 %)	
Nakagawa et al. (2008)	116			24 (20.7 %)		Depressed pts
Simon et al. (2004b)	360			67 (18.8 %)		BD-I pts
Simon et al. (2004b)	115			14 (12.2 %)		BD-II pts
Tamam and Ozpoyraz (2002)	70			10 (14.3 %)		BD-I pts
Yerevanian et al. (2001)	35	MDD	98	3 (8.6 %)	3 (3.0 %)	Mostly BD-II pts
Pooled	*3,504*			*410 (11.7 %)*		
		MDD	*294*		*66 (22.4 %)*	

MDD major depressive disorder, *Schiz* schizophrenia, *Gen pop* general population

Okan Ibiloglu and Caykoylu 2011; Koyuncu et al. 2010; Simon et al. 2004b) and 1.5–62.3 % life time (Yerevanian et al. 2001; Tamam and Ozpoyraz 2002; Pini et al. 1997, 2003; Krishnan 2005; Simon et al. 2004b; Altshuler et al. 2010; Azorin et al. 2009; Zutshi et al. 2006; Magalhaes et al. 2010; Szadoczky et al. 1998; Dilsaver et al. 2008; Coryell et al. 2009; Craig et al. 2002; Slama et al. 2004; Henry et al. 2003; Nakagawa et al. 2008; Levander et al. 2007; Chen and Dilsaver 1995; Kawa et al. 2005). Probably, depending on the composition of the study sample, the frequency of OCD is lower in BD in comparison to unipolar depression (Kruger et al. 1995).

Reversely, BD is observed in 10.3–16 % of OCD patients with the majority of these cases (up to two-thirds) being BD-II (Perugi et al. 1997; Timpano et al. 2012; Darby et al. 2011; Hantouche et al. 2002; Maina et al. 2007). However, some rates reported are so low that they suggest BD is not more frequent in OCD than in controls (Nestadt et al. 2009). This might be probably to the fact that the distribution of bipolarity among OCD patients is not homogenous with only female OCD patients manifesting also BD (Grabe et al. 2001). When spectrums instead of distinct disorders are concerned, a significant overlap between the bipolar spectrum and the obsessive spectrum is observed (Angst et al. 2005).

An illness chart, generally suggests that OCD has an early onset and precedes BD onset in half to two-thirds of patients, while in the vast majority the course is chronic and fluctuating (Zutshi et al. 2007; Issler et al. 2005). The similarity between cross-sectional and lifetime rates is in support of the idea that OCD is a chronic condition when comorbid with BD; however, this might not be entirely true since OC symptoms improve significantly during periods of acute mania (Zutshi et al. 2007), and this improvement is so great that often no cases of OCD are detected during periods of acute mania (Magalhaes et al. 2010). Other authors argue that an episodic course appears to be typical of OCD when comorbid with BD (Perugi et al. 1997, 2002; Zutshi et al. 2007; Tukel et al. 2006; Strakowski et al. 1998). According to these suggestions, bipolarity has a pathoplastic effect on OCD (Strakowski et al. 1998; Mahasuar et al. 2011), and probably, in neurobiology, the OC symptoms are neurobiologically related more to BD mechanisms rather than to OCD (Zutshi et al. 2007). There seems that OC symptoms cycle in phase with BD symptomatology, and the rule is that in the absence of mood symptoms OC symptoms also disappear (Strakowski et al. 1998). It is important to mention that switching to mania or hypomania during treatment of OCD with antidepressants has been reported (White et al. 1986; Steiner 1991; Vieta and Bernardo 1992; Rihmer et al. 1996; Perugi et al. 2002).

Comorbid OCD and BD are related with a more gradual onset of OC symptoms (Perugi et al. 1997); higher rate of depressive episodes (Perugi et al. 1997, 2002; Zutshi et al. 2007; Mahasuar et al. 2011); higher general anxiety (Perugi et al. 2002; Zutshi et al. 2007; Tukel et al. 2006); better insight (Tukel et al. 2006); more frequent history of suicide attempts (Magalhaes et al. 2010; Mahasuar et al. 2011; Kruger et al. 2000), rapid cycling and alcohol, nicotine, coffee and substance dependence (Perugi et al. 2002; Magalhaes et al. 2010); and more frequent hospitalizations (Mahasuar et al. 2011) as well as greater overall severity of the clinical picture and global disability (Mahasuar et al. 2011; Tukel et al. 2006) although OC symptoms might be less severe (Zutshi et al. 2007). In BD patients with comorbid OC, there are reports suggesting a higher frequency of narcissistic and antisocial personality disorders (Maina et al. 2007) and a high family loading for mood disorders (Zutshi et al. 2007). OC symptoms are characterized by a significantly higher rate of sexual, religious and symmetry/exactness obsessions, more ordering/arranging compulsions and a significantly lower rate of checking rituals (Perugi et al. 1997, 2002; Tukel et al. 2006). There is only one study which reports that there was no difference between BD patients with and without comorbid OCD concerning age, sex, education, marital status, polarity, age of BD onset, presence of psychotic symptoms, presence of rapid cycling, history of suicide attempts, first episode type and predominant episode type (Koyuncu et al. 2010).

The reported rates concerning the presence of OCD in BD patients are shown in detail in Table 10.7. The pooled rate suggests that cross-sectionally 8.2 % of BD patients suffer from OCD. This rate is similar to that reported in the unipolar depression group and almost half of that reported in patients with schizophrenia. The pooled lifetime rate for OCD in BD patients is 8.8 % and identical to the cross-sectional rate, suggesting a chronic course for OCD in BD patients. It is more three times higher than the rate observed in the control population and similar to that reported in unipolar depressive patients (Table 10.8).

10.1.3 Comorbid Attention Deficit Hyperactivity Disorder (ADHD)

ADHD is usually considered to be a paediatric disorder; however, its characteristics often persist for the whole life span. It is considered to constitute either an early sign or a risk factor for the development of other mental disorders.

The research on comorbidity of BD with ADHD started after the results of epidemiological studies in children and adolescents which suggested a high comorbid appearance (Biederman et al. 1996). The current book focuses mainly on adult BD, and in this frame the comorbidity of ADHD with BD will be discussed for adult patients only, except for those issues whose understanding demands to consider also paediatric ADHD.

First, it is important to point out that diagnosing ADHD in adults can be a challenge. Hyperactivity and externalizing behaviours tend to decrease with age (Nierenberg et al. 2005), while the high comorbidity with major depression, BD, anxiety disorders and alcohol and substance abuse obscures the clinical picture (Fischer et al. 2007; Kessler et al. 2006). At least 80 % of adults with ADHD suffer from a second mental disorder, with one-fourth to one-third suffering from depression (Fischer et al. 2007; Biederman et al. 1993). Thus, ADHD is frequently not diagnosed, and it has been reported that only one in ten adults ADHD is diagnosed and appropriately treated (Faraone and Antshel 2008).

Specifically, concerning the coexistence with BD, it is believed that patients with comorbid ADHD/BD are under-diagnosed and under-treated (Klassen et al. 2010).

Table 10.8 Cross-sectional and lifetime rates of OCD comorbidity in BD patients

Study	*N*	Control population	*N*	Prevalence in BD *N*(%)	Prevalence in control *N*%	Comments
Cross-sectional rates						
Bellani et al. (2012)	205	MDD	105	28 (13.7 %)	2 (1.9 %)	
Boylan et al. (2004)	138			12 (8.7 %)		
Ciapparelli et al. (2007)	56	Schiz	98	10 (17.8 %)	20 (20.4 %)	BD with psychotic features
Cosoff and Hafner (1998)	20	Schiz	60	6 (30 %)	8 (13.3 %)	
Dell'Osso et al. (2011)	508			21 (4.1 %)		
Kruger et al. (1995)	37	MDD	105	13 (35.1 %)	37 (35.2 %)	BD-I inpatients
Mantere et al. (2006)	191	MDD	269	4 (2.1 %)	18 (6.7 %)	Acute BD pts
McElroy et al. (2001)	288			22 (7.6 %)		STANLEY
Okan Ibiloglu and Caykoylu (2011)	50			3 (6.0 %)		BD-I
Okan Ibiloglu and Caykoylu (2011)	46			7 (15.2 %)		BD-II
Otto et al. (2006)	918			62 (6.8 %)		STEP-BD. >75 % BD-I, half in recovery, ~25 % depressed
Simon et al. (2004b)	360			24 (67 %)		BD-I
Simon et al. (2004b)	115			3 (2.6 %)		BD-II
Strakowski et al. (1992)	41			3 (7.3 %)		First-episode manic/mixed inpatients
Tamam and Ozpoyraz (2002)	70			23 (32.9 %)		BD-I
Zutshi et al. (2006)	80	Controls	50	20 (25 %)	1 (2 %)	Remitted BD
Koyuncu et al. (2010)	185			22 (11.9 %)		
Koyuncu et al. (2010)	13			3 (23.1 %)		
Kruger et al. (2000)	143			10 (7 %)		
Pashinian et al. (2006)	56			1 (1.8 %)		

(continued)

Table 10.8 (continued)

Study	*N*	Control population	*N*	Prevalence in BD *N*(%)	Prevalence in control *N*%	Comments
Vieta et al. (2001)	129			2 (1.6 %)		BD-I first manic episode patients
Pooled	*3,649*			*299 (8.2 %)*		BD-I patients in remission
		MDD	*479*		*57 (11.9 %)*	
		Schiz	*158*		*28 (17.7 %)*	
		Controls	*50*		*1 (2.0 %)*	
Lifetime rates						
Altshuler et al. (2010)	711			68 (9.6 %)		>80 % BD-I Stanley
Azorin et al. (2009)	1,090			16 (1.5 %)		Manic acutely hospitalized
Chen and Dilsaver (1995)	168			35 (20.8 %)		ECA
Coryell et al. (2009)	427			11 (2.6 %)		Lifetime
Craig et al. (2002)	138	MDD with psychosis	87	3 (2.2 %)	5 (5.8 %)	BD with psychosis
Dilsaver et al. (2008)	69	MDD	118	43 (62.3 %)	22 (18.6 %)	Latinos
Henry et al. (2003)	318			9 (2.8 %)		75 % BD-I, half psychotic currently or lifetime
Kawa et al. (2005)	211			17 (8 %)		
Levander et al. (2007)	350			48 (13.7 %)		Stanley, 2/3 with alcohol use
McElroy et al. (2001)	288			27 (9.38)		STANLEY
Nakagawa et al. (2008)	116			8 (6,9 %)		Depressed
Pini et al. (1997)	24	MDD	38	5 (20.1 %)	5 (13.2 %)	BD depression
Robins and Regier (1991)	168	Gen pop	18,571	35 (20.8 %)	483 (2.6 %)	ECA
Simon et al. (2004b)	360			39 (10,8 %)		BD-I
Simon et al. (2004b)	115			8 (7.0 %)		BD-II

Slama et al. (2004)	301			9 (3.0 %)		Pts in remission
Szadoczky et al. (1998)	149	MDD	443	5 (3.4 %)	29 (6.5 %)	Epidemiological
Tamam and Ozpoyraz (2002)	70			27 (38.6 %)		BD-I
Yerevanian et al. (2001)	35	MDD	98	5 (14.3 %)	6 (6.1 %)	Lifetime, mostly BD-II
Zutshi et al. (2006)	80	Controls	50	28 (35.0 %)	1 (2.0 %)	Remitted BD
Magalhaes et al. (2010)	259			32 (12.4 %)		
Pooled	*5,447*			*478 (8.8 %)*		
		MDD	*784*		*67 (8.5 %)*	
		Gen pop	*18,621*		*484 (2.6 %)*	

MDD major depressive disorder, *Schiz* schizophrenia, *Gen pop* general population

This comorbidity is complex and of unclear nature (Sachs et al. 2000), but also sometimes there is an artificial inflation of comorbidity because of overlapping symptomatology (Pataki and Carlson 2013). This overlapping between the clinical pictures of BD and ADHD constitutes a significant problem in everyday clinical practice. It is important to have in mind that periodicity, decreased need for sleep, psychotic symptoms, hallucinations and inflated self-esteem are not elements of the clinical picture of ADHD and can be used in the differential diagnosis (Wingo and Ghaemi 2007; Kent and Craddock 2003). Essentially, the problem of differential diagnosis lies in the differentiation between severe ADHD with mood lability and mania/hypomania (Barkley and Fischer 2010). The only paper which studied the use or exclusion of overlapping symptoms reported that although the majority of patients kept the same diagnosis irrespective of criteria used, a significant minority, maybe up to 20–30 % of patients did not (Milberger et al. 1995). To make things even more complex, two-thirds of patients with comorbid ADHD and BD suffer also from an anxiety disorder (Tamam et al. 2008).

The literature suggests that the prevalence of ADHD in adult BD patients ranges from 3.2 to 30 % (Sachs et al. 2000; Wingo and Ghaemi 2007; Perugi et al. 2013; Nierenberg et al. 2005; McIntyre et al. 2010b; Weber et al. 2011; Sentissi et al. 2008; Tamam et al. 2006, 2008; Merikangas et al. 2011; Kessler et al. 2006). The studies do not differentiate between cross-sectional and lifetime rates. In adult subjects with childhood ADHD which did not persist into adulthood, the rate of BD was higher and equal to 10–34.1 % (Tamam et al. 2006, 2008; Winokur et al. 1993; Carlson et al. 2002; Sachs et al. 2000; Bernardi et al. 2010). A significant proportion of BD patients (up to 25 %) has received treatment with stimulants in the past because of the presence of ADHD or refractory depression, but it is interesting that less than half of them received also a concurrent mood stabilizer (Wingo and Ghaemi 2008). This supports the hypothesis that the wide use of stimulants in North America for the treatment of children with ADHD might induce an earlier-onset BD (DelBello et al. 2001); however, this hypothesis has not been confirmed, and even a protective effect for stimulants has been reported (Tillman and Geller 2006).

Reversely up to 5.1–47 % of adult ADHD patients suffer from BD (Park et al. 2011; Secnik et al. 2005; Wilens et al. 2003; McGough et al. 2005; Faraone et al. 2006b) and approximately 28 % of ADHD children will manifest BD-I during early adulthood (Tillman and Geller 2006). The range of rates for adult ADHD patients alone is narrower and much lower and equal to 1.5–4.4 % (Biederman and Faraone 2005; Faraone et al. 2006a; Kessler et al. 2006).

Comorbid ADHD is associated with earlier age at illness onset (Sachs et al. 2000; Nierenberg et al. 2005; McIntyre et al. 2010b; Tamam et al. 2006), more frequent mixed episodes vs. pure manic (Perugi et al. 2013), more frequent early onset of substance abuse (in up to 90 % of patients) (Wilens et al. 1997), a higher number of psychiatric comorbidities (Wilens et al. 2009; McIntyre et al. 2010b), decreased quality of life (McIntyre et al. 2010b) and worse course of bipolar disorder and greater burden of other psychiatric comorbid conditions (Klassen et al. 2010; Perugi et al. 2013; Pataki and Carlson 2013; Nierenberg et al. 2005; Bernardi et al. 2010; Ruggero et al. 2010; Carlson et al. 2012; Ryden et al. 2009). Two conflicting reports on the type of BD exist. The first suggested that the vast majority of patients with this specific comorbidity (almost 90 %) belong to the BD-II type (Wilens et al. 2003), while the second one suggested they are more often BD-I (Nierenberg et al. 2005).

Family studies are equivocal. One review suggested there is no relationship between BD and ADHD (Duffy 2012), while another review concluded the opposite (Skirrow et al. 2012). There are studies which suggest that there is a strong connection between ADHD and BD and the comorbid condition runs in families, with over 20 % of offspring or BD parents manifesting ADHD. These particular studies included BD patients with a more severe form of the disorder and high comorbidity, and therefore their conclusions might not be generalizable (Chang et al. 2000; Singh et al. 2007; Hirshfeld-Becker et al. 2006; Henin et al. 2005; Birmaher et al. 2009, 2010; Faraone et al. 1997, 2001).

As mentioned before, the nature of BD/ADHD comorbidity is complex and of unclear nature; however, a familial aggregation seems probably, and this points towards a developmental neurobiological association between ADHD and BD, going beyond symptomatic similarities (Skirrow et al. 2012). On the other hand, the careful review of all available data across different domains of research suggests that most findings are equivocal concerning the true nature of this comorbidity (Wingo and Ghaemi 2007).

The reported rates concerning the presence of ADHD in BD patients are shown in detail in Table 10.9. The pooled rate suggests that 6 % of BD patients suffer from ADHD. There is no separation in cross-sectional and lifetime rates.

10.1.4 Comorbid Complicated Grief (CG)

The vast majority of BD patients also report a lifetime history of a significant loss. This issue has not been adequately studied, and there is only one publication on 120 patients, 103 of whom (86 %) reported such a significant loss, and one-quarter met diagnostic criteria for CG. These patients were also more likely to manifest comorbid panic disorder, alcohol abuse and increased rate of lifetime suicide attempts, greater functional impairment and poorer social support (Simon et al. 2005).

10.1.5 Comorbid Eating Disorders

Any eating disorder (ED) is seen in 0–21 % of BD patients (Cassano et al. 1998; Dittmann et al. 2002; Edmonds et al. 1998; MacQueen et al. 2003; Mantere et al. 2006, 2010; McElroy et al. 1995, 2001, 2011; Wildes et al. 2008; Seixas et al. 2012; Pashinian et al. 2006) and especially in females (Seixas et al. 2012). Reversely two-thirds of patients with ED also suffer from BD (Simpson et al. 1992). Furthermore, close to half of BD patients report significant loss of control concerning food consumption (Wildes et al. 2008). It seems that when the ED spectrum is studied along with the BD spectrum, comorbidity and clinical correlates become stronger and more meaningful (McElroy et al. 2005).

Table 10.9 Cross-sectional and lifetime rates of ADHD comorbidity in BD patients

Study	*N*	Control population	*N*	Prevalence in BD *N*(%)	Prevalence in control *N*%	Comments
Sentissi et al. (2008)	73			22 (30.1 %)		Euthymic pts
Tamam et al. (2006)	44			7 (15.9 %)		Euthymic BD-I pts
Tamam et al. (2008)	159			26 (16.4 %)		Pts remission
Weber et al. (2011)	27,054			854 (3.2 %)		National Hospital Discharge Survey (NHDS)
McIntyre et al. (2010b)	176	MDD	213	31 (17.6 %)	11 (5.2 %)	
Nierenberg et al. (2005)	1,000			95 (9.5 %)		STEP-BD
Merikangas et al. (2011)	721			199 (27.6 %)		World mental health survey
Perugi et al. (2013)	96			19 (19.8 %)		
Sachs et al. (2000)	56			8 (14.3 %)		Childhood-onset ADHD
Kessler et al. (2006)	3,199			678 (21.2 %)		Epidemiological study
Pooled	*32,578*			*1,939 (6.0 %)*		

MDD major depressive disorder

Concerning specific ED, around 8.8–12.9 % of BD patients are also suffering from binge eating disorder (BED) (Bellani et al. 2012; Kruger et al. 1996; McElroy et al. 2011, 2013; Schoofs et al. 2011; Krishnan 2005; Fornaro et al. 2010; Angst 1998). Around two times, these rates manifest subthreshold BED, and 42.3 % of patients with comorbid BED and BD are obese (McElroy et al. 2013; Kruger et al. 1996). Reversely in 9.3 % of BED patients, BD is also present (Javaras et al. 2008). Menstrual cycle significantly influences BED by worsening it prior to menses. It is reported that 80 % of BD-BED patients noticed regular weight gain prior to menses (Schoofs et al. 2011). Anorexia nervosa (AN) is seen in 0–3.1 % of BD patients, and more frequent in younger ones (Dell'Osso et al. 2011; Fogarty et al. 1994; McElroy et al. 2001, 2011; Pini et al. 1999; Seixas et al. 2012; Fornaro et al. 2010). It might be absent during periods of mania (Fogarty et al. 1994). Bulimia nervosa (BN) is seen in 1.4–7.5 % of BD patients (Baldassano et al. 2005; McElroy et al. 2001, 2011; Pini et al. 1999; Strakowski et al. 1992, 1993; Vieta et al. 2001; Seixas et al. 2012; Fornaro et al. 2010) and up to 7–12 % in bipolar females (Baldassano et al. 2005; Strakowski et al. 1992; Schuckit et al. 1996). Reversely, BN patients are at a 4.5 times higher risk to also suffer from BD (Lunde et al. 2009). Most if not all BN-BD patients are female (Ramacciotti et al. 2005; Seixas et al. 2012).

Several studies report that BD-ED patients have specific clinical features. Female patients with ED have an earlier onset of BD and an increased number of mood episodes, predominantly depressive (Mantere et al. 2010; Brietzke et al. 2011). Rapid cycling and comorbid drug abuse might be more common in BED-BD patients (Brietzke et al. 2011; Fornaro et al. 2010) After controlling for obesity, BED was found to correlate with suicidality, psychosis, mood instability, anxiety disorder comorbidity and substance abuse comorbidity (Brietzke et al. 2011; McElroy et al. 2013). Reversely, after controlling for BED status, obesity was found to correlate with greater general medical comorbidity, but lower substance abuse comorbidity (McElroy et al. 2013). The correlation of ED with BD subtype and especially with BD-II is controversial, and data are inconclusive (McElroy et al. 2011; Simpson et al. 1992).

There are some but rather limited data suggesting the familial coaggregation of eating disorders with BD (Mangweth et al. 2003; Ramacciotti et al. 2005).

The reported rates concerning the presence of eating disorders in BD patients are shown in detail in Table 10.10. The pooled rates suggest that any eating disorder is present in 9.6 % of BD patients, anorexia in 2.4 %, bulimia in 4.4 % and binge eating disorder in 9.6 %. All these rates are significantly higher than those seen in the general population.

10.1.6 Various Other Comorbid Conditions

A number of other psychiatric conditions can be found as comorbid in BD patients. For these conditions, the literature is poor, and data are scarce.

One study reported that one-third of BD patients manifest a comorbid behavioural addiction (three times higher rate in comparison to controls), with

Table 10.10 Cross-sectional and lifetime rates of eating disorders comorbidity in BD patients

Study	*N*	Control population	*N*	Prevalence in BD *N*(%)	Prevalence in control *N*%	Comments
Any eating disorder						
Cassano et al. (1998)	47			3 (6.4 %)		BD-I pts with psychotic features
Dittmann et al. (2002)	108			10 (9.4 %)		BD-I pts, lifetime rates
Dittmann et al. (2002)	38			0 (0.0 %)		BD-II pts, lifetime rates
Edmonds et al. (1998)	64			4 (6.3 %)		
MacQueen et al. (2003)	139			21 (15.1 %)		
Mantere et al. (2006)	191	MDD	269	15 (7.9 %)	2 (0.7 %)	Acute BD pts, cross-sectional rates
Mantere et al. (2010)	191			12 (8.3 %)		Half depressed, cross-sectional rates
McElroy et al. (1995)	71			6 (8.5 %)		BD-I pts, acute mania
McElroy et al. (2001)	288			4 (1.4 %)		STANLEY foundation data, cross-sectional rates
McElroy et al. (2001)	288			17 (5.9 %)		STANLEY foundation data, lifetime rates
Wildes et al. (2008)	81			17 (21.0 %)		
Seixas et al. (2012)	356			19 (5.3 %)		
Pashinian et al. (2006)	56			8 (14.3 %)		
McElroy et al. (2011)	875			125 (14.3 %)		Lifetime rate
Pooled	*2,793*			*269 (9.6 %)*		
Anorexia nervosa						
Dell'Osso et al. (2011)	508			9 (1.6 %)		Cross-sectional rates
Seixas et al. (2012)	356			11 (3.1 %)		
Fogarty et al. (1994)	22			0 (0.0 %)		Epidemiological study on 3,258 general population subjects, identified 22 manic pts
McElroy et al. (2001)	288			0 (0.0 %)		STANLEY foundation data, cross-sectional rates
McElroy et al. (2001)	288			6 (2.1 %)		STANLEY foundation data, lifetime rates

McElroy et al. (2011)	875			27 (3.1 %)		Lifetime rate
Pini et al. (1999)	125			3 (2.4 %)		BD-I
Pooled	2,337			56 (2.4 %)		
Bulimia nervosa						
Baldassano et al. (2005)	482			36 (7.5 %)		STEP-BD pts, 12 % rate in females
Seixas et al. (2012)	356			8 (2.2 %)		
McElroy et al. (2001)	288			4 (1.4 %)		STANLEY foundation data
McElroy et al. (2001)	288			11 (3.8 %)		STANLEY foundation data
Pini et al. (1999)	125			5 (4.0 %)		BD-I
Strakowski et al. (1992)	41			3 (7.3 %)		12 % rate in females
Strakowski et al. (1993)	60			4 (6.6 %)		BD-I, first episode of mania
McElroy et al. (2011)	875			42 (4.8 %)		Lifetime rate
Vieta et al. (2001)	129			3 (2.3 %)		BD-I pts in remission
Pooled	*2,644*			*116 (4.4 %)*		
Binge eating						
Bellani et al. (2012)	205	MDD	105	25 (12.2 %)	5 (4.8 %)	Cross-sectional rates
McElroy et al. (2011)	875			77 (8.8 %)		Lifetime rate
Kruger et al. (1996)	62			8 (12.9 %)		
McElroy et al. (2013)	717			68 (9.5 %)		
Pooled	*1,859*			*178 (9.6 %)*		

MDD major depressive disorder

pathological gambling, compulsive buying and sexual and work addictions being the most important (Di Nicola et al. 2010).

Tourette's disorder seems to be more frequent among BD patients in comparison to the general population, with a four times higher risk; however, this comorbidity is not adequately studied (Robertson 2006; Kerbeshian et al. 1995). Similarly, impulse control disorders seem to correlate with BD with the overlapping of symptoms being a significant problem for the differential diagnosis (McElroy et al. 1996). The risk of firesetting could be five times higher in BD in comparison to the general population (Blanco et al. 2010). Shoplifting is also prevalent (Blanco et al. 2008).

Premenstrual syndrome (PMS) and premenstrual dysphoric disorder (PMDD) are frequent in BD and especially in BD-II patients. The reverse is also true with PMS and PMDD patients being at an increased risk to develop BD-I (Cirillo et al. 2012).

One study suggested that mania was observed in 4.2 % of somatization patients (Brown et al. 1990).

10.1.7 Comorbid Psychiatric Disorders and BD-II

There are some studies suggesting that there is no differences in comorbidity between patients with BD-I vs. BD-II (Koyuncu et al. 2010; Vieta et al. 2000; McElroy et al. 2001, 2011); however, other studies strongly support the higher comorbidity rate in BD-II (especially anxiety and eating disorders) along with a higher familial load especially in first-degree relatives and in relationship with substance abuse (Mantere et al. 2006; Baek et al. 2011; Mula et al. 2008a; Judd et al. 2003; Rihmer et al. 2001).

10.2 Medical Comorbidity

10.2.1 General Medical Comorbidity

General medical comorbidity has been recognized as an important problem especially for BD patients. They are reported to have up to four times higher health care costs in comparison to patients without mental disorders, and a significant determinant of this is medical comorbidity (Bryant-Comstock et al. 2002; Stender et al. 2002; Gardner et al. 2006; Centorrino et al. 2009). It is disappointing that despite the above well-known issues, it is usual that medical conditions remain under-recognized and under-treated in the real world, and as a consequence, the life expectancy for patients with BD is approximately 30 % lower than that of the general population, and it is lower also in comparison to other mental disorders (Fagiolini and Goracci 2009; Alstrom 1942; Babigian and Odoroff 1969). This is not only because medical comorbidity increases the already great burden of the bipolar illness but also because BD patients are less likely to receive proper care and diagnosis, like the rest of the population. The presence of stigma and their own lack of cooperation are largely responsible for this (Morriss and Mohammed 2005). Even when properly diagnosed and appropriately treated, their adherence is problematic, and the overall outcome is generally less favourable. Additionally, their care is more complex and expensive, with more frequent use of health services and more hospitalizations because of their somatic problems (Sullivan et al. 2006). These have a significant impact on the patients' quality of life, but the increased mortality is even more important. The decrease in life expectancy is primarily due to premature cardiovascular mortality (Colton and Manderscheid 2006). In this frame, it is embarrassing that some pharmacological interventions put the patient at a higher risk for the manifestation of specific somatic disorders, especially cardiovascular.

Depending on the study sample, 11.5–75.7 % of BD patients are reported to manifest some somatic comorbidity with cardiovascular, endocrinological, gastrointestinal disorders and pain being the most prevalent (Beyer et al. 2005; Carney and Jones 2006; Douzenis et al. 2012; Feldman et al. 2012; Kilbourne et al. 2004; Magalhaes et al. 2012; McIntyre et al. 2006a; Oreski et al. 2012; Subramaniam et al. 2013; Weber et al. 2011; Strakowski et al. 1992, 1994; Perron et al. 2009; Krishnan 2005; Castelo et al. 2012; Kemp et al. 2013; McIntyre et al. 2007b). At least some specific medical conditions like thyroid disease, migraine, and obesity appear to be more frequent in females (Carney and Jones 2006). This high medical comorbidity seems to lead to an overall worse long-term course and outcome (Thompson et al. 2006; McIntyre et al. 2006a) and greater disability (Perron et al. 2009). There is one study disputing the effect of medical comorbidity on the overall outcome (Strakowski et al. 1992), but other studies further confirm it and suggest that this effect is not generic, but on the contrary it is a specific effect of each specific somatic comorbidity on outcome and disability (Pirraglia et al. 2009) as well as of age and duration of illness (Soreca et al. 2008, 2009). Inpatient data suggest that hypothyroidism, viral hepatitis, obesity and various diseases of the skin and subcutaneous tissue and of the nervous, respiratory and musculoskeletal systems are found significantly more often in BD patients. The relative risk for these somatic disorders varies from 1.5 to 4 depending on the specific illness and the population under study (Weber et al. 2011; Chou et al. 2013; Laursen et al. 2011), and there is some stronger relationship to depressive symptoms (Thompson et al. 2006; Kemp et al. 2013). Multiple somatic comorbidity seems to be the rule rather than the exception with BD patients suffering from an average of 2.7 or more medical conditions (Soreca et al. 2009; Kilbourne et al. 2009b; McIntyre et al. 2006a). Unfortunately, up to 70 % of them might be unaware of their somatic problems (Feldman et al. 2012). Psychiatric comorbidity further increases the risk for the presence of somatic disorders (Daratha et al. 2012; Kemp et al. 2013; Magalhaes et al. 2012), and probably this is partially mediated by the high stress load BD patients experience (McIntyre et al. 2007b). A gender effect could be present in at least some of these comorbidities especially thyroid disease (Arnold 2003).

The link between BD and medical conditions is not known; however, probably medical comorbidity is not solely the secondary result of the overall burden of BD, but it is highly likely that at least some conditions like diabetes mellitus and autoimmune disorders to share aetiopathogenetic mechanisms, probably of an immunoinflammatory nature in the frame of 'stress-sensitive' medical disorders (Altamura et al. 2011; Soreca et al. 2009).

As expected, the treatment of these multiple comorbidities is even more difficult, and several principles exist to manage the increasingly complex problems. Central are the establishment of the diagnosis, the risk assessment, determining the appropriate setting for the treatment, planning for the long-term management, determining the sequence of treatments since simultaneous treatments might be problematic and detailed assessment of the different faces of the outcome with the use of psychometric and neuropsychological tools and laboratory testing (McIntyre et al. 2012; Ramasubbu et al. 2012; Soreca et al. 2008). More specifically, cardiovascular disorder appears to be the most consistent cause of premature mortality in BD (Roshanaei-Moghaddam and Katon 2009). Since cardiovascular disease has known and modifiable risk factors, the improvement of the general health of BD patients and the increase of their life expectancy appear to be achievable goals though very difficult ones.

The reported rates concerning the presence of any medical comorbidity in BD patients are shown in detail in Table 10.11. The pooled rates suggest that any medical comorbidity is present in half of BD patients. This rate is similar to the rate reported for patients with schizophrenia and double of what is reported concerning the general population.

10.2.2 Metabolic Syndrome and Related Medical Conditions

10.2.2.1 Obesity

Obesity is a condition defined as body mass index (BMI) above 30 or waist circumference over 102 cm (40 in.) in men and 88 cm (35 in.) in women and waist-to-hip ratio >0.9 for men and >0.85 for women. Waist circumference might be a better index concerning central (abdominal) obesity which is considered to be more medically problematic. A problem is that other cut-off points are also used in various studies to define obesity (e.g. BMI >25 or waist circumference >105 cm).

Although the epidemiological data are inconclusive, obesity is a frequent problem in mental patients, and this is especially true concerning BD. Whether obesity constitutes a problem specific for BD or mental disorders in general is a matter of debate, because obesity is also highly frequent in the general population (McElroy et al. 2002) and weight loss is reported in a minority of BD-I patients (Carney and Jones 2006). Obesity has been reported as a significant health issue concerning the whole bipolar spectrum population with 90 % of severely obese patients belonging to that spectrum and BD-II being the most usual diagnosis (Alciati et al. 2007, 2011).

The reported prevalence of obesity in BD varies from 1.4 to 55.4 % (Kim et al. 2009; Sicras et al. 2008; McIntyre et al. 2010c; Kemp et al. 2010, 2013; Guo et al. 2006; Carney and Jones 2006; Krishnan 2005; Salvi et al. 2008; Weber et al. 2011; Petry et al. 2008; McIntyre et al. 2007a; McElroy et al. 2002, 2004, 2013; Elmslie et al. 2000, 2001; Mather et al. 2009; Maina et al. 2008; Fagiolini et al. 2002; Calkin

Table 10.11 Cross-sectional and lifetime rates of any medical comorbidity in BD patients

Study	*N*	Control population	*N*	Prevalence in BD *N*(%)	Prevalence in control *N*%	Comments
Beyer et al. (2005)	1,379			607 (44.0 %)		Duke University Medical Center outpatient clinical database, 2/3 manic and 1/3 depressed cross-sectional data
Carney and Jones (2006)	3,557	In- and outpatients	726,262	2,694 (75.7 %)	328,886 (45.3 %)	BD-I pts from the Wellmark Blue Cross/Blue Shield (BC/BS) of Iowa administrative claims data
Douzenis et al. (2012)	228			120 (52.6 %)		Inpatients, cross-sectional data
Feldman et al. (2012)	61			7 (11.5 %)		Acute bipolar depression, from the NCT00276965 trial
Feldman et al. (2012)	17			3 (17.6 %)		Anxious BD pts from the NCT01172652 trial
Kilbourne et al. (2004)	4,310	VA national cohort	3,408,760	980 (22.7 %)	678,512 (19.9 %)	VA national patient population, cross-sectional data
Magalhaes et al. (2012)	3,399			1,998 (58.8 %)		STEP-BD data
McIntyre et al. (2006a)	938	Gen pop	35,848	603 (64.3 %)	17,386 (48.5 %)	Canadian Community Health Survey, lifetime rates
Oreski et al. (2012)	97	Schiz	192	65 (67.0 %)	97 (50.5 %)	Inpatient records
Subramaniam et al. (2013)	88			46 (52.3 %)		BD-I pts
Strakowski et al. (1992)	41			9 (21.9 %)		
Perron et al. (2009)	1,548			502 (32.4 %)		BD-I pts
Pooled	*15,663*			*7,634 (48.7 %)*		
		Gen pop	*4,171,062*		*1,024,881 (24.6 %)*	

Schiz schizophrenia

et al. 2009; Chwastiak et al. 2011; Muller-Oerlinghausen et al. 1979; Fiedorowicz et al. 2008, 2011; Birkenaes et al. 2007), and this high variability of results makes conclusions difficult. Reversely, in morbidly obese patients, BD is diagnosed at a rate of 2.8–11 % (Black et al. 1992; Britz et al. 2000; Simon et al. 2006).

Medication seems to have a significant impact (McIntyre 2002; Keck and McElroy 2003). Lithium (Vendsborg et al. 1976; Sachs et al. 2006) and valproate (Dinesen et al. 1984; Pylvanen et al. 2002; Swann 2001) can cause weight gain. It has been reported that patients on lithium gain weight in contrast to patients under lamotrigine (Bowden et al. 2006; Muller-Oerlinghausen et al. 1979; Atmaca et al. 2002; Vendsborg et al. 1976) and weight gain during lithium treatment has shown to lead to poor adherence (Gitlin et al. 1989). Treatment with antipsychotics and especially with those belonging to the second generation has also been related to weight gain (Henderson et al. 2000; Simpson 2005; Volavka et al. 2002; Zipursky et al. 2005; Nasrallah 2003). It seems that most of weight gain happens during the acute phase and not during the maintenance (Fagiolini et al. 2002).

Beyond iatrogenic effects, individuals with bipolar disorder often adopt unhealthy lifestyles, may have poor diets and receive inadequate exercise (Kilbourne et al. 2007).

Patients with a more chronic course and longer duration manifest higher rates of overweight and obesity (Calkin et al. 2009; Maina et al. 2008) with depressive episodes being responsible for most of this effect (Maina et al. 2008; Keck and McElroy 2003; Fagiolini et al. 2002). There does not seem to be a significant effect of gender (Maina et al. 2008; Elmslie et al. 2000, 2001) although women with obesity and extreme obesity seem to be more likely to have atypical major depressive episodes in their bipolar illness (Pickering et al. 2007). Substance abuse is inversely related with obesity in BD patients (McIntyre et al. 2007a). The comorbidity of eating disorders can partially but not completely explain the prevalence of overweight and obesity in BD patients (Maina et al. 2008) since in these patients, preference for carbohydrate consumption and low levels of physical activity and exercise are seen very often (Keck and McElroy 2003).

The reported rates concerning the presence of obesity in BD patients are shown in detail in Table 10.12. The pooled rates suggest that obesity is present in 15 % of BD patients, and this rate is 30 % higher than the reported in unipolar depressed patients and four to five times higher than the respected rate in the general population.

10.2.2.2 Dyslipidaemia

Dyslipidaemia could concern the presence of hypertriglyceridaemia (above 150 mg/dL) or low HDL-C (<40 mg/dL in men and <50 mg/dL in women). The first report on the presence of higher lipid levels in the blood of BD patients was published in the late 1960s (Brandrup and Randrup 1967). The rates vary greatly probably because of different definitions and methods utilized. For example, one method of assessing the rates is to monitor antilipidaemic prescriptions. One such study reported that around 16 % of BD and patients with schizophrenia were receiving such medication but only 10 % of controls (Bai et al. 2013).

Table 10.12 Rates of obesity in BD patients

Study	*N*	Control population	*N*	Prevalence in BD *N*(%)	Prevalence in control *N*%	Comments
Birkenaes et al. (2007)	110	Gen pop	18,770	27 (24.5)	2,647 (14.1 %)	
Calkin et al. (2009)	276			108 (39.1 %)		Tertiary care patients, 2/3 BD-I
Carney and Jones (2006)	3,557	In- and outpatients	726,262	163 (4.6 %)	7,828 (1.1 %)	BD-I, Wellmark Blue Cross/Blue Shield (BC/BS) of Iowa administrative claims data
Carney and Jones (2006)	3,557	Gen pop	726,262	163 (4.6 %)	7,828 (1.1 %)	BD-I medical registry
Chwastiak et al. (2011)	9,522			3,733 (39.2 %)		Epidemiological
Elmslie et al. (2000)	89	Controls	445	17 (19.1 %)	52 (11.7 %)	BD-I euthymic
Fagiolini et al. (2002)	50			16 (32.0 %)		BD-I
Fagiolini et al. (2003)	175			62 (35.4 %)		BD-I
Fagiolini et al. (2005)	171			84 (49.1 %)		BD-I
Fiedorowicz et al. (2008)	161			77 (47.8 %)		2/3 BD-I
Fiedorowicz et al. (2011)	135	MDD	524	40 (29.6 %)	57 (10.9 %)	Epidemiological
Guo et al. (2006)	6,178			533 (8,6 %)		Health-care database
Kemp et al. (2010)	125			63 (50.4 %)		RCT patients
Kemp et al. (2013)	260			96 (36.9 %)		Lithium Treatment—Moderate-Dose Use Study (LiTMUS)
Kemp et al. (2013)	260			96 (36.9 %)		Lithium Treatment—Moderate-Dose Use Study (LiTMUS)
Kim et al. (2009)	184			56 (30.4 %)		BD-I inpatients, 2/3 manic
Maina et al. (2008)	76	OCD	65	1 (1.4 %)	0 (0.0 %)	Half BD-I
Mather et al. (2009)	885			192 (21.7 %)		Epidemiological
McElroy et al. (2002)	644			135 (21.0 %)		

(continued)

Table 10.12 (continued)

Study	*N*	Control population	*N*	Prevalence in BD *N*(%)	Prevalence in control *N*%	Comments
McElroy et al. (2013)	717			307 (42.8 %)		
McIntyre et al. (2007a)	938	Gen pop	36,046	520 (55.4 %)	17,158 (47.6 %)	BD-I Canadian Community Health Survey
McIntyre et al. (2010c)	99			37 (41.1 %)		Euthymic patients, diabetic excluded
Salvi et al. (2008)	99			50 (50.0 %)		
Sicras et al. (2008)	178	Gen pop	85,850	41 (23.0 %)	9,701 (11.3 %)	Health-care database
Thompson et al. (2006)	174			58 (33.3 %)		BD-I
Wang et al. (2006)	267			29 (10.9 %)		BD-I STEP-BD
Wang et al. (2006)	97			24 (24.7 %)		BD-II STEP-BD
Weber et al. (2011)	27,054	Gen pop	2,325,247	1,668 (6.2 %)	96,949 (4.2 %)	US hospital discharges between 1979 and 2006
Pooled	*56,038*			*8,396 (15.0 %)*		
		Gen pop	*3,918,882*		*142,163 (3.6 %)*	

MDD major depressive disorder, *OCD* obsessive–compulsive disorder, *Gen pop* general population

Overall the literature reports that any kind of dyslipidaemia is present in 0.9–57.5 % of BD patients (Salvi et al. 2008, 2011; Kim et al. 2009; Chang et al. 2009; Sicras et al. 2008; McIntyre et al. 2010c; Kemp et al. 2010; Guo et al. 2006; Garcia-Portilla et al. 2008; Fiedorowicz et al. 2008; Centorrino et al. 2009; Oreski et al. 2012; Fenn et al. 2005; Weber et al. 2011; Kilbourne et al. 2004; Carney and Jones 2006; Lin et al. 2007; Fagiolini et al. 2005; Kemp et al. 2013). Second-generation antipsychotics constitute a major factor for the development of hyperlipidaemia in BD patients (Huang and Chen 2005; Henderson 2001; Henderson et al. 2000; Osser et al. 1999).

The reported rates concerning the presence of dyslipidaemia in BD patients are shown in detail in Table 10.13. The pooled rates suggest that dyslipidaemia is present in 17.2 % of BD patients, and this rate is probably similar to the rate reported concerning patients with schizophrenia and tenfold higher than the respected rate in the general population.

10.2.2.3 Diabetes Mellitus (DM)

DM is defined as fasting blood glucose ≥100 mg/dL. The first reports concerning a possible increased prevalence of DM in BD patients were published in the early twentieth century (Raphael and Parsons 1921; Kasanin 1926). Again one method to calculate the rates of DM is to count antidiabetic prescriptions. One such study reported that around 10 % of BD and patients with schizophrenia were receiving such medication but only 6 % of controls (Bai et al. 2013). The literature suggests that 1.1–43.5 % of BD patients suffer from DM (Ramsey et al. 2010; Beyer et al. 2005; Carney and Jones 2006; Cassidy et al. 1999; Centorrino et al. 2009; Chang et al. 2009; Chien et al. 2010; Fagiolini et al. 2005; Fenn et al. 2005; Fiedorowicz et al. 2008, 2011; Garcia-Portilla et al. 2008; Guo et al. 2006; Hirschfeld et al. 2003; Kemp et al. 2010, 2013; Kilbourne et al. 2004; Kim et al. 2009; Laursen et al. 2011; Lin et al. 2007; McIntyre et al. 2006a; Oreski et al. 2012; Regenold et al. 2002; Ruzickova et al. 2003; Salvi et al. 2008, 2011; Subramaniam et al. 2013; Thompson et al. 2006; van Winkel et al. 2008a; Weber et al. 2011). In BD-II, the mean rate is around 10 % (Krishnan 2005). The range of reported rates is significant, and although the results are suggestive of the presence of increased rate in BD patients in comparison to the general population, the conclusions are problematic.

It has been reported that the age at first hospitalization and duration of illness are not related to the development of DM in BD patients (Cassidy et al. 1999). Impaired glucose metabolism, insulin resistance and diabetes mellitus are related to treatment with lithium (Hermida et al. 1994), valproic acid (Dinesen et al. 1984; Pylvanen et al. 2002) and second-generation antipsychotics (Henderson 2001; Henderson et al. 2000; Guo et al. 2006; Lambert et al. 2005; Ollendorf et al. 2004; Sernyak et al. 2005; Gianfrancesco et al. 2003).

The reported rates concerning the presence of DM in BD patients are shown in detail in Table 10.14. The pooled rates suggest that DM is present in 9.8 % of BD patients, and this rate is probably similar to the rate reported concerning patients with schizophrenia, unipolar depression and the general population.

Table 10.13 Rates of dyslipidemia in BD patients

Study	*N*	Control population	*N*	Prevalence in BD *N*(%)	Prevalence in control *N*%	Comments
Carney and Jones (2006)	3,557	Other patients	726,262	438 (12.3 %)	55,495 (7.6 %)	Wellmark Blue Cross/Blue Shield (BC/BS) of Iowa administrative claims data, BD-I pts
Centorrino et al. (2009)	28,531	Gen pop	85,593	5,861 (20.5 %)	14,170 (16.6 %)	Health-care data
Chang et al. (2009)	117			43 (36.8 %)		
Fagiolini et al. (2005)	171			70 (40.9 %)		
Fenn et al. (2005)	290			65 (22.4 %)		Inpatients, mostly BD-I
Fenn et al. (2005)	290			81 (27.9 %)		Inpatients, mostly BD-I
Fiedorowicz et al. (2008)	73			42 (57.5 %)		2/3 BD-I pts
Garcia-Portilla et al. (2008)	194			66 (30.0 %)		
Guo et al. (2006)	6,178			86 (1.4 %)		Health-care database
Kemp et al. (2010)	125			39 (31.2 %)		RCT pts
Kemp et al. (2013)	264			81 (30.7 %)		Lithium Treatment—Moderate Dose Use Study (LiTMUS) study
Kemp et al. (2013)	263			50 (19.0 %)		Lithium Treatment—Moderate-Dose Use Study (LiTMUS) study
Kilbourne et al. (2004)	4,310	VA national cohort	3,408,760	973 (22.6 %)	0 (0.0 %)	VA national patient population
Kim et al. (2009)	184			38 (20.7 %)		BD-I inpatients, 2/3 manic
Lin et al. (2007)	2,289	Gen pop	16,413	20 (0.9 %)	48 (0.3 %)	All sample underwent appendectomy
McIntyre et al. (2010c)	99			33 (38.8 %)		Euthymic pts, diabetic excluded
Oreski et al. (2012)	97	Schiz	192	49 (50.5 %)	86 (44.8 %)	Inpatient records
Salvi et al. (2008)	99			35 (37.4 %)		Inpatients

Salvi et al. (2011)	200			68 (34.0 %)		2/3 BD-II pts
Sicras et al. (2008)	178	Gen pop	85,850	41 (23.0 %)	9,701 (11.3 %)	Health-care database
Weber et al. (2011)	27,054	Gen pop	2,325,247	999 (3.7 %)	132,389 (5.7 %)	US hospital discharges between 1979 and 2006
Pooled	*47,509*			*8,179 (17.2 %)*		
		Gen pop	*4,322,878*		*79,414 (1.8 %)*	

Schiz schizophrenia, *Gen pop* general population

Table 10.14 Rates of diabetes mellitus in BD patients

Study	*N*	Control population	*N*	Prevalence in BD *N*(%)	Prevalence in control *N*%	Comments
Beyer et al. (2005)	1,379			59 (4.3 %)		BD-I, Duke University Medical Center outpatient clinical database, 2/3 manic and 1/3 depressed
Carney and Jones (2006)	3,557	In- and outpatients	726,262	63 (1.8)	4,401 (0.6)	BD-I, Wellmark Blue Cross/Blue Shield (BC/BS) of Iowa administrative claims data, diabetes, complicated
Carney and Jones (2006)	3,557	In- and outpatients	726,262	146 (4.1)	17,205 (2.4)	Wellmark Blue Cross/Blue Shield (BC/BS) of Iowa administrative claims data, diabetes, uncomplicated
Cassidy et al. (1999)	345			34 (9.9 %)		BD-I inpatients representative of US general population
Centorrino et al. (2009)	28,531	Gen pop	85,593	3,663 (12.8 %)	5,955 (7.0 %)	Health-care data
Chang ct al. (2009)	117			16 (13.7 %)		
Chien et al. (2010)	1,848	Gen pop	764,579	199 (10.8 %)	42,591 (5.6 %)	National medical claims database
(Fagiolini et al. (2005)	171			14 (8.2 %)		
Fenn et al. (2005)	290			5 (1.7 %)		Inpatients mostly BD-I, DM-I
Fenn et al. (2005)	290			24 (8.3 %)		Inpatients mostly BD-I, DM-II
Fiedorowicz et al. (2008)	142			43 (30.3 %)		2/3 BD-I
Fiedorowicz et al. (2011)	135	MDD	524	8 (5,9 %)	47 (9,0 %)	Epidemiological data
Garcia-Portilla et al. (2008)	194			23 (11.9 %)		
Guo et al. (2006)	6,178			920 (14.9 %)		Health-care database
Hirschfeld et al. (2003)	2,134	Gen pop	83,224	156 (7.3 %)	5,826 (7.0 %)	Epidemiological data
Kemp et al. (2010)	125			11 (8.8 %)		RCT patients
Kemp et al. (2013)	259			50 (19.3 %)		Lithium Treatment—Moderate-Dose Use Study (LiTMUS) study

Kilbourne et al. (2004)	4,310	VA national cohort	3,408,760	743 (17.2 %)	532,926 (15.6 %)	VA national patient population
Kim et al. (2009)	184			80 (43.5 %)		BD-I inpatients, 2/3 manic
Laursen et al. (2011)	6,215	Gen pop	2,428,518	74 (1.2 %)	12,950 (0.5 %)	Population-based cohort study
Lin et al. (2007)	2,289	Gen pop	16,413	101 (4.4 %)	363 (2.2 %)	All sample underwent appendectomy
McIntyre et al. (2006a)	938	Gen pop	35,848	40 (4.3 %)	1,721 (4.8 %)	Canadian Community Health Survey
Oreski et al. (2012)	97	Schiz	192	9 (9.3 %)	8 (4.2 %)	Inpatient records
Regenold et al. (2002)	136			35 (25.73 %)		Inpatients, BD-I, DM-II
Ruzickova et al. (2003)	222			26 (11.7 %)		¾ BD-I pts
Salvi et al. (2008)	99			11 (11.1 %)		Inpatients
Salvi et al. (2011)	200			21 (10.5 %)		2/3 BD-II pts
Subramaniam et al. (2013)	88			3 (3.4 %)		BD-I pts
Thompson et al. (2006)	174			2 (1.1 %)		BD-I pts
van Winkel et al. (2008a)	60			4 (6.7 %)		
Weber et al. (2011)	27,054	Gen pop	2,325,247	1,962 (7.3 %)	262,382 (10.0 %)	US hospital discharges between 1979 and 2006
Ramsey et al. (2010)	58	Gen pop	1,339	2 (3.4 %)	64 (4.8 %)	Epidemiological Catchment Area
Pooled	*87,529*			*8,547 (9.8 %)*		
		Gen pop	*9,875,783*		*886,384 (9.0 %)*	

Schiz schizophrenia, *Gen pop* general population

10.2.2.4 Hypertension

Hypertension is defined as the presence of a systolic blood pressure ≥130 mmHg and a diastolic blood pressure ≥85 mmHg. The literature suggests a rate of 2.4–67.5 % in BD patients, and conclusions are difficult (Ramsey et al. 2010; Huang et al. 2009; Carney and Jones 2006; Centorrino et al. 2009; Chang et al. 2009; Fagiolini et al. 2005; Fenn et al. 2005; Fiedorowicz et al. 2008, 2011; Garcia-Portilla et al. 2008; Guo et al. 2006; Hirschfeld et al. 2003; Johannessen et al. 2006; Kemp et al. 2010, 2013; Kilbourne et al. 2004; Lin et al. 2007; McIntyre et al. 2006a, 2010c; Perron et al. 2009; Salvi et al. 2008, 2011; Subramaniam et al. 2013; Weber et al. 2011; Beyer et al. 2005; Douzenis et al. 2012).

The reported rates concerning the presence of hypertension in BD patients are shown in detail in table 10.15. The pooled rates suggest that hypertension is present in 14.7 % of BD patients, and this rate is probably similar to the rate reported concerning patients with unipolar depression and the general population.

10.2.2.5 Comorbid Metabolic Syndrome

The term metabolic syndrome refers to a cluster of risk factors for cardiovascular disease, diabetes mellitus and premature mortality (Gans 2006) and is best defined according to the Third Report of the US National Cholesterol Education Program Expert Panel on Detection, Evaluation, and Treatment of High Blood Cholesterol in Adults (ATP-III) which considers abdominal adiposity, hypertension, impaired fasting glucose or diabetes mellitus and atherogenic dyslipidaemia as its principal components (National Cholesterol Education Program (NCEP) Expert Panel on Detection, Evaluation, and Treatment of High Blood Cholesterol in Adults (Adult Treatment Panel III) 2002). The prevalence of the metabolic syndrome in the western world is approximately 15–25 % in the general population, it increases with age, and it is more frequent among women (Ford et al. 2002; Hu et al. 2004; Laaksonen et al. 2002).

The literature suggests that the rate of metabolic syndrome in BD patients ranges from 0.37 % to 66.6 % (Taylor et al. 2010; Cardenas et al. 2008; Centorrino et al. 2009; Chang et al. 2009; Correll et al. 2008; Fagiolini et al. 2005; Fiedorowicz et al. 2008; Garcia-Portilla et al. 2008; John et al. 2009; Kemp et al. 2010, 2013; McIntyre et al. 2010c; Salvi et al. 2008, 2011; Sicras et al. 2008; van Winkel et al. 2008a, b; Vuksan-Cusa et al. 2009; Yumru et al. 2007; Jakovljevic et al. 2007). One study reported the respected rate for schizoaffective disorder bipolar type to be 42.4 % (Basu et al. 2004).

The prevailing conclusion is that it is increased in BD patients. Disparate estimates are reported ranging from comparability to approximately two- to threefold greater than the general population, and this seems to be a worldwide fact (McIntyre et al. 2005, 2010a). It is important to note that as patients spend more time in BD, the rates of the metabolic syndrome increase dramatically and this happens at a rate which implies it is rather an effect of the disease (and its correlating features including treatment) rather than of increasing age (Salvi et al. 2012; Taylor and MacQueen 2006).

Comorbid medical conditions such as diabetes, hypertension, dyslipidaemia and obesity are under-diagnosed and under-treated in hospitalized psychiatric patients compared with the non-psychiatric population. The attitude of psychiatrists is rather

Table 10.15 Rates of hypertension in BD patients

Study	*N*	Control population	*N*	Prevalence in BD *N*(%)	Prevalence in control *N*%	Comments
Carney and Jones (2006)	3,557	In- and outpatients	726,262	645 (18.1 %)	66,575 (9.2 %)	BD-I, Wellmark Blue Cross/Blue Shield (BC/BS) of Iowa administrative claims data
Centorrino et al. (2009)	28,531	Gen pop	85,593	6,418 (22.5 %)	14,787 (17.3 %)	Health-care data
Chang et al. (2009)	117			11 (9.4 %)		
Douzenis et al. (2012)	228			34 (14.9 %)		Inpatients
Fagiolini et al. (2005)	171			67 (39.2 %)		
Fenn et al. (2005)	290			94 (32.4 %)		Inpatients mostly BD-I
Fiedorowicz et al. (2008)	166			112 (67.5 %)		2/3 BD-I
Fiedorowicz et al. (2011)	135	MDD	524	38 (28,1 %)	144 (27,5 %)	Epidemiological
Garcia-Portilla et al. (2008)	194			39 (20.1 %)		
Guo et al. (2006)	6,178			1,460 (23,6 %)		Health-care database
Hirschfeld et al. (2003)	2,134	Gen pop	83,224	327 (15.3 %)	10,237 (12,3 %)	Epidemiological
Johannessen et al. (2006)	25,339	Gen pop	113,698	602 (2.4 %)	2,375 (2.1 %)	Nationwide register study; BD diagnosis should had preceded that of hypertension
Kemp et al. (2010)	125			8 (6.4 %)		RCT patients
Kemp et al. (2013)	264			114 (44.0 %)		Lithium Treatment—Moderate-Dose Use Study (LiTMUS)
Kilbourne et al. (2004)	4,310	VA national cohort	3,408,760	1,500 (34.8 %)	1,256,034 (36.8 %)	VA national patient population
Lin et al. (2007)	2,289	Gen pop	16,413	105 (4.6 %)	359 (2.2 %)	All sample underwent appendectomy
McIntyre et al. (2006a)	938	Gen pop	35,848	98 (10.4 %)	5,341 (14.9 %)	Canadian Community Health Survey
McIntyre et al. (2010c)	99			28 (29.7 %)		Euthymic patients, diabetic excluded

(continued)

Table 10.15 (continued)

Study	*N*	Control population	*N*	Prevalence in BD *N*(%)	Prevalence in control *N*%	Comments
Perron et al. (2009)	1,548	Gen pop	41,545	377 (24,3 %)	7,889 (19 %)	National Epidemiologic Survey on Alcohol and Related Conditions (NESARC)
Salvi et al. (2008)	99			42 (40.0 %)		Inpatients
Salvi et al. (2011)	200			106 (53.0 %)		2/3 BD-II
Subramaniam et al. (2013)	88			12 (13.6 %)		BD-I
Weber et al. (2011)	27,054	Gen pop	2,325,247	3,692 (13.6 %)	389,633 (16.8 %)	US hospital discharges
Huang et al. (2009)	41,557	MDD	76 430	5,436 (13.1 %)	7,719 (10.1 %)	Health registry
Ramsey et al. (2010)	58	Gen pop	1,339	15 (25.9 %)	316 (23.6 %)	ECA
Pooled	*145,669*			*21,454 (14.7 %)*		
		Gen pop	*6,837,929*		*1,753,546 (25.6 %)*	
		MDD	*76,954*		*7,863 (10.2 %)*	

MDD major depressive disorder, *Gen pop* general population problematic with only half of them ever having diagnosed metabolic syndrome in their patients and less than three-quarters believing that it poses their patients at a significant health risk (Bauer et al. 2008). Subsequently it is well documented that patients with mental illness in general have significantly less preventive intervention during hospitalization (Briskman et al. 2012). In this frame, it is extremely important to mention that at least some metabolic syndrome cases are due to medication (Sicras-Mainar et al. 2008; Cardenas et al. 2008).

The reported rates concerning the presence of metabolic syndrome in BD patients are shown in detail in Table 10.16. The pooled rates suggest that the metabolic syndrome is present in 29.5 % of BD patients, and this rate is probably similar to the rate reported concerning patients with schizophrenia and double for that in the general population.

10.2.3 Comorbid Vascular Disease

Whether there is a true temporal association between BD and cardiovascular comorbidity is unknown, as is the nature of any such association (Weiner et al. 2011). According to early studies, cardiovascular disease was very common, was appearing at a younger age in BD patients (Slater 1938; Bumke 1928) and was the leading cause of mortality among BD patients (Derby 1933; Alstrom 1942; Tsuang et al. 1980; Weeke et al. 1987; Weeke and Vaeth 1986; Sharma and Markar 1994; Laursen et al. 2007; Osby et al. 2001).

The possible excess cardiovascular mortality associated with schizophrenia and BD in comparison to the general population is attributed in part to an increased risk of the modifiable coronary heart disease risk factors: obesity, smoking, diabetes, hypertension and dyslipidaemia. Antipsychotic medication and possibly other psychotropic medication like antiepileptics and antidepressants can induce weight gain or worsen other metabolic cardiovascular risk factors. Smoking is more common in those with BD, even when compared to other serious mental illnesses (Lasser et al. 2000). BD patients may have limited access to general health care with less opportunity for cardiovascular risk screening and prevention than would be expected in a non-psychiatric population (De Hert et al. 2009). The observations concerning a higher cardiovascular morbidity and mortality in BD patients precede the era of modern pharmacotherapeutics, and thus the twofold risk in these patients should be considered as primary (Weiner et al. 2011). Maybe BD-I patients manifest higher mortality rates due to cardiovascular disease in comparison to BD-II and unipolar depressives (Angst et al. 2002).

10.2.3.1 Heart Disease

The literature suggests that circulatory disease in general has a prevalence of 13–22.7 % in BD patients (Ramsey et al. 2010; Oreski et al. 2012; Beyer et al. 2005) and in the same patients a variety of heart disorders including congestive heart failure, valvular disease and arrhythmias are reported to be more frequent in comparison to the general population (Carney and Jones 2006). More specifically, any

Table 10.16 Rates of the metabolic syndrome in BD patients

Study	*N*	Control population	*N*	Prevalence in BD *N*(%)	Prevalence in control *N*%	Comments
Cardenas et al. (2008)	98			48 (49.0 %)		90 % males
Centorrino et al. (2009)	28,531	Gen pop	85,593	105 (0.37 %)	136 (0.2 %)	Health-care data
Chang et al. (2009)	117			20 (17.1 %)		
Correll et al. (2008)	74	Schizophrenia	111	32 (43.2 %)	51 (45.9 %)	
Fagiolini et al. (2005)	171			51 (29.8 %)		
Fiedorowicz et al. (2008)	125			45 (36.0 %)		2/3 BD-I pts
Garcia-Portilla et al. (2008)	194			39 (20.1 %)		
John et al. (2009)	39	Schizophrenia	92	26 (66.6 %)	47 (51.1 %)	
Kemp et al. (2010)	125			45 (36.0 %)		RCT pts
Kemp et al. (2013)	264			79 (29.9 %)		Lithium Treatment—Moderate-Dose Use Study (LiTMUS) study
McIntyre et al. (2010c)	99			31 (32.6 %)		Euthymic pts, diabetic excluded
Salvi et al. (2008)	99			25 (25.3 %)		Inpatients
Salvi et al. (2011)	200			53 (26.5 %)		2/3 BD-II pts
Sicras et al. (2008)	178	Gen pop	85,850	44 (24.7 %)	12,362 (14.4 %)	Health-care database
van Winkel et al. (2008a)	60			10 (16.7 %)		
van Winkel et al. (2008b)	112	Schizophrenia	503	26 (23.2 %)	145 (28.8 %)	
Vuksan-Cusa et al. (2009)	40			11 (27.5 %)		
Yumru et al. (2007)	125			40 (32 %)		BD-I Health-care database
Pooled	*2,120*			*625 (29.5 %)*		
		Gen pop	*85,850*		*12,362 (14.4 %)*	
		Schiz	*614*		*196 (31.9 %)*	

Schiz schizophrenia, *Gen pop* general population

cardiovascular disease is reported to affect 2.7–48.6 % (Beyer et al. 2005; Fenn et al. 2005; Fiedorowicz et al. 2011; Guo et al. 2006; Kemp et al. 2013; Magalhaes et al. 2012; McIntyre et al. 2006a; Oreski et al. 2012; Perron et al. 2009; Ramsey et al. 2010; Subramaniam et al. 2013; Thompson et al. 2006), arrhythmias 2.8–17.9 % (Carney and Jones 2006; Fenn et al. 2005; Perron et al. 2009), congestive heart failure 0.5–4.9 % (Carney and Jones 2006; Kilbourne et al. 2004; Laursen et al. 2011; Ramsey et al. 2010; Strakowski et al. 1992), ischaemic heart disease 0.4–18 % (Ramsey et al. 2010; Huang et al. 2009; Carney and Jones 2006; Guo et al. 2006; Fiedorowicz et al. 2011; Centorrino et al. 2009; Fenn et al. 2005; Kilbourne et al. 2004; Laursen et al. 2011; Perron et al. 2009) and peripheral vascular disease 0.3–2.9 % of BD patients (Kilbourne et al. 2004; Laursen et al. 2011; Carney and Jones 2006).

Reversely, hospital registries suggest that approximately 2 % of hospitalized patients with acute myocardial infarction also suffer from BD (Abrams et al. 2009). Vascular risks factors were greater and current cholesterol levels higher in the late-onset group (Cassidy and Carroll 2002). Controlling for behavioural factors diminished, but did not eliminate, the impact of heart disease on mortality in BD patients (Kilbourne et al. 2009a). It is interesting that while cardiovascular morbidity might be similar to the general population, mortality is several times higher (Laursen et al. 2009).

The reported rates concerning the presence of cardiovascular disease in BD patients are shown in detail in Table 10.17. The pooled rates suggest that any cardiovascular disease is present in 7.6 % of BD patients, and this rate is probably similar to the rate reported concerning patients with schizophrenia and unipolar depression and double of that in the general population. Arrhythmia is present in 7.5 % of BD patients, and this rate is several times higher than the respective in the general population. On the contrary, congestive heart failure is present at a lower rate in comparison to the general population (1.5 % vs. 2.5 %). The pooled rate for the ischaemic heart disease is 3.3 % of BD patients and is probably several times higher than the reported rate in the general population.

10.2.4 Comorbid Neurological Conditions

Any neurological condition is diagnosed from 10.7 % cross-sectionally to 37.9 % lifetime in BD-I inpatients (Fattal et al. 2007; Beyer et al. 2005; Fenn et al. 2005). There is a variety of neurological syndromes which have been reported to coexist with BD, but the rates depend on the quality and composition of the study sample (Beyer et al. 2005; Kemp et al. 2013; Magalhaes et al. 2012; Oreski et al. 2012; Strakowski et al. 1992; Carney and Jones 2006; Subramaniam et al. 2013; Carta et al. 2012; Shanmugiah et al. 2008; Weber et al. 2011).

The rate of headache is probably similar to that seen in the general population (Kilbourne et al. 2004), but in BD-I the rate is reported to be as high as 20–25 % and four times higher in comparison to other patient groups (Carney and Jones 2006; Thompson et al. 2006). In BD-I inpatients, the rate of head trauma is 1 %

Table 10.17 Rates of cardiovascular disease in BD patients

Study	*N*	Control population	*N*	Prevalence in BD *N*(%)	Prevalence in control *N*%	Comments
Any cardiovascular disease						
Beyer et al. (2005)	1,379			179 (13.0 %)		Duke University Medical Center outpatient clinical database, 2/3 manic and 1/3 depressed pts
Fenn et al. (2005)	290			141 (48.6 %)		Inpatients, mostly BD-I, lifetime rate
Fenn et al. (2005)	290			101 (34.8 %)		Inpatients mostly BD-I, cross-sectional rate
Fiedorowicz et al. (2011)	135	MDD	524	12 (8,9 %)	57 (10,9 %)	Epidemiological data
Guo et al. (2006)	6,178			189 (3,1 %)		Health-care database
Kemp et al. (2013)	264			30 (11.4 %)		Lithium Treatment—Moderate-Dose Use Study (LiTMUS), any heart disease
Kemp et al. (2013)	261			44 (16.9 %)		Lithium Treatment—Moderate-Dose Use Study (LiTMUS), any cardiovascular disease
Magalhaes et al. (2012)	3,399			398 (11.7 %)		STEP-BD
McIntyre et al. (2006a)	938	Gen pop	35,848	41 (4.4 %)	1,936 (5.4 %)	Canadian Community Health Survey
Oreski et al. (2012)	97	Schiz	192	22 (22.7 %)	14 (7.3 %)	Inpatient records
Perron et al. (2009)	1,548	Gen pop	41,545	41 (2.7 %)	785 (1.9 %)	National Epidemiologic Survey on Alcohol and Related Conditions (NESARC)
Ramsey et al. (2010)	58	Gen pop	1,339	5 (8.6 %)	57 (4.3 %)	ECA
Subramaniam et al. (2013)	88			6 (6.8 %)		BD-I pts
Thompson et al. (2006)	174			32 (18.4 %)		BD-I pts
Pooled	*14,545*			*1,110 (7.6 %)*		
		Gen pop	*78,732*		*2,778 (3.5 %)*	

Arrhythmias						
Carney and Jones (2006)	3,557	In- and outpatients	726,262	116 (3.3 %)	8,740 (1.2 %)	BD-I pts, Wellmark Blue Cross/Blue Shield (BC/BS) of Iowa administrative claims data
Fenn et al. (2005)	290			8 (2.8 %)		Inpatients, mostly BD-I pts, cross-sectional
Fenn et al. (2005)	290			11 (3.8 %)		Inpatients, mostly BD-I pts, lifetime
Perron et al. (2009)	1,548	Gen pop	41,545	277 (17.9 %)	2,368 (5.7 %)	National Epidemiologic Survey on Alcohol and Related Conditions (NESARC)
Pooled	*5,395*			*404 (7.5 %)*		
		Gen pop	*767,807*		*12,108 (1.6 %)*	
Congestive heart failure						
Carney and Jones (2006)	3,557	In- and outpatients	726,262	43 (1.2 %)	3,117 (0.4 %)	BD-I Wellmark Blue Cross/Blue Shield (BC/BS) of Iowa administrative claims data
Kilbourne et al. (2004)	4,310	VA national cohort	3,408,760	136 (3.2 %)	161,171 (4.7 %)	VA national patient population
Laursen et al. (2011)	6,215	Gen pop	2,428,518	28 (0.5 %)	3,065 (0.1 %)	Population-based cohort study
Ramsey et al. (2010)	58	Gen pop	1,339	1 (1.7 %)	9 (6.7 %)	ECA
Strakowski et al. (1992)	41			2 (4.9 %)		First-episode acute mania
Pooled	*14,181*			*210 (1.5 %)*		
		Gen pop	*6,564,879*		*167,362 (2.5 %)*	

(continued)

Table 10.17 (continued)

Study	*N*	Control population	*N*	Prevalence in BD *N*(%)	Prevalence in control *N*%	Comments
Ischaemic heart disease						
Carney and Jones (2006)	3,557	In- and outpatients	726,262	135 (3.8 %)	13,567 (1.9 %)	BD-I, Wellmark Blue Cross/Blue Shield (BC/BS) of Iowa administrative claims data
Centorrino et al. (2009)	28,531	Gen pop	85,593	670 (2.3 %)	893 (1.0 %)	Health-care data
Fenn et al. (2005)	290			28 (9.7 %)		Inpatients mostly BD-I pts, coronary artery disease, cross-sectional
Fenn et al. (2005)	290			35 (12.1 %)		Inpatients mostly BD-I pts, coronary artery disease, cross-sectional, lifetime
Fenn et al. (2005)	290			6 (2.1 %)		Inpatients mostly BD-I pts, in process to establish coronary artery disease, cross-sectional
Fenn et al. (2005)	290			11 (3.8 %)		Inpatients mostly BD-I pts, coronary artery disease, lifetime
Guo et al. (2006)	6,178			40 (0,6 %)		Health-care database
Huang et al. (2009)	41,557	MDD	76,430	1,434 (3.5 %)	2,232 (2.9 %)	Health registry
Kilbourne et al. (2004)	4,310	VA national cohort	3,408,760	455 (10.6 %)	560,626 (16.4 %)	VA national patient population
Laursen et al. (2011)	6,215	Gen pop	2,428,518	23 (0.4 %)	6,156 (0.3 %)	Population-based cohort study
Perron et al. (2009)	1,548	Gen pop	41,545	278 (18 %)	2,381 (5,7 %)	National Epidemiologic Survey on Alcohol and Related Conditions (NESARC)
Perron et al. (2009)	1,548	Gen pop	41,545	18 (1.2 %)	386 (0,9 %)	National Epidemiologic Survey on Alcohol and Related Conditions (NESARC)

Ramsey et al. (2010)	58	Gen pop	1,339	4 (6.9 %)	50 (3.7 %)	ECA
Pooled	*93,792*			*3,092 (3.3 %)*		
		Gen pop	*2,682,969*		*9,866 (0.4 %)*	
Peripheral vascular disease						
Kilbourne et al. (2004)	4,310	VA national cohort	3,408,760	126 (2.9 %)	132,153 (3.9 %)	VA national patient population
Laursen et al. (2011)	6,215	Gen pop	2,428,518	18 (0.3 %)	7,443 (0.3 %)	Population-based cohort study
Carney and Jones (2006)	3,557	In- and outpatients	726,262	42 (1.2 %)	2,519 (0.4 %)	BD-I
						Wellmark Blue Cross/Blue Shield (BC/BS) of Iowa administrative claims data
Various cardiovascular disorders						
Carney and Jones (2006)	3,557	In- and outpatients	726,262	2 (0.1 %)	426 (0.1 %)	BD-I
						Pulmonary circulation dis, Wellmark Blue Cross/Blue Shield (BC/BS) of Iowa administrative claims data
Carney and Jones (2006)	3,557	In- and outpatients	726,262	68 (1.9 %)	5,517 (0.8 %)	BD-I
						Valvular disease current
						Wellmark Blue Cross/Blue Shield (BC/BS) of Iowa administrative claims data

Schiz schizophrenia, *MDD* major depressive disorder, *Gen pop* general population cross-sectionally and 7.6 % lifetime (Fenn et al. 2005). The rate of dementia is similar to that of the general population concerning Alzheimer's disease but double concerning other dementias, probably because of the higher prevalence of cardiovascular risk factors in BD patients (Kilbourne et al. 2004; Laursen et al. 2011). High rates of locomotor disorder and Parkinson's disease have also been reported, but the data are limited (Oreski et al. 2012; Weber et al. 2011; Kilbourne et al. 2004).

One of the most frequent findings in brain MRI scan of BD patients is white matter hyperintensities. Their role in the aetiopathogenesis of BD is not well understood. They do not seem to constitute a primary risk factor or endophenotype for BD, and probably they reflect the presence of medical comorbidities (e.g. migraine, cerebrovascular disease, multiple sclerosis, etc.) (Gunde et al. 2011; Ahearn et al. 1998; Iacovides and Andreoulakis 2011).

10.2.4.1 Stroke

Stroke is a vascular disease, and thus it is expected to manifest increased rates in BD patients, since they also manifest higher rates of several risk factors for the development of any vascular disease. The literature concerning stroke in BD patients is limited; however, the reported rates so far are more or less similar to those of the general population. Cross-sectionally, 0.2–1.9 % of BD patients suffer from stroke (Kilbourne et al. 2004; Fenn et al. 2005; Carney and Jones 2006; Laursen et al. 2011), and the lifetime prevalence is reported to be equal to 2.8 % (Fenn et al. 2005). However, it is obvious that these rates significantly depend on the composition of the sample and conclusions are difficult. The list of published studies with stroke rates in BD patients are shown in Table 10.18.

10.2.4.2 Migraine

Migraine is a very common disorder, affecting probably 15 % of the population, with female rates being double than those of males (Vos et al. 2012). It is considered to be a neurovascular disorder (Bartleson and Cutrer 2010), and it is characterized by the recurrence of painful and non-painful episodic phenomena and a variety of neurological manifestations. It is chronic in the sense that acute episodes tend to recur and have a significant global burden on the whole life of the patient. Migraine is considered to be a highly heterogenous disease both in terms of pathophysiology as well as in terms of resulting disability. In most cases, it occurs with a multifactorial inherited character and with a significant association to other neurological diseases (e.g. epilepsy, cerebrovascular disorders and stroke, mitochondrial diseases), cardiovascular disorders and especially mental disorders (anxiety, mood and personality disorders). It is interesting to note that the comorbid presence of hypertension and mental disorders often facilitates changes in the migraine pattern, changing it from an episodic towards a chronic character (Lipton 2009; Radat and Swendsen 2005). Typically, migraine is thought to correlate with certain personality features like perfectionism, neuroticism, repressed aggression and depression; however, the cause and effect of this relationship remains elusive.

The relationship of migraine with mood disorders has been extensively studied, but depression has been the dominant focus. Probably bipolar cases have been

Table 10.18 Rates of stroke in BD patients

Study	*N*	Control population	*N*	Prevalence in BD *N*(%)	Prevalence in control *N*%	Comments
Kilbourne et al. (2004)	4,310	VA national cohort	3,408,760	73 (1.7 %)	72,793 (2.1 %)	VA national patient population
Fenn et al. (2005)	290			4 (1.4 %)		Inpatients mostly BD-I
Carney and Jones (2006)	3,557	In- and outpatients	726,262	66 (1.9 %)	3,187 (0.4 %)	BD-I, Wellmark Blue Cross/Blue Shield (BC/BS) of Iowa administrative claims data
Laursen et al. (2011)	6,215	Gen pop	2,428,518	15 (0.2 %)	2,054 (0.1 %)	Population-based cohort study
Fenn et al. (2005)	290			8 (2.8 %)		Inpatients mostly BD-I, lifetime rate

Gen pop general population

included in depressive samples, but these studies cannot give information concerning BD. Migraine with aura has been reported to correlate more robustly with psychiatric comorbidity in comparison to migraine without aura, and this seems to concern also comorbidity with BD (Radat and Swendsen 2005; Ortiz et al. 2010). However, the findings to support a link between migraine and BD are inconsistent. The literature suggests the rate of BD in migraine patients ranges from 5 to 10 % (Antonaci et al. 2011; Breslau et al. 1991, 1994; Baskin and Smitherman 2009). The literature is conflicting with some studies reporting no association at all (Swartz et al. 2000), while others report a significant correlation with migraine patients manifesting several times higher rates of BD in comparison to the general population and probably around 17 % (Holland et al. 2011; Chen et al. 2012; Jette et al. 2008; Ratcliffe et al. 2009; Hamelsky and Lipton 2006; Merikangas et al. 1990; Breslau 1998). In patients with migraine, the prevailing type of bipolar illness is BD-II, probably accompanied by high levels of anxiety (Fasmer and Oedegaard 2001; Fasmer 2001; Ortiz et al. 2010).

In patients with BD, the rate of migraine is reported to be 4.7–76.9 % (Blehar et al. 1998; Cassidy et al. 1957; Hirschfeld et al. 2003; Holland et al. 2011; Kemp et al. 2013; Marchesi et al. 1989; McIntyre et al. 2006a, b; Nguyen and Low 2013; Ortiz et al. 2010; Ratcliffe et al. 2009; Weber et al. 2011; Calabrese et al. 2003; Fasmer 2001; Low et al. 2003; Mahmood et al. 1999).

It seems that in the vast majority of patients the onset of migraine precedes that of BD (Ortiz et al. 2010). In BD patients, the type of BD plays a role also, with very low rates for BD-I (<20 %) and around 1/3–3/4 of BD-II patients manifesting migraine sometime in their lives (Low et al. 2003; Fasmer 2001; Ortiz et al. 2010).

It has been reported that the clinical and family history characteristics of unipolar depressed patients with migraine resemble those of BD-II and therefore the presence of migraine should be considered to be a bipolar feature when seen in unipolar patients (Oedegaard and Fasmer 2005).

The list of studies reporting the rates of migraine in BD patients is shown in Table 10.19. The pooled rate is 6.3 % and seems to be fivefold higher from the rate of migraine reported in the general population.

10.2.4.3 Epilepsy

Epilepsy is considered to relate to psychosis, but comorbidity rates are not accurately known. Patients with epilepsy are reported to be at a two- to sixfold higher risk to manifest BD (Ottman et al. 2011; Ettinger et al. 2005; de Oliveira et al. 2010; Clarke et al. 2012; Adelow et al. 2012; Mula et al. 2009) although there are reports suggesting that BD in epileptic patients has a rate similar to that seen in the general population (Harden and Goldstein 2002; Mula et al. 2008b).

In patients with BD, the lifetime rates of epilepsy is 4.9–8.3 % (Hirschfeld et al. 2003; Fenn et al. 2005), and it is higher than cross-sectional rates which are reported to range between 0.5 % and 4.1 % (Kemp et al. 2013; Oreski et al. 2012; Weber et al. 2011; Fenn et al. 2005; Strakowski et al. 1992).

The nature of this comorbidity is elusive. Often, interictal manic symptoms are reportedly in people with epilepsy (Barry 2003), and some of the symptoms

Table 10.19 Rates of migraine in BD patients

Study	*N*	Control population	*N*	Prevalence in BD *N*(%)	Prevalence in control *N*%	Comments
Blehar et al. (1998)	327			69 (21.1 %)		
Calabrese et al. (2003)	1,167	Gen pop	1,283	280 (24.0 %)	141 (11.0 %)	
Cassidy et al. (1957)	100			49 (49.0 %)		
Fasmer (2001)	14	MDD	35	2 (1.42 %)	16 (45.7 %)	BD-I inpatients
Fasmer (2001)	13	MDD	35	10 (76.9 %)	16 (45.7 %)	BD-II inpatients
Hirschfeld et al. (2003)	2,134	Gen pop	83,224	499 (23.4 %)	8,406 (10.1 %)	Epidemiological data
Holland et al. (2011)	169			8 (4.7 %)		
Kemp et al. (2013)	261			64 (24.5 %)		Lithium Treatment—Moderate-Dose Use Study (LiTMUS)
Low et al. (2003)	108			43 (39.8 %)		
Mahmood et al. (1999)	81			21 (25.9 %)		
Marchesi et al. (1989)	30			6 (20.0 %)		
McIntyre et al. (2006b)	1,054			79 (7.5 %)		Canadian Community Health Survey
McIntyre et al. (2006a, b)	938	Gen pop	36,046	233 (24.8 %)	3,713 (10.3 %)	Canadian Community Health Survey
Nguyen and Low (2013)	888	Gen pop	32,102	216 (24.3 %)	2,985 (9.3 %)	Canadian Community Health Survey
Ortiz et al. (2010)	323			79 (24.5 %)		2/3 BD-I pts
Ratcliffe et al. (2009)	40			11 (27.5 %)		Epidemiological data
Weber et al. (2011)	27,054	Gen pop	2,325,247	530 (1.9 %)	16,383 (0.7 %)	US hospital discharges between 1979 and 2006
Pooled	*34,701*			*2,199 (6.3 %)*		
		Gen pop	*2,477,902*		*31,628 (1.3 %)*	

Gen pop general population

attributed to a distinct 'epileptic personality' may be attributable to features of a BD. While more than 10 % of epileptic patients might fulfil some type of BD diagnostic criteria, less than 2 % can be considered to suffer from 'real' BD since in most cases, bipolar symptoms are related to phenotype copies of BD (e.g. peri-ictal manifestations or the forced normalization phenomenon) or they represent treatment-emergent adverse effects or even surgery complications (Mula 2010; Mula et al. 2008b).

The list of studies reporting the rates of epilepsy in BD patients is shown in Table 10.20. The pooled rate is 0.9 % and seems to be double in comparison to the rate of epilepsy reported in the general population, but maybe lower to the rate reported in patients with schizophrenia.

10.2.5 Infectious Diseases

10.2.5.1 Hepatitis B and C (HCV)

Hepatitis B is reported to affect 4.5 % of BD patients during lifetime (Fenn et al. 2005).

Patients with HCV are 1.5 times more likely to suffer also from BD in comparison to controls (Butt et al. 2006). Similarly BD patients seems to suffer more frequently from HCV although the rates reported are confusing and range widely from 1.9 to 58.9 % (Kemp et al. 2013; Weber et al. 2011; Fenn et al. 2005; Kilbourne et al. 2004; Beyer et al. 2005; Matthews et al. 2008). The pooled rate for HCV is 10.1 % and is almost tenfold higher in comparison to the general population rate (Table 10.21).

10.2.5.2 Human Immunodeficiency Virus (HIV)

The rate of HIV infection in BD patients is reported to be 0.1–2.8 % (Beyer et al. 2005, 2007; Fenn et al. 2005; Laursen et al. 2011; Carney and Jones 2006; Kilbourne et al. 2004). This is higher than the respected rate of the general population. Reversely, in patients with HIV, BD is diagnosed in 8.1 % and this is up to fourtimes higher than the rate observed in the general population. Two-thirds of BD patients (4–5 %) were reported to suffer from BD-I (de Sousa Gurgel et al. 2013; Kilbourne et al. 2001; Lyketsos et al. 1993). It is encouraging that maybe patients with AIDS and comorbid psychiatric disorders might receive better care than expected (Goulet et al. 2000); however, often they fail to seek help early in the course of the disease and might manifest more often dementia (Lyketsos et al. 1993). Overall, the comorbidity of BD with HIV is related with poor adherence and worse outcome (Badiee et al. 2012).

The pooled rate for HIV infection in BD patients is 0.7 %, and it is similar to that reported in unipolar depressed patients but several times higher from that reported in the general population (Table 10.21).

The relationship of BD with hepatitis and HIV infection exists probably because of the high prevalence of risk-taking behaviours in BD patients, especially concerning sexual activity and substance abuse. Not only it is reported that the

Table 10.20 Rates of epilepsy in BD patients

Study	Control population	*N*	Prevalence in BD *N*(%)	Prevalence in control *N*%	*N*	Comments
Fenn et al. (2005)			12 (4.1 %)		290	Inpatients mostly BD-I current
Fenn et al. (2005)			24 (8.3 %)		290	Inpatients mostly BD-I, lifetime
Hirschfeld et al. (2003)	Gen pop	83,224	105 (4.9 %)	999 (1.2 %)	2,134	Epidemiological, lifetime
Kemp et al. (2013)			8 (3.1 %)		258	Lithium Treatment—Moderate-Dose Use Study (LiTMUS)
Oreski et al. (2012)	Schiz	192	1 (1.0 %)	8 (4.2 %)	97	Inpatient records
Strakowski et al. (1992)			1 (2.4 %)		41	Temp lobe epilepsy, first-episode mania
Weber et al. (2011)	Gen pop	2,325,247	136 (0.5 %)	9,133 (3.9 %)	27,054	US hospital discharges between 1979 and 2006
Pooled			*275 (0.9 %)*		*29,874*	
	Gen pop	*2,408,471*		*10,132 (0.4 %)*		

Gen pop general population

Table 10.21 Rates of hepatitis B and C and HIV infection in BD patients

Study	*N*	Control population	*N*	Prevalence in BD *N*(%)	Prevalence in control *N*%	Comments
Hepatitis B						
Fenn et al. (2005)	290			9 (3.1 %)		Inpatients mostly BD-I, hepatitis B, cross-sectional rate
Fenn et al. (2005)	290			13 (4.5 %)		Inpatients mostly BD-I, hepatitis B, lifetime rate
Hepatitis C						
Beyer et al. (2005)	1,379			26 (1.9 %)		BD-I pts, Duke University Medical Center outpatient clinical database, 2/3 manic and 1/3 depressed, hepatitis C, cross-sectional rate
Fenn et al. (2005)	290			39 (13.4 %)		Inpatients mostly BD-I, hepatitis C, cross-sectional rate
Fenn et al. (2005)	290			45 (15.5 %)		Inpatients mostly BD-I, hepatitis C, lifetime rate
Kemp et al. (2013)	262			11 (4.2 %)		Lithium Treatmcnt—Moderate-Dose Use Study (LiTMUS)
Kilbourne et al. (2004)	4,310	VA national cohort	3,408,760	252 (5.8 %)	38,312 (1.1 %)	VA national patient population, hepatitis C, cross-sectional study
Matthews et al. (2008)	5,026	MDD	4,724	3,006 (59.8 %)	3,860 (81.7 %)	VISN 20 Consumer Health Information and Performance Sets (CHIPS) Data Warehouse
Weber et al. (2011)	27,054	Gen pop	2,325,247	553 (2.0 %)	23,397 (1.0 %)	US hospital discharges between 1979 and 2006
Pooled	*38,321*			*3,893 (10.1 %)*		
			5,734,007		*61,709 (1.1 %)*	

HIV						
Beyer et al. (2005)	1,379			39 (2.8 %)		BD-I pts, Duke University Medical Center outpatient clinical database, 2/3 manic and 1/3 depressed pts
Beyer et al. (2007)	1,213	MDD	5,621	32 (2.6 %)	79 (1.4 %)	Outpatients
Carney and Jones (2006)	3,557	In- and outpatients	726,262	5 (0.1)	99 (0.0)	Wellmark Blue Cross/Blue Shield (BC/BS) of Iowa administrative claims data, BD-I pts
Fenn et al. (2005)	290			4 (1.4 %)		Inpatients mostly BD-I, cross-sectional rate
Fenn et al. (2005)	290			5 (1.7 %)		Inpatients, mostly BD-I, lifetime rate
Kilbourne et al. (2004)	4,310	VA national cohort	3,408,760	35 (0.8 %)	18,364 (0.5 %)	VA national patient population
Laursen et al. (2011)	6,215	Gen pop	2,428,518	3 (0.0 %)	901 (0.0 %)	Population-based cohort study
Pooled	*17,254*			*123 (0.7 %)*		
			6,563,540		*19,364 (0.0 %)*	

Gen pop general population, *MDD* major depressive disorder coexistence of substance abuse raises the rate dramatically (Beyer et al. 2007), but even more, substance abuse might be the crucial factor without the existence of an independent association between serious mental illness and the risk of HIV infection (Prince et al. 2012).

10.2.6 Cancer

The rates for any cancer in BD patients range from 0.2 to 7.5 % (Kilbourne et al. 2004; Kemp et al. 2013; Magalhaes et al. 2012; McGinty et al. 2012; Oreski et al. 2012; McIntyre et al. 2006a; Beyer et al. 2005; Laursen et al. 2011; Carney and Jones 2006). They seem to concern all organ systems (Carney and Jones 2006), and no racial differences are evident (McGinty et al. 2012). The various rates for specific types vary from negligible concerning leukaemia to 2.5 % for breast cancer (Laursen et al. 2011; McGinty et al. 2012; Kilbourne et al. 2004; Carney and Jones 2006; Fenn et al. 2005).

The list of studies with cancer rates in BD are shown in Table 10.22. The pooled rate for any cancer in BD is 1.8 %, and it is 1.5-fold higher than that observed in the general population and similar to that seen in patients with schizophrenia. Prostate cancer has a pooled rate of 1.4 %, while the rates of other specific cancers are shown in Table 10.22.

Overall the literature suggests that BD patients are roughly in a double risk of developing cancer in comparison to the general population. Probably this is because several risk factors for cancer are disproportionately prevalent in BD patients. The high rates of smoking, low rates of childbearing, increased prolactin levels, the sedentary lifestyle, the diet high in fat and low in fruits and vegetables as well as other risk factors could be the main reason for the increase in cancer rates in BD patients.

10.2.7 Endocrinological Disorders

Any endocrinological disorder is seen in 13.6–28.6 % of BD patients (Fenn et al. 2005; Beyer et al. 2005; Kemp et al. 2013; Oreski et al. 2012). The major problem concerns the thyroid gland, probably not only because of treatment with lithium. Any thyroid disorder is seen in 6.5–15.1 % of BD patients (Kemp et al. 2013; Oreski et al. 2012; Thompson et al. 2006; Magalhaes et al. 2012; McIntyre et al. 2006a; Kilbourne et al. 2004; Krishnan 2005). Hypothyroidism is seen in 0.3–9.2 % (Valle et al. 1999; Fenn et al. 2005), while hypothyroidism in 2.4–13 % of BD patients (Strakowski et al. 1992; Valle et al. 1999; Weber et al. 2011; Carney and Jones 2006; Fenn et al. 2005). Endocrinological disorders and especially hypothyroidism might adversely influence the outcome of BD.

The rates of endocrinological disorders are shown in Table 10.23. The pooled rates suggest that any endocrinological disorder is seen in 17.6 %. Any thyroid disorder is seen in 10.2 % of BD patients, and this rate is very much higher than the respected in the general population and double of that reported in schizophrenia.

Table 10.22 Rates of cancer in BD patients

Study	*N*	Control population	*N*	Prevalence in BD *N*(%)	Prevalence in control *N*%	Comments
Any cancer						
Beyer et al. (2005)	1,379			39 (2.8 %)		BD-I, Duke University Medical Center outpatient clinical database, 2/3 manic and 1/3 depressed, cross-sectional
Carney and Jones (2006)	3,557	In- and outpatients	726,262	21 (0.6)	2,994 (0.4 %)	BD-I, Wellmark Blue Cross/Blue Shield (BC/BS) of Iowa administrative claims data, metastatic cancer, cross-sectional rates
Carney and Jones (2006)	3,557	In- and outpatients	726,262	98 (2.8)	12,341 (1.7 %)	BD-I Wellmark Blue Cross/Blue Shield (BC/BS) of Iowa administrative claims, nonmetastatic cancer, cross-sectional rates
Kemp et al. (2013)	261			7 (2.7 %)		Lithium Treatment—Moderate-Dose Use Study (LiTMUS)
Laursen et al. (2011)	6,215	Gen pop	2,428,518	85 (1.4 %)	26,048 (1.1 %)	Population-based cohort study, any cancer, cross-sectional rates
Laursen et al. (2011)	6,215	Gen pop	2,428,518	10 (0.2 %)	4,798 (0.2 %)	Population-based cohort study, metastatic solid tumour, cross-sectional rates
Magalhaes et al. (2012)	3,399			34 (1.0 %)		STEP-BD
McGinty et al. (2012)	1,002			75 (7.5 %)		Maryland Medicaid adult beneficiaries with serious mental illness
McIntyre et al. (2006a)	938	Gen pop	35,848	12 (1.3 %)	717 (2.0 %)	Canadian Community Health Survey, lifetime
Oreski et al. (2012)	97	Schiz	192	5 (5.2 %)	4 (2.1 %)	Inpatient records
Pooled	*20,405*		*3,916,890*	*376 (1.8 %)*		
			3,916,890		*42,100 (1.1 %)*	

(continued)

Table 10.22 (continued)

Study	*N*	Control population	*N*	Prevalence in BD *N*(%)	Prevalence in control *N*%	Comments
Prostate						
Carney and Jones (2006)	3,557	In- and outpatients	726,262	60 (4.3 %)	6,393 (1.9 %)	BD-I, Wellmark Blue Cross/Blue Shield (BC/BS) of Iowa administrative claims data, prostatic benign hyperplasia current
Fenn et al. (2005)	290			2 (0.7 %)		Inpatients mostly BD-I, cross-sectional rate
Fenn et al. (2005)	290			5 (1.7 %)		Inpatients mostly BD-I, lifetime rate
Fenn et al. (2005)	290			14 (4.8 %)		Inpatients mostly BD-I, prostatic benign hyperplasia, cross-sectional
Fenn et al. (2005)	290			22 (7.6 %)		Inpatients mostly BD-I, prostatic benign hypertrophy, lifetime
Kilbourne et al. (2004)	4,310	VA national cohort	3,408,760	68 (1.6 %)	106,195 (3.1 %)	VA national patient population, cross-sectional
Kilbourne et al. (2004)	4,310	VA national cohort	3,408,760	43 (1.0 %)	307,160 (9.0 %)	VA national patient population, prostatic benign hyperplasia, cross-sectional
McGinty et al. (2012)	369			1 (0.3 %)		Maryland Medicaid adult beneficiaries with serious mental illness
Pooled	*5,259*			*76 (1.4 %)*		
Other types						
Laursen et al. (2011)	6,215	Gen pop	2,428,518	2 (0.0 %)	885 (0.0 %)	Population-based cohort study, leukaemia current
McGinty et al. (2012)	633	Schiz		16 (2.5 %)		Maryland Medicaid adult beneficiaries with serious mental illness, the breast
McGinty et al. (2012)	1,002	Schiz		11 (1.1 %)		Maryland Medicaid adult beneficiaries with serious mental illness, the colon

McGinty et al. (2012)	1,002	Schiz		13 (1.3 %)		Maryland Medicaid adult beneficiaries with serious mental illness, the lung
Kilbourne et al. (2004)	4,310	VA national cohort	3,408,760	14 (0.3 %)	29,637 (0.9 %)	VA national patient population, the lung current
Carney and Jones (2006)	3,557	In- and outpatients	726,262	7 (0.2)	1,401 (0.2)	BD-I, Wellmark Blue Cross/Blue Shield (BC/BS) of Iowa administrative claims data, lymphoma current
Laursen et al. (2011)	6,215	Gen pop	2,428,518	5 (0.1 %)	2,195 (0.1 %)	Population-based cohort study, lymphoma current
Kilbourne et al. (2004)	4,310	VA national cohort	3,408,760	50 (1.2 %)	0 (0.0 %)	VA national patient population, skin cancer current

Gen pop general population, *Schiz* schizophrenia

Table 10.23 Rates of endocrinological disorders in BD patients

Study	*N*	Control population	*N*	Prevalence in BD *N*(%)	Prevalence in control *N*%	Comments
Any endocrinological dis						
Beyer et al. (2005)	1,379			187 (13.6 %)		Duke University Medical Center outpatient clinical database, 2/3 manic and 1/3 depressed pts, cross-sectional
Fenn et al. (2005)	290			66 (22.8 %)		Inpatients mostly BD-I cross-sectional
Fenn et al. (2005)	290			83 (28.6 %)		Inpatients mostly BD-I, lifetime
Kemp et al. (2013)	264			66 (25.0 %)		Lithium Treatment—Moderate-Dose Use Study (LiTMUS)
Oreski et al. (2012)	97	Schiz	192	22 (22.7 %)	18 (9.4 %)	Inpatient records
Pooled	*2,030*			*358 (17.6 %)*		
Any thyroid dis						
Kemp et al. (2013)	261			17 (6.5 %)		Lithium Treatment—Moderate-Dose Use Study (LiTMUS)
Kilbourne et al. (2004)	4,310	VA national cohort	3,408,760	303 (7.0 %)	0 (0.0 %)	VA national patient population, cross-sectional
Magalhaes et al. (2012)	3,399			513 (15.1 %)		STEP-BD
McIntyre et al. (2006a)	938	Gen pop	35,848	69 (7.4 %)	2,007 (5.6 %)	Canadian Community Health Survey, lifetime
Oreski et al. (2012)	97	Schiz	192	13 (13.4 %)	13 (6.8 %)	Inpatient records
Thompson et al. (2006)	174			22 (12.6 %)		BD-I pts, cross-sectional
Pooled	*9,179*			*937 (10.2 %)*		
		Gen pop	*3,444,608*		*2,020 (0.1 %)*	

Hyperthyroidism						
Fenn et al. (2005)	290			1 (0.3 %)		Inpatients mostly BD-I, cross-sectional
Fenn et al. (2005)	290			5 (1.7 %)		Inpatients mostly BD-I, lifetime
Valle et al. (1999)	54			5 (9.2 %)		Lithium-naïve pts
Hypothyroidism						
Carney and Jones (2006)	3,557	In- and outpatients	726,262	340 (9.6 %)	18,168 (2.5 %)	BD-I, Wellmark Blue Cross/Blue Shield (BC/BS) of Iowa administrative claims data, cross-sectional
Fenn et al. (2005)	290			29 (10.0 %)		Inpatients mostly BD-I pts, cross-sectional
Fenn et al. (2005)	290			40 (13.8 %)		Inpatients mostly BD-I pts, lifetime
Strakowski et al. (1992)	41			1 (2.4 %)		First-episode manic pts
Valle et al. (1999)	54			5 (9.2 %)		Lithium-naïve pts
Weber et al. (2011)	27,054			1,936 (7.2 %)		US hospital discharges between 1979 and 2006
Pooled	*30,996*			*2,311 (7.5 %)*		

Gen pop general population, *Schiz* schizophrenia

Hypothyroidism is seen in 7.5 % of BD patients, and it is probably much higher than the rate in the general population.

10.2.8 Gastroenterological Disorders

A variety of gastroenterological problems and conditions are reported in BD patients at higher than expected rates. Cross-sectionally 7.3–33.9 % are reported to suffer from any gastroenterological disorder (Beyer et al. 2005; Thompson et al. 2006; Oreski et al. 2012; Fenn et al. 2005), and the respected rate might be around 33 % for lifetime rates (Fenn et al. 2005). Any liver disease is reported in 0.3–21 % (Kemp et al. 2013; Perron et al. 2009; Fenn et al. 2005; Carney and Jones 2006; Fuller et al. 2011; Laursen et al. 2011), cirrhosis (mostly because of alcohol abuse) in 0.9–2.1 % (Perron et al. 2009; Fuller et al. 2011; Fenn et al. 2005), gastritis in 0.3–15 % (Perron et al. 2009; Fenn et al. 2005; Kilbourne et al. 2004) and peptic ulcer in 0.9–22 % (Goodwin et al. 2009; Perron et al. 2009; Subramaniam et al. 2013; McIntyre et al. 2006a; Fenn et al. 2005; Magalhaes et al. 2012; Carney and Jones 2006; Laursen et al. 2011). Other gastroenterological disorders are reported also like Crohn's disease (McIntyre et al. 2006a) and oesophageal varices (Fenn et al. 2005), incontinence (Fenn et al. 2005) and gastrointestinal fluid and electrolyte disorders (Carney and Jones 2006).

A list with the studies reporting the rates of comorbid gastroenterological disorders is shown in Table 10.24. Pooled rates suggest that liver disease is present in 7.5 % of BD patients and this is much higher than the expected in the general population and similar to that seen in schizophrenia. Peptic ulcer is seen in 3.6 % of BD patients, and this rate is seven times higher than that in the general population.

10.2.9 Disorders of the Blood

Any disorder of the blood is seen in 1.5–3.8 % of BD patients (Beyer et al. 2005; Fenn et al. 2005), anaemia of any kind in 0.5–6.4 % (Kemp et al. 2013; Carney and Jones 2006; Kilbourne et al. 2004) and coagulopathy in 1.1 % of BD patients (Carney and Jones 2006).

10.2.10 Respiratory System Disorders

Respiratory disorders are also more prevalent in BD patients in comparison to the general population, and vice versa. In asthma patients, BD has a prevalence of almost 5 % (Goodwin et al. 2003, 2010). In BD patients, a variety of comorbid medical problems of the respiratory system exist. Probably 1–24.1 % of them suffer from any respiratory problem (Laursen et al. 2011; Carney and Jones 2006; Douzenis et al. 2012; Fenn et al. 2005; Beyer et al. 2005; Kemp et al. 2013; Oreski et al. 2012; Thompson et al. 2006; Subramaniam et al. 2013). Asthma is present in

Table 10.24 Rates of gastroenterological disorders in BD patients

Study	*N*	Control population	*N*	Prevalence in BD *N*(%)	Prevalence in control *N*%	Comments
Any gastroenterological dis						
Beyer et al. (2005)	1,379			101 (7.3 %)		Duke University Medical Center outpatient clinical database, BD-I 2/3 manic and 1/3 depressed, cross-sectional rate
Fenn et al. (2005)	290			52 (17.9 %)		Inpatients mostly BD-I, cross-sectional rate
Fenn et al. (2005)	290			114 (39.3 %)		Inpatients mostly BD-I pts, lifetime
Oreski et al. (2012)	97	Schiz	192	16 (16.5 %)	21 (10.9 %)	Inpatient records
Thompson et al. (2006)	174			59 (33.9 %)		BD-I, cross-sectional rate
Cirrhosis						
Fenn et al. (2005)	290			5 (1.7 %)		Inpatients mostly BD-I, alcoholic, cross-sectional rate
Fenn et al. (2005)	290			6 (2.1 %)		Inpatients mostly BD-I, alcoholic, lifetime
Fuller et al. (2011)	5,319	Schiz	6,521	85 (1.6 %)	104 (1.6 %)	VISN 20 Consumer Health Information and Performance Set Data Warehouse, alcohol
Perron et al. (2009)	1,548	Gen pop	41,545	14 (0,9 %)	87 (0,2 %)	National Epidemiologic Survey on Alcohol and Related Conditions (NESARC)
Gastritis						
Fenn et al. (2005)	290			1 (0.3 %)		Inpatients mostly BD-I, gastritis and alcohol, cross-sectional rate

(continued)

Table 10.24 (continued)

Study	*N*	Control population	*N*	Prevalence in BD *N*(%)	Prevalence in control *N*%	Comments
Fenn et al. (2005)	290			2 (0.7 %)		Inpatients mostly BD-I, alcohol and gastritis, lifetime
Kilbourne et al. (2004)	4,310	VA national cohort	3,408,760	284 (6.6 %)	169,721 (5.0 %)	VA national patient population, gastritis, cross-sectional rate
Perron et al. (2009)	1,548	Gen pop	41,545	232 (15.0 %)	2,464 (5,9 %)	National Epidemiologic Survey on Alcohol and Related Conditions (NESARC)
Liver disease						
Carney and Jones (2006)	3,557	In- and outpatients	726,262	39 (1.1 %)	1,281 (0.2 %)	BD-I, Wellmark Blue Cross/Blue Shield (BC/BS) of Iowa administrative claims data, cross-sectional rate
Fenn ct al. (2005)	290			49 (16.9 %)		Inpatients mostly BD-I, cross-sectional rate
Fenn et al. (2005)	290			61 (21.0 %)		Inpatients mostly BD-I pts, lifetime
Fuller et al. (2011)	5,319	Schiz	6,521	1,144 (21.5 %)	1,461 (22.4 %)	VISN 20 Consumer Health Information and Performance Set Data Warehouse
Kemp et al. (2013)	263			10 (3.8 %)		Lithium Treatment—Moderate-Dose Use Study (LiTMUS)
Laursen et al. (2011)	6,215	Gen pop	2,428,518	18 (0.3 %)	1,582 (0.1 %)	Population-based cohort study, cross-sectional rate
Laursen et al. (2011)	6,215	Gen pop	2,428,518	82 (1.3 %)	6,647 (0.3 %)	Population-based cohort study, lifetime rate
Perron et al. (2009)	1,548	Gen pop	41,545	30 (1.9 %)	220 (0.5 %)	National Epidemiologic Survey on Alcohol and Related Conditions (NESARC)

Pooled	*17,192*			*1,290 (7.5 %)*		
		Gen pop	*3,196,325*		*3,083 (0.1 %)*	
Peptic ulcer						
Carney and Jones (2006)	3,557	In- and outpatients	726,262	31 (0.9)	1,515 (0.2)	BD-I pts, Wellmark Blue Cross/ Blue Shield (BC/BS) of Iowa administrative claims data, cross-sectional rate
Fenn et al. (2005)	290			13 (4.5 %)		Inpatients mostly BD-I, cross-sectional rate
Fenn et al. (2005)	290			36 (12.4 %)		Inpatients mostly BD-I pts, lifetime
Goodwin et al. (2009)	1,411			31 (2.2 %)		National Epidemiologic Survey of Alcohol and Related Conditions
Laursen et al. (2011)	6,215	Gen pop	2,428,518	62 (1.0 %)	13,458 (0.6 %)	Population-based cohort study, cross-sectional rate
Magalhaes et al. (2012)	3,399			217 (6.4 %)		STEP-BD
McIntyre et al. (2006a)	938	Gen pop	35,848	101 (10.8 %)	1,398 (3.9 %)	Canadian Community Health Survey, lifetime
Perron et al. (2009)	1,548	Gen pop	41,545	141 (9.1 %)	1,039 (2.5 %)	National Epidemiologic Survey on Alcohol and Related Conditions (NESARC)
Subramaniam et al. (2013)	88			4 (4.5 %)		BD-I pts
Pooled	*17,736*			*636 (3.6 %)*		
		Gen pop	*3,232,173*		*17,410 (0.5 %)*	

(continued)

Table 10.24 (continued)

Study	*N*	Control population	*N*	Prevalence in BD *N*(%)	Prevalence in control *N*%	Comments
Other gastroenterological dis						
Carney and Jones (2006)	3,557	In- and outpatients	726,262	216 (6.1)	7,632 (1.1)	BD-I, Wellmark Blue Cross/Blue Shield (BC/BS) of Iowa administrative claims data, gastrointestinal fluid and electrolyte disorders, cross-sectional rate
Fenn et al. (2005)	290			2 (0.7 %)		Inpatients mostly BD-I, current oesophageal varices
Fenn et al. (2005)	290			3 (1.0 %)		Inpatients mostly BD-I, lifetime, oesophageal varices
Fenn et al. (2005)	290			5 (1.7 %)		Inpatients mostly BD-I, incontinence current
Fenn et al. (2005)	290			8 (2.8 %)		Inpatients mostly BD-I, incontinence, lifetime
McIntyre et al. (2006a)	938	Gen pop	35,848	38 (4.1 %)	968 (2.7 %)	Canadian Community Health Survey, Crohn's disease, lifetime

Gen pop general population, *Schiz* schizophrenia

2.9–18.3 % (Calabrese et al. 2003; Carney and Jones 2006; Fenn et al. 2005; Hirschfeld et al. 2003; Kemp et al. 2013; Kilbourne et al. 2004; McIntyre et al. 2006a; Weber et al. 2011). Chronic obstructive pulmonary disorder (COPD) is present in 2.2–10.6 % (Hirschfeld et al. 2003; Kilbourne et al. 2004; Fenn et al. 2005; Guo et al. 2006; Lin et al. 2007; Beyer et al. 2005). The rate for sleep apnoea is reported to be 1.7 % cross-sectionally and 3.4 % lifetime (Fenn et al. 2005), and chronic bronchitis is found in 7.9 % of BD patients (McIntyre et al. 2006a), pneumonia in 7.3 % (Strakowski et al. 1992) and history of pulmonary embolism in 0.8 % (Strudsholm et al. 2005). In a bipolar spectrum perspective, subjects at high risk for sleep apnoea were reported to have increased scores on measures of both depression and mania, even when sleep items were not counted in the total scores (Soreca et al. 2012).

The list of published studies reporting rates of comorbid respiratory disorders is shown in Table 10.25. The pooled rate of any respiratory disorder is 7 %, more than triple of that seen in the general population. The respected rate for asthma is 7.4 %, three times higher than that of the general population and that of COPD is 5.4 % and probably similar to that of general population.

10.2.11 Various Comorbid Medical Disorders

10.2.11.1 Dermatological Disorders

Any dermatological disorder is seen in 2–13.2 % cross-sectionally (Fenn et al. 2005; Douzenis et al. 2012; Beyer et al. 2005; Thompson et al. 2006) and in 20.3 % of BD patients lifetime (Fenn et al. 2005). Eczema and psoriasis are seen each in 0.5 % of BD patients which is roughly double of what expected in the general population (Weber et al. 2011). From a reverse angle, patients with psoriasis have double rates of BD (1.1 % vs. 0.5 %), in comparison to controls (Han et al. 2011).

The pooled rate concerning any comorbid dermatological disorder is equal to 4.2 % (Table 10.26).

10.2.11.2 Immunological Disorders

There are reports in the literature suggesting the presence of an immune/inflammatory imbalance in BD. Several laboratory findings of inflammatory factors have been reported (Barbosa et al. 2012), and one of the robust findings concerns the rate of positive TPO-Abs, which is almost double in BD patients in comparison to controls. On the basis of this, a twin study suggested there is a fundamental relationship in the aetiopathogenesis of autoimmune thyroiditis and BD (Vonk et al. 2007).

In accord with the above, it has been proposed that a history of autoimmune disorders including Guillain–Barre syndrome, Crohn's disease and autoimmune hepatitis seems to constitute a 'risk factor' for the latter development of BD (Eaton et al. 2010).

In terms of epidemiology, patients with fibromyalgia have extremely high rates of BD, and maybe up to three-quarters of fibromyalgia patients are also suffering from BD (Alciati et al. 2012; Arnold et al. 2006; Carta et al. 2006). The literature on

Table 10.25 Rates of respiratory disorders in BD patients

Study	*N*	Control population	*N*	Prevalence in BD *N*(%)	Prevalence in control *N*%	Comments
Any respiratory dis						
Beyer et al. (2005)	1,379			101 (7.3 %)		Duke University Medical Center outpatient clinical database, 2/3 manic and 1/3 depressed, cross-sectional
Carney and Jones (2006)	3,557	In- and outpatients	726,262	458 (12.9 %)	25,894 (3.6 %)	BD-I, Wellmark Blue Cross/Blue Shield (BC/BS) of Iowa administrative claims data chronic, cross-sectional
Douzenis et al. (2012)	228			16 (7.1 %)		Inpatients, cross-sectional
Fenn et al. (2005)	290			38 (13.1 %)		Inpatients mostly BD-I pts, cross-sectional
Fenn et al. (2005)	290			70 (24.1 %)		Inpatients mostly BD-I pts, lifetime
Kemp et al. (2013)	264			71 (26.9 %)		Lithium Treatment—Moderate-Dose Use Study (LiTMUS)
Laursen et al. (2011)	6,215	Gen pop	2,428,518	126 (2.0 %)	38,653 (1.6 %)	Population-based cohort study, cross-sectional
Oreski et al. (2012)	97	Schiz	192	1 (1.0 %)	8 (4.2 %)	Inpatient records
Subramaniam et al. (2013)	88			13 (14.8 %)		BD-I pts
Thompson et al. (2006)	174			41 (23.6 %)		BD-I pts, cross-sectional
Pooled	*12,292*			*865 (7.0 %)*		
		Gen pop	*3,154,780*		*64,547 (2.0 %)*	
Asthma						
Calabrese et al. (2003)	1,167	Gen pop	1,283	198 (17.0 %)	128 (10.0 %)	Lifetime
Carney and Jones (2006)	3,557	In- and outpatients	726,262	261 (7.3 %)	12,542 (1.7 %)	BD-I, Wellmark Blue Cross/Blue Shield (BC/BS) of Iowa administrative claims data, cross-sectional

Fenn et al. (2005)	290			9 (3.1 %)		Inpatients mostly BD-I, cross-sectional
Fenn et al. (2005)	290			16 (5.5 %)		Inpatients mostly BD-I, lifetime
Hirschfeld et al. (2003)	2,134	Gen pop	83,224	391 (18.3 %)	7,740 (9.3 %)	Epidemiological, lifetime
Kemp et al. (2013)	263			38 (14.4 %)		Lithium Treatment—Moderate-Dose Use Study (LiTMUS)
Kilbourne et al. (2004)	4,310	VA national cohort	3,408,760	127 (2.9 %)	85,278 (2.5 %)	VA national patient population, cross-sectional
McIntyre et al. (2006a)	938	Gen pop	35,848	149 (15.9 %)	2,975 (8.3 %)	Canadian Community Health Survey, lifetime
Weber et al. (2011)	27,054			1,751 (6.7 %)		US hospital discharges between 1979 and 2006
Pooled	*39,713*			*2,924 (7.4 %)*		
		Gen pop	*4,255,377*		*108,663 (2.6 %)*	
COPD						
Beyer et al. (2005)	1,379			84 (6.1 %)		BD-I pts
Fenn et al. (2005)	290			23 (7.9 %)		Inpatients mostly BD-I pts, cross-sectional
Fenn et al. (2005)	290			26 (9.0 %)		Inpatients mostly BD-I pts, lifetime
Guo et al. (2006)	6,178			258 (4.2 %)		Health-care database, cross-sectional
Hirschfeld et al. (2003)	2,134	Gen pop	83,224	47 (2.2 %)	1,248 (1.5 %)	Epidemiological, lifetime
Kilbourne et al. (2004)	4,310	VA national cohort	3,408,760	455 (10.6 %)	318,861 (9.4 %)	VA national patient population, cross-sectional
Lin et al. (2007)	2,289	Gen pop	16,413	23 (1.0 %)	102 (0.6 %)	All sample underwent appendectomy, cross-sectional
Pooled	*16,580*			*890 (5.4 %)*		
		Gen pop	*3,508,397*		*320,211 (9.1 %)*	

(continued)

Table 10.25 (continued)

Study	*N*	Control population	*N*	Prevalence in BD *N*(%)	Prevalence in control *N*%	Comments
Various						
Fenn et al. (2005)	290			5 (1.7 %)		Inpatients mostly BD-I pts, sleep apnoea, cross-sectional
Fenn et al. (2005)	290			10 (3.4 %)		Inpatients mostly BD-I pts, sleep apnoea, lifetime
McIntyre et al. (2006a)	938	Gen pop	35,848	74 (7.9 %)	1,111 (3.1 %)	Canadian Community Health Survey, chronic bronchitis, lifetime
Strakowski et al. (1992)	41			3 (7.3 %)		First-episode manic pts, pneumonia
Strudsholm et al. (2005)	25,834	Gen pop	117,815	214 (0.8 %)	699 (0.6 %)	Danish Psychiatric Central Research Register, pulmonary embolism, lifetime

Gen pop general population, *Schiz* schizophrenia

Table 10.26 Rates of dermatological disorders in BD patients

Study	*N*	Control population	*N*	Prevalence in BD *N*(%)	Prevalence in control *N*%	Comments
Any dermatological dis						
Beyer et al. (2005)	1,379			28 (2.0 %)		BD-I pts, Duke University Medical Center outpatient clinical database, 2/3 manic and 1/3 depressed pts
Douzenis et al. (2012)	228			16 (7.1 %)		Inpatients
Fenn et al. (2005)	290			20 (6.9 %)		Inpatients mostly BD-I, cross-sectional rate
Fenn et al. (2005)	290			59 (20.3 %)		Inpatients mostly BD-I, lifetime rate
Thompson et al. (2006)	174			23 (13.2 %)		BD-I
Pooled	2,071			87 (4.2 %)		
Specific dermatological dis						
Weber et al. (2011)	27,054	Gen pop	2,325,247	144 (0.5 %)	4,427 (0.2 %)	US hospital discharges between 1979 and 2006, eczema
Weber et al. (2011)	27,054	Gen pop	2,325,247	135 (0.5 %)	4,390 (0.2 %)	US hospital discharges between 1979 and 2006, psoriasis

Gen pop general population

comorbidity of BD with various allergies suggest that although the risk of BD in patients with allergies is 1.5–2 in comparison to the normal populations (Patten and Williams 2007), there might be a bias in the methodology of the reported results and the overall comorbidity rate is not different from that seen in the general population, but the presence of BD reduces the chance of correct diagnosis and treatment of allergies (Goodwin et al. 2012). Up to 2.8 % of BD patients also suffer from fibromyalgia and another 3.8 % from chronic fatigue syndrome at some time in their lives, while 2.7 % suffer from rheumatoid arthritis. There rates are two to three times higher to those expected in the general population (McIntyre et al. 2006a; Carney and Jones 2006). A list of studies with rates of comorbid immunological disorders is shown in Table 10.27.

10.2.11.3 Musculoskeletal Disorders

BD could be related to a variety of musculoskeletal disorders since several risk factors leading to them are highly prevalent among BD patients. It is well known that bone metabolism is related to nutritional alterations, polydipsia, smoking and endocrinological disorders including medication-induced hyperprolactinaemia. Lithium, carbamazepine and valproate can also affect bone density (Misra et al. 2004).

Any disorder of the musculoskeletal system is seen in 10.7–49.7 % of BD patients (Thompson et al. 2006; Fenn et al. 2005; Beyer et al. 2005; Kemp et al. 2013). More specifically, it has been reported that 1–30.7 % of BD patients suffer from some type of arthritis cross-sectionally or lifetime (Perron et al. 2009; Weber et al. 2011; Kilbourne et al. 2004; McIntyre et al. 2006a; Carney and Jones 2006; Fenn et al. 2005; Guo et al. 2006). Up to one-quarter of BD patients complain of backache (Carney and Jones 2006; Kilbourne et al. 2004), 13 % report hip problems (Kilbourne et al. 2004), and close to one-third some kind of chronic pain syndrome (Goldstein et al. 2009; Subramaniam et al. 2013). For most of these conditions, the rates are twofold higher than those reported for the general population.

A list of studies with rates of comorbid musculoskeletal disorders is shown in Table 10.28. The pooled rates suggest that any musculoskeletal disorder is present in 16.7 % of BD patients. The pooled rates for arthritis are probably misleading, and the most probable rate is around 14 %, and it is similar to that reported in the general population.

10.2.11.4 Genitourinary Disorders

Any genitourinary disorder is reported in 3.7–24.7 % of BD patients (Kemp et al. 2013; Fenn et al. 2005; Beyer et al. 2005; Thompson et al. 2006). Cross-sectionally, there are reported menstruation problems in 12.8 %, endometriosis in 1.7 %, inflammatory disease of the ovary in 8.1 %, cystitis in 1.3 %, mammary dysplasia in 4.8 % (Carney and Jones 2006), complication of gestational pregnancy and childbirth in 0.4 % (Beyer et al. 2005) and various gynaecologic problems in 2.1 % (Oreski et al. 2012). In patients with polycystic ovary syndrome, the rate of BD is 11.1 %, that is, several times higher than that of the general population (Rassi et al. 2010). The list of studies with specific rates is shown in Table 10.29.

Table 10.27 Rates of immunological disorders in BD patients

Study	*N*	Control population	*N*	Prevalence in BD *N*(%)	Prevalence in control *N*%	Comments
Any autoimmune dis						
Fenn et al. (2005)	290			4 (1.4 %)		Inpatients mostly BD-I, current
Fenn et al. (2005)	290			7 (2.4 %)		Inpatients mostly BD-I, lifetime
Allergies						
Calabrese et al. (2003)	1,167	Gen pop	1,283	490 (42 %)	372 (29.0 %)	Lifetime
Hirschfeld et al. (2003)	2,134	Gen pop	83,224	864 (40.5 %)	22,138 (26.6 %)	Epidemiological, lifetime
Hirschfeld et al. (2003)	2,134	Gen pop	83,224	864 (40.5 %)	22,138 (26.6 %)	Epidemiological
Various autoimmune dis						
McIntyre et al. (2006a)	938	Gen pop	35,848	36 (3.8 %)	394 (1.1 %)	Canadian Community Health Survey, chronic fatigue syndrome, lifetime
McIntyre et al. (2006a)	938	Gen pop	35,848	26 (2.8 %)	502 (1.4 %)	Canadian Community Health Survey, fibromyalgia, lifetime
Carney and Jones (2006)	3,557	In- and outpatients	726,262	97 (2.7)	9,407 (1.3)	BD-I Wellmark Blue Cross/Blue Shield (BC/BS) of Iowa administrative claims data, rheumatoid arthritis, current

Gen pop general population

Table 10.28 Rates of musculoskeletal disorders in BD patients

Study	*N*	Control population	*N*	Prevalence in BD *N*(%)	Prevalence in control *N*%	Comments
Any musculoskeletal dis						BD-I pts, cross-sectional
Beyer et al. (2005)	1,379			141 (10.7 %)		Duke University Medical Center outpatient clinical database, 2/3 manic and 1/3 depressed, cross-sectional
Fenn et al. (2005)	290			68 (23.4 %)		Inpatients mostly BD-I, cross-sectional
Fenn et al. (2005)	290			144 (49.7 %)		Inpatients mostly BD-I, lifetime
Kemp et al. (2013)	264			87 (33.0 %)		Lithium Treatment—Moderate-Dose Use Study (LiTMUS)
Thompson et al. (2006)	174			56 (31.2 %)		
Pooled	*2,107*			*352 (16.7 %)*		
Arthritis						
Carney and Jones (2006)	3,557	In- and outpatients	726,262	200 (5.6)	15,939 (2.2)	BD-I, Wellmark Blue Cross/Blue Shield (BC/BS) of Iowa administrative claims data, cross-sectional
Fenn et al. (2005)	290			33 (11.4 %)		Inpatients mostly BD-I, cross-sectional
Fenn et al. (2005)	290			46 (15.9 %)		Inpatients mostly BD-I, lifetime
Guo et al. (2006)	6,178			200 (3.2 %)		Health-care database, cross-sectional
Kilbourne et al. (2004)	4,310	VA national cohort	3,408,760	677 (15.7 %)	549,603 (16.1 %)	VA national patient population, cross-sectional
McIntyre et al. (2006a)	938	Gen pop	35,848	193 (20.6 %)	6,238 (17.4 %)	Canadian Community Health Survey, lifetime

Perron et al. (2009)	1,548	Gen pop	41,545	476 (30.7 %)	8,691 (20.9 %)	National Epidemiologic Survey on Alcohol and Related Conditions (NESARC)
Weber et al. (2011)	27,054	Gen pop	2,325,247	272 (1.0 %)	13,818 (0.6 %)	US hospital discharges between 1979 and 2006
Various musculoskeletal dis						
Carney and Jones (2006)	3,557	In- and outpatients	726,262	919 (25.8)	96,201 (13.3)	Backache, BD-I, Wellmark Blue Cross/ Blue Shield (BC/BS) of Iowa administrative claims data, cross-sectional
Goldstein et al. (2009)	883	Gen pop	42,210	219 (24.8 %)	5,023 (11.9 %)	National Epidemiologic Survey on Alcohol and Related Conditions
Kilbourne et al. (2004)	4,310	VA national cohort	3,408,760	565 (13.1 %)	0 (0.0 %)	VA national patient population, hip problems, cross-sectional
Kilbourne et al. (2004)	4,310	VA national cohort	3,408,760	10 (0.2 %)	19,855 (0.6 %)	VA national patient population, spinal cord injury, cross-sectional
Kilbourne et al. (2004)	4,310	VA national cohort	3,408,760	663 (15.4 %)	361,868 (10.6 %)	VA national patient population, lower back pain, cross-sectional
Laursen et al. (2011)	6,215	Gen pop	2,428,518	21 (0.3 %)	18,154 (0.7 %)	Population-based cohort study, connective tissue disease, cross-sectional
Subramaniam et al. (2013)	88			25 (28.4 %)		BD-I pts, pain chronic

Gen pop general population

Table 10.29 Rates of genitourinary disorders in BD patients

Study	*N*	Control population	*N*	Prevalence in BD *N*(%)	Prevalence in control *N*%	Comments
Any genitourinary dis						
Beyer et al. (2005)	1,379			51 (3.7 %)		BD-I pts, Duke University Medical Center outpatient clinical database, 2/3 manic and 1/3 depressed, current
Fenn et al. (2005)	290			26 (9.0 %)		Inpatients mostly BD-I, cross-sectional
Fenn et al. (2005)	290			62 (21.4 %)		Inpatients mostly BD-I, lifetime
Kemp et al. (2013)	264			45 (17.0 %)		Lithium Treatment—Moderate-Dose Use Study (LiTMUS)
Thompson et al. (2006)	174			43 (24.7 %)		BD-I pts, cross-sectional
Specific genitourinary dis						
Beyer et al. (2005)	1,379			5 (0.4 %)		BD-I pts, Duke University Medical Center outpatient clinical database, 2/3 manic and 1/3 depressed and complications of pregnancy, childbirth and the puerperium, cross-sectional
Carney and Jones (2006)	3,557	In- and outpatients	726,262	277 (12.8 %)	19,330 (5.1 %)	BD-I pts, Wellmark Blue Cross/Blue Shield (BC/BS) of Iowa administrative claims data, menstruation disorders, cross-sectional
Carney and Jones (2006)	3,557	In- and outpatients	726,262	37 (1.7 %)	2,359 (0.6 %)	BD-I pts, Wellmark Blue Cross/Blue Shield (BC/BS) of Iowa administrative claims data, endometriosis, cross-sectional
Carney and Jones (2006)	3,557	In- and outpatients	726,262	174 (8.1 %)	9,676 (2.5 %)	BD-I pts, Wellmark Blue Cross/Blue Shield (BC/BS) of Iowa administrative claims data, inflammatory disease of the ovary, cross-sectional
Carney and Jones (2006)	3,557	In- and outpatients	726,262	28 (1.3 %)	1,094 (0.3 %)	BD-I pts, Wellmark Blue Cross/Blue Shield (BC/BS) of Iowa administrative claims data, cystitis, cross-sectional
Carney and Jones (2006)	3,557	In- and outpatients	726,262	103 (4.8 %)	11,385 (3.0 %)	BD-I pts, Wellmark Blue Cross/Blue Shield (BC/BS) of Iowa administrative claims data, mammary dysplasia, cross-sectional
Oreski et al. (2012)	97	Schiz	192	2 (2.1 %)	7 (3.6 %)	Inpatient records, gynaecologic disorders

Gen pop general population, *Schiz* schizophrenia

10.2.11.5 Renal Disorders

Renal disorders are important for BD patients since lithium exerts renal toxicity. Any renal disorder is reported to be present in 0.7–6.6 % of BD patients, and probably this is several times higher from what is expected in the general population (Kemp et al. 2013; Fenn et al. 2005; Lin et al. 2007; Laursen et al. 2011). Renal failure is reported cross-sectionally in 0.8–1.3 % of BD patients, and the rate is probably similar to that of the general population (Kilbourne et al. 2004; Carney and Jones 2006). The co-segregation in this family suggests a close proximity between genes for the two disorders. The two known loci of medullary cystic kidney disease are in regions of chromosomes 1 and 16 that have been previously linked to bipolar disorder and schizophrenia. This family may be a useful resource for positional cloning of bipolar candidate genes (Kimmel et al. 2005). The list of studies with specific rates is shown in Table 10.30.

10.2.11.6 Various Other Comorbid Medical Disorders

Various types of accidents and injuries are reported in 11.9–40.9 % of BD patients (Carney and Jones 2006; Kilbourne et al. 2004), otolaryngologic disorders in 9 % cross-sectionally and 23.1 % lifetime (Fenn et al. 2005) and cataract in 1.8 % lifetime (McIntyre et al. 2006a). Any type of pancreatitis is reported in 3.8 % of BD patients cross-sectionally (Kilbourne et al. 2004), infectious aetiology in 0.6 % (Carney and Jones 2006) and alcoholic pancreatitis 0.7 % cross-sectionally and 1.7 % lifetime (Fenn et al. 2005).

Approximately 2.2–3 % of intensive care unit patients suffer also from BD, but this did not seem to increase overall mortality during the next month (Abrams et al. 2010a, b). The rate of BD in systemic lupus erythematosus is reported to be as high as 6 % (Bachen et al. 2009). The list of studies with specific rates is shown in Table 10.31.

10.3 Genetics and Endophenotypes

Comorbidity can be better understood and interpreted by using family studies (Wickramaratne and Weissman 1993), since the pattern of comorbidity seen in families gives important clues on the true relationship between clinical syndromes. In this frame, family studies suggest a genetic relationship between anxiety disorders and BD (Klein and Depue 1985; Dilsaver and White 1986). Some authors suggested that the genetic heterogeneity of BD is the cause of comorbidity with generalized anxiety (MacKinnon et al. 2003a, b) and panic attacks (MacKinnon et al. 1997, 2002; Doughty et al. 2004) and thus they are a core feature of some BD patients rather than comorbid conditions per se. Essentially this means that BD with panic attacks is more or less a separate disorder, since the two clinical pictures tend to appear together in the relatives of BD probands. In previous studies of the National Institute of Mental Health (NIMH) Genetics Initiative Bipolar Disorder Consortium, familial aggregation was described for panic disorder (MacKinnon et al. 1997, 2002), specific phobia and OCD (Potash et al. 2007), but these analyses did not control for different rates of diagnoses among sites or for additional comorbidity

Table 10.30 Rates of renal disorders in BD patients

Study	*N*	Control population	*N*	Prevalence in BD *N*(%)	Prevalence in control *N*%	Comments
Any renal dis						
Fenn et al. (2005)	290			7 (2.4 %)		Inpatients mostly BD-I, cross-sectional
Fenn et al. (2005)	290			19 (6.6 %)		Inpatients mostly BD-I, lifetime
Kemp et al. (2013)	264			6 (2.3 %)		Lithium Treatment—Moderate-Dose Use Study (LiTMUS)
Laursen et al. (2011)	6,215	Gen pop	2,428,518	44 (0.7 %)	6,085 (0.3 %)	Population-based cohort study, cross-sectional
Lin et al. (2007)	2,289	Gen pop	16,413	72 (3.1 %)	76 (0.5 %)	All sample underwent appendectomy, cross-sectional
Renal failure						
Kilbourne et al. (2004)	4,310	VA national cohort	3,408,760	58 (1.3 %)	58,109 (1.7 %)	VA national patient population, cross-sectional
Carney and Jones (2006)	3,557	In- and outpatients	726,262	30 (0.8 %)	1,514 (0.2 %)	BD-I, Wellmark Blue Cross/Blue Shield (BC/BS) of Iowa administrative claims data, cross-sectional

Gen pop general population

Table 10.31 Rates of various medical disorders in BD patients

Study	*N*	Control population	*N*	Prevalence in BD *N*(%)	Prevalence in control *N*%	Comments
Carney and Jones (2006)	3,557	In- and outpatients	726,262	1,453 (40.9)	145,431 (20.0)	BD-I pts, Wellmark Blue Cross/Blue Shield (BC/BS) of Iowa administrative claims data, accidents and injuries, cross-sectional
Carney and Jones (2006)	3,557	In- and outpatients	726,262	21 (0.6 %)	1,058 (0.2 %)	BD-I pts, Wellmark Blue Cross/Blue Shield (BC/BS) of Iowa administrative claims data, pancreatitis viral/infectious, cross-sectional
Fenn et al. (2005)	290			26 (9.0 %)		Inpatients mostly BD-I, otolaryngologic disorders, cross-sectional
Fenn et al. (2005)	290			67 (23.1 %)		Inpatients mostly BD-I, otolaryngologic disorders, lifetime
Fenn et al. (2005)	290			2 (0.7 %)		Inpatients mostly BD-I, alcoholic pancreatitis, cross-sectional
Fenn et al. (2005)	290			5 (1.7 %)		Inpatients mostly BD-I, alcoholic pancreatitis, lifetime
Kilbourne et al. (2004)	4,310	VA national cohort	3,408,760	514 (11.9 %)	0 (0.0 %)	VA national patient population, accidents/injuries, cross-sectional
Kilbourne et al. (2004)	4,310	VA national cohort	3,408,760	162 (3.8 %)	0 (0.0 %)	VA national patient population, pancreatitis, cross-sectional
McIntyre et al. (2006a)	938	Gen pop	35,848	17 (1.8 %)	1,685 (4.7 %)	Canadian Community Health Survey, cataract, lifetime

Gen pop general population

among the anxiety disorders. The data concerning specific phobia are equivocal (Goes et al. 2012). Familial panic attacks seem to increase the likelihood of rapid cycling (MacKinnon et al. 2003b), and this contributes to the possibility there is a separate cluster of patients. Even a genetic link has been proposed (Logue et al. 2009). A similar proposal has been put forwards for anxiety comorbidity in general (Wozniak et al. 2002).

The distribution of trait anxiety scores in the family members and controls based on their genetic proximity to affected individuals, and diagnostic status suggests that trait anxiety could be an endophenotype in these BD-I families (Contreras et al. 2010). In high-risk offspring of BP parents, anxiety syndromes typically precede the onset of mood syndromes (Duffy et al. 2007; Sala et al. 2010) and often persist throughout adulthood (Mantere et al. 2010). Overall the data are still inconclusive on the true relationship of anxiety and BD (Doughty et al. 2004).

There are studies which suggest that there is a strong connection between ADHD and BD and the comorbid condition runs in families, with over 20 % of offspring or BD parents manifesting ADHD. These particular studies included BD patients with a more severe form of the disorder and high comorbidity, and therefore their conclusions might not be generalizable (Chang et al. 2000; Singh et al. 2007; Hirshfeld-Becker et al. 2006; Henin et al. 2005; Birmaher et al. 2009, 2010; Faraone et al. 1997, 2001). If a familial aggregation is accepted, this points towards a developmental neurobiological association between ADHD and BD, going beyond symptomatic similarities (Skirrow et al. 2012). On the other hand, the careful review of all available data across different domains of research suggests that most findings are equivocal concerning the true nature of this comorbidity and this is also reflected in systematic reviews on this issue (Wingo and Ghaemi 2007; Duffy 2012; Skirrow et al. 2012).

Both patients with unipolar depression and with BD, when they have family history of BD, are reported to be at a three- to fourfold higher risk to suffer also from migraine. This might not be the case concerning a family history of unipolar depression (Dilsaver et al. 2009). Epilepsy seems also to aggregate with psychosis in families (Clarke et al. 2012).

It is of extreme interest that antithyroid antibodies seem to manifest a familial aggregation with BD. One study reported that the TPO-Abs were positive in 27 % of the bipolar index twins, 29 % of the monozygotic bipolar co-twins, 27 % of the monozygotic non-bipolar co-twins, 25 % of the dizygotic bipolar co-twins, 17 % of the dizygotic non-bipolar co-twins and 16 % of the control twins. These findings might suggest that a form of autoimmune thyroiditis might be related to BD but more important to the genetic vulnerability to develop the disorder, thus constituting a potential biomarker and endophenotype (Vonk et al. 2007).

References

Abrams TE, Vaughan-Sarrazin M, Rosenthal GE (2009) Psychiatric comorbidity and mortality after acute myocardial infarction. Circ Cardiovasc Qual Outcome 2(3):213–220. doi:10.1161/CIRCOUTCOMES.108.829143, CIRCOUTCOMES.108.829143 [pii]

Abrams TE, Vaughan-Sarrazin M, Rosenthal GE (2010a) Influence of psychiatric comorbidity on surgical mortality. Arch Surg 145(10):947–953. doi:10.1001/archsurg.2010.190, 145/10/947 [pii]

Abrams TE, Vaughan-Sarrazin M, Rosenthal GE (2010b) Preexisting comorbid psychiatric conditions and mortality in nonsurgical intensive care patients. Am J Crit Care 19(3):241–249. doi:10.4037/ajcc2010967, 19/3/241 [pii]

Adelow C, Andersson T, Ahlbom A, Tomson T (2012) Hospitalization for psychiatric disorders before and after onset of unprovoked seizures/epilepsy. Neurology 78(6):396–401. doi:10.1212/WNL.0b013e318245f461, WNL.0b013e318245f461 [pii]

Ahearn EP, Steffens DC, Cassidy F, Van Meter SA, Provenzale JM, Seldin MF, Weisler RH, Krishnan KR (1998) Familial leukoencephalopathy in bipolar disorder. Am J Psychiatry 155(11):1605–1607

Alciati A, D'Ambrosio A, Foschi D, Corsi F, Mellado C, Angst J (2007) Bipolar spectrum disorders in severely obese patients seeking surgical treatment. J Affect Disord 101(1–3):131–138. doi:10.1016/j.jad.2006.11.008, S0165-0327(06)00483-6 [pii]

Alciati A, Gesuele F, Rizzi A, Sarzi-Puttini P, Foschi D (2011) Childhood parental loss and bipolar spectrum in obese bariatric surgery candidates. Int J Psychiatry Med 41(2):155–171

Alciati A, Sarzi-Puttini P, Batticciotto A, Torta R, Gesuele F, Atzeni F, Angst J (2012) Overactive lifestyle in patients with fibromyalgia as a core feature of bipolar spectrum disorder. Clin Exp Rheumatol 30(6 Suppl 74):122–128. doi:6652 [pii]

Alstrom C (1942) Mortality in mental hospitals. Acta Psychiatr Neurol 17:1–42

Altamura AC, Serati M, Albano A, Paoli RA, Glick ID, Dell'Osso B (2011) An epidemiologic and clinical overview of medical and psychopathological comorbidities in major psychoses. Eur Arch Psychiatry Clin Neurosci 261(7):489–508. doi:10.1007/s00406-011-0196-4

Altshuler LL, Kupka RW, Hellemann G, Frye MA, Sugar CA, McElroy SL, Nolen WA, Grunze H, Leverich GS, Keck PE, Zermeno M, Post RM, Suppes T (2010) Gender and depressive symptoms in 711 patients with bipolar disorder evaluated prospectively in the Stanley Foundation bipolar treatment outcome network. Am J Psychiatry 167(6):708–715. doi:10.1176/appi.ajp.2009.09010105, appi.ajp.2009.09010105 [pii]

Angst J (1998) The emerging epidemiology of hypomania and bipolar II disorder. J Affect Disord 50(2–3):143–151. doi:S0165-0327(98)00142-6 [pii]

Angst F, Stassen HH, Clayton PJ, Angst J (2002) Mortality of patients with mood disorders: follow-up over 34–38 years. J Affect Disord 68(2–3):167–181. doi:S0165032701003779 [pii]

Angst J, Gamma A, Endrass J, Hantouche E, Goodwin R, Ajdacic V, Eich D, Rossler W (2005) Obsessive-compulsive syndromes and disorders: significance of comorbidity with bipolar and anxiety syndromes. Eur Arch Psychiatry Clin Neurosci 255(1):65–71. doi:10.1007/s00406-005-0576-8

Antonaci F, Nappi G, Galli F, Manzoni GC, Calabresi P, Costa A (2011) Migraine and psychiatric comorbidity: a review of clinical findings. J Headache Pain 12(2):115–125. doi:10.1007/s10194-010-0282-4

Arnold LM (2003) Gender differences in bipolar disorder. Psychiatr Clin North Am 26(3):595–620

Arnold LM, Hudson JI, Keck PE, Auchenbach MB, Javaras KN, Hess EV (2006) Comorbidity of fibromyalgia and psychiatric disorders. J Clin Psychiatry 67(8):1219–1225

Atmaca M, Kuloglu M, Tezcan E, Ustundag B (2002) Weight gain and serum leptin levels in patients on lithium treatment. Neuropsychobiology 46(2):67. doi:65414 [pii]

Azorin JM, Kaladjian A, Adida M, Hantouche EG, Hameg A, Lancrenon S, Akiskal HS (2009) Psychopathological correlates of lifetime anxiety comorbidity in bipolar I patients: findings from a French national cohort. Psychopathology 42(6):380–386. doi:10.1159/000241193, 000241193 [pii]

Babigian HM, Odoroff CL (1969) The mortality experience of a population with psychiatric illness. Am J Psychiatry 126(4):470–480

Bachen EA, Chesney MA, Criswell LA (2009) Prevalence of mood and anxiety disorders in women with systemic lupus erythematosus. Arthritis Rheum 61(6):822–829. doi:10.1002/art.24519

Badiee J, Riggs PK, Rooney AS, Vaida F, Grant I, Atkinson JH, Moore DJ (2012) Approaches to identifying appropriate medication adherence assessments for HIV infected individuals with comorbid bipolar disorder. AIDS Patient Care STDS 26(7):388–394. doi:10.1089/apc.2011.0447

Baek JH, Park DY, Choi J, Kim JS, Choi JS, Ha K, Kwon JS, Lee D, Hong KS (2011) Differences between bipolar I and bipolar II disorders in clinical features, comorbidity, and family history. J Affect Disord 131(1–3):59–67. doi:10.1016/j.jad.2010.11.020, S0165-0327(10)00717-2 [pii]

Bai YM, Su TP, Chen MH, Chen TJ, Chang WH (2013) Risk of developing diabetes mellitus and hyperlipidemia among patients with bipolar disorder, major depressive disorder, and schizophrenia: a 10-year nationwide population-based prospective cohort study. J Affect Disord. doi:10.1016/j.jad.2013.02.019, S0165-0327(13)00178-X [pii]

Baldassano CF, Marangell LB, Gyulai L, Ghaemi SN, Joffe H, Kim DR, Sagduyu K, Truman CJ, Wisniewski SR, Sachs GS, Cohen LS (2005) Gender differences in bipolar disorder: retrospective data from the first 500 STEP-BD participants. Bipolar Disord 7(5):465–470. doi:10.1111/j.1399-5618.2005.00237.x, BDI237 [pii]

Barbosa IG, Rocha NP, de Miranda AS, Magalhaes PV, Huguet RB, de Souza LP, Kapczinski F, Teixeira AL (2012) Increased levels of adipokines in bipolar disorder. J Psychiatr Res 46(3):389–393. doi:10.1016/j.jpsychires.2011.11.010, S0022-3956(11)00276-7 [pii]

Barkley RA, Fischer M (2010) The unique contribution of emotional impulsiveness to impairment in major life activities in hyperactive children as adults. J Am Acad Child Adolesc Psychiatry 49(5):503–513. doi:00004583-201005000-00011 [pii]

Barry JJ (2003) The recognition and management of mood disorders as a comorbidity of epilepsy. Epilepsia 44(Suppl 4):30–40. doi:4005 [pii]

Bartleson JD, Cutrer FM (2010) Migraine update. Diagnosis and treatment. Minn Med 93(5):36–41

Baskin SM, Smitherman TA (2009) Migraine and psychiatric disorders: comorbidities, mechanisms, and clinical applications. Neurol Sci 30(Suppl 1):S61–S65. doi:10.1007/s10072-009-0071-5

Basu R, Brar JS, Chengappa KN, John V, Parepally H, Gershon S, Schlicht P, Kupfer DJ (2004) The prevalence of the metabolic syndrome in patients with schizoaffective disorder–bipolar subtype. Bipolar Disord 6(4):314–318. doi:10.1111/j.1399-5618.2004.00126.x, BDI126 [pii]

Bauer M, Lecrubier Y, Suppes T (2008) Awareness of metabolic concerns in patients with bipolar disorder: a survey of European psychiatrists. Eur Psychiatry 23(3):169–177. doi:10.1016/j.eurpsy.2007.10.007, S0924-9338(07)01423-X [pii]

Bellani M, Hatch JP, Nicoletti MA, Ertola AE, Zunta-Soares G, Swann AC, Brambilla P, Soares JC (2012) Does anxiety increase impulsivity in patients with bipolar disorder or major depressive disorder? J Psychiatr Res 46(5):616–621. doi:10.1016/j.jpsychires.2012.01.016, S0022-3956(12)00027-1 [pii]

Bernardi S, Cortese S, Solanto M, Hollander E, Pallanti S (2010) Bipolar disorder and comorbid attention deficit hyperactivity disorder. A distinct clinical phenotype? Clinical characteristics and temperamental traits. World J Biol Psychiatry 11(4):656–666. doi:10.3109/15622971003653238

Beyer J, Kuchibhatla M, Gersing K, Krishnan KR (2005) Medical comorbidity in a bipolar outpatient clinical population. Neuropsychopharmacology 30(2):401–404. doi:10.1038/sj.npp.1300608, 1300608 [pii]

Beyer JL, Taylor L, Gersing KR, Krishnan KR (2007) Prevalence of HIV infection in a general psychiatric outpatient population. Psychosomatics 48(1):31–37. doi:10.1176/appi.psy.48.1.31, 48/1/31 [pii]

Biederman J, Faraone SV (2005) Attention-deficit hyperactivity disorder. Lancet 366(9481):237–248. doi:10.1016/S0140-6736(05)66915-2, S0140-6736(05)66915-2 [pii]

Biederman J, Faraone SV, Spencer T, Wilens T, Norman D, Lapey KA, Mick E, Lehman BK, Doyle A (1993) Patterns of psychiatric comorbidity, cognition, and psychosocial functioning in adults with attention deficit hyperactivity disorder. Am J Psychiatry 150(12):1792–1798

Biederman J, Faraone S, Mick E, Wozniak J, Chen L, Ouellette C, Marrs A, Moore P, Garcia J, Mennin D, Lelon E (1996) Attention-deficit hyperactivity disorder and juvenile mania: an overlooked comorbidity? J Am Acad Child Adolesc Psychiatry 35(8):997–1008. doi:10.1097/00004583-199608000-00010, S0890-8567(09)62493-X [pii]

Birkenaes AB, Opjordsmoen S, Brunborg C, Engh JA, Jonsdottir H, Ringen PA, Simonsen C, Vaskinn A, Birkeland KI, Friis S, Sundet K, Andreassen OA (2007) The level of cardiovascular risk factors in bipolar disorder equals that of schizophrenia: a comparative study. J Clin Psychiatry 68(6):917–923

Birmaher B, Axelson D, Monk K, Kalas C, Goldstein B, Hickey MB, Obreja M, Ehmann M, Iyengar S, Shamseddeen W, Kupfer D, Brent D (2009) Lifetime psychiatric disorders in school-aged offspring of parents with bipolar disorder: the Pittsburgh Bipolar Offspring study. Arch Gen Psychiatry 66(3):287–296. doi:10.1001/archgenpsychiatry.2008.546, 66/3/287 [pii]

Birmaher B, Axelson D, Goldstein B, Monk K, Kalas C, Obreja M, Hickey MB, Iyengar S, Brent D, Shamseddeen W, Diler R, Kupfer D (2010) Psychiatric disorders in preschool offspring of parents with bipolar disorder: the Pittsburgh Bipolar Offspring Study (BIOS). Am J Psychiatry 167(3):321–330. doi:10.1176/appi.ajp.2009.09070977, appi.ajp.2009.09070977 [pii]

Bisserbe JC, Weiller E, Boyer P, Lepine JP, Lecrubier Y (1996) Social phobia in primary care: level of recognition and drug use. Int Clin Psychopharmacol 11(Suppl 3):25–28

Black DW, Goldstein RB, Mason EE (1992) Prevalence of mental disorder in 88 morbidly obese bariatric clinic patients. Am J Psychiatry 149(2):227–234

Blanco C, Grant J, Petry NM, Simpson HB, Alegria A, Liu SM, Hasin D (2008) Prevalence and correlates of shoplifting in the United States: results from the National Epidemiologic Survey on Alcohol and Related Conditions (NESARC). Am J Psychiatry 165(7):905–913. doi:10.1176/appi.ajp.2008.07101660, appi.ajp.2008.07101660 [pii]

Blanco C, Alegria AA, Petry NM, Grant JE, Simpson HB, Liu SM, Grant BF, Hasin DS (2010) Prevalence and correlates of fire-setting in the United States: results from the National Epidemiologic Survey on Alcohol and Related Conditions (NESARC). J Clin Psychiatry 71(9):1218–1225. doi:10.4088/JCP.08m04812gry

Blehar MC, DePaulo JR Jr, Gershon ES, Reich T, Simpson SG, Nurnberger JI Jr (1998) Women with bipolar disorder: findings from the NIMH Genetics Initiative sample. Psychopharmacol Bull 34(3):239–243

Bowden CL, Calabrese JR, Ketter TA, Sachs GS, White RL, Thompson TR (2006) Impact of lamotrigine and lithium on weight in obese and nonobese patients with bipolar I disorder. Am J Psychiatry 163(7):1199–1201. doi:10.1176/appi.ajp.163.7.1199, 163/7/1199 [pii]

Bowen R, South M, Hawkes J (1994) Mood swings in patients with panic disorder. Can J Psychiatry 39(2):91–94

Boylan KR, Bieling PJ, Marriott M, Begin H, Young LT, MacQueen GM (2004) Impact of comorbid anxiety disorders on outcome in a cohort of patients with bipolar disorder. J Clin Psychiatry 65(8):1106–1113

Brandrup E, Randrup A (1967) A controlled investigation of plasma lipids in manic-depressives. Br J Psychiatry 113(502):987–992

Breslau N (1998) Psychiatric comorbidity in migraine. Cephalalgia 18(Suppl 22):56–58, discussion 58–61

Breslau N, Davis GC, Andreski P (1991) Migraine, psychiatric disorders, and suicide attempts: an epidemiologic study of young adults. Psychiatry Res 37(1):11–23

Breslau N, Merikangas K, Bowden CL (1994) Comorbidity of migraine and major affective disorders. Neurology 44(10 Suppl 7):S17–S22

Brietzke E, Moreira CL, Toniolo RA, Lafer B (2011) Clinical correlates of eating disorder comorbidity in women with bipolar disorder type I. J Affect Disord 130(1–2):162–165. doi:10.1016/j.jad.2010.10.020, S0165-0327(10)00634-8 [pii]

Briskman I, Bar G, Boaz M, Shargorodsky M (2012) Impact of co-morbid mental illness on the diagnosis and management of patients hospitalized for medical conditions in a general hospital. Int J Psychiatry Med 43(4):339–348

Britz B, Siegfried W, Ziegler A, Lamertz C, Herpertz-Dahlmann BM, Remschmidt H, Wittchen HU, Hebebrand J (2000) Rates of psychiatric disorders in a clinical study group of adolescents

with extreme obesity and in obese adolescents ascertained via a population based study. Int J Obes Relat Metab Disord 24(12):1707–1714
Brown FW, Golding JM, Smith GR Jr (1990) Psychiatric comorbidity in primary care somatization disorder. Psychosom Med 52(4):445–451
Bryant-Comstock L, Stender M, Devercelli G (2002) Health care utilization and costs among privately insured patients with bipolar I disorder. Bipolar Disord 4(6):398–405. doi:1o148 [pii]
Bumke O (1928) Handbuch der Geisteskrankheiten. Julius Springer Verlag, Berlin
Butt AA, Evans R, Skanderson M, Shakil AO (2006) Comorbid medical and psychiatric conditions and substance abuse in HCV infected persons on dialysis. J Hepatol 44(5):864–868. doi:10.1016/j.jhep.2006.01.024, S0168-8278(06)00069-9 [pii]
Calabrese JR, Hirschfeld RM, Reed M, Davies MA, Frye MA, Keck PE, Lewis L, McElroy SL, McNulty JP, Wagner KD (2003) Impact of bipolar disorder on a U.S. community sample. J Clin Psychiatry 64(4):425–432
Calkin C, van de Velde C, Ruzickova M, Slaney C, Garnham J, Hajek T, O'Donovan C, Alda M (2009) Can body mass index help predict outcome in patients with bipolar disorder? Bipolar Disord 11(6):650–656. doi:10.1111/j.1399-5618.2009.00730.x, BDI730 [pii]
Cardenas J, Frye MA, Marusak SL, Levander EM, Chirichigno JW, Lewis S, Nakelsky S, Hwang S, Mintz J, Altshuler LL (2008) Modal subcomponents of metabolic syndrome in patients with bipolar disorder. J Affect Disord 106(1–2):91–97. doi:10.1016/j.jad.2007.05.030, S0165-0327(07)00216-9 [pii]
Carlson GA, Bromet EJ, Driessens C, Mojtabai R, Schwartz JE (2002) Age at onset, childhood psychopathology, and 2-year outcome in psychotic bipolar disorder. Am J Psychiatry 159(2): 307–309
Carlson GA, Kotov R, Chang SW, Ruggero C, Bromet EJ (2012) Early determinants of four-year clinical outcomes in bipolar disorder with psychosis. Bipolar Disord 14(1):19–30. doi:10.1111/j.1399-5618.2012.00982.x
Carney CP, Jones LE (2006) Medical comorbidity in women and men with bipolar disorders: a population-based controlled study. Psychosom Med 68(5):684–691. doi:10.1097/01.psy.0000237316.09601.88.68/5/684 [pii]
Carta MG, Cardia C, Mannu F, Intilla G, Hardoy MC, Anedda C, Ruggero V, Fornasier D, Cacace E (2006) The high frequency of manic symptoms in fibromyalgia does influence the choice of treatment? Clin Pract Epidemiol Ment Health 2:36. doi:10.1186/1745-0179-2-36, 1745-0179-2-36 [pii]
Carta M, Mura G, Sorbello O, Farina G, Demelia L (2012) Quality of life and psychiatric symptoms in Wilson's disease: the relevance of bipolar disorders. Clin Pract Epidemiol Ment Health 8:102–109. doi:10.2174/1745017901208010102, CPEMH-8-102 [pii]
Cassano GB, Pini S, Saettoni M, Rucci P, Dell'Osso L (1998) Occurrence and clinical correlates of psychiatric comorbidity in patients with psychotic disorders. J Clin Psychiatry 59(2):60–68
Cassidy F, Carroll BJ (2002) Vascular risk factors in late onset mania. Psychol Med 32(2):359–362
Cassidy WL, Flanagan NB, Spellman M, Cohen ME (1957) Clinical observations in manic-depressive disease; a quantitative study of one hundred manic-depressive patients and fifty medically sick controls. J Am Med Assoc 164(14):1535–1546
Cassidy F, Forest K, Murry E, Carroll BJ (1998a) A factor analysis of the signs and symptoms of mania. Arch Gen Psychiatry 55(1):27–32
Cassidy F, Murry E, Forest K, Carroll BJ (1998b) Signs and symptoms of mania in pure and mixed episodes. J Affect Disord 50(2–3):187–201. doi:S0165-0327(98)00016-0 [pii]
Cassidy F, Ahearn E, Carroll BJ (1999) Elevated frequency of diabetes mellitus in hospitalized manic-depressive patients. Am J Psychiatry 156(9):1417–1420
Castelo MS, Hyphantis TN, Macedo DS, Lemos GO, Machado YO, Kapczinski F, McIntyre RS, Carvalho AF (2012) Screening for bipolar disorder in the primary care: a Brazilian survey. J Affect Disord 143(1–3):118–124. doi:10.1016/j.jad.2012.05.040, S0165-0327(12)00395-3 [pii]

Centorrino F, Mark TL, Talamo A, Oh K, Chang J (2009) Health and economic burden of metabolic comorbidity among individuals with bipolar disorder. J Clin Psychopharmacol 29(6):595–600. doi:10.1097/JCP.0b013e3181bef8a6, 00004714-200912000-00014 [pii]

Chang KD, Steiner H, Ketter TA (2000) Psychiatric phenomenology of child and adolescent bipolar offspring. J Am Acad Child Adolesc Psychiatry 39(4):453–460. doi:10.1097/00004583-200004000-00014, S0890-8567(09)66188-8 [pii]

Chang HH, Chou CH, Chen PS, Gean PW, Huang HC, Lin CY, Yang YK, Lu RB (2009) High prevalence of metabolic disturbances in patients with bipolar disorder in Taiwan. J Affect Disord 117(1–2):124–129. doi:10.1016/j.jad.2008.12.018, S0165-0327(08)00511-9 [pii]

Chen YW, Dilsaver SC (1995) Comorbidity of panic disorder in bipolar illness: evidence from the Epidemiologic Catchment Area Survey. Am J Psychiatry 152(2):280–282

Chen YC, Tang CH, Ng K, Wang SJ (2012) Comorbidity profiles of chronic migraine sufferers in a national database in Taiwan. J Headache Pain 13(4):311–319. doi:10.1007/s10194-012-0447-4

Chien IC, Chang KC, Lin CH, Chou YJ, Chou P (2010) Prevalence of diabetes in patients with bipolar disorder in Taiwan: a population-based national health insurance study. Gen Hosp Psychiatry 32(6):577–582. doi:10.1016/j.genhosppsych.2010.09.005, S0163-8343(10)00187-8 [pii]

Chou SP, Huang B, Goldstein R, Grant BF (2013) Temporal associations between physical illnesses and mental disorders-Results from the Wave 2 National Epidemiologic Survey on Alcohol and Related Conditions (NESARC). Compr Psychiatry. doi:10.1016/j.comppsych.2012.12.020, S0010-440X(13)00017-5 [pii]

Chwastiak LA, Rosenheck RA, Kazis LE (2011) Association of psychiatric illness and obesity, physical inactivity, and smoking among a national sample of veterans. Psychosomatics 52(3):230–236. doi:10.1016/j.psym.2010.12.009, S0033-3182(10)00032-0 [pii]

Ciapparelli A, Paggini R, Marazziti D, Carmassi C, Bianchi M, Taponecco C, Consoli G, Lombardi V, Massimetti G, Dell'osso L (2007) Comorbidity with axis I anxiety disorders in remitted psychotic patients 1 year after hospitalization. CNS Spectr 12(12):913–919

Cirillo PC, Passos RB, Bevilaqua MC, Lopez JR, Nardi AE (2012) Bipolar disorder and premenstrual syndrome or premenstrual dysphoric disorder comorbidity: a systematic review. Rev Bras Psiquiatr 34(4):467–479. doi:S1516-44462012000400015 [pii]

Clarke MC, Tanskanen A, Huttunen MO, Clancy M, Cotter DR, Cannon M (2012) Evidence for shared susceptibility to epilepsy and psychosis: a population-based family study. Biol Psychiatry 71(9):836–839. doi:10.1016/j.biopsych.2012.01.011, S0006-3223(12)00050-9 [pii]

Colton CW, Manderscheid RW (2006) Congruencies in increased mortality rates, years of potential life lost, and causes of death among public mental health clients in eight states. Prev Chronic Dis 3(2):A42. doi:A42 [pii]

Contreras J, Hare E, Pacheco A, Escamilla M, Raventos H (2010) Is subclinical anxiety an endophenotype for bipolar I patients? A study from a Costa Rican sample. J Affect Disord 122(3):267–272. doi:10.1016/j.jad.2009.07.017, S0165-0327(09)00337-1 [pii]

Conus P, Cotton S, Abdel-Baki A, Lambert M, Berk M, McGorry PD (2006) Symptomatic and functional outcome 12 months after a first episode of psychotic mania: barriers to recovery in a catchment area sample. Bipolar Disord 8(3):221–231. doi:10.1111/j.1399-5618.2006.00315.x, BDI315 [pii]

Correll CU, Frederickson AM, Kane JM, Manu P (2008) Equally increased risk for metabolic syndrome in patients with bipolar disorder and schizophrenia treated with second-generation antipsychotics. Bipolar Disord 10(7):788–797. doi:10.1111/j.1399-5618.2008.00625.x, BDI625 [pii]

Coryell W, Solomon DA, Fiedorowicz JG, Endicott J, Schettler PJ, Judd LL (2009) Anxiety and outcome in bipolar disorder. Am J Psychiatry 166(11):1238–1243. doi:10.1176/appi.ajp.2009.09020218, appi.ajp.2009.09020218 [pii]

Cosoff SJ, Hafner RJ (1998) The prevalence of comorbid anxiety in schizophrenia, schizoaffective disorder and bipolar disorder. Aust N Z J Psychiatry 32(1):67–72

Craig T, Hwang MY, Bromet EJ (2002) Obsessive-compulsive and panic symptoms in patients with first-admission psychosis. Am J Psychiatry 159(4):592–598

Daratha KB, Barbosa-Leiker C, HB M, Short R, Layton ME, McPherson S, Dyck DG, McFarland BH, Tuttle KR (2012) Co-occurring mood disorders among hospitalized patients and risk for subsequent medical hospitalization. Gen Hosp Psychiatry 34(5):500–505. doi:10.1016/j.genhosppsych.2012.05.001, S0163-8343(12)00144-2 [pii]

Darby L, Agius M, Zaman R (2011) Co-morbidity of bipolar affective disorder and obsessive compulsive disorder in a Bedford community psychiatry team. Psychiatr Danub 23(Suppl 1):S130–S133

Das A (2013) Anxiety disorders in bipolar I mania: prevalence, effect on illness severity, and treatment implications. Indian J Psychol Med 35(1):53–59. doi:10.4103/0253-7176.112202, IJPsyM-35-53 [pii]

De Hert M, Dekker JM, Wood D, Kahl KG, Holt RI, Moller HJ (2009) Cardiovascular disease and diabetes in people with severe mental illness position statement from the European Psychiatric Association (EPA), supported by the European Association for the Study of Diabetes (EASD) and the European Society of Cardiology (ESC). Eur Psychiatry 24(6):412–424. doi:10.1016/j.eurpsy.2009.01.005, S0924-9338(09)00017-0 [pii]

de Oliveira GN, Kummer A, Salgado JV, Portela EJ, Sousa-Pereira SR, David AS, Teixeira AL (2010) Psychiatric disorders in temporal lobe epilepsy: an overview from a tertiary service in Brazil. Seizure 19(8):479–484. doi:10.1016/j.seizure.2010.07.004, S1059-1311(10)00153-6 [pii]

de Sousa Gurgel W, da Silva Carneiro AH, Barreto Reboucas D, Negreiros de Matos KJ, Silva Leitao TD, Gomes de Matos ESF, Affective Disorders Study Group G (2013) Prevalence of bipolar disorder in a HIV-infected outpatient population. AIDS Care. doi:10.1080/09540121.2013.779625

DelBello MP, Soutullo CA, Hendricks W, Niemeier RT, McElroy SL, Strakowski SM (2001) Prior stimulant treatment in adolescents with bipolar disorder: association with age at onset. Bipolar Disord 3(2):53–57

Dell'Osso B, Buoli M, Bortolussi S, Camuri G, Vecchi V, Altamura AC (2011) Patterns of axis I comorbidity in relation to age in patients with bipolar disorder: a cross-sectional analysis. J Affect Disord 130(1–2):318–322. doi:10.1016/j.jad.2010.10.008, S0165-0327(10)00622-1 [pii]

Derby I (1933) Manic-depressive "exhaustion" deaths: an analysis of "exhaustion" case histories. Psychiatr Q 7:436–449

Di Nicola M, Tedeschi D, Mazza M, Martinotti G, Harnic D, Catalano V, Bruschi A, Pozzi G, Bria P, Janiri L (2010) Behavioural addictions in bipolar disorder patients: role of impulsivity and personality dimensions. J Affect Disord 125(1–3):82–88. doi:10.1016/j.jad.2009.12.016, S0165-0327(09)00568-0 [pii]

Dilsaver SC, Chen YW (2003) Social phobia, panic disorder and suicidality in subjects with pure and depressive mania. J Affect Disord 77(2):173–177. doi:S0165032702001143 [pii]

Dilsaver SC, White K (1986) Affective disorders and associated psychopathology: a family history study. J Clin Psychiatry 47(4):162–169

Dilsaver SC, Chen YW, Swann AC, Shoaib AM, Tsai-Dilsaver Y, Krajewski KJ (1997) Suicidality, panic disorder and psychosis in bipolar depression, depressive-mania and pure-mania. Psychiatry Res 73(1–2):47–56

Dilsaver SC, Benazzi F, Akiskal KK, Akiskal HS (2008) Differential patterns of lifetime multiple anxiety disorder comorbidity between Latino adults with bipolar I and major depressive disorders. Bull Menninger Clin 72(2):130–148. doi:10.1521/bumc.2008.72.2.130 [pii]

Dilsaver SC, Benazzi F, Oedegaard KJ, Fasmer OB, Akiskal HS (2009) Is a family history of bipolar disorder a risk factor for migraine among affectively ill patients? Psychopathology 42(2):119–123. doi:10.1159/000204762, 000204762 [pii]

Dinesen H, Gram L, Andersen T, Dam M (1984) Weight gain during treatment with valproate. Acta Neurol Scand 70(2):65–69

Dittmann S, Biedermann NC, Grunze H, Hummel B, Scharer LO, Kleindienst N, Forsthoff A, Matzner N, Walser S, Walden J (2002) The Stanley Foundation Bipolar Network: results of the naturalistic follow-up study after 2.5 years of follow-up in the German centres. Neuropsychobiology 46(Suppl 1):2–9. doi:68018. 68018 [pii]

Doughty CJ, Wells JE, Joyce PR, Olds RJ, Walsh AE (2004) Bipolar-panic disorder comorbidity within bipolar disorder families: a study of siblings. Bipolar Disord 6(3):245–252. doi:10.1111/j.1399-5618.2004.00120.x, BDI120 [pii]

Douzenis A, Seretis D, Nika S, Nikolaidou P, Papadopoulou A, Rizos EN, Christodoulou C, Tsopelas C, Mitchell D, Lykouras L (2012) Factors affecting hospital stay in psychiatric patients: the role of active comorbidity. BMC Health Serv Res 12:166. doi:10.1186/1472-6963-12-166, 1472-6963-12-166 [pii]

Duffy A (2012) The nature of the association between childhood ADHD and the development of bipolar disorder: a review of prospective high-risk studies. Am J Psychiatry 169(12):1247–1255. doi:10.1176/appi.ajp.2012.11111725, 1461100 [pii]

Duffy A, Alda M, Crawford L, Milin R, Grof P (2007) The early manifestations of bipolar disorder: a longitudinal prospective study of the offspring of bipolar parents. Bipolar Disord 9(8):828–838. doi:10.1111/j.1399-5618.2007.00421.x, BDI421 [pii]

Eaton WW, Pedersen MG, Nielsen PR, Mortensen PB (2010) Autoimmune diseases, bipolar disorder, and non-affective psychosis. Bipolar Disord 12(6):638–646. doi:10.1111/j.1399-5618.2010.00853.x

Edmonds LK, Mosley BJ, Admiraal AJ, Olds RJ, Romans SE, Silverstone T, Walsh AE (1998) Familial bipolar disorder: preliminary results from the Otago Familial Bipolar Genetic Study. Aust N Z J Psychiatry 32(6):823–829

El-Mallakh RS, Hollifield M (2008) Comorbid anxiety in bipolar disorder alters treatment and prognosis. Psychiatr Q 79(2):139–150. doi:10.1007/s11126-008-9071-5

Elmslie JL, Silverstone JT, Mann JI, Williams SM, Romans SE (2000) Prevalence of overweight and obesity in bipolar patients. J Clin Psychiatry 61(3):179–184

Elmslie JL, Mann JI, Silverstone JT, Williams SM, Romans SE (2001) Determinants of overweight and obesity in patients with bipolar disorder. J Clin Psychiatry 62(6):486–491, quiz 492–483

Ettinger AB, Reed ML, Goldberg JF, Hirschfeld RM (2005) Prevalence of bipolar symptoms in epilepsy vs other chronic health disorders. Neurology 65(4):535–540. doi:10.1212/01.wnl.0000172917.70752.05, 65/4/535 [pii]

Fagiolini A, Goracci A (2009) The effects of undertreated chronic medical illnesses in patients with severe mental disorders. J Clin Psychiatry 70(Suppl 3):22–29. doi:10.4088/JCP.7075su1c.04

Fagiolini A, Frank E, Houck PR, Mallinger AG, Swartz HA, Buysse DJ, Ombao H, Kupfer DJ (2002) Prevalence of obesity and weight change during treatment in patients with bipolar I disorder. J Clin Psychiatry 63(6):528–533

Fagiolini A, Kupfer DJ, Houck PR, Novick DM, Frank E (2003) Obesity as a correlate of outcome in patients with bipolar I disorder. Am J Psychiatry 160(1):112–117

Fagiolini A, Frank E, Scott JA, Turkin S, Kupfer DJ (2005) Metabolic syndrome in bipolar disorder: findings from the Bipolar Disorder Center for Pennsylvanians. Bipolar Disord 7(5):424–430. doi:10.1111/j.1399-5618.2005.00234.x, BDI234 [pii]

Faraone SV, Antshel KM (2008) Diagnosing and treating attention-deficit/hyperactivity disorder in adults. World Psychiatry 7(3):131–136

Faraone SV, Biederman J, Mennin D, Wozniak J, Spencer T (1997) Attention-deficit hyperactivity disorder with bipolar disorder: a familial subtype? J Am Acad Child Adolesc Psychiatry 36(10):1378–1387; discussion 1387–1390. doi:10.1097/00004583-199710000-00020, S0890-8567(09)63280-9 [pii]

Faraone SV, Biederman J, Monuteaux MC (2001) Attention deficit hyperactivity disorder with bipolar disorder in girls: further evidence for a familial subtype? J Affect Disord 64(1):19–26. doi:S0165-0327(00)00213-5 [pii]

Faraone SV, Biederman J, Mick E (2006a) The age-dependent decline of attention deficit hyperactivity disorder: a meta-analysis of follow-up studies. Psychol Med 36(2):159–165. doi:10.1017/S003329170500471X, S003329170500471X [pii]

Faraone SV, Biederman J, Spencer T, Mick E, Murray K, Petty C, Adamson JJ, Monuteaux MC (2006b) Diagnosing adult attention deficit hyperactivity disorder: are late onset and subthreshold diagnoses valid? Am J Psychiatry 163(10):1720–1729. doi:10.1176/appi.ajp.163.10.1720, 163/10/1720 [pii], quiz 1859

Fasmer OB (2001) The prevalence of migraine in patients with bipolar and unipolar affective disorders. Cephalalgia 21(9):894–899. doi:279 [pii]

Fasmer OB, Oedegaard KJ (2001) Clinical characteristics of patients with major affective disorders and comorbid migraine. World J Biol Psychiatry 2(3):149–155

Fattal O, Link J, Quinn K, Cohen BH, Franco K (2007) Psychiatric comorbidity in 36 adults with mitochondrial cytopathies. CNS Spectr 12(6):429–438

Feinstein A (1970) The pre-therapeutic classification of co-morbidity in chronic disease. J Chronic Dis 23:455–468

Feldman NS, Gwizdowski IS, Fischer EG, Yang H, Suppes T (2012) Co-occurrence of serious or undiagnosed medical conditions with bipolar disorder preventing clinical trial randomization: a case series. J Clin Psychiatry 73(6):874–877. doi:10.4088/JCP.11m07331

Fenn HH, Bauer MS, Altshuler L, Evans DR, Williford WO, Kilbourne AM, Beresford TP, Kirk G, Stedman M, Fiore L (2005) Medical comorbidity and health-related quality of life in bipolar disorder across the adult age span. J Affect Disord 86(1):47–60. doi:10.1016/j.jad.2004.12.006, S0165-0327(04)00442-2 [pii]

Feske U, Frank E, Mallinger AG, Houck PR, Fagiolini A, Shear MK, Grochocinski VJ, Kupfer DJ (2000) Anxiety as a correlate of response to the acute treatment of bipolar I disorder. Am J Psychiatry 157(6):956–962

Fiedorowicz JG, Palagummi NM, Forman-Hoffman VL, Miller DD, Haynes WG (2008) Elevated prevalence of obesity, metabolic syndrome, and cardiovascular risk factors in bipolar disorder. Ann Clin Psychiatry 20(3):131–137. doi:10.1080/10401230802177722, 795040456 [pii]

Fiedorowicz JG, He J, Merikangas KR (2011) The association between mood and anxiety disorders with vascular diseases and risk factors in a nationally representative sample. J Psychosom Res 70(2):145–154. doi:10.1016/j.jpsychores.2010.07.010, S0022-3999(10)00308-9 [pii]

Fischer AG, Bau CH, Grevet EH, Salgado CA, Victor MM, Kalil KL, Sousa NO, Garcia CR, Belmonte-de-Abreu P (2007) The role of comorbid major depressive disorder in the clinical presentation of adult ADHD. J Psychiatr Res 41(12):991–996. doi:10.1016/j.jpsychires.2006.09.008, S0022-3956(06)00200-7 [pii]

Fogarty F, Russell JM, Newman SC, Bland RC (1994) Epidemiology of psychiatric disorders in Edmonton. Mania. Acta Psychiatr Scand Suppl 376:16–23

Ford ES, Giles WH, Dietz WH (2002) Prevalence of the metabolic syndrome among US adults: findings from the third National Health and Nutrition Examination Survey. JAMA 287(3):356–359. doi:jbr10281 [pii]

Fornaro M, Perugi G, Gabrielli F, Prestia D, Mattei C, Vinciguerra V, Fornaro P (2010) Lifetime co-morbidity with different subtypes of eating disorders in 148 females with bipolar disorders. J Affect Disord 121(1–2):147–151. doi:10.1016/j.jad.2009.06.007, S0165-0327(09)00265-1 [pii]

Frank E, Cyranowski JM, Rucci P, Shear MK, Fagiolini A, Thase ME, Cassano GB, Grochocinski VJ, Kostelnik B, Kupfer DJ (2002) Clinical significance of lifetime panic spectrum symptoms in the treatment of patients with bipolar I disorder. Arch Gen Psychiatry 59(10):905–911. doi:yoa20445 [pii]

Freeman MP, Freeman SA, McElroy SL (2002) The comorbidity of bipolar and anxiety disorders: prevalence, psychobiology, and treatment issues. J Affect Disord 68(1):1–23. doi:S0165032700002998 [pii]

Fuller BE, Rodriguez VL, Linke A, Sikirica M, Dirani R, Hauser P (2011) Prevalence of liver disease in veterans with bipolar disorder or schizophrenia. Gen Hosp Psychiatry 33(3):232–237. doi:10.1016/j.genhosppsych.2011.03.006, S0163-8343(11)00114-9 [pii]

Gans RO (2006) The metabolic syndrome, depression, and cardiovascular disease: interrelated conditions that share pathophysiologic mechanisms. Med Clin North Am 90(4):573–591. doi:10.1016/j.mcna.2006.05.002, S0025-7125(06)00040-X [pii]

Gao K, Tolliver BK, Kemp DE, Verduin ML, Ganocy SJ, Bilali S, Brady KT, Shim SS, Findling RL, Calabrese JR (2008) Differential interactions between comorbid anxiety disorders and substance use disorder in rapid cycling bipolar I or II disorder. J Affect Disord 110(1–2): 167–173. doi:10.1016/j.jad.2007.12.229, S0165-0327(07)00661-1 [pii]

Garcia-Portilla MP, Saiz PA, Benabarre A, Sierra P, Perez J, Rodriguez A, Livianos L, Torres P, Bobes J (2008) The prevalence of metabolic syndrome in patients with bipolar disorder. J Affect Disord 106(1–2):197–201. doi:10.1016/j.jad.2007.06.002, S0165-0327(07)00226-1 [pii]

Gardner HH, Kleinman NL, Brook RA, Rajagopalan K, Brizee TJ, Smeeding JE (2006) The economic impact of bipolar disorder in an employed population from an employer perspective. J Clin Psychiatry 67(8):1209–1218

Gaudiano BA, Miller IW (2005) Anxiety disorder comorbidity in bipolar I disorder: relationship to depression severity and treatment outcome. Depress Anxiety 21(2):71–77. doi:10.1002/da.20053

Gianfrancesco F, White R, Wang RH, Nasrallah HA (2003) Antipsychotic-induced type 2 diabetes: evidence from a large health plan database. J Clin Psychopharmacol 23(4):328–335. doi:10.1097/01.jcp.0000085404.08426.3a

Gitlin MJ, Cochran SD, Jamison KR (1989) Maintenance lithium treatment: side effects and compliance. J Clin Psychiatry 50(4):127–131

Goes FS, McCusker MG, Bienvenu OJ, Mackinnon DF, Mondimore FM, Schweizer B, Depaulo JR, Potash JB (2012) Co-morbid anxiety disorders in bipolar disorder and major depression: familial aggregation and clinical characteristics of co-morbid panic disorder, social phobia, specific phobia and obsessive-compulsive disorder. Psychol Med 42(7):1449–1459. doi:10.1017/S0033291711002637, S0033291711002637 [pii]

Goldstein BI, Levitt AJ (2007) Prevalence and correlates of bipolar I disorder among adults with primary youth-onset anxiety disorders. J Affect Disord 103(1–3):187–195. doi:10.1016/j.jad.2007.01.029, S0165-0327(07)00049-3 [pii]

Goldstein BI, Levitt AJ (2008) The specific burden of comorbid anxiety disorders and of substance use disorders in bipolar I disorder. Bipolar Disord 10(1):67–78. doi:10.1111/j.1399-5618.2008.00461.x, BDI461 [pii]

Goldstein BI, Houck PR, Karp JF (2009) Factors associated with pain interference in an epidemiologic sample of adults with bipolar I disorder. J Affect Disord 117(3):151–156. doi:10.1016/j.jad.2009.01.011, S0165-0327(09)00031-7 [pii]

Gonzalez-Pinto A, Galan J, Martin-Carrasco M, Ballesteros J, Maurino J, Vieta E (2012) Anxiety as a marker of severity in acute mania. Acta Psychiatr Scand 126(5):351–355. doi:10.1111/j.1600-0447.2012.01882.x

Goodwin RD, Hamilton SP (2002) The early-onset fearful panic attack as a predictor of severe psychopathology. Psychiatry Res 109(1):71–79. doi:S0165178101003572 [pii]

Goodwin RD, Hoven CW (2002) Bipolar-panic comorbidity in the general population: prevalence and associated morbidity. J Affect Disord 70(1):27–33. doi:S0165032701003986 [pii]

Goodwin RD, Jacobi F, Thefeld W (2003) Mental disorders and asthma in the community. Arch Gen Psychiatry 60(11):1125–1130. doi:10.1001/archpsyc.60.11.1125, 60/11/1125 [pii]

Goodwin RD, Keyes KM, Stein MB, Talley NJ (2009) Peptic ulcer and mental disorders among adults in the community: the role of nicotine and alcohol use disorders. Psychosom Med 71(4):463–468. doi:10.1097/PSY.0b013e3181988137, PSY.0b013e3181988137 [pii]

Goodwin RD, Pagura J, Cox B, Sareen J (2010) Asthma and mental disorders in Canada: impact on functional impairment and mental health service use. J Psychosom Res 68(2):165–173. doi:10.1016/j.jpsychores.2009.06.005, S0022-3999(09)00231-1 [pii]

Goodwin RD, Galea S, Perzanowski M, Jacobi F (2012) Impact of allergy treatment on the association between allergies and mood and anxiety in a population sample. Clin Exp Allergy 42(12):1765–1771. doi:10.1111/j.1365-2222.2012.04042.x

Goulet JL, Molde S, Constantino J, Gaughan D, Selwyn PA (2000) Psychiatric comorbidity and the long-term care of people with AIDS. J Urban Health 77(2):213–221

Grabe HJ, Meyer C, Hapke U, Rumpf HJ, Freyberger HJ, Dilling H, John U (2001) Lifetime-comorbidity of obsessive-compulsive disorder and subclinical obsessive-compulsive disorder in Northern Germany. Eur Arch Psychiatry Clin Neurosci 251(3):130–135

Gunde E, Blagdon R, Hajek T (2011) White matter hyperintensities: from medical comorbidities to bipolar disorders and back. Ann Med 43(8):571–580. doi:10.3109/07853890.2011.595733

Guo JJ, Keck PE Jr, Corey-Lisle PK, Li H, Jiang D, Jang R, L'Italien GJ (2006) Risk of diabetes mellitus associated with atypical antipsychotic use among patients with bipolar disorder: a retrospective, population-based, case-control study. J Clin Psychiatry 67(7):1055–1061

Hamelsky SW, Lipton RB (2006) Psychiatric comorbidity of migraine. Headache 46(9):1327–1333. doi:10.1111/j.1526-4610.2006.00576.x, HED576 [pii]

Han C, Lofland JH, Zhao N, Schenkel B (2011) Increased prevalence of psychiatric disorders and health care-associated costs among patients with moderate-to-severe psoriasis. J Drugs Dermatol 10(8):843–850

Hantouche EG, Kochman F, Demonfaucon C, Barrot I, Millet B, Lancrenon S, Akiskal HS (2002) Bipolar obsessive-compulsive disorder: confirmation of results of the "ABC-OCD" survey in 2 populations of patient members versus non-members of an association. Encéphale 28(1):21–28

Harden CL, Goldstein MA (2002) Mood disorders in patients with epilepsy: epidemiology and management. CNS Drugs 16(5):291–302. doi:160502 [pii]

Henderson DC (2001) Clozapine: diabetes mellitus, weight gain, and lipid abnormalities. J Clin Psychiatry 62(Suppl 23):39–44

Henderson DC, Cagliero E, Gray C, Nasrallah RA, Hayden DL, Schoenfeld DA, Goff DC (2000) Clozapine, diabetes mellitus, weight gain, and lipid abnormalities: a five-year naturalistic study. Am J Psychiatry 157(6):975–981

Henin A, Biederman J, Mick E, Sachs GS, Hirshfeld-Becker DR, Siegel RS, McMurrich S, Grandin L, Nierenberg AA (2005) Psychopathology in the offspring of parents with bipolar disorder: a controlled study. Biol Psychiatry 58(7):554–561. doi:10.1016/j.biopsych.2005.06.010, S0006-3223(05)00716-X [pii]

Henry C, Van den Bulke D, Bellivier F, Etain B, Rouillon F, Leboyer M (2003) Anxiety disorders in 318 bipolar patients: prevalence and impact on illness severity and response to mood stabilizer. J Clin Psychiatry 64(3):331–335

Hermida OG, Fontela T, Ghiglione M, Uttenthal LO (1994) Effect of lithium on plasma glucose, insulin and glucagon in normal and streptozotocin-diabetic rats: role of glucagon in the hyperglycaemic response. Br J Pharmacol 111(3):861–865

Himmelhoch JM (1998) Social anxiety, hypomania and the bipolar spectrum: data, theory and clinical issues. J Affect Disord 50(2–3):203–213. doi:S0165-0327(98)00139-6 [pii]

Himmelhoch JM, Garfinkel ME (1986) Sources of lithium resistance in mixed mania. Psychopharmacol Bull 22(3):613–620

Hirschfeld RM, Calabrese JR, Weissman MM, Reed M, Davies MA, Frye MA, Keck PE Jr, Lewis L, McElroy SL, McNulty JP, Wagner KD (2003) Screening for bipolar disorder in the community. J Clin Psychiatry 64(1):53–59

Hirshfeld-Becker DR, Biederman J, Henin A, Faraone SV, Dowd ST, De Petrillo LA, Markowitz SM, Rosenbaum JF (2006) Psychopathology in the young offspring of parents with bipolar disorder: a controlled pilot study. Psychiatry Res 145(2–3):155–167. doi:10.1016/j.psychres.2005.08.026, S0165-1781(05)00376-8 [pii]

Holland J, Agius M, Zaman R (2011) Prevalence of co-morbid bipolar disorder and migraine in a regional hospital psychiatric outpatient department. Psychiatr Danub 23(Suppl 1):S23–S24

Hu G, Qiao Q, Tuomilehto J, Balkau B, Borch-Johnsen K, Pyorala K (2004) Prevalence of the metabolic syndrome and its relation to all-cause and cardiovascular mortality in nondiabetic European men and women. Arch Intern Med 164(10):1066–1076. doi:10.1001/archinte.164.10.1066, 164/10/1066 [pii]

Huang TL, Chen JF (2005) Serum lipid profiles and schizophrenia: effects of conventional or atypical antipsychotic drugs in Taiwan. Schizophr Res 80(1):55–59. doi:10.1016/j.schres.2005.05.001, S0920-9964(05)00191-X [pii]

Huang KL, Su TP, Chen TJ, Chou YH, Bai YM (2009) Comorbidity of cardiovascular diseases with mood and anxiety disorder: a population based 4-year study. Psychiatry Clin Neurosci 63(3):401–409. doi:10.1111/j.1440-1819.2009.01974.x, PCN1974 [pii]

Iacovides A, Andreoulakis E (2011) Bipolar disorder and resembling special psychopathological manifestations in multiple sclerosis: a review. Curr Opin Psychiatry 24(4):336–340. doi:10.1097/YCO.0b013e328347341d

Issler CK, Amaral JA, Tamada RS, Schwartzmann AM, Shavitt RG, Miguel EC, Lafer B (2005) Clinical expression of obsessive-compulsive disorder in women with bipolar disorder. Rev Bras Psiquiatr 27(2):139–142. doi:S1516-44462005000200013 [pii]. /S1516-44462005000200013

Jakovljevic M, Crncevic Z, Ljubicic D, Babic D, Topic R, Saric M (2007) Mental disorders and metabolic syndrome: a fatamorgana or warning reality? Psychiatr Danub 19(1–2):76–86

Javaras KN, Pope HG, Lalonde JK, Roberts JL, Nillni YI, Laird NM, Bulik CM, Crow SJ, McElroy SL, Walsh BT, Tsuang MT, Rosenthal NR, Hudson JI (2008) Co-occurrence of binge eating disorder with psychiatric and medical disorders. J Clin Psychiatry 69(2):266–273. doi:ej07m03211 [pii]

Jette N, Patten S, Williams J, Becker W, Wiebe S (2008) Comorbidity of migraine and psychiatric disorders–a national population-based study. Headache 48(4):501–516. doi:10.1111/j.1526-4610.2007.00993.x, HED993 [pii]

Johannessen L, Strudsholm U, Foldager L, Munk-Jorgensen P (2006) Increased risk of hypertension in patients with bipolar disorder and patients with anxiety compared to background population and patients with schizophrenia. J Affect Disord 95(1–3):13–17. doi:10.1016/j.jad.2006.03.027, S0165-0327(06)00220-5 [pii]

John AP, Koloth R, Dragovic M, Lim SC (2009) Prevalence of metabolic syndrome among Australians with severe mental illness. Med J Aust 190(4):176–179. doi:joh10319_fm [pii]

Johnson JG, Cohen P, Brook JS (2000) Associations between bipolar disorder and other psychiatric disorders during adolescence and early adulthood: a community-based longitudinal investigation. Am J Psychiatry 157(10):1679–1681

Judd LL, Kessler RC, Paulus MP, Zeller PV, Wittchen HU, Kunovac JL (1998) Comorbidity as a fundamental feature of generalized anxiety disorders: results from the National Comorbidity Study (NCS). Acta Psychiatr Scand Suppl 393:6–11

Judd LL, Akiskal HS, Schettler PJ, Coryell W, Maser J, Rice JA, Solomon DA, Keller MB (2003) The comparative clinical phenotype and long term longitudinal episode course of bipolar I and II: a clinical spectrum or distinct disorders? J Affect Disord 73(1–2):19–32, doi:S0165032702003245 [pii]

Kasanin J (1926) The blood sugar curve in mental disease. Arch Neurol Psychiatry 16:414–419

Kauer-Sant'Anna M, Frey BN, Andreazza AC, Cereser KM, Gazalle FK, Tramontina J, da Costa SC, Santin A, Kapczinski F (2007) Anxiety comorbidity and quality of life in bipolar disorder patients. Can J Psychiatry 52(3):175–181

Kawa I, Carter JD, Joyce PR, Doughty CJ, Frampton CM, Wells JE, Walsh AE, Olds RJ (2005) Gender differences in bipolar disorder: age of onset, course, comorbidity, and symptom presentation. Bipolar Disord 7(2):119–125. doi:10.1111/j.1399-5618.2004.00180.x, BDI180 [pii]

Keck PE, McElroy SL (2003) Bipolar disorder, obesity, and pharmacotherapy-associated weight gain. J Clin Psychiatry 64(12):1426–1435

Keck PE Jr, McElroy SL, Strakowski SM, West SA, Hawkins JM, Huber TJ, Newman RM, DePriest M (1995) Outcome and comorbidity in first- compared with multiple-episode mania. J Nerv Ment Dis 183(5):320–324

Keck PE Jr, McElroy SL, Strakowski SM, West SA, Sax KW, Hawkins JM, Bourne ML, Haggard P (1998) 12-month outcome of patients with bipolar disorder following hospitalization for a manic or mixed episode. Am J Psychiatry 155(5):646–652

Keller MB (2006) Prevalence and impact of comorbid anxiety and bipolar disorder. J Clin Psychiatry 67(Suppl 1):5–7

Kemp DE, Calabrese JR, Tran QV, Pikalov A, Eudicone JM, Baker RA (2010) Metabolic syndrome in patients enrolled in a clinical trial of aripiprazole in the maintenance treatment of bipolar I disorder: a post hoc analysis of a randomized, double-blind, placebo-controlled trial. J Clin Psychiatry 71(9):1138–1144. doi:10.4088/JCP.09m05159gre

Kemp DE, Sylvia LG, Calabrese JR, Nierenberg AA, Thase ME, Reilly-Harrington NA, Ostacher MJ, Leon AC, Ketter TA, Friedman ES, Bowden CL, Rabideau DJ, Pencina M, Iosifescu DV

(2013) General medical burden in bipolar disorder: findings from the LiTMUS comparative effectiveness trial. Acta Psychiatr Scand. doi:10.1111/acps.12101

Kent L, Craddock N (2003) Is there a relationship between attention deficit hyperactivity disorder and bipolar disorder? J Affect Disord 73(3):211–221. doi:S016503270200927 [pii]

Kerbeshian J, Burd L, Klug MG (1995) Comorbid Tourette's disorder and bipolar disorder: an etiologic perspective. Am J Psychiatry 152(11):1646–1651

Kessler RC, McGonagle KA, Zhao S, Nelson CB, Hughes M, Eshleman S, Wittchen HU, Kendler KS (1994) Lifetime and 12-month prevalence of DSM-III-R psychiatric disorders in the United States. Results from the National Comorbidity Survey. Arch Gen Psychiatry 51(1):8–19

Kessler RC, Rubinow DR, Holmes C, Abelson JM, Zhao S (1997) The epidemiology of DSM-III-R bipolar I disorder in a general population survey. Psychol Med 27(5):1079–1089

Kessler RC, Stang P, Wittchen HU, Stein M, Walters EE (1999) Lifetime co-morbidities between social phobia and mood disorders in the US National Comorbidity Survey. Psychol Med 29(3):555–567

Kessler RC, Adler L, Barkley R, Biederman J, Conners CK, Demler O, Faraone SV, Greenhill LL, Howes MJ, Secnik K, Spencer T, Ustun TB, Walters EE, Zaslavsky AM (2006) The prevalence and correlates of adult ADHD in the United States: results from the National Comorbidity Survey Replication. Am J Psychiatry 163(4):716–723. doi:10.1176/appi.ajp.163.4.716, 163/4/716 [pii]

Kessler RC, Merikangas KR, Wang PS (2007) Prevalence, comorbidity, and service utilization for mood disorders in the United States at the beginning of the twenty-first century. Annu Rev Clin Psychol 3:137–158. doi:10.1146/annurev.clinpsy.3.022806.091444

Kilbane EJ, Gokbayrak NS, Galynker I, Cohen L, Tross S (2009) A review of panic and suicide in bipolar disorder: does comorbidity increase risk? J Affect Disord 115(1–2):1–10. doi:10.1016/j.jad.2008.09.014, S0165-0327(08)00374-1 [pii]

Kilbourne AM, Justice AC, Rabeneck L, Rodriguez-Barradas M, Weissman S (2001) General medical and psychiatric comorbidity among HIV-infected veterans in the post-HAART era. J Clin Epidemiol 54(Suppl 1):S22–S28. doi:S0895435601004437 [pii]

Kilbourne AM, Cornelius JR, Han X, Pincus HA, Shad M, Salloum I, Conigliaro J, Haas GL (2004) Burden of general medical conditions among individuals with bipolar disorder. Bipolar Disord 6(5):368–373. doi:10.1111/j.1399-5618.2004.00138.x, BDI138 [pii]

Kilbourne AM, Rofey DL, McCarthy JF, Post EP, Welsh D, Blow FC (2007) Nutrition and exercise behavior among patients with bipolar disorder. Bipolar Disord 9(5):443–452. doi:10.1111/j.1399-5618.2007.00386.x, BDI386 [pii]

Kilbourne AM, Morden NE, Austin K, Ilgen M, McCarthy JF, Dalack G, Blow FC (2009a) Excess heart-disease-related mortality in a national study of patients with mental disorders: identifying modifiable risk factors. Gen Hosp Psychiatry 31(6):555–563. doi:10.1016/j.genhosppsych.2009.07.008, S0163-8343(09)00141-8 [pii]

Kilbourne AM, Perron BE, Mezuk B, Welsh D, Ilgen M, Bauer MS (2009b) Co-occurring conditions and health-related quality of life in patients with bipolar disorder. Psychosom Med 71(8):894–900. doi:10.1097/PSY.0b013e3181b49948, PSY.0b013e3181b49948 [pii]

Kim B, Kim S, McIntyre RS, Park HJ, Kim SY, Joo YH (2009) Correlates of metabolic abnormalities in bipolar I disorder at initiation of acute phase treatment. Psychiatry Investig 6(2):78–84. doi:10.4306/pi.2009.6.2.78

Kimmel RJ, Kovacs I, Vrabel C, Wood B, Schalling M, Kelsoe JR (2005) Cosegregation of bipolar disorder and autosomal-dominant medullary cystic kidney disease in a large family. Am J Psychiatry 162(10):1972–1974. doi:10.1176/appi.ajp.162.10.1972, 162/10/1972 [pii]

Kinley DJ, Walker JR, Enns MW, Sareen J (2011) Panic attacks as a risk for later psychopathology: results from a nationally representative survey. Depress Anxiety 28(5):412–419. doi:10.1002/da.20809

Klassen LJ, Katzman MA, Chokka P (2010) Adult ADHD and its comorbidities, with a focus on bipolar disorder. J Affect Disord 124(1–2):1–8. doi:10.1016/j.jad.2009.06.036, S0165-0327(09)00317-6 [pii]

Klein DN, Depue RA (1985) Obsessional personality traits and risk for bipolar affective disorder: an offspring study. J Abnorm Psychol 94(3):291–297

Koyuncu A, Tukel R, Ozyildirim I, Meteris H, Yazici O (2010) Impact of obsessive-compulsive disorder comorbidity on the sociodemographic and clinical features of patients with bipolar disorder. Compr Psychiatry 51(3):293–297. doi:10.1016/j.comppsych.2009.07.006, S0010-440X(09)00085-6 [pii]

Krishnan KR (2005) Psychiatric and medical comorbidities of bipolar disorder. Psychosom Med 67(1):1–8. doi:10.1097/01.psy.0000151489.36347.18, 67/1/1 [pii]

Kruger S, Cooke RG, Hasey GM, Jorna T, Persad E (1995) Comorbidity of obsessive compulsive disorder in bipolar disorder. J Affect Disord 34(2):117–120. doi:10.016503279500008B [pii]

Kruger S, Shugar G, Cooke RG (1996) Comorbidity of binge eating disorder and the partial binge eating syndrome with bipolar disorder. Int J Eat Disord 19(1):45–52. doi:10.1002/(SICI)1098-108X(199601)19:1<45::AID-EAT6>3.0.CO;2-W [pii]

Kruger S, Braunig P, Cooke RG (2000) Comorbidity of obsessive-compulsive disorder in recovered inpatients with bipolar disorder. Bipolar Disord 2(1):71–74

Kupka RW, Nolen WA, Altshuler LL, Denicoff KD, Frye MA, Leverich GS, Keck PE Jr, McElroy SL, Rush AJ, Suppes T, Post RM (2001) The Stanley Foundation Bipolar Network. 2. Preliminary summary of demographics, course of illness and response to novel treatments. Br J Psychiatry Suppl 41:s177–s183

Kupka RW, Nolen WA, Post RM, McElroy SL, Altshuler LL, Denicoff KD, Frye MA, Keck PE Jr, Leverich GS, Rush AJ, Suppes T, Pollio C, Drexhage HA (2002) High rate of autoimmune thyroiditis in bipolar disorder: lack of association with lithium exposure. Biol Psychiatry 51(4):305–311. doi:S0006322301012173 [pii]

Laaksonen DE, Lakka HM, Niskanen LK, Kaplan GA, Salonen JT, Lakka TA (2002) Metabolic syndrome and development of diabetes mellitus: application and validation of recently suggested definitions of the metabolic syndrome in a prospective cohort study. Am J Epidemiol 156(11):1070–1077

Lambert BL, Chou CH, Chang KY, Tafesse E, Carson W (2005) Antipsychotic exposure and type 2 diabetes among patients with schizophrenia: a matched case-control study of California Medicaid claims. Pharmacoepidemiol Drug Saf 14(6):417–425. doi:10.1002/pds.1092

Lasser K, Boyd JW, Woolhandler S, Himmelstein DU, McCormick D, Bor DH (2000) Smoking and mental illness: a population-based prevalence study. JAMA 284(20):2606–2610. doi:joc00268 [pii]

Laursen TM, Munk-Olsen T, Nordentoft M, Mortensen PB (2007) Increased mortality among patients admitted with major psychiatric disorders: a register-based study comparing mortality in unipolar depressive disorder, bipolar affective disorder, schizoaffective disorder, and schizophrenia. J Clin Psychiatry 68(6):899–907

Laursen TM, Munk-Olsen T, Agerbo E, Gasse C, Mortensen PB (2009) Somatic hospital contacts, invasive cardiac procedures, and mortality from heart disease in patients with severe mental disorder. Arch Gen Psychiatry 66(7):713–720. doi:10.1001/archgenpsychiatry.2009.61, 66/7/713 [pii]

Laursen TM, Munk-Olsen T, Gasse C (2011) Chronic somatic comorbidity and excess mortality due to natural causes in persons with schizophrenia or bipolar affective disorder. PLoS One 6(9):e24597. doi:10.1371/journal.pone.0024597, PONE-D-11-09662 [pii]

Lee JH, Dunner DL (2008) The effect of anxiety disorder comorbidity on treatment resistant bipolar disorders. Depress Anxiety 25(2):91–97. doi:10.1002/da.20279

Lensi P, Cassano GB, Correddu G, Ravagli S, Kunovac JL, Akiskal HS (1996) Obsessive-compulsive disorder. Familial-developmental history, symptomatology, comorbidity and course with special reference to gender-related differences. Br J Psychiatry 169(1):101–107

Levander E, Frye MA, McElroy S, Suppes T, Grunze H, Nolen WA, Kupka R, Keck PE Jr, Leverich GS, Altshuler LL, Hwang S, Mintz J, Post RM (2007) Alcoholism and anxiety in bipolar illness: differential lifetime anxiety comorbidity in bipolar I women with and without alcoholism. J Affect Disord 101(1–3):211–217. doi:10.1016/j.jad.2006.11.023, S0165-0327(06)00505-2 [pii]

Leverich GS, Altshuler LL, Frye MA, Suppes T, Keck PE Jr, McElroy SL, Denicoff KD, Obrocea G, Nolen WA, Kupka R, Walden J, Grunze H, Perez S, Luckenbaugh DA, Post RM (2003) Factors associated with suicide attempts in 648 patients with bipolar disorder in the Stanley Foundation Bipolar Network. J Clin Psychiatry 64(5):506–515

Lin HC, Tsai SY, Lee HC (2007) Increased risk of developing stroke among patients with bipolar disorder after an acute mood episode: a six-year follow-up study. J Affect Disord 100(1–3): 49–54. doi:10.1016/j.jad.2006.09.016, S0165-0327(06)00401-0 [pii]

Lipton RB (2009) Tracing transformation: chronic migraine classification, progression, and epidemiology. Neurology 72(5 Suppl):S3–S7. doi:10.1212/WNL.0b013e3181974b19, 72/5_Supplement_1/S3 [pii]

Logue MW, Durner M, Heiman GA, Hodge SE, Hamilton SP, Knowles JA, Fyer AJ, Weissman MM (2009) A linkage search for joint panic disorder/bipolar genes. Am J Med Genet B Neuropsychiatr Genet 150B(8):1139–1146. doi:10.1002/ajmg.b.30939

Low NC, Du Fort GG, Cervantes P (2003) Prevalence, clinical correlates, and treatment of migraine in bipolar disorder. Headache 43(9):940–949. doi:03184 [pii]

Lunde AV, Fasmer OB, Akiskal KK, Akiskal HS, Oedegaard KJ (2009) The relationship of bulimia and anorexia nervosa with bipolar disorder and its temperamental foundations. J Affect Disord 115(3):309–314. doi:10.1016/j.jad.2008.10.012, S0165-0327(08)00398-4 [pii]

Lyketsos CG, Hanson AL, Fishman M, Rosenblatt A, McHugh PR, Treisman GJ (1993) Manic syndrome early and late in the course of HIV. Am J Psychiatry 150(2):326–327

MacKinnon DF, McMahon FJ, Simpson SG, McInnis MG, DePaulo JR (1997) Panic disorder with familial bipolar disorder. Biol Psychiatry 42(2):90–95. doi:10.1016/S0006-3223(96)00299-5, S0006-3223(96)00299-5 [pii]

MacKinnon DF, Zandi PP, Cooper J, Potash JB, Simpson SG, Gershon E, Nurnberger J, Reich T, DePaulo JR (2002) Comorbid bipolar disorder and panic disorder in families with a high prevalence of bipolar disorder. Am J Psychiatry 159(1):30–35

MacKinnon DF, Zandi PP, Gershon E, Nurnberger JI Jr, Reich T, DePaulo JR (2003a) Rapid switching of mood in families with multiple cases of bipolar disorder. Arch Gen Psychiatry 60(9):921–928. doi:10.1001/archpsyc.60.9.921, 60/9/921 [pii]

MacKinnon DF, Zandi PP, Gershon ES, Nurnberger JI Jr, DePaulo JR Jr (2003b) Association of rapid mood switching with panic disorder and familial panic risk in familial bipolar disorder. Am J Psychiatry 160(9):1696–1698

MacQueen GM, Marriott M, Begin H, Robb J, Joffe RT, Young LT (2003) Subsyndromal symptoms assessed in longitudinal, prospective follow-up of a cohort of patients with bipolar disorder. Bipolar Disord 5(5):349–355. doi:048 [pii]

Magalhaes PV, Kapczinski NS, Kapczinski F (2010) Correlates and impact of obsessive-compulsive comorbidity in bipolar disorder. Compr Psychiatry 51(4):353–356. doi:10.1016/j.comppsych.2009.11.001, S0010-440X(09)00132-1 [pii]

Magalhaes PV, Kapczinski F, Nierenberg AA, Deckersbach T, Weisinger D, Dodd S, Berk M (2012) Illness burden and medical comorbidity in the Systematic Treatment Enhancement Program for Bipolar Disorder. Acta Psychiatr Scand 125(4):303–308. doi:10.1111/j.1600-0447.2011.01794.x

Mahasuar R, Janardhan Reddy YC, Math SB (2011) Obsessive-compulsive disorder with and without bipolar disorder. Psychiatry Clin Neurosci 65(5):423–433. doi:10.1111/j.1440-1819.2011.02247.x

Mahmood T, Romans S, Silverstone T (1999) Prevalence of migraine in bipolar disorder. J Affect Disord 52(1–3):239–241

Maina G, Albert U, Pessina E, Bogetto F (2007) Bipolar obsessive-compulsive disorder and personality disorders. Bipolar Disord 9(7):722–729. doi:10.1111/j.1399-5618.2007.00508.x, BDI508 [pii]

Maina G, Salvi V, Vitalucci A, D'Ambrosio V, Bogetto F (2008) Prevalence and correlates of overweight in drug-naive patients with bipolar disorder. J Affect Disord 110(1–2):149–155. doi:10.1016/j.jad.2007.12.233, S0165-0327(07)00425-9 [pii]

Maj M (2005) "Psychiatric comorbidity": an artefact of current diagnostic systems? Br J Psychiatry 186:182–184. doi:10.1192/bjp.186.3.182, 186/3/182 [pii]

Mangweth B, Hudson JI, Pope HG, Hausmann A, De Col C, Laird NM, Beibl W, Tsuang MT (2003) Family study of the aggregation of eating disorders and mood disorders. Psychol Med 33(7):1319–1323

Mantere O, Melartin TK, Suominen K, Rytsala HJ, Valtonen HM, Arvilommi P, Leppamaki S, Isometsa ET (2006) Differences in axis I and II comorbidity between bipolar I and II disorders and major depressive disorder. J Clin Psychiatry 67(4):584–593

Mantere O, Isometsa E, Ketokivi M, Kiviruusu O, Suominen K, Valtonen HM, Arvilommi P, Leppamaki S (2010) A prospective latent analyses study of psychiatric comorbidity of DSM-IV bipolar I and II disorders. Bipolar Disord 12(3):271–284. doi:10.1111/j.1399-5618.2010.00810.x, BDI810 [pii]

Marchesi C, De Ferri A, Petrolini N, Govi A, Manzoni GC, Coiro V, De Risio C (1989) Prevalence of migraine and muscle tension headache in depressive disorders. J Affect Disord 16(1):33–36

Mather AA, Cox BJ, Enns MW, Sareen J (2009) Associations of obesity with psychiatric disorders and suicidal behaviors in a nationally representative sample. J Psychosom Res 66(4):277–285. doi:10.1016/j.jpsychores.2008.09.008, S0022-3999(08)00429-7 [pii]

Matthews AM, Huckans MS, Blackwell AD, Hauser P (2008) Hepatitis C testing and infection rates in bipolar patients with and without comorbid substance use disorders. Bipolar Disord 10(2):266–270. doi:10.1111/j.1399-5618.2007.00472.x, BDI472 [pii]

McElroy SL, Strakowski SM, Keck PE Jr, Tugrul KL, West SA, Lonczak HS (1995) Differences and similarities in mixed and pure mania. Compr Psychiatry 36(3):187–194. doi:0010-440X(95)90080-F [pii]

McElroy SL, Pope HG Jr, Keck PE Jr, Hudson JI, Phillips KA, Strakowski SM (1996) Are impulse-control disorders related to bipolar disorder? Compr Psychiatry 37(4):229–240. doi:S0010-440X(96)90001-2 [pii]

McElroy SL, Altshuler LL, Suppes T, Keck PE Jr, Frye MA, Denicoff KD, Nolen WA, Kupka RW, Leverich GS, Rochussen JR, Rush AJ, Post RM (2001) Axis I psychiatric comorbidity and its relationship to historical illness variables in 288 patients with bipolar disorder. Am J Psychiatry 158(3):420–426

McElroy SL, Frye MA, Suppes T, Dhavale D, Keck PE Jr, Leverich GS, Altshuler L, Denicoff KD, Nolen WA, Kupka R, Grunze H, Walden J, Post RM (2002) Correlates of overweight and obesity in 644 patients with bipolar disorder. J Clin Psychiatry 63(3):207–213

McElroy SL, Kotwal R, Malhotra S, Nelson EB, Keck PE, Nemeroff CB (2004) Are mood disorders and obesity related? A review for the mental health professional. J Clin Psychiatry 65(5):634–651, quiz 730

McElroy SL, Kotwal R, Keck PE Jr, Akiskal HS (2005) Comorbidity of bipolar and eating disorders: distinct or related disorders with shared dysregulations? J Affect Disord 86(2–3):107–127. doi:10.1016/j.jad.2004.11.008, S0165-0327(04)00436-7 [pii]

McElroy SL, Frye MA, Hellemann G, Altshuler L, Leverich GS, Suppes T, Keck PE, Nolen WA, Kupka R, Post RM (2011) Prevalence and correlates of eating disorders in 875 patients with bipolar disorder. J Affect Disord 128(3):191–198. doi:10.1016/j.jad.2010.06.037, S0165-0327(10)00465-9 [pii]

McElroy SL, Crow S, Biernacka JM, Winham S, Geske J, Barboza AB, Prieto ML, Chauhan M, Seymour LR, Mori N, Frye MA (2013) Clinical phenotype of bipolar disorder with comorbid binge eating disorder. J Affect Disord. doi:10.1016/j.jad.2013.05.024, S0165-0327(13)00383-2 [pii]

McGinty EE, Zhang Y, Guallar E, Ford DE, Steinwachs D, Dixon LB, Keating NL, Daumit GL (2012) Cancer incidence in a sample of Maryland residents with serious mental illness. Psychiatr Serv 63(7):714–717. doi:10.1176/appi.ps.201100169, 1204715 [pii]

McGough JJ, Smalley SL, McCracken JT, Yang M, Del'Homme M, Lynn DE, Loo S (2005) Psychiatric comorbidity in adult attention deficit hyperactivity disorder: findings from multiplex families. Am J Psychiatry 162(9):1621–1627. doi:10.1176/appi.ajp.162.9.1621, 162/9/1621 [pii]

McIntyre RS (2002) Psychotropic drugs and adverse events in the treatment of bipolar disorders revisited. J Clin Psychiatry 63(Suppl 3):15–20

McIntyre RS, Konarski JZ, Misener VL, Kennedy SH (2005) Bipolar disorder and diabetes mellitus: epidemiology, etiology, and treatment implications. Ann Clin Psychiatry 17(2):83–93

McIntyre RS, Konarski JZ, Soczynska JK, Wilkins K, Panjwani G, Bouffard B, Bottas A, Kennedy SH (2006a) Medical comorbidity in bipolar disorder: implications for functional outcomes and health service utilization. Psychiatr Serv 57(8):1140–1144. doi:10.1176/appi.ps.57.8.1140, 57/8/1140 [pii]

McIntyre RS, Konarski JZ, Wilkins K, Bouffard B, Soczynska JK, Kennedy SH (2006b) The prevalence and impact of migraine headache in bipolar disorder: results from the Canadian Community Health Survey. Headache 46(6):973–982. doi:10.1111/j.1526-4610.2006.00469.x, HED469 [pii]

McIntyre RS, McElroy SL, Konarski JZ, Soczynska JK, Bottas A, Castel S, Wilkins K, Kennedy SH (2007a) Substance use disorders and overweight/obesity in bipolar I disorder: preliminary evidence for competing addictions. J Clin Psychiatry 68(9):1352–1357

McIntyre RS, Soczynska JK, Beyer JL, Woldeyohannes HO, Law CW, Miranda A, Konarski JZ, Kennedy SH (2007b) Medical comorbidity in bipolar disorder: re-prioritizing unmet needs. Curr Opin Psychiatry 20(4):406–416. doi:10.1097/YCO.0b013e3281938102, 00001504-200707000-00017 [pii]

McIntyre RS, Danilewitz M, Liauw SS, Kemp DE, Nguyen HT, Kahn LS, Kucyi A, Soczynska JK, Woldeyohannes HO, Lachowski A, Kim B, Nathanson J, Alsuwaidan M, Taylor VH (2010a) Bipolar disorder and metabolic syndrome: an international perspective. J Affect Disord 126(3):366–387. doi:10.1016/j.jad.2010.04.012, S0165-0327(10)00348-4 [pii]

McIntyre RS, Kennedy SH, Soczynska JK, Nguyen HT, Bilkey TS, Woldeyohannes HO, Nathanson JA, Joshi S, Cheng JS, Benson KM, Muzina DJ (2010b) Attention-deficit/hyperactivity disorder in adults with bipolar disorder or major depressive disorder: results from the international mood disorders collaborative project. Prim Care Companion J Clin Psychiatry 12(3). doi:10.4088/PCC.09m00861gry, PCC.09 m00861 [pii]

McIntyre RS, Woldeyohannes HO, Soczynska JK, Miranda A, Lachowski A, Liauw SS, Grossman T, Lourenco MT, Kim B, Alsuwaidan MT, Kennedy SH (2010b) The rate of metabolic syndrome in euthymic Canadian individuals with bipolar I/II disorder. Adv Ther 27(11):828–836. doi:10.1007/s12325-010-0072-z

McIntyre RS, Rosenbluth M, Ramasubbu R, Bond DJ, Taylor VH, Beaulieu S, Schaffer A (2012) Managing medical and psychiatric comorbidity in individuals with major depressive disorder and bipolar disorder. Ann Clin Psychiatry 24(2):163–169. doi:acp_2402g [pii]

Merikangas KR, Angst J, Isler H (1990) Migraine and psychopathology. Results of the Zurich cohort study of young adults. Arch Gen Psychiatry 47(9):849–853

Merikangas KR, Jin R, He JP, Kessler RC, Lee S, Sampson NA, Viana MC, Andrade LH, Hu C, Karam EG, Ladea M, Medina-Mora ME, Ono Y, Posada-Villa J, Sagar R, Wells JE, Zarkov Z (2011) Prevalence and correlates of bipolar spectrum disorder in the world mental health survey initiative. Arch Gen Psychiatry 68(3):241-251. doi:10.1001/archgenpsychiatry.2011.12. 68/3/241 [pii]

Milberger S, Biederman J, Faraone SV, Murphy J, Tsuang MT (1995) Attention deficit hyperactivity disorder and comorbid disorders: issues of overlapping symptoms. Am J Psychiatry 152(12):1793–1799

Misra M, Papakostas GI, Klibanski A (2004) Effects of psychiatric disorders and psychotropic medications on prolactin and bone metabolism. J Clin Psychiatry 65(12):1607–1618, quiz 1590, 1760–1601

Moor S, Crowe M, Luty S, Carter J, Joyce PR (2012) Effects of comorbidity and early age of onset in young people with Bipolar Disorder on self harming behaviour and suicide attempts. J Affect Disord 136(3):1212–1215. doi:10.1016/j.jad.2011.10.018, S0165-0327(11)00667-7 [pii]

Morriss R, Mohammed FA (2005) Metabolism, lifestyle and bipolar affective disorder. J Psychopharmacol 19(6 Suppl):94–101. doi:10.1177/0269881105058678, 19/6_suppl/94 [pii]

Mueser KT, Salyers MP, Rosenberg SD, Goodman LA, Essock SM, Osher FC, Swartz MS, Butterfield MI (2004) Interpersonal trauma and posttraumatic stress disorder in patients with severe mental illness: demographic, clinical, and health correlates. Schizophr Bull 30(1):45–57

Mula M (2010) The clinical spectrum of bipolar symptoms in epilepsy: a critical reappraisal. Postgrad Med 122(4):17–23. doi:10.3810/pgm.2010.07.2171

Mula M, Pini S, Monteleone P, Iazzetta P, Preve M, Tortorella A, Amato E, Di Paolo L, Conversano C, Rucci P, Cassano GB, Maj M (2008a) Different temperament and character dimensions correlate with panic disorder comorbidity in bipolar disorder and unipolar depression. J Anxiety Disord 22(8):1421–1426. doi:10.1016/j.janxdis.2008.02.004, S0887-6185(08)00056-X [pii]

Mula M, Schmitz B, Jauch R, Cavanna A, Cantello R, Monaco F, Trimble MR (2008b) On the prevalence of bipolar disorder in epilepsy. Epilepsy Behav 13(4):658–661. doi:10.1016/j.yebeh.2008.08.002, S1525-5050(08)00252-7 [pii]

Mula M, Jauch R, Cavanna A, Collimedaglia L, Barbagli D, Gaus V, Kretz R, Viana M, Cantello R, Monaco F, Schmitz B (2009) Manic/hypomanic symptoms and quality of life measures in patients with epilepsy. Seizure 18(7):530–532. doi:10.1016/j.seizure.2009.05.008, S1059-1311(09)00105-8 [pii]

Muller-Oerlinghausen B, Passoth PM, Poser W, Pudel V (1979) Impaired glucose tolerance in long-term lithium-treated patients. Int Pharmacopsychiatry 14(6):350–362

Nakagawa A, Grunebaum MF, Sullivan GM, Currier D, Ellis SP, Burke AK, Brent DA, Mann JJ, Oquendo MA (2008) Comorbid anxiety in bipolar disorder: does it have an independent effect on suicidality? Bipolar Disord 10(4):530–538. doi:10.1111/j.1399-5618.2008.00590.x, BDI590 [pii]

Nasrallah HA (2003) Factors in antipsychotic drug selection: tolerability considerations. CNS Spectr 8(11 Suppl 2):23–25

Neria Y, Bromet EJ, Sievers S, Lavelle J, Fochtmann LJ (2002) Trauma exposure and posttraumatic stress disorder in psychosis: findings from a first-admission cohort. J Consult Clin Psychol 70(1):246–251

Nery-Fernandes F, Quarantini LC, Galvao-De-Almeida A, Rocha MV, Kapczinski F, Miranda-Scippa A (2009) Lower rates of comorbidities in euthymic bipolar patients. World J Biol Psychiatry 10(4 Pt 2):474–479. doi:10.1080/15622970802688929, 910761991 [pii]

Nestadt G, Di CZ, Riddle MA, Grados MA, Greenberg BD, Fyer AJ, McCracken JT, Rauch SL, Murphy DL, Rasmussen SA, Cullen B, Pinto A, Knowles JA, Piacentini J, Pauls DL, Bienvenu OJ, Wang Y, Liang KY, Samuels JF, Roche KB (2009) Obsessive-compulsive disorder: subclassification based on co-morbidity. Psychol Med 39(9):1491–1501. doi:10.1017/S0033291708004753, S0033291708004753 [pii]

Neves FS, Malloy-Diniz LF, Correa H (2009) Suicidal behavior in bipolar disorder: what is the influence of psychiatric comorbidities? J Clin Psychiatry 70(1):13–18. doi:ej08m04037 [pii]

Nguyen TV, Low NC (2013) Comorbidity of migraine and mood episodes in a nationally representative population-based sample. Headache 53(3):498–506. doi:10.1111/j.1526-4610.2012.02264.x

Nierenberg AA, Miyahara S, Spencer T, Wisniewski SR, Otto MW, Simon N, Pollack MH, Ostacher MJ, Yan L, Siegel R, Sachs GS (2005) Clinical and diagnostic implications of lifetime attention-deficit/hyperactivity disorder comorbidity in adults with bipolar disorder: data from the first 1000 STEP-BD participants. Biol Psychiatry 57(11):1467–1473. doi:10.1016/j.biopsych.2005.01.036, S0006-3223(05)00113-7 [pii]

Oedegaard KJ, Fasmer OB (2005) Is migraine in unipolar depressed patients a bipolar spectrum trait? J Affect Disord 84(2–3):233–242. doi:10.1016/j.jad.2003.11.007, S0165032703003197 [pii]

Okan Ibiloglu A, Caykoylu A (2011) The comorbidity of anxiety disorders in bipolar I and bipolar II patients among Turkish population. J Anxiety Disord 25(5):661–667. doi:10.1016/j.janxdis.2011.02.008, S0887-6185(11)00031-4 [pii]

Olfson M, Guardino M, Struening E, Schneier FR, Hellman F, Klein DF (2000) Barriers to the treatment of social anxiety. Am J Psychiatry 157(4):521–527

Ollendorf DA, Joyce AT, Rucker M (2004) Rate of new-onset diabetes among patients treated with atypical or conventional antipsychotic medications for schizophrenia. MedGenMed 6(1):5. doi:466800 [pii]

Oreski I, Jakovljevic M, Aukst-Margetic B, Orlic ZC, Vuksan-Cusa B (2012) Comorbidity and multimorbidity in patients with schizophrenia and bipolar disorder: similarities and differences. Psychiatr Danub 24(1):80–85

Ortiz A, Cervantes P, Zlotnik G, van de Velde C, Slaney C, Garnham J, Turecki G, O'Donovan C, Alda M (2010) Cross-prevalence of migraine and bipolar disorder. Bipolar Disord 12(4): 397–403. doi:10.1111/j.1399-5618.2010.00832.x, BDI832 [pii]

Osby U, Brandt L, Correia N, Ekbom A, Sparen P (2001) Excess mortality in bipolar and unipolar disorder in Sweden. Arch Gen Psychiatry 58(9):844–850. doi:yoa20257 [pii]

Osser DN, Najarian DM, Dufresne RL (1999) Olanzapine increases weight and serum triglyceride levels. J Clin Psychiatry 60(11):767–770

Ottman R, Lipton RB, Ettinger AB, Cramer JA, Reed ML, Morrison A, Wan GJ (2011) Comorbidities of epilepsy: results from the Epilepsy Comorbidities and Health (EPIC) survey. Epilepsia 52(2):308–315. doi:10.1111/j.1528-1167.2010.02927.x

Otto MW, Perlman CA, Wernicke R, Reese HE, Bauer MS, Pollack MH (2004) Posttraumatic stress disorder in patients with bipolar disorder: a review of prevalence, correlates, and treatment strategies. Bipolar Disord 6(6):470–479. doi:10.1111/j.1399-5618.2004.00151.x, BDI151 [pii]

Otto MW, Simon NM, Wisniewski SR, Miklowitz DJ, Kogan JN, Reilly-Harrington NA, Frank E, Nierenberg AA, Marangell LB, Sagduyu K, Weiss RD, Miyahara S, Thas ME, Sachs GS, Pollack MH (2006) Prospective 12-month course of bipolar disorder in out-patients with and without comorbid anxiety disorders. Br J Psychiatry 189:20–25. doi:10.1192/bjp.bp.104.007773, 189/1/20 [pii]

Park S, Cho MJ, Chang SM, Jeon HJ, Cho SJ, Kim BS, Bae JN, Wang HR, Ahn JH, Hong JP (2011) Prevalence, correlates, and comorbidities of adult ADHD symptoms in Korea: results of the Korean epidemiologic catchment area study. Psychiatry Res 186(2–3):378–383. doi:10.1016/j.psychres.2010.07.047, S0165-1781(10)00479-8 [pii]

Pashinian A, Faragian S, Levi A, Yeghiyan M, Gasparyan K, Weizman R, Weizman A, Fuchs C, Poyurovsky M (2006) Obsessive-compulsive disorder in bipolar disorder patients with first manic episode. J Affect Disord 94(1–3):151–156. doi:10.1016/j.jad.2006.03.022, S0165-0327(06)00167-4 [pii]

Pataki C, Carlson GA (2013) The comorbidity of ADHD and bipolar disorder: any less confusion? Curr Psychiatry Rep 15(7):372. doi:10.1007/s11920-013-0372-5

Patten SB, Williams JV (2007) Self-reported allergies and their relationship to several Axis I disorders in a community sample. Int J Psychiatry Med 37(1):11–22

Pecknold JC, Fleury D (1986) Alprazolam-induced manic episode in two patients with panic disorder. Am J Psychiatry 143(5):652–653

Perron BE, Howard MO, Nienhuis JK, Bauer MS, Woodward AT, Kilbourne AM (2009) Prevalence and burden of general medical conditions among adults with bipolar I disorder: results from the National Epidemiologic Survey on Alcohol and Related Conditions. J Clin Psychiatry 70(10):1407–1415. doi:10.4088/JCP.08m04586yel

Perugi G, Akiskal HS, Pfanner C, Presta S, Gemignani A, Milanfranchi A, Lensi P, Ravagli S, Cassano GB (1997) The clinical impact of bipolar and unipolar affective comorbidity on obsessive-compulsive disorder. J Affect Disord 46(1):15–23. doi:S0165-0327(97)00075-X [pii]

Perugi G, Akiskal HS, Ramacciotti S, Nassini S, Toni C, Milanfranchi A, Musetti L (1999) Depressive comorbidity of panic, social phobic, and obsessive-compulsive disorders re-examined: is there a bipolar II connection? J Psychiatr Res 33(1):53–61. doi:S0022-3956(98)00044-2 [pii]

Perugi G, Frare F, Toni C, Mata B, Akiskal HS (2001) Bipolar II and unipolar comorbidity in 153 outpatients with social phobia. Compr Psychiatry 42(5):375–381. doi:10.1053/comp.2001.26270, S0010-440X(01)24652-5 [pii]

Perugi G, Toni C, Frare F, Travierso MC, Hantouche E, Akiskal HS (2002) Obsessive-compulsive-bipolar comorbidity: a systematic exploration of clinical features and treatment outcome. J Clin Psychiatry 63(12):1129–1134

Perugi G, Ceraudo G, Vannucchi G, Rizzato S, Toni C, Dell'osso L (2013) Attention deficit/hyperactivity disorder symptoms in Italian bipolar adult patients: a preliminary report. J Affect Disord 149(1–3):430–434. doi:10.1016/j.jad.2012.12.010, S0165-0327(12)00843-9 [pii]

Petry NM, Barry D, Pietrzak RH, Wagner JA (2008) Overweight and obesity are associated with psychiatric disorders: results from the National Epidemiologic Survey on Alcohol and Related Conditions. Psychosom Med 70(3):288–297. doi:10.1097/PSY.0b013e3181651651, PSY.0b013e3181651651 [pii]

Pickering RP, Grant BF, Chou SP, Compton WM (2007) Are overweight, obesity, and extreme obesity associated with psychopathology? Results from the national epidemiologic survey on alcohol and related conditions. J Clin Psychiatry 68(7):998–1009

Pini S, Cassano GB, Simonini E, Savino M, Russo A, Montgomery SA (1997) Prevalence of anxiety disorders comorbidity in bipolar depression, unipolar depression and dysthymia. J Affect Disord 42(2–3):145–153. doi:S0165-0327(96)01405-X [pii]

Pini S, Dell'Osso L, Mastrocinque C, Marcacci G, Papasogli A, Vignoli S, Pallanti S, Cassano G (1999) Axis I comorbidity in bipolar disorder with psychotic features. Br J Psychiatry 175:467–471

Pini S, Dell'Osso L, Amador XF, Mastrocinque C, Saettoni M, Cassano GB (2003) Awareness of illness in patients with bipolar I disorder with or without comorbid anxiety disorders. Aust N Z J Psychiatry 37(3):355–361. doi:1188 [pii]

Pini S, Maser JD, Dell'Osso L, Abelli M, Muti M, Gesi C, Cassano GB (2006) Social anxiety disorder comorbidity in patients with bipolar disorder: a clinical replication. J Anxiety Disord 20(8):1148–1157. doi:10.1016/j.janxdis.2006.03.006, S0887-6185(06)00042-9 [pii]

Pirraglia PA, Biswas K, Kilbourne AM, Fenn H, Bauer MS (2009) A prospective study of the impact of comorbid medical disease on bipolar disorder outcomes. J Affect Disord 115(3):355–359. doi:10.1016/j.jad.2008.09.020, S0165-0327(08)00393-5 [pii]

Post RM, Rubinow DR, Uhde TW, Roy-Byrne PP, Linnoila M, Rosoff A, Cowdry R (1989) Dysphoric mania. Clinical and biological correlates. Arch Gen Psychiatry 46(4):353–358

Potash JB, Toolan J, Steele J, Miller EB, Pearl J, Zandi PP, Schulze TG, Kassem L, Simpson SG, Lopez V, MacKinnon DF, McMahon FJ (2007) The bipolar disorder phenome database: a resource for genetic studies. Am J Psychiatry 164(8):1229–1237. doi:10.1176/appi.ajp.2007.06122045, 164/8/1229 [pii]

Prince JD, Walkup J, Akincigil A, Amin S, Crystal S (2012) Serious mental illness and risk of new HIV/AIDS diagnoses: an analysis of Medicaid beneficiaries in eight states. Psychiatr Serv 63(10):1032–1038. doi:10.1176/appi.ps.201100342, 1305600 [pii]

Provencher MD, Guimond AJ, Hawke LD (2012) Comorbid anxiety in bipolar spectrum disorders: a neglected research and treatment issue? J Affect Disord 137(1–3):161–164. doi:10.1016/j.jad.2011.12.001, S0165-0327(11)00761-0 [pii]

Pylvanen V, Knip M, Pakarinen A, Kotila M, Turkka J, Isojarvi JI (2002) Serum insulin and leptin levels in valproate-associated obesity. Epilepsia 43(5):514–517. doi:epi31501 [pii]

Radat F, Swendsen J (2005) Psychiatric comorbidity in migraine: a review. Cephalalgia 25(3):165–178. doi:10.1111/j.1468-2982.2004.00839.x, CHA839 [pii]

Ramacciotti CE, Paoli RA, Marcacci G, Piccinni A, Burgalassi A, Dell'Osso L, Garfinkel PE (2005) Relationship between bipolar illness and binge-eating disorders. Psychiatry Res 135(2):165–170. doi:10.1016/j.psychres.2004.04.014, S0165-1781(05)00093-4 [pii]

Ramasubbu R, Beaulieu S, Taylor VH, Schaffer A, McIntyre RS (2012) The CANMAT task force recommendations for the management of patients with mood disorders and comorbid medical conditions: diagnostic, assessment, and treatment principles. Ann Clin Psychiatry 24(1):82–90. doi:acp_2401h [pii]

Ramsey CM, Leoutsakos JM, Mayer LS, Eaton WW, Lee HB (2010) History of manic and hypomanic episodes and risk of incident cardiovascular disease: 11.5 year follow-up from the Baltimore Epidemiologic Catchment Area Study. J Affect Disord 125(1–3):35–41. doi:10.1016/j.jad.2009.12.024, S0165-0327(10)00003-0 [pii]

Raphael T, Parsons J (1921) Blood sugar studies in dementia praecox and manic-depressive insanity. Arch Neurol Psychiatry 5:681–709

Rassi A, Veras AB, dos Reis M, Pastore DL, Bruno LM, de Avila MA, Bruno RV, Nardi AE (2010) Prevalence of psychiatric disorders in patients with polycystic ovary syndrome. Compr Psychiatry 51(6):599–602. doi:10.1016/j.comppsych.2010.02.009, S0010-440X(10)00012-X [pii]

Ratcliffe GE, Enns MW, Jacobi F, Belik SL, Sareen J (2009) The relationship between migraine and mental disorders in a population-based sample. Gen Hosp Psychiatry 31(1):14–19. doi:10.1016/j.genhosppsych.2008.09.006, S0163-8343(08)00167-9 [pii]

Regenold WT, Thapar RK, Marano C, Gavirneni S, Kondapavuluru PV (2002) Increased prevalence of type 2 diabetes mellitus among psychiatric inpatients with bipolar I affective and schizoaffective disorders independent of psychotropic drug use. J Affect Disord 70(1):19–26. doi:S0165032701004566 [pii]

Rihmer Z, Barsi J, Belso N, Pestality P, Gyorgy S (1996) Antidepressant-induced hypomania in obsessive-compulsive disorder. Int Clin Psychopharmacol 11(3):203–205

Rihmer Z, Szadoczky E, Furedi J, Kiss K, Papp Z (2001) Anxiety disorders comorbidity in bipolar I, bipolar II and unipolar major depression: results from a population-based study in Hungary. J Affect Disord 67(1–3):175–179. doi:S0165032701003093 [pii]

Robertson MM (2006) Mood disorders and Gilles de la Tourette's syndrome: an update on prevalence, etiology, comorbidity, clinical associations, and implications. J Psychosom Res 61(3):349–358. doi:10.1016/j.jpsychores.2006.07.019, S0022-3999(06)00344-8 [pii]

Robins L, Regier D (1991) Psychiatric disorders in America: the Epidemiologic Catchment Area study. Free Press, New York

Roshanaei-Moghaddam B, Katon W (2009) Premature mortality from general medical illnesses among persons with bipolar disorder: a review. Psychiatr Serv 60(2):147–156. doi:10.1176/appi.ps.60.2.147, 60/2/147 [pii]

Ruggero CJ, Carlson GA, Kotov R, Bromet EJ (2010) Ten-year diagnostic consistency of bipolar disorder in a first-admission sample. Bipolar Disord 12(1):21–31. doi:10.1111/j.1399-5618.2009.00777.x, BDI777 [pii]

Ruzickova M, Slaney C, Garnham J, Alda M (2003) Clinical features of bipolar disorder with and without comorbid diabetes mellitus. Can J Psychiatry 48(7):458–461

Ryden E, Thase ME, Straht D, Aberg-Wistedt A, Bejerot S, Landen M (2009) A history of childhood attention-deficit hyperactivity disorder (ADHD) impacts clinical outcome in adult bipolar patients regardless of current ADHD. Acta Psychiatr Scand 120(3):239–246. doi:10.1111/j.1600-0447.2009.01399.x, ACP1399 [pii]

Sachs GS, Baldassano CF, Truman CJ, Guille C (2000) Comorbidity of attention deficit hyperactivity disorder with early- and late-onset bipolar disorder. Am J Psychiatry 157(3):466–468

Sachs G, Bowden C, Calabrese JR, Ketter T, Thompson T, White R, Bentley B (2006) Effects of lamotrigine and lithium on body weight during maintenance treatment of bipolar I disorder. Bipolar Disord 8(2):175–181. doi:10.1111/j.1399-5618.2006.00308.x, BDI308 [pii]

Sala R, Axelson DA, Castro-Fornieles J, Goldstein TR, Ha W, Liao F, Gill MK, Iyengar S, Strober MA, Goldstein BI, Yen S, Hower H, Hunt J, Ryan ND, Dickstein D, Keller MB, Birmaher B (2010) Comorbid anxiety in children and adolescents with bipolar spectrum disorders: prevalence and clinical correlates. J Clin Psychiatry 71(10):1344–1350. doi:10.4088/JCP.09m05845gre

Salvi V, Albert U, Chiarle A, Soreca I, Bogetto F, Maina G (2008) Metabolic syndrome in Italian patients with bipolar disorder. Gen Hosp Psychiatry 30(4):318–323. doi:10.1016/j.genhosppsych.2008.04.009, S0163-8343(08)00072-8 [pii]

Salvi V, D'Ambrosio V, Rosso G, Bogetto F, Maina G (2011) Age-specific prevalence of metabolic syndrome in Italian patients with bipolar disorder. Psychiatry Clin Neurosci 65(1):47–54. doi:10.1111/j.1440-1819.2010.02160.x

Salvi V, D'Ambrosio V, Bogetto F, Maina G (2012) Metabolic syndrome in Italian patients with bipolar disorder: a 2-year follow-up study. J Affect Disord 136(3):599–603. doi:10.1016/j.jad.2011.10.025, S0165-0327(11)00674-4 [pii]

Sasson Y, Chopra M, Harrari E, Amitai K, Zohar J (2003) Bipolar comorbidity: from diagnostic dilemmas to therapeutic challenge. Int J Neuropsychopharmacol 6(2):139–144. doi:10.1017/S1461145703003432, S1461145703003432 [pii]

Savino M, Perugi G, Simonini E, Soriani A, Cassano GB, Akiskal HS (1993) Affective comorbidity in panic disorder: is there a bipolar connection? J Affect Disord 28(3):155–163

Schaffer A, Cairney J, Cheung A, Veldhuizen S, Levitt A (2006) Community survey of bipolar disorder in Canada: lifetime prevalence and illness characteristics. Can J Psychiatry 51(1):9–16

Schneier FR, Johnson J, Hornig CD, Liebowitz MR, Weissman MM (1992) Social phobia. Comorbidity and morbidity in an epidemiologic sample. Arch Gen Psychiatry 49(4):282–288

Schoofs N, Chen F, Braunig P, Stamm T, Kruger S (2011) Binge eating disorder and menstrual cycle in unmedicated women with bipolar disorder. J Affect Disord 129(1–3):75–78. doi:10.1016/j.jad.2010.08.016, S0165-0327(10)00550-1 [pii]

Schuckit MA, Tipp JE, Anthenelli RM, Bucholz KK, Hesselbrock VM, Nurnberger JI Jr (1996) Anorexia nervosa and bulimia nervosa in alcohol-dependent men and women and their relatives. Am J Psychiatry 153(1):74–82

Schurhoff F, Bellivier F, Jouvent R, Mouren-Simeoni MC, Bouvard M, Allilaire JF, Leboyer M (2000) Early and late onset bipolar disorders: two different forms of manic-depressive illness? J Affect Disord 58(3):215–221. doi:S0165032799001111 [pii]

Secnik K, Swensen A, Lage MJ (2005) Comorbidities and costs of adult patients diagnosed with attention-deficit hyperactivity disorder. Pharmacoeconomics 23(1):93–102. doi:2318 [pii]

Seixas C, Miranda-Scippa A, Nery-Fernandes F, Andrade-Nascimento M, Quarantini LC, Kapczinski F, Oliveira IR (2012) Prevalence and clinical impact of eating disorders in bipolar patients. Rev Bras Psiquiatr 34(1):66–70. doi:S1516-44462012000100012 [pii]

Sentissi O, Navarro JC, De Oliveira H, Gourion D, Bourdel MC, Bayle FJ, Olie JP, Poirier MF (2008) Bipolar disorders and quality of life: the impact of attention deficit/hyperactivity disorder and substance abuse in euthymic patients. Psychiatry Res 161(1):36–42. doi:10.1016/j.psychres.2007.06.016, S0165-1781(07)00198-9 [pii]

Sernyak MJ, Gulanski B, Rosenheck R (2005) Undiagnosed hyperglycemia in patients treated with atypical antipsychotics. J Clin Psychiatry 66(11):1463–1467

Shanmugiah A, Sinha S, Taly AB, Prashanth LK, Tomar M, Arunodaya GR, Reddy JY, Khanna S (2008) Psychiatric manifestations in Wilson's disease: a cross-sectional analysis. J Neuropsychiatry Clin Neurosci 20(1):81–85. doi:10.1176/appi.neuropsych.20.1.81, 20/1/81 [pii]

Sharma R, Markar HR (1994) Mortality in affective disorder. J Affect Disord 31(2):91–96

Sholomskas AJ (1990) Mania in a panic disorder patient treated with fluoxetine. Am J Psychiatry 147(8):1090–1091

Sicras A, Rejas J, Navarro R, Serrat J, Blanca M (2008) Metabolic syndrome in bipolar disorder: a cross-sectional assessment of a Health Management Organization database. Bipolar Disord 10(5):607–616. doi:10.1111/j.1399-5618.2008.00599.x, BDI599 [pii]

Sicras-Mainar A, Blanca-Tamayo M, Rejas-Gutierrez J, Navarro-Artieda R (2008) Metabolic syndrome in outpatients receiving antipsychotic therapy in routine clinical practice: a cross-sectional assessment of a primary health care database. Eur Psychiatry 23(2):100–108. doi:10.1016/j.eurpsy.2007.07.005, S0924-9338(07)01362-4 [pii]

Simon NM, Otto MW, Weiss RD, Bauer MS, Miyahara S, Wisniewski SR, Thase ME, Kogan J, Frank E, Nierenberg AA, Calabrese JR, Sachs GS, Pollack MH (2004a) Pharmacotherapy for bipolar disorder and comorbid conditions: baseline data from STEP-BD. J Clin Psychopharmacol 24(5):512–520. doi:00004714-200410000-00007 [pii]

Simon NM, Otto MW, Wisniewski SR, Fossey M, Sagduyu K, Frank E, Sachs GS, Nierenberg AA, Thase ME, Pollack MH (2004b) Anxiety disorder comorbidity in bipolar disorder patients: data from the first 500 participants in the Systematic Treatment Enhancement Program for Bipolar Disorder (STEP-BD). Am J Psychiatry 161(12):2222–2229. doi:10.1176/appi.ajp.161.12.2222, 161/12/2222 [pii]

Simon NM, Pollack MH, Fischmann D, Perlman CA, Muriel AC, Moore CW, Nierenberg AA, Shear MK (2005) Complicated grief and its correlates in patients with bipolar disorder. J Clin Psychiatry 66(9):1105–1110

Simon GE, Von Korff M, Saunders K, Miglioretti DL, Crane PK, van Belle G, Kessler RC (2006) Association between obesity and psychiatric disorders in the US adult population. Arch Gen Psychiatry 63(7):824–830. doi:10.1001/archpsyc.63.7.824, 63/7/824 [pii]

Simpson GM (2005) Atypical antipsychotics and the burden of disease. Am J Manag Care 11 (8 Suppl):S235–S241. doi:2953 [pii]

Simpson SG, al-Mufti R, Andersen AE, DePaulo JR JR Jr (1992) Bipolar II affective disorder in eating disorder inpatients. J Nerv Ment Dis 180(11):719–722

Singh JB, Zarate CA Jr (2006) Pharmacological treatment of psychiatric comorbidity in bipolar disorder: a review of controlled trials. Bipolar Disord 8(6):696–709. doi:10.1111/j.1399-5618.2006.00371.x, BDI371 [pii]

Singh MK, DelBello MP, Stanford KE, Soutullo C, McDonough-Ryan P, McElroy SL, Strakowski SM (2007) Psychopathology in children of bipolar parents. J Affect Disord 102(1–3):131–136. doi:10.1016/j.jad.2007.01.004, S0165-0327(07)00004-3 [pii]

Skirrow C, Hosang GM, Farmer AE, Asherson P (2012) An update on the debated association between ADHD and bipolar disorder across the lifespan. J Affect Disord 141(2–3):143–159. doi:10.1016/j.jad.2012.04.003, S0165-0327(12)00234-0 [pii]

Slama F, Bellivier F, Henry C, Rousseva A, Etain B, Rouillon F, Leboyer M (2004) Bipolar patients with suicidal behavior: toward the identification of a clinical subgroup. J Clin Psychiatry 65(8):1035–1039

Slater EZ (1938) ur Erbpathoogie des manisch-depressiven Irreseins. Die Eltern und Kinder von Manisch-Depressiven. (Hereditary pathology of manic-depressive illness. Parents and offspring of manicdepressives). Z Gesamte Neurol Psychiatr (163):1–47

Soreca I, Fagiolini A, Frank E, Houck PR, Thompson WK, Kupfer DJ (2008) Relationship of general medical burden, duration of illness and age in patients with bipolar I disorder. J Psychiatr Res 42(11):956–961. doi:10.1016/j.jpsychires.2007.10.009, S0022-3956(07)00183-5 [pii]

Soreca I, Frank E, Kupfer DJ (2009) The phenomenology of bipolar disorder: what drives the high rate of medical burden and determines long-term prognosis? Depress Anxiety 26(1):73–82. doi:10.1002/da.20521

Soreca I, Levenson J, Lotz M, Frank E, Kupfer DJ (2012) Sleep apnea risk and clinical correlates in patients with bipolar disorder. Bipolar Disord 14(6):672–676. doi:10.1111/j.1399-5618.2012.01044.x

Sorvaniemi M, Hintikka J (2005) Recorded psychiatric comorbidity with bipolar disorder–a Finnish hospital discharge register study. Nord J Psychiatry 59(6):531–533. doi:10.1080/08039480500360773, VL0375G732718418 [pii]

Steiner W (1991) Fluoxetine-induced mania in a patient with obsessive-compulsive disorder. Am J Psychiatry 148(10):1403–1404

Stender M, Bryant-Comstock L, Phillips S (2002) Medical resource use among patients treated for bipolar disorder: a retrospective, cross-sectional, descriptive analysis. Clin Ther 24(10):1668–1676. doi:S0149291802800704 [pii]

Strakowski SM, Tohen M, Stoll AL, Faedda GL, Goodwin DC (1992) Comorbidity in mania at first hospitalization. Am J Psychiatry 149(4):554–556

Strakowski SM, Stoll AL, Tohen M, Faedda GL, Goodwin DC (1993) The Tridimensional Personality Questionnaire as a predictor of six-month outcome in first episode mania. Psychiatry Res 48(1):1–8

Strakowski SM, MeElroy SL, Keck PW Jr, West SA (1994) The co-occurrence of mania with medical and other psychiatric disorders. Int J Psychiatry Med 24(4):305–328

Strakowski SM, Sax KW, McElroy SL, Keck PE Jr, Hawkins JM, West SA (1998) Course of psychiatric and substance abuse syndromes co-occurring with bipolar disorder after a first psychiatric hospitalization. J Clin Psychiatry 59(9):465–471

Strudsholm U, Johannessen L, Foldager L, Munk-Jorgensen P (2005) Increased risk for pulmonary embolism in patients with bipolar disorder. Bipolar Disord 7(1):77–81. doi:10.1111/j.1399-5618.2004.00176.x, BDI176 [pii]

Subramaniam M, Abdin E, Vaingankar JA, Chong SA (2013) Prevalence, correlates, comorbidity and severity of bipolar disorder: results from the Singapore Mental Health Study. J Affect Disord 146(2):189–196. doi:10.1016/j.jad.2012.09.002, S0165-0327(12)00621-0 [pii]

Sullivan G, Han X, Moore S, Kotrla K (2006) Disparities in hospitalization for diabetes among persons with and without co-occurring mental disorders. Psychiatr Serv 57(8):1126–1131. doi:10.1176/appi.ps.57.8.1126, 57/8/1126 [pii]

Swann AC (2001) Major system toxicities and side effects of anticonvulsants. J Clin Psychiatry 62(Suppl 14):16–21

Swartz KL, Pratt LA, Armenian HK, Lee LC, Eaton WW (2000) Mental disorders and the incidence of migraine headaches in a community sample: results from the Baltimore Epidemiologic Catchment area follow-up study. Arch Gen Psychiatry 57(10):945–950. doi:yoa9175 [pii]

Szadoczky E, Papp Z, Vitrai J, Rihmer Z, Furedi J (1998) The prevalence of major depressive and bipolar disorders in Hungary. Results from a national epidemiologic survey. J Affect Disord 50(2–3):153–162. doi:S0165-0327(98)00056-1 [pii]

Tamam L, Ozpoyraz N (2002) Comorbidity of anxiety disorder among patients with bipolar I disorder in remission. Psychopathology 35(4):203–209. doi:63824 [pii]

Tamam L, Tuglu C, Karatas G, Ozcan S (2006) Adult attention-deficit hyperactivity disorder in patients with bipolar I disorder in remission: preliminary study. Psychiatry Clin Neurosci 60(4):480–485. doi:10.1111/j.1440-1819.2006.01535.x, PCN1535 [pii]

Tamam L, Karakus G, Ozpoyraz N (2008) Comorbidity of adult attention-deficit hyperactivity disorder and bipolar disorder: prevalence and clinical correlates. Eur Arch Psychiatry Clin Neurosci 258(7):385–393. doi:10.1007/s00406-008-0807-x

Taylor V, MacQueen G (2006) Associations between bipolar disorder and metabolic syndrome: a review. J Clin Psychiatry 67(7):1034–1041

Taylor CT, Hirshfeld-Becker DR, Ostacher MJ, Chow CW, LeBeau RT, Pollack MH, Nierenberg AA, Simon NM (2008) Anxiety is associated with impulsivity in bipolar disorder. J Anxiety Disord 22(5):868–876. doi:10.1016/j.janxdis.2007.09.001, S0887-6185(07)00171-5 [pii]

Taylor V, McKinnon MC, Macdonald K, Jaswal G, Macqueen GM (2010) Adults with mood disorders have an increased risk profile for cardiovascular disease within the first 2 years of treatment. Can J Psychiatry 55(6):362–368

National Cholesterol Education Program (NCEP) Expert Panel on Detection, Evaluation, and Treatment of High Blood Cholesterol in Adults (Adult Treatment Panel III) (2002) Third report of the National Cholesterol Education Program (NCEP) expert panel on detection, evaluation, and treatment of high blood cholesterol in adults (adult treatment panel III) final report. Circulation 106(25):3143–3421

Thompson WK, Kupfer DJ, Fagiolini A, Scott JA, Frank E (2006) Prevalence and clinical correlates of medical comorbidities in patients with bipolar I disorder: analysis of acute-phase data from a randomized controlled trial. J Clin Psychiatry 67(5):783–788

Tillman R, Geller B (2006) Controlled study of switching from attention-deficit/hyperactivity disorder to a prepubertal and early adolescent bipolar I disorder phenotype during 6-year prospective follow-up: rate, risk, and predictors. Dev Psychopathol 18(4):1037–1053. doi:10.1017/S0954579406060512, S0954579406060512 [pii]

Timpano KR, Rubenstein LM, Murphy DL (2012) Phenomenological features and clinical impact of affective disorders in OCD: a focus on the bipolar disorder and OCD connection. Depress Anxiety 29(3):226–233. doi:10.1002/da.20908

Tohen M, Zarate CA Jr, Hennen J, Khalsa HM, Strakowski SM, Gebre-Medhin P, Salvatore P, Baldessarini RJ (2003) The McLean-Harvard First-Episode Mania Study: prediction of recovery and first recurrence. Am J Psychiatry 160(12):2099–2107

Tohen M, Calabrese J, Vieta E, Bowden C, Gonzalez-Pinto A, Lin D, Xu W, Corya S (2007) Effect of comorbid anxiety on treatment response in bipolar depression. J Affect Disord 104 (1–3):137–146. doi:10.1016/j.jad.2007.03.014, S0165-0327(07)00122-X [pii]

Toniolo RA, Caetano SC, da Silva PV, Lafer B (2009) Clinical significance of lifetime panic disorder in the course of bipolar disorder type I. Compr Psychiatry 50(1):9–12. doi:10.1016/j.comppsych.2008.06.001, S0010-440X(08)00085-0 [pii]

Tsuang MT, Woolson RF, Fleming JA (1980) Causes of death in schizophrenia and manic-depression. Br J Psychiatry 136:239–242

Tukel R, Meteris H, Koyuncu A, Tecer A, Yazici O (2006) The clinical impact of mood disorder comorbidity on obsessive-compulsive disorder. Eur Arch Psychiatry Clin Neurosci 256(4): 240–245. doi:10.1007/s00406-006-0632-z

Valle J, Ayuso-Gutierrez JL, Abril A, Ayuso-Mateos JL (1999) Evaluation of thyroid function in lithium-naive bipolar patients. Eur Psychiatry 14(6):341–345. doi:S0924-9338(99)00158-3 [pii]

van Winkel R, De Hert M, Van Eyck D, Hanssens L, Wampers M, Scheen A, Peuskens J (2008a) Prevalence of diabetes and the metabolic syndrome in a sample of patients with bipolar disorder. Bipolar Disord 10(2):342–348. doi:10.1111/j.1399-5618.2007.00520.x, BDI520 [pii]

van Winkel R, van Os J, Celic I, Van Eyck D, Wampers M, Scheen A, Peuskens J, De Hert M (2008b) Psychiatric diagnosis as an independent risk factor for metabolic disturbances: results from a comprehensive, naturalistic screening program. J Clin Psychiatry 69(8):1319–1327. doi:ej08m04030 [pii]

Vendsborg PB, Bech P, Rafaelsen OJ (1976) Lithium treatment and weight gain. Acta Psychiatr Scand 53(2):139–147

Vieta E, Bernardo M (1992) Antidepressant-induced mania in obsessive-compulsive disorder. Am J Psychiatry 149(9):1282–1283

Vieta E, Colom F, Martinez-Aran A, Benabarre A, Reinares M, Gasto C (2000) Bipolar II disorder and comorbidity. Compr Psychiatry 41(5):339–343. doi:S0010440X00254321 [pii]

Vieta E, Colom F, Corbella B, Martinez-Aran A, Reinares M, Benabarre A, Gasto C (2001) Clinical correlates of psychiatric comorbidity in bipolar I patients. Bipolar Disord 3(5):253–258. doi:030504 [pii]

Volavka J, Czobor P, Sheitman B, Lindenmayer JP, Citrome L, McEvoy JP, Cooper TB, Chakos M, Lieberman JA (2002) Clozapine, olanzapine, risperidone, and haloperidol in the treatment of patients with chronic schizophrenia and schizoaffective disorder. Am J Psychiatry 159(2):255–262

Vonk R, van der Schot AC, Kahn RS, Nolen WA, Drexhage HA (2007) Is autoimmune thyroiditis part of the genetic vulnerability (or an endophenotype) for bipolar disorder? Biol Psychiatry 62(2):135–140. doi:10.1016/j.biopsych.2006.08.041, S0006-3223(06)01112-7 [pii]

Vos T, Flaxman AD, Naghavi M, Lozano R, Michaud C, Ezzati M, Shibuya K, Salomon JA, Abdalla S, Aboyans V, Abraham J, Ackerman I, Aggarwal R, Ahn SY, Ali MK, Alvarado M, Anderson HR, Anderson LM, Andrews KG, Atkinson C, Baddour LM, Bahalim AN, Barker-Collo S, Barrero LH, Bartels DH, Basanez MG, Baxter A, Bell ML, Benjamin EJ, Bennett D, Bernabe E, Bhalla K, Bhandari B, Bikbov B, Bin Abdulhak A, Birbeck G, Black JA, Blencowe H, Blore JD, Blyth F, Bolliger I, Bonaventure A, Boufous S, Bourne R, Boussinesq M, Braithwaite T, Brayne C, Bridgett L, Brooker S, Brooks P, Brugha TS, Bryan-Hancock C, Bucello C, Buchbinder R, Buckle G, Budke CM, Burch M, Burney P, Burstein R, Calabria B, Campbell B, Canter CE, Carabin H, Carapetis J, Carmona L, Cella C, Charlson F, Chen H, Cheng AT, Chou D, Chugh SS, Coffeng LE, Colan SD, Colquhoun S, Colson KE, Condon J, Connor MD, Cooper LT, Corriere M, Cortinovis M, de Vaccaro KC, Couser W, Cowie BC, Criqui MH, Cross M, Dabhadkar KC, Dahiya M, Dahodwala N, Damsere-Derry J, Danaei G, Davis A, De Leo D, Degenhardt L, Dellavalle R, Delossantos A, Denenberg J, Derrett S, Des

Jarlais DC, Dharmaratne SD, Dherani M, Diaz-Torne C, Dolk H, Dorsey ER, Driscoll T, Duber H, Ebel B, Edmond K, Elbaz A, Ali SE, Erskine H, Erwin PJ, Espindola P, Ewoigbokhan SE, Farzadfar F, Feigin V, Felson DT, Ferrari A, Ferri CP, Fevre EM, Finucane MM, Flaxman S, Flood L, Foreman K, Forouzanfar MH, Fowkes FG, Franklin R, Fransen M, Freeman MK, Gabbe BJ, Gabriel SE, Gakidou E, Ganatra HA, Garcia B, Gaspari F, Gillum RF, Gmel G, Gosselin R, Grainger R, Groeger J, Guillemin F, Gunnell D, Gupta R, Haagsma J, Hagan H, Halasa YA, Hall W, Haring D, Haro JM, Harrison JE, Havmoeller R, Hay RJ, Higashi H, Hill C, Hoen B, Hoffman H, Hotez PJ, Hoy D, Huang JJ, Ibeanusi SE, Jacobsen KH, James SL, Jarvis D, Jasrasaria R, Jayaraman S, Johns N, Jonas JB, Karthikeyan G, Kassebaum N, Kawakami N, Keren A, Khoo JP, King CH, Knowlton LM, Kobusingye O, Koranteng A, Krishnamurthi R, Lalloo R, Laslett LL, Lathlean T, Leasher JL, Lee YY, Leigh J, Lim SS, Limb E, Lin JK, Lipnick M, Lipshultz SE, Liu W, Loane M, Ohno SL, Lyons R, Ma J, Mabweijano J, MacIntyre MF, Malekzadeh R, Mallinger L, Manivannan S, Marcenes W, March L, Margolis DJ, Marks GB, Marks R, Matsumori A, Matzopoulos R, Mayosi BM, McAnulty JH, McDermott MM, McGill N, McGrath J, Medina-Mora ME, Meltzer M, Mensah GA, Merriman TR, Meyer AC, Miglioli V, Miller M, Miller TR, Mitchell PB, Mocumbi AO, Moffitt TE, Mokdad AA, Monasta L, Montico M, Moradi-Lakeh M, Moran A, Morawska L, Mori R, Murdoch ME, Mwaniki MK, Naidoo K, Nair MN, Naldi L, Narayan KM, Nelson PK, Nelson RG, Nevitt MC, Newton CR, Nolte S, Norman P, Norman R, O'Donnell M, O'Hanlon S, Olives C, Omer SB, Ortblad K, Osborne R, Ozgediz D, Page A, Pahari B, Pandian JD, Rivero AP, Patten SB, Pearce N, Padilla RP, Perez-Ruiz F, Perico N, Pesudovs K, Phillips D, Phillips MR, Pierce K, Pion S, Polanczyk GV, Polinder S, Pope CA 3rd, Popova S, Porrini E, Pourmalek F, Prince M, Pullan RL, Ramaiah KD, Ranganathan D, Razavi H, Regan M, Rehm JT, Rein DB, Remuzzi G, Richardson K, Rivara FP, Roberts T, Robinson C, De Leon FR, Ronfani L, Room R, Rosenfeld LC, Rushton L, Sacco RL, Saha S, Sampson U, Sanchez-Riera L, Sanman E, Schwebel DC, Scott JG, Segui-Gomez M, Shahraz S, Shepard DS, Shin H, Shivakoti R, Singh D, Singh GM, Singh JA, Singleton J, Sleet DA, Sliwa K, Smith E, Smith JL, Stapelberg NJ, Steer A, Steiner T, Stolk WA, Stovner LJ, Sudfeld C, Syed S, Tamburlini G, Tavakkoli M, Taylor HR, Taylor JA, Taylor WJ, Thomas B, Thomson WM, Thurston GD, Tleyjeh IM, Tonelli M, Towbin JA, Truelsen T, Tsilimbaris MK, Ubeda C, Undurraga EA, van der Werf MJ, van Os J, Vavilala MS, Venketasubramanian N, Wang M, Wang W, Watt K, Weatherall DJ, Weinstock MA, Weintraub R, Weisskopf MG, Weissman MM, White RA, Whiteford H, Wiersma ST, Wilkinson JD, Williams HC, Williams SR, Witt E, Wolfe F, Woolf AD, Wulf S, Yeh PH, Zaidi AK, Zheng ZJ, Zonies D, Lopez AD, Murray CJ, AlMazroa MA, Memish ZA (2012) Years lived with disability (YLDs) for 1160 sequelae of 289 diseases and injuries 1990–2010: a systematic analysis for the Global Burden of Disease Study 2010. Lancet 380(9859):2163–2196. doi:10.1016/S0140-6736(12)61729-2, S0140-6736(12)61729-2 [pii]

Vuksan-Cusa B, Marcinko D, Nad S, Jakovljevic M (2009) Differences in cholesterol and metabolic syndrome between bipolar disorder men with and without suicide attempts. Prog Neuropsychopharmacol Biol Psychiatry 33(1):109–112. doi:10.1016/j.pnpbp.2008.10.017, S0278-5846(08)00321-7 [pii]

Wang PW, Sachs GS, Zarate CA, Marangell LB, Calabrese JR, Goldberg JF, Sagduyu K, Miyahara S, Ketter TA (2006) Overweight and obesity in bipolar disorders. J Psychiatr Res 40(8): 762–764. doi:10.1016/j.jpsychires.2006.01.007, S0022-3956(06)00022-7 [pii]

Weber NS, Fisher JA, Cowan DN, Niebuhr DW (2011) Psychiatric and general medical conditions comorbid with bipolar disorder in the National Hospital Discharge Survey. Psychiatr Serv 62(10):1152–1158. doi:10.1176/appi.ps.62.10.1152, 62/10/1152 [pii]

Weeke A, Vaeth M (1986) Excess mortality of bipolar and unipolar manic-depressive patients. J Affect Disord 11(3):227–234

Weeke A, Juel K, Vaeth M (1987) Cardiovascular death and manic-depressive psychosis. J Affect Disord 13(3):287–292

Weiller E, Bisserbe JC, Boyer P, Lepine JP, Lecrubier Y (1996) Social phobia in general health care: an unrecognised undertreated disabling disorder. Br J Psychiatry 168(2):169–174

Weiner M, Warren L, Fiedorowicz JG (2011) Cardiovascular morbidity and mortality in bipolar disorder. Ann Clin Psychiatry 23(1):40–47. doi:acp_2301f [pii]

White K, Keck PE Jr, Lipinski J (1986) Serotonin-uptake inhibitors in obsessive-compulsive disorder: a case report. Compr Psychiatry 27(3):211–214

Wickramaratne PJ, Weissman MM (1993) Using family studies to understand comorbidity. Eur Arch Psychiatry Clin Neurosci 243(3–4):150–157

Wildes JE, Marcus MD, Fagiolini A (2008) Prevalence and correlates of eating disorder comorbidity in patients with bipolar disorder. Psychiatry Res 161(1):51–58. doi:10.1016/j.psychres.2007.09.003, S0165-1781(07)00328-9 [pii]

Wilens TE, Biederman J, Mick E, Faraone SV, Spencer T (1997) Attention deficit hyperactivity disorder (ADHD) is associated with early onset substance use disorders. J Nerv Ment Dis 185(8):475–482

Wilens TE, Biederman J, Wozniak J, Gunawardene S, Wong J, Monuteaux M (2003) Can adults with attention-deficit/hyperactivity disorder be distinguished from those with comorbid bipolar disorder? Findings from a sample of clinically referred adults. Biol Psychiatry 54(1):1–8. doi:S0006322302016669 [pii]

Wilens TE, Biederman J, Faraone SV, Martelon M, Westerberg D, Spencer TJ (2009) Presenting ADHD symptoms, subtypes, and comorbid disorders in clinically referred adults with ADHD. J Clin Psychiatry 70(11):1557–1562. doi:10.4088/JCP.08m04785pur

Wingo AP, Ghaemi SN (2007) A systematic review of rates and diagnostic validity of comorbid adult attention-deficit/hyperactivity disorder and bipolar disorder. J Clin Psychiatry 68(11):1776–1784

Wingo AP, Ghaemi SN (2008) Frequency of stimulant treatment and of stimulant-associated mania/hypomania in bipolar disorder patients. Psychopharmacol Bull 41(4):37–47

Winokur G, Coryell W, Endicott J, Akiskal H (1993) Further distinctions between manic-depressive illness (bipolar disorder) and primary depressive disorder (unipolar depression). Am J Psychiatry 150(8):1176–1181

Wittchen HU, Zhao S, Kessler RC, Eaton WW (1994) DSM-III-R generalized anxiety disorder in the National Comorbidity Survey. Arch Gen Psychiatry 51(5):355–364

Wozniak J, Biederman J, Monuteaux MC, Richards J, Faraone SV (2002) Parsing the comorbidity between bipolar disorder and anxiety disorders: a familial risk analysis. J Child Adolesc Psychopharmacol 12(2):101–111. doi:10.1089/104454602760219144

Yerevanian BI, Koek RJ, Ramdev S (2001) Anxiety disorders comorbidity in mood disorder subgroups: data from a mood disorders clinic. J Affect Disord 67(1–3):167–173. doi:S0165032701004487 [pii]

Young LT, Cooke RG, Robb JC, Levitt AJ, Joffe RT (1993) Anxious and non-anxious bipolar disorder. J Affect Disord 29(1):49–52

Young S, Pfaff D, Lewandowski KE, Ravichandran C, Cohen BM, Ongur D (2013) Anxiety disorder comorbidity in bipolar disorder, schizophrenia and schizoaffective disorder. Psychopathology 46(3):176–185. doi:10.1159/000339556, 000339556 [pii]

Yumru M, Savas HA, Kurt E, Kaya MC, Selek S, Savas E, Oral ET, Atagun I (2007) Atypical antipsychotics related metabolic syndrome in bipolar patients. J Affect Disord 98(3):247–252. doi:10.1016/j.jad.2006.08.009, S0165-0327(06)00343-0 [pii]

Zipursky RB, Gu H, Green AI, Perkins DO, Tohen MF, McEvoy JP, Strakowski SM, Sharma T, Kahn RS, Gur RE, Tollefson GD, Lieberman JA (2005) Course and predictors of weight gain in people with first-episode psychosis treated with olanzapine or haloperidol. Br J Psychiatry 187:537–543. doi:10.1192/bjp.187.6.537, 187/6/537 [pii]

Zutshi A, Reddy YC, Thennarasu K, Chandrashekhar CR (2006) Comorbidity of anxiety disorders in patients with remitted bipolar disorder. Eur Arch Psychiatry Clin Neurosci 256(7):428–436. doi:10.1007/s00406-006-0658-2

Zutshi A, Kamath P, Reddy YC (2007) Bipolar and nonbipolar obsessive-compulsive disorder: a clinical exploration. Compr Psychiatry 48(3):245–251. doi:10.1016/j.comppsych.2006.12.005, S0010-440X(06)00145-3 [pii]

Classification and Epidemiology 11

11.1 Classification

11.1.1 General Considerations

The principle of classification is that it is a reductionist process by which complex phenomena can be grouped into categories on the basis of objective and stringent criteria. Often the criteria are less reliable and valid than expected or needed; however, many researchers follow the opinion of Claude Lévi-Strauss (1908–2009) that 'any classification is better than no classification at all'. On the other hand, classification itself has an impact on nosology since it often gives birth to interest groups of experts and followers and it might trigger vicious circles concerning their survival. Once classification follows a specific path, a radical change is often difficult if not impossible and this is evident from the way modern classification systems move on from previous to the next edition.

Classification as a tool was glorified in the nineteenth century after the successful classification of plants and animals and the fact that it was that process that eventually led to the evolution theory by Charles Darwin. Medicine and especially psychiatry adopted this new tool as it did with most other successful tools from other fields of science, and particularly with the efforts of Emil Kraepelin, the first solid classification of mental diseases started to emerge.

It is an unfortunate fact that current psychiatric classification is based exclusively on the clinical picture and no objective laboratory input independent from the clinical picture is available like in the rest of medicine. Thus, currently the grouping and classification of mental disorders is based on shared phenomenological characteristics.

Therefore, classification in psychiatry was and still is a matter of controversy and it is likely to remain this way in the near future. Not only how mental disorders should be classified is a matter of debate, but even, at a more fundamental level, a matter of debate is whether the classification approach and its tools are relevant at all in psychiatry and mental illness.

K.N. Fountoulakis, *Bipolar Disorder: An Evidence-Based Guide to Manic Depression*, DOI 10.1007/978-3-642-37216-2_11

No matter how reliable or valid a classification in psychiatry is, there are certain advantages from its application. It facilitates communication among health professionals, it helps defining mental disorders and in this way it facilitates clinical practice and research and also the keeping of medical archives and statistics and supports administrative and legal issues. However, it should be noted that since the establishment of current classification systems in the international psychiatric community, social, ideological, political and economic forces has increasingly voiced opinions regarding the classification of mental disorders and in many cases it seems that they exerted at least some influence.

One of the most controversial issues is of course fundamental: the definition of mental illness itself. A definition of mental disorder appeared for the first time in DSM-III with focus on distress and impairment. The definition was further elaborated in the following DSM editions with the addition of the concept of dysfunction and risk for a number of adverse situations and outcomes, including loss of freedom or death. It is important to note that especially for BD, the impairment/distress criterion is problematic because patients could be elated, happy and not distressed at all and maybe with a higher-than-usual functioning and sharp thinking at least for specific periods and during hypomanic episodes. Thus, it is known that periods of hypomania are often perceived as periods of full recovery or normal happiness and cannot be traced even by experienced clinicians.

Apart from these conceptual problems, linguistic, cultural and 'nationalistic' issues make an internationally accepted classification a major challenge (Sartorius 1978, 1988).

11.1.2 Contemporary Classification Systems

A history of the efforts to identify and classify mental disorders and especially BD can be found in the first chapter of the current book, which deals with the history of BD. It is not within the scope of this chapter to include a thorough analysis and description of the history of modern classification systems; however, a brief focused overview is necessary.

Throughout the nineteenth century, there were various attempts to create a meaningful classification system in medicine in general and in psychiatry in particular. The first important classification system in the USA appeared in 1917 and was developed by the American Medico-Psychological Association, while in 1948 the World Health Organization (WHO) revised the International List of Causes of Death and renamed it to Manual of the International Statistical Classification of Diseases, Injuries, and Causes of Death, 6th edition (ICD-6). ICD-7 followed in 1957, ICD-8 in 1968, ICD-9 in 1975 and ICD-10 in 1990 (WHO 1992). The 11th edition (ICD-11) is scheduled to appear in the next year or two.

In the ICD-6 edition, a classification of mental disorders was included for the first time under the title 'Mental, Psychoneurotic, and Personality Disorders'. In 1951 the US Public Health Service undertook an initiative in collaboration with the American Psychiatric Association which led 1 year later to the publication of the 1st edition of the Diagnostic and Statistical Manual of Mental Disorders (DSM-I). DSM-II followed in 1968 and DSM-III in 1980, DSM-III-R in 1987, DSM-IV in 1994 and its text revision in 2000, while the current version DSM-5 was published in 2013 (American Psychiatric Association 2013).

In ICD, the classification of mental and behavioural disorders comprises 1 of the 21 chapters (Chap. 5, F00–F99), while there is also another chapter (Chap. 6, G00–G99) which includes neurological disorders with some overlapping with Chap. 5. In 1975 the ICD 'family' of classifications were born and included the International Nomenclature of Diseases (IND); the International Classification of Functioning, Disability and Health (ICF); and the Classification of Mental Disorders for Use in Primary Health Care (PHC/ICD-10) (WHO 1994). Another important decision, which was taken in 1975, was to incorporate brief descriptions of the categories of mental disorders to guide and assist the diagnosis made by a mental health professional but not to help the lay coder.

On the other hand, a major contribution of the DSM was the multiaxial classification and the development of operationalized criteria for the diagnosis for the first time in DSM-III. ICD followed by adopting the operationalized criteria approach in a special ICD-10 edition for research purposes.

Overall, the DSM appears to rely on a more solid base of evidence in comparison to the ICD which often relies on consensus among specialists from different countries and different approaches. The history of the evolution of contemporary classification systems reveals that there was a revival of diagnostic thinking in the 1950s with the introduction of DSM-III. This occurred partly because psychiatry and psychiatrists wished to remain within the discipline of medicine and partially because the dawn of the era of psychopharmacology was demanding an operationalized and reliable system of diagnosis, classification and reporting.

11.1.3 Contemporary Classification of BD and Related Disorders

Contemporary classification systems (ICD and DSM) do not follow the concept of the 'bipolar spectrum' and are much cautious and reserved towards many suggestions and approaches which were described in detail in the specific chapters of the current book. Their approach is based on the definition of the manic and of the depressive episode with some important differences between them.

In ICD-10, BD is included in the chapter 'mood (affective) disorders' (F30–F39) and the ICD classification is shown in Table 11.1. However, for the first time, in DSM-5, bipolar disorders were separated from unipolar depression and now they both have their own separate chapter (Table 11.2). In previous editions of the DSM, they were both grouped under the chapter 'mood disorders'. The 'bipolar' chapter includes BD and cyclothymia, while the 'depression' chapter includes disruptive mood dysregulation disorder, major depressive disorder, persistent depressive disorder (dysthymia) and premenstrual dysphoric disorder. Both chapters include 'unspecified', 'other' and 'due to' categories.

Table 11.1 Classification of mood (affective) disorders according to ICD-10

F30–F39	*Mood [affective] disorders*
F30	*Manic episode*
F30.0	Hypomania
F30.1	Mania without psychotic symptoms
F30.2	Mania with psychotic symptoms
F30.8	Other manic episodes
F30.9	Manic episode, unspecified
F31	*Bipolar affective disorder*
F31.0	Bipolar affective disorder, current episode hypomanic
F31.1	Bipolar affective disorder, current episode manic without psychotic symptoms
F31.2	Bipolar affective disorder, current episode manic with psychotic symptoms
F31.3	Bipolar affective disorder, current episode mild or moderate depression
0.30	Without somatic syndrome
0.31	With somatic syndrome
F31.4	Bipolar affective disorder, current episode severe depression without psychotic symptoms
F31.5	Bipolar affective disorder, current episode severe depression with psychotic symptoms
F31.6	Bipolar affective disorder, current episode mixed
F31.7	Bipolar affective disorder, currently in remission
F31.8	Other bipolar affective disorders
F31.9	Bipolar affective disorder, unspecified
F32	*Depressive episode*
F32.0	Mild depressive episode
0.00	Without somatic syndrome
0.01	With somatic syndrome
F32.1	Moderate depressive episode
0.10	Without somatic syndrome
0.11	With somatic syndrome
F32.2	Severe depressive episode without psychotic symptoms
F32.3	Severe depressive episode with psychotic symptoms
F32.8	Other depressive episodes
F32.9	Depressive episode, unspecified
F34.0	*Cyclothymia*
F38.00	*Mixed affective episode*

BD-II disorder was first introduced in DSM-IV in 1994 and is not part of the ICD-10 diagnostic list. However, hypomania is accepted as a diagnostic entity in ICD-10 (F30.0), but it is considered simply a low-severity mania. It is also important to note that hypomania is the only mental condition that could be related to improved functioning rather than impairment. It is excluded if the level of impairment is too severe.

Table 11.2 Classification of bipolar disorders according to DSM-5

		BD-I
		Current or most recent episode manic
296.41	(F31.11)	Mild
296.42	(F31.12)	Moderate
296.43	(F31.13)	Severe
296.44	(F31.2)	With psychotic features
296.45	(F31.73)	In partial remission
296.46	(F31.74)	In full remission
296.40	(F31.9)	Unspecified
296.40	(F31.0)	*Current or most recent episode hypomanic*
296.45	(F31.73)	In partial remission
296.46	(F31.74)	In full remission
296.40	(F31.9)	Unspecified
		Current or most recent episode depressed
296.51	(F31.31)	Mild
296.52	(F31.32)	Moderate
296.53	(F31.4)	Severe
296.54	(F31.5)	With psychotic features
296.55	(F31.75)	In partial remission
296.56	(F31.76)	In full remission
296.50	(F31.9)	Unspecified
296.7	(F31.9)	*Current or most recent episode unspecified*
296.89	(F31.81)	**BD-II**
		Specify current or most recent episode:
		Hypomanic
		Depressed
		Specify course if full criteria for a mood episode are not currently met:
		In partial remission
		In full remission
		Specify severity if full criteria for a mood episode are not currently met:
		Mild
		Moderate
		Severe
301.13	(F34.0)	**Cyclothymic disorder**
		Specify if: with anxious distress
		Substance/medication-induced bipolar and related disorder
		Specify if:
		Onset during intoxication
		Onset during withdrawal

(continued)

Table 11.2 (continued)

293.83		**Bipolar and related disorder due to another medical condition**
		Specify if:
	(F06.33)	With manic features
	(F06.33)	With manic- or hypomanic-like episode
	(F06.34)	With mixed features
296.89	(F31.89)	Other specified bipolar and related disorder
296.80	(F31.9)	Unspecified bipolar and related disorder

Specifiers: anxious distress, mixed features, rapid cycling, melancholic features, atypical features, mood-congruent/incongruent psychotic features, catatonia, peripartum onset, seasonal pattern

In ICD-10 a 'mixed affective episode' (F38.0) is defined as an affective episode of at least 2 weeks duration which is characterized by either a mixture or a rapid alternation (usually within a few hours) of hypomanic, manic and depressive symptoms. Thus, the ICD includes under the definition of 'mixed' at least some of the very fast ultrarapid cycling cases.

A radical change was the abolishment of the concept of 'mixed' episodes by DSM-5. In previous versions of DSM, mixed episodes were defined as the coexistence of full-blown manic and depressive episodes simultaneously. Although such a coexistence is rather rare and difficult, almost one-third of patients recruited in pharmaceutical trials of acute mania were diagnosed as 'mixed'. Thus, there exist ample data, although neither properly analysed nor published. Instead of the diagnosis of mixed episodes, DSM-5 introduced the 'mixed features specifier' concept. According to this, a mood episode (either manic or depressed) has mixed features if at least three criteria of the opposite pole (from a specific list) coexist.

It is of prime importance for conceptual reasons but especially for practical pharmacological treatment considerations to mention that this 'mixed features' specifier is also included in the 'unipolar' chapter. Taken verbatim and in combination with strict labelling for the use of medication treatment, this means that a major depressive episode with mixed features without a hypomanic or manic episode in the past should be treated with antidepressants, also double acting ones, without the concomitant use of an antimanic agent. This is a matter of debate, with public health and maybe also with legal consequences.

Another important change in the DSM-5 is the introduction of 'anxious distress' specifier which demands the presence of at least two criteria from a list of five (tension, restlessness, concentration difficulties, worry, fear of losing control).

The ICD-10 classification accepts the presence of 'somatic syndrome' which seems analogous, but it is not identical to 'melancholic features' of DSM-5 (Fountoulakis et al. 1999). The 'atypical features', 'rapid cycling' and 'anxious distress' are described in DSM-5 but not in ICD-10. Also ICD-10 does not differentiate psychotic symptoms into 'mood congruent' vs. 'mood incongruent'. The other specifiers, 'catatonia', 'peripartum onset' and 'seasonal pattern', are not included in the ICD-10 either. It is important to note that ICD-10 recognizes catatonia only in the frame of schizophrenia.

A brief comparison of the two classification systems can be found in Table 11.3.

Table 11.3 Comparison of ICD-10 and DSM-5 concerning the classification of bipolar disorders

ICD-10	DSM-5
A single mood (affective) disorders chapter	Two chapters: bipolar vs. depression chapters
No BD subtypes	BD-I vs. BD-II
Hypomanic is part of manic episode	Hypomanic is distinct from manic
No specifiers concerning remission status	In partial/full remission
Mixed episode	Mixed features specifier
Somatic syndrome	Melancholic features specifier
No specifiers	Anxious distress
	Rapid cycling
	Atypical features
	Mood-congruent/incongruent psychotic features
	Catatonia
	Peripartum onset
	Seasonal pattern

11.2 Epidemiology of BD

Common clinical sense strongly suggests that mood disorders are among the most frequent psychiatric illnesses both in the community and in psychiatric settings (Muller-Oerlinghausen et al. 2002; Royal Australian and New Zealand College of Psychiatrists Clinical Practice Guidelines Team for Bipolar Disorder 2004; Oakley Browne et al. 2006). Their rates are increasing partially because their misdiagnosing as schizophrenia cases is decreasing. However, whether this is correct or not and what is the magnitude of the rates can be shown only with epidemiological studies. In addition community-based epidemiological studies in the field of psychiatry provide several important and clinically useful pieces of information on the prevalence and other characteristics (e.g. risk factors, social correlates and use of health care) of mood disorders that cannot be extrapolated from everyday clinical practice. This is impossible simply because inpatient and outpatient samples constitute the most severe and complicated cases and since many patients do not seek treatment at all. Thus, in- and outpatients as samples are not representative of the natural population of bipolar patients and the findings from research on them cannot be generalized without reservation.

Technically, epidemiological studies can be divided into three types: descriptive (registering rates), analytic (exploring risk factors) and experimental (testing associations). Most of the literature on BD belongs to the first two types and especially to the descriptive type.

In the last few decades, there was an increasing interest in psychiatric epidemiology which among other things was the result of the improvement in methodology because of the introduction of operational criteria and well-defined psychiatric diagnostic categories.

Another important development was the availability of reliable and valid instruments for use in epidemiological surveys and especially suitable for use by lay interviewers. These are the Diagnostic Interview Schedule (DIS) (Robins et al. 1981), the Composite International Diagnostic Interview Schedule (CIDI) (Robins et al. 1988), the Mini International Diagnostic Interview (MINI) (Sheehan et al. 1998) and the Schedule for Clinical Assessment in Neuropsychiatry (SCAN) (Wing et al. 1990).

Usual problems and limitations that accompany research on psychiatric epidemiology include the fact that each mental disorder separately has a very small prevalence (almost always below 5 %) and thus large numbers of people (thousands) from the general population ought to be investigated. In order for this to be possible, structured interviews are applied by non-clinicians. As a consequence, the data are of low quality and only a few questions can be answered with reasonable reliability and validity. Many issues might not be able to be investigated at all. Other problems are the changing of diagnostic criteria and the small but important differences between the two major classification systems, age-specific issues since the incidence of bipolar disorder may be increasing disproportionately in younger individuals (Parker et al. 2006) and of course nonresponse or refusal to participate in the survey. This last problem is accompanied by the question whether refusal is random or not.

Especially concerning BD, a point which plays a major role in the shaping of the figures is the definition of hypomania and of mixed, irritable or dysphoric forms of manic episodes. This is further complicated because of the presence of inaccurate recall and the low sensitivity of the interview instruments concerning subthreshold symptomatology and nonclassical clinical pictures (Kessler et al. 1997b).

The most important epidemiological studies are reviewed below and their results are summarized in Table 11.4

11.2.1 The Amish Study

The Amish study (Egeland et al. 1983; Hostetter et al. 1983; Egeland and Hostetter 1983) was unique in the sense that it was conducted in a population which was culturally and genetically homogenous (N=12,500). Interestingly, it reported similar prevalence rates between unipolar depression and bipolar illness and also similar rates between genders. It is impressive that 79 % of patients with BD-I were previously diagnosed as suffering from schizophrenia.

11.2.2 The Epidemiological Catchment Area (ECA)

The ECA was conducted in 1980–1984 (Regier et al. 1984, 1988, 1993; Bourdon et al. 1992; Eaton et al. 1981). It assessed 18,571 persons (59 % females) from five geographical sites in the USA, aged 18–65, with the DIS which was applied by lay

Table 11.4 Summary table of epidemiological data from selected studies

			BD-I				BD-II			Bipolar spectrum
			Prevalence		Incidence		Prevalence			Prevalence
Study	Country	Time period	Lifetime	Annual	Annual	Age at onset	Lifetime	Annual	Age at onset	Lifetime
Amish study[a]	USA	1976–1980								
ECA	USA	1980–1984	0.8	0.6	3.2	18	0.5			6.4
NCS	USA	1990–1992	1.7	1.3		21				
NCS-R	USA	2005	1.0	0.6		19	1.1	0.8	20	4.4
CNCG	Canada	1988	0.6			22				
	Puerto Rico	1987	0.6			18				
	Germany	1992	0.5			25				
	Taiwan	1989	0.3			22				
	South Korea	1990	0.4			18				
	New Zealand	1989	1.5							
Zurich study	Switzerland	1978–1982		0.7						5.5
Shatin study[b]	Hong Kong	1984–1986	0.15							
Nottingham study[b]	UK	1992–1994			2.5					
Netherlands study[b]	Netherlands	1996–1999	2.0		2.7					
Australia study[b]	Australia	2004		0.5						
Butajira study	Ethiopia	2005	0.5			22[c]				

(continued)

Table 11.4 (continued)

			BD-I				BD-II			Bipolar spectrum
			Prevalence		Incidence		Prevalence			Prevalence
Study	Country	Time period	Lifetime	Annual	Annual	Age at onset	Lifetime	Annual	Age at onset	Lifetime
Irish study	Ireland	1995–2000			2.2					
Hirschfeld et al.	USA	2003								3.7
Merikangas et al.	Various	2011	0.6	0.4			0.4	0.3		2.4
Various studies	Various		0.2–1.9	1.3	2.2		0.5–2	0.2		3–8.3

Incidence per 100,000 residents
[a]Results not compatible with current table
[b]The rates reported concern combined BD-I and BD-II
[c]Mean age

interviewers. Persons living in institutions (prisons, boarding houses, etc.) were included. The response rate was 76 %. Its results suggested a lifetime prevalence of 0.8 % for BD-I (0.3–1.2 %) and an annual prevalence 0.6 % (0.2–1 %) with similar prevalence for males and females. The annual incidence was 0.4 % (0.1–0.6 %) of cases which corresponds to approximately 3.2 (0.8–4.8) per 100,000 residents. The median age at onset was 18 years. A reanalysis of the ECA data with the addition of subthreshold bipolarity produced a total lifetime prevalence of 6.4 % with 0.5 % being a lifetime prevalence of BD-II (Judd and Akiskal 2003).

11.2.3 The National Comorbidity Survey (NCS)

The NCS was conducted in 1990–1992 and included 8,098 persons aged 15–54 years old, from across the USA (Kessler et al. 1993, 1994a, b, 1995, 1996, 1997a; Magee et al. 1996; Kendler et al. 1996; Warner et al. 1995; Wittchen et al. 1994; Blazer et al. 1994). The study utilized the UM-CIDI applied by lay interviewers and the response rate was 84 %. In 2005 a replication study, the NCS-R, was conducted in 9,282 persons assessed by professional interviewers (Kessler et al. 2004, 2005a, b, 2012a, b; Nierenberg et al. 2010; Angst et al. 2010; Merikangas et al. 2007; Kessler and Merikangas 2004). In both studies, only persons living in the community were included.

The results of the NCS suggested a lifetime prevalence of 1.7 % for BD-I and an annual prevalence of 1.3 % with similar prevalence for males and females. The median age at onset was 21 years. Data on BD-II were not reported because this diagnosis was considered unreliable.

The results of the NCS-R suggested a lifetime prevalence of 1.0 % for BD-I and an annual prevalence of 0.6 % with again similar prevalence for males and females. The median age at onset was 19 years. Concerning BD-II the lifetime prevalence was 1.1 % and the annual prevalence was 0.8 % with similar prevalence for males and females. The median age at onset was 20 years. There was a small difference between males and females in the BD-II rates with female rates being slightly higher.

11.2.4 The Cross-National Collaborative Group (CNCG)

The CNCG was created after the success of the ECA and included BD data from seven countries (USA, Canada, Puerto Rico, Germany, Taiwan, South Korea and New Zealand) which were gathered between the years 1980–1992 (Weissman et al. 1996). The ECA data were used concerning the USA, while only data from Edmonton were used for Canada (Orn et al. 1988), Munich for Germany (Wittchen et al. 1992) and Christchurch for New Zealand (Oakley-Browne et al. 1989; Wells et al. 1989). The data from Puerto Rico (Canino et al. 1987), Taiwan (Hwu et al. 1989) and South Korea (Lee et al. 1990a, b) were more representative of the populations of these countries.

The target population was 48,012,018 and the persons interviewed were 41,425, that is, a ratio of 1:1,159. The combined analysis was restricted to persons aged 18–64 years old.

The rates seemed moderately consistent cross-nationally. Men had higher rates in Korea. The rates by country are shown in Table 11.4.

11.2.5 Zurich Switzerland

This study was launched in the early 1980s and included persons from the canton of Zurich alone. Only those persons at high risk to develop mental disorders plus matched controls were selected (Angst et al. 1984, 2005; Wicki and Angst 1991). In total 4,547 persons aged 19–20 were assessed and reassessed four more times until the age of 34. The interview included the semi-structured interview SPIKE, administered by a clinical psychologist. That study reported an annual prevalence of BD-I of 0.7 % and a lifetime prevalence of the bipolar spectrum of 5.5 %.

11.2.6 Shatin, Hong Kong

The Shatin study was a community survey and took place in 1984–1986. It included 7,229 aged 18–64 years old who were assessed with the DIS. The Shatin was a new city and the population recently moved there and was not representative of the general population of the area. Probably it did not include any mentally ill people like an older community. The lifetime prevalence for BD was very low (0.15 %) and similar between males and females (Chen et al. 1993).

11.2.7 Nottingham, UK

The Nottingham study included only first referrals to general adult psychiatric clinics over the period 1992–1994 (Brewin et al. 1997). All cases were assessed with the SCAN and the SANS. Those cases which were not referred to a hospital were not included; thus, the registration is incomplete and biased towards more severe cases. The rates were calculated against a population of 397,048 residents of the general population. The 2-year incidence rate reported for BD was 0.005 % which corresponds to an annual incidence of 2.5 per 100,000.

11.2.8 The Netherlands Study

This was a prospective study which included 7,067 persons aged 18–64 years old from the general population (Regeer et al. 2002; Bijl et al. 2002; ten Have et al. 2002). There were three follow-up assessments during the years 1996–1999 with the CIDI. The results originally suggested a lifetime prevalence of BD equal to

2.4 %, which was reduced to 2.0 % after reassessment by a clinician. The annual incidence was equal to 2.7 per 100,000. There was no significant difference between males and females.

11.2.9 The Australian Study

The Australian National Survey included 10,641 persons from the general population and accessed them with the CIDI. The year prevalence of euphoric BD (combined BD-I and BD-II) was 0.5 % (Mitchell et al. 2004).

11.2.10 The Butajira Study

This study took part in the Butajira district in Ethiopia in a predominantly treatment naive population. It included a door-to-door screening of the entire adult population aged 15–49 years old. Eventually out of 83,387 of registered population, 68,378 were successfully screened with the CIDI and key informant method during the first step. The second step included confirmatory SCAN interviews. The results reported a lifetime prevalence of BD-I disorder of 0.5 % with the rate being 0.6 % for males and 0.3 % for females. The mean age of cases was 29.5 years, with no significant sex difference. The mean age of first recognition of illness was 22.0 years. There was no significant sex difference in the age at onset of manic or depressive phases. During the survey only 7.1 % of the cases were undergoing treatment (Negash et al. 2005).

11.2.11 The Merikangas et al. 2011 Study

A more recent cross-sectional, face-to-face, household survey assessed 61,392 community adults in 11 countries in the Americas, Europe and Asia with the CIDI and reported that the lifetime prevalence was 0.6 % for BD-I and 0.4 % for BD-II, while the year prevalence was 0.4 and 0.3 %, respectively (Merikangas et al. 2011)

11.2.12 Other Smaller Studies

There are a number of smaller studies with sample sizes below 5,000. They include one study from Iceland on 2,396 persons in their mid-1950s, which reported a lifetime prevalence of 0.2 % for BD-I and 0.5 % for BD-II (Stefansson et al. 1991). Another study from Hungary in 2,953 persons from GP registries, aged 18–64 years old, reported a lifetime prevalence of BD-I equal to 1.5 % and of BD-II equal to 2 %. The onset was traced at the age of 17.9 for females and 22 for males (Szadoczky et al. 1998). A study from Florence, Italy, on a community sample of 1,000 persons from the registries of GPs reported an annual prevalence of 1.3 % for BD-I and

0.2 % for BD-II. A number of methodological issues, including the fact that only mood disorders were probed during this survey, limit the usefulness of the results (Faravelli et al. 1990). A 10-year birth cohort study from Israel assessed 2,741 persons with the use of the SADS and interview by a psychiatrist. The results suggested a 6-month prevalence of 0.7 % for BD-I and 0.9 % for BD-II, with no difference between genders (Levav et al. 1993). One unpublished study from Ireland in 29,542 persons reported an annual incidence of 2.2 per 100,000 residents (Goodwin and Jamison 2007). A study from Norway in 2,066 persons aged 18–65 years old with the use of the CIDI reported an annual prevalence of 0.9 % and a lifetime prevalence of 1.6 % (Kringlen et al. 2001). A study from Sao Paulo, Brazil, in 1,464 persons with the CIDI reported an annual prevalence of 0.5 % and lifetime of 1 % with no differences between genders (Andrade et al. 2002). Finally a study from Chile in 2,978 persons with the use of the CIDI reported an annual prevalence of 1.4 % and a lifetime of 1.9 % with the lifetime rates being higher for females (2.2 vs. 1.5) (Vicente et al. 2006).

11.2.13 Epidemiology of the Bipolar Spectrum

The issue of the bipolar spectrum and its clinical as well as treatment consequences has been discussed in Chap. 6 of the current book. However, there are no rigorous data on its prevalence and the prevalence of softer bipolar clinical cases in general.

Still, there are several studies which try to chart the epidemiology of bipolar spectrum cases. One study from Israel reported a 6-month prevalence equal to 2.6 % (Levav et al. 1993) and another study from Italy reported an annual prevalence equal to 3.4 % (Faravelli and Incerpi 1985). Several other studies from the USA (Hirschfeld et al. 2003a, b; Oliver and Simmons 1985; Weissman and Myers 1978; Judd and Akiskal 2003; Kessler et al. 2006), Italy (Faravelli et al. 2006), Hungary (Szadoczky et al. 1998), Germany (Heun and Maier 1993), Switzerland (Angst et al. 1984, 2005; Wicki and Angst 1991; Angst 1998) and Brazil (Moreno and Andrade 2005) reported that in the adult population the lifetime prevalence of the bipolar spectrum is between 3 and 8.3 %.

The rates reported by these studies are both impressive and important since they suggest that the prevalence of the bipolar spectrum is many times higher than that of classic BD-I and BD-II. The problem is that the more the criteria are broadened, the higher the rates are rising, but also the diagnosis becomes less reliable. The largest of these studies came from the USA, assessed 85,000 persons with the MDQ and reported a lifetime prevalence equal to 3.7 % (Hirschfeld et al. 2003a, b). A similar rate was reported by the NCS-R which reported a combined lifetime rate of 4.4 % (BD-I 1.4 %, BD-II 1.6 % and bipolar subthreshold 1.4 %) (Kessler et al. 2006).

A more recent cross-sectional, face-to-face, household survey assessed 61,392 community adults in 11 countries in the Americas, Europe and Asia with the CIDI and reported that the lifetime prevalence for subthreshold BD was 1.4 % and for bipolar spectrum 2.4 %. The year prevalence was 0.8 % for subthreshold BD and 1.5 % for the bipolar spectrum. It is interesting that the USA had the highest prevalence of bipolar spectrum illness (4.4 %), while India had the lowest (0.1 %). The difference is so big that it raises important fundamental questions (Merikangas et al. 2011).

11.2.14 Conclusions on Epidemiology

According to the WHO, BD affected an estimated 29.5 million persons worldwide in 2004 (WHO 2008). The available data suggest that the life prevalence of BD-I is around 1 %, with probably a similar rate concerning BD-II. The complete bipolar spectrum probably has lifetime prevalence around 5 %. There are no striking differences between genders. However, these figures should be considered as only indicative, since important discrepancies exist among studies and countries.

The rather small difference between annual and lifetime rates suggests BD is both an episodic but also a chronic mental disorder with high recurrence rates. The changing rates with time, with a trend for increase, might reflect, at least partially, the increasing substance abuse and also the increasing use of antidepressants in the treatment of bipolar depression.

The various studies from around the world suggest that the age at onset is late adolescence or early adulthood, around the age of 18–20. It has been reported that childhood-onset BD occurs with prevalence estimates of 0.1–2.5 % in paediatric samples (Merikangas et al. 2012; Stringaris et al. 2010) with approximately one-fourth of BD patients having the onset before the age of 13 (Perlis et al. 2004). This might be more common in the USA than in Europe (Post et al. 2008) and among other things suggests caution in the use of stimulants for the treatment of children with ADHD.

Epidemiological data on comorbidity were presented in Chap. 11 and on clinical issues (relapse, chronicity, substance abuse, neurocognitive deficit, disability, etc.) in other specific chapters.

References

American Psychiatric Association (2013) Diagnostic and statistical manual of mental disorders, 5th edn, DSM-5. American Psychiatric Association, Washington, DC

Andrade L, Walters EE, Gentil V, Laurenti R (2002) Prevalence of ICD-10 mental disorders in a catchment area in the city of Sao Paulo, Brazil. Soc Psychiatry Psychiatr Epidemiol 37(7):316–325. doi:10.1007/s00127-002-0551-x

Angst J (1998) The emerging epidemiology of hypomania and bipolar II disorder. J Affect Disord 50(2–3):143–151

Angst J, Dobler-Mikola A, Binder J (1984) The Zurich study–a prospective epidemiological study of depressive, neurotic and psychosomatic syndromes. I. Problem, methodology. Eur Arch Psychiatry Neurol Sci 234(1):13–20

Angst J, Gamma A, Neuenschwander M, Ajdacic-Gross V, Eich D, Rossler W, Merikangas KR (2005) Prevalence of mental disorders in the Zurich Cohort Study: a twenty year prospective study. Epidemiol Psichiatr Soc 14(2):68–76

Angst J, Cui L, Swendsen J, Rothen S, Cravchik A, Kessler RC, Merikangas KR (2010) Major depressive disorder with subthreshold bipolarity in the National Comorbidity Survey Replication. Am J Psychiatry 167(10):1194–1201. doi:10.1176/appi.ajp.2010.09071011

Royal Australian and New Zealand College of Psychiatrists Clinical Practice Guidelines Team for Bipolar Disorder (2004) Australian and New Zealand clinical practice guidelines for the treatment of bipolar disorder. Aust N Z J Psychiatry 38(5):280–305. doi:10.1111/j.1440-1614.2004.01356.x

Bijl RV, De Graaf R, Ravelli A, Smit F, Vollebergh WA, Netherlands Mental Health S Incidence (2002) Gender and age-specific first incidence of DSM-III-R psychiatric disorders in the general population. Results from the Netherlands Mental Health Survey and Incidence Study (NEMESIS). Soc Psychiatry Psychiatr Epidemiol 37(8):372–379. doi:10.1007/s00127-002-0566-3

Blazer DG, Kessler RC, McGonagle KA, Swartz MS (1994) The prevalence and distribution of major depression in a national community sample: the National Comorbidity Survey. Am J Psychiatry 151(7):979–986

Bourdon KH, Rae DS, Locke BZ, Narrow WE, Regier DA (1992) Estimating the prevalence of mental disorders in U.S. adults from the Epidemiologic Catchment Area Survey. Public Health Rep 107(6):663–668

Brewin J, Cantwell R, Dalkin T, Fox R, Medley I, Glazebrook C, Kwiecinski R, Harrison G (1997) Incidence of schizophrenia in Nottingham. A comparison of two cohorts, 1978–80 and 1992–94. Br J Psychiatry 171:140–144

Canino GJ, Bird HR, Shrout PE, Rubio-Stipec M, Bravo M, Martinez R, Sesman M, Guevara LM (1987) The prevalence of specific psychiatric disorders in Puerto Rico. Arch Gen Psychiatry 44(8):727–735

Chen CN, Wong J, Lee N, Chan-Ho MW, Lau JT, Fung M (1993) The Shatin community mental health survey in Hong Kong. II. Major findings. Arch Gen Psychiatry 50(2):125–133

Eaton WW, Regier DA, Locke BZ, Taube CA (1981) The epidemiologic catchment area program of the National Institute of Mental Health. Public Health Rep 96(4):319–325

Egeland JA, Hostetter AM (1983) Amish Study, I: affective disorders among the Amish, 1976–1980. Am J Psychiatry 140(1):56–61

Egeland JA, Hostetter AM, Eshleman SK 3rd (1983) Amish Study, III: the impact of cultural factors on diagnosis of bipolar illness. Am J Psychiatry 140(1):67–71

Faravelli C, Incerpi G (1985) Epidemiology of affective disorders in Florence. Preliminary results. Acta Psychiatr Scand 72(4):331–333

Faravelli C, Guerrini Degl'Innocenti B, Aiazzi L, Incerpi G, Pallanti S (1990) Epidemiology of mood disorders: a community survey in Florence. J Affect Disord 20(2):135–141

Faravelli C, Rosi S, Alessandra Scarpato M, Lampronti L, Amedei SG, Rana N (2006) Threshold and subthreshold bipolar disorders in the Sesto Fiorentino study. J Affect Disord 94(1–3):111–119. doi:10.1016/j.jad.2006.01.031

Fountoulakis KN, Iacovides A, Nimatoudis I, Kaprinis G, Ierodiakonou C (1999) Comparison of the diagnosis of melancholic and atypical features according to DSM-IV and somatic syndrome according to ICD-10 in patients suffering from major depression. Eur Psychiatry 14(8):426–433

Goodwin F, Jamison K (2007) Manic-depressive illness, 2nd edn. Oxford University Press, New York

Heun R, Maier W (1993) The distinction of bipolar II disorder from bipolar I and recurrent unipolar depression: results of a controlled family study. Acta Psychiatr Scand 87(4):279–284

Hirschfeld RM, Calabrese JR, Weissman MM, Reed M, Davies MA, Frye MA, Keck PE Jr, Lewis L, McElroy SL, McNulty JP, Wagner KD (2003a) Screening for bipolar disorder in the community. J Clin Psychiatry 64(1):53–59

Hirschfeld RM, Holzer C, Calabrese JR, Weissman M, Reed M, Davies M, Frye MA, Keck P, McElroy S, Lewis L, Tierce J, Wagner KD, Hazard E (2003b) Validity of the mood disorder questionnaire: a general population study. Am J Psychiatry 160(1):178–180

Hostetter AM, Egeland JA, Endicott J (1983) Amish Study, II: consensus diagnoses and reliability results. Am J Psychiatry 140(1):62–66

Hwu HG, Yeh EK, Chang LY (1989) Prevalence of psychiatric disorders in Taiwan defined by the Chinese diagnostic interview schedule. Acta Psychiatr Scand 79(2):136–147

Judd LL, Akiskal HS (2003) The prevalence and disability of bipolar spectrum disorders in the US population: re-analysis of the ECA database taking into account subthreshold cases. J Affect Disord 73(1–2):123–131

Kendler KS, Gallagher TJ, Abelson JM, Kessler RC (1996) Lifetime prevalence, demographic risk factors, and diagnostic validity of nonaffective psychosis as assessed in a US community sample. The National Comorbidity Survey. Arch Gen Psychiatry 53(11):1022–1031

Kessler RC, Merikangas KR (2004) The National Comorbidity Survey Replication (NCS-R): background and aims. Int J Methods Psychiatr Res 13(2):60–68

Kessler RC, McGonagle KA, Swartz M, Blazer DG, Nelson CB (1993) Sex and depression in the National Comorbidity Survey. I: lifetime prevalence, chronicity and recurrence. J Affect Disord 29(2–3):85–96

Kessler RC, McGonagle KA, Nelson CB, Hughes M, Swartz M, Blazer DG (1994a) Sex and depression in the National Comorbidity Survey. II: cohort effects. J Affect Disord 30(1):15–26

Kessler RC, McGonagle KA, Zhao S, Nelson CB, Hughes M, Eshleman S, Wittchen HU, Kendler KS (1994b) Lifetime and 12-month prevalence of DSM-III-R psychiatric disorders in the United States. Results from the National Comorbidity Survey. Arch Gen Psychiatry 51(1):8–19

Kessler RC, Sonnega A, Bromet E, Hughes M, Nelson CB (1995) Posttraumatic stress disorder in the National Comorbidity Survey. Arch Gen Psychiatry 52(12):1048–1060

Kessler RC, Nelson CB, McGonagle KA, Liu J, Swartz M, Blazer DG (1996) Comorbidity of DSM-III-R major depressive disorder in the general population: results from the US National Comorbidity Survey. Br J Psychiatry Suppl 30:17–30

Kessler RC, Anthony JC, Blazer DG, Bromet E, Eaton WW, Kendler K, Swartz M, Wittchen HU, Zhao S (1997a) The US National Comorbidity Survey: overview and future directions. Epidemiol Psichiatr Soc 6(1):4–16

Kessler RC, Rubinow DR, Holmes C, Abelson JM, Zhao S (1997b) The epidemiology of DSM-III-R bipolar I disorder in a general population survey. Psychol Med 27(5):1079–1089

Kessler RC, Berglund P, Chiu WT, Demler O, Heeringa S, Hiripi E, Jin R, Pennell BE, Walters EE, Zaslavsky A, Zheng H (2004) The US National Comorbidity Survey Replication (NCS-R): design and field procedures. Int J Methods Psychiatr Res 13(2):69–92

Kessler RC, Berglund P, Demler O, Jin R, Merikangas KR, Walters EE (2005a) Lifetime prevalence and age-of-onset distributions of DSM-IV disorders in the National Comorbidity Survey Replication. Arch Gen Psychiatry 62(6):593–602. doi:10.1001/archpsyc.62.6.593

Kessler RC, Chiu WT, Demler O, Merikangas KR, Walters EE (2005b) Prevalence, severity, and comorbidity of 12-month DSM-IV disorders in the National Comorbidity Survey Replication. Arch Gen Psychiatry 62(6):617–627. doi:10.1001/archpsyc.62.6.617

Kessler RC, Akiskal HS, Angst J, Guyer M, Hirschfeld RM, Merikangas KR, Stang PE (2006) Validity of the assessment of bipolar spectrum disorders in the WHO CIDI 3.0. J Affect Disord 96(3):259–269. doi:10.1016/j.jad.2006.08.018

Kessler RC, Avenevoli S, Costello EJ, Georgiades K, Green JG, Gruber MJ, He JP, Koretz D, McLaughlin KA, Petukhova M, Sampson NA, Zaslavsky AM, Merikangas KR (2012a) Prevalence, persistence, and sociodemographic correlates of DSM-IV disorders in the National Comorbidity Survey replication adolescent supplement. Arch Gen Psychiatry 69(4):372–380. doi:10.1001/archgenpsychiatry.2011.160

Kessler RC, Avenevoli S, Costello J, Green JG, Gruber MJ, McLaughlin KA, Petukhova M, Sampson NA, Zaslavsky AM, Merikangas KR (2012b) Severity of 12-month DSM-IV disorders in the National Comorbidity Survey replication adolescent supplement. Arch Gen Psychiatry 69(4):381–389. doi:10.1001/archgenpsychiatry.2011.1603

Kringlen E, Torgersen S, Cramer V (2001) A Norwegian psychiatric epidemiological study. Am J Psychiatry 158(7):1091–1098

Lee CK, Kwak YS, Yamamoto J, Rhee H, Kim YS, Han JH, Choi JO, Lee YH (1990a) Psychiatric epidemiology in Korea. Part I: gender and age differences in Seoul. J Nerv Ment Dis 178(4):242–246

Lee CK, Kwak YS, Yamamoto J, Rhee H, Kim YS, Han JH, Choi JO, Lee YH (1990b) Psychiatric epidemiology in Korea. Part II: urban and rural differences. J Nerv Ment Dis 178(4):247–252

Levav I, Kohn R, Dohrenwend BP, Shrout PE, Skodol AE, Schwartz S, Link BG, Naveh G (1993) An epidemiological study of mental disorders in a 10-year cohort of young adults in Israel. Psychol Med 23(3):691–707

Magee WJ, Eaton WW, Wittchen HU, McGonagle KA, Kessler RC (1996) Agoraphobia, simple phobia, and social phobia in the National Comorbidity Survey. Arch Gen Psychiatry 53(2):159–168

Merikangas KR, Akiskal HS, Angst J, Greenberg PE, Hirschfeld RM, Petukhova M, Kessler RC (2007) Lifetime and 12-month prevalence of bipolar spectrum disorder in the National Comorbidity Survey replication. Arch Gen Psychiatry 64(5):543–552. doi:10.1001/archpsyc.64.5.543

Merikangas KR, Jin R, He JP, Kessler RC, Lee S, Sampson NA, Viana MC, Andrade LH, Hu C, Karam EG, Ladea M, Medina-Mora ME, Ono Y, Posada-Villa J, Sagar R, Wells JE, Zarkov Z (2011) Prevalence and correlates of bipolar spectrum disorder in the world mental health survey initiative. Arch Gen Psychiatry 68(3):241–251. doi:10.1001/archgenpsychiatry.2011.12

Merikangas KR, Cui L, Kattan G, Carlson GA, Youngstrom EA, Angst J (2012) Mania with and without depression in a community sample of US adolescents. Arch Gen Psychiatry 69(9):943–951. doi:10.1001/archgenpsychiatry.2012.38

Mitchell PB, Slade T, Andrews G (2004) Twelve-month prevalence and disability of DSM-IV bipolar disorder in an Australian general population survey. Psychol Med 34(5):777–785

Moreno DH, Andrade LH (2005) The lifetime prevalence, health services utilization and risk of suicide of bipolar spectrum subjects, including subthreshold categories in the Sao Paulo ECA study. J Affect Disord 87(2–3):231–241. doi:10.1016/j.jad.2005.04.010

Muller-Oerlinghausen B, Berghofer A, Bauer M (2002) Bipolar disorder. Lancet 359(9302):241–247

Negash A, Alem A, Kebede D, Deyessa N, Shibre T, Kullgren G (2005) Prevalence and clinical characteristics of bipolar I disorder in Butajira, Ethiopia: a community-based study. J Affect Disord 87(2–3):193–201. doi:10.1016/j.jad.2005.03.011

Nierenberg AA, Akiskal HS, Angst J, Hirschfeld RM, Merikangas KR, Petukhova M, Kessler RC (2010) Bipolar disorder with frequent mood episodes in the National Comorbidity Survey replication (NCS-R). Mol Psychiatry 15(11):1075–1087. doi:10.1038/mp.2009.61

Oakley Browne MA, Wells JE, Scott KM (2006) Te Rau Hinengaro: the New Zealand mental health survey. Ministry of Health, Wellington

Oakley-Browne MA, Joyce PR, Wells JE, Bushnell JA, Hornblow AR (1989) Christchurch Psychiatric Epidemiology Study, Part II: six month and other period prevalences of specific psychiatric disorders. Aust N Z J Psychiatry 23(3):327–340

Oliver JM, Simmons ME (1985) Affective disorders and depression as measured by the diagnostic interview schedule and the Beck depression inventory in an unselected adult population. J Clin Psychol 41(4):469–477

Orn H, Newman SC, Bland RC (1988) Design and field methods of the Edmonton survey of psychiatric disorders. Acta Psychiatr Scand Suppl 338:17–23

Parker G, Brotchie H, Fletcher K (2006) An increased proportional representation of bipolar disorder in younger depressed patients: analysis of two clinical databases. J Affect Disord 95(1–3):141–144. doi:10.1016/j.jad.2006.04.024

Perlis RH, Miyahara S, Marangell LB, Wisniewski SR, Ostacher M, DelBello MP, Bowden CL, Sachs GS, Nierenberg AA, Investigators S-B (2004) Long-term implications of early onset in bipolar disorder: data from the first 1000 participants in the systematic treatment enhancement program for bipolar disorder (STEP-BD). Biol Psychiatry 55(9):875–881. doi:10.1016/j.biopsych.2004.01.022

Post RM, Luckenbaugh DA, Leverich GS, Altshuler LL, Frye MA, Suppes T, Keck PE, McElroy SL, Nolen WA, Kupka R, Grunze H, Walden J (2008) Incidence of childhood-onset bipolar illness in the USA and Europe. Br J Psychiatry 192(2):150–151. doi:10.1192/bjp.bp.107.037820

Regeer EJ, Rosso ML, ten Have M, Vollebergh W, Nolen WA (2002) Prevalence of bipolar disorder: a further study in The Netherlands. Bipolar Disord 4(Suppl 1):37–38

Regier DA, Myers JK, Kramer M, Robins LN, Blazer DG, Hough RL, Eaton WW, Locke BZ (1984) The NIMH epidemiologic catchment area program. Historical context, major objectives, and study population characteristics. Arch Gen Psychiatry 41(10):934–941

Regier DA, Boyd JH, Burke JD Jr, Rae DS, Myers JK, Kramer M, Robins LN, George LK, Karno M, Locke BZ (1988) One-month prevalence of mental disorders in the United States. Based on five epidemiologic catchment area sites. Arch Gen Psychiatry 45(11):977–986

Regier DA, Farmer ME, Rae DS, Myers JK, Kramer M, Robins LN, George LK, Karno M, Locke BZ (1993) One-month prevalence of mental disorders in the United States and sociodemographic characteristics: the epidemiologic catchment area study. Acta Psychiatr Scand 88(1):35–47

Robins LN, Helzer JE, Croughan J, Ratcliff KS (1981) National Institute of Mental Health diagnostic interview schedule. Its history, characteristics, and validity. Arch Gen Psychiatry 38(4):381–389

Robins LN, Wing J, Wittchen HU, Helzer JE, Babor TF, Burke J, Farmer A, Jablenski A, Pickens R, Regier DA et al (1988) The Composite International Diagnostic interview. An epidemiologic Instrument suitable for use in conjunction with different diagnostic systems and in different cultures. Arch Gen Psychiatry 45(12):1069–1077

Sartorius N (1978) Diagnosis and classification: cross cultural and international perspectives. Ment Health Soc 5(1–2):79–85

Sartorius N (1988) International perspectives of psychiatric classification. Br J Psychiatry Suppl 1:9–14

Sheehan DV, Lecrubier Y, Sheehan KH, Amorim P, Janavs J, Weiller E, Hergueta T, Baker R, Dunbar GC (1998) The Mini-International Neuropsychiatric Interview (M.I.N.I.): the development and validation of a structured diagnostic psychiatric interview for DSM-IV and ICD-10. J Clin Psychiatry 59(Suppl 20):22–33; quiz 34–57

Stefansson JG, Lindal E, Bjornsson JK, Guomundsdottir A (1991) Lifetime prevalence of specific mental disorders among people born in Iceland in 1931. Acta Psychiatr Scand 84(2):142–149

Stringaris A, Santosh P, Leibenluft E, Goodman R (2010) Youth meeting symptom and impairment criteria for mania-like episodes lasting less than four days: an epidemiological enquiry. J Child Psychol Psychiatry 51(1):31–38. doi:10.1111/j.1469-7610.2009.02129.x

Szadoczky E, Papp Z, Vitrai J, Rihmer Z, Furedi J (1998) The prevalence of major depressive and bipolar disorders in Hungary. Results from a national epidemiologic survey. J Affect Disord 50(2–3):153–162

ten Have M, Vollebergh W, Bijl R, Nolen WA (2002) Bipolar disorder in the general population in The Netherlands (prevalence, consequences and care utilisation): results from The Netherlands Mental Health Survey and Incidence Study (NEMESIS). J Affect Disord 68(2–3):203–213

Vicente B, Kohn R, Rioseco P, Saldivia S, Levav I, Torres S (2006) Lifetime and 12-month prevalence of DSM-III-R disorders in the Chile psychiatric prevalence study. Am J Psychiatry 163(8):1362–1370. doi:10.1176/appi.ajp.163.8.1362

Warner LA, Kessler RC, Hughes M, Anthony JC, Nelson CB (1995) Prevalence and correlates of drug use and dependence in the United States. Results from the National Comorbidity Survey. Arch Gen Psychiatry 52(3):219–229

Weissman MM, Myers JK (1978) Affective disorders in a US urban community: the use of research diagnostic criteria in an epidemiological survey. Arch Gen Psychiatry 35(11):1304–1311

Weissman MM, Bland RC, Canino GJ, Faravelli C, Greenwald S, Hwu HG, Joyce PR, Karam EG, Lee CK, Lellouch J, Lepine JP, Newman SC, Rubio-Stipec M, Wells JE, Wickramaratne PJ, Wittchen H, Yeh EK (1996) Cross-national epidemiology of major depression and bipolar disorder. JAMA 276(4):293–299

Wells JE, Bushnell JA, Hornblow AR, Joyce PR, Oakley-Browne MA (1989) Christchurch Psychiatric Epidemiology Study, Part I: methodology and lifetime prevalence for specific psychiatric disorders. Aust N Z J Psychiatry 23(3):315–326

WHO (1992) The ICD-10 classification of mental and behavioural disorders – clinical descriptions and diagnostic guidelines. World Health Organization, Geneva

WHO (1994) Diagnostic and management guidelines for mental disorders in primary health care. Hogrefe & Huber, Seattle

WHO (2008) The global burden of disease 2004: update. World Health Organization, Geneva

Wicki W, Angst J (1991) The Zurich Study. X. Hypomania in a 28- to 30-year-old cohort. Eur Arch Psychiatry Clin Neurosci 240(6):339–348

Wing JK, Babor T, Brugha T, Burke J, Cooper JE, Giel R, Jablenski A, Regier D, Sartorius N (1990) SCAN. Schedules for clinical assessment in neuropsychiatry. Arch Gen Psychiatry 47(6):589–593

Wittchen HU, Essau CA, von Zerssen D, Krieg JC, Zaudig M (1992) Lifetime and six-month prevalence of mental disorders in the Munich follow-up study. Eur Arch Psychiatry Clin Neurosci 241(4):247–258

Wittchen HU, Zhao S, Kessler RC, Eaton WW (1994) DSM-III-R generalized anxiety disorder in the National Comorbidity Survey. Arch Gen Psychiatry 51(5):355–364

Disability and Overall Burden Related with Bipolar Disorder

12

12.1 Disability

12.1.1 Overview and Definitions

The concept of disability is complex and has been revised several times in the past. It is defined as the consequence of an impairment which might be physical, cognitive, mental or sensory and could be either developmental or acquired. Combinations also occur. The consequences of any impairment could be loss of function or limitations in participation in various activities and in completing tasks (World Health Organization 2014).

One important issue is that often, especially concerning people suffering from mental illness, stigma and prejudice plays an important role (usually through exclusion and isolation) in the development of disability, and this role might be stronger than the effect of the illness per se. It is reasonable that a general and global correlation exists between disability and poverty. A direct causality is probable but the direction is not stable; more often there is a vicious circle between them (World Health Organization 2011).

The World Health Organization (WHO) published The International Classification of Functioning, Disability and Health (ICF), which lists nine broad domains of functioning (learning and applying knowledge; general tasks and demands; communication; basic physical mobility; domestic life and self-care; interpersonal interactions and relationships; community, social and civic life; employment; and other major life areas) (World Health Organization 2001).

A number of different approaches and models apply in the concept and definition of disability. The medical model considers disability as a problem which is directly caused by a health condition and demands medical treatment. The social model considers disability as a problem created by the social environment rather than the condition of the health of the individual. The social model includes an ideological dimension and suggests that elimination of disability and its consequences is a human right of prime importance for the society. The spectrum model suggests that

K.N. Fountoulakis, *Bipolar Disorder: An Evidence-Based Guide to Manic Depression*, DOI 10.1007/978-3-642-37216-2_12

disability should be defined according to thresholds set on a continuum of disability on multiple domains, while the moral model suggests that people are morally responsible for their own disability. The tragedy/charity model considers disabled people as victims of circumstance who are deserving of pity. An integrated pragmatic model is the expert/professional model which usually starts from the medical model but goes on to investigate and encompass all relevant sources and aspects of disability. Other models include the legitimacy model, the social adapted model, the economic model, the empowering model, the market model and the consumer model. All models are asymmetrical; most models perceive the disabled person as a passive client of intervention, while on the contrary, the moral model attributes unrealistic responsibility on the disabled individual. The empowering, market and the consumer model place the disabled person at the centre with the right to informed choice and decision (Langtree 2014).

12.1.2 Disability in BD Patients

Mood disorders constitute the most frequent causes of morbidity and mortality in developed countries according to WHO (World Health Organization 1999), while self-inflicting injuries constitute the sixth leading cause of death in adults in low- and middle-income countries and the second in high-income countries (Lopez 2005). Mood disorders compromise quality of life and ability to work and are the cause of chronic impairment to a greater degree in comparison to many widespread severe disorders including cardiovascular diseases (Ogilvie et al. 2005).

The extremes of mood manifested by BD patients and the accompanied changes in energy, volition, motives and psychomotor activity make BD one of the most disabling medical conditions with a devastating effect in general health, work, family and personal relationships, education and quality of life (Dore and Romans 2001; Simon 2003; Huxley and Baldessarini 2007; Pope et al. 2007). The complex nature of BD complicates the measurement of impairment (Dean et al. 2004); however, already in 1990, BD was included among the ten more disabling conditions in terms of disability-adjusted life years (DALYs) by the WHO (Murray and Lopez 1996).

Although the last few decades, there are available efficacious treatments for BD; often syndromal or symptomatic recovery does not go together with functional recovery. This means that in spite of the fact that patients recover in clinical terms, frequently they do not return to their functioning level as it was before getting ill. This was clearly shown even for patients at the earliest stage of the illness, in a 2-year follow-up study on BD patients who were hospitalized on their first manic episode with psychotic symptoms. One study reported that although almost 80 % of patients were symptom-free or mildly symptomatic, only 43 % were employed, and only 21 % were working at their expected level of employment. Approximately 30 % were unable to work (Dion et al. 1988). Another study reported that although 97 % of patients had achieved syndromal recovery at endpoint, only 37 % achieved functional recovery (Tohen et al. 2000). In a third study, 62.3 % of patients had met criteria for full remission of mood symptoms, but simultaneously another 62.3 % of the patients had at least moderate disability (Kauer-Sant'Anna et al. 2009). It is evident that the majority of BD patients do not achieve complete functional recovery and are in need of ongoing psychosocial rehabilitation (Pradhan et al. 1999).

Overall BD is associated with significant impairment in work, family and social life, and the impairment is present not only during the acute phases of the illness (Sanchez-Moreno et al. 2009). The literature suggests that at least some degree of disability is present during the majority of long-term follow-up. In one study, impairment was found in the majority of assessments, corresponding to 54–59 % of the time, including 19–23 % with moderate and 7–9 % of the time with severe overall impairment. However, it seems that severe disability occurred for a substantial percentage of time only in the specific area of work role function. BD-I patients were reported to be completely unable to carry out work role functions during 30 % of the time, which was significantly more in comparison to BD-II (20 %) and unipolar depression (21 %) (Judd et al. 2008).

Impairment in work seems to be a basic and widespread disability in BD patients. In comparison with healthy subjects, BD-I patients reported lower levels of work productivity, more frequent outpatient visits and more prescribed medication. They were more likely to miss work; to have worked reduced hours due to medical or mental health issues; to receive disability payments; to have been involved in a crime, be uninsured or covered by Medicare; or to have been fired or laid off (McMorris et al. 2009). Disability pension and benefits are an important element which often determines things instead of being determined by them. It is a fact that disability benefits are rarely awarded when a person is working. Moreover, receipt of disability benefits increases the likelihood that a person with BD will be receiving health-care benefits, and, in many cases, those benefits provide greater access to treatment compared to health-care insurance received through an employer or through unemployment health coverage. Thus, for many patients, the incentives to work run counter to access to treatment among people with BD (Elinson et al. 2007).

It is important to note that at least some BD patients manifest fundamental problems concerning their overall abilities and functioning. For example, it seems that despite comparable IQ levels, patients with BD completed fewer years of education in comparison to controls. In one study, although over 60 % of both groups entered college, only 16 % of BD patients received a college degree. In contrast 47 % of the comparison sample completed college. Educational attainment did not differ between subgroups of patients with earlier vs. later illness onset, nor as a function of comorbid substance abuse (Glahn et al. 2006). Despite similar levels of education, BD patients had lower social and occupational function than the general population, and no association was found between education and disability for BD patients (Schoeyen et al. 2011a). It seems that other factors than severity of illness play a role for education and work abilities in BD patients (Schoeyen et al. 2011b).

12.1.2.1 Prevalence of Disability in BD Patients

The literature suggests that the majority of BD patients manifest some kind of chronic disability. Taking into consideration the episodic nature of the disease, the prevalence of disability should be considered both in terms of the percentage of individuals affected and in terms of the percentage of the time in their lives they spend with disability. The episodic nature of the illness along with its progress and its different forms make the severity of disability to fluctuate, and thus, the epidemiological approach is complex and inherently incomplete.

It has been reported that the disability affecting at least one area of life (e.g. work, social life or family life) is present in 52–54 % of the patients, while in 37 %, the disability affects at least two areas (Gutierrez-Rojas et al. 2010). In accord with this, it has been also reported that specifically BD-I patients are completely unable to carry out work role functions during 30 % of the time, while BD-II were also unable for 20 % of their time (Judd et al. 2008). Similarly, another study found that almost two-thirds of BD patients had at least moderate disability, but the percentage fell to one-fourth after successful treatment after 6 months (Kauer-Sant'Anna et al. 2009).

The prevailing picture is that two-thirds are reported to be impaired, with one-third being moderately impaired and one-third severely (Magliano et al. 2009). Cross-sectionally one-third of patients manifest severe dysfunction at work (Kusznir et al. 2000).

12.1.2.2 Clinical Correlates of Disability in BD Patients

An important first observation is that the type of BD determines the degree of disability, with BD-I patients experiencing significantly more disability in comparison to BD-II patients (Judd et al. 2008). There seems to be a differential effect of different types of symptoms, with depressive symptoms causing significant psychosocial impairment in both BD-I and BD-II patients, while hypomanic symptoms in BD-II patients are not only non-disabling, but they may even enhance functioning. Also manic symptoms in BD-I patients are causing significant psychosocial impairment. In general, psychosocial disability fluctuates in parallel with changes in affective symptom severity (Judd et al. 2005), but overall in many aspects, BD-I and BD-II patients do not differ much in terms of disability (Judd and Akiskal 2003).

The second important observation is that overall, disability is correlated more with depressive symptoms even when subsyndromal (Judd et al. 2005; Wingo et al. 2010; Simon et al. 2007; Kauer-Sant'Anna et al. 2009; Sanchez-Moreno et al. 2009; Gutierrez-Rojas et al. 2010; Rosa et al. 2011; Bowden and Krishnan 2004; Bauer et al. 2009; Bowie et al. 2010; Marangell 2004; Mur et al. 2009), although there is a general effect of any current psychopathology (Rosa et al. 2011; Ozer et al. 2002). This is especially true for social and family functioning (Wingo et al. 2010). Only work disability seems to be significantly associated not only with current depressive symptoms but also with previous repeated manic episodes, and hospitalizations and inversely with the educational attainment (Gutierrez-Rojas et al. 2010). A generalized impairment is present also during periods of euthymia (Sanchez-Moreno et al. 2009; Rosa et al. 2011; Judd et al. 2005).

A number of additional factors have been reported to correlate with disability. Females seem to preserve social functioning more than men (Morgan et al. 2005). More severe disability is related with disrupted biological rhythms (Giglio et al.

2010), a comorbid substance abuse (Tohen et al. 1998), history of psychotic symptoms (Tohen et al. 1990, 2000), subsyndromal residual symptoms (Gitlin et al. 1995; Martinez-Aran et al. 2002; Marangell 2004; MacQueen et al. 2001) and the stage of the illness (Tohen et al. 1990; MacQueen et al. 2000; Dion et al. 1988; O'Connell et al. 1991). Also a significant role is played by a younger age of onset (Tohen et al. 2000) especially in combination with low premorbid functioning (Reznik and Sirota 1999; Cannon et al. 1997).

However, there are some reports which did not find any relationship between clinical variables and psychosocial outcome (Martinez-Aran et al. 2004; MacQueen et al. 2001; Coryell et al. 1998; Goldberg et al. 1995; Keck et al. 1998; Harrow et al. 1990), and the functional outcome was not better in studies in which patients have very low levels of residual symptomatology (MacQueen et al. 1997; Tohen et al. 2000; Dion et al. 1988). Thus, some authors suggest that the neurocognitive disorder is what mediates the effect (Chakrabarti and Gill 2002; Wilson and Crowe 2009; Coryell et al. 1998).

12.1.2.3 The Impact of the Neurocognitive Deficit on Impairment and Disability

Neurocognitive dysfunction is not routinely assessed in BD patients, and only a few studies investigate it and correlate it with the resulting psychosocial impairment and disability (Goldberg et al. 1993). Recently its effect has been recognized to such an extent that it has been proposed that functional disability may be restricted to a subgroup of cognitively impaired BD patients with a deficit in their executive function (Altshuler et al. 2008).

There are a number of studies which reported a strong relationship between neurocognitive impairment and overall psychosocial functioning (Atre-Vaidya et al. 1998; Zubieta et al. 2001; Martinez-Aran et al. 2002, 2004; Tohen et al. 1990; Dickerson et al. 2001; Sanchez-Moreno et al. 2009; Levy et al. 2010). In BD-I patients, changes in the composite neurocognitive score over 1 year and deficits in the visual/motor processing domain predicted functioning or disability changes over follow-up period (Tabares-Seisdedos et al. 2008). Both impairment at work and interpersonal relationships seem to depend on neurocognition and mediated by adaptive and social competence (Bowie et al. 2010).

More specifically, the psychosocial functioning was reported to significantly correlate with processing speed (Mur et al. 2009; Burdick et al. 2010), abstract thinking (Burdick et al. 2010) and verbal memory and executive function measures even in euthymic patients (Martinez-Aran et al. 2002, 2007).

Impairment at work was found to correlate with difficulty remembering long-term information (Martinez-Aran et al. 2002) as well as with inhibitory control, spatial working memory, generalized verbal learning and memory deficits even in euthymic patients (Martinez-Aran et al. 2004; Burdick et al. 2010). These are indicative of a deficit in frontal executive functions and specifically in the encoding and retrieval of verbal information. Also self-reported concentration problems and years of education were reported to predict work performance (Gilbert et al. 2010).

It is important to note that attention and concentration problems seem not to be responsible for the poor psychosocial functioning (Martinez-Aran et al. 2002, 2007).

There is one report which suggests no relationship between the neurocognitive function and impairment, but it suffers from methodological problems (Ferrier et al. 1999).

12.1.2.4 The Role of Medication on Impairment and Disability

Since medication is the backbone of the treatment of BD, the correct usage of agents is expected to lead to better outcome. It is unfortunate however that the available treatments have limitations in their capacity to improve the functioning and reduce the disability of BD patients.

On the other hand, pharmacological treatment often has adverse effects which in turn could have a negative impact not only on the quality of life of patients but also on functioning itself (Zarate et al. 2000).

It is known (see relevant chapters of this book) that there is no specific beneficial effect of treatment on the neurocognitive deficit, and moreover, there seems not to be any difference in the neurocognitive performance between patients taking lithium, antidepressants or antipsychotics compared with patients who did not take those medications. However, there are reports which suggesting that number of drugs has an adverse effect on the psychosocial outcome even in euthymic BD patients (Martinez-Aran et al. 2007; Goldberg et al. 1996; Dean et al. 2004). However, since these studies are uncontrolled and naturalistic in essence, it is unclear whether it is the medications per se that exert this adverse effect or the patients who are in a need for more aggressive pharmacological treatment are more impaired.

12.1.2.5 Comparison with Disability Caused by Other Mental Disorders

It is almost by definition that BD is considered to have a better outcome in comparison to schizophrenia. Kraepelin introduced this approach, and it was one of the major criteria to distinguish between manic-depression and 'dementia praecox' (Kraepelin 1921). Since then the literature suggests that in BD the impairment is less stable and chronic in comparison to schizophrenia although the utilization of services is greater by BD patients (Morgan et al. 2005). It is reported that in patients with schizophrenia, global functioning 1 year later was predicted by a composite neurocognitive score and verbal memory, motor speed and vocabulary, while residual clinical symptoms did not seem to play a role. On the contrary, in BD-I patients, residual depressive symptoms, psychosis, premorbid adjustment and the deficit in the visual/motor processing domain all together were predictors of functioning (Tabares-Seisdedos et al. 2008).

There is a line of research suggesting the deficit in BD is greater in comparison with unipolar depression (Judd et al. 2008), while schizoaffective disorders occupy a position between mood disorders and schizophrenia (Marneros et al. 1990).

However, there is a chance the difference is because of the presence of a severely impaired group (pronounced negative syndrome) within the large population affected with schizophrenia (Bellack et al. 1989). In accord with this, many studies suggest there is no difference in terms of disability between BD, unipolar depression and schizophrenia (Pini et al. 2005).

12.2 Quality of Life

Quality of life (QoL) is another complex concept which to a significant extent is ill defined and vague. The term is often used to essentially denote 'life satisfaction' which however is quite a different concept and largely depends on the individual's mood. Therefore, in order to comprehend what the literature really suggests, one needs to see in depth the methodology and the psychometric tools used in each study. A core problematic issue is that almost by definition depression is related to low life satisfaction and wellbeing while mania and hypomania exactly the opposite.

Overall, QoL is reported to correlate with current depressive symptoms either threshold or subthreshold (Ozer et al. 2002; Michalak et al. 2008; Depp et al. 2006), although one study suggested that it is neurocognitive impairment rather than depressive or manic symptoms which is responsible for the low sense of wellbeing in BD patients (Depp et al. 2006, 2009). The presence of psychotic symptoms also deteriorates QoL (Depp et al. 2006). When euthymic, at least some BD patients might have QoL similar to that of the general population (Chand et al. 2004).

It is evident that the perception of the QoL, in and outside the family, is altered for the patient (Morselli et al. 2004), with daily hassles contributing significantly to its deterioration (Chand et al. 2004). Wellbeing and perception of general health is lower in BD patients even when euthymic in comparison to the general population (Depp et al. 2006).

The literature is somewhat inconsistent but overall suggests that euthymic BD patients have better QoL in comparison to patients with stable schizophrenia (Michalak et al. 2008; Chand et al. 2004), similar or worse to that of unipolar depression and anxiety disorders and similar or worse to those patients with other chronic nonmental illnesses (Michalak et al. 2008; Dean et al. 2004). However, when not euthymic, BD patients might have a sense of wellbeing and general health similar to patients with schizophrenia, and additionally more medical comorbidity (Depp et al. 2006). It appears that QOL is poorer in bipolar disorder than in other mood disorders and anxiety disorders, but that schizophrenia might compromise QOL more severely than bipolar disorder. Existing data also suggest that for patients with bipolar disorder, QOL is negatively associated with depression (Michalak et al. 2008).

12.3 Caregiver and Family Burden

Like most mental disorders, BD besides making patients suffer, it has also a deep impact on the lives of caregivers and the family (Platt 1985; Brodaty and Green 2002; Lowery et al. 2000; Murray and Lopez 1996). The old belief that it is the family and its members who cause the mental disease in one of the family members has been replaced by exactly the opposite concept, that is, the illness of one particular family member causes distress and puts the rest of the family members at risk for the deterioration of their mental and somatic health (Tantum 1989).

However, in psychiatry, in both the literature and in the everyday clinical practice, almost all the medical attention is focused on the patient, while caregivers and family are largely neglected. However, keeping the caregivers and family in good shape is of great importance since the support they provide is considered to be a positive prognostic factor and an essential contributor to the wellbeing of the patient.

There are several reasons why family members should be also at the focus of medical care. Apart from the everyday burden they experience because of the illness of a family member, some other family members may share a genetic predisposition for psychiatric morbidity which in turn may constitute them vulnerable to experiencing higher levels of stress as a consequence of their relative's illness.

'Caregiving' is more specific and narrower as a concept than simply being the member of a family with an ill relative. It refers to the provision of actual assistance in response to the specific everyday and long-term needs of the patient and his illness. On the other hand, the concept of 'family burden' applies to all family members whether they are or not involved in the provision of practical assistance to the patient (Sales 2003; Poulin et al. 2010).

Although the stress–coping together with the stress–vulnerability model constitute fundamental approaches in the understanding of caregiver burden (Leclerc et al. 1997), there seems to be additional features which compose the complete picture of the experience of caregivers and families (Szmukler et al. 1996). The overall caregiver and family burden has been classified into two broad categories, the 'objective' and the 'subjective' burden (Hoenig and Hamilton 1966). 'Objective' burden refers to externally identifiable and quantifiable events (divorce, hospitalizations, economic problems, etc.) (Fadden et al. 1987), while 'subjective' burden refers to the personal feelings and psychological condition of the caregiver (Grad and Sainbury 1963; Grad and Sainsbury 1963; Hoenig and Hamilton 1966, 1969; Platt 1985; Fadden et al. 1987).

According to the classification of caregivers by Platt (1985), three gross categories exist: the effective caregivers (no health problems, low stress, adaptive coping), the burdened caregivers (high level of stress and less adaptive coping) and finally the stigmatized caregivers (healthy, stressed due to perceived stigma, effective coping). According to Katon, among caregivers the level of stress is correlated with the condition of their health, and those caregivers with the higher degree of caregiving burden also had poor physical and mental health (Katon 1984). It has been reported that caregivers of BD patients used a wide variety of coping strategies, both problem and emotion focused, with problem-focused coping strategies being more common (Chakrabarti and Gill 2002).

12.3.1 Prevalence of Caregiver Burden

More than 90 % of family members reported severe subjective (rated by relative) and objective burden (rated by interviewer) at admission; none of them was free of burden. At the time of follow-up, about one-quarter (23.5 %) and two-thirds

(64.7 %) of family members did not experience any objective and subjective burden, respectively; subjective and objective family burden was moderate in about one-third (35.3 %) and a half (52.9 %), respectively. None of the family members reported severe burden subjectively, while the objective burden was rated to be severe in a quarter (23.5 %) of family members (Maji et al. 2011). Overall, the literature suggests that nearly all caregivers of BD patients report at least moderate burden (Chakrabarti and Gill 2002; Cook et al. 1994; Perlick et al. 1999, 2007b).

At baseline, 93 % of caregivers reported moderate or greater distress in at least one burden domain. As a group, caregiver illness beliefs (illness awareness, perception of patient and family control) explained an additional 18–28 % of variance in burden experienced beyond the effects of the patient's clinical state and history (Perlick et al. 1999).

Eighty-nine percent, 52 %, and 61 % of caregivers, respectively, experienced moderate or higher burden in relation to patient problem behaviours, role dysfunction or disruption of household routine. High-burden caregivers reported more physical health problems, depressive symptoms, health-risk behaviour and health service use and less social support than less-burden caregivers. They also provided more financial support to their bipolar relative (Perlick et al. 2007b).

12.3.2 Objective Burden

The role of the caregiver of a person with BD is demanding both in psychological as well as in physical terms, it is distressing and burdensome and can affect health and QoL (Struening et al. 2001; Chakrabarti et al. 1992; Perlick et al. 1999; Dore and Romans 2001). In turn, the consequences of caregiver's burden can affect the overall outcome of BD itself in a variety of ways, including treatment adherence and overall lifestyle (Perlick et al. 2001, 2004), putting the patient and his family in a vicious cycle.

It seems that higher caregiver burden is related to patient-related factors like the chronicity of the disease and high levels of impairment (Chakrabarti et al. 1992), but also it seems to be correlated also with the caregiver beliefs and knowledge about the illness (Perlick et al. 1999) as well as the caregiver's personality and subsequent adoption of specific coping styles (Chakrabarti and Gill 2002). Disruptions include changes to household, social and leisure activities, employment and finances (Fadden et al. 1987; Dore and Romans 2001). Disruptions to household management are not a source of major burden in comparison to the disruption of interpersonal relationships especially during periods of acute episodes (Brodie and Leff 1971). Most caregivers, especially partner caregivers experience significant disruption in social activities and leisure pursuits. Not only coexistence and living together becomes difficult and hard but also divorces or separations are common as a result of the burden, and in turn, this has an adverse effect on the course of the illness leading to a worse psychosocial outcome (Goodwin et al. 1990; Dore and Romans 2001).

The literature suggests that caregiver burden is related to most recent events related with the patient, and in this frame, it also implicates feelings of inadequacy and guilt concerning the failure to assist the patient to avoid these events (Perlick et al. 1999; Vieta 2005).

The most frequently distressing behaviours for caregivers are reported to be hyperactivity, irritability and withdrawal but also aggressive or violent behaviour and impulsive spending. Depression and suicidality also cause significant burden (Perlick et al. 1999; Targum et al. 1981; Dore and Romans 2001). It is important to note that several behaviours are mistakenly considered by both the family and the mental health professionals to be the product of 'character' or 'personality' rather than the disease (Lam et al. 2005). These groups of 'personality-like behaviours' are extremely burdensome for the caregivers and very difficult to cope with both in objective terms but also psychologically and should be the target of specific intervention in the family (Dore and Romans 2001).

Although caregivers were rarely obliged to change the nature of their work, three quarters of those working outside home had to reduce their hours of work or take time off work during acute episodes. More than one-fourth experienced a reduction in income (Dore and Romans 2001), and 89, 52 and 61 % of them, respectively, experienced moderate or higher burden in relation to patient problem behaviours, role dysfunction or disruption of household routine (Perlick et al. 2007b). They are also often unable to accept full-time jobs or the particular job they would prefer with profound consequences on their career. The direct financial contributions for family members are also significant and add to the economic burden of the family (Simon 2002).

Special cases are parents with BD. These patients find it difficult to fulfil their role and obligations as parents, especially concerning teaching their children to be moderate and to have limits and self-control. Parenting was complicated by the intense feelings and loosening of limits the patients often experience and frequently in relationship with the raising of children. The issue does not involve only the objective incapacity but also the subjective feelings of guilt and inadequacy as well as the perceived stigma and its consequence for the children (Wilson and Crowe 2009; Link et al. 1997, 2001; Corrigan and Wassel 2008).

12.3.3 Subjective Burden

The composition of the caregiver population is important because it determines the quality and type of burden and detects the measures and interventions needed. It has been shown that the majority are family members (37 % parents, 32 % a partner and 24 % another relative) (Dore and Romans 2001). One of the first changes that take place in the relationship between caregiver and patient is the transformation of its nature with the existing spousal, family or friendship relationships initially superimposing on the caregiver–patient relationship only to be absorbed later as time passes and disease progresses. The nature and quality of this relationship will be determined by social circumstances and culturally situated health beliefs which eventually will also determine to a significant extent the experience of burden (Ogilvie et al. 2005).

Especially concerning recent events related with the disease, the caregivers suffer from feelings of guilt and inadequacy because they feel that they failed in their efforts to support and protect the patient and to keep him under proper treatment.

They are also scared of a possible relapse when the disorder is stabilized (Reinares et al. 2006; Perlick et al. 1999; Vieta 2005).

Often the psychological state of the patient 'contaminates' the caregiver, and it has been reported that caregivers suffer more when the patient is depressive rather than manic, although this could be the results of a number of accompanying features (e.g. depression is more chronic than mania) (Reinares et al. 2006; Ostacher et al. 2008). This in turn affects the patient's recovery by adding stress to the living environment. It has been reported that the caregivers of BD patients have high levels of expressed emotion, including critical, hostile or over-involved attitudes (Honig et al. 1997; O'Connell et al. 1991; Priebe et al. 1989; Huxley and Baldessarini 2007; Ogilvie et al. 2005). These feelings of despair, sadness, helplessness and hopelessness, as well as guilt for contributing to the illness or anger and rejection of the patient all might contribute to the deterioration of the QoL of the caregiver and even the deterioration of his mental and physical health (Tantum 1989). The vicious cycle includes also the psychological condition of caregivers themselves since nearly 70 % of them were distressed mainly by the way the illness had affected their own mental health and everyday life (Reinares et al. 2006). Levels of depression vary with whether the caregiver is a spouse or a parent (Chessick et al. 2007).

There is a different way parents and partners cope with specific issues. For example, parents are stressed more with a patient with a history of suicidal behaviour since they seem to blame themselves and feel responsible for their child's mental health history, while partners feel responsible for the late onset of suicidality probably because they feel they had pushed the patient towards suicide (Goldstein et al. 2002).

Eventually the mental health of caregivers might deteriorate, and if the stress is high, they could develop depression and increase use of mental health services (Perlick et al. 2005, 2007a, b, 2008; Steele et al. 2009; Gallagher and Mechanic 1996; Eisdorfer 1991). The literature includes several efforts to assess the levels of stress (Lam et al. 2005; Goossens et al. 2008; Hill et al. 1998; Tranvag and Kristoffersen 2008), anxiety (Goldstein et al. 2002; Perlick et al. 2005) and depression (Tranvag and Kristoffersen 2008; Perlick et al. 2007b, 2008; Bernhard et al. 2006), while one paper measured caregiver psychotic symptoms (Goldstein et al. 2002).

It is clear that a strong relationship between depressive symptoms and caregiver burden is present (Perlick et al. 2004), but the direction of causality and the association between illness severity and burden cannot be easily assessed. Often it seems that the caregiver burden predicts patient relapse (Perlick et al. 2001).

Caregivers often face problems because of aggressive and violent behaviours (17 %), odd behaviours (10 %), overactivity, overtalkativeness, impulsive spends (each 4 %) and suicidal ideation and attempts. Often the police is involved either because the patient has broken the law or because the caregivers have asked its intervention. It has been reported that the police had intervened at least once in two-thirds of the patients during an acute episode. Involuntary admissions to hospitals are not uncommon and constitute a significant point of bitter conflict with the patients. The vast majority of caregivers (81 %) reported that they are distressed by the changes in the relationship with the patient during acute episodes with two-thirds of caregivers reporting that the distress was severe. With remission of the acute phase, it seems that the relationship improves and 80 % of caregivers report satisfactory close relationships during euthymic phases. It is interesting that half of them believe that the disease brought them closer with the patient. Relationships seem to be overall better when the caregiver is female and the patient male (Dore and Romans 2001). However, even after remission, a degree of psychosocial impairment persists, and this constitutes a burdensome experience for caregivers and families that, in turn, can adversely affect the long-term course and outcome for the patient (Perlick et al. 2001; McPherson et al. 1992). Delayed return to work and usual activities after the resolution of the acute phase adds to burden (Sachs et al. 2007).

Marriage is a special case and determines a distinct form of caregiving. The literature is rather restricted and some authors suggest that marriage is largely not compatible with caregiving since it is destabilized by the illness (Greene et al. 1976), especially because of manic symptoms (Janowsky et al. 1970) with separation or divorce being frequent (DiNicola 1989; McPherson et al. 1992; Kessler et al. 1998). An additional source of burden and of tension between partners is the possibility that the illness is inheritable. It seems that only about half of partners were aware BD could be inherited prior to the birth of their children (Dore and Romans 2001). The literature is conflicting on this matter; however, it seems that the majority of partners when learning about this possibility did not reconsider marriage or decide not to have children (Trippitelli et al. 1998; Dore and Romans 2001). It is important to note that patients do not seem to realize the above issues and their implications (Targum et al. 1981).

Some authors report on the potential positive aspects of caregiving and of the perceived benefits. Often caregivers report feelings of gratification, love and pride, self-confidence, inner strength and maturity and they also describe important life lessons learned (Veltman et al. 2002; Bauer et al. 2012).

12.3.4 Influence of Sociodemographic Factors on Caregiver Burden

Although no clear differences have been consistently found concerning race, religion or ethnic group, there are some data suggesting that sociodemographic and cultural factors have an effect on burden, which is however not adequately studied. An early study suggested that gender of the patient, religion, education, occupation, family type and size and the locus of control of both patients and relatives did not influence the extent of burden significantly (Chakrabarti et al. 1992); however, subsequent research suggested that the levels of depression in caregivers varied with whether the caregiver was a spouse or a parent, with parents more heavily afflicted (Chessick et al. 2007). Also female caregivers were reported to suffer more from problems regarding quality of relationship with the patient, while male caregivers experienced more constraints on their own autonomy, uncertainty concerning their judgement of patients' capacity and uncertainty because of the changing symptoms of illness (Bauer et al. 2010).

It has been reported that black caregivers tended to report less burden than whites which were similar to Hispanics, and this could not be explained by any usually considered protective mechanism (e.g. social support, religious involvement, illness attributions) (Stueve et al. 1997).

12.3.5 Special Topics Related to Caregiver Burden

12.3.5.1 Suicidality

Suicidality constitutes a cardinal source of stress and burden worldwide (Pompili et al. 2009), since it combines a number of unusual features, including permanent loss of a love one; theoretically it is preventable and the caregiver feels responsible for that (Chessick et al. 2009), and ultimately it is beyond comprehension for the average healthy person. Taking the responsibility for the life of the patient seems to be a burden so heavy that the caregiver cannot bear for prolonged periods of time without a significant impact (Perlick et al. 2008).

BD is characterized among others by increased suicidality, both in terms of completed suicide but also for frequent and persistent suicidal ideation (Goodwin et al. 1990; Angst et al. 2005; Guze and Robins 1970), and this is of course a significant source of distress for caregivers of BD patients (Perlick et al. 1999; Targum et al. 1981; Dore and Romans 2001; Fadden et al. 1987). Additionally, suicidality is correlated with a distinct surrounding psychopathology, and this could be the source of additional burden (Ostacher et al. 2008; Kennedy et al. 2007; Altshuler et al. 2002).

When the patient has either current ideation or lifetime history of suicidal attempts, the caregiver is reported to suffer from a deterioration of his general health. The magnitude of burden it causes depends on the relationship with the patient, with parents of patients experiencing more burden than spouses (Chessick et al. 2007; Allen et al. 2005).

12.3.5.2 Violence Towards the Caregiver

BD is a mental disorder which is related more than other disorders with bursts of violence especially during acute manic or mixed episodes (Raveendranathan et al. 2012). Especially when combined with overall verbal and physical aggression and behavioural disinhibition, it constitutes a major source of distress for caregivers and the family as a whole (Currier and Allen 2000; Amore et al. 2008).

The literature on the impact of violence and aggression on caregivers of BD patients is limited, but it is reasonable to assume that the ability of family members to predict the bursts of violence could help in preventing them or at least decrease their impact (Raveendranathan et al. 2012; Dore and Romans 2001). It is positive that most caregivers and family members consider acts of violence to be part of the disease and its symptoms rather than under the direct control and responsibility of the patient (Dore and Romans 2001).

Violence and aggression towards the caregiver is frequent with almost half of them having such an experience. At least one in four had experienced a serious act. Far higher is the percentage of caregivers and family members who were afraid that they will be victims of violent acts during an acute episode. It is important to note that violence seems to be more common towards partners than other caregivers and family members and does not seem to be determined by the gender of the patient (Dore and Romans 2001). It is interesting that violence does not seem to have an effect on the caregiver's mental health appeared (Dore and Romans 2001). From a reverse point of view, it seems that violence is more frequently targeting the close environment and not strangers. It is reported that family members were the victims of violence in 70 % of these violent episodes while 81 % were somehow provoked (Raveendranathan et al. 2012).

However, predicting violence is rather difficult. Interestingly, family members identified three quarters of the patients as irritable only prior to the episode but not in general (Raveendranathan et al. 2012). Only previous history of violence plus male sex, substance abuse and positive symptoms seem to be strong predictive factors (Amore et al. 2008).

12.3.6 Comparison with Burden Caused by Other Disorders

Research results suggest that BD causes more objective burden on caregivers than unipolar depression (Heru and Ryan 2004; Ogilvie et al. 2005; Chakrabarti et al. 1992) and similar degree of burden in comparison to caregivers of patients with schizophrenia although the latter tend to experience caregiving in a more negative way (Nehra et al. 2005; Grover et al. 2012; Chadda et al. 2007). It is unclear whether they tend to use similar types of coping strategies as one study suggests (Chadda et al. 2007) since another one reported that problem-focused coping strategies were more common in caregivers of BD patients and emotion-focused strategies in caregivers of patients with schizophrenia (Chakrabarti and Gill 2002).

However, in contrast to the latter, one study reported those caregivers of BD patients who have higher scores on neuroticism which is a temperament trait associated with depression and anxiety used a more coercive coping style (expressing anger, using physical force, etc.) in comparison to caregivers of patients with schizophrenia (Nehra et al. 2005, 2006).

Probably the cluster of symptoms and the constellation of behaviours are more important concerning the development of disability and caregiver burden than diagnosis per se. Manic symptoms are considered very much burdensome by caregivers followed by positive and negative symptoms. In caregivers of BD patients, manic symptomatology was considered to be more problematic in comparison to what caregivers of patients with schizophrenia reported. Mental health professionals seem to miss the burden caused by positive and negative symptoms in BD patients (Mueser et al. 1996).

Finally, one study found that caregivers of patients with BD had more financial cost burden than other caregivers (Dore and Romans 2001).

12.3.7 Interventions

Since it has been confirmed that caregivers of BD patients often seek mental health care, proper training of mental health professionals and development of specific services seem important to deal with this need (Ogilvie et al. 2005; Perlick et al. 2005; Lam et al.

2005; Hill et al. 1998). Some authors investigated support services available for parents of youth with BD, and the conclusion was rather disappointing (Nadkarni and Fristad 2012). Taking into consideration the specific needs of different groups and their attitude is important in order to develop suitable interventions. For example, it has been shown that male caregivers drop out at higher rates in comparison to female caregivers. This might mean that specific engagement strategies are required to engage younger male caregivers which are at risk to experience high level of burden (Perlick et al. 2001).

A basic target of intervention to reduce caregiver and family burden would be to help in identifying the rewards of caregiving. This could lead to the improvement of caregiving abilities and improve coping with distressful and challenging situations, and consequently reducing the global caregiver burden (Veltman et al. 2002). Also it is important to identify and modify all these burdensome aspects of living with and care for the patient (Reinares et al. 2006). Generally, the interventions to reduce caregiver burden could be grouped under simple interventions at the clinician's level (e.g. assessment of burden, psychoeducational and elementary support interventions) and the more complex interventions such as family interventions (Pompili et al. 2014). There are also short-term interventions that can be provided at the time of acute hospitalization for families of BD patients and are reported to reduce caregiver burden (Heru and Ryan 2004).

There are specific modules developed to tackle specific issues. For example, family-focused therapy (FFT) has also been adapted to treat suicidal symptoms in the patients with BD, and in this frame, family members, caregivers and patients are educated to have open discussions concerning all issues including suicidality and related prodromal symptoms (Chessick et al. 2009; Miklowitz and Taylor 2006; Miklowitz et al. 2003). Such interventions could relieve caregiver distress, and also it might reduce the risk of future suicide attempts (Practice guideline for the assessment and treatment of patients with suicidal behaviors 2003).

Promoting the autonomy of the patient and reducing the caregiver's responsibility level for the patient's treatment should be crucial goals of psychosocial treatment (Reinares et al. 2006). Burden was reported to be higher when the relatives had poor psychological support and help in emergencies by the social network (Magliano et al. 2009). The various interventions on caregivers were shown to improve caregiver quality of life and interpersonal relationships within the family (Fristad et al. 2003; Fristad 2006; Corring 2002; Cuijpers 1999; Dixon et al. 2001; Johnson 2000) and certainly reduce the subjective burden but not the objective burden (Perlick et al. 2010; Reinares et al. 2004).

Finally, it is reasonable to assume that improving the training of mental health professionals working with caregivers and families can make patient outcomes better and reduce caregiver distress (Ogilvie et al. 2005). However, the need for better and in-depth understanding of the nature of caregiver burden is needed.

12.3.8 Caregiver Burden and Patient Outcome

It is not only logical to assume that when caregivers of BD patients less experience a high burden, the overall patient outcome is adversely affected, but also there are research data to support this (Perlick et al. 2001). The relationship is strong and is probably mediated through the caregiver and family burden effect on the patient's treatment adherence (Perlick et al. 2004).

Not only the longitudinal course can be predicted by caregiver burden but also in an impressive way, the caregiver burden reported during periods of acute relapse seems to predict the short-term outcome (Perlick et al. 2001).

A delicate issue is that caregiving, direct and indirect financial cost, burden and patient outcome are all intercorrelated, and in this frame, it is important to understand which costs are more than others associated with the worsening of burden in order to become the focus of intervention of any type, both psychological and politico-economical (Wolff et al. 2006).

12.4 Cost

More than half of the veterans (56 %) reported significant out-of-pocket costs. This was more likely among patients who were married, younger, homeless, with private insurance, without service-connected disabilities and who reported access difficulties (McCarthy et al. 2010).

Patients with BD seem to be the most costly in terms of overall medical and psychological care in comparison to other mental patients and one of the most costly categories of patients in the whole field of medicine. It is very difficult to obtain meaningful costs in terms of absolute numbers because of the changing price of medication and services as well as the changes in health policy. Also the episodic nature of the disease has a profound effect on the methodology to calculate the cost. It is quite different to calculate the cost on the basis of the period immediately after a hospitalization and different to calculate on the basis of prolonged random periods of time. For example, one study reported that the mean direct costs incurred over the 3-month period following hospitalization was 22,297 euros, with 98.6 % of those costs due to hospitalization (Olie and Levy 2002). This is clearly misleading as a general picture.

Often the estimations are theoretical and are based on a lot of assumptions and of questionable value, like a recent estimation with a comparison of in- and outpatient treatment strategies based on lithium or valproate plus psychosocial intervention (Chisholm et al. 2005). However, a comparison with other medical and mental conditions is absolutely valuable and important.

In order to be able to estimate the costs in a realistic way and also be able to device interventions to reduce them, a prerequisite is to know enough of the natural course of the illness and the need for intervention at each point. It is also important to have in mind that different countries not only have different health systems, but they also differ in their mentality of how treatment should be done.

Thus, it is important to have in mind that in France the proportion of manic episodes requiring hospitalization is probably around 63 %, with an average length of stay of 32.4 days. Following this reasoning, the hospitalization-related costs alone were estimated to be around three billion euros for the year 1999 (de Zelicourt et al. 2003). For the same period (1999–2000), in the UK, the annual National Health Service (NHS) cost concerning the managing of BD was estimated to be 199 million pounds sterling. Hospital admissions accounted for 35 %. Additionally, the annual direct non-health-care cost was estimated to be 86 million pounds sterling annually, and the indirect societal cost was estimated to be 1,770 million pounds sterling annually. The sum of the about costs suggests that for the years 1999–2000, the total annual cost to UK society attributable to BD was estimated to be two billion pounds sterling with only 10 % of this cost being attributable to NHS resource use, 4 % to non-health-care resource use and 86 % to indirect costs (Das Gupta and Guest 2002). However, another UK study estimated for the same time period that the UK national cost of BD was 4.59 billion pounds sterling, with hospitalization during acute episodes representing the largest component (Fajutrao et al. 2009).

One attempt to calculate the direct and absolute cost of medical service and prescription claims in the USA for the years 2004–2005, for 28,531 BD patients, also compared the data for 1 year with data for 85,593 age- and sex-matched control patients with no mental health disorders and no psychotropic medication use. Patients with BD had a significantly higher prevalence of metabolic comorbidities than the general population (37 % vs. 30 %; $p<0.0001$), and annual medical service treatment costs for metabolic conditions were twice that of the control cohort (531 USD vs. 233 USD; $p<0.0001$). Prescription medication costs for metabolic conditions were higher as well, with bipolar cohort per-patient costs of 571 USD vs. 301 USD for the control cohort ($p<0.0001$). Also BD patients had significantly (four times up) higher overall medical service and prescription drug costs than those of the control cohort (12,764 USD vs. 3,140 USD; $p<0.0001$) (Centorrino et al. 2009).

Thus, according to the above reports, the cost of hospitalization alone in France was comparable to the total societal cost in the UK, while the service and medication usage alone in the USA 5 years later was double or more than the two above-mentioned costs. Ten years later (2009), the estimated direct and indirect costs of BD-I and BD-II disorders were 30.7 and 120.3 billion USD, respectively, raising the estimated total economic burden imposed by BD to 151.0 billion USD, that is, approximately ten times higher in comparison to the total societal cost in the UK 10 years before. One important observation of this study was that while the indirect cost increased in proportion with the increase in the prevalence of BD, the direct costs escalated out of proportion (Dilsaver 2010). The costs reported from Australia (2005) are more in accord with those reported from the USA (Fisher et al. 2007), while the costs reported from USA for the years around 1990 were three to four times lower (Kleinman et al. 2003). The annual NHS cost of BD for the years 2009–2010 was estimated to be 342 million pound sterlings, with hospitalizations accounting for 60 %, outpatient and community mental health 26.7 % and medication in primary care 7.4 % of the overall direct costs of care (Young et al. 2011). This latter study is in accord with one of the two earlier ones (Das Gupta and Guest 2002) but also suggests that the direct NHS costs almost doubled within a decade at least in absolute numbers.

The data are reasonably conclusive and suggest that BD is the most expensive mental health-care diagnosis, both for patients with BD and for their insurance plans. It is reported that all comparisons between employees with BD and those employees without, with other mental disorders, and employees with no mental disorders revealed that the cost related with BD was significantly higher. The only exception was sick leave cost which was similar with patients with any mental disorder. It is interesting that BD is the most costly disorder in nearly every health benefits category, with a small minority of patients (2.4 %) accounting for 20 % of the total costs, and this difference was due to medical comorbidity costs (Brook et al. 2006). Additionally, employees with BD were reported to miss an average of 18.9 workdays annually, while employees without BD missed 7.4 days annually ($p<0.05$) (Gardner et al. 2006). Also BD patients had more job insecurity because of absenteeism (McIntyre et al. 2008). The costs because of absence from work seem to correlate significantly with treatment adherence (Bagalman et al. 2010). A study on insured persons reported that while only 3.0 % were identified as having BD, they accounted for 12.4 % of total plan expenditures. Also it reported that BD patients incurred annual out-of-pocket expenses of 568 USD, more than double in comparison to the 232 USD of out-of-pocket expenses incurred by all claimants. The inpatient hospital admission rate for BD patients was also higher (39.1 %) in comparison to 4.5 % for all other mental health-care claimants and so were the payments for covered medical services (Peele et al. 2003).

The distribution of the costs is of prime importance. The big difference in the costs is caused not because of the treatment of the primary mental diagnosis but because of comorbid somatic conditions. BD patients are not only reported to receive an average of 15 CNS drug prescriptions per person, at an average cost of 582 USD in comparison to 1 CNS drug prescription with an average cost of 33 USD per person. In BD patients, medical encounters accounted for 45.8 % of costs, while the respected rate in non-bipolar patients was 4.2 % of costs (Stender et al. 2002).

Conclusively, the literature is robust in suggesting that BD is the most expensive mental disorder both for insurances as well as for patients and their families. Not only the psychiatric treatment is complex and expensive but also the treatment of somatic comorbidities is extremely costly. Differences in the health-care systems and the availability of services determine the costs and their distribution in a different way from country to country.

12.5 Stigma

Stigma is a problem which is present in many situations in human society, and especially it is widespread in medicine. However, in psychiatry it is where stigma causes disproportionally many problems and affects the lives of millions of people. In mental health, it is not the exception, but on the contrary, it is rather frequent that stigma rather than the illness itself is responsible for most of impairment and disability directly or indirectly.

It is important to have in mind that the stigma of mental illness was reported to be prevalent among caregivers of BD patients no matter whether the symptomatology was active or in remission (Gonzalez et al. 2007a). One study reported that the prevalent opinions concerning the illness and its aetiology among relatives were split into two opposite views: One was ‘it is Satan’s work’ (35.8 %) and the other ‘it is a natural illness’ (23.2 %). Other similarly conflicting opinions were ‘genetic’

(9.5 %), 'witchcraft' (10.5 %) and 'curse by enemies' (10.5 %). Interestingly these opinions were similar to the opinion of cancer and infertility caregivers, but it seems that in general psychiatric caregivers had higher frequency of anger and stigma (Ohaeri and Fido 2001). Concerning the nature of stigma, four themes were identified: stigma expectations and experiences, sense of self/identity, judicious disclosure, and moving beyond internalized stigma (Michalak et al. 2011).

It seems that perceived stigma is positively associated with depressive symptoms in the caregiver and reduced social support and avoidance account for most of that relationship (Perlick et al. 2007a). In patients the self-perceived stigma correlates with lower functioning, being on disability benefit and current mood symptoms (Vazquez et al. 2010). Stigma seems to accumulate in minorities with BD patients who are members of ethnic/racial minority groups who continue to receive less intensive specialized mental health treatment than do European American patients in the USA; however, interestingly, this did not seem to affect the overall outcome and disability which were similar (Gonzalez et al. 2007b).

References

Allen MH, Chessick CA, Miklowitz DJ, Goldberg JF, Wisniewski SR, Miyahara S, Calabrese JR, Marangell L, Bauer MS, Thomas MR, Bowden CL, Sachs GS (2005) Contributors to suicidal ideation among bipolar patients with and without a history of suicide attempts. Suicide Life Threat Behav 35(6):671–680

Altshuler LL, Gitlin MJ, Mintz J, Leight KL, Frye MA (2002) Subsyndromal depression is associated with functional impairment in patients with bipolar disorder. J Clin Psychiatry 63(9):807–811

Altshuler LL, Bearden CE, Green MF, van Gorp W, Mintz J (2008) A relationship between neurocognitive impairment and functional impairment in bipolar disorder: a pilot study. Psychiatry Res 157(1–3):289–293. doi:10.1016/j.psychres.2007.01.001, S0165-1781(07)00003-0 [pii]

Amore M, Menchetti M, Tonti C, Scarlatti F, Lundgren E, Esposito W, Berardi D (2008) Predictors of violent behavior among acute psychiatric patients: clinical study. Psychiatry Clin Neurosci 62(3):247–255. doi:10.1111/j.1440-1819.2008.01790.x

Angst J, Angst F, Gerber-Werder R, Gamma A (2005) Suicide in 406 mood-disorder patients with and without long-term medication: a 40 to 44 years' follow-up. Arch Suicide Res 9(3):279–300

Atre-Vaidya N, Taylor MA, Seidenberg M, Reed R, Perrine A, Glick-Oberwise F (1998) Cognitive deficits, psychopathology, and psychosocial functioning in bipolar mood disorder. Neuropsychiatry Neuropsychol Behav Neurol 11(3):120–126

Bagalman E, Yu-Isenberg KS, Durden E, Crivera C, Dirani R, Bunn WB 3rd (2010) Indirect costs associated with nonadherence to treatment for bipolar disorder. J Occup Environ Med 52(5):478–485. doi:10.1097/JOM.0b013e3181db811d

Bauer M, Glenn T, Grof P, Rasgon NL, Marsh W, Sagduyu K, Alda M, Lewitzka U, Sasse J, Kozuch-Krolik E, Whybrow PC (2009) Frequency of subsyndromal symptoms and employment status in patients with bipolar disorder. Soc Psychiatry Psychiatr Epidemiol 44(7):515–522. doi:10.1007/s00127-008-0464-4

Bauer R, Gottfriedsen GU, Binder H, Dobmeier M, Cording C, Hajak G, Spiessl H (2010) Burden of caregivers of patients with bipolar affective disorders. Am J Orthopsychiatry 81(1):139–148. doi:10.1111/j.1939-0025.2010.01081.x

Bauer R, Koepke F, Sterzinger L, Spiessl H (2012) Burden, rewards, and coping–the ups and downs of caregivers of people with mental illness. J Nerv Ment Dis 200(11):928–934. doi:10.1097/NMD.0b013e31827189b1

Bellack AS, Morrison RL, Mueser KT, Wade J (1989) Social competence in schizoaffective disorder, bipolar disorder, and negative and non-negative schizophrenia. Schizophr Res 2(4–5): 391–401, 0920-9964(89)90032-7 [pii]

Bernhard B, Schaub A, Kummler P, Dittmann S, Severus E, Seemuller F, Born C, Forsthoff A, Licht RW, Grunze H (2006) Impact of cognitive-psychoeducational interventions in bipolar patients and their relatives. Eur Psychiatry 21(2):81–86. doi:10.1016/j.eurpsy.2005.09.007

Bowden CL, Krishnan AA (2004) Pharmacotherapy for bipolar depression: an economic assessment. Expert Opin Pharmacother 5(5):1101–1107. doi:10.1517/14656566.5.5.1101

Bowie CR, Depp C, McGrath JA, Wolyniec P, Mausbach BT, Thornquist MH, Luke J, Patterson TL, Harvey PD, Pulver AE (2010) Prediction of real-world functional disability in chronic mental disorders: a comparison of schizophrenia and bipolar disorder. Am J Psychiatry 167(9):1116–1124. doi:10.1176/appi.ajp.2010.09101406, appi.ajp.2010.09101406 [pii]

Brodaty H, Green A (2002) Who cares for the carer? The often forgotten patient. Aust Fam Physician 31(9):833–836

Brodie HK, Leff MJ (1971) Bipolar depression–a comparative study of patient characteristics. Am J Psychiatry 127(8):1086–1090

Brook RA, Rajagopalan K, Kleinman NL, Smeeding JE, Brizee TJ, Gardner HH (2006) Incurring greater health care costs: risk stratification of employees with bipolar disorder. Prim Care Companion J Clin Psychiatry 8(1):17–24

Burdick KE, Goldberg JF, Harrow M (2010) Neurocognitive dysfunction and psychosocial outcome in patients with bipolar I disorder at 15-year follow-up. Acta Psychiatr Scand 122(6):499–506. doi:10.1111/j.1600-0447.2010.01590.x, ACP1590 [pii]

Cannon M, Jones P, Gilvarry C, Rifkin L, McKenzie K, Foerster A, Murray RM (1997) Premorbid social functioning in schizophrenia and bipolar disorder: similarities and differences. Am J Psychiatry 154(11):1544–1550

Centorrino F, Mark TL, Talamo A, Oh K, Chang J (2009) Health and economic burden of metabolic comorbidity among individuals with bipolar disorder. J Clin Psychopharmacol 29(6):595–600. doi:10.1097/JCP.0b013e3181bef8a6, 00004714-200912000-00014 [pii]

Chadda RK, Singh TB, Ganguly KK (2007) Caregiver burden and coping: a prospective study of relationship between burden and coping in caregivers of patients with schizophrenia and bipolar affective disorder. Soc Psychiatry Psychiatr Epidemiol 42(11):923–930. doi:10.1007/s00127-007-0242-8

Chakrabarti S, Gill S (2002) Coping and its correlates among caregivers of patients with bipolar disorder: a preliminary study. Bipolar Disord 4(1):50–60

Chakrabarti S, Kulhara P, Verma SK (1992) Extent and determinants of burden among families of patients with affective disorders. Acta Psychiatr Scand 86(3):247–252

Chand PK, Mattoo SK, Sharan P (2004) Quality of life and its correlates in patients with bipolar disorder stabilized on lithium prophylaxis. Psychiatry Clin Neurosci 58(3):311–318. doi:10.1111/j.1440-1819.2004.01237.x PCN1237

Chessick CA, Perlick DA, Miklowitz DJ, Kaczynski R, Allen MH, Morris CD, Marangell LB (2007) Current suicide ideation and prior suicide attempts of bipolar patients as influences on caregiver burden. Suicide Life Threat Behav 37(4):482–491. doi:10.1521/suli.2007.37.4.482

Chessick CA, Perlick DA, Miklowitz DJ, Dickinson LM, Allen MH, Morris CD, Gonzalez JM, Marangell LB, Cosgrove V, Ostacher M (2009) Suicidal ideation and depressive symptoms among bipolar patients as predictors of the health and well-being of caregivers. Bipolar Disord 11(8):876–884. doi:10.1111/j.1399-5618.2009.00765.x

Chisholm D, van Ommeren M, Ayuso-Mateos JL, Saxena S (2005) Cost-effectiveness of clinical interventions for reducing the global burden of bipolar disorder. Br J Psychiatry 187:559–567. doi:10.1192/bjp.187.6.559, 187/6/559 [pii]

Cook JA, Lefley HP, Pickett SA, Cohler BJ (1994) Age and family burden among parents of offspring with severe mental illness. Am J Orthopsychiatry 64(3):435–447

Corrigan PW, Wassel A (2008) Understanding and influencing the stigma of mental illness. J Psychosoc Nurs Ment Health Serv 46(1):42–48

Corring DJ (2002) Quality of life: perspectives of people with mental illnesses and family members. Psychiatr Rehabil J 25(4):350–358

Coryell W, Turvey C, Endicott J, Leon AC, Mueller T, Solomon D, Keller M (1998) Bipolar I affective disorder: predictors of outcome after 15 years. J Affect Disord 50(2–3):109–116
Cuijpers P (1999) The effects of family intervention on relatives' burden: a meta-analysis. J Ment Health 8:275–285
Currier GW, Allen MH (2000) Emergency psychiatry: physical and chemical restraint in the psychiatric emergency service. Psychiatr Serv 51(6):717–719
Das Gupta R, Guest JF (2002) Annual cost of bipolar disorder to UK society. Br J Psychiatry 180:227–233
de Zelicourt M, Dardennes R, Verdoux H, Gandhi G, Khoshnood B, Chomette E, Papatheodorou ML, Edgell ET, Even C, Fagnani F (2003) Frequency of hospitalisations and inpatient care costs of manic episodes: in patients with bipolar I disorder in France. Pharmacoeconomics 21(15):1081–1090, 21152 [pii]
Dean BB, Gerner D, Gerner RH (2004) A systematic review evaluating health-related quality of life, work impairment, and healthcare costs and utilization in bipolar disorder. Curr Med Res Opin 20(2):139–154. doi:10.1185/030079903125002801
Depp CA, Davis CE, Mittal D, Patterson TL, Jeste DV (2006) Health-related quality of life and functioning of middle-aged and elderly adults with bipolar disorder. J Clin Psychiatry 67(2):215–221
Depp CA, Mausbach BT, Eyler LT, Palmer BW, Cain AE, Lebowitz BD, Patterson TL, Jeste DV (2009) Performance-based and subjective measures of functioning in middle-aged and older adults with bipolar disorder. J Nerv Ment Dis 197(7):471–475. doi:10.1097/NMD.0b013e3181ab5c9b, 00005053-200907000-00001 [pii]
Dickerson FB, Sommerville J, Origoni AE, Ringel NB, Parente F (2001) Outpatients with schizophrenia and bipolar I disorder: do they differ in their cognitive and social functioning? Psychiatry Res 102(1):21–27
Dilsaver SC (2010) An estimate of the minimum economic burden of bipolar I and II disorders in the United States: 2009. J Affect Disord 129(1–3):79–83. doi:10.1016/j.jad.2010.08.030, S0165-0327(10)00566-5 [pii]
DiNicola VF (1989) The child's predicament in families with a mood disorder. Research findings and family interventions. Psychiatr Clin North Am 12(4):933–949
Dion GL, Tohen M, Anthony WA, Waternaux CS (1988) Symptoms and functioning of patients with bipolar disorder six months after hospitalization. Hosp Community Psychiatry 39(6): 652–657
Dixon L, Stewart B, Burland J, Delahanty J, Lucksted A, Hoffman M (2001) Pilot study of the effectiveness of the family-to-family education program. Psychiatr Serv 52(7):965–967
Dore G, Romans SE (2001) Impact of bipolar affective disorder on family and partners. J Affect Disord 67(1–3):147–158, S0165032701004505 [pii]
Eisdorfer C (1991) Caregiving: an emerging risk factor for emotional and physical pathology. Bull Menn Clin 55(2):238–247
Elinson L, Houck P, Pincus HA (2007) Working, receiving disability benefits, and access to mental health care in individuals with bipolar disorder. Bipolar Disord 9(1–2):158–165. doi:10.1111/j.1399-5618.2007.00431.x, BDI431 [pii]
Fadden G, Bebbington P, Kuipers L (1987) The burden of care: the impact of functional psychiatric illness on the patient's family. Br J Psychiatry 150:285–292
Fajutrao L, Locklear J, Priaulx J, Heyes A (2009) A systematic review of the evidence of the burden of bipolar disorder in Europe. Clin Pract Epidemiol Ment Health 5:3. doi:10.1186/1745-0179-5-3, 1745-0179-5-3 [pii]
Ferrier IN, Stanton BR, Kelly TP, Scott J (1999) Neuropsychological function in euthymic patients with bipolar disorder. Br J Psychiatry 175:246–251
Fisher LJ, Goldney RD, Dal Grande E, Taylor AW, Hawthorne G (2007) Bipolar disorders in Australia. A population-based study of excess costs. Soc Psychiatry Psychiatr Epidemiol 42(2):105–109. doi:10.1007/s00127-006-0133-4
Fristad MA (2006) Psychoeducational treatment for school-aged children with bipolar disorder. Dev Psychopathol 18(4):1289–1306. doi:10.1017/S0954579406060627
Fristad MA, Goldberg-Arnold JS, Gavazzi SM (2003) Multi-family psychoeducation groups in the treatment of children with mood disorders. J Marital Fam Ther 29(4):491–504

Gallagher SK, Mechanic D (1996) Living with the mentally ill: effects on the health and functioning of other household members. Soc Sci Med 42(12):1691–1701, 0277953695002960 [pii]

Gardner HH, Kleinman NL, Brook RA, Rajagopalan K, Brizee TJ, Smeeding JE (2006) The economic impact of bipolar disorder in an employed population from an employer perspective. J Clin Psychiatry 67(8):1209–1218

Giglio LM, Magalhaes PV, Kapczinski NS, Walz JC, Kapczinski F (2010) Functional impact of biological rhythm disturbance in bipolar disorder. J Psychiatr Res 44(4):220–223. doi:10.1016/j.jpsychires.2009.08.003, S0022-3956(09)00176-9 [pii]

Gilbert AM, Olino TM, Houck P, Fagiolini A, Kupfer DJ, Frank E (2010) Self-reported cognitive problems predict employment trajectory in patients with bipolar I disorder. J Affect Disord 124(3):324–328. doi:10.1016/j.jad.2009.11.012, S0165-0327(09)00505-9 [pii]

Gitlin MJ, Swendsen J, Heller TL, Hammen C (1995) Relapse and impairment in bipolar disorder. Am J Psychiatry 152(11):1635–1640

Glahn DC, Bearden CE, Bowden CL, Soares JC (2006) Reduced educational attainment in bipolar disorder. J Affect Disord 92(2–3):309–312. doi:10.1016/j.jad.2006.01.025, S0165-0327(06)00046-2 [pii]

Goldberg TE, Gold JM, Greenberg R, Griffin S, Schulz SC, Pickar D, Kleinman JE, Weinberger DR (1993) Contrasts between patients with affective disorders and patients with schizophrenia on a neuropsychological test battery. Am J Psychiatry 150(9):1355–1362

Goldberg JF, Harrow M, Grossman LS (1995) Course and outcome in bipolar affective disorder: a longitudinal follow-up study. Am J Psychiatry 152(3):379–384

Goldberg JF, Harrow M, Leon AC (1996) Lithium treatment of bipolar affective disorders under naturalistic followup conditions. Psychopharmacol Bull 32(1):47–54

Goldstein TR, Miklowitz DJ, Richards JA (2002) Expressed emotion attitudes and individual psychopathology among the relatives of bipolar patients. Fam Process 41(4):645–657

Gonzalez JM, Perlick DA, Miklowitz DJ, Kaczynski R, Hernandez M, Rosenheck RA, Culver JL, Ostacher MJ, Bowden CL (2007a) Factors associated with stigma among caregivers of patients with bipolar disorder in the STEP-BD study. Psychiatr Serv 58(1):41–48. doi:10.1176/appi.ps.58.1.41-a, 58/1/41-a [pii]

Gonzalez JM, Thompson P, Escamilla M, Araga M, Singh V, Farrelly N, Thase ME, Miklowitz DJ, Bowden CL (2007b) Treatment characteristics and illness burden among European Americans, African Americans, and Latinos in the first 2,000 patients of the systematic treatment enhancement program for bipolar disorder. Psychopharmacol Bull 40(1):31–46

Goodwin FK, Jamison KR, Goodwin F (1990) Suicide. In: Goodwin FK, Jamison KR (eds) Manic-depressive illness. Oxford University Press, New York, pp 227–244

Goossens PJ, Van Wijngaarden B, Knoppert-van Der Klein EA, Van Achterberg T (2008) Family caregiving in bipolar disorder: caregiver consequences, caregiver coping styles, and caregiver distress. Int J Soc Psychiatry 54(4):303–316

Grad J, Sainbury M (1963) Evaluating a community care service. In: Freeman H, Farndale J (eds) Trends in mental health services. Pergamon Press, Oxford

Grad J, Sainsbury P (1963) Mental illness and the family. Lancet 1(7280):544–547

Greene BL, Lustig N, Lee RR (1976) Marital therapy when one spouse has a primary affective disorder. Am J Psychiatry 133(7):827–830

Grover S, Chakrabarti S, Aggarwal M, Avasthi A, Kulhara P, Sharma S, Khehra N (2012) Comparative study of the experience of caregiving in bipolar affective disorder and schizophrenia. Int J Soc Psychiatry 58(6):614–622. doi:10.1177/0020764011419054

Gutierrez-Rojas L, Jurado D, Gurpegui M (2010) Factors associated with work, social life and family life disability in bipolar disorder patients. Psychiatry Res 186(2–3):254–260. doi:10.1016/j.psychres.2010.06.020, S0165-1781(10)00362-8 [pii]

Guze SB, Robins E (1970) Suicide and primary affective disorders. Br J Psychiatry 117(539):437–438

Harrow M, Goldberg JF, Grossman LS, Meltzer HY (1990) Outcome in manic disorders. A naturalistic follow-up study. Arch Gen Psychiatry 47(7):665–671

Heru AM, Ryan CE (2004) Burden, reward and family functioning of caregivers for relatives with mood disorders: 1-year follow-up. J Affect Disord 83(2–3):221–225. doi:10.1016/j.jad.2004.04.013

Hill RG, Shepherd G, Hardy P (1998) In sickness and in health: the experiences of friends and relatives caring for people with manic depression. J Ment Health 7:611–620
Hoenig J, Hamilton MW (1966) The schizophrenic patient in the community and his effect on the household. Int J Soc Psychiatry 12(3):165–176
Hoenig J, Hamilton M (1969) The desegregation of the mentally ill. Routledge and Keegan-Paul, London
Honig A, Hofman A, Rozendaal N, Dingemans P (1997) Psycho-education in bipolar disorder: effect on expressed emotion. Psychiatry Res 72(1):17–22, S0165-1781(97)00072-3 [pii]
Huxley N, Baldessarini RJ (2007) Disability and its treatment in bipolar disorder patients. Bipolar Disord 9(1–2):183–196. doi:10.1111/j.1399-5618.2007.00430.x
Janowsky DS, Leff M, Epstein RS (1970) Playing the manic game. Interpersonal maneuvers of the acutely manic patient. Arch Gen Psychiatry 22(3):252–261
Johnson ED (2000) Differences among families coping with serious mental illness: a qualitative analysis. Am J Orthopsychiatry 70(1):126–134
Judd LL, Akiskal HS (2003) The prevalence and disability of bipolar spectrum disorders in the US population: re-analysis of the ECA database taking into account subthreshold cases. J Affect Disord 73(1–2):123–131, S0165032702003324 [pii]
Judd LL, Akiskal HS, Schettler PJ, Endicott J, Leon AC, Solomon DA, Coryell W, Maser JD, Keller MB (2005) Psychosocial disability in the course of bipolar I and II disorders: a prospective, comparative, longitudinal study. Arch Gen Psychiatry 62(12):1322–1330. doi:10.1001/archpsyc.62.12.1322, 62/12/1322 [pii]
Judd LL, Schettler PJ, Solomon DA, Maser JD, Coryell W, Endicott J, Akiskal HS (2008) Psychosocial disability and work role function compared across the long-term course of bipolar I, bipolar II and unipolar major depressive disorders. J Affect Disord 108(1–2):49–58. doi:10.1016/j.jad.2007.06.014, S0165-0327(07)00333-3 [pii]
Katon W (1984) Depression: relationship to somatization and chronic medical illness. J Clin Psychiatry 45(3 Pt 2):4–12
Kauer-Sant'Anna M, Bond DJ, Lam RW, Yatham LN (2009) Functional outcomes in first-episode patients with bipolar disorder: a prospective study from the Systematic Treatment Optimization Program for Early Mania project. Compr Psychiatry 50(1):1–8. doi:10.1016/j.comppsych.2008.05.013, S0010-440X(08)00084-9 [pii]
Keck PE Jr, McElroy SL, Strakowski SM, West SA, Sax KW, Hawkins JM, Bourne ML, Haggard P (1998) 12-month outcome of patients with bipolar disorder following hospitalization for a manic or mixed episode. Am J Psychiatry 155(5):646–652
Kennedy N, Foy K, Sherazi R, McDonough M, McKeon P (2007) Long-term social functioning after depression treated by psychiatrists: a review. Bipolar Disord 9(1–2):25–37. doi:10.1111/j.1399-5618.2007.00326.x
Kessler RC, Walters EE, Forthofer MS (1998) The social consequences of psychiatric disorders, III: probability of marital stability. Am J Psychiatry 155(8):1092–1096
Kleinman L, Lowin A, Flood E, Gandhi G, Edgell E, Revicki D (2003) Costs of bipolar disorder. Pharmacoeconomics 21(9):601–622, 2191 [pii]
Kraepelin E (1921) Manic-depressive insanity and paranoia. Livingstone, Edinburgh
Kusznir A, Cooke RG, Young LT (2000) The correlates of community functioning in patients with bipolar disorder. J Affect Disord 61(1–2):81–85, S0165-0327(99)00193-7 [pii]
Lam D, Donaldson C, Brown Y, Malliaris Y (2005) Burden and marital and sexual satisfaction in the partners of bipolar patients. Bipolar Disord 7(5):431–440. doi:10.1111/j.1399-5618.2005.00240.x
Langtree I (2014) Definitions of the models of disability. http://www.disabled-world.com/definitions/disability-models.php. 2014
Leclerc C, Lesage A, Ricard N (1997) Relevance of the stress-coping paradigm in the elaboration of a stress management model for schizophrenics. Sante Ment Que 22(2):233–256
Levy B, Medina AM, Hintz K, Weiss RD (2010) Ecologically valid support for the link between cognitive and psychosocial functioning in bipolar disorder. Psychiatry Res 185(3):353–357. doi:10.1016/j.psychres.2010.06.010, S0165-1781(10)00352-5 [pii]

Link BG, Struening EL, Rahav M, Phelan JC, Nuttbrock L (1997) On stigma and its consequences: evidence from a longitudinal study of men with dual diagnoses of mental illness and substance abuse. J Health Soc Behav 38(2):177–190

Link BG, Struening EL, Neese-Todd S, Asmussen S, Phelan JC (2001) Stigma as a barrier to recovery: the consequences of stigma for the self-esteem of people with mental illnesses. Psychiatr Serv 52(12):1621–1626

Lopez AD (2005) The evolution of the global burden of disease framework for disease, injury and risk factor quantification: developing the evidence base for national, regional and global public health action. Glob Health 1(1):5. doi:10.1186/1744-8603-1-5

Lowery K, Mynt P, Aisbett J, Dixon T, O'Brien J, Ballard C (2000) Depression in the carers of dementia sufferers: a comparison of the carers of patients suffering from dementia with Lewy bodies and the carers of patients with Alzheimer's disease. J Affect Disord 59(1):61–65, S0165-0327(99)00123-8 [pii]

MacQueen GM, Young LT, Robb JC, Cooke RG, Joffe RT (1997) Levels of functioning and well-being in recovered psychotic versus nonpsychotic mania. J Affect Disord 46(1):69–72

MacQueen GM, Young LT, Robb JC, Marriott M, Cooke RG, Joffe RT (2000) Effect of number of episodes on wellbeing and functioning of patients with bipolar disorder. Acta Psychiatr Scand 101(5):374–381

MacQueen GM, Young LT, Joffe RT (2001) A review of psychosocial outcome in patients with bipolar disorder. Acta Psychiatr Scand 103(3):163–170

Magliano L, Orrico A, Fiorillo A, Del Vecchio H, Castiello G, Malangone C, De Rosa C, Capuano V, Maj M, Torchio E, Franzoi V, Pingani L, Curti C, Spanarello S, Scattina M, Fuchs H, Test GR, Ferrigno J, Minciotti E, Innocente P, Bardicchia F, Galli A, La Rovere R, Maroncelli M, Iapichino S, Pannozzo M, Nuccetelli F, Di Nunzio R, Armellino R, Palladino C, Delcuratolo V, Cadoni M, Cannas A, Caniglia A, Cudia M (2009) Family burden in bipolar disorders: results from the Italian Mood Disorders Study (IMDS). Epidemiol Psichiatr Soc 18(2):137–146

Maji KR, Sood M, Sagar R, Khandelwal SK (2011) A follow-up study of family burden in patients with bipolar affective disorder. Int J Soc Psychiatry. doi:10.1177/0020764010390442, 0020764010390442 [pii]

Marangell LB (2004) The importance of subsyndromal symptoms in bipolar disorder. J Clin Psychiatry 65(Suppl 10):24–27

Marneros A, Deister A, Rohde A (1990) Psychopathological and social status of patients with affective, schizophrenic and schizoaffective disorders after long-term course. Acta Psychiatr Scand 82(5):352–358

Martinez-Aran A, Vieta E, Colom F, Reinares M, Benabarre A, Torrent C, Goikolea JM, Corbella B, Sanchez-Moreno J, Salamero M (2002) Neuropsychological performance in depressed and euthymic bipolar patients. Neuropsychobiology 46(Suppl 1):16–21

Martinez-Aran A, Vieta E, Colom F, Torrent C, Sanchez-Moreno J, Reinares M, Benabarre A, Goikolea JM, Brugue E, Daban C, Salamero M (2004) Cognitive impairment in euthymic bipolar patients: implications for clinical and functional outcome. Bipolar Disord 6(3):224–232. doi:10.1111/j.1399-5618.2004.00111.x

Martinez-Aran A, Vieta E, Torrent C, Sanchez-Moreno J, Goikolea JM, Salamero M, Malhi GS, Gonzalez-Pinto A, Daban C, Alvarez-Grandi S, Fountoulakis K, Kaprinis G, Tabares-Seisdedos R, Ayuso-Mateos JL (2007) Functional outcome in bipolar disorder: the role of clinical and cognitive factors. Bipolar Disord 9(1–2):103–113. doi:10.1111/j.1399-5618.2007.00327.x

McCarthy JF, Valenstein M, Zivin K, Zeber JE, Kilbourne AM (2010) Access-related measures and out-of-system utilization among veterans with bipolar disorder. Psychiatr Serv 61(10):1035–1038. doi:10.1176/appi.ps.61.10.1035, 61/10/1035 [pii]

McIntyre RS, Wilkins K, Gilmour H, Soczynska JK, Konarksi JZ, Miranda A, Woldeyohannes HO, Vagic D, Alsuwaidan M, Kennedy SH (2008) The effect of bipolar I disorder and major depressive disorder on workforce function. Chronic Dis Can 28(3):84–91

McMorris BJ, Downs KE, Panish JM, Dirani R (2009) Workplace productivity, employment issues, and resource utilization in patients with bipolar I disorder. J Med Econ 13(1):23–32. doi:10.3111/13696990903475833

McPherson HM, Dore GM, Loan PA, Romans SE (1992) Socioeconomic characteristics of a Dunedin sample of bipolar patients. N Z Med J 105(933):161–162

Michalak EE, Murray G, Young AH, Lam RW (2008) Burden of bipolar depression: impact of disorder and medications on quality of life. CNS Drugs 22(5):389–406, 2253 [pii]

Michalak E, Livingston JD, Hole R, Suto M, Hale S, Haddock C (2011) 'It's something that I manage but it is not who I am': reflections on internalized stigma in individuals with bipolar disorder. Chronic Illn 7(3):209–224. doi:10.1177/1742395310395959, 1742395310395959 [pii]

Miklowitz DJ, Taylor DO (2006) Family-focused treatment of the suicidal bipolar patient. Bipolar Disord 8(5 Pt 2):640–651

Miklowitz DJ, George EL, Richards JA, Simoneau TL, Suddath RL (2003) A randomized study of family-focused psychoeducation and pharmacotherapy in the outpatient management of bipolar disorder. Arch Gen Psychiatry 60(9):904–912. doi:10.1001/archpsyc.60.9.904

Morgan VA, Mitchell PB, Jablensky AV (2005) The epidemiology of bipolar disorder: sociodemographic, disability and service utilization data from the Australian National Study of Low Prevalence (Psychotic) Disorders. Bipolar Disord 7(4):326–337. doi:10.1111/j.1399-5618.2005.00229.x, BDI229 [pii]

Morselli PL, Elgie R, Cesana BM (2004) GAMIAN-Europe/BEAM survey II: cross-national analysis of unemployment, family history, treatment satisfaction and impact of the bipolar disorder on life style. Bipolar Disord 6(6):487–497. doi:10.1111/j.1399-5618.2004.00160.x

Mueser KT, Webb C, Pfeiffer M, Gladis M, Levinson DF (1996) Family burden of schizophrenia and bipolar disorder: perceptions of relatives and professionals. Psychiatr Serv 47(5):507–511

Mur M, Portella MJ, Martinez-Aran A, Pifarre J, Vieta E (2009) Influence of clinical and neuropsychological variables on the psychosocial and occupational outcome of remitted bipolar patients. Psychopathology 42(3):148–156. doi:10.1159/000207456, 000207456 [pii]

Murray CJL, Lopez AD (eds) (1996) The global burden of disease. A comprehensive assessment of the mortality and disability from diseases, injuries and risk factors in 1990 and projected to 2020. Harvard School of Public Health on behalf of the World Health Organisation, and the World Bank, Boston

Nadkarni RB, Fristad MA (2012) Stress and support for parents of youth with bipolar disorder. Isr J Psychiatry Relat Sci 49(2):104–110

Nehra R, Chakrabarti S, Kulhara P, Sharma R (2005) Caregiver-coping in bipolar disorder and schizophrenia–a re-examination. Soc Psychiatry Psychiatr Epidemiol 40(4):329–336. doi:10.1007/s00127-005-0884-3

Nehra R, Chakrabarti S, Pradhan BK, Khehra N (2006) Comparison of cognitive functions between first- and multi-episode bipolar affective disorders. J Affect Disord 93(1–3):185–192. doi:10.1016/j.jad.2006.03.013, S0165-0327(06)00139-X [pii]

O'Connell RA, Mayo JA, Flatow L, Cuthbertson B, O'Brien BE (1991) Outcome of bipolar disorder on long-term treatment with lithium. Br J Psychiatry 159:123–129

Ogilvie AD, Morant N, Goodwin GM (2005) The burden on informal caregivers of people with bipolar disorder. Bipolar Disord 7(Suppl 1):25–32. doi:10.1111/j.1399-5618.2005.00191.x

Ohaeri JU, Fido AA (2001) The opinion of caregivers on aspects of schizophrenia and major affective disorders in a Nigerian setting. Soc Psychiatry Psychiatr Epidemiol 36(10):493–499

Olie JP, Levy E (2002) Manic episodes: the direct cost of a three-month period following hospitalisation. Eur Psychiatry 17(5):278–286, S0924933802006806 [pii]

Ostacher MJ, Nierenberg AA, Iosifescu DV, Eidelman P, Lund HG, Ametrano RM, Kaczynski R, Calabrese J, Miklowitz DJ, Sachs GS, Perlick DA (2008) Correlates of subjective and objective burden among caregivers of patients with bipolar disorder. Acta Psychiatr Scand 118(1):49–56. doi:10.1111/j.1600-0447.2008.01201.x

Ozer S, Ulusahin A, Batur S, Kabakci E, Saka MC (2002) Outcome measures of interepisode bipolar patients in a Turkish sample. Soc Psychiatry Psychiatr Epidemiol 37(1):31–37

Peele PB, Xu Y, Kupfer DJ (2003) Insurance expenditures on bipolar disorder: clinical and parity implications. Am J Psychiatry 160(7):1286–1290

Perlick D, Clarkin JF, Sirey J, Raue P, Greenfield S, Struening E, Rosenheck R (1999) Burden experienced by care-givers of persons with bipolar affective disorder. Br J Psychiatry 175:56–62

Perlick D, Rosenheck RR, Clarkin JF, Raue P, Sirey J (2001) Impact of family burden and patient symptom status on clinical outcome in bipolar affective disorder. J Nerv Ment Dis 189(1): 31–37

Perlick D, Rosenheck RA, Clarkin JF, Maciejewski PK, Sirey J, Struening E, Link BG (2004) Impact of family burden and affective response on clinical outcome among patients with bipolar disorder. Psychiatr Serv 55(9):1029–1035. doi:10.1176/appi.ps.55.9.1029

Perlick D, Hohenstein JM, Clarkin JF, Kaczynski R, Rosenheck RA (2005) Use of mental health and primary care services by caregivers of patients with bipolar disorder: a preliminary study. Bipolar Disord 7(2):126–135. doi:10.1111/j.1399-5618.2004.00172.x

Perlick D, Miklowitz DJ, Link BG, Struening E, Kaczynski R, Gonzalez J, Manning LN, Wolff N, Rosenheck RA (2007a) Perceived stigma and depression among caregivers of patients with bipolar disorder. Br J Psychiatry 190:535–536. doi:10.1192/bjp.bp.105.020826

Perlick D, Rosenheck RA, Miklowitz DJ, Chessick C, Wolff N, Kaczynski R, Ostacher M, Patel J, Desai R (2007b) Prevalence and correlates of burden among caregivers of patients with bipolar disorder enrolled in the systematic treatment enhancement program for bipolar disorder. Bipolar Disord 9(3):262–273. doi:10.1111/j.1399-5618.2007.00365.x

Perlick D, Rosenheck RA, Miklowitz DJ, Kaczynski R, Link B, Ketter T, Wisniewski S, Wolff N, Sachs G (2008) Caregiver burden and health in bipolar disorder: a cluster analytic approach. J Nerv Ment Dis 196(6):484–491. doi:10.1097/NMD.0b013e3181773927

Perlick DA, Miklowitz DJ, Lopez N, Chou J, Kalvin C, Adzhiashvili V, Aronson A (2010) Family-focused treatment for caregivers of patients with bipolar disorder. Bipolar Disord 12(6):627–637. doi:10.1111/j.1399-5618.2010.00852.x

Pini S, de Queiroz V, Pagnin D, Pezawas L, Angst J, Cassano GB, Wittchen HU (2005) Prevalence and burden of bipolar disorders in European countries. Eur Neuropsychopharmacol 15(4):425–434. doi:10.1016/j.euroneuro.2005.04.011, S0924-977X(05)00074-X [pii]

Platt S (1985) Measuring the burden of psychiatric illness on the family: an evaluation of some rating scales. Psychol Med 15(2):383–393

Pompili M, Rihmer Z, Innamorati M, Lester D, Girardi P, Tatarelli R (2009) Assessment and treatment of suicide risk in bipolar disorders. Expert Rev Neurother 9(1):109–136. doi:10.1586/14737175.9.1.109

Pompili M, Harnic D, Gonda X, Forte A, Dominici G, Innamorati M, Fountoulakis KN, Serafini G, Sher L, Janiri L, Rihmer Z, Amore M, Girardi P (2014) Impact of living with bipolar patients: making sense of caregivers' burden. World J Psychiatry 4(1):1–12. doi:10.5498/wjp.v4.i1.1

Pope M, Dudley R, Scott J (2007) Determinants of social functioning in bipolar disorder. Bipolar Disord 9(1–2):38–44. doi:10.1111/j.1399-5618.2007.00323.x

Poulin MJ, Brown SL, Ubel PA, Smith DM, Jankovic A, Langa KM (2010) Does a helping hand mean a heavy heart? Helping behavior and well-being among spouse caregivers. Psychol Aging 25(1):108–117. doi:10.1037/a0018064

Practice guideline for the assessment and treatment of patients with suicidal behaviors (2003) Am J Psychiatry 160(11 Suppl):1–60

Pradhan SC, Sinha VK, Singh TB (1999) Psycho-social dysfunctions in patients after recovery from mania and depression. Int J Rehabil Res 22(4):303–309

Priebe S, Wildgrube C, Muller-Oerlinghausen B (1989) Lithium prophylaxis and expressed emotion. Br J Psychiatry 154:396–399

Raveendranathan D, Chandra PS, Chaturvedi SK (2012) Violence among psychiatric inpatients: a victim's perspective. East Asian Arch Psychiatry 22(4):141–145

Reinares M, Vieta E, Colom F, Martinez-Aran A, Torrent C, Comes M, Goikolea JM, Benabarre A, Sanchez-Moreno J (2004) Impact of a psychoeducational family intervention on caregivers of stabilized bipolar patients. Psychother Psychosom 73(5):312–319. doi:10.1159/00007884878848

Reinares M, Vieta E, Colom F, Martinez-Aran A, Torrent C, Comes M, Goikolea JM, Benabarre A, Daban C, Sanchez-Moreno J (2006) What really matters to bipolar patients' caregivers: sources of family burden. J Affect Disord 94(1–3):157–163. doi:10.1016/j.jad.2006.04.022

Reznik I, Sirota P (1999) Premorbid social functioning with schizophrenia and bipolar disorder. Am J Psychiatry 156(6):986

Rosa AR, Reinares M, Michalak EE, Bonnin CM, Sole B, Franco C, Comes M, Torrent C, Kapczinski F, Vieta E (2011) Functional impairment and disability across mood states in bipolar disorder. Value Health 13(8):984–988. doi:10.1111/j.1524-4733.2010.00768.x, VHE768 [pii]

Sachs GS, Nierenberg AA, Calabrese JR, Marangell LB, Wisniewski SR, Gyulai L, Friedman ES, Bowden CL, Fossey MD, Ostacher MJ, Ketter TA, Patel J, Hauser P, Rapport D, Martinez JM, Allen MH, Miklowitz DJ, Otto MW, Dennehy EB, Thase ME (2007) Effectiveness of adjunctive antidepressant treatment for bipolar depression. N Engl J Med 356(17):1711–1722. doi:10.1056/NEJMoa064135

Sales E (2003) Family burden and quality of life. Qual Life Res 12(Suppl 1):33–41

Sanchez-Moreno J, Martinez-Aran A, Tabares-Seisdedos R, Torrent C, Vieta E, Ayuso-Mateos JL (2009) Functioning and disability in bipolar disorder: an extensive review. Psychother Psychosom 78(5):285–297. doi:10.1159/000228249, 000228249 [pii]

Schoeyen HK, Birkenaes AB, Vaaler AE, Auestad BH, Malt UF, Andreassen OA, Morken G (2011a) Bipolar disorder patients have similar levels of education but lower socio-economic status than the general population. J Affect Disord 129(1–3):68–74, S0165-0327(10)00546-X [pii]

Schoeyen HK, Vaaler AE, Auestad BH, Malt UF, Melle I, Andreassen OA, Morken G (2011b) Despite clinical differences, bipolar disorder patients from acute wards and outpatient clinics have similar educational and disability levels compared to the general population. J Affect Disord 132(1–2):209–215. doi:10.1016/j.jad.2011.02.025, S0165-0327(11)00079-6 [pii]

Simon GE (2002) Why we care about the economic and social burden of bipolar disorder. In: Maj M, Akiskal H, Lopez- Ibor JJ, Sartorius N (eds) Bipolar disorder-WPA series on evidence and experience in psychiatry. Wiley, London, pp 474–476

Simon GE (2003) Social and economic burden of mood disorders. Biol Psychiatry 54(3):208–215, S0006322303004207 [pii]

Simon GE, Bauer MS, Ludman EJ, Operskalski BH, Unutzer J (2007) Mood symptoms, functional impairment, and disability in people with bipolar disorder: specific effects of mania and depression. J Clin Psychiatry 68(8):1237–1245

Steele A, Maruyama N, Galynker I (2009) Psychiatric symptoms in caregivers of patients with bipolar disorder: a review. J Affect Disord 121(1–2):10–21. doi:10.1016/j.jad.2009.04.020, S0165-0327(09)00171-2 [pii]

Stender M, Bryant-Comstock L, Phillips S (2002) Medical resource use among patients treated for bipolar disorder: a retrospective, cross-sectional, descriptive analysis. Clin Ther 24(10):1668–1676, S0149291802800704 [pii]

Struening EL, Perlick DA, Link BG, Hellman F, Herman D, Sirey JA (2001) Stigma as a barrier to recovery: The extent to which caregivers believe most people devalue consumers and their families. Psychiatr Serv 52(12):1633–1638

Stueve A, Vine P, Struening EL (1997) Perceived burden among caregivers of adults with serious mental illness: comparison of black, Hispanic, and white families. Am J Orthopsychiatry 67(2):199–209

Szmukler GI, Burgess P, Herrman H, Benson A, Colusa S, Bloch S (1996) Caring for relatives with serious mental illness: the development of the experience of caregiving inventory. Soc Psychiatry Psychiatr Epidemiol 31(3–4):137–148

Tabares-Seisdedos R, Balanza-Martinez V, Sanchez-Moreno J, Martinez-Aran A, Salazar-Fraile J, Selva-Vera G, Rubio C, Mata I, Gomez-Beneyto M, Vieta E (2008) Neurocognitive and clinical predictors of functional outcome in patients with schizophrenia and bipolar I disorder at one-year follow-up. J Affect Disord 109(3):286–299. doi:10.1016/j.jad.2007.12.234, S0165-0327(08)00015-3 [pii]

Tantum D (1989) Familial factors in psychiatric disorder. Curr Opin Psychiatry 2:296–301

Targum SD, Dibble ED, Davenport YB, Gershon ES (1981) The family attitudes questionnaire. Patients' and spouses' views of bipolar illness. Arch Gen Psychiatry 38(5):562–568

Tohen M, Waternaux CM, Tsuang MT (1990) Outcome in mania. A 4-year prospective follow-up of 75 patients utilizing survival analysis. Arch Gen Psychiatry 47(12):1106–1111

Tohen M, Greenfield SF, Weiss RD, Zarate CA Jr, Vagge LM (1998) The effect of comorbid substance use disorders on the course of bipolar disorder: a review. Harv Rev Psychiatry 6(3):133–141

Tohen M, Hennen J, Zarate CM Jr, Baldessarini RJ, Strakowski SM, Stoll AL, Faedda GL, Suppes T, Gebre-Medhin P, Cohen BM (2000) Two-year syndromal and functional recovery in 219 cases of first-episode major affective disorder with psychotic features. Am J Psychiatry 157(2): 220–228

Tranvag O, Kristoffersen K (2008) Experience of being the spouse/cohabitant of a person with bipolar affective disorder: a cumulative process over time. Scand J Caring Sci 22(1):5–18. doi:10.1111/j.1471-6712.2007.00562.x

Trippitelli CL, Jamison KR, Folstein MF, Bartko JJ, DePaulo JR (1998) Pilot study on patients' and spouses' attitudes toward potential genetic testing for bipolar disorder. Am J Psychiatry 155(7):899–904

Vazquez GH, Kapczinski F, Magalhaes PV, Cordoba R, Lopez Jaramillo C, Rosa AR, Sanchez De Carmona M, Tohen M (2010) Stigma and functioning in patients with bipolar disorder. J Affect Disord 130(1-2):323–327. doi:10.1016/j.jad.2010.10.012, S0165-0327(10)00626-9 [pii]

Veltman A, Cameron J, Stewart DE (2002) The experience of providing care to relatives with chronic mental illness. J Nerv Ment Dis 190(2):108–114

Vieta E (2005) Improving treatment adherence in bipolar disorder through psychoeducation. J Clin Psychiatry 66(Suppl 1):24–29

Wilson L, Crowe M (2009) Parenting with a diagnosis bipolar disorder. J Adv Nurs 65(4):877–884. doi:10.1111/j.1365-2648.2008.04954.x

Wingo AP, Baldessarini RJ, Compton MT, Harvey PD (2010) Correlates of recovery of social functioning in types I and II bipolar disorder patients. Psychiatry Res 177(1–2):131–134. doi:10.1016/j.psychres.2010.02.020, S0165-1781(10)00094-6 [pii]

Wolff N, Perlick DA, Kaczynski R, Calabrese J, Nierenberg A, Miklowitz DJ (2006) Modeling costs and burden of informal caregiving for persons with bipolar disorder. J Ment Health Policy Econ 9(2):99–110

World Health Organization (1999) Annual report. World Health Organization, Geneva

World Health Organization (2001) International classification of functioning, disability and health. WHO, Geneva

World Health Organization (2011) World report on disability. WHO, Geneva

World Health Organization (2014) Disability. http://www.who.int/topics/disabilities/en/. 2014

Young AH, Rigney U, Shaw S, Emmas C, Thompson JM (2011) Annual cost of managing bipolar disorder to the UK healthcare system. J Affect Disord 133(3):450–456. doi:10.1016/j.jad.2011.06.016, S0165-0327(11)00335-1 [pii]

Zarate CA Jr, Tohen M, Land M, Cavanagh S (2000) Functional impairment and cognition in bipolar disorder. Psychiatry Q 71(4):309–329

Zubieta JK, Huguelet P, O'Neil RL, Giordani BJ (2001) Cognitive function in euthymic bipolar I disorder. Psychiatry Res 102(1):9–20

Aetiopathogenesis of Bipolar Disorder 13

BD was traditionally conceptualized in the frame of mood (affective) disorders until its separation from unipolar depression by DSM-5. This long history caused much of the research to focus indiscriminately on 'mood disorders' by pooling together bipolar and unipolar patients in study samples. Bipolar depression was not studied separately from unipolar for too long, and mania was not the intensive focus of research.

Therefore, the aetiopathogenesis of BD was considered as related with that of unipolar depression rather than with that of schizophrenia. Most experts agree that mood disorders have both endogenous and exogenous components and in most patients they are both present. This approach is a sharp rejection of the 'historical dualism' suggested by Rene Descartes in the seventeenth century and theoretically has its roots in the 'psychobiology' of Adolf Meyer (1866–1950) which used the term to emphasize that psychological and biological factors interact in the development of mental disorders. The bio-psychosocial model, proposed by George L. Engel (1913–1999) (Engel 1977, 1980), provides a non-specific but inclusive theoretical framework in order to host all variables suggested by various approaches to cause depression.

However, such an approach is obsolete today because the need is for specific and accurate models and predictions and not for general frameworks. It is a problem that in psychiatry such an advanced understanding is lacking not only for BD but for mental disorders in general.

13.1 Social Theories

All the literature on social theories for mood disorders refer essentially to unipolar depression, and much of it is often generalized to include bipolar depression although such an approach is probably mistaken. Social theories are attractive to lay people especially since along with many psychological theories, they attribute mood disorders to adverse life events. However, even in the frame of unipolar

K.N. Fountoulakis, *Bipolar Disorder: An Evidence-Based Guide to Manic Depression*, DOI 10.1007/978-3-642-37216-2_13

depression, this assumption is far from being proven (Harkness and Luther 2001; Paykel et al. 1984). But the sensitization of stress-responsive neurobiological systems as a possible consequence of early adverse experience has been more solidly implicated in the pathophysiology of mood and anxiety disorders. A history of childhood abuse per se may be related to increased neuroendocrine stress reactivity, which is further enhanced when additional trauma is experienced in adulthood (Heim et al. 2002).

Depressed patients were reported to have higher perceptions of day-to-day stressors (hassles), reduced perception of uplifting events, excessive reliance on emotion-focused coping strategies and diminished quality of life in comparison to controls, and this can be considered in the frame of an early sensitization procedure. Among depressed patients the hassles, coping styles and some elements of quality of life were related to symptom severity, as well as treatment resistance (Ravindran et al. 2002). However, it is questionable whether this is a true fact or these patients (which have higher personality psychopathology and interpersonal rejection sensitivity) tend to over-report life events (Fountoulakis et al. 2006).

Thus, many authors insist that psychosocial factors are relatively unimportant in the subsequent course of severe and recurrent depressions, in contrast to their contribution to onset of such depressions and subsequent outcome of milder depressions (Paykel et al. 1996; Thomson and Hendrie 1972). This could be especially valid concerning bipolar depression which is longitudinally characterized by more 'endogenous' and psychotic features.

13.2 Psychological Theories

The literature on psychological theories for BD is limited. Most of the researchers had focused so far on the unipolar types depression and mood instability; therefore, there is no clear psychodynamic (or similar) theory concerning mania.

The only available specific theory implies that mania has the same cause with depression and they are both related with the loss of a loved object. The difference is that while depression emerges from the introjection of the lost object, mania is the result of the attempt to avoid depression. Essentially mania constitutes a defence against an underlying depression and utilizes a number of defence mechanisms like omnipotence, denial, idealization and contempt. In this frame, the euphoric state of the patient is understood as a tendency to extinguish any unpleasant aspects of reality and to disregard for the problems of reality, even if the situation is tragic. Thus, mixed episodes are easily psychodynamically understood, since the manic elements seen in depressed patients are considered to be defences. Overall this hypothesis corresponds more to 'elation' but not to mania, and there are no empirical studies to support the suggestion that a stressful event precedes the onset of acute mania.

Some authors stress the repetitive maladaptive patterns in the family, including avoidance of affect, unrealistic standards of conformity and displaced parental low self-esteem (Davenport et al. 1979), but such approaches lack specificity and probably refer to a generic family and personality dysfunction which is more or less common in most mental disorders (Kutcher et al. 1992). Some reports include problematic methodology and study samples, and the results are difficult to interpret (Loeb and Loeb 1992; Louet et al. 2010) or are based on the study of isolated cases (Steggles 2012).

The psychological theories on the aetiopathogenesis of depression are more elaborated, and they cover a wide variety of concepts and hypotheses. All of them were derived from observations in patients with conditions including reactive and characterological depression, personality disorders and unipolar depression, and they assume that more or less all these conditions emerge from a common or similar background. The most important psychological theories for depression are listed below:

13.2.1 Aggression-Turned-Inward Model

It has been proposed by Sigmund Freud and Karl Abraham on the basis of a 'metaphor' from physics to psychology ('hydraulic mind'). According to this model, during the oral phase (i.e. during the 12th–18th months of life) disturbances in the relationship between the infant and the mother establish a vulnerability to develop depression. Then during the adult life, a real or imaginary loss leads to depression as the result of aggressive impulses turned inward and directed against the ambivalently loved internalized object which had been lost. The aim of that turned-inward aggression was supposed to be the punishment of the love object which fails to fulfil the patient's need to be loved. It is therefore accompanied by guilt which could lead to suicidal behaviour. Later other authors proposed somewhat different versions of this model. The drawbacks of this model include that it represents a relatively closed circuit independent of the outside world, while the clinical fact is that many depressed patients openly express anger and hostility against others which is reduced after treatment and that there is no evidence supporting the concept that expressing anger outwards has a therapeutic effect in the treatment of clinical depression.

13.2.2 Object Loss

The term refers to traumatic separation from significant objects of attachment. However, according to empirical research data, only a minority of no more than 10 % of people experiencing bereavement will eventually manifest clinical depression. Thus, the model includes two steps: an early one which includes the development of vulnerability because of a significant loss during childhood and a second step during which this vulnerability interacts with a significant loss during adult life and eventually leads to clinical depression. This model fits better the data in comparison to the aggression turned inward and has some support from studies on primates although the latter point to a broad psychopathology rather than specifically depression.

13.2.3 Loss of Self-Esteem

Depression is considered to originate from the inability of the ego to give up unattainable goals and ideals resulting in a collapse of self-esteem. This model suggests that the narcissistic injury that destroys the patient's self-esteem comes from the internalized values of the ego rather than the hydraulic pressure deriving from the id as proposed by the aggression-turned-inward model. In this frame the loss of self-esteem has a sociocultural and existential dimension, and thus, this theory is to a significant extent testable. The drawback of this theory is that both persons with low and high self-esteem can develop depression or mania without any significant differences among them.

13.2.4 Cognitive Model

The cognitive model was developed by Aaron Beck and suggests that thinking in a negative way is the core of clinical depression. According to this, depression is conceptualized in the frame of the 'cognitive triad'. This triad proposes that patients conceive the self, the environment and the future in a negative depressive way (helplessness, negativism and hopelessness). In the core there seems to be bias in the way of thinking of the person. This is the cause of an interpretation of any experiences in a profound negative attributional style (mental schemata) which is considered to be global, internal and stable. This bias in the way of thinking is because of overgeneralization, magnification of negative events with a simultaneous minimization of positive events, arbitrary inference and selective abstraction. Systematic errors in thinking allow the persistence of negative schemas despite contradictory evidence. The major drawback of this model is the fact that it is based on retrospective observations of depressed patients; thus, the negative triad could be simply part of the clinical picture or subclinical manifestations of depression and not the cause of it. The major advantage is that it led to the first testable and practical psychotherapeutic approach which seems to be effective in a specific subgroup of patients.

13.2.5 Learned Helplessness Model

This model is based on animal experiments and proposes that the depressive attitude is learned during past situations in which the person was not able to terminate or avoid undesirable or traumatic events. However, it seems that the learned helplessness paradigm is more general and refers to a broader mental condition (e.g. social behaviour, posttraumatic stress disorder, etc.). It seems that past events could shape a personality profile which includes passivity, lack of hostility and self-blame. However, this line of thinking could lead to the notion that depression and the behaviours accompanying it should be considered to be a result of a masochistic lifestyle with manipulative behavioural patterns in order to handle interpersonal issues. Even more, recent animal research has implicated the importance of genetic factors in the vulnerability to learning to behave helplessly.

13.2.6 Depression and Reinforcement

According to the reinforcement model, the behaviours characteristic for depression develop because of a lack of appropriate rewards and with receipt of non-contingent rewards. This theory bridges personality, low self-esteem and learned helplessness with the human social environment; however, it seems more appropriate for the interpretation of social issues than clinical depression. A psychotherapeutic approach aiming to improve the patient's social skills is based on this theory.

13.3 Neurobiology of BD

13.3.1 Neuroanatomy of BD

A first step in understanding the neurobiology of BD would be to adequately explore and understand the neurobiology of emotions. However, in spite of the tremendous development of clinical neurosciences during the last 20 years, emotions and their disorders are still not satisfactorily understood.

There are many brain structures which are supposed to associate with the experience of mood and production of normal affect and emotions. Grossly, they form two complementary neural networks referred to as the ventral and the dorsal systems. The ventral system includes the amygdala, insula, ventral striatum, ventral anterior cingulate cortex (ACC) and the prefrontal cortex (PFC) and subserves the identification of the emotional significance of a stimulus, the production of affective states and also the automatic regulation of emotional responses (Swanda et al. 2000). The dorsal system includes the hippocampus, the dorsal ACC and PFC and subserves the conscious regulation of affective states and subsequent behaviour (Davidson and Irwin 1999). A simplified neurobiological model may propose that 'mood' derives probably from processes largely taking part in the amygdala and the insula, while 'emotion' is generated mainly in the anterior cingulate cortex (ACC) and more specifically in area 25 (Anderson and Phelps 2002). However, its regulation is likely to implicate area 24 and the dorsolateral prefrontal cortex (DLPFC). In between, 'mood' and 'emotion' lies the 'affect' which is at least partially generated in the ACC and partially in other brain areas including the prefrontal cortex (PFC).

Both psychological and biological aetiological factors converge in the diencephalic substrates of pleasure and reward (Akiskal and McKinney 1973), and the corresponding conceptual model (Figs. 13.1 and 13.2) links the central chemistry and physiology of structures that generate mood and reward mechanisms, memory storage and retrieval, as well as motor responses and behavioural disturbances which are characteristic of BD (Fountoulakis et al. 2008a). Among the structures involved in this model, the ACC and amygdala are thought to play a key role in the integration of emotional and cognitive dimensions mainly during the depressive phases of BD. The CC is a heterogeneous structure in terms of cytoarchitecture and function (Fig. 13.2). Its role on the neurophysiological basis of emotional expression and affective regulation is considered of major importance. For instance, damage of this

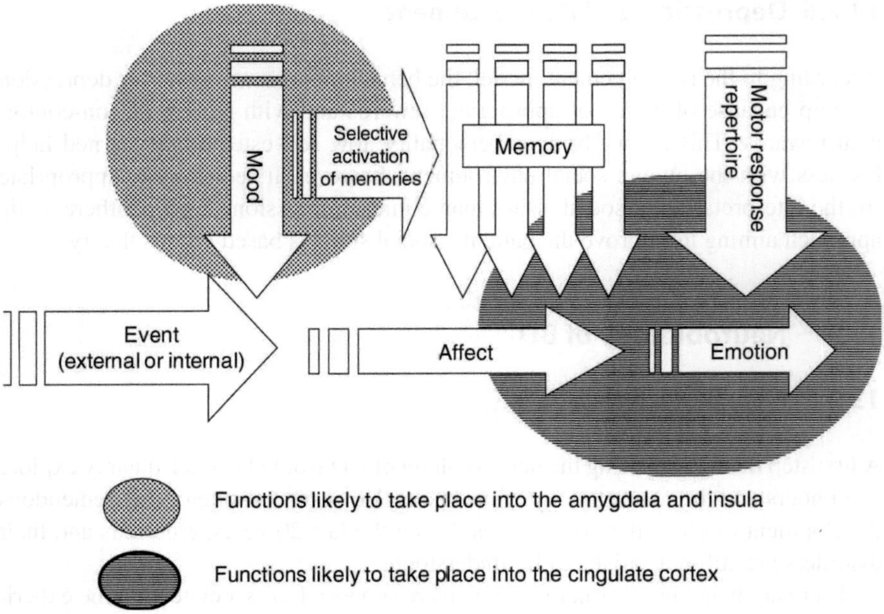

Fig. 13.1 A very simplified model for mood affect and emotion in response to stimuli. The model does not include the plethora of existing feedback (Reprinted with permission from Fountoulakis et al. (2008a))

Fig. 13.2 The areas of the cingulate cortex implicated in the production of affect (Reprinted with permission from Fountoulakis et al. (2008a))

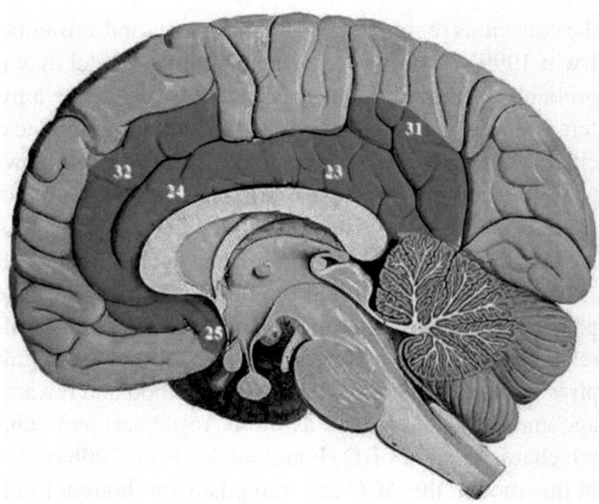

area has been associated with impaired pain regulation, akinetic mutism and apathy and indifference to pain (Chow and Cummings 2000).

Mood disorders may involve a dysfunctional coordination of limbic-cortical connections, with dorsal structures being responsible for neurocognitive disorders, ventral structures for somatic symptoms and the rostral ACC for the coordination of them (Tekin and Cummings 2002). Most of the current neuroanatomical and functional observations in ACC, mostly in its subgenual part (areas 25 and part of 24), argue in favour of a mixed neurodevelopmental and neurodegenerative process contributing in the pathophysiology of mood disorders.

13.3.1.1 Structural Neuroimaging

The presence of volumetric changes in the brains of BD patients is definitely known since approximately 20 years, and they have been interpreted according to two major theories. The first implies the presence of neurodevelopmental abnormalities which are independent of the severity or the long-term course of the disease or the response to treatment. Alternatively, they may reflect neurodegenerative changes related to the chronicity of the disorder. Both conceptions are supported by research data which showed that volume decrease in this area is present as early as the prodromal phase but seems to increase with the duration of illness (Farrow et al. 2005; Hajek et al. 2005; Hirayasu et al. 1999; Kaur et al. 2005; Lyoo et al. 2006; Lagopoulos et al. 2012; Strakowski et al. 2002). Thus, a volumetric decrease seems to be present and it might have some prognostic value.

The literature so far suggests that patients with BD manifest an enlargement of the third and lateral ventricles (Soares et al. 2005), white matter hyperintensities (Moore et al. 2001; Silverstone et al. 2003; Marlinge et al. 2014) and reduced grey matter in the prefrontal cortex, the hippocampus and the cerebellum (Moorhead et al. 2007; Soares et al. 2005; Blumberg et al. 2006) as well as a volume reduction in the left cingulate cortex (CC) (Bruno et al. 2006; Lyoo et al. 2006) or the right CC (McDonald et al. 2004). Some studies suggest the volumetric reduction in the CC is bilateral (Bearden et al. 2007; Coyle et al. 2006; Doris et al. 2004; Lochhead et al. 2004). There is a large body of literature pointing to a specific vulnerability of the left anterior CC (ACC) and in particular its subgenual part (sgACC) (Atmaca et al. 2007; Lyoo et al. 2004; Sassi et al. 2004) or left posterior CC (PCC) (Hirayasu et al. 1999; Houenou et al. 2007; Wilke et al. 2004). However, some studies report a right or bilateral ACC (Bruno et al. 2004; Cannon et al. 2006a) or a left or bilateral PCC volume decrease (Farrow et al. 2005; Kaur et al. 2005; Lim et al. 1999; Lochhead et al. 2004). Although, it should be noted that there is some degree of heterogeneity among studies concerning the specific areas which manifest atrophy or lesions, in general the findings concern the prefrontal, cingulate and subgenual cortices; the fusiform gyrus; and the left hippocampus (Lim et al. 2013; Javadapour et al. 2007; Fountoulakis et al. 2008a).

Histologically, volume loss may reflect grey or white matter changes. There are reports suggesting a grey matter loss in the CC bilaterally (Lim et al. 1999; Doris et al. 2004) or specifically in the left CC (Wilke et al. 2004; Drevets et al. 1997; Lyoo et al. 2004) which could be progressive (Farrow et al. 2005). Loss of macromolecular density was reported for the right sgACC and adjacent white matter in BD patients compared to controls (Bruno et al. 2004), while the use of diffusion tensor imaging tractography (DT-MRI) documented a significantly increased number of reconstructed fibres between the left sgACC and left amygdalo-hippocampal complex in BD patients compared to healthy controls (Houenou et al. 2007). Another DT-MRI study reported significantly shorter white matter tracts in the genu, body and splenium of the corpus callosum compared to healthy controls. Additionally,

BD patients exhibited reduced fibre density in the genu and body of the corpus callosum and in the inferior longitudinal fasciculus bilaterally. In the left uncinate fasciculus, however, BD subjects exhibited significantly greater fibre density than healthy controls (Torgerson et al. 2013).

While in schizophrenia a loss of brain volume is evident already at onset, in BD this happens latter. This is especially true concerning grey matter, while on the contrary, the loss of white mater volume might happen first and be present already at onset (Berk et al. 2010; Vita et al. 2009; Bora et al. 2010; Strakowski et al. 1993). Therefore, it is possible that white matter pathology is the prominent finding during the early stages (Lim et al. 2013; Lin et al. 2013), while grey matter loss follows years later (Arango et al. 2012).

The decrease in volume is generally correlated with the number of episodes (Strakowski et al. 2002), and these findings are considered to be associated with a poor prognosis (Moore et al. 2001; Silverstone et al. 2003).

On the other hand, there are reports suggesting that there was no difference in grey matter loss in BD patients in comparison to controls and there was also no effect of the number of episodes (Brambilla et al. 2002; Lopez-Larson et al. 2002; Zimmerman et al. 2006; Zipursky et al. 1997; Nery et al. 2009). It is interesting that in contrast to the rest of the literature, an increase in the size of the amygdala (Blumberg et al. 2006) and the grey matter density in the ACC of BD patients have been reported (Adler et al. 2007; Bearden et al. 2007) thus raising doubts about the presence of a widely present neurodevelopmental abnormality in BD. Also, in spite of findings concerning specific regions, it seems that the total brain volume remains stable, and this puts forward a number of problems concerning the methods of quantification of brain volume and other methodological issues (Fountoulakis et al. 2008a).

There are evidences that at least three variables might influence the volumetric changes in BD: the presence of cognitive decline (Bruno et al. 2006), response to treatment (Sassi et al. 2004; Cannon et al. 2006a; Atmaca et al. 2007; Bearden et al. 2007) and genetic background (McDonald et al. 2004), but overall the literature on neuroimaging data at different stages of BD is limited and most of the data are cross-sectional (Lim et al. 2013; Balanza-Martinez et al. 2005) which make generalizable conclusions difficult.

13.3.1.2 Neuropathological Data

A significant part of the total contribution on the neuropathology of BD is based on the material provided by the Stanley Neuropathology Consortium (Cotter et al. 2002; Knable 1999; Raedler et al. 1999; Torrey et al. 2005; Webster et al. 2005; Zavitsanou et al. 2004, 2005).

The validity of histological findings depends on the quality of the material available, staining procedures and number of sections within each area. An additional variable to consider is a possible pharmacological effect on brain microstructure (Fountoulakis et al. 2008a). For instance, an early neuropathological study showed a preferential concentration of lithium in the retrosplenial CC (corresponding to BA 23 and 31) and caudate nucleus suggesting a differential regional impact of this molecule in BD (Spirtes 1976). Not surprisingly, to date there are no convincing evidence supporting neuronal or glial loss in BD.

Macroscopically, one study reported a 20 % reduction in the volume of area 24 in BD patients compared to controls. However, because of the small study sample, the difference was not significant. The authors did not find changes in the number or size of neurons in area sg24 in BD cases. The reduction in glial number (41 %) was statistical significant only in the familial BD subgroup (bilaterally) (Ongur et al. 1998). Two other studies reported no differences in the size of cell bodies; however, they also reported a 27 % reduction in the density of non-pyramidal neurons in layer II of the ACC in BD patients. In sporadic cases without chronic drug treatment, it has been reported that the mean total and laminar cortical thicknesses as well as mean pyramidal neuron size were significantly decreased in sg Brodmann area (BA) 24 in BD patients (Bouras et al. 2001). Another study reported a decreased clustering of neurons in the BA 24c bilaterally in BD patients, and the neuronal somal size was reduced in layer V (16 %), and neuronal density was increased in layer VI in (63 %) (Chana et al. 2003). An increase in density of 2,3-dioxygenase-immunoreactive glial cells in both grey and white matter of the ACC was also reported (Miller et al. 2006).

A number of independent studies failed to identify differences in glial density or neuronal size in BD compared to controls (Benes et al. 2000, 2001; Cotter et al. 2001).

A meta-analysis reported a decreased density (31 %) of non-pyramidal neurons bilaterally in layer II of the ACC in BD patients. They reported no differences in glial numbers with 2D cell counting, but significant glial reduction in layers III, V and VI when using 3D cell counting (Todtenkopf et al. 2005). Western blot data did not add further clarity since studies reported decreased levels (32 %) of glial fibrillary acidic protein (GFAP) mRNA in the white but not grey matter of ACC, area 24b (bilaterally) in BD patients (Torrey et al. 2005; Webster et al. 2005).

Interestingly, it has been reported that proteins related to the number and functioning of synapses such as synaptophysin, complexin II and growth-associated protein-43 (GAP-43) may be reduced in the BA 24a and 24b of the ACC of BD patients. On the contrary, there were no differences in complexin I and beta-actin levels between BD and controls (Eastwood and Harrison 2001). Since synaptophysin is a marker of synaptic density and GAP-43 is a marker of insult-induced plasticity, these findings suggest a loss of synapses with impaired remodelling. The reduction of complexin II but not I suggests a progressive destruction of excitatory rather than inhibitory synapses (Auer et al. 2000).

Exploring the hypothesis that glutamatergic inputs onto gamma-aminobutyric acid interneurons via the N-methyl-d-aspartate (NMDA) receptor are altered in the ACC in schizophrenia and BD, Woo et al. reported that the density of all GAD(67) mRNA-containing neurons was decreased by 35 % in layer II of the ACC. This decrease reached 60 % for GAD(67) mRNA-containing neurons that co-expressed NR(2A)mRNA (Woo et al. 2004).

To test the hypothesis that apoptosis could play a role in BD-related neuronal pathology, the Klenow method for in situ end-labelling of single-stranded DNA breaks was applied to the ACC from 18 healthy controls, 18 patients with schizophrenia and 10 with BD. Here again, the results did not reveal any reduction in BD patients (Benes et al. 2003). In contrast, apolipoprotein D protein levels showed a 57 % increase in BA 24 (Thomas et al. 2003). Moreover, there is evidence indicating that there is more DNA fragmentation in cells showing no detectable GAD67 mRNA in patients with BD than controls. These findings suggest that non-GABAergic cells may be selectively vulnerable to oxidative stress in patients with BD (Buttner et al. 2007).

A recent review focused on the medial prefrontal cortex (mPFC) network and reported the presence of a volume decrease with reductions in neuronal size and/or changes in neuronal density, reductions in glial cell density and changes in gene expression. These findings point to both white and grey matter loss probably on the basis of a reduction in the cell counts of specific subpopulations of GABAergic interneurons (Savitz et al. 2014).

13.3.2 Functional Studies

13.3.2.1 Functional Neuroimaging

Unfortunately the functional neuroimaging studies are usually restricted to the depressive phase of the illness simply because when patients are in an acute manic phase, it is very difficult to provide the level of collaboration needed to apply this kind of examination.

One of the rare studies on mania reported an increased activity in the left dorsal ACC (BA 24 and 32) and postulated the presence of a state-dependent activation of a left fronto-striatal neural system that includes the ACC and the caudate nucleus (Blumberg et al. 2000). Another study was in accord with this observation and also showed a decreased metabolism in the left sgACC (BA 25 and part of 24) during the depressed phase in familial BD (Drevets et al. 1997). This latter finding may partly reflect the concomitant grey matter volume reduction that reached 39 % in this area. In contrast, a PET analysis in 27 medication-free, mildly to severely depressed BD patients revealed that the psychomotor–anhedonia symptom cluster correlated with increased metabolism in the right ACC raising the question of interhemispheric differences in ACC involvement in BD (Dunn et al. 2002). Besides the already mentioned methodological limitations, the impact of psychopharmacological treatment on metabolic values at rest is a key parameter to consider when interpreting these data. For instance, the administration of lithium or valproate is associated with increased metabolism in right pregenual ACC in BD-II patients as compared to controls (Mah et al. 2007).

Activation data in untreated BD patients could be divided into two main categories: those obtained with classical neuropsychological tests and those corresponding to emotionally significant situations. Neuropsychological activation studies mainly included working memory, executive function and attention paradigms. Functional MRI results were quite variable in respect to possible trait- related changes. For instance, while performing a 2-back visuospatial working memory task, children and adolescents with stable BD showed an increased activation of the ACC bilaterally compared to controls (Chang et al. 2004). In contrast, negative or discrepant data were obtained after activation using the Stroop interference task (Gruber et al.

2004). In terms of state-related changes, increased metabolic rates were found in the left dorsal ACC using PET in manic patients during tests involving decision-making and sustained attention (Rubinsztein et al. 2001). In the same line, SPECT data pointed to the relationship between poor executive function performance and increased CC metabolism in unmedicated manic patients (Benabarre et al. 2005). However, most fMRI studies still support the hypofrontality hypothesis in mania (Altshuler et al. 2005; Blumberg et al. 2003; Roth et al. 2006).

Emotional activation in BD led to strikingly discrepant trait- and state-dependent fMRI patterns. During the visualization of positively valenced pictures, familial euthymic BD patients had greater activation in the left ACC, while during the visualization of negatively valenced pictures, they displayed a decreased activation in the right PCC compared to controls (Chang et al. 2004). Euthymic BD patients exhibited an increased activity in the right pregenual ACC in response to both angry and happy faces compared to neutral faces (Pavuluri et al. 2007). Conversely, a fMRI study of ten euthymic patients with BD-I and ten age- and gender-matched healthy subjects during a modified word-based memory task designed to implicitly evoke negative, positive or no affective changes showed a significantly greater ACC and PCC activation by both negative and positive affects in healthy subjects as compared to patients in response (Malhi et al. 2007). During an emotional and nonemotional go/no-go test, euthymic BD patients displayed an increased activity in the left dorsal ACC (BA 24) and right PCC (BA 23) when inhibiting emotional compared to neutral stimuli (Wessa et al. 2007).

Patients with mania had attenuated subjective rating of the intensity of sad facial expressions that was associated with decreased activation in the sgACC and bilateral amygdala and increased activation in the PCC and posterior insula (Lennox et al. 2004). Importantly, the rostral ACC response to emotional faces was decreased in unmedicated, but not in medicated, manic patients compared to controls pointing to the possibility that mood-stabilizing medications may reverse functional abnormalities in BD (Blumberg et al. 2005). This is further supported by recent PET/SPECT studies on the induction of negative emotions in BD. Both at baseline and after transient sadness induction, euthymic BD patients had an increase in dorsal ACC (BA 24a) and a decrease in the left PCC (BA 24 and 31) rCBF compared to controls. Depressed patients showed only a decrease in the right PCC (BA 31) (Kruger et al. 2003). A subsequent PET study utilizing the same method in nine euthymic lithium responders and nine healthy siblings revealed that induced sadness increases rCBF in the ACC in all subjects. The siblings' pattern of rCBF changes was similar to that of the lithium-treated patients and included an increased rCBF in the dorsal and rostral ACC (BA 24a/b) (Kruger et al. 2006).

13.3.2.2 Impact of Pharmacological Treatment on Activation Patterns

It is a very difficult task to isolate the effect of pharmacological treatment on metabolic patterns in BD patients. However, most contributions confirm the well-known confounding influence of most psychotropic agents. Overall, the literature suggests that medicated BD patients exhibit greater activation in the ACC in comparison to drug-free BD patients (Strakowski et al. 2005).

Concerning lithium, the double-blind acute withdrawal of lithium was associated with a marked decrease of perfusion in limbic areas and mainly in the ACC. Interestingly, half of patients developed manic symptoms during the placebo phase, which was accompanied by a relative increase of perfusion in the superior ACC (Goodwin et al. 1997). During treatment, lithium-treated patients displayed an increased activation of BA 24a, whereas valproate treatment seems to decrease the metabolic rates in this area (Kruger et al. 2006). However, proton magnetic resonance spectroscopy (1H MRS) indicated that acute lithium treatment is associated with a significant reduction in the myoinositol/creatine ratio. This decrement was also present in lithium responders when analysed separately from nonresponders (Davanzo et al. 2001).

A PET study on ten depressed BD patients and ten controls suggests that the administration of high-dose levothyroxine treatment adjunctive to ongoing medication (antidepressants and mood stabilizers) reduced the significantly higher activity in the right sgACC (areas 25 and part of 24) measured before treatment in BP depressed patients compared to controls. In contrast to that observed in subcortical structures, this decrease did not correlate with symptom improvement (Bauer et al. 2005).

An MRS study of glutamate+glutamine/creatine ratio (Glx/Cr) in the ACC of ten untreated manic and eight risperidone-treated BD children suggested that untreated children had a lower Glx/Cr (Moore et al. 2007a). Another MRS study evaluated the status of the ACC at baseline and after an open trial of lamotrigine in 23 BD depressed patients and 12 control subjects. It revealed that baseline CSF-corrected absolute concentrations of Glx, glutamate (Glu) and creatine+phosphocreatine (Cr) were significantly higher in BD depressed subjects vs. healthy controls. The nonmelancholic subtype had significantly higher baseline Glx and Glu levels than the melancholic subtype. Remission with lamotrigine was associated with a significant decrease in glutamine (Gln) concentrations (Frye et al. 2007). A third MRS study exploring again the Glu and Glx levels in the ACC of 22 (15 medicated and 7 unmedicated) children and adolescents with BD vs. ten healthy controls suggests that untreated BD patients have significantly lower glutamine levels than controls or medicated patients. In the light of the cardinal role of glial cells in glutamate metabolism, these results suggest the presence of an abnormality in ACC glia in untreated children and adolescents with BD (Moore et al. 2007b).

13.3.3 Neurotransmitters and Receptors

Data coming from animal experiments and models implicate the limbic–diencephalic brain in mood disorders and more specifically neurons containing serotonin and noradrenaline. Historically the monoamine deficiency hypothesis is based on data from the study of the cerebrospinal fluid (CSF) metabolites. According to this theory, there is a monoamine deficiency, especially norepinephrine (NE), in depression. Later, studies illustrated that this theory should also include serotonin (5-HT), leading to a broader theory regarding neurotransmission disorder in the central nervous system (CNS) (Schildkraut 1965; Maas 1975; Van Praag and Leijnse 1963).

Later, the cholinergic–noradrenergic imbalance hypothesis (Davidson 1972; Tarsy et al. 1972; Janowsky et al. 1972) included acetylcholine in a broader model for mood disorders. More complex models include state changes (depending on the polarity of the mood episode) in the excitatory amino acid function in specific areas of the cortex (Fountoulakis et al. 2008a).

However, in spite of decades of extensive research, there is no definite proof for either a deficiency or an excess of either the quantity or the overall functioning of biogenic amines in specific brain structures. Even when these abnormalities were documented, it has been shown that they are neither necessary nor sufficient for the occurrence of mood disorders. In contrast, it seems that the neurotransmitter disorders recognized until today refer to a broader behavioural dysfunction which includes behavioural disinhibition, obsessive–compulsive symptoms, anxiety, eating disorders and substance and alcohol abuse as well as personality disorders. This is not peculiar since most classic animal models are in essence post-traumatic stress models and most biological psychoendocrinological markers are markers of stress-related somatic reactions. Recent research explores disturbances at the level of second messengers and close to DNA function with variable success but no definite conclusions.

Using a 5-HT radioligand in 18 depressed, unmedicated BD patients and 37 controls, the same group showed that in BD, the mean 5-HT binding is increased in the dorsal CC. Most importantly, the presence of anxiety symptoms (and mainly obsessions and compulsions) correlated positively with 5-HT binding in the dorsal CC. BD suicide attempters displayed an increased 5-HT binding in ACC compared to both controls and BD non-attempters (Cannon et al. 2006b). A more recent PET study of 11 unmedicated BD patients revealed that they had significantly lower dopamine transporter (DAT) availability relative to healthy controls in the dorsal caudate bilaterally (Anand et al. 2011).

Another PET study assessed the binding potential of muscarinic M2 receptors in 16 unmedicated BD patients in depressive phase vs. 17 unipolar patients and 23 controls. BD patients had a lower mean ACC M2 receptor binding compared to both unipolar depressive patients and controls. The authors suggested that this reduction could be explained by a reduction in M2 receptor density or affinity. Alternatively, it could indicate an elevation in endogenous acetylcholine levels in BD patients compared to the other two groups (Cannon et al. 2006a). Negative autoradiographic data were mainly published for M1 and M4 receptors (Zavitsanou et al. 2004, 2005) with the marked exception of a significant effect of suicide on [(3)H]pirenzepine binding in the ACC in BD (Zavitsanou et al. 2004).

While for unipolar depression the antidepressant effect on serotonin pathways is considered to be both a necessary and a sufficient condition for the achievement of the treatment response, this is not the case with bipolar depression. It is true however that the neurobiology of bipolar depression still remains elusive and the assumption that serotonin has a dominant role comes from the belief that unipolar and bipolar depression share at least some neurobiologic substrates. However, the monoamine hypothesis for unipolar depression is based mainly on treatment data (TCAs and SSRIs), and these treatments have no proven efficacy against bipolar depression.

One of the theories that exist so far suggested that the 5-HT-1A receptor is the most likely target (Yatham et al. 2005). However, the data available today do not support such an assumption, since that receptor is activated by aripiprazole, lamotrigine, ziprasidone and other compounds which are proven not to be efficacious (Fountoulakis et al. 2008a, b; Fountoulakis and Vieta 2008; Fountoulakis et al. 2007; Vieta et al. 2010). A second model reviewed both the clinical treatment data as well as the preclinical properties of those agents with proven efficacy against bipolar depression vs. those with proven non-efficacy (Fountoulakis et al. 2012). The results suggested that the stronger predictors for antidepressant efficacy in bipolar depression were norepinephrine alpha-1, dopamine D1 and histamine antagonism. However, while they seem to be a necessary condition, they don't seem to be sufficient, since they characterize agents without bipolar antidepressant efficacy. The second stronger cluster of predictor activities includes 5-HT2A, muscarinic and dopamine D2 and D3 antagonism, 5-HT-1A agonism and norepinephrine reuptake inhibition. All the above properties characterize both quetiapine and the OFC and seem to be a unique combination not shared by any of the drugs without bipolar antidepressant efficacy.

The importance of the blockade of dopamine receptors is an open question; it could simply be the consequence of the presence of antipsychotic properties in both quetiapine and the OFC. These antipsychotic/antimanic properties could constitute an important element for an agent to succeed in an RCT on bipolar depression, since they might protect from manic switches and subsequently from dropouts (which was largely the cause for the failure of venlafaxine).

Eventually this model suggests that norepinephrine reuptake and 5-HT-1A agonism are at the centre and closer to the core deficit and points out that serotonin reuptake is not a sufficient condition for antidepressant efficacy in bipolar depression, and this is in sharp contrast with unipolar depression. Although 5-HT-1A activation is necessary, it is not sufficient. Another core conclusion is that norepinephrine activity is more important.

A line of research is also in accord with the results and conclusions of the current review. The literature suggests that both serotonin and norepinephrine are lower in the locus ceruleus of bipolar patients who died from suicide (Wiste et al. 2008) and that norepinephrine might play a more important role than serotonin in the pathophysiology of bipolar disorder (Young et al. 1994). It has been proposed that the antidepressant activity of quetiapine is mediated, at least in part, by its metabolite N-desalkylquetiapine through norepinephrine reuptake inhibition and partial 5-HT(1A) agonism (Jensen et al. 2008). Also, chronic administration of olanzapine alone significantly increased firing of locus ceruleus (LC) neurons, while chronic administration of fluoxetine alone significantly reduced firing of LC neurons. It seems that in the combination condition (OFC), olanzapine was able to block the fluoxetine-induced suppression of the LC, and a significant increase in LC activity was observed (Seager et al. 2004, 2005).

Similarly, there are no evidences supporting a significant involvement of the human endogenous cannabinoid system (Burnet and Harrison 2000; Koethe et al. 2007; Peckys and Hurd 2001).

The GABA is considered to be a promising target of research for the elucidation of the pathophysiology of BD but also for the development of novel treatment approaches (Fountoulakis et al. 2012).

A possible deficit in GABA and developmental/synaptic neurochemical systems in BD has been sustained by the detailed analysis of Torrey et al. who assessed up to 100 RNA, protein and other neurochemical markers in a single set of 60 post-mortem brains including 15 from patients with BD (Torrey et al. 2005). Nine post-mortem studies attempted to explore whether changes in receptor densities may influence the expression of key inhibitory or excitatory pathways in BD brains. The density of GABAergic terminals was significantly reduced in all four layers of BA 24 bilaterally. This reduction was most significant in layers II (27.8 %) and III (37.2 %) (Benes et al. 2000, 2001). The study of GABA neurons containing NMDA 2A subunit mRNA in the anterior cingulate cortex (ACC) suggested that their numerical density was decreased by 60 % in layer 2 in patients with BD (Woo et al. 2004). The same researchers reported that in the ACC the subset of GABA interneurons that contained the calcium-binding protein calbindin (with preferential localization to layer 2) was either increased in density or had become more frequently NR2A expressing in patients with schizophrenia compared with the normal control subjects and subjects with BD (Woo et al. 2008b).

The use of calcium-binding proteins (CBPs) parvalbumin (PV), calretinin (CR) and calbindin-D28K (CB) as markers of cortical gamma aminobutyric acid (GABA) neurotransmission in BD did not confirm the involvement of GABA inhibitory circuits in this disorder (Cotter et al. 2002). In the same line, a recent GAD immunocytochemical analysis did not identify differences between BD and controls rendering unlikely a deficit of GABA synthesis in bipolar patients (Bielau et al. 2007).

State-related biochemical changes were also analysed with proton MRS studies. The comparison of ACC choline (Cho) and myoinositol (MI) levels in 9 BD patients taking either lithium or valproate, and 14 controls revealed that BD depression severity correlated positively with Cho/creatine–phosphocreatine (Cr-PCr) in the left CC. No clinical or drug-related changes were observed for the MI/Cr–PCr ratio in this study (Moore et al. 2000) as well as in a similar one (Bertolino et al. 2003). In contrast, significantly higher MI levels and MI/Cr–PCr ratio as well as N-acetyl-L-aspartate (NAA) and glutamate–glutamine metabolite levels were measured in 10 depressed BD patients as compared to 10 patients with intermittent explosive disorder and 13 controls (Davanzo et al. 2003). In line with this observation, mania has been associated with reduced glutamate/glutamine levels in the ACC (Moore et al. 2007a). In terms of trait-related changes, euthymic BD patients receiving lithium treatment for at least 4 weeks showed no significant difference in the ACC NAA/Cr and Cho/Cr ratio compared to controls. However, chronic administration of psychotropic drugs could have had an independent effect on NAA/Cr. In conclusion, these results suggest that NAA, which is a putative marker of neuronal density and a measure of neuronal viability and integrity, could be reduced in the ACC of BD patients, and medication might be able to reverse this deficit. They also suggest that mania may be associated with reduced glutamate/glutamine levels in the ACC. Medication acts here as a confounding factor again.

In the use of in situ radioligand binding and autoradiography to measure neurochemical markers in the prefrontal cortex (PFC) Brodmann area (BA), nine revealed an age-related decrease in NMDA receptor density in control subjects that was absent in schizophrenia and BD (Dean et al. 2001). Two other studies suggested that in the PFC, glutamatergic regulation via the subunit 2A-containing NMDA receptors does not appear to be altered in bipolar disorder in contrast to schizophrenia (Bitanihirwe et al. 2010; Woo et al. 2008a). This was confirmed by a study from another research group, which reported decreased NR1 expression in the dorsolateral prefrontal cortex of bipolar patients and no changes of NR2B or NR2D. Although the NR1 is obligatory, receptor autoradiography revealed no alterations in receptor binding, indicating no change in total receptor number. These authors also measured associated postsynaptic density (PSD) protein (PSD95, neurofilament light (NF-L) and SAP102) transcripts and reported reduced NF-L expression in schizophrenia and reduced SAP102 expression in bipolar disorder restricted to small cells of layer II and large cells of layer III. Taken all together these data suggest abnormal receptor stoichiometry (Beneyto and Meador-Woodruff 2008). The same research group had previously reported the NR3A mRNA was significantly decreased by 12 % in bipolar disorder relative to the comparison group in the dorsolateral prefrontal cortex (Mueller and Meador-Woodruff 2004).

The situ hybridization to assess hippocampal expression of the transcripts encoding NMDA receptor subunits NR1, 2A, 2B, 2C and 2D and the transcripts for the NMDA receptor-associated PSD proteins PSD95, PSD93, NF-L and SAP102 revealed a significant decrease in the expression of transcripts for NR1 and NR2A subunits and SAP102 in BD but no changes in schizophrenia (McCullumsmith et al. 2007). However, peculiarly, the same group reports negative or conflicting results concerning the hippocampus (Beneyto et al. 2007). Another research group did not confirm the reduction in the NR1 specifically in the hippocampal dentate gyrus, but did find a decrease in PSD-95 in the dentate molecular layer (Toro and Deakin 2005). The use of in situ radioligand binding with semiquantitative autoradiography, to measure the density of [3H]MK-801, [3H]CGP39653 (that bind to NMDA receptors), [3H]AMPA and [3H]kainate binding in hippocampi, suggested that in subjects with BD there were significant decreases in the density of [3H]MK-801 binding in the cornu ammonis as well as the pyramidal and polymorphic layers of the subiculum. There were no changes in the densities of [3H]AMPA or [3H]kainate binding in these subjects (Scarr et al. 2003).

In the perirhinal cortex, a decreased expression of NR1 and NR2B is reported (Beneyto et al. 2007); however, another research group did not find any changes in NR1 or PSD-95 in the orbitofrontal cortex (OFC) of bipolar patients (Toro and Deakin 2005).

The investigation of the NR1 subunit in superior temporal cortex (STC) using radioligand binding of [(3)H]L-689,560 to the glycine site and quantitative immunoblotting techniques revealed an increased receptor density in schizophrenia and decrease in bipolar and depressive disorders (Nudmamud-Thanoi and Reynolds 2004).

In the striatum an expression of transcripts encoding PSD-95 and SAP-102 is reported in BD, while no significant changes in NF-L and PSD-93 mRNAs were observed (Kristiansen and Meador-Woodruff 2005). In the thalamus, no changes in

NR1 and NR2A-D were found; however, there was a decreased NF-L, PSD95 and SAP102 transcripts in the thalamus of patients with BD (Clinton and Meador-Woodruff 2004).

Genetic studies suggest a relationship of genes encoding the 1, 2A and 2B subunits of the NMDA receptor with bipolar illness implying a hypoglutamatergic state in bipolar patients. However, the studies are few and have not been replicated. Neuropathological studies suggest a possible decrease in the density of NMDA receptor and more consistently a reduced NMDA-mediated glutamatergic activity in patients with BD. The literature suggests a reduction of NMDA density in the PFC as well as abnormal NMDA composition. In the ACC a reduction of 2A subunit is reported. In the hippocampus data are conflicting concerning the NMDA density, but they confirm a functional hypoactivity specific for this kind of receptors. No changes in density, only functional hypoactivity was reported for the thalamus. Lithium seems to reduce NMDA activity possibly through reduced phosphorylation of this receptor.

Thus, the literature might suggest BD is related with slower NMDA kinetics because of lower contribution of NR2A subunits. This could serve to bridge neurodevelopmental hypotheses for the development of BD and neuropharmacological data. Slower kinetics might make NMDA receptors incapable of dealing with the increased speed of stimuli during manic episodes leading to disorganization (Fountoulakis et al. 2012).

A number of biological markers have been developed so far to assist the diagnosis and assessment of depression, but no one is proved so far strong enough for use in clinical practice. The dexamethasone-suppression test (DST) has been widely used for the study of hypothalamus–pituitary–adrenal (HPA) axis disorders in patients with depression (Green and Kane 1983; Evans and Golden 1987; Stokes et al. 1984). It requires the oral administration of 1 mg dexamethasone (a synthetic glucocorticoid) at 23:00 on day 1 and the assessment of cortisol levels at the same time, at 08:00, at 16:00 and at 23:00 on day 2. A cortisol value of 5 μg/dl, in at least one measurement in day 2, is considered to be the cut-off point between normal (suppressors) and pathological (non-suppressors). Longer protocols requiring higher dosage for dexamethasone and a 24 h long assessment have also been suggested. The test presents a 67 % sensitivity and 96 % specificity in the diagnosis of melancholy in psychiatric inpatients. The results of the up-to-date research efforts report that DST presents results that are probably related with the severity of depression and the patient's family history. Other psychoendocrinological markers are the TRH stimulation test (blunted thyroid-stimulating hormone response to thyrotropin-releasing hormone) (Musselman and Nemeroff 1996; Kendler et al. 2000) and the fluramine and d-fenfluramine challenge tests which (Siever et al. 1984; Fessler et al. 1984; Quattrone et al. 1979; Garattini et al. 1987; Di Renzo et al. 1989; Rowland and Carlton 1986) are supposed to reflect central serotonin activity (administration of 30 mg of the d-fenfluramine orally and measurement of prolactin plasma levels at the baseline and 60′, 120′, 180′, 240′ and 300′ after the administration), blunted growth hormone (GH) response to the a2-adrenergic receptor agonist clonidine (an index of noradrenergic dysregulation) and others. A non-endocrinological marker is based on EEG and concerns the observation that depressed patients are phase advanced in many biological rhythms, especially concerning the latency to the first rapid eye movement in sleep (shortened REM latency) (Kupfer 1976).

A possible comprehensive model could suggest that mood patients have a deficit in the adequate mobilization of neurotransmitters when facing continued or repeated stress, and as a result, through a 'kindling' effect (Kendler et al. 2000; Post and Silberstein 1994; Post et al. 1984, 1988, 1992; Post and Weiss 1989, 1998) the mood change is intense, prolonged and not self-limited and tends to be triggered by progressively unimportant events and finally automatically.

13.3.4 Genetic Studies

The role of genetics in the development of BD is well known, and there is significant support in the literature from family, twin and adoption studies. It is also known that the mechanisms through witch genetic factors play a role are complex, probably with several of them interacting with the environment.

Not only the genes involved are multiple but also the mode of transmission seems to be complex; thus, BD is not a Mendelian disease (Andreassen et al. 2013). On the contrary it seems that it manifests significant genetic heterogeneity. Methodological issues also exist and perplex the problem but emerging technologies promise to solve at least some of the problems. Research is rapidly moving towards the utilization of genome-wide association scan (GWAS) studies (Segurado et al. 2003).

So far one of the greatest problems is that studies suffer from poor replicability and explain only a small portion of the genetic variance (around 70–80 %). Overall mood disorders have a reduced penetrance (less than 100 %) which increases with age. Little is known about the role of epigenetics and imprinting in BD.

Overall, family studies indicate a morbid risk of BD in first-degree relatives of bipolar probands that ranges between 3 and 8 % that is significantly higher in comparison to the general population. It is interesting to note that unipolar depression is the most common mood disorder in families of bipolar probands, while the reverse does not happen. Patients with BD are more likely to marry a person who also has a mood disorder (assortative mating). This leads to families with higher load than expected. Twin studies often pool together unipolar and bipolar disorders and report a two to four times higher risk for monozygotic twins in comparison to dizygotic. When BD is contrasted with unipolar depression the genetic load appears to be higher for BD. Again, as in family studies, unipolar depression is the most common mood disorder in monozygotic co-twins of bipolar probands. Concerning adoption studies, only a few exist and their results are inconclusive (Kelsoe 2009).

The analysis of genetic data to elucidate the mechanism of genetic transmission has not given robust results yet probably because the data are inconsistent. Most findings so far have not been replicated. Essentially all models of transmission that have been tested were rejected. The presence of multiple genes and simultaneously of multiple modes of transmission is the probable answer. It is fortunate that genetic research is one of the hottest and fastest developing areas of research on BD. On the other hand it is unfortunate that the fruits are yet to come. Often weak findings are reported (Badner et al. 2012). A meta-analysis reported that six pathways (corticotropin-releasing hormone signalling, cardiac beta-adrenergic signalling, phospholipase C signalling, glutamate receptor signalling, endothelin 1 signalling and cardiac hypertrophy signalling) and nine genes (CACNA1C, DTNA, FOXP1, GNG2, ITPR2, LSAMP, NPAS3, NCOA2 and NTRK3) were found to relate with BD (Nurnberger et al. 2014). Another review concluded that the expression profiles of BD-associated genes do not explain the majority of structural abnormalities observed in BD (McCarthy et al. 2014).

A GWAS study in 1461 BD patients reported that after genotyping for 372,193 single nucleotide polymorphisms (SNPs), the strongest results concerned myosin5B (MYO5B) and tetraspanin-8 (TSPAN8) and possibly the epidermal growth factor receptor (EGFR), but the results failed to replicate. Further analysis with the use of controls from the Wellcome Trust Case Control study reported that the results pointed to SNPs related with the voltage-dependent calcium channel, L-type, alpha 1C subunit (CACNA1C) gene (Sklar et al. 2008; Wellcome Trust Case Control 2007). Another GWAS confirmed the involvement of ion channel structural and regulatory genes, including voltage-gated ion channels and the broader ion channel group that comprises both voltage- and ligand-gated channels in the pathogenesis of BD (Askland et al. 2009).

In accord with the above are a number of studies concerning the genes related with NMDA receptors (Mundo et al. 2003; Itokawa et al. 2003; Avramopoulos et al. 2007; Martucci et al. 2006; Fountoulakis et al. 2012). These studies suggested that BD is associated with an abnormal structure of the NMDA receptor because of lower contribution of NR2A subunits, with predominance of more immature forms resulting in disordered receptor properties and slower kinetics. These slower kinetics might make NMDA receptors incapable of dealing with the increased speed of stimuli during manic episodes leading to disorganization (Fountoulakis et al. 2012).

A number of special issues have also been the focus of genetic research. It has been suggested that some genes are less specific and contribute to multiple phenotypes giving rise to the bipolar spectrum (Kelsoe 2003). There are data suggesting that the hyperthymic temperament relates to chromosomes 1q44, 2p16, 6q16 and 14q23; the dysthymic to chromosomes 3p21 and 13q34; and the irritable to chromosome 6q24 (Greenwood et al. 2013a). Also it has been reported that irritable mania results from a distinct set of genes in comparison to euphoric mania, including a region on chromosome 13q31 (Greenwood et al. 2013b). Comorbidity is another issue with migraine being at the centre (Oedegaard et al. 2010). The genetic distinction between BD and other disorders was also the focus of research. It seems that BD and unipolar depression share some common genetic substrate, while at the same time BD-I and BD-II are not genetically identical. There is also a genetic overlap between BD and schizophrenia (Fountoulakis et al. 2012; Cross-Disorder Group of the Psychiatric Genomics et al. 2013; Andreassen et al. 2013).

References

Adler CM, DelBello MP, Jarvis K, Levine A, Adams J, Strakowski SM (2007) Voxel-based study of structural changes in first-episode patients with bipolar disorder. Biol Psychiatry 61(6):776–781. doi:10.1016/j.biopsych.2006.05.042

Akiskal HS, McKinney WT Jr (1973) Depressive disorders: toward a unified hypothesis. Science 182(4107):20–29

Altshuler LL, Bookheimer SY, Townsend J, Proenza MA, Eisenberger N, Sabb F, Mintz J, Cohen MS (2005) Blunted activation in orbitofrontal cortex during mania: a functional magnetic resonance imaging study. Biol Psychiatry 58(10):763–769. doi:10.1016/j.biopsych.2005.09.012

Anand A, Barkay G, Dzemidzic M, Albrecht D, Karne H, Zheng QH, Hutchins GD, Normandin MD, Yoder KK (2011) Striatal dopamine transporter availability in unmedicated bipolar disorder. Bipolar Disord 13(4):406–413. doi:10.1111/j.1399-5618.2011.00936.x

Anderson AK, Phelps EA (2002) Is the human amygdala critical for the subjective experience of emotion? Evidence of intact dispositional affect in patients with amygdala lesions. J Cogn Neurosci 14(5):709–720. doi:10.1162/08989290260138618

Andreassen OA, Thompson WK, Schork AJ, Ripke S, Mattingsdal M, Kelsoe JR, Kendler KS, O'Donovan MC, Rujescu D, Werge T, Sklar P, Psychiatric Genomics C, Bipolar D, Schizophrenia Working G, Roddey JC, Chen CH, McEvoy L, Desikan RS, Djurovic S, Dale AM (2013) Improved detection of common variants associated with schizophrenia and bipolar disorder using pleiotropy-informed conditional false discovery rate. PLoS Genet 9(4):e1003455. doi:10.1371/journal.pgen.1003455

Arango C, Rapado-Castro M, Reig S, Castro-Fornieles J, Gonzalez-Pinto A, Otero S, Baeza I, Moreno C, Graell M, Janssen J, Parellada M, Moreno D, Bargallo N, Desco M (2012) Progressive brain changes in children and adolescents with first-episode psychosis. Arch Gen Psychiatry 69(1):16–26. doi:10.1001/archgenpsychiatry.2011.150

Askland K, Read C, Moore J (2009) Pathways-based analyses of whole-genome association study data in bipolar disorder reveal genes mediating ion channel activity and synaptic neurotransmission. Hum Genet 125(1):63–79. doi:10.1007/s00439-008-0600-y

Atmaca M, Ozdemir H, Cetinkaya S, Parmaksiz S, Belli H, Poyraz AK, Tezcan E, Ogur E (2007) Cingulate gyrus volumetry in drug free bipolar patients and patients treated with valproate or valproate and quetiapine. J Psychiatr Res 41(10):821–827. doi:10.1016/j.jpsychires.2006.07.006

Auer DP, Putz B, Kraft E, Lipinski B, Schill J, Holsboer F (2000) Reduced glutamate in the anterior cingulate cortex in depression: an in vivo proton magnetic resonance spectroscopy study. Biol Psychiatry 47(4):305–313

Avramopoulos D, Lasseter VK, Fallin MD, Wolyniec PS, McGrath JA, Nestadt G, Valle D, Pulver AE (2007) Stage II follow-up on a linkage scan for bipolar disorder in the Ashkenazim provides suggestive evidence for chromosome 12p and the GRIN2B gene. Genet Med 9(11):745–751. doi:10.1097/GIM.0b013e318159a37c

Badner JA, Koller D, Foroud T, Edenberg H, Nurnberger JI Jr, Zandi PP, Willour VL, McMahon FJ, Potash JB, Hamshere M, Grozeva D, Green E, Kirov G, Jones I, Jones L, Craddock N, Morris D, Segurado R, Gill M, Sadovnick D, Remick R, Keck P, Kelsoe J, Ayub M, MacLean A, Blackwood D, Liu CY, Gershon ES, McMahon W, Lyon GJ, Robinson R, Ross J, Byerley W (2012) Genome-wide linkage analysis of 972 bipolar pedigrees using single-nucleotide polymorphisms. Mol Psychiatry 17(8):818–826. doi:10.1038/mp.2011.89

Balanza-Martinez V, Tabares-Seisdedos R, Selva-Vera G, Martinez-Aran A, Torrent C, Salazar-Fraile J, Leal-Cercos C, Vieta E, Gomez-Beneyto M (2005) Persistent cognitive dysfunctions in bipolar I disorder and schizophrenic patients: a 3-year follow-up study. Psychother Psychosom 74(2):113–119. doi:10.1159/000083170

Bauer M, London ED, Rasgon N, Berman SM, Frye MA, Altshuler LL, Mandelkern MA, Bramen J, Voytek B, Woods R, Mazziotta JC, Whybrow PC (2005) Supraphysiological doses of levothyroxine alter regional cerebral metabolism and improve mood in bipolar depression. Mol Psychiatry 10(5):456–469. doi:10.1038/sj.mp.4001647

Bearden CE, Thompson PM, Dalwani M, Hayashi KM, Lee AD, Nicoletti M, Trakhtenbroit M, Glahn DC, Brambilla P, Sassi RB, Mallinger AG, Frank E, Kupfer DJ, Soares JC (2007) Greater cortical gray matter density in lithium-treated patients with bipolar disorder. Biol Psychiatry 62(1):7–16. doi:10.1016/j.biopsych.2006.10.027

Benabarre A, Vieta E, Martinez-Aran A, Garcia-Garcia M, Martin F, Lomena F, Torrent C, Sanchez-Moreno J, Colom F, Reinares M, Brugue E, Valdes M (2005) Neuropsychological disturbances and cerebral blood flow in bipolar disorder. Aust N Z J Psychiatry 39(4):227–234. doi:10.1111/j.1440-1614.2004.01558.x

Benes FM, Todtenkopf MS, Logiotatos P, Williams M (2000) Glutamate decarboxylase(65)-immunoreactive terminals in cingulate and prefrontal cortices of schizophrenic and bipolar brain. J Chem Neuroanat 20(3–4):259–269

Benes FM, Vincent SL, Todtenkopf M (2001) The density of pyramidal and nonpyramidal neurons in anterior cingulate cortex of schizophrenic and bipolar subjects. Biol Psychiatry 50(6):395–406

Benes FM, Walsh J, Bhattacharyya S, Sheth A, Berretta S (2003) DNA fragmentation decreased in schizophrenia but not bipolar disorder. Arch Gen Psychiatry 60(4):359–364. doi:10.1001/archpsyc.60.4.359

Beneyto M, Meador-Woodruff JH (2008) Lamina-specific abnormalities of NMDA receptor-associated postsynaptic protein transcripts in the prefrontal cortex in schizophrenia and bipolar disorder. Neuropsychopharmacology 33(9):2175–2186. doi:10.1038/sj.npp.1301604

Beneyto M, Kristiansen LV, Oni-Orisan A, McCullumsmith RE, Meador-Woodruff JH (2007) Abnormal glutamate receptor expression in the medial temporal lobe in schizophrenia and mood disorders. Neuropsychopharmacology 32(9):1888–1902. doi:10.1038/sj.npp.1301312

Berk M, Hallam K, Malhi GS, Henry L, Hasty M, Macneil C, Yucel M, Pantelis C, Murphy B, Vieta E, Dodd S, McGorry PD (2010) Evidence and implications for early intervention in bipolar disorder. J Ment Health 19(2):113–126. doi:10.3109/09638230903469111

Bertolino A, Frye M, Callicott JH, Mattay VS, Rakow R, Shelton-Repella J, Post R, Weinberger DR (2003) Neuronal pathology in the hippocampal area of patients with bipolar disorder: a study with proton magnetic resonance spectroscopic imaging. Biol Psychiatry 53(10):906–913

Bielau H, Steiner J, Mawrin C, Trubner K, Brisch R, Meyer-Lotz G, Brodhun M, Dobrowolny H, Baumann B, Gos T, Bernstein HG, Bogerts B (2007) Dysregulation of GABAergic neurotransmission in mood disorders: a postmortem study. Ann N Y Acad Sci 1096:157–169. doi:10.1196/annals.1397.081

Bitanihirwe BK, Lim MP, Woo TU (2010) N-methyl-D-aspartate receptor expression in parvalbumin-containing inhibitory neurons in the prefrontal cortex in bipolar disorder. Bipolar Disord 12(1):95–101. doi:10.1111/j.1399-5618.2009.00785.x

Blumberg HP, Stern E, Martinez D, Ricketts S, de Asis J, White T, Epstein J, McBride PA, Eidelberg D, Kocsis JH, Silbersweig DA (2000) Increased anterior cingulate and caudate activity in bipolar mania. Biol Psychiatry 48(11):1045–1052

Blumberg HP, Leung HC, Skudlarski P, Lacadie CM, Fredericks CA, Harris BC, Charney DS, Gore JC, Krystal JH, Peterson BS (2003) A functional magnetic resonance imaging study of bipolar disorder: state- and trait-related dysfunction in ventral prefrontal cortices. Arch Gen Psychiatry 60(6):601–609. doi:10.1001/archpsyc.60.6.601

Blumberg HP, Donegan NH, Sanislow CA, Collins S, Lacadie C, Skudlarski P, Gueorguieva R, Fulbright RK, McGlashan TH, Gore JC, Krystal JH (2005) Preliminary evidence for medication effects on functional abnormalities in the amygdala and anterior cingulate in bipolar disorder. Psychopharmacology (Berl) 183(3):308–313. doi:10.1007/s00213-005-0156-7

Blumberg HP, Krystal JH, Bansal R, Martin A, Dziura J, Durkin K, Martin L, Gerard E, Charney DS, Peterson BS (2006) Age, rapid-cycling, and pharmacotherapy effects on ventral prefrontal cortex in bipolar disorder: a cross-sectional study. Biol Psychiatry 59(7):611–618. doi:10.1016/j.biopsych.2005.08.031

Bora E, Fornito A, Yucel M, Pantelis C (2010) Voxelwise meta-analysis of gray matter abnormalities in bipolar disorder. Biol Psychiatry 67(11):1097–1105. doi:10.1016/j.biopsych.2010.01.020

Bouras C, Kovari E, Hof PR, Riederer BM, Giannakopoulos P (2001) Anterior cingulate cortex pathology in schizophrenia and bipolar disorder. Acta Neuropathol 102(4):373–379

Brambilla P, Nicoletti MA, Harenski K, Sassi RB, Mallinger AG, Frank E, Kupfer DJ, Keshavan MS, Soares JC (2002) Anatomical MRI study of subgenual prefrontal cortex in bipolar and unipolar subjects. Neuropsychopharmacology 27(5):792–799. doi:10.1016/S0893-133X(02)00352-4

Bruno SD, Barker GJ, Cercignani M, Symms M, Ron MA (2004) A study of bipolar disorder using magnetization transfer imaging and voxel-based morphometry. Brain 127(Pt 11):2433–2440. doi:10.1093/brain/awh274

Bruno SD, Papadopoulou K, Cercignani M, Cipolotti L, Ron MA (2006) Structural brain correlates of IQ changes in bipolar disorder. Psychol Med 36(5):609–618. doi:10.1017/S0033291706007112

Burnet PW, Harrison PJ (2000) Substance P (NK1) receptors in the cingulate cortex in unipolar and bipolar mood disorder and schizophrenia. Biol Psychiatry 47(1):80–83

Buttner N, Bhattacharyya S, Walsh J, Benes FM (2007) DNA fragmentation is increased in non-GABAergic neurons in bipolar disorder but not in schizophrenia. Schizophr Res 93(1–3):33–41. doi:10.1016/j.schres.2007.01.030

Cannon DM, Carson RE, Nugent AC, Eckelman WC, Kiesewetter DO, Williams J, Rollis D, Drevets M, Gandhi S, Solorio G, Drevets WC (2006a) Reduced muscarinic type 2 receptor binding in subjects with bipolar disorder. Arch Gen Psychiatry 63(7):741–747. doi:10.1001/archpsyc.63.7.741

Cannon DM, Ichise M, Fromm SJ, Nugent AC, Rollis D, Gandhi SK, Klaver JM, Charney DS, Manji HK, Drevets WC (2006b) Serotonin transporter binding in bipolar disorder assessed using [11C]DASB and positron emission tomography. Biol Psychiatry 60(3):207–217. doi:10.1016/j.biopsych.2006.05.005

Chana G, Landau S, Beasley C, Everall IP, Cotter D (2003) Two-dimensional assessment of cytoarchitecture in the anterior cingulate cortex in major depressive disorder, bipolar disorder, and schizophrenia: evidence for decreased neuronal somal size and increased neuronal density. Biol Psychiatry 53(12):1086–1098

Chang K, Adleman NE, Dienes K, Simeonova DI, Menon V, Reiss A (2004) Anomalous prefrontal-subcortical activation in familial pediatric bipolar disorder: a functional magnetic resonance imaging investigation. Arch Gen Psychiatry 61(8):781–792. doi:10.1001/archpsyc.61.8.781

Chow T, Cummings J (2000) Neuropsychiatry: clinical assessment and approach to diagnosis. In: Sadock B, Sadock V (eds) Comprehensive textbook of psychiatry. Lippincott Williams & Wilkins, Philadelphia

Clinton SM, Meador-Woodruff JH (2004) Abnormalities of the NMDA receptor and associated intracellular molecules in the thalamus in schizophrenia and bipolar disorder. Neuropsychopharmacology 29(7):1353–1362. doi:10.1038/sj.npp.1300451

Cotter D, Mackay D, Landau S, Kerwin R, Everall I (2001) Reduced glial cell density and neuronal size in the anterior cingulate cortex in major depressive disorder. Arch Gen Psychiatry 58(6):545–553

Cotter D, Landau S, Beasley C, Stevenson R, Chana G, MacMillan L, Everall I (2002) The density and spatial distribution of GABAergic neurons, labelled using calcium binding proteins, in the anterior cingulate cortex in major depressive disorder, bipolar disorder, and schizophrenia. Biol Psychiatry 51(5):377–386

Coyle TR, Kochunov P, Patel RD, Nery FG, Lancaster JL, Mangin JF, Riviere D, Pillow DR, Davis GJ, Nicoletti MA, Serap Monkul E, Fox PT, Soares JC (2006) Cortical sulci and bipolar disorder. Neuroreport 17(16):1739–1742. doi:10.1097/01.wnr.0000239957.53072.f0

Cross-Disorder Group of the Psychiatric Genomics C, Lee SH, Ripke S, Neale BM, Faraone SV, Purcell SM, Perlis RH, Mowry BJ, Thapar A, Goddard ME, Witte JS, Absher D, Agartz I, Akil H, Amin F, Andreassen OA, Anjorin A, Anney R, Anttila V, Arking DE, Asherson P, Azevedo MH, Backlund L, Badner JA, Bailey AJ, Banaschewski T, Barchas JD, Barnes MR, Barrett TB, Bass N, Battaglia A, Bauer M, Bayes M, Bellivier F, Bergen SE, Berrettini W, Betancur C, Bettecken T, Biederman J, Binder EB, Black DW, Blackwood DH, Bloss CS, Boehnke M, Boomsma DI, Breen G, Breuer R, Bruggeman R, Cormican P, Buccola NG, Buitelaar JK, Bunney WE, Buxbaum JD, Byerley WF, Byrne EM, Caesar S, Cahn W, Cantor RM, Casas M, Chakravarti A, Chambert K, Choudhury K, Cichon S, Cloninger CR, Collier DA, Cook EH, Coon H, Cormand B, Corvin A, Coryell WH, Craig DW, Craig IW, Crosbie J, Cuccaro ML,

Curtis D, Czamara D, Datta S, Dawson G, Day R, De Geus EJ, Degenhardt F, Djurovic S, Donohoe GJ, Doyle AE, Duan J, Dudbridge F, Duketis E, Ebstein RP, Edenberg HJ, Elia J, Ennis S, Etain B, Fanous A, Farmer AE, Ferrier IN, Flickinger M, Fombonne E, Foroud T, Frank J, Franke B, Fraser C, Freedman R, Freimer NB, Freitag CM, Friedl M, Frisen L, Gallagher L, Gejman PV, Georgieva L, Gershon ES, Geschwind DH, Giegling I, Gill M, Gordon SD, Gordon-Smith K, Green EK, Greenwood TA, Grice DE, Gross M, Grozeva D, Guan W, Gurling H, De Haan L, Haines JL, Hakonarson H, Hallmayer J, Hamilton SP, Hamshere ML, Hansen TF, Hartmann AM, Hautzinger M, Heath AC, Henders AK, Herms S, Hickie IB, Hipolito M, Hoefels S, Holmans PA, Holsboer F, Hoogendijk WJ, Hottenga JJ, Hultman CM, Hus V, Ingason A, Ising M, Jamain S, Jones EG, Jones I, Jones L, Tzeng JY, Kahler AK, Kahn RS, Kandaswamy R, Keller MC, Kennedy JL, Kenny E, Kent L, Kim Y, Kirov GK, Klauck SM, Klei L, Knowles JA, Kohli MA, Koller DL, Konte B, Korszun A, Krabbendam L, Krasucki R, Kuntsi J, Kwan P, Landen M, Langstrom N, Lathrop M, Lawrence J, Lawson WB, Leboyer M, Ledbetter DH, Lee PH, Lencz T, Lesch KP, Levinson DF, Lewis CM, Li J, Lichtenstein P, Lieberman JA, Lin DY, Linszen DH, Liu C, Lohoff FW, Loo SK, Lord C, Lowe JK, Lucae S, MacIntyre DJ, Madden PA, Maestrini E, Magnusson PK, Mahon PB, Maier W, Malhotra AK, Mane SM, Martin CL, Martin NG, Mattheisen M, Matthews K, Mattingsdal M, McCarroll SA, McGhee KA, McGough JJ, McGrath PJ, McGuffin P, McInnis MG, McIntosh A, McKinney R, McLean AW, McMahon FJ, McMahon WM, McQuillin A, Medeiros H, Medland SE, Meier S, Melle I, Meng F, Meyer J, Middeldorp CM, Middleton L, Milanova V, Miranda A, Monaco AP, Montgomery GW, Moran JL, Moreno-De-Luca D, Morken G, Morris DW, Morrow EM, Moskvina V, Muglia P, Muhleisen TW, Muir WJ, Muller-Myhsok B, Murtha M, Myers RM, Myin-Germeys I, Neale MC, Nelson SF, Nievergelt CM, Nikolov I, Nimgaonkar V, Nolen WA, Nothen MM, Nurnberger JI, Nwulia EA, Nyholt DR, O'Dushlaine C, Oades RD, Olincy A, Oliveira G, Olsen L, Ophoff RA, Osby U, Owen MJ, Palotie A, Parr JR, Paterson AD, Pato CN, Pato MT, Penninx BW, Pergadia ML, Pericak-Vance MA, Pickard BS, Pimm J, Piven J, Posthuma D, Potash JB, Poustka F, Propping P, Puri V, Quested DJ, Quinn EM, Ramos-Quiroga JA, Rasmussen HB, Raychaudhuri S, Rehnstrom K, Reif A, Ribases M, Rice JP, Rietschel M, Roeder K, Roeyers H, Rossin L, Rothenberger A, Rouleau G, Ruderfer D, Rujescu D, Sanders AR, Sanders SJ, Santangelo SL, Sergeant JA, Schachar R, Schalling M, Schatzberg AF, Scheftner WA, Schellenberg GD, Scherer SW, Schork NJ, Schulze TG, Schumacher J, Schwarz M, Scolnick E, Scott LJ, Shi J, Shilling PD, Shyn SI, Silverman JM, Slager SL, Smalley SL, Smit JH, Smith EN, Sonuga-Barke EJ, St Clair D, State M, Steffens M, Steinhausen HC, Strauss JS, Strohmaier J, Stroup TS, Sutcliffe JS, Szatmari P, Szelinger S, Thirumalai S, Thompson RC, Todorov AA, Tozzi F, Treutlein J, Uhr M, van den Oord EJ, Van Grootheest G, Van Os J, Vicente AM, Vieland VJ, Vincent JB, Visscher PM, Walsh CA, Wassink TH, Watson SJ, Weissman MM, Werge T, Wienker TF, Wijsman EM, Willemsen G, Williams N, Willsey AJ, Witt SH, Xu W, Young AH, Yu TW, Zammit S, Zandi PP, Zhang P, Zitman FG, Zollner S, International Inflammatory Bowel Disease Genetics C, Devlin B, Kelsoe JR, Sklar P, Daly MJ, O'Donovan MC, Craddock N, Sullivan PF, Smoller JW, Kendler KS, Wray NR (2013) Genetic relationship between five psychiatric disorders estimated from genome-wide SNPs. Nat Genet 45(9):984–994. doi:10.1038/ng.2711

Davanzo P, Thomas MA, Yue K, Oshiro T, Belin T, Strober M, McCracken J (2001) Decreased anterior cingulate myo-inositol/creatine spectroscopy resonance with lithium treatment in children with bipolar disorder. Neuropsychopharmacology 24(4):359–369. doi:10.1016/S0893-133X(00)00207-4

Davanzo P, Yue K, Thomas MA, Belin T, Mintz J, Venkatraman TN, Santoro E, Barnett S, McCracken J (2003) Proton magnetic resonance spectroscopy of bipolar disorder versus intermittent explosive disorder in children and adolescents. Am J Psychiatry 160(8):1442–1452

Davenport YB, Adland ML, Gold PW, Goodwin FK (1979) Manic-depressive illness: psychodynamic features of multigenerational families. Am J Orthopsychiatry 49(1):24–35

Davidson J (1972) Cholinergic-adrenergic hypothesis of mania and depression. Lancet 2(7789): 1249

Davidson RJ, Irwin W (1999) The functional neuroanatomy of emotion and affective style. Trends Cogn Sci 3(1):11–21

Dean B, Pavey G, McLeod M, Opeskin K, Keks N, Copolov D (2001) A change in the density of [(3)H]flumazenil, but not [(3)H]muscimol binding, in Brodmann's Area 9 from subjects with bipolar disorder. J Affect Disord 66(2–3):147–158

Di Renzo G, Amoroso S, Taglialatela M, Canzoniero L, Basile V, Fatatis A, Annunziato L (1989) Pharmacological characterization of serotonin receptors involved in the control of prolactin secretion. Eur J Pharmacol 162(2):371–373

Doris A, Belton E, Ebmeier KP, Glabus MF, Marshall I (2004) Reduction of cingulate gray matter density in poor outcome bipolar illness. Psychiatry Res 130(2):153–159. doi:10.1016/j.pscychresns.2003.09.002

Drevets WC, Price JL, Simpson JR Jr, Todd RD, Reich T, Vannier M, Raichle ME (1997) Subgenual prefrontal cortex abnormalities in mood disorders. Nature 386(6627):824–827. doi:10.1038/386824a0

Dunn RT, Kimbrell TA, Ketter TA, Frye MA, Willis MW, Luckenbaugh DA, Post RM (2002) Principal components of the beck depression inventory and regional cerebral metabolism in unipolar and bipolar depression. Biol Psychiatry 51(5):387–399

Eastwood SL, Harrison PJ (2001) Synaptic pathology in the anterior cingulate cortex in schizophrenia and mood disorders. A review and a Western blot study of synaptophysin, GAP-43 and the complexins. Brain Res Bull 55(5):569–578

Engel GL (1977) The need for a new medical model: a challenge for biomedicine. Science 196(4286):129–136

Engel GL (1980) The clinical application of the biopsychosocial model. Am J Psychiatry 137(5):535–544

Evans DL, Golden R (1987) The dexamethasone suppression test: a review. In: Loosen P, Nemeroff C (eds) Handbook of clinical psychoneuroendocrinology. Wiley, New York, pp 313–335

Farrow TF, Whitford TJ, Williams LM, Gomes L, Harris AW (2005) Diagnosis-related regional gray matter loss over two years in first episode schizophrenia and bipolar disorder. Biol Psychiatry 58(9):713–723. doi:10.1016/j.biopsych.2005.04.033

Fessler RG, Deyo SN, Meltzer HY, Miller RJ (1984) Evidence that the medial and dorsal raphe nuclei mediate serotonergically-induced increases in prolactin release from the pituitary. Brain Res 299(2):231–237

Fountoulakis KN, Vieta E (2008) Treatment of bipolar disorder: a systematic review of available data and clinical perspectives. Int J Neuropsychopharmacol 11(7):999–1029. doi:10.1017/S1461145708009231

Fountoulakis KN, Iacovides A, Kaprinis S, Kaprinis G (2006) Life events and clinical subtypes of major depression: a cross-sectional study. Psychiatry Res 143(2–3):235–244. doi:10.1016/j.psychres.2005.09.018

Fountoulakis KN, Vieta E, Siamouli M, Valenti M, Magiria S, Oral T, Fresno D, Giannakopoulos P, Kaprinis GS (2007) Treatment of bipolar disorder: a complex treatment for a multi-faceted disorder. Ann Gen Psychiatry 6:27. doi:10.1186/1744-859X-6-27

Fountoulakis KN, Giannakopoulos P, Kovari E, Bouras C (2008a) Assessing the role of cingulate cortex in bipolar disorder: neuropathological, structural and functional imaging data. Brain Res Rev 59(1):9–21. doi:10.1016/j.brainresrev.2008.04.005

Fountoulakis KN, Grunze H, Panagiotidis P, Kaprinis G (2008b) Treatment of bipolar depression: an update. J Affect Disord 109(1–2):21–34. doi:10.1016/j.jad.2007.10.016

Fountoulakis KN, Kelsoe JR, Akiskal H (2012) Receptor targets for antidepressant therapy in bipolar disorder: an overview. J Affect Disord 138(3):222–238. doi:10.1016/j.jad.2011.04.043

Frye MA, Watzl J, Banakar S, O'Neill J, Mintz J, Davanzo P, Fischer J, Chirichigno JW, Ventura J, Elman S, Tsuang J, Walot I, Thomas MA (2007) Increased anterior cingulate/medial prefrontal cortical glutamate and creatine in bipolar depression. Neuropsychopharmacology 32(12):2490–2499. doi:10.1038/sj.npp.1301387

Garattini S, Mennini T, Samanin R (1987) From fenfluramine racemate to d-fenfluramine. Specificity and potency of the effects on the serotoninergic system and food intake. Ann N Y Acad Sci 499:156–166

Goodwin GM, Cavanagh JT, Glabus MF, Kehoe RF, O'Carroll RE, Ebmeier KP (1997) Uptake of 99mTc-exametazime shown by single photon emission computed tomography before and after lithium withdrawal in bipolar patients: associations with mania. Br J Psychiatry 170:426–430

Green HS, Kane JM (1983) The dexamethasone suppression test in depression. Clin Neuropharmacol 6(1):7–24

Greenwood TA, Badner JA, Byerley W, Keck PE, McElroy SL, Remick RA, Sadovnick AD, Akiskal HS, Kelsoe JR (2013a) Heritability and genome-wide SNP linkage analysis of temperament in bipolar disorder. J Affect Disord 150(3):1031–1040. doi:10.1016/j.jad.2013.05.035

Greenwood TA, Bipolar Genome Study C, Kelsoe JR (2013b) Genome-wide association study of irritable vs. elated mania suggests genetic differences between clinical subtypes of bipolar disorder. PLoS One 8(1):e53804. doi:10.1371/journal.pone.0053804

Gruber SA, Rogowska J, Yurgelun-Todd DA (2004) Decreased activation of the anterior cingulate in bipolar patients: an fMRI study. J Affect Disord 82(2):191–201. doi:10.1016/j.jad.2003.10.010

Hajek T, Carrey N, Alda M (2005) Neuroanatomical abnormalities as risk factors for bipolar disorder. Bipolar Disord 7(5):393–403. doi:10.1111/j.1399-5618.2005.00238.x

Harkness KL, Luther J (2001) Clinical risk factors for the generation of life events in major depression. J Abnorm Psychol 110(4):564–572

Heim C, Newport DJ, Wagner D, Wilcox MM, Miller AH, Nemeroff CB (2002) The role of early adverse experience and adulthood stress in the prediction of neuroendocrine stress reactivity in women: a multiple regression analysis. Depress Anxiety 15(3):117–125. doi:10.1002/da.10015

Hirayasu Y, Shenton ME, Salisbury DF, Kwon JS, Wible CG, Fischer IA, Yurgelun-Todd D, Zarate C, Kikinis R, Jolesz FA, McCarley RW (1999) Subgenual cingulate cortex volume in first-episode psychosis. Am J Psychiatry 156(7):1091–1093

Houenou J, Wessa M, Douaud G, Leboyer M, Chanraud S, Perrin M, Poupon C, Martinot JL, Paillere-Martinot ML (2007) Increased white matter connectivity in euthymic bipolar patients: diffusion tensor tractography between the subgenual cingulate and the amygdalo-hippocampal complex. Mol Psychiatry 12(11):1001–1010. doi:10.1038/sj.mp.4002010

Itokawa M, Yamada K, Iwayama-Shigeno Y, Ishitsuka Y, Detera-Wadleigh S, Yoshikawa T (2003) Genetic analysis of a functional GRIN2A promoter (GT)n repeat in bipolar disorder pedigrees in humans. Neurosci Lett 345(1):53–56

Janowsky DS, El-Yousefo MK, Davis JM, Sekerke HJ (1972) A cholinergic-adrenergic hypothesis of mania and depression. Lancet 2(7778):632–635

Javadapour A, Malhi GS, Ivanovski B, Chen X, Wen W, Sachdev P (2007) Increased anterior cingulate cortex volume in bipolar I disorder. Aust N Z J Psychiatry 41(11):910–916. doi:10.1080/00048670701634978

Jensen NH, Rodriguiz RM, Caron MG, Wetsel WC, Rothman RB, Roth BL (2008) N-desalkylquetiapine, a potent norepinephrine reuptake inhibitor and partial 5-HT1A agonist, as a putative mediator of quetiapine's antidepressant activity. Neuropsychopharmacology 33(10):2303–2312. doi:10.1038/sj.npp.1301646

Kaur S, Sassi RB, Axelson D, Nicoletti M, Brambilla P, Monkul ES, Hatch JP, Keshavan MS, Ryan N, Birmaher B, Soares JC (2005) Cingulate cortex anatomical abnormalities in children and adolescents with bipolar disorder. Am J Psychiatry 162(9):1637–1643. doi:10.1176/appi.ajp.162.9.1637

Kelsoe JR (2003) Arguments for the genetic basis of the bipolar spectrum. J Affect Disord 73(1–2):183–197

Kelsoe J (2009) Mood disorders: genetics. In: Sadock B, Sadock V, Ruiz P (eds) Kaplan & Sadock's comprehensive textbook of psychiatry, 9th edn. Lippincott Williams & Wilkins, Philadelphia

Kendler KS, Thornton LM, Gardner CO (2000) Stressful life events and previous episodes in the etiology of major depression in women: an evaluation of the "kindling" hypothesis. Am J Psychiatry 157(8):1243–1251

Knable MB (1999) Schizophrenia and bipolar disorder: findings from studies of the Stanley Foundation Brain Collection. Schizophr Res 39(2):149–152; discussion 163

Koethe D, Llenos IC, Dulay JR, Hoyer C, Torrey EF, Leweke FM, Weis S (2007) Expression of CB1 cannabinoid receptor in the anterior cingulate cortex in schizophrenia, bipolar disorder, and major depression. J Neural Transm 114(8):1055–1063. doi:10.1007/s00702-007-0660-5

Kristiansen LV, Meador-Woodruff JH (2005) Abnormal striatal expression of transcripts encoding NMDA interacting PSD proteins in schizophrenia, bipolar disorder and major depression. Schizophr Res 78(1):87–93. doi:10.1016/j.schres.2005.06.012

Kruger S, Seminowicz D, Goldapple K, Kennedy SH, Mayberg HS (2003) State and trait influences on mood regulation in bipolar disorder: blood flow differences with an acute mood challenge. Biol Psychiatry 54(11):1274–1283

Kruger S, Alda M, Young LT, Goldapple K, Parikh S, Mayberg HS (2006) Risk and resilience markers in bipolar disorder: brain responses to emotional challenge in bipolar patients and their healthy siblings. Am J Psychiatry 163(2):257–264. doi:10.1176/appi.ajp.163.2.257

Kupfer DJ (1976) REM latency: a psychobiologic marker for primary depressive disease. Biol Psychiatry 11(2):159–174

Kutcher S, Marton P, Szalai J, Kennedy B (1992) Specificity of psychoanalytic hypotheses regarding the onset of adolescent psychoses: an empirical test of a psychodynamic model. J Am Acad Child Adolesc Psychiatry 31(4):699–701. doi:10.1097/00004583-199207000-00018; discussion 701–792

Lagopoulos J, Hermens DF, Naismith SL, Scott EM, Hickie IB (2012) Frontal lobe changes occur early in the course of affective disorders in young people. BMC Psychiatry 12:4. doi:10.1186/1471-244X-12-4

Lennox BR, Jacob R, Calder AJ, Lupson V, Bullmore ET (2004) Behavioural and neurocognitive responses to sad facial affect are attenuated in patients with mania. Psychol Med 34(5): 795–802

Lim KO, Rosenbloom MJ, Faustman WO, Sullivan EV, Pfefferbaum A (1999) Cortical gray matter deficit in patients with bipolar disorder. Schizophr Res 40(3):219–227

Lim CS, Baldessarini RJ, Vieta E, Yucel M, Bora E, Sim K (2013) Longitudinal neuroimaging and neuropsychological changes in bipolar disorder patients: review of the evidence. Neurosci Biobehav Rev 37(3):418–435. doi:10.1016/j.neubiorev.2013.01.003

Lin A, Reniers RL, Wood SJ (2013) Clinical staging in severe mental disorder: evidence from neurocognition and neuroimaging. Br J Psychiatry Suppl 54:s11–s17. doi:10.1192/bjp.bp.112.119156

Lochhead RA, Parsey RV, Oquendo MA, Mann JJ (2004) Regional brain gray matter volume differences in patients with bipolar disorder as assessed by optimized voxel-based morphometry. Biol Psychiatry 55(12):1154–1162. doi:10.1016/j.biopsych.2004.02.026

Loeb LR, Loeb FF Jr (1992) A psychodynamic approach to the early diagnosis of manic-depressive disorder in adolescence. Adolesc Psychiatry 18:348–364

Lopez-Larson MP, DelBello MP, Zimmerman ME, Schwiers ML, Strakowski SM (2002) Regional prefrontal gray and white matter abnormalities in bipolar disorder. Biol Psychiatry 52(2):93–100

Louet E, Consoli A, Lucanto R, Duplant N, Bailly-Salin MJ, Lemoigne A, Martin M, Mayer C, Thompson C, Gollier-Briant F, Laurent C, Brunelle J, Bodeau N, Cohen D (2010) Psychodynamic-oriented psychological assessment predicts evolution to schizophrenia at 8-year follow-up in adolescents hospitalized for a manic/mixed episode: interest of an overall subjective rating. J Physiol Paris 104(5):257–262. doi:10.1016/j.jphysparis.2010.08.004

Lyoo IK, Kim MJ, Stoll AL, Demopulos CM, Parow AM, Dager SR, Friedman SD, Dunner DL, Renshaw PF (2004) Frontal lobe gray matter density decreases in bipolar I disorder. Biol Psychiatry 55(6):648–651. doi:10.1016/j.biopsych.2003.10.017

Lyoo IK, Sung YH, Dager SR, Friedman SD, Lee JY, Kim SJ, Kim N, Dunner DL, Renshaw PF (2006) Regional cerebral cortical thinning in bipolar disorder. Bipolar Disord 8(1):65–74. doi:10.1111/j.1399-5618.2006.00284.x

Maas JW (1975) Biogenic amines and depression. Biochemical and pharmacological separation of two types of depression. Arch Gen Psychiatry 32(11):1357–1361

Mah L, Zarate CA Jr, Singh J, Duan YF, Luckenbaugh DA, Manji HK, Drevets WC (2007) Regional cerebral glucose metabolic abnormalities in bipolar II depression. Biol Psychiatry 61(6):765–775. doi:10.1016/j.biopsych.2006.06.009

Malhi GS, Lagopoulos J, Owen AM, Ivanovski B, Shnier R, Sachdev P (2007) Reduced activation to implicit affect induction in euthymic bipolar patients: an fMRI study. J Affect Disord 97(1–3): 109–122. doi:10.1016/j.jad.2006.06.005

Marlinge E, Bellivier F, Houenou J (2014) White matter alterations in bipolar disorder: potential for drug discovery and development. Bipolar Disord 16(2):97–112. doi:10.1111/bdi.12135
Martucci L, Wong AH, De Luca V, Likhodi O, Wong GW, King N, Kennedy JL (2006) N-methyl-D-aspartate receptor NR2B subunit gene GRIN2B in schizophrenia and bipolar disorder: polymorphisms and mRNA levels. Schizophr Res 84(2–3):214–221. doi:10.1016/j.schres.2006.02.001
McCarthy MJ, Liang S, Spadoni AD, Kelsoe JR, Simmons AN (2014) Whole brain expression of bipolar disorder associated genes: structural and genetic analyses. PLoS One 9(6):e100204. doi:10.1371/journal.pone.0100204
McCullumsmith RE, Kristiansen LV, Beneyto M, Scarr E, Dean B, Meador-Woodruff JH (2007) Decreased NR1, NR2A, and SAP102 transcript expression in the hippocampus in bipolar disorder. Brain Res 1127(1):108–118. doi:10.1016/j.brainres.2006.09.011
McDonald C, Bullmore ET, Sham PC, Chitnis X, Wickham H, Bramon E, Murray RM (2004) Association of genetic risks for schizophrenia and bipolar disorder with specific and generic brain structural endophenotypes. Arch Gen Psychiatry 61(10):974–984. doi:10.1001/archpsyc.61.10.974
Miller CL, Llenos IC, Dulay JR, Weis S (2006) Upregulation of the initiating step of the kynurenine pathway in postmortem anterior cingulate cortex from individuals with schizophrenia and bipolar disorder. Brain Res 1073–1074:25–37. doi:10.1016/j.brainres.2005.12.056
Moore CM, Breeze JL, Gruber SA, Babb SM, Frederick BB, Villafuerte RA, Stoll AL, Hennen J, Yurgelun-Todd DA, Cohen BM, Renshaw PF (2000) Choline, myo-inositol and mood in bipolar disorder: a proton magnetic resonance spectroscopic imaging study of the anterior cingulate cortex. Bipolar Disord 2(3 Pt 2):207–216
Moore PB, Shepherd DJ, Eccleston D, Macmillan IC, Goswami U, McAllister VL, Ferrier IN (2001) Cerebral white matter lesions in bipolar affective disorder: relationship to outcome. Br J Psychiatry J Ment Sci 178:172–176
Moore CM, Biederman J, Wozniak J, Mick E, Aleardi M, Wardrop M, Dougherty M, Harpold T, Hammerness P, Randall E, Lyoo IK, Renshaw PF (2007a) Mania, glutamate/glutamine and risperidone in pediatric bipolar disorder: a proton magnetic resonance spectroscopy study of the anterior cingulate cortex. J Affect Disord 99(1–3):19–25. doi:10.1016/j.jad.2006.08.023
Moore CM, Frazier JA, Glod CA, Breeze JL, Dieterich M, Finn CT, Frederick B, Renshaw PF (2007b) Glutamine and glutamate levels in children and adolescents with bipolar disorder: a 4.0-T proton magnetic resonance spectroscopy study of the anterior cingulate cortex. J Am Acad Child Adolesc Psychiatry 46(4):524–534. doi:10.1097/chi.0b013e31802f5f2c
Moorhead TW, McKirdy J, Sussmann JE, Hall J, Lawrie SM, Johnstone EC, McIntosh AM (2007) Progressive gray matter loss in patients with bipolar disorder. Biol Psychiatry 62(8):894–900. doi:10.1016/j.biopsych.2007.03.005
Mueller HT, Meador-Woodruff JH (2004) NR3A NMDA receptor subunit mRNA expression in schizophrenia, depression and bipolar disorder. Schizophr Res 71(2–3):361–370. doi:10.1016/j.schres.2004.02.016
Mundo E, Tharmalingham S, Neves-Pereira M, Dalton EJ, Macciardi F, Parikh SV, Bolonna A, Kerwin RW, Arranz MJ, Makoff AJ, Kennedy JL (2003) Evidence that the N-methyl-D-aspartate subunit 1 receptor gene (GRIN1) confers susceptibility to bipolar disorder. Mol Psychiatry 8(2):241–245. doi:10.1038/sj.mp.4001218
Musselman DL, Nemeroff CB (1996) Depression and endocrine disorders: focus on the thyroid and adrenal system. Br J Psychiatry Suppl 30:123–128
Nery FG, Chen HH, Hatch JP, Nicoletti MA, Brambilla P, Sassi RB, Mallinger AG, Keshavan MS, Soares JC (2009) Orbitofrontal cortex gray matter volumes in bipolar disorder patients: a region-of-interest MRI study. Bipolar Disord 11(2):145–153. doi:10.1111/j.1399-5618.2009.00662.x
Nudmamud-Thanoi S, Reynolds GP (2004) The NR1 subunit of the glutamate/NMDA receptor in the superior temporal cortex in schizophrenia and affective disorders. Neurosci Lett 372(1–2):173–177. doi:10.1016/j.neulet.2004.09.035
Nurnberger JI Jr, Koller DL, Jung J, Edenberg HJ, Foroud T, Guella I, Vawter MP, Kelsoe JR, Psychiatric Genomics Consortium Bipolar G (2014) Identification of pathways for bipolar disorder: a meta-analysis. JAMA Psychiatry 71(6):657–664. doi:10.1001/jamapsychiatry.2014.176

Oedegaard KJ, Greenwood TA, Lunde A, Fasmer OB, Akiskal HS, Kelsoe JR, Consortium NGIBD (2010) A genome-wide linkage study of bipolar disorder and co-morbid migraine: replication of migraine linkage on chromosome 4q24, and suggestion of an overlapping susceptibility region for both disorders on chromosome 20p11. J Affect Disord 122(1–2):14–26. doi:10.1016/j.jad.2009.06.014
Ongur D, Drevets WC, Price JL (1998) Glial reduction in the subgenual prefrontal cortex in mood disorders. Proc Natl Acad Sci U S A 95(22):13290–13295
Pavuluri MN, O'Connor MM, Harral E, Sweeney JA (2007) Affective neural circuitry during facial emotion processing in pediatric bipolar disorder. Biol Psychiatry 62(2):158–167. doi:10.1016/j.biopsych.2006.07.011
Paykel ES, Rao BM, Taylor CN (1984) Life stress and symptom pattern in out-patient depression. Psychol Med 14(3):559–568
Paykel ES, Cooper Z, Ramana R, Hayhurst H (1996) Life events, social support and marital relationships in the outcome of severe depression. Psychol Med 26(1):121–133
Peckys D, Hurd YL (2001) Prodynorphin and kappa opioid receptor mRNA expression in the cingulate and prefrontal cortices of subjects diagnosed with schizophrenia or affective disorders. Brain Res Bull 55(5):619–624
Post RM, Silberstein SD (1994) Shared mechanisms in affective illness, epilepsy, and migraine. Neurology 44(10 Suppl 7):S37–S47
Post RM, Weiss SR (1989) Sensitization, kindling, and anticonvulsants in mania. J Clin Psychiatry 50(Suppl):23–30; discussion 45–47
Post RM, Weiss SR (1998) Sensitization and kindling phenomena in mood, anxiety, and obsessive-compulsive disorders: the role of serotonergic mechanisms in illness progression. Biol Psychiatry 44(3):193–206
Post RM, Weiss SR, Pert A (1984) Differential effects of carbamazepine and lithium on sensitization and kindling. Prog Neuropsychopharmacol Biol Psychiatry 8(3):425–434
Post RM, Weiss SR, Pert A (1988) Implications of behavioral sensitization and kindling for stress-induced behavioral change. Adv Exp Med Biol 245:441–463
Post RM, Susan R, Weiss B (1992) Sensitization, kindling, and carbamazepine: an update on their implications for the course of affective illness. Pharmacopsychiatry 25(1):41–43. doi:10.1055/s-2007-1014386
Quattrone A, Schettini G, di Renzo G, Tedeschi G, Preziosi P (1979) Effect of midbrain raphe lesion or 5,7-dihydroxytryptamine treatment on the prolactin-releasing action of quipazine and D-fenfluramine in rats. Brain Res 174(1):71–79
Raedler TJ, Knable MB, Lafargue T, Urbina RA, Egan MF, Pickar D, Weinberger DR (1999) In vivo determination of striatal dopamine D2 receptor occupancy in patients treated with olanzapine. Psychiatry Res 90(2):81–90
Ravindran AV, Matheson K, Griffiths J, Merali Z, Anisman H (2002) Stress, coping, uplifts, and quality of life in subtypes of depression: a conceptual frame and emerging data. J Affect Disord 71(1–3):121–130
Roth RM, Koven NS, Randolph JJ, Flashman LA, Pixley HS, Ricketts SM, Wishart HA, Saykin AJ (2006) Functional magnetic resonance imaging of executive control in bipolar disorder. Neuroreport 17(11):1085–1089. doi:10.1097/01.wnr.0000227979.06013.57
Rowland NE, Carlton J (1986) Neurobiology of an anorectic drug: fenfluramine. Prog Neurobiol 27(1):13–62
Rubinsztein JS, Fletcher PC, Rogers RD, Ho LW, Aigbirhio FI, Paykel ES, Robbins TW, Sahakian BJ (2001) Decision-making in mania: a PET study. Brain 124(Pt 12):2550–2563
Sassi RB, Brambilla P, Hatch JP, Nicoletti MA, Mallinger AG, Frank E, Kupfer DJ, Keshavan MS, Soares JC (2004) Reduced left anterior cingulate volumes in untreated bipolar patients. Biol Psychiatry 56(7):467–475. doi:10.1016/j.biopsych.2004.07.005
Savitz JB, Price JL, Drevets WC (2014) Neuropathological and neuromorphometric abnormalities in bipolar disorder: view from the medial prefrontal cortical network. Neurosci Biobehav Rev 42:132–147. doi:10.1016/j.neubiorev.2014.02.008
Scarr E, Pavey G, Sundram S, MacKinnon A, Dean B (2003) Decreased hippocampal NMDA, but not kainate or AMPA receptors in bipolar disorder. Bipolar Disord 5(4):257–264

Schildkraut JJ (1965) The catecholamine hypothesis of affective disorders: a review of supporting evidence. Am J Psychiatry 122(5):509–522

Seager MA, Huff KD, Barth VN, Phebus LA, Rasmussen K (2004) Fluoxetine administration potentiates the effect of olanzapine on locus coeruleus neuronal activity. Biol Psychiatry 55(11):1103–1109. doi:10.1016/j.biopsych.2004.02.012

Seager MA, Barth VN, Phebus LA, Rasmussen K (2005) Chronic coadministration of olanzapine and fluoxetine activates locus coeruleus neurons in rats: implications for bipolar disorder. Psychopharmacology (Berl) 181(1):126–133. doi:10.1007/s00213-005-2198-2

Segurado R, Detera-Wadleigh SD, Levinson DF, Lewis CM, Gill M, Nurnberger JI Jr, Craddock N, DePaulo JR, Baron M, Gershon ES, Ekholm J, Cichon S, Turecki G, Claes S, Kelsoe JR, Schofield PR, Badenhop RF, Morissette J, Coon H, Blackwood D, McInnes LA, Foroud T, Edenberg HJ, Reich T, Rice JP, Goate A, McInnis MG, McMahon FJ, Badner JA, Goldin LR, Bennett P, Willour VL, Zandi PP, Liu J, Gilliam C, Juo SH, Berrettini WH, Yoshikawa T, Peltonen L, Lonnqvist J, Nothen MM, Schumacher J, Windemuth C, Rietschel M, Propping P, Maier W, Alda M, Grof P, Rouleau GA, Del-Favero J, Van Broeckhoven C, Mendlewicz J, Adolfsson R, Spence MA, Luebbert H, Adams LJ, Donald JA, Mitchell PB, Barden N, Shink E, Byerley W, Muir W, Visscher PM, Macgregor S, Gurling H, Kalsi G, McQuillin A, Escamilla MA, Reus VI, Leon P, Freimer NB, Ewald H, Kruse TA, Mors O, Radhakrishna U, Blouin JL, Antonarakis SE, Akarsu N (2003) Genome scan meta-analysis of schizophrenia and bipolar disorder, part III: bipolar disorder. Am J Hum Genet 73(1):49–62. doi:10.1086/376547

Siever LJ, Murphy DL, Slater S, de la Vega E, Lipper S (1984) Plasma prolactin changes following fenfluramine in depressed patients compared to controls: an evaluation of central serotonergic responsivity in depression. Life Sci 34(11):1029–1039

Silverstone T, McPherson H, Li Q, Doyle T (2003) Deep white matter hyperintensities in patients with bipolar depression, unipolar depression and age-matched control subjects. Bipolar Disord 5(1):53–57

Sklar P, Smoller JW, Fan J, Ferreira MA, Perlis RH, Chambert K, Nimgaonkar VL, McQueen MB, Faraone SV, Kirby A, de Bakker PI, Ogdie MN, Thase ME, Sachs GS, Todd-Brown K, Gabriel SB, Sougnez C, Gates C, Blumenstiel B, Defelice M, Ardlie KG, Franklin J, Muir WJ, McGhee KA, MacIntyre DJ, McLean A, VanBeck M, McQuillin A, Bass NJ, Robinson M, Lawrence J, Anjorin A, Curtis D, Scolnick EM, Daly MJ, Blackwood DH, Gurling HM, Purcell SM (2008) Whole-genome association study of bipolar disorder. Mol Psychiatry 13(6):558–569. doi:10.1038/sj.mp.4002151

Soares JC, Kochunov P, Monkul ES, Nicoletti MA, Brambilla P, Sassi RB, Mallinger AG, Frank E, Kupfer DJ, Lancaster J, Fox P (2005) Structural brain changes in bipolar disorder using deformation field morphometry. Neuroreport 16(6):541–544

Spirtes MA (1976) Lithium levels in monkey and human brain after chronic, therapeutic, oral dosage. Pharmacol Biochem Behav 5(2):143–147

Steggles GR (2012) The process of recovery of a schizoaffectively disordered mind: a psychoanalytic theory of the functional psychoses, the psychodynamic pentapointed cognitive construct theory. BMJ Case Rep. doi:10.1136/bcr-2012-006683

Stokes PE, Stoll PM, Koslow SH, Maas JW, Davis JM, Swann AC, Robins E (1984) Pretreatment DST and hypothalamic-pituitary-adrenocortical function in depressed patients and comparison groups. A multicenter study. Arch Gen Psychiatry 41(3):257–267

Strakowski SM, Wilson DR, Tohen M, Woods BT, Douglass AW, Stoll AL (1993) Structural brain abnormalities in first-episode mania. Biol Psychiatry 33(8–9):602–609

Strakowski SM, DelBello MP, Zimmerman ME, Getz GE, Mills NP, Ret J, Shear P, Adler CM (2002) Ventricular and periventricular structural volumes in first- versus multiple-episode bipolar disorder. Am J Psychiatry 159(11):1841–1847

Strakowski SM, Adler CM, Holland SK, Mills NP, DelBello MP, Eliassen JC (2005) Abnormal FMRI brain activation in euthymic bipolar disorder patients during a counting Stroop interference task. Am J Psychiatry 162(9):1697–1705. doi:10.1176/appi.ajp.162.9.1697

Swanda R, Haaland K, LaRue A (2000) Clinical neuropsychology and intellectual assessment of adults. In: Sadock B, Sadock V (eds) Comprehensive textbook of psychiatry. Lippincott Williams & Wilkins, Philadelphia, pp 689–702

Tarsy D, Leopold N, Sax DS (1972) Cholinergic-adrenergic hypothesis of mania and depression. Lancet 2(7787):1153

Tekin S, Cummings JL (2002) Frontal-subcortical neuronal circuits and clinical neuropsychiatry: an update. J Psychosom Res 53(2):647–654

Thomas EA, Dean B, Scarr E, Copolov D, Sutcliffe JG (2003) Differences in neuroanatomical sites of apoD elevation discriminate between schizophrenia and bipolar disorder. Mol Psychiatry 8(2):167–175. doi:10.1038/sj.mp.4001223

Thomson KC, Hendrie HC (1972) Environmental stress in primary depressive illness. Arch Gen Psychiatry 26(2):130–132

Todtenkopf MS, Vincent SL, Benes FM (2005) A cross-study meta-analysis and three-dimensional comparison of cell counting in the anterior cingulate cortex of schizophrenic and bipolar brain. Schizophr Res 73(1):79–89. doi:10.1016/j.schres.2004.08.018

Torgerson CM, Irimia A, Leow AD, Bartzokis G, Moody TD, Jennings RG, Alger JR, Van Horn JD, Altshuler LL (2013) DTI tractography and white matter fiber tract characteristics in euthymic bipolar I patients and healthy control subjects. Brain Imag Behav 7(2):129–139. doi:10.1007/s11682-012-9202-3

Toro C, Deakin JF (2005) NMDA receptor subunit NRI and postsynaptic protein PSD-95 in hippocampus and orbitofrontal cortex in schizophrenia and mood disorder. Schizophr Res 80(2–3):323–330. doi:10.1016/j.schres.2005.07.003

Torrey EF, Barci BM, Webster MJ, Bartko JJ, Meador-Woodruff JH, Knable MB (2005) Neurochemical markers for schizophrenia, bipolar disorder, and major depression in postmortem brains. Biol Psychiatry 57(3):252–260. doi:10.1016/j.biopsych.2004.10.019

Van Praag M, Leijnse B (1963) Die Bedeutung Dermonoamineoxydashemmung als Antidepressives Prinzip I. Psychopharmacologia 4(1):1–14

Vieta E, Locklear J, Gunther O, Ekman M, Miltenburger C, Chatterton ML, Astrom M, Paulsson B (2010) Treatment options for bipolar depression: a systematic review of randomized, controlled trials. J Clin Psychopharmacol 30(5):579–590. doi:10.1097/JCP.0b013e3181f15849

Vita A, De Peri L, Sacchetti E (2009) Gray matter, white matter, brain, and intracranial volumes in first-episode bipolar disorder: a meta-analysis of magnetic resonance imaging studies. Bipolar Disord 11(8):807–814. doi:10.1111/j.1399-5618.2009.00759.x

Webster MJ, O'Grady J, Kleinman JE, Weickert CS (2005) Glial fibrillary acidic protein mRNA levels in the cingulate cortex of individuals with depression, bipolar disorder and schizophrenia. Neuroscience 133(2):453–461. doi:10.1016/j.neuroscience.2005.02.037

Wellcome Trust Case Control C (2007) Genome-wide association study of 14,000 cases of seven common diseases and 3,000 shared controls. Nature 447(7145):661–678. doi:10.1038/nature05911

Wessa M, Houenou J, Paillere-Martinot ML, Berthoz S, Artiges E, Leboyer M, Martinot JL (2007) Fronto-striatal overactivation in euthymic bipolar patients during an emotional go/nogo task. Am J Psychiatry 164(4):638–646. doi:10.1176/appi.ajp.164.4.638

Wilke M, Kowatch RA, DelBello MP, Mills NP, Holland SK (2004) Voxel-based morphometry in adolescents with bipolar disorder: first results. Psychiatry Res 131(1):57–69. doi:10.1016/j.pscychresns.2004.01.004

Wiste AK, Arango V, Ellis SP, Mann JJ, Underwood MD (2008) Norepinephrine and serotonin imbalance in the locus coeruleus in bipolar disorder. Bipolar Disord 10(3):349–359. doi:10.1111/j.1399-5618.2007.00528.x

Woo TU, Walsh JP, Benes FM (2004) Density of glutamic acid decarboxylase 67 messenger RNA-containing neurons that express the N-methyl-D-aspartate receptor subunit NR2A in the anterior cingulate cortex in schizophrenia and bipolar disorder. Arch Gen Psychiatry 61(7):649–657. doi:10.1001/archpsyc.61.7.649

Woo TU, Kim AM, Viscidi E (2008a) Disease-specific alterations in glutamatergic neurotransmission on inhibitory interneurons in the prefrontal cortex in schizophrenia. Brain Res 1218:267–277. doi:10.1016/j.brainres.2008.03.092

Woo TU, Shrestha K, Lamb D, Minns MM, Benes FM (2008b) N-methyl-D-aspartate receptor and calbindin-containing neurons in the anterior cingulate cortex in schizophrenia and bipolar disorder. Biol Psychiatry 64(9):803–809. doi:10.1016/j.biopsych.2008.04.034

Yatham LN, Goldstein JM, Vieta E, Bowden CL, Grunze H, Post RM, Suppes T, Calabrese JR (2005) Atypical antipsychotics in bipolar depression: potential mechanisms of action. J Clin Psychiatry 66(Suppl 5):40–48

Young LT, Warsh JJ, Kish SJ, Shannak K, Hornykeiwicz O (1994) Reduced brain 5-HT and elevated NE turnover and metabolites in bipolar affective disorder. Biol Psychiatry 35(2):121–127

Zavitsanou K, Katsifis A, Mattner F, Huang XF (2004) Investigation of m1/m4 muscarinic receptors in the anterior cingulate cortex in schizophrenia, bipolar disorder, and major depression disorder. Neuropsychopharmacology 29(3):619–625. doi:10.1038/sj.npp.1300367

Zavitsanou K, Katsifis A, Yu Y, Huang XF (2005) M2/M4 muscarinic receptor binding in the anterior cingulate cortex in schizophrenia and mood disorders. Brain Res Bull 65(5):397–403. doi:10.1016/j.brainresbull.2005.02.007

Zimmerman ME, DelBello MP, Getz GE, Shear PK, Strakowski SM (2006) Anterior cingulate subregion volumes and executive function in bipolar disorder. Bipolar Disord 8(3):281–288. doi:10.1111/j.1399-5618.2006.00298.x

Zipursky RB, Seeman MV, Bury A, Langevin R, Wortzman G, Katz R (1997) Deficits in gray matter volume are present in schizophrenia but not bipolar disorder. Schizophr Res 26(2–3):85–92

14 Psychometric and Neuropsychological Assessment

14.1 Introduction

While the diagnosis can be made on the basis of an unstructured interview, and this is the way mostly followed in everyday clinical practice, the quantification of symptomatology and of various deficits is quite a different issue. Although the clinical opinion can give a rough impression of the 'quality' of the clinical picture and its 'severity', and most important how they change from one time point to another, such estimations are largely idiosyncratic.

The psychometric and neuropsychological tools do exactly that. They quantify the clinical picture and are useful for keeping records, facilitating communication between clinicians, monitoring patients over time and providing of reliable data for statistical and administrative purposes since health-care administrators and insurances are increasingly demanding standardized assessment and reporting to justify the need for services or to assess the quality of the provided care. Additionally, the use of psychometric and neuropsychological tools is the backbone of modern psychiatric research, and the average clinician should be familiar with at least the basic principles of psychometrics and the basic tools in order to be able to follow the advances in the field.

In practical terms, rating scales offer some practical advantages, like saving valuable physician time in carefully selected patients, since self-report questionnaires can be filled in the waiting room or other type of testing can be done by nurses or technicians. Also it is not unusual that patients answer easier to paper and pencil testing concerning 'sensitive' topics, e.g. sexuality, in comparison with the face-to-face interview. However, it is an important, although a very frequent, mistake many clinicians do, when the diagnostic decision is uncertain, to utilize psychometric testing for additional confirmation or information. The clinician should have in mind that unfortunately, psychiatry has not yet access to an equivalent of a true laboratory testing, which is independent of clinical assessment, the way the rest of medicine has. It is doubtful that the rating scale can elicit information that an experienced clinician cannot elicit with a face-to-face unstructured interview. What the

K.N. Fountoulakis, *Bipolar Disorder: An Evidence-Based Guide to Manic Depression*, DOI 10.1007/978-3-642-37216-2_14

psychometric and neuropsychological tools do is that they constitute a standardized protocol for the registration of symptoms, signs and deficits.

In general, the rating scales are divided into two broad categories: self-report and administered by an interviewer. Further, concerning of their task, they are divided in those that give information to assist the diagnosis of a specific disorder, and therefore they have a cut-off score which suggests the presence or absence of diagnosis and those that simply quantify a psychometric feature either normal or pathological. Many tools claim to do both but almost always they are better suited to do either.

The individual items vary in format and the most common ways to answer them is either bimodal (usually yes/no or true/false) or a Likert scale, which is an ordinal scale with three to seven points that measures severity, intensity, frequency or other attributes. When a Likert scale is used, the levels are usually partially or fully anchored, and an explanation or a meaning is assigned for each level.

The two principal properties of a psychometric or neuropsychological tool are reliability (a scale should be consistent and repeatable in terms of different raters, different times or different conditions) and validity (a scale should truly measure what it is supposed to measure and not something similar, e.g. depression not anxiety).

14.2 Psychometric Tools

There is a large number of psychometric tools available for the assessment of various aspects of the clinical symptomatology of mood disorders and the clinician can choose which one to use on the basis of his training and specific needs. A basic list can be found in Table 14.1.

14.2.1 Depression Rating Scales

The rating of depression can be done both on the basis of self-report and also on the basis of an interview, since usually there is insight and the patient is able to describe his inner experience. The literature suggests there is no significant difference among the various self-administered instruments assessing depression in terms of performance, and overall sensitivity is around 84 % and specificity around 72 % (Mulrow et al. 1995; Fountoulakis et al. 2007).

14.2.1.1 The Hamilton Depression Rating Scale (HAM-D) (Hamilton 1960)

The HAM-D is worldwide the most well-known and frequently used scale to quantify depression. There are several versions but the most often used are the 17- and the 21-item versions. It is based on an interview by a trained examiner and a structured interview is also available. This is the most widely known and used scale worldwide. Some of the items it includes are assessing somatic symptoms, anxiety or physiological function. Medication adverse events might contaminate many of them. These characteristics make its application in the somatically ill and the elderly

Table 14.1 List of psychiatric rating scales by field of assessment

Domain	Tool
Mania	Young Mania Rating Scale (YMRS)
	Bech–Rafaelsen Mania Rating Scale (MRS)
	Hypomania/Mania Symptom Checklist (HCL-32)
Depression	Hamilton Depression Rating Scale (HAM-D)
	Mondgomery–Asberg Depression Rating Scale (MADRS)
	Beck Depression Inventory (BDI-I and BDI-II)
	Zung Depression Rating Scale (ZDRS)
	Geriatric Depression Scale (GDS)
	Center for Epidemiological Studies-Depression (CES-D)
Anxiety	Hamilton Anxiety Scale (HAM-A)
	Panic Disorder Severity Scale (PDSS)
	Yale–Brown Obsessive–Compulsive Scale (YBOCS)
	State–Trait Anxiety Inventory (STAI)
Psychotic features	Brief Psychiatric Rating Scale (BPRS)
	Positive and Negative Symptoms Scale (PANSS)
	The Scale for the Assessment of Positive Symptoms and the Scale for the Assessment of Negative Symptoms (SAPS/SANS)
Temperament and personality	Temperament Evaluation of the Memphis, Pisa, Paris, and San Diego Autoquestionnaire (TEMPS-A)
	Temperament and Character Inventory (TCI)
	NEO-Personality Inventory-3rd edition (NEO-PI-3)
	Minnesota Multiphasic Personality Inventory 2nd edition (MMPI-2)
Disability/general	Visual analog scale (VAS)
	Clinical Global Impression (CGI)
	Global Disability Scale (Glo.Di.S)
	Sheehan Disability Scale (SDS)
	Global Assessment of Functioning (GAF)
	Global Assessment of Relational Functioning (GARF)
	Social and Occupational Functioning Assessment Scale (SOFAS)
	SF-36
Multiple assessment tools	Mood Disorder Questionnaire (MDQ)
	Brief Psychiatric Rating Scale (BPRS)
Adverse events scales	The Systematic Assessment of Treatment-Emergent Events (SAFTEE)
	Abnormal Involuntary Movement Scale (AIMS)
	UKU-SERS Scale
	Simpson–Angus Rating Scale for Extrapyramidal Side Effects
Substance abuse scales	CAGE
	Alcohol Use Disorders Identification Test (AUDIT)
	Addiction Severity Index (ASI)
	Drug Abuse Screening Test (DAST)

(continued)

Table 14.1 (continued)

Domain	Tool
Other	Risk Assessment for Suicidality Scale (RASS)
	Scale to the Unawareness of Mental Disorder (SUMD)
	Drug Attitude Inventory-30 items version (DAI-30)
	Insight and Treatment Attitudes Questionnaire (ITAQ)
	Sleep Disorders Questionnaire (SDQ)
	Internet Addiction Scale (IAS)
	Arizona Sexual Experiences Scale (ASEX)
	Social Support Questionnaire (SSQ)
	Caregiver Burden Scale (CBS)

somewhat problematic. Overall the scale does not correspond to the concept of depression as we consider it today and as it is defined according to contemporary classification systems. Many aspects of depression (e.g. atypical or mixed features) are not assessed.

The scale takes less than half hour to be administered and both reliability and validity appear to be good. There is a huge body of data and experience from its use in a variety of tasks, including pharmaceutical trials.

14.2.1.2 Montgomery–Asberg Depression Rating Scale (MADRS) (Montgomery and Asberg 1979)

The MADRS was developed almost explicitly for use in pharmaceutical clinical trials and therefore the items it includes are those who are more sensitive to medication treatment. It does not assess depression in a global way and misses much of symptomatology, as it is designed for use in younger and somatically healthy patients. It includes only ten items and its rating is based on an interview, although a self-report version also exists. It takes probably 15 min to administer and exerts very good reliability and validity and notably high sensitivity to change.

14.2.1.3 Beck Depression Inventory (BDI-I) (Beck et al. 1961, 1996)

The BDI is based on the cognitive theory for depression proposed by Aaron Beck. It includes 21 items; it is self-report and assesses behaviour, thought content and the cognitive aspect of depression but avoids many aspect of symptomatology. It is widely used and a revised version (BDI-II) which is adjusted to contemporary classification (with the inclusion of somatic symptoms) is also available.

The scale can be completed in less than 10 min. Although the overall reliability is good, there is a problem with lower than expected test–retest reliability which essentially might reflect changes in the underlying symptoms.

14.2.1.4 Zung Depression Rating Scale (ZDRS) (Zung 1965)

The ZDRS is an old self-report scale which reflects an older concept of depression which was widely accepted during the 1960s and might not produce reliable and valid results in somatic patients and geriatric populations. It also under-assesses atypical depressive patients. However, both reliability and validity are good.

14.2.1.5 **Geriatric Depression Scale (GDS)** (Yesavage et al. 1982)

It is the first scale especially designed for use in elderly populations. It is a self-report scale; however, sometimes it is necessary to administer it through an interviewer. It exists in a 30-item and a 15-item form. It focuses mainly on the psychological concern of the patient and the way he/she perceives life, avoiding the assessment of somatic complaints.

14.2.1.6 **Center for Epidemiological Studies-Depression Scale (CES-D) (Radloff** 1977)

The CES-D is a self-report instrument and one of the most widely used. It seems that it is least affected by somatic disorders and handicaps. It consists of 20 items. The validity of the CES-D might be compromised when used with somatic patients or elderly individuals, and modifications for its use in these populations have been recommended. Both reliability and validity are high and extensive literature on its use is available.

14.2.2 Mania Rating Scales

Mania has quality issues similar to psychotic episodes, including limited or lack of insight, hostility and lack of cooperation as well as agitation all of which make self-reporting problematic. Therefore, both the two major mania scales are interview based. There is at least one hypomania scale (HCL-32) which is self-report.

14.2.2.1 **Young Mania Rating Scale (YMRS) (Young et al.** 1978)

The YMRS is applied by a trained interviewer and includes 11 items. It takes less than 30 min to apply. It has good reliability and validity and it is supported by a large literature. It is useful in both clinical practice and research and it has been proved sensitive to change.

14.2.2.2 **The Bech–Rafaelsen Mania Rating Scale (MRS)** (Bech et al. 1978)

It consists of 11 items and assesses the severity of mania in bipolar patients. It is rated by an examiner. Its reliability and validity are reported to be good. It is not used as widely or as often as the YMRS and the supporting literature is limited.

14.2.2.3 **Hypomania/Mania Symptom Checklist (HCL-32) (Angst et al.** 2005)

The HCL-32 is a checklist of 32 manic or hypomanic symptoms. It is self-report instrument in contrast to the YMRS and the MRS, and it is especially useful in the screening for BD-II and bipolar spectrum disorders. It has satisfactory reliability and validity.

14.2.3 Anxiety Rating Scales

Anxiety is a concept which covers many disorders in contemporary classification. It exists in the frame of individual disorders (e.g. panic disorder, generalized anxiety disorder, etc.) or as a transnosological constellation of symptoms (e.g. the anxiety specifier in mood disorders). The anxiety disorders are characterized by different temporal properties. For example, panic disorder is episodic with attacks of short duration while generalized anxiety disorder is more chronic. Some forms are mainly cognitive while some others are mainly somatic and neurovegetative. Anxiety as an accompanying feature of BD can take any form, from a distinct disorder to a subtle specifier. However, these specific characteristics of anxiety are important in order to determine the scale which best fits the needs of the study or the individual patient. Obsessive convulsive disorder (OCD) is no longer classified in anxiety disorders according to DSM but a related scale is listed here in accord with the ICD classification. Anxiety scales can be self-reported because like depressive scales, they depend on subjective descriptions of inner states and insight and cooperation are good.

14.2.3.1 Hamilton Anxiety Rating Scale (HAM-A) (Hamilton 1959)

The HAM-A is the sister scale of the HAM-D. Therefore, it presents many of the same advantages and disadvantages including a global assessment of anxious symptomatology which however is not in accord with the concepts adopted by contemporary classification systems. It covers 'worry' in a limited way while on the contrary it includes many somatic items. It does not assess episodic anxiety in the form of panic attacks. It is interview-based and so far no detailed guidelines for its application exist.

14.2.3.2 Panic Disorder Severity Scale (PDSS) (Shear et al. 1997)

The PDSS is specifically designed to assess anxiety in the frame of panic attacks. It includes seven items and its development was partially based on the Yale–Brown obsessive–compulsive scale. Originally the scale was developed to be used on the basis of an interview but a self-report version is also available. Reliability and validity are acceptable and it seems to be sensitive to change.

14.2.3.3 Yale–Brown Obsessive–Compulsive Scale (YBOCS) (Goodman et al. 1989a, b)

The YBOCS was developed to measure the severity of symptoms in OCD. It includes ten items and it is based on a clinical interview but a self-report version is also available. It takes approximately 15 min to complete. Although data are rather limited, the reliability and validity appear to be good.

14.2.3.4 State–Trait Anxiety Inventory-Form Y (STAI-Y) (Spielberger 1966, 1970, 1972, 1976, 1979)

The STAI-Y is a self-rating scale for the assessment of state and trait anxiety. State anxiety (S-anxiety) refers to the subjective and transitory feeling of tension, nervousness and worry and may be characterized by activation of the autonomous nervous system, at a given moment. Trait anxiety (T-anxiety) refers to relatively stable individual differences in anxiety proneness as a personality trait, that is, in the tendency to perceive and respond to stressful situations with elevations in the intensity of state anxiety (S-anxiety) reactions. In general, the STAI measures anxiety as a feature of the general population; thus, it is expected its scores to follow the normal distribution. However, it is widely used in the assessment of patient populations. The STAI is reported to be reliable and valid and has been used extensively in research and clinical practice and comprises separate self-report scales for measuring state and trait anxiety, consistent with the definitions given above. The S-anxiety scale consists of 20 statements that evaluate how the respondent feels 'right now, at this moment'. The T-anxiety scale consists of 20 statements that evaluate how the respondent feels 'generally'.

14.2.4 Psychotic Symptoms Rating Scales

The assessment and quantification of psychotic symptoms constitute a challenge. Psychotic patients often have limited insight, poor judgment and collaboration and behaviour problems (e.g. agitation) which make assessment difficult. As a rule, psychotic symptoms are reliably rated only through an interview performed by a trained clinician and rarely or never with self-report instruments.

14.2.4.1 The Brief Psychiatric Rating Scale (BPRS) (Zanello et al. 2013; Gabbard et al. 1987; Flemenbaum and Zimmermann 1973)

The BPRS was developed in the 1960s as a short comprehensive scale for the measuring of the severity of all aspects of psychiatric symptomatology but mainly of psychotic symptoms. The standard version includes 18 items and it is applied by a trained interviewer. Its administration takes approximately half hour and a semi-structured interview is available. Reliability and validity are reported to be good although the scale is somewhat old-fashioned and does not conform with contemporary classification systems. It has been used extensively for decades in research studies concerning schizophrenia.

14.2.4.2 The Positive and Negative Syndrome Scale (PANSS) (Kay et al. 1987)

The PANSS was developed in the late 1980s and includes 30 items which compose three subscales: positive symptoms, negative symptoms and general psychopathology. It is applied on the basis of an interview by a trained clinician and takes approximately 45 min to complete. It has become the standard tool for the assessing of patients with schizophrenia and other psychotic disorders. It has high reliability and validity.

14.2.4.3 The Scale for the Assessment of Positive Symptoms and the Scale for the Assessment of Negative Symptoms (SAPS/SANS) (Andreasen et al. 1995)

The SAPS and the SANS were developed to provide a detailed assessment of positive and negative symptoms of schizophrenia. They can be used separately or in combination. Each one includes 30 items. A trained clinician is necessary for their application. Each scale demands approximately half hour for its application. Both have excellent reliability and validity and one of their strongest points is the precise description of each item plus detailed guidelines for the application. Probably they are more complicated and difficult to apply in comparison to the PANSS and this is the reason they are not preferred.

14.2.5 Disability and General Assessment

Disability is a complex concept which is discussed in detail in Chap. 10. The available instruments to quantify it are also complex and they often mix symptoms with subjective feelings and objective dysfunction and impairment. A tool to assess the general impression of the condition of the patient usually mixes a number of information and eventually arrives at a scoring which often reflects the rater's impression concerning the severity of the illness. Partially this concept is covered in the chapter which discusses 'staging' (Chap. 15).

14.2.5.1 Visual Analogue Scale (VAS) (Rosenthal et al. 1987)

The VAS constitutes a very simple method, according to which, the examiner or the patient himself is asked to determine the quantity of the symptomatology, according to a specific question, on a bar 100 mm in length. One end of the bar is defined as 'lack of ….' (0 mm) and the opposite one as 'profound ….' (100 mm). The distance from the beginning (in mm or in %) is considered as the 'degree' of the symptom or of the issue under assessment. This method has been in existence since 1921. Today, it is considered somewhat outdated and not suitable for research purposes, but still it is useful in order to rate issues pertaining to the inner experience of the patient, or too complex constructs, although in the latter case a single aspect seems to dominate the opinion of the ratter.

14.2.5.2 Clinical Global Impression (CGI) (Guy 1976)

The CGI is essentially a group of simple scales rather than a single scale. They are rated by an interviewer and were developed to assess mainly symptom severity and change usually as treatment response. The most frequently used are Clinical Global Impression- Severity scale (CGI-S) and the Clinical Global Impression- Improvement scale (CGI-I). However, various modifications exist on the basis of different definition of the target to be rated, e.g. the Clinical Global Impression-Overall Bipolar Severity (CGI-BP).

14.2.5.3 General Assessment of Functioning (GAF) (Patterson and Lee 1995), General Assessment of Relational Functioning (GARF) and Social and Occupational Functioning Assessment Scale (SOFAS) (Morosini et al. 2000)

These are a family of scales introduced by the DSM classification system. They are rated by an interviewer and assess global functioning in the psychological (GAF), family, social (GARF) and occupational domain (SOFAS). They utilize a continuum from 0 to 100 similar in many ways to a VAS. They represent a non-specific way to quantify various domains of interest but they are of unknown (possibly low) reliability and validity.

14.2.5.4 Short Form-36 Items (SF-36) (McHorney et al. 1993)

The SF-36 is a self-report scale which is often used as a measure of quality of life but in fact it is a general measure of health status from the patient's point of view. This means that the scale registers the subjective view of the patient which is often independent of the presence or absence of specific diseases. It consists of 36 items and focuses on the person's functioning in relationship to somatic problems and psychological distress over the last month. It takes less than 15 min to administer. Although it has shown high reliability and validity, the interpretation its scores should be done very carefully and always by taking into consideration the special characteristics of the study sample or the individual person.

14.2.5.5 Global Disability Scale (Glo.Di.S) (Fountoulakis et al. 2012a)

The Glo.Di.S was developed on a concept similar of that of the WHO-DAS and the World Health Organization concerning disability. It includes 25 items assessing different aspects of disability which are grouped in factors explaining (everyday functioning, social and interpersonal functioning, severity and mental disability). Reliability is very high (Cronbach's alpha 0.95). The Glo.Di.S. has the potential to serve as a reliable and valid tool for assessing functioning and disability, but the literature is still limited. Further research is needed to prove that it could be useful across countries and populations and whether it provides data that are culturally meaningful and comparable. It can be used in surveys and in clinical research settings, and it can generate information of use in evaluating health needs and the effectiveness of interventions to reduce disability and improve health.

14.2.6 Temperament and Personality Inventories

Issues pertaining to temperament are discussed in Chap. 5 and to personality in Chap. 8. Below the most widely used questionnaires to assess temperament, character and personality are listed along with a brief description. All are self-report questionnaires with high reliability and strong theoretical background.

14.2.6.1 The Temperament Evaluation of the Memphis, Pisa, Paris, and San Diego Autoquestionnaire (TEMPS-A) (Akiskal et al. 2005)

The TEMPS was developed as a semi-structured TEMPS-I, administered in interview format and as a self-rating autoquestionnaire, the TEMPS-A with 109 (for men) or 110 (for women) items. It is based on Hagop Akiskal's theory on the affective components of temperament and their relationship to mood disorders and creativity. This approach resulted in an operationalized definition of the five affective temperaments (depressive, hyperthymic, irritable, cyclothymic and anxious) which are reflected in the five subscales of the TEMPS-A. The TEMPS-A is different from the TCI and the NEO-PI-3 in that it frames questions in the language of affectivity and is rooted in an evolutionary biologic perspective and its clinical validity has been recently supported on a genetic basis.

14.2.6.2 NEO-Personality Inventory-3rd Edition (NEO-PI-3) (Costa and McCrae 1997)

The NEO-PI-3 is a personality inventory which is based on the five factor theory of personality dimensions (big five). It includes 240 items which are grouped in five major traits (extraversion, agreeableness, conscientiousness, neuroticism and openness to experience). Below each trait there are six facets. Its development was based in principal on a psycholinguistic approach, and therefore it reflects concepts and ideas that exist in everyday human language but not complex scientific constructs. There are also shorter versions. There is a big literature support concerning its reliability and validity.

14.2.6.3 Temperament and Character Inventory (TCI) (Cloninger et al. 1993)

The TCI was developed as a questionnaire to explore the neurobiological foundation for personality, according to the theories of Robert Cloninger. Originally it had been suggested that the temperaments as defined by the Cloninger theory correspond to dopaminergic, serotonergic and noradrenergic activity. More recent studies have linked them to genes. The TCI includes the assessment of complex inner experience which is avoided by the NEO-PI-3 and attempts to dig into complex concepts. It too has high reliability and validity and a bulk of supportive literature.

14.2.6.4 Minnesota Multiphasic Personality Inventory 2nd Edition (MMPI-2) (Butcher et al. 1991)

The MMPI is the personality questionnaire most widely used in both clinical practice and research. Its second edition includes 567 items and is used in a variety of settings and aims, from clinical practice to screen job candidates. It takes approximately 2 h to complete. The MMPI was developed completely and exclusively in an empirical way from a large pool of items. There is no solid theory behind its development; however, various studies on its structure revealed clusters of items corresponding to human behaviours. It is considered to assess the more 'state' aspect of personality in contrast to the TEMPS, TCI and NEO-PI-3 which assess more stable aspects of temperament and personality.

14.2.7 Adverse Events Scales

There are a number of scales which have been developed to assess the adverse effects from medication treatment. There are two types: those who assess movement disorders and EPS in particular and those who cover a broad variety of adverse events.

14.2.7.1 The Systematic Assessment of Treatment-Emergent Events (SAFTEE) (Levine and Schooler 1986)

The SAFTEE has two versions, a general inquiry form (SAFTEE-GI) and a detailed specific inquiry form (SAFTEE-SI). The later includes a formal review of symptoms. The questions used are focused on the novelty of the symptoms and avoid implying any relationship to medication. The SAFTEE form utilizes specified terms which are listed by organ system to register the answers and guides the interviewer in a specific way to proceed. It has good reliability and validity and it is useful also in clinical practice as a structured way to assess adverse events.

14.2.7.2 Abnormal Involuntary Movement Scale (AIMS) (Abnormal Involuntary Movement Scale (AIMS) 1988; Lane et al. 1985)

The AIMS registers dyskinetic symptoms in patients taking antipsychotics. It includes 12 items but formally a total score is not calculated. It takes less than 10 min to administer and manifests excellent reliability and validity.

14.2.7.3 Simpson–Angus Rating Scale for Extrapyramidal Side Effects (Simpson and Angus 1970)

The Simpson–Angus rating scale was developed to monitor the effects of antipsychotics. It includes ten items and it focuses on the assessment of drug-induced parkinsonism. It takes approximately 10 min to administer and manifests good reliability and validity.

14.2.7.4 UKU-SERS (Lingjaerde et al. 1987)

The UKU-SERS provides a global and comprehensive side-effect profile with well-defined and operationalized items. It covers most known adverse events caused by psychotropic agents. It includes 48 items and takes approximately half an hour to administer, but it demands experienced trained clinicians for its application. The reliability and validity are both satisfactory. A patient-rated version is also available.

14.2.8 Substance Use Scales

The assessment of substance use disorders can be greatly facilitated with the use of self-report scales for a number of reasons, including saving time for the clinician and making the patient feeling more comfortable with reporting his abuse and dependence problems.

14.2.8.1 CAGE (Ewing 1984)

The CAGE was developed as a very brief screen for significant alcohol problems. It is an acronym for the four questions that comprise the instrument (cut-annoyed-guilt-eye opener). It can be administered in less than a minute, either orally or on paper. It is of unknown reliability but validity is very good, but it cannot identify early cases.

14.2.8.2 Alcohol Use Disorders Identification Test (AUDIT) (Saunders et al. 1993)

The AUDIT was developed by the WHO as a brief screening instrument for the early detection of hazardous and harmful alcohol use. It assesses alcohol use for the last year and currently. It includes ten items and can be applied in less than 5 min by a lay interviewer. It includes an optional clinical screening part involving a physical examination and blood tests. It has good reliability and validity and focuses on the early detection rather than the diagnosis.

14.2.8.3 Addiction Severity Index (ASI) (McLellan et al. 1992)

The ASI was developed to assess functional impairment due to alcohol or drug use problems. It includes 142 items which register both subjective patient reports as well as observations made by the interviewer. It covers the last month but also the lifetime of the patient, it takes more than an hour to apply and in principal it requires a trained clinician to administer. Its reliability and validity are reported to be good.

14.2.8.4 Drug Abuse Screening Test (DAST)

The DAST is an adaptation of the Michigan Alcohol Screening Test (MAST) and was developed as a screening and assessment instrument for drug abuse. It includes 20 items, it assesses lifetime drug use and it is sensitive to change at the lifetime scale but not for shorter periods. Its administration takes less than 10 min. Reliability and validity are reported to be good.

14.2.9 Other Rating Scales

A number of other rating scales exist, developed to assess a variety of topics and symptoms. These include the Risk Assessment for Suicidality Scale (RASS) (Fountoulakis et al. 2012b), the Scale to the Unawareness of Mental Disorder (SUMD), the Drug Attitude Inventory-30 items version (DAI-30), the Sleep Disorders Questionnaire (SDQ), the Arizona Sexual Experiences Scale (ASEX) and others.

14.3 Neuropsychological Tools

It is probably true that in most parts of the world, the training of the average psychiatrist focuses little on the ways of assessing in depth and detail the neurocognitive deficit. Therefore, the use of neuropsychological tools is almost the standard way to investigate this domain of symptomatology. An additional reason is that there is a long tradition of charting and quantification of the neurocognitive impairment across a variety of psychiatric and neurological disorders with the use of sophisticated tools.

The application of most of these tools requires some degree of special training since the interviewer should be familiar with neurocognitive function and its domains as well as their interplay. It is not unusual for an anxious geriatric patient to obtain a dementia-like MMSE score if the rater is inexperienced and applies the instrument in a cookbook fashion.

The most often used neuropsychological tests in everyday clinical practice is the Mini Mental Status Examination (MMSE) (Folstein et al. 1975), the Wechsler Memory Scale-Revised (D'Elia et al. 1989) the Trail Making Test (Reitan 1971) and the Clock Drawing Test (Sunderland et al. 1989). The general intelligence (IQ) can be measured with the Wechsler Adult Intelligence Scale- – Revised (WAIS-R) which includes two subscales: verbal and performance. The Verbal Fluency Test demands the patient to name as many objects and animals is able to, within a time frame of 1 min.

In Table 14.2 a list of cognitive domains and the test most useful in the assessment of each domain are given.

Table 14.2 List of neuropsychological tools by domain of assessment

Domain	Tool
General screening tests	Mini Mental State Examination (MMSE) Cambridge Cognitive Examination (CAMCOG)
Premorbid IQ	Single-word reading score from the North American Adult Reading Test (NAART) Wide Range Achievement Test (WRAT) Vocabulary subtest score from the Wechsler Adult Intelligence Scale (WAIS)
Current IQ	Wechsler Adult Intelligence Scale (WAIS)
Psychomotor and mental speed	Digit Symbol Substitution Test (DSST) Trail Making Test-A (TMT-A) Reaction time tests
Attention	Continuous Performance Test (CPT) Digits Forward
Working memory	Digits Backward
Verbal memory	
Learning	California Verbal Learning Test (CVLT)
Short delayed recall	Rey Auditory Verbal Learning Test (RAVLT)
Long delayed recall	Wechsler Memory Scale-Logical Memory (WMS-LM)
Recognition	Free recall
Nonverbal memory	Rey Complex Figure Test (RCFT)—Immediate and delayed recall Wechsler Memory Scale-Visual Reproduction (WMS-VR)
Visuospatial function	Block design Rey Complex Figure Test (RCFT)—copy
Language/verbal fluency	Controlled Oral Word Association Test (COWA-FAS) Animal Naming (AN)
Executive function	Wisconsin Card Sorting Test (WCST)—Categories achieved and perseverative errors Stroop Color Word Test (SCWT) Trail Making Test-B (TMT-B)
Social cognition and theory of mind	Benton Facial Recognition Test (BFRT) Faces Test (FT) Eyes Test (ET) Hinting Task (HT) False belief and deception tasks Picture sequencing Character intention tasks Faux pas

References

Abnormal Involuntary Movement Scale (AIMS) (1988) Psychopharmacol Bull 24(4):781–783

Akiskal HS, Akiskal KK, Haykal RF, Manning JS, Connor PD (2005) TEMPS-A: progress towards validation of a self-rated clinical version of the temperament evaluation of the Memphis, Pisa, Paris, and San Diego autoquestionnaire. J Affect Disord 85(1–2):3–16. doi:10.1016/j.jad.2004.12.001, S0165-0327(04)00397-0 [pii]

Andreasen NC, Arndt S, Miller D, Flaum M, Nopoulos P (1995) Correlational studies of the scale for the assessment of negative symptoms and the scale for the assessment of positive symptoms: an overview and update. Psychopathology 28(1):7–17

Angst J, Adolfsson R, Benazzi F, Gamma A, Hantouche E, Meyer TD, Skeppar P, Vieta E, Scott J (2005) The HCL-32: towards a self-assessment tool for hypomanic symptoms in outpatients. J Affect Disord 88(2):217–233. doi:10.1016/j.jad.2005.05.011

Bech P, Rafaelsen OJ, Kramp P, Bolwig TG (1978) The mania rating scale: scale construction and inter-observer agreement. Neuropharmacology 17(6):430–431

Beck AT, Ward CH, Mendelson M, Mock J, Erbaugh J (1961) An inventory for measuring depression. Arch Gen Psychiatry 4:561–571

Beck AT, Steer RA, Ball R, Ranieri W (1996) Comparison of Beck depression inventories -IA and -II in psychiatric outpatients. J Pers Assess 67(3):588–597

Butcher JN, Graham JR, Fowler RD (1991) Special series: the MMPI-2. J Pers Assess 57(2):203–204. doi:10.1207/s15327752jpa5702_1

Cloninger CR, Svrakic DM, Przybeck TR (1993) A psychobiological model of temperament and character. Arch Gen Psychiatry 50(12):975–990

Costa PT Jr, McCrae RR (1997) Stability and change in personality assessment: the revised NEO personality inventory in the year 2000. J Pers Assess 68(1):86–94

D'Elia L, Satz P, Schretlen D (1989) Wechsler memory scale: a critical appraisal of the normative studies. J Clin Exp Neuropsychol 11(4):551–568

Ewing JA (1984) Detecting alcoholism. The CAGE questionnaire. JAMA 252(14):1905–1907

Flemenbaum A, Zimmermann RL (1973) Inter- and intra-rater reliability of the brief psychiatric rating scale. Psychol Rep 32(3):783–792

Folstein MF, Folstein SE, McHugh PR (1975) "Mini-mental state". A practical method for grading the cognitive state of patients for the clinician. J Psychiatr Res 12(3):189–198, 0022-3956(75)90026-6 [pii]

Fountoulakis KN, Bech P, Panagiotidis P, Siamouli M, Kantartzis S, Papadopoulou A, Papadopoulou M, Kaprinis S, Kourila E, Iacovides A, St Kaprinis G (2007) Comparison of depressive indices: reliability, validity, relationship to anxiety and personality and the role of age and life events. J Affect Disord 97(1–3):187–195. doi:10.1016/j.jad.2006.06.015, S0165-0327(06)00283-7 [pii]

Fountoulakis KN, Lekka E, Kouidi E, Chouvarda I, Deligiannis A, Maglaveras N (2012a) Development of the global disability scale (Glo.Di.S): preliminary results. Ann Gen Psychiatry 11(1):14

Fountoulakis KN, Pantoula E, Siamouli M, Moutou K, Gonda X, Rihmer Z, Iacovides A, Akiskal H (2012b) Development of the risk assessment suicidality scale (RASS): a population-based study. J Affect Disord 138(3):449–457. doi:10.1016/j.jad.2011.12.045

Gabbard GO, Coyne L, Kennedy LL, Beasley C, Deering CD, Schroder P, Larson J, Cerney MS (1987) Interrater reliability in the use of the brief psychiatric rating scale. Bull Menninger Clin 51(6):519–531

Goodman WK, Price LH, Rasmussen SA, Mazure C, Delgado P, Heninger GR, Charney DS (1989a) The Yale-Brown obsessive compulsive scale. II. Validity. Arch Gen Psychiatry 46(11):1012–1016

Goodman WK, Price LH, Rasmussen SA, Mazure C, Fleischmann RL, Hill CL, Heninger GR, Charney DS (1989b) The Yale-Brown obsessive compulsive scale. I. Development, use, and reliability. Arch Gen Psychiatry 46(11):1006–1011

Guy W (1976) ECDEU assessment manual for psychopharmacology. US Department of Health, Education, and Welfare Public Health Service Alcohol, Drug Abuse, and Mental Health Administration, Rockville

Hamilton M (1959) The assessment of anxiety states by rating. Br J Med Psychol 32(1):50–55

Hamilton M (1960) A rating scale for depression. J Neurol Neurosurg Psychiatry 23:56–62

Kay SR, Fiszbein A, Opler LA (1987) The positive and negative syndrome scale (PANSS) for schizophrenia. Schizophr Bull 13(2):261–276

Lane RD, Glazer WM, Hansen TE, Berman WH, Kramer SI (1985) Assessment of tardive dyskinesia using the abnormal involuntary movement scale. J Nerv Ment Dis 173(6):353–357

Levine J, Schooler NR (1986) SAFTEE: a technique for the systematic assessment of side effects in clinical trials. Psychopharmacol Bull 22(2):343–381

Lingjaerde O, Ahlfors UG, Bech P, Dencker SJ, Elgen K (1987) The UKU side effect rating scale. A new comprehensive rating scale for psychotropic drugs and a cross-sectional study of side effects in neuroleptic-treated patients. Acta Psychiatr Scand Suppl 334:1–100

McHorney CA, Ware JE Jr, Raczek AE (1993) The MOS 36-item short-form health survey (SF-36): II. Psychometric and clinical tests of validity in measuring physical and mental health constructs. Med Care 31(3):247–263

McLellan AT, Kushner H, Metzger D, Peters R, Smith I, Grissom G, Pettinati H, Argeriou M (1992) The fifth edition of the addiction severity index. J Subst Abuse Treat 9(3):199–213

Montgomery SA, Asberg M (1979) A new depression scale designed to be sensitive to change. Br J Psychiatry 134:382–389

Morosini PL, Magliano L, Brambilla L, Ugolini S, Pioli R (2000) Development, reliability and acceptability of a new version of the DSM-IV social and occupational functioning assessment scale (SOFAS) to assess routine social functioning. Acta Psychiatr Scand 101(4):323–329

Mulrow C, Williams J, Gerety M, Ramirez G, Montiel O, Kerber C (1995) Case-finding instruments for depression in primary care settings. Ann Intern Med 123:913–921

Patterson DA, Lee MS (1995) Field trial of the global assessment of functioning scale–modified. Am J Psychiatry 152(9):1386–1388

Radloff L (1977) The CES-D scale: a self-report depression scale for research in the general population. Appl Psychol Meas 1:385–401

Reitan RM (1971) Trail making test results for normal and brain-damaged children. Percept Mot Skills 33(2):575–581

Rosenthal MP, Goldfarb NI, Carlson BL, Sagi PC, Balaban DJ (1987) Assessment of depression in a family practice center. J Fam Pract 25(2):143–149

Saunders JB, Aasland OG, Babor TF, de la Fuente JR, Grant M (1993) Development of the alcohol use disorders identification test (AUDIT): WHO collaborative project on early detection of persons with harmful alcohol consumption–II. Addiction 88(6):791–804

Shear MK, Brown TA, Barlow DH, Money R, Sholomskas DE, Woods SW, Gorman JM, Papp LA (1997) Multicenter collaborative panic disorder severity scale. Am J Psychiatry 154(11):1571–1575

Simpson GM, Angus JW (1970) A rating scale for extrapyramidal side effects. Acta Psychiatr Scand Suppl 212:11–19

Spielberger CD (1966) Theory and research on anxiety. In: Spielberger CD (ed) Anxiety and behavior. Academic, New York

Spielberger CD (1972) Anxiety as an emotional state. In: CDS (ed) Anxiety: current trends in theory and research, vol 1. Academic, New York

Spielberger CD (1976) The nature and measurement of anxiety. In: CDSRD-G (ed) Cross-cultural anxiety. Hemisphere/Wiley, Washington, DC

Spielberger CD (1979) Preliminary manual for the State-Trait Personality Inventory (STPI). University of South Florida

Spielberger CD, Gorsuch RL, Lushene RE (1970) Manual for the state-trait anxiety inventory (self-evaluation questionnaire). Consulting Psychologists Press, Palo Alto

Sunderland T, Hill JL, Mellow AM, Lawlor BA, Gundersheimer J, Newhouse PA, Grafman JH (1989) Clock drawing in Alzheimer's disease. A novel measure of dementia severity. J Am Geriatr Soc 37(8):725–729

Yesavage JA, Brink TL, Rose TL, Lum O, Huang V, Adey M, Leirer VO (1982) Development and validation of a geriatric depression screening scale: a preliminary report. J Psychiatr Res 17(1):37–49

Young RC, Biggs JT, Ziegler VE, Meyer DA (1978) A rating scale for mania: reliability, validity and sensitivity. Br J Psychiatry 133:429–435
Zanello A, Berthoud L, Ventura J, Merlo MC (2013) The brief psychiatric rating scale (version 4.0) factorial structure and its sensitivity in the treatment of outpatients with unipolar depression. Psychiatry Res 210(2):626–633. doi:10.1016/j.psychres.2013.07.001
Zung WW (1965) A self-rating depression scale. Arch Gen Psychiatry 12:63–70

Staging of Bipolar Disorder

15

15.1 The Concept of Staging

After the revolution which was brought with the introduction of operationalized diagnostic criteria by contemporary classification systems, the reliability and the validity of psychiatric diagnosis were greatly improved. Following the improvement in categorical diagnosis, two new needs emerge. The first is to explore all aspects of symptomatology and quantify severity. This is a function addressed with the use of psychometric and neuropsychological tools. There is much improvement in this field although much remains to be done (see Chap. 14). The second and still unfulfilled need is to define and rate seriousness, progression, changes in physiology and damage made and the extent and the specific characteristics of the disease. 'Staging' is the term which defines this procedure and it can provide the clinician with a valuable tool to assist the treatment design.

The field in medicine where staging is most successful and enjoys great importance is that of clinical oncology. In cancer treatment, staging is a valuable tool which determines the treatment strategy and suggests the prognosis.

It is common that psychiatrists constantly use some kind of a staging system; however, all of these systems are informal and they derive from subjective and anecdotal personal clinical experience. A true scientific staging system would constitute a heuristic tool intending to position the patient on a gradient of stages from 'unsymptomatic but at risk' to 'end stage'.

In 1993, there was the first formal proposal for the staging of mental illness (Fava and Kellner 1993). Several attempts followed (McGorry 2007) and 20 years later, a significant literature on the feasibility of staging and usefulness and its limits in psychiatry is available (Cosci and Fava 2013; McGorry 2007, 2010a, b; McGorry et al. 2006, 2007, 2010; Yung and McGorry 1996, 2007; Vieta et al. 2011).

It is important to note that in psychiatry, the diagnostic reliability and validity does not lead to predictive validity in the majority of cases (Hickie et al. 2013). Different diagnoses might have similar prognosis and overlapping treatments and persons with the same diagnosis might have different prognosis and need radically

K.N. Fountoulakis, *Bipolar Disorder: An Evidence-Based Guide to Manic Depression*, DOI 10.1007/978-3-642-37216-2_15

different treatments. Staging is one of the concepts which come to fill the gap between diagnosis and prognosis.

The concept of staging if and when applied has a number of implications. Almost by definition, it suggests that early stages are easier to treat while later stages are rather refractory to treatment. Thus, these later stages might need the application of treatment options with more adverse events and higher risk and less overall benefit (Post et al. 2010).

15.2 Staging of BD

It is reasonable to assume that staging can be applied to any illness or disorder that tends to progress. Although there is an old debate whether BD is static or progressing, the predominant approach today is that it is progressive at least to the extent other mental disorders are and not as benign as thought in the past. A description of its long-term course is discussed in Chap. 3 of the current book.

A reliable staging model is long in place concerning schizophrenia (Insel 2010), but staging is still a matter of debate concerning mood disorders. The 'kindling effect' was an early effort on this direction and probably works well for unipolar depression (Kendler et al. 2000; Post 1992; Segal et al. 1996); however, BD is rather too complex so that a single factor, procedure or approach could be sufficient for its staging. Probably a single model of early and very late stages of BD is viable (McGorry et al. 2008; Baldessarini et al. 2014), but things become rather complex in the middle.

Furthermore, often things are not as simple and straightforward as they seem or we wish them to be. Some authors generalize the finding for trials on the usefulness of early identification of the prodromal symptoms of relapse (Perry et al. 1999) to suggest that a similar strategy would be appropriate and beneficial for the prodromal stage of the disease, but this is a completely different issue.

Additionally, a factor which complicates the staging concept itself as well as the staging models is the effect of medication. It is certain that medication reduces symptoms, but it is uncertain whether there are medications which are truly neuroprotective in the neurobiological sense. There are some authors who argue that lithium might be such an agent, but the data are inconclusive, especially when it is combined with typical antipsychotics (Fountoulakis et al. 2008c). On the other hand, it is certain that many pharmacological agents exert severe adverse effects on the general somatic health of patients thus perplexing their overall picture and maybe perplexing the staging. Even if we set aside the fact that the prodromal phase as we consider it today lacks both specificity and sensitivity, it is unknown whether early treatment (during childhood or adolescence) with any of the agents in use today will benefit or actually worsen the overall outcome of the disease since preventive efficacy is unknown and adverse effects probable.

15.2.1 Clinical Determinants of BD Staging

The earliest research contribution to the effort of staging BD was the description of the stages of mania in the early 1970s (see Chap. 2). Carlson and Goodwin not only

Table 15.1 List of the multiple clinical aspects of manic–depressive illness

1. Manic episodes
2. Depressive episodes
3. Mixed episodes
4. Subthreshold manic symptoms
5. Subthreshold depressive symptoms
6. 'Mixed' states and 'roughening'
7. Mood lability/cyclothymia/'personality-like' behaviour
8. Psychotic features
9. Predominant polarity
10. Frequency of episodes/rapid cycling
11. Neurocognitive disorder
12. Drug/alcohol abuse
13. Behavioural dependencies (e.g. gambling)
14. Comorbid anxiety and other mental disorders
15. Comorbid somatic disorders
16. Self-destructive behaviour and suicidality
17. Functional deficit and disability

described discrete stages in the development and course of acute mania, but also they described a 'rollback phenomenon', that is, the clinical condition improves by manifesting the same stages but at a reverse order (Carlson and Goodwin 1973). Fava and colleagues proposed a somewhat different staging model for acute mania which included a prodromal personality-like stage, one hypomania and one mania without psychotic features stages and a psychotic mania stage (Fava and Kellner 1993). However, the description or the staging of acute episodes has a minor influence on the staging of the complete picture and the long-term course of BD.

If one takes the whole constellation of features and symptoms of BD into consideration (Table 15.1), he will realize that a staging system should include all these features and consider their position in the long-term course of the disorder and their relationship to treatment response, overall outcome and disability. The major features are acute major mood episodes, subthreshold and personality-like symptoms, psychotic features, predominant polarity, frequency, the neurocognitive deficit and comorbidity.

It seems that manic and depressive episodes load BD patients each with a different kind of burden and they push different pathways in the advancement of the disease. Mixed episodes sometimes resemble manic and sometimes resemble depressive episodes. Probably the predominant polarity, after several years, eventually turns to be depressive in the majority of patients (Alessandra et al. 2013; Garcia-Lopez et al. 2009; Popovic and Vieta 2013), while subsyndromal depressive symptoms dominate the inter-episode intervals, often since the beginning of the illness. Thus, depression is usually always present while the tendency to relapse into a manic episode seems to wane with the advancement of the disease. Even subsyndromal depressive symptoms cause significant disability (Judd and Akiskal 2003) and they put the patient at a three-time higher risk to relapse (Judd et al. 2008). Therefore, it seems it is depression that is mainly responsible for the burden of the disease (Judd et al. 2002, 2003; Goodwin and Jamison 2007).

Later in the course of the illness, with repeated acute episodes and with the increasing duration of the disease, the neurocognitive functioning worsens (Lewandowski et al. 2011; Clark et al. 2002; Cavanagh et al. 2002; Lebowitz et al. 2001; Zubieta et al. 2001; Denicoff et al. 1999; El-Badri et al. 2001; Reinares et al. 2010). One study reported that good vs. poor outcome groups, corresponding to early and late stages of BD, differed in terms of two underlying dimensions: illness severity and neurocognitive function (Reinares et al. 2013). More precisely it seems that manic episodes as well as psychotic features are those which load the patient with most of the neurocognitive deficit (Lewandowski et al. 2011). Depressive episodes also increase the neurocognitive impairment but to a lesser extent in comparison to manic episodes (Robinson and Ferrier 2006). There are data implying that the neurocognitive deficit might not progress after a specific stage (Strejilevich and Martino 2013).

Psychotic features seem to be a very important element which is related more with manic episodes. However, even in the frame of bipolar depression, psychotic features constitute a stable trait which tends to repeat itself across episodes (Helms and Smith 1983; Nelson et al. 1984; Aronson et al. 1988a, b).

The place of cyclothymia and dysthymia on this life-chart-based staging method is unknown, although cyclothymia is used in the already proposed staging models as an early prodromal phase (Cosci and Fava 2013; Berk et al. 2007a, b).

Rapid cycling is a complicated issue. Probably rapid cycling patients experience a higher number of major mood episodes in comparison to non-rapid cyclers, and this adds to the overall burden. The role of the number of episodes has been solidly proven by a number of authors (Torres et al. 2010; Vieta et al. 2013; Lopez-Jaramillo et al. 2010; Rosa et al. 2012; Post et al. 2003, 2010; Tohen et al. 2010; McGorry 2010a) and this is also the conclusion from an analysis of STEP-BD data which suggested that the number of previous episodes can be used as a reliable and valid proxy of staging (Magalhaes et al. 2012a). On the other hand, it seems that rapid cycling is state rather than trait and might not be valid as a long-term indicator (Carvalho et al. 2014). It is not known whether rapid cycling disappears as a process or it is overwhelmed by the domination of other stronger features, e.g. chronic unremitted depression. Chronic depression also determines to a significant extent the overall refractoriness, mainly because the available treatment options for bipolar depression are limited in comparison with those against mania (Fountoulakis et al. 2008b, 2011; Fountoulakis and Vieta 2008; Fountoulakis 2009).

Probably the only reliable prodromal syndrome is the presence of clinical anxiety in high-risk adolescents which increases the age-adjusted risk for the development of mood disorder from 40 to 85 % (HR = 2.6) with a similar increase in the risk for comorbid substance abuse during or after the development of the acute mood episode (Duffy et al. 2010).

A graphic representation of the important clinical features and their longitudinal possible relationship to the stages of BD is shown in Fig. 15.1. Probably the curves presented in this figure include also oscillations, but this feature was omitted for the sake of simplicity. On the basis of clinical data, it seems that three major stages can be identified, in addition to the at-risk and prodromal phase. The first stage includes a rather benign course with acute episodes of balanced polarity without psychotic features, good neurocognitive function, good response to treatment and also probably spontaneous remission. Important elements at this stage are the low frequency of inter-episode residual symptoms and good overall functioning without disability. On

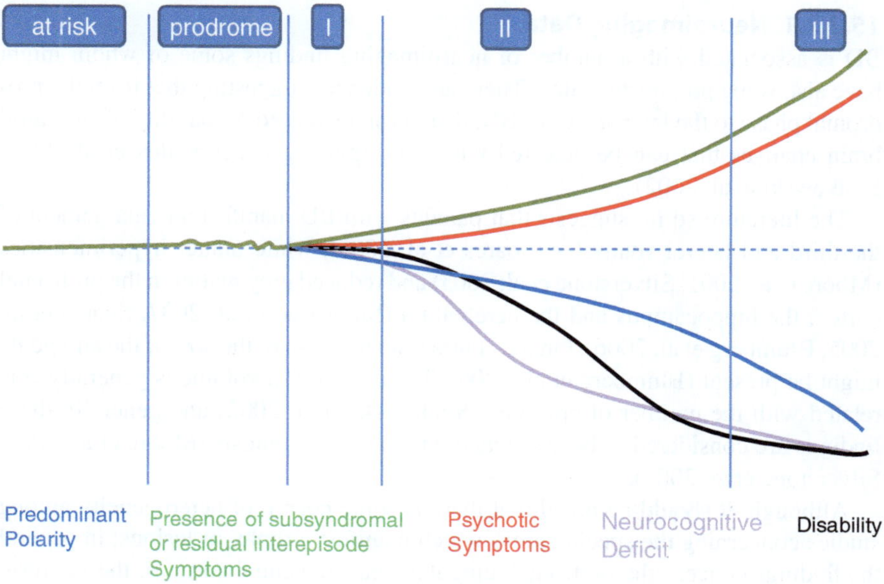

Fig. 15.1 A graphic representation of the important clinical features and their longitudinal possible relationship to the stages of BD. Probably the curves presented in this figure include also oscillations, but this feature was omitted for the sake of simplicity

the contrary, the third (last) stage is probably characterized by depressive predominant polarity with chronic refractory unremitted depression often with psychotic features, accompanied by a significant neurocognitive deficit and severe overall disability. Probably severe somatic comorbidity is present also, but this remains to be shown. These are in accord with research data which support the validity of the early vs. late stages in terms of differences in functioning and disability (Kapczinski et al. 2014; Rosa et al. 2012, 2014; Scott et al. 2013; Hamilton et al. 2011).

The middle stage is characterized by variability and probably it is composed by many different trajectories which reflect different combinations of clinical features and courses as well as comorbidities. Since many patients seek professional help only after they enter this stage, future research should focus mainly on this as well as in at-risk persons and the prodromal phase. One should have in mind that so far research has shown that risk factors and prodromal symptoms are non-specific and with low predictive value, maybe with the exception of anxiety in adolescents with positive family history (Fava 1999; McNamara et al. 2010).

15.2.2 Neurobiological Determinants of BD Staging

The neurobiology of BD is not well studied and the literature is rather limited in comparison to schizophrenia and unipolar depression. However, there is at least some data which suggests that a number of biomarkers differ in early- and late-stage BD (Kapczinski et al. 2009a).

15.2.2.1 Neuroimaging Data

BD is associated with a number of neuroimaging findings some of whom might have also some prognostic value. There are evidences suggesting that from the prodromal phase to the later stages of BD, there is an increased probability of structural brain changes that can be detected with neuroimaging (Lagopoulos et al. 2012; Strakowski et al. 2002).

The literature so far suggests that patients with BD manifest an enlargement of the third and lateral ventricles (Soares et al. 2005), white matter hyperintensities (Moore et al. 2001; Silverstone et al. 2003) and reduced grey matter in the prefrontal cortex, the hippocampus and the cerebellum (Moorhead et al. 2007; Soares et al. 2005; Blumberg et al. 2006). On the contrary an increase in the size of the amygdala might be present (Blumberg et al. 2006). The decrease in volume is generally correlated with the number of episodes (Strakowski et al. 2002) and generally these findings are considered to be associated with a poor prognosis (Moore et al. 2001; Silverstone et al. 2003).

Although, it should be noted that there is some degree of heterogeneity among studies concerning the specific areas which manifest atrophy or lesions; in general the findings concern the prefrontal, cingulate and subgenual cortices; the fusiform gyrus; and the left hippocampus (Lin et al. 2013; Javadapour et al. 2007; Fountoulakis et al. 2008a). On the other hand, there are reports suggesting that there was no difference in grey matter loss in BD patients in comparison to controls and there was also no effect of the number of episodes (Nery et al. 2009). In spite of findings concerning specific regions, it seems that the total brain volume remains stable, and this puts forward a number of problems concerning the methods of quantification of brain volume and other methodological issues (Fountoulakis et al. 2008a).

It is interesting that while in schizophrenia a loss of brain volume is evident already at onset, in BD this happens later. This is especially true concerning grey matter, while on the contrary, the loss of white mater volume might happen first and be present already at onset (Berk et al. 2010; Vita et al. 2009; Bora et al. 2010; Strakowski et al. 1993). Therefore, it is possible that white matter pathology is the prominent finding during the early stages (Lin et al. 2013), while grey matter loss follows years later (Arango et al. 2012).

Overall, the literature on neuroimaging data at different stages of BD is limited and most of the data are cross-sectional (Lim et al. 2013; Balanza-Martinez et al. 2005).

15.2.2.2 Neurochemical Data

The debate on the usefulness of peripheral biomarkers in psychiatry is several decades old; however, they are still considered to be important because they are conceptualized as mediators of allostasis and neurodegeneration (Juster et al. 2010; Kapczinski et al. 2008b; Berk 2009; Berk et al. 2011b).

Generally, it has been hypothesized that cellular mechanisms of resilience to stress are less efficient at later stages of BD (Fries et al. 2012). Research data suggest the levels of brain-derived neurotrophic factor (BDNF) (Cunha et al. 2008), neurotrophin-3 and neurotrophin-4 (NT3 and NT4) (Walz et al. 2007, 2009) and glial cell line-derived neurotrophic factor (GDNF) (Rosa et al. 2006) levels are reduced in BD patients.

An important study measured BDNF, tumour necrosis factor (TNF)-alpha and interleukin-6 and interleukin-10 levels in 60 BD-I patients and 60 matched healthy controls. It reported that BDNF was negatively correlated with the length of illness and was decreased only in the patients at the late stages of the disease. All the interleukins and TNF-alpha were increased already since the early stages, but interleukin-6 was not increased during the later stages. Also BDNF and interleukin-6 showed a relative decrease at the later stages in comparison to the earlier stages. TNF-alpha showed a further increase at the later stage. It seems that the decreases in the BDNF levels in BD patients are also age related (Yatham et al. 2009). Another study confirmed the finding that the levels of interleukin-10 decline in the late stages of BD (Rosa et al. 2014). These results are suggestive of a failure of those mechanisms responsible for the defence against the toxic effects of inflammation (i.e. BDNF) at later stages, while on the contrary, the inflammatory process persists (Kauer-Sant'Anna et al. 2009).

Further exploration of this sample also revealed a significant increase in 3-nitrotyrosine levels among all patients. The activity of glutathione S-transferase and reductase was increased only in the late-stage patients. Glutathione peroxidase activity and carbonyl content did not differ among the groups. These data are in accord with a possible tyrosine nitration-induced damage in BD patients that is present already since the early stages of the illness. The increased activity of glutathione S-transferase and reductase at later stages might suggest the activation of a compensatory mechanism (Andreazza et al. 2009). Also, serum thiobarbituric acid reactive substances and BDNF levels were found to be negatively correlated one to the other in BD patients but not in controls, suggesting that the lowering of BDNF levels in acute episodes occurs in parallel with increased oxidative stress, suggesting that such changes occur in an orchestrated fashion (Kapczinski et al. 2008a). The comparison of these patients to sepsis patients revealed almost similar levels of toxicity (Kapczinski et al. 2011). In partial disagreement with the above, a study in 115 BD patients and 25 first-degree relatives reported that increased interleukin-6 was associated with the late stages of the disease (Grande et al. 2014).

Similar conclusions were found by a study in 130 BD patients and 130 controls which reported that BD patients had significantly higher levels of inflammatory cytokines, including soluble interleukin-6 receptor (sIL-6R), soluble interleukin-2 receptor, C-reactive protein (CRP), soluble tumour necrosis factor receptor type 1 (sTNF-R1), soluble P-selectin receptor (sP-selectin) and monocyte chemotactic protein-1 (MCP-1). BD-II patients had lower levels of sTNF-R1 in comparison to BD-I. Also depressed patients had significantly lower levels of sTNF-R1 than the patients in manic/hypomanic episode and euthymic patients. These results in combination with the clinical data mentioned previously might suggest a role for sTNF-R1 in the staging of BD (Bai et al. 2014).

Two studies supported the hypothesis that mainly mania is associated with a proinflammatory state. The first one investigated serum high-sensitivity C-reactive protein (hsCRP) in manic, depressed and euthymic BD patients in comparison to controls and reported that the serum hsCRP levels were increased in manic patients in comparison to euthymic and depressed BD patients and controls. These results are in accord with clinical data suggesting a specific neurotoxic effect of acute manic episodes (Cunha et al. 2008). In accord with this, the comparison of 61 BD patients with 25 controls in terms TNF-alpha, interleukin-2, interleukin-4, interleukin-6, interleukin-10 and IFN-gamma revealed that during mania interleukin-2, interleukin-4 and interleukin-6 were increased in BD patients in comparison with controls while depressed patients manifested an increase only in interleukin-6 levels and euthymic patients only in interleukin-4 (Brietzke et al. 2009).

The failure of protective mechanisms at later stages was confirmed by a meta-analysis which reported a correlation between the age and length of illness and serum BDNF (Fernandes et al. 2011). However, it seems that in spite of the more or less proper functioning of neuroprotective mechanisms during the early stages of BD, damage might start early. The assessment of serum protein carbonyl content (PCC) and thiobarbituric acid reactive substances (TBARS) suggested that BD patients had higher PCC levels than healthy subjects which is suggestive of a protein oxidative damage since the early stages (Magalhaes et al. 2012b). In another study the glial activity was assessed by measuring serum S100B content; the oxidative stress was assessed using serum TBARS and activities of antioxidant enzymes in BD patients during different episodes of the disease. The results showed that there was a significant increase of serum S100B during episodes of mania and depression, but not in euthymic patients. Superoxide dismutase (SOD) activity, as well the SOD/glutathione peroxidase plus catalase ratio, was also increased in manic and depressed patients. On the other hand, TBARS levels were increased in BD patients regardless of the phase of the disorder. These findings suggest a potential oxidative damage in BD patients with the mechanism being active mainly during the active phases of the illness but not during the euthymic phase. Such changes appear to relate to astrocyte function, as indicated by serum S100B elevation and thus they can also be related theoretically to brain MRI findings (Andreazza et al. 2007a).

The development of a 'systemic toxicity index' suggested that neurotoxicity was similar in patients under an acute manic or depressive episode and higher than in euthymic patients. The latter were similar to controls (Kapczinski et al. 2010; Magalhaes et al. 2011). An interesting finding was that the overall toxicity seemed to be attenuated in patients under medication treatment (Magalhaes et al. 2011). Another study reported that the levels of only SOD, catalase (CAT), alpha-linolenic acid and eicosapentaenoic acid (EPA) were significantly lower in BD patients, whereas glutathione peroxidase (GPx) was not (Ranjekar et al. 2003).

There is also a line of research indicating a significant damage in the DNA of BD patients in comparison to controls. The measuring of urinary excretion of 8-oxo-7,8-dihydro-2′-deoxyguanosine (8-oxodG) and 8-oxo-7,8-dihydroguanosine (8-oxoGuo) which are both markers of oxidatively generated DNA and RNA damage in 37 rapid cycling BD patients and in 40 age- and gender-matched controls revealed that the excretion of both was 40 % elevated in euthymic BD patients in comparison to controls. These results support the presence of an increased oxidatively generated damage to nucleosides in BD patients (Munkholm et al. 2014). Additionally the comparison of BD patients and controls in terms of the leukocyte mitochondrial DNA (mtDNA) revealed that the copy number was significantly lower in the BD group suggesting that BD patients had significantly higher mitochondrial oxidative damage which was also positively correlated with age (Chang et al. 2014). Similarly, the investigation of 32 BD-I outpatients and 32 controls for DNA damage with the single cell gel electrophoresis comet assay revealed that there was an increased frequency of DNA damage in BD patients relative to controls, which correlated with the severity of symptoms of both depression and mania (Andreazza et al. 2007b). The measurement of the telomere length in 44 chronic mood patients and 44 controls revealed that the telomere length was significantly shorter in patients, representing as much as 10 years of accelerated ageing (Simon et al. 2006).

Overall, it seems there is considerable literature to support the hypothesis that in BD patients an inflammatory process exists, and it is combined at later stages with a deterioration of neurotrophic factors efficacy. The data so far imply that there is a combination of inflammation, oxidative stress, apoptosis and impairment in neurogenesis. This combination could result in the anatomical changes already mentioned above, probably via pro-apoptotic pathways, and the overall result is correlated with the number of mood episodes which exert a cumulative effect (Brietzke and Kapczinski 2008; Kapczinski et al. 2008b; Post et al. 2003). There are limited data supporting the idea that successful treatment could be neuroprotective and it could attenuate the neurostructural changes and postpone or even halt the progress on the disease (Berk et al. 2014).

So far there is one RCT which has shown the utility of the glutathione precursor N-acetyl cysteine which is a substance which might reinforce the role of the pathways of neuroprotection and neurogenesis (Berk et al. 2008).

15.2.3 Treatment Data Supporting the Staging Approach

The results of the European Mania in Bipolar Longitudinal Evaluation of Medication (EMBLEM) study which included 3,115 BD patients reported that significantly more first-episode patients achieved complete symptomatic and functional recovery in comparison to those patients with multiple episodes (Tohen et al. 2010).

A post hoc analysis reported that patients at an early stage benefited from caregiver psychoeducation by having longer time to recurrence, while there were no significant benefits from caregiver psychoeducation in patients at later stages (Reinares et al. 2010). Overall, this seems to be a generalized effect concerning psychotherapy in BD patients (Reinares et al. 2013; Scott et al. 2006) with 10–12 previous episodes probably constituting the cut-off. On the contrary, it seems that functional remediation could be more suitable for patients in advanced stages (Torrent et al. 2013).

The analysis of the pooled data from mania, depression and maintenance studies of olanzapine suggested that the response rates for the mania and maintenance studies ranged from 52 to 69 % and 10–50 %, respectively, for individuals with one to five previous episodes and from 29 to 59 % and 11–40 % for individuals with >5 previous episodes. For the depression studies, response rates were significantly higher for the one to five group for two measures only and the difference was less robust (Berk et al. 2011a). Similarly further studies support the suggestion that lithium and olanzapine appear to be more efficacious during the early phases of the BD (Swann et al. 1999; Ketter et al. 2006) and maybe that higher lithium levels might be necessary to achieve a therapeutic effect after three or more mood episodes (Gelenberg et al. 1989).

15.3 Existing Models for the Staging of BD

There are five major staging models proposed concerning BD (Berk et al. 2007a, b; Kapczinski et al. 2009b; Post 2010; Frank et al. 2014; Cosci and Fava 2013; Post et al. 2012). In summary they are shown in Table 15.2 together with the possible accompanied clinical, neurobiological and treatment data as well as disability status.

15.3.1 The Model of Berk et al. (2007a, b)

Stage 0: *asymptomatic at-risk stage*

This stage refers to the period before the manifestation of any kind of symptomatology. It concerns persons loaded with potent risk factors for the development of BD, including family history of either BD or unipolar depression, history of pregnancy or obstetric complications, winter–spring birth, childbirth, early traumatic events and childhood history of physical or sexual abuse. Biological risk factors (endophenotypes) include circadian rhythms, response to sleep deprivation, white matter hyperintensities, response to psychostimulants, cholinergic sensitivity, P300 event-related potential abnormalities and changes in peripheral mononuclear cells. A history of substance abuse constitutes an additional risk factor.

Stage 1a and 1b: *prodrome*

During this stage, the patient experiences the onset of subthreshold symptoms (dysthymia, cyclothymia) or mood fluctuations and a variety of comorbid conditions and behavioural problems. Unfortunately and in spite of various proposals, currently there are no specific symptoms in the frame of depressive symptomatology to denote the onset of BD. The most promising seem to be the refractoriness to antidepressants and antidepressant-induced mania, hypomania or agitation. An additional problem is that this stage is not specific for BD.

Stage 2: *first-episode mood disorder*

At this point a formal diagnosis is made and proper treatment is essential. Unfortunately the first episode is most often depressive and the diagnosis of unipolar depression is put. This delays proper treatment until a manic or hypomanic episode emerges. Currently it is impossible to differentiate bipolar from unipolar depression in a reliable and valid way.

Stage 3b: *recurrence*

At this stage the diagnosis is firm, episodes alternate and polarity slowly turns into depressive. Response to treatment is variable and so is residual inter-episode symptomatology.

Table 15.2 A summary of the existing models for the staging of BD against the clinical, neurobiological and treatment data and disability as discussed in the current chapter

Stage	Berk et al.	Kapczinski et al.	Cosci and Fava	Post et al.	Frank et al.	Findings
At-risk	Stage 0: asymptomatic at-risk stage	Latent phase	–	Stage I–II	Stage 0	*Clinical*: asymptomatic *Neurobiology*: genes *Treatment*: unknown *Disability*: absent
Prodrome	Stage 1a and 1b: prodrome	–	Stage 1	Stage III	Stage 1a, b	*Clinical*: non-specific symptoms, anxiety *Neurobiology*: white matter hyperintensities *Treatment*: unknown *Disability*: absent
First episode	Stage 2: first-episode mood disorder	Stage I	Stage 2	Stage IV	Stage 2	*Clinical*: acute mania or major depression *Neurobiology*: white matter loss, inflammation mechanisms activated, neuroprotective mechanisms intact *Treatment*: good response to medication, psychoeducation recommended *Disability*: absent
Early phase	Stage 3b: recurrence	Stage I	Mainly stage 2, partially stage 3	Stage V	Stage 3a, b	*Clinical*: acute episodes of either pole, without or with minimal residual symptoms *Neurobiology*: white matter loss, probably grey matter loss, inflammation mechanisms activated, neuroprotective mechanisms relatively but not entirely intact *Treatment*: good response to medication, psychoeducation recommended *Disability*: mild

(continued)

Table 15.2 (continued)

Stage	Berk et al.	Kapczinski et al.	Cosci and Fava	Post et al.	Frank et al.	Findings
Middle phase	Stage 3b: recurrence	Stage II	Stage 3 and 4	Stage VI	Stage 3a, b	*Clinical*: acute episodes of either pole with significant residual symptoms, psychotic symptoms, neurocognitive decline *Neurobiology*: both white and grey matter loss. Inflammation process active, neuroprotective mechanisms gradually declining. Possible DNA damage *Treatment*: variable response to medication. Unknown which psychotherapy is more suitable *Disability*: moderate
Late phase	Stage 4: treatment resistance	Stage III and IV	Stage 3 and 4	Stage VII–VIII	Stage 4	*Clinical*: predominant depressive polarity, possibly with mixed and psychotic features, severe neurocognitive deficit *Neurobiology*: both white and grey matter loss, inflammation process active, neuroprotective mechanisms failing, DNA damage *Treatment*: refractoriness, recommendation for functional remediation *Disability*: severe

Stage 4: treatment resistance

The definition of treatment resistance is complex (Fountoulakis 2012); however, it seems that with the passing years and accumulation of episodes, BD patients develop a type of resistance to treatment. The duration of episodes is prolonged and residual symptoms (especially depressive) is the rule rather than the exception.

15.3.2 The Model of Kapczinski et al. (2009b)

Latent phase

This model puts significant emphasis in family history and more specifically on the genetic loading of individuals. Thus, it defines a first phase which includes asymptomatic persons at risk for developing BD. The recommended intervention is to avoid environmental factors which supposedly interact with genes to produce psychopathology.

Stage I

This model does not include a prodrome stage with subsyndromal symptoms. It proceeds to stage I which is characterized by full remission of episodes without any residual symptoms between episodes. This suggests a benign course of the illness and/or excellent response to treatment.

Stage II

This stage is characterized by the presence of inter-episode symptoms and comorbidities. Response to treatment is less good and impairment starts emerging.

Stage III

This stage is characterized by neurocognitive impairment and significant functional disability. Response to treatment is poor and complex strategies are needed.

Stage IV

Severe disability and neurocognitive impairment; unable to live alone.

15.3.3 The Model of Post et al. (Post 2010; Post et al. 2012)

Stage I

Initial vulnerability based on genetic or environmental impact

Stage II

The well-interval

Stage III

The prodrome

Stage IV

Illness onset with the occurrence of a full-blown episode

Stage V
Episode recurrence

Stage VI
Illness progression

Stage VII
Treatment refractoriness

Stage VIII
Late- or end-stage illness with catastrophic social, neurocognitive and medical deterioration and inability to care for oneself

15.3.4 The Model of Cosci and Fava (2013)

Stage 1
This stage corresponds to a prodromal phase and includes mild or non-specific symptoms of mood disorder and/or cyclothymia

Stage 2
It includes the development of full-blown major depressive or manic/hypomanic episodes

Stage 3
Concerns the presence of residual phase symptoms with marked neurocognitive deficit and disability in spite of treatment

Stage 4
Refers to refractoriness to treatment with the emergence of acute episodes despite mood-stabilizing treatment

15.3.5 The Model of Frank et al. (2014)

Stage 0
This state refers to an increased risk of BD in asymptomatic patients.

Stage 1a
This includes the presence of mild or non-specific symptoms.

Stage 1b
It refers to ultra-high risk. There are moderate but subthreshold symptoms present, with neurocognitive impairment and functional decline.

Stage 2
First full-blown episode of BD. Presence of neurocognitive deficits and functional decline.

Stage 3a
Incomplete remission from first episode.

Stage 3b
Includes the recurrence or relapse of psychotic or mood symptoms, but with good response to treatment. Presence of residual symptoms or neurocognition below the best level achieved following remission from first episode.

Stage 4
Severe, chronic illness with significant disability.

15.4 The Future of Staging of BD

A summary of the existing models for the staging of BD against the clinical, neurobiological, treatment data and disability as discussed in the current chapter is shown in Table 15.2.

There is broad consensus that staging of BD could be proven valuable both in the prevention and in the development of more efficacious and appropriate treatment of BD (McIntyre and Correll 2014); however, there is important controversy as to how far we can go on the basis of existing data.

Although there is some support for the proposed staging models, the research base is thin, the heterogeneity of the data is significant and the studies include small numbers. A number of vicious logical cycles could be in place. Most of the data are cross-sectional (Kapczinski et al. 2014) and the need for a transdiagnostic and longitudinal research approach is prominent (Lin et al. 2013).

The data so far support the presence of an asymptomatic at-risk phase and of a non-specific prodromal phase. This prodromal phase seems to be common for a number of mental disorders and prediction is impossible on the basis of current knowledge. The literature is also supportive of the presence of an early stage of the full-blown illness, during which the episodes are well defined, there are no or very few inter-episode residual symptoms, there is good response to treatment and there is little disability. It is also in support for the presence of a late stage which is associated with a more chronic and refractory disease, probably with depressive predominant polarity, psychotic features and significant disability. It is disappointing that there is little research on the treatment effect at late stages (Berk et al. 2012).

Future research should utilize a longitudinal prospective design in order to chart in detail the clinical picture (including neurocognitive function and disability) as well as the neurobiological changes that occur in the long-term course of BD and their relationship with the response to treatment. Such an approach will provide with valuable information on how to best stage BD and how to best design the therapeutic intervention.

References

Alessandra MA, Colom F, Pacchiarotti I, Murru A, Scott J, Valenti M, Mazzarini L, Mar Bonnin CD, Jose SM, Serretti A, Vieta E (2013) Treatment strategies according to clinical features in a naturalistic cohort study of bipolar patients: a principal component analysis of lifetime pharmacological and biophysic treatment options. Eur Neuropsychopharmacol 23(4):263–275

Andreazza AC, Cassini C, Rosa AR, Leite MC, de Almeida LM, Nardin P, Cunha AB, Ceresér KM, Santin A, Gottfried C, Salvador M, Kapczinski F, Goncalves CA (2007a) Serum S100B and antioxidant enzymes in bipolar patients. J Psychiatr Res 41(6):523–529. doi:10.1016/j.jpsychires.2006.07.013

Andreazza AC, Frey BN, Erdtmann B, Salvador M, Rombaldi F, Santin A, Goncalves CA, Kapczinski F (2007b) DNA damage in bipolar disorder. Psychiatry Res 153(1):27–32. doi:10.1016/j.psychres.2006.03.025

Andreazza AC, Kapczinski F, Kauer-Sant'Anna M, Walz JC, Bond DJ, Goncalves CA, Young LT, Yatham LN (2009) 3-Nitrotyrosine and glutathione antioxidant system in patients in the early and late stages of bipolar disorder. J Psychiatry Neurosci 34(4):263–271

Arango C, Rapado-Castro M, Reig S, Castro-Fornieles J, Gonzalez-Pinto A, Otero S, Baeza I, Moreno C, Graell M, Janssen J, Parellada M, Moreno D, Bargallo N, Desco M (2012) Progressive brain changes in children and adolescents with first-episode psychosis. Arch Gen Psychiatry 69(1):16–26. doi:10.1001/archgenpsychiatry.2011.150

Aronson TA, Shukla S, Gujavarty K, Hoff A, DiBuono M, Khan E (1988a) Relapse in delusional depression: a retrospective study of the course of treatment. Compr Psychiatry 29(1):12–21

Aronson TA, Shukla S, Hoff A, Cook B (1988b) Proposed delusional depression subtypes: preliminary evidence from a retrospective study of phenomenology and treatment course. J Affect Disord 14(1):69–74

Bai YM, Su TP, Tsai SJ, Wen-Fei C, Li CT, Pei-Chi T, Mu-Hong C (2014) Comparison of inflammatory cytokine levels among type I/type II and manic/hypomanic/euthymic/depressive states of bipolar disorder. J Affect Disord 166:187–192. doi:10.1016/j.jad.2014.05.009

Balanza-Martinez V, Tabares-Seisdedos R, Selva-Vera G, Martinez-Aran A, Torrent C, Salazar-Fraile J, Leal-Cercos C, Vieta E, Gomez-Beneyto M (2005) Persistent cognitive dysfunctions in bipolar I disorder and schizophrenic patients: a 3-year follow-up study. Psychother Psychosom 74(2):113–119. doi:10.1159/000083170

Baldessarini RJ, Tondo L, Visioli C (2014) First-episode types in bipolar disorder: predictive associations with later illness. Acta Psychiatr Scand 129(5):383–392. doi:10.1111/acps.12204

Berk M (2009) Neuroprogression: pathways to progressive brain changes in bipolar disorder. Int J Neuropsychopharmacol 12(4):441–445. doi:10.1017/S1461145708009498

Berk M, Conus P, Lucas N, Hallam K, Malhi GS, Dodd S, Yatham LN, Yung A, McGorry P (2007a) Setting the stage: from prodrome to treatment resistance in bipolar disorder. Bipolar Disord 9(7):671–678. doi:10.1111/j.1399-5618.2007.00484.x

Berk M, Hallam KT, McGorry PD (2007b) The potential utility of a staging model as a course specifier: a bipolar disorder perspective. J Affect Disord 100(1–3):279–281. doi:10.1016/j.jad.2007.03.007

Berk M, Copolov DL, Dean O, Lu K, Jeavons S, Schapkaitz I, Anderson-Hunt M, Bush AI (2008) N-acetyl cysteine for depressive symptoms in bipolar disorder–a double-blind randomized placebo-controlled trial. Biol Psychiatry 64(6):468–475. doi:10.1016/j.biopsych.2008.04.022

Berk M, Hallam K, Malhi GS, Henry L, Hasty M, Macneil C, Yucel M, Pantelis C, Murphy B, Vieta E, Dodd S, McGorry PD (2010) Evidence and implications for early intervention in bipolar disorder. J Ment Health 19(2):113–126. doi:10.3109/09638230903469111

Berk M, Brnabic A, Dodd S, Kelin K, Tohen M, Malhi GS, Berk L, Conus P, McGorry PD (2011a) Does stage of illness impact treatment response in bipolar disorder? Empirical treatment data and their implication for the staging model and early intervention. Bipolar Disord 13(1):87–98. doi:10.1111/j.1399-5618.2011.00889.x

Berk M, Kapczinski F, Andreazza AC, Dean OM, Giorlando F, Maes M, Yucel M, Gama CS, Dodd S, Dean B, Magalhaes PV, Amminger P, McGorry P, Malhi GS (2011b) Pathways underlying

neuroprogression in bipolar disorder: focus on inflammation, oxidative stress and neurotrophic factors. Neurosci Biobehav Rev 35(3):804–817. doi:10.1016/j.neubiorev.2010.10.001
Berk M, Berk L, Udina M, Moylan S, Stafford L, Hallam K, Goldstone S, McGorry PD (2012) Palliative models of care for later stages of mental disorder: maximizing recovery, maintaining hope, and building morale. Aust N Z J Psychiatry 46(2):92–99. doi:10.1177/0004867411432072
Berk M, Berk L, Dodd S, Cotton S, Macneil C, Daglas R, Conus P, Bechdolf A, Moylan S, Malhi GS (2014) Stage managing bipolar disorder. Bipolar Disord 16(5):471–477. doi:10.1111/bdi.12099
Blumberg HP, Krystal JH, Bansal R, Martin A, Dziura J, Durkin K, Martin L, Gerard E, Charney DS, Peterson BS (2006) Age, rapid-cycling, and pharmacotherapy effects on ventral prefrontal cortex in bipolar disorder: a cross-sectional study. Biol Psychiatry 59(7):611–618. doi:10.1016/j.biopsych.2005.08.031
Bora E, Fornito A, Yucel M, Pantelis C (2010) Voxelwise meta-analysis of gray matter abnormalities in bipolar disorder. Biol Psychiatry 67(11):1097–1105. doi:10.1016/j.biopsych.2010.01.020
Brietzke E, Kapczinski F (2008) TNF-alpha as a molecular target in bipolar disorder. Prog Neuro-Psychopharmacol Biol Psychiatry 32(6):1355–1361. doi:10.1016/j.pnpbp.2008.01.006
Brietzke E, Stertz L, Fernandes BS, Kauer-Sant'anna M, Mascarenhas M, Escosteguy Vargas A, Chies JA, Kapczinski F (2009) Comparison of cytokine levels in depressed, manic and euthymic patients with bipolar disorder. J Affect Disord 116(3):214–217. doi:10.1016/j.jad.2008.12.001
Carlson GA, Goodwin FK (1973) The stages of mania. A longitudinal analysis of the manic episode. Arch Gen Psychiatry 28(2):221–228
Carvalho AF, Dimellis D, Gonda X, Vieta E, McLntyre RS, Fountoulakis KN (2014) Rapid cycling in bipolar disorder: a systematic review. J Clin Psychiatry 75(6):e578–e586. doi:10.4088/JCP.13r08905
Cavanagh JT, Van Beck M, Muir W, Blackwood DH (2002) Case-control study of neurocognitive function in euthymic patients with bipolar disorder: an association with mania. Br J Psychiatry 180:320–326
Chang CC, Jou SH, Lin TT, Liu CS (2014) Mitochondrial DNA variation and increased oxidative damage in euthymic patients with bipolar disorder. Psychiatry Clin Neurosci 68(7):551–557. doi:10.1111/pcn.12163
Clark L, Iversen SD, Goodwin GM (2002) Sustained attention deficit in bipolar disorder. Br J Psychiatry 180:313–319
Cosci F, Fava GA (2013) Staging of mental disorders: systematic review. Psychother Psychosom 82(1):20–34. doi:10.1159/000342243
Cunha AB, Andreazza AC, Gomes FA, Frey BN, da Silveira LE, Goncalves CA, Kapczinski F (2008) Investigation of serum high-sensitive C-reactive protein levels across all mood states in bipolar disorder. Eur Arch Psychiatry Clin Neurosci 258(5):300–304. doi:10.1007/s00406-007-0797-0
Denicoff KD, Ali SO, Mirsky AF, Smith-Jackson EE, Leverich GS, Duncan CC, Connell EG, Post RM (1999) Relationship between prior course of illness and neuropsychological functioning in patients with bipolar disorder. J Affect Disord 56(1):67–73, S0165-0327(99)00028-2 [pii]
Duffy A, Alda M, Hajek T, Sherry SB, Grof P (2010) Early stages in the development of bipolar disorder. J Affect Disord 121(1–2):127–135. doi:10.1016/j.jad.2009.05.022
El-Badri SM, Ashton CH, Moore PB, Marsh VR, Ferrier IN (2001) Electrophysiological and cognitive function in young euthymic patients with bipolar affective disorder. Bipolar Disord 3(2):79–87
Fava GA (1999) Subclinical symptoms in mood disorders: pathophysiological and therapeutic implications. Psychol Med 29(1):47–61
Fava GA, Kellner R (1993) Staging: a neglected dimension in psychiatric classification. Acta Psychiatr Scand 87(4):225–230
Fernandes BS, Gama CS, Cereser KM, Yatham LN, Fries GR, Colpo G, de Lucena D, Kunz M, Gomes FA, Kapczinski F (2011) Brain-derived neurotrophic factor as a state-marker of mood episodes in bipolar disorders: a systematic review and meta-regression analysis. J Psychiatr Res 45(8):995–1004. doi:10.1016/j.jpsychires.2011.03.002
Fountoulakis KN (2009) An update of evidence-based treatment of bipolar depression: where do we stand? Curr Opin Psychiatry 23(1):19–24. doi:10.1097/YCO.0b013e328333e132

Fountoulakis KN (2012) Refractoriness in bipolar disorder: definitions and evidence-based treatment. CNS Neurosci Ther 18(3):227–237. doi:10.1111/j.1755-5949.2011.00259.x

Fountoulakis KN, Vieta E (2008) Treatment of bipolar disorder: a systematic review of available data and clinical perspectives. Int J Neuropsychopharmacol 11(7):999–1029. doi:10.1017/S1461145708009231, S1461145708009231 [pii]

Fountoulakis KN, Giannakopoulos P, Kovari E, Bouras C (2008a) Assessing the role of cingulate cortex in bipolar disorder: neuropathological, structural and functional imaging data. Brain Res Rev 59(1):9–21. doi:10.1016/j.brainresrev.2008.04.005

Fountoulakis KN, Grunze H, Panagiotidis P, Kaprinis G (2008b) Treatment of bipolar depression: an update. J Affect Disord 109(1-2):21–34. doi:10.1016/j.jad.2007.10.016, S0165-0327(07)00378-3 [pii]

Fountoulakis KN, Vieta E, Bouras C, Notaridis G, Giannakopoulos P, Kaprinis G, Akiskal H (2008c) A systematic review of existing data on long-term lithium therapy: neuroprotective or neurotoxic? Int J Neuropsychopharmacol 11(2):269–287. doi:10.1017/S1461145707007821

Fountoulakis KN, Kelsoe JR, Akiskal H (2011) Receptor targets for antidepressant therapy in bipolar disorder: an overview. J Affect Disord 138(3):222–238. doi:10.1016/j.jad.2011.04.043, S0165-0327(11)00210-2 [pii]

Frank E, Nimgaonkar VL, Phillips ML, Kupfer DJ (2014) All the world's a (clinical) stage: rethinking bipolar disorder from a longitudinal perspective. Mol Psychiatry. doi:10.1038/mp.2014.71

Fries GR, Pfaffenseller B, Stertz L, Paz AV, Dargel AA, Kunz M, Kapczinski F (2012) Staging and neuroprogression in bipolar disorder. Curr Psychiatry Rep 14(6):667–675. doi:10.1007/s11920-012-0319-2

Garcia-Lopez A, De Dios-Perrino C, Ezquiaga E (2009) Polarity of the first episode and predominant polarity in a cohort of bipolar outpatients. Eur Neuropsychopharmacol 19:S571

Gelenberg AJ, Kane JM, Keller MB, Lavori P, Rosenbaum JF, Cole K, Lavelle J (1989) Comparison of standard and low serum levels of lithium for maintenance treatment of bipolar disorder. N Engl J Med 321(22):1489–1493. doi:10.1056/NEJM198911303212201

Goodwin F, Jamison K (2007) Manic-depressive illness, 2nd edn. Oxford University Press, New York

Grande I, Magalhaes PV, Chendo I, Stertz L, Panizutti B, Colpo GD, Rosa AR, Gama CS, Kapczinski F, Vieta E (2014) Staging bipolar disorder: clinical, biochemical, and functional correlates. Acta Psychiatr Scand 129(6):437–444. doi:10.1111/acps.12268

Hamilton BA, Naismith SL, Scott EM, Purcell S, Hickie IB (2011) Disability is already pronounced in young people with early stages of affective disorders: data from an early intervention service. J Affect Disord 131(1–3):84–91. doi:10.1016/j.jad.2010.10.052

Helms PM, Smith RE (1983) Recurrent psychotic depression. Evidence of diagnostic stability. J Affect Disord 5(1):51–54

Hickie IB, Scott J, Hermens DF, Scott EM, Naismith SL, Guastella AJ, Glozier N, McGorry PD (2013) Clinical classification in mental health at the cross-roads: which direction next? BMC Med 11:125. doi:10.1186/1741-7015-11-125

Insel TR (2010) Rethinking schizophrenia. Nature 468(7321):187–193. doi:10.1038/nature09552

Javadapour A, Malhi GS, Ivanovski B, Chen X, Wen W, Sachdev P (2007) Increased anterior cingulate cortex volume in bipolar I disorder. Aust N Z J Psychiatry 41(11):910–916. doi:10.1080/00048670701634978

Judd LL, Akiskal HS (2003) The prevalence and disability of bipolar spectrum disorders in the US population: re-analysis of the ECA database taking into account subthreshold cases. J Affect Disord 73(1–2):123–131

Judd LL, Akiskal HS, Schettler PJ, Endicott J, Maser J, Solomon DA, Leon AC, Rice JA, Keller MB (2002) The long-term natural history of the weekly symptomatic status of bipolar I disorder. Arch Gen Psychiatry 59(6):530–537, yoa20425 [pii]

Judd LL, Akiskal HS, Schettler PJ, Coryell W, Endicott J, Maser JD, Solomon DA, Leon AC, Keller MB (2003) A prospective investigation of the natural history of the long-term weekly symptomatic status of bipolar II disorder. Arch Gen Psychiatry 60(3):261–269, yoa20225 [pii]

Judd LL, Schettler PJ, Akiskal HS, Coryell W, Leon AC, Maser JD, Solomon DA (2008) Residual symptom recovery from major affective episodes in bipolar disorders and rapid episode relapse/recurrence. Arch Gen Psychiatry 65(4):386–394. doi:10.1001/archpsyc.65.4.386, 65/4/386 [pii]

Juster RP, McEwen BS, Lupien SJ (2010) Allostatic load biomarkers of chronic stress and impact on health and cognition. Neurosci Biobehav Rev 35(1):2–16. doi:10.1016/j.neubiorev.2009.10.002

Kapczinski F, Frey BN, Andreazza AC, Kauer-Sant'Anna M, Cunha AB, Post RM (2008a) Increased oxidative stress as a mechanism for decreased BDNF levels in acute manic episodes. Rev Bras Psiquiatr 30(3):243–245

Kapczinski F, Vieta E, Andreazza AC, Frey BN, Gomes FA, Tramontina J, Kauer-Sant'anna M, Grassi-Oliveira R, Post RM (2008b) Allostatic load in bipolar disorder: implications for pathophysiology and treatment. Neurosci Biobehav Rev 32(4):675–692. doi:10.1016/j.neubiorev.2007.10.005

Kapczinski F, Dias VV, Kauer-Sant'Anna M, Brietzke E, Vazquez GH, Vieta E, Berk M (2009a) The potential use of biomarkers as an adjunctive tool for staging bipolar disorder. Prog Neuro-Psychopharmacol Biol Psychiatry 33(8):1366–1371. doi:10.1016/j.pnpbp.2009.07.027

Kapczinski F, Dias VV, Kauer-Sant'Anna M, Frey BN, Grassi-Oliveira R, Colom F, Berk M (2009b) Clinical implications of a staging model for bipolar disorders. Expert Rev Neurother 9(7):957–966. doi:10.1586/ern.09.31

Kapczinski F, Dal-Pizzol F, Teixeira AL, Magalhaes PV, Kauer-Sant'Anna M, Klamt F, Pasquali MA, Quevedo J, Gama CS, Post R (2010) A systemic toxicity index developed to assess peripheral changes in mood episodes. Mol Psychiatry 15(8):784–786. doi:10.1038/mp.2009.112

Kapczinski F, Dal-Pizzol F, Teixeira AL, Magalhaes PV, Kauer-Sant'Anna M, Klamt F, Moreira JC, de Bittencourt Pasquali MA, Fries GR, Quevedo J, Gama CS, Post R (2011) Peripheral biomarkers and illness activity in bipolar disorder. J Psychiatr Res 45(2):156–161. doi:10.1016/j.jpsychires.2010.05.015

Kapczinski F, Magalhaes PV, Balanza-Martinez V, Dias VV, Frangou S, Gama CS, Gonzalez-Pinto A, Grande I, Ha K, Kauer-Sant'Anna M, Kunz M, Kupka R, Leboyer M, Lopez-Jaramillo C, Post RM, Rybakowski JK, Scott J, Strejilevitch S, Tohen M, Vazquez G, Yatham L, Vieta E, Berk M (2014) Staging systems in bipolar disorder: an International Society for Bipolar Disorders Task Force report. Acta Psychiatrica Scand. doi:10.1111/acps.12305

Kauer-Sant'Anna M, Kapczinski F, Andreazza AC, Bond DJ, Lam RW, Young LT, Yatham LN (2009) Brain-derived neurotrophic factor and inflammatory markers in patients with early- vs. late-stage bipolar disorder. Int J Neuropsychopharmacol 12(4):447–458. doi:10.1017/S1461145708009310

Kendler KS, Thornton LM, Gardner CO (2000) Stressful life events and previous episodes in the etiology of major depression in women: an evaluation of the "kindling" hypothesis. Am J Psychiatry 157(8):1243–1251

Ketter TA, Houston JP, Adams DH, Risser RC, Meyers AL, Williamson DJ, Tohen M (2006) Differential efficacy of olanzapine and lithium in preventing manic or mixed recurrence in patients with bipolar I disorder based on number of previous manic or mixed episodes. J Clin Psychiatry 67(1):95–101

Lagopoulos J, Hermens DF, Naismith SL, Scott EM, Hickie IB (2012) Frontal lobe changes occur early in the course of affective disorders in young people. BMC Psychiatry 12:4. doi:10.1186/1471-244X-12-4

Lebowitz BK, Shear PK, Steed MA, Strakowski SM (2001) Verbal fluency in mania: relationship to number of manic episodes. Neuropsychiatr Neuropsychol Behav Neurol 14(3):177–182

Lewandowski KE, Cohen BM, Ongur D (2011) Evolution of neuropsychological dysfunction during the course of schizophrenia and bipolar disorder. Psychol Med 41(2):225–241. doi:10.1017/S0033291710001042, S0033291710001042 [pii]

Lim CS, Baldessarini RJ, Vieta E, Yucel M, Bora E, Sim K (2013) Longitudinal neuroimaging and neuropsychological changes in bipolar disorder patients: review of the evidence. Neurosci Biobehav Rev 37(3):418–435. doi:10.1016/j.neubiorev.2013.01.003

Lin A, Reniers RL, Wood SJ (2013) Clinical staging in severe mental disorder: evidence from neurocognition and neuroimaging. Br J Psychiatry Suppl 54:s11–s17. doi:10.1192/bjp.bp.112.119156

Lopez-Jaramillo C, Lopera-Vasquez J, Gallo A, Ospina-Duque J, Bell V, Torrent C, Martinez-Aran A, Vieta E (2010) Effects of recurrence on the cognitive performance of patients with bipolar I disorder: implications for relapse prevention and treatment adherence. Bipolar Disord 12(5):557–567. doi:10.1111/j.1399-5618.2010.00835.x

Magalhaes PV, Jansen K, Pinheiro RT, Klamt F, Teixeira AL, da Silva RA, Kapczinski F (2011) Systemic toxicity in early-stage mood disorders. J Psychiatr Res 45(10):1407–1409. doi:10.1016/j.jpsychires.2011.05.008

Magalhaes PV, Dodd S, Nierenberg AA, Berk M (2012a) Cumulative morbidity and prognostic staging of illness in the Systematic Treatment Enhancement Program for Bipolar Disorder (STEP-BD). Aust N Z J Psychiatry 46(11):1058–1067. doi:10.1177/0004867412460593

Magalhaes PV, Jansen K, Pinheiro RT, Colpo GD, da Motta LL, Klamt F, da Silva RA, Kapczinski F (2012b) Peripheral oxidative damage in early-stage mood disorders: a nested population-based case-control study. Int J Neuropsychopharmacol 15(8):1043–1050. doi:10.1017/S1461145711001532

McGorry PD (2007) Issues for DSM-V: clinical staging: a heuristic pathway to valid nosology and safer, more effective treatment in psychiatry. Am J Psychiatry 164(6):859–860. doi:10.1176/appi.ajp.164.6.859

McGorry PD (2010a) Risk syndromes, clinical staging and DSM V: new diagnostic infrastructure for early intervention in psychiatry. Schizophr Res 120(1–3):49–53. doi:10.1016/j.schres.2010.03.016

McGorry PD (2010b) Staging in neuropsychiatry: a heuristic model for understanding, prevention and treatment. Neurotox Res 18(3–4):244–255. doi:10.1007/s12640-010-9179-x

McGorry PD, Hickie IB, Yung AR, Pantelis C, Jackson HJ (2006) Clinical staging of psychiatric disorders: a heuristic framework for choosing earlier, safer and more effective interventions. Aust N Z J Psychiatry 40(8):616–622. doi:10.1111/j.1440-1614.2006.01860.x

McGorry PD, Purcell R, Hickie IB, Yung AR, Pantelis C, Jackson HJ (2007) Clinical staging: a heuristic model for psychiatry and youth mental health. Med J Aust 187(7 Suppl):S40–S42

McGorry PD, Killackey E, Yung A (2008) Early intervention in psychosis: concepts, evidence and future directions. World Psychiatry 7(3):148–156

McGorry PD, Nelson B, Goldstone S, Yung AR (2010) Clinical staging: a heuristic and practical strategy for new research and better health and social outcomes for psychotic and related mood disorders. Can J Psychiatry 55(8):486–497

McIntyre RS, Correll C (2014) Predicting and preventing bipolar disorder: the need to fundamentally advance the strategic approach. Bipolar Disord 16(5):451–454. doi:10.1111/bdi.12216

McNamara RK, Nandagopal JJ, Strakowski SM, DelBello MP (2010) Preventative strategies for early-onset bipolar disorder: towards a clinical staging model. CNS Drugs 24(12):983–996. doi:10.2165/11539700-000000000-00000

Moore PB, Shepherd DJ, Eccleston D, Macmillan IC, Goswami U, McAllister VL, Ferrier IN (2001) Cerebral white matter lesions in bipolar affective disorder: relationship to outcome. Br J Psychiatry 178:172–176

Moorhead TW, McKirdy J, Sussmann JE, Hall J, Lawrie SM, Johnstone EC, McIntosh AM (2007) Progressive gray matter loss in patients with bipolar disorder. Biol Psychiatry 62(8):894–900. doi:10.1016/j.biopsych.2007.03.005

Munkholm K, Poulsen HE, Kessing LV, Vinberg M (2014) Elevated levels of urinary markers of oxidatively generated DNA and RNA damage in bipolar disorder. Bipolar Disord. doi:10.1111/bdi.12245

Nelson WH, Khan A, Orr WW Jr (1984) Delusional depression. Phenomenology, neuroendocrine function, and tricyclic antidepressant response. J Affect Disord 6(3–4):297–306

Nery FG, Chen HH, Hatch JP, Nicoletti MA, Brambilla P, Sassi RB, Mallinger AG, Keshavan MS, Soares JC (2009) Orbitofrontal cortex gray matter volumes in bipolar disorder patients: a region-of-interest MRI study. Bipolar Disord 11(2):145–153. doi:10.1111/j.1399-5618.2009.00662.x

Perry A, Tarrier N, Morriss R, McCarthy E, Limb K (1999) Randomised controlled trial of efficacy of teaching patients with bipolar disorder to identify early symptoms of relapse and obtain treatment. BMJ 318(7177):149–153

Popovic D, Vieta E (2013) Clinical implications of polarity index of drugs in maintenance treatment of bipolar disorder: a naturalistic study. Eur Neuropsychopharmacol 23:S68–S69

Post RM (1992) Transduction of psychosocial stress into the neurobiology of recurrent affective disorder. Am J Psychiatry 149(8):999–1010

Post RM (2010) Mechanisms of illness progression in the recurrent affective disorders. Neurotox Res 18(3–4):256–271. doi:10.1007/s12640-010-9182-2

Post RM, Denicoff KD, Leverich GS, Altshuler LL, Frye MA, Suppes TM, Rush AJ, Keck PE Jr, McElroy SL, Luckenbaugh DA, Pollio C, Kupka R, Nolen WA (2003) Morbidity in 258 bipolar outpatients followed for 1 year with daily prospective ratings on the NIMH life chart method. J Clin Psychiatry 64(6):680–690; quiz 738–789

Post RM, Altshuler LL, Frye MA, Suppes T, Keck PE Jr, McElroy SL, Leverich GS, Luckenbaugh DA, Rowe M, Pizzarello S, Kupka RW, Grunze H, Nolen WA (2010) Complexity of pharmacologic treatment required for sustained improvement in outpatients with bipolar disorder. J Clin Psychiatry 71(9):1176–1186. doi:10.4088/JCP.08m04811yel; quiz 1252–1273

Post RM, Fleming J, Kapczinski F (2012) Neurobiological correlates of illness progression in the recurrent affective disorders. J Psychiatr Res 46(5):561–573. doi:10.1016/j.jpsychires.2012.02.004

Ranjekar PK, Hinge A, Hegde MV, Ghate M, Kale A, Sitasawad S, Wagh UV, Debsikdar VB, Mahadik SP (2003) Decreased antioxidant enzymes and membrane essential polyunsaturated fatty acids in schizophrenic and bipolar mood disorder patients. Psychiatry Res 121(2):109–122

Reinares M, Colom F, Rosa AR, Bonnin CM, Franco C, Sole B, Kapczinski F, Vieta E (2010) The impact of staging bipolar disorder on treatment outcome of family psychoeducation. J Affect Disord 123(1–3):81–86. doi:10.1016/j.jad.2009.09.009

Reinares M, Papachristou E, Harvey P, Mar Bonnin C, Sanchez-Moreno J, Torrent C, Ayuso-Mateos JL, Ploubidis GB, Vieta E, Frangou S (2013) Towards a clinical staging for bipolar disorder: defining patient subtypes based on functional outcome. J Affect Disord 144(1–2):65–71. doi:10.1016/j.jad.2012.06.005

Robinson LJ, Ferrier IN (2006) Evolution of cognitive impairment in bipolar disorder: a systematic review of cross-sectional evidence. Bipolar Disord 8(2):103–116. doi:10.1111/j.1399-5618.2006.00277.x, BDI277 [pii]

Rosa AR, Frey BN, Andreazza AC, Cereser KM, Cunha AB, Quevedo J, Santin A, Gottfried C, Goncalves CA, Vieta E, Kapczinski F (2006) Increased serum glial cell line-derived neurotrophic factor immunocontent during manic and depressive episodes in individuals with bipolar disorder. Neurosci Lett 407(2):146–150. doi:10.1016/j.neulet.2006.08.026

Rosa AR, Gonzalez-Ortega I, Gonzalez-Pinto A, Echeburua E, Comes M, Martinez-Aran A, Ugarte A, Fernandez M, Vieta E (2012) One-year psychosocial functioning in patients in the early vs. late stage of bipolar disorder. Acta Psychiatr Scand 125(4):335–341. doi:10.1111/j.1600-0447.2011.01830.x

Rosa AR, Magalhaes PV, Czepielewski L, Sulzbach MV, Goi PD, Vieta E, Gama CS, Kapczinski F (2014) Clinical staging in bipolar disorder: focus on cognition and functioning. J Clin Psychiatry 75(5):e450–e456. doi:10.4088/JCP.13m08625

Scott J, Paykel E, Morriss R, Bentall R, Kinderman P, Johnson T, Abbott R, Hayhurst H (2006) Cognitive-behavioural therapy for severe and recurrent bipolar disorders: randomised controlled trial. Br J Psychiatry 188:313–320. doi:10.1192/bjp.188.4.313

Scott J, Leboyer M, Hickie I, Berk M, Kapczinski F, Frank E, Kupfer D, McGorry P (2013) Clinical staging in psychiatry: a cross-cutting model of diagnosis with heuristic and practical value. Br J Psychiatry 202(4):243–245. doi:10.1192/bjp.bp.112.110858

Segal ZV, Williams JM, Teasdale JD, Gemar M (1996) A cognitive science perspective on kindling and episode sensitization in recurrent affective disorder. Psychol Med 26(2):371–380

Silverstone T, McPherson H, Li Q, Doyle T (2003) Deep white matter hyperintensities in patients with bipolar depression, unipolar depression and age-matched control subjects. Bipolar Disord 5(1):53–57

Simon NM, Smoller JW, McNamara KL, Maser RS, Zalta AK, Pollack MH, Nierenberg AA, Fava M, Wong KK (2006) Telomere shortening and mood disorders: preliminary support for a chronic stress model of accelerated aging. Biol Psychiatry 60(5):432–435. doi:10.1016/j.biopsych.2006.02.004

Soares JC, Kochunov P, Monkul ES, Nicoletti MA, Brambilla P, Sassi RB, Mallinger AG, Frank E, Kupfer DJ, Lancaster J, Fox P (2005) Structural brain changes in bipolar disorder using deformation field morphometry. Neuroreport 16(6):541–544

Strakowski SM, Wilson DR, Tohen M, Woods BT, Douglass AW, Stoll AL (1993) Structural brain abnormalities in first-episode mania. Biol Psychiatry 33(8–9):602–609

Strakowski SM, DelBello MP, Zimmerman ME, Getz GE, Mills NP, Ret J, Shear P, Adler CM (2002) Ventricular and periventricular structural volumes in first- versus multiple-episode bipolar disorder. Am J Psychiatry 159(11):1841–1847

Strejilevich SA, Martino DJ (2013) Cognitive function in adulthood and elderly euthymic bipolar patients: a comparison to test models of cognitive evolution. J Affect Disord 150(3):1188–1191. doi:10.1016/j.jad.2013.05.012

Swann AC, Bowden CL, Calabrese JR, Dilsaver SC, Morris DD (1999) Differential effect of number of previous episodes of affective disorder on response to lithium or divalproex in acute mania. Am J Psychiatry 156(8):1264–1266

Tohen M, Vieta E, Gonzalez-Pinto A, Reed C, Lin D, European Mania in Bipolar Longitudinal Evaluation of Medication Advisory B (2010) Baseline characteristics and outcomes in patients with first episode or multiple episodes of acute mania. J Clin Psychiatry 71(3):255–261. doi:10.4088/JCP.08m04580

Torrent C, Bonnin Cdel M, Martinez-Aran A, Valle J, Amann BL, Gonzalez-Pinto A, Crespo JM, Ibanez A, Garcia-Portilla MP, Tabares-Seisdedos R, Arango C, Colom F, Sole B, Pacchiarotti I, Rosa AR, Ayuso-Mateos JL, Anaya C, Fernandez P, Landin-Romero R, Alonso-Lana S, Ortiz-Gil J, Segura B, Barbeito S, Vega P, Fernandez M, Ugarte A, Subira M, Cerrillo E, Custal N, Menchon JM, Saiz-Ruiz J, Rodao JM, Isella S, Alegria A, Al-Halabi S, Bobes J, Galvan G, Saiz PA, Balanza-Martinez V, Selva G, Fuentes-Dura I, Correa P, Mayoral M, Chiclana G, Merchan-Naranjo J, Rapado-Castro M, Salamero M, Vieta E (2013) Efficacy of functional remediation in bipolar disorder: a multicenter randomized controlled study. Am J Psychiatry 170(8):852–859. doi:10.1176/appi.ajp.2012.12070971

Torres IJ, DeFreitas VG, DeFreitas CM, Kauer-Sant'Anna M, Bond DJ, Honer WG, Lam RW, Yatham LN (2010) Neurocognitive functioning in patients with bipolar I disorder recently recovered from a first manic episode. J Clin Psychiatry 71(9):1234–1242. doi:10.4088/JCP.08m04997yel

Vieta E, Reinares M, Rosa AR (2011) Staging bipolar disorder. Neurotox Res 19(2):279–285. doi:10.1007/s12640-010-9197-8

Vieta E, Popovic D, Rosa AR, Sole B, Grande I, Frey BN, Martinez-Aran A, Sanchez-Moreno J, Balanza-Martinez V, Tabares-Seisdedos R, Kapczinski F (2013) The clinical implications of cognitive impairment and allostatic load in bipolar disorder. E Psychiatry 28(1):21–29. doi:10.1016/j.eurpsy.2011.11.007

Vita A, De Peri L, Sacchetti E (2009) Gray matter, white matter, brain, and intracranial volumes in first-episode bipolar disorder: a meta-analysis of magnetic resonance imaging studies. Bipolar Disord 11(8):807–814. doi:10.1111/j.1399-5618.2009.00759.x

Walz JC, Andreazza AC, Frey BN, Cacilhas AA, Cereser KM, Cunha AB, Weyne F, Stertz L, Santin A, Goncalves CA, Kapczinski F (2007) Serum neurotrophin-3 is increased during manic and depressive episodes in bipolar disorder. Neurosci Lett 415(1):87–89. doi:10.1016/j.neulet.2007.01.002

Walz JC, Magalhaes PV, Giglio LM, Cunha AB, Stertz L, Fries GR, Andreazza AC, Kapczinski F (2009) Increased serum neurotrophin-4/5 levels in bipolar disorder. J Psychiatr Res 43(7):721–723. doi:10.1016/j.jpsychires.2008.10.005

Yatham LN, Kapczinski F, Andreazza AC, Trevor Young L, Lam RW, Kauer-Sant'anna M (2009) Accelerated age-related decrease in brain-derived neurotrophic factor levels in bipolar disorder. Int J Neuropsychopharmacol 12(1):137–139. doi:10.1017/S1461145708009449

Yung AR, McGorry PD (1996) The prodromal phase of first-episode psychosis: past and current conceptualizations. Schizophr Bull 22(2):353–370

Yung AR, McGorry PD (2007) Prediction of psychosis: setting the stage. Br J Psychiatry Suppl 51:s1–s8. doi:10.1192/bjp.191.51.s1

Zubieta JK, Huguelet P, O'Neil RL, Giordani BJ (2001) Cognitive function in euthymic bipolar I disorder. Psychiatry Res 102(1):9–20, S0165-1781(01)00242-6 [pii]

Biological Therapies 16

16.1 General Background

Bipolar disorder is complex, with different facets and stages, and it is not exactly known how this affects the everyday clinical practice. Its treatment is also complex, and unfortunately the hard data are insufficient to support all decisions. Reports at the case report level do exist, but they should not be considered sufficient (Fountoulakis et al. 2004b, 2007a). Rigorously collected data are available only for a limited number of agents and for selected aspects of the disease (Fountoulakis 2008, 2010b, 2012a; Fountoulakis et al. 2004a, 2005, 2007b, 2008a, 2012b; Nivoli et al. 2011). There are a number of issues which are still open to discussion. These include the definition of maintenance and of refractoriness (Fountoulakis 2012b) but mainly what is the most appropriate sequence of steps in the long-term treatment (Fountoulakis and Vieta 2008). The current chapter will systematically review the hard pharmaceutical data on the treatment of BD. As it will focus on efficacy data specifically for BD, only a brief description of the most important agents or groups of agents and their adverse events will be made, since these can be found easily in other books and sources.

16.1.1 Lithium

Lithium is a rather rare chemical element with atomic number 3 and its symbol is 'Li'. It belongs to the alkali metal group, and it is the lightest metal and the least dense solid element. Two stable lithium isotopes can be found in nature. It is soft, silver white and highly reactive and inflammable. Because of this, in nature it always occurs in pegmatitic minerals, is present in ocean water and usually and is obtained from brines and clays.

It was discovered in 1800 by the Brazilian chemist and statesman José Bonifácio de Andrada e Silva (1763–1838) in a mine on the island of Utö, Sweden, in the form of petalite ($LiAlSi_4O_{10}$). After extensive research on petalite, in 1817 Johan August

K.N. Fountoulakis, *Bipolar Disorder: An Evidence-Based Guide to Manic Depression*, DOI 10.1007/978-3-642-37216-2_16

Arfwedson (1792–1841) identified a new element which the head of the laboratory Jöns Jakob Berzelius (1779–1848) gave the name 'lithion' or 'lithina', from the Greek word 'lithos' (stone) and from the Greek word λιθος (transliterated as lithos, meaning 'stone'). The pure element was isolated in 1821 by William Thomas Brande (1788–1866) by electrolysis of lithium oxide. The method of electrolysis made large quantities of lithium available, and the commercial production and usage begun in the late nineteenth century. Lithium has several important applications in industry, ranging from glass and ceramics to lithium batteries and high-tech weapons. Today most lithium is used in batteries.

Although trace amounts exist in all organisms, there are no known physiological functions for lithium, and live organisms can survive without it. In spite of this, lithium has been used as medication already since the late nineteenth century.

In 1847 Alfred Baring Garrod (1819–1907) announced that he had discovered uric acid in the blood of gouty patients. Since at least in the laboratory, lithium could dissolve uric acid crystals isolated from the kidneys, and using lithium to dissolve urate in the body seemed a logical step. Garrod discovered that gouty uric acid deposits in finger joints are soluble in vitro in a lithium solution, and Alexander Ure (early nineteenth century–1866) in 1843 introduced lithium into medicine by showing that in vitro a uric acid bladder stone lost weight in a lithium carbonate solution. It is interesting that according to the works of Armand Trousseau (1801–1867) in France and Alexander Haig in the UK, mania and depression are related to the uric acid nosology (brain gout). Although Garrod made lithium treatment of gout widely known in 1859, unfortunately it was proven that the levels of lithium needed to dissolve urate in the body were toxic (Marmol 2008; Shorter 2009; Johnson and Amdisen 1983; Strobusch and Jefferson 1980). Following these observations and suggestions, a number of beverages included lithium as their component in the late nineteenth and early twentieth century (Fig. 16.1). Charles Leiper Grigg (1868–1940) introduced a lemon-lime soft drink in 1929 under the label 'Bib-Label Lithiated Lemon-Lime Soda' which soon changed to 7 Up (Fig. 16.2). However by 1948 lithium has been removed from

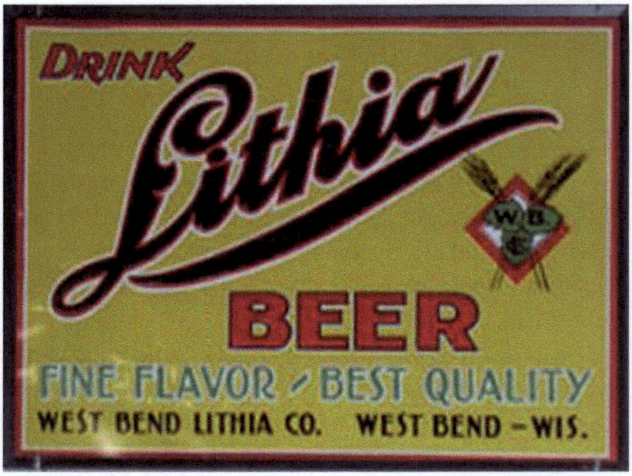

Fig. 16.1 Example of beverages which included lithium as their component in the late nineteenth and early twentieth century

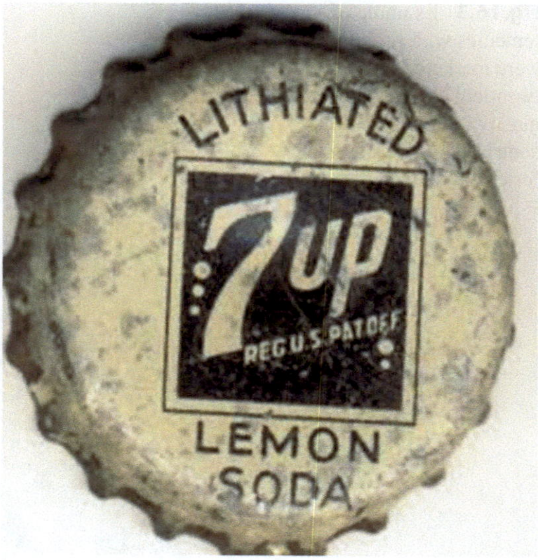

Fig. 16.2 The original 7 Up-included lithium

all beverages because of cases of toxicity, and its free marketing was prohibited (Marmol 2008). In parallel, a number of remedies with lithium were marketed in the early twentieth century (Figs. 16.3 and 16.4) and were mostly indicated for the control of renal calculi and 'uric acid diathesis' (Shorter 2009).

The first psychiatric indication for lithium came from Silas Weir Mitchell (1829–1914), a neurologist from Philadelphia, in 1870. Mitchell recommended lithium as an anticonvulsant and hypnotic (Mitchell 1870) and letter for 'general nervousness' (Mitchell 1877). Already in 1871, William Alexander Hammond (1828–1900) was maybe the first to prescribe a modern and effective psychotropic agent, and this was lithium (Mitchell and Hadzi-Pavlovic 2000). At that time, he was the professor of Diseases of the Mind and Nervous System at the Bellevue Hospital Medical College in New York. The Danish psychiatrist Carl Lange (1834–1900) used lithium in the treatment of recurrent brief depression in 1886, while his brother, Frederik Lange (1842–1907), used lithium in the treatment of 35 melancholic depressive patients (including some milder forms of BD) in 1894 (Lenox and Watson 1994).

However in spite of encouraging results, by the turn of the twentieth century, the 'brain gout' theory of mood disorders disappeared as a medical entity, and the use of lithium in psychiatry was abandoned.

After the WWII, in 1949 in the Bundoora Repatriation Hospital, a veterans hospital in a suburb of Melbourne, the Australian John Cade (1912–1980) injected urine from patients with schizophrenia to guinea pigs to test the hypothesis that mania is caused by intoxication by a normal body element circulating in excess, while melancholia is the corresponding deprative condition. He used lithium urate as control and observed it caused the rodents to be tranquilized. In fact it is possible that the animals were lethargic because of lithium toxicity, and this seems to be the case with the patients of William Alexander Hammond, since the dosages reported by both researchers lead to lithium intoxication. In 1949 Cade reported positive

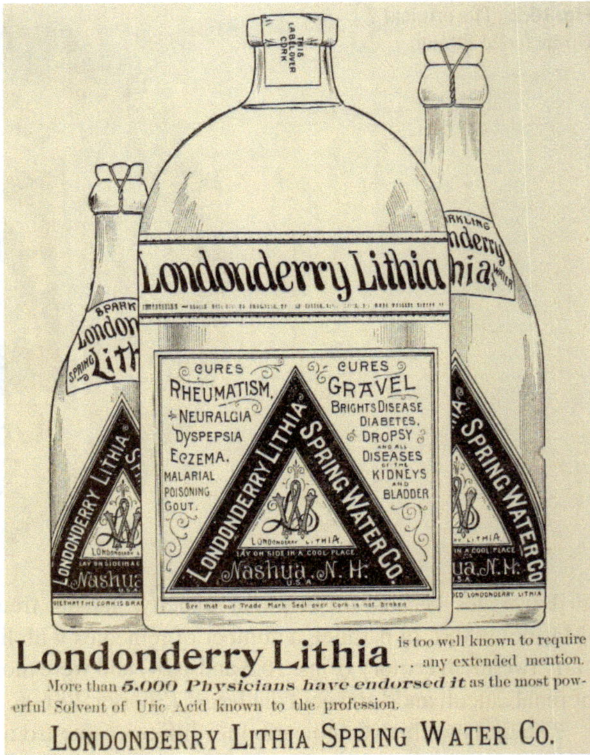

Fig. 16.3 Example of remedies with lithium which were marketed in the early twentieth century and were mostly indicated for the control of renal calculi and 'uric acid diathesis'

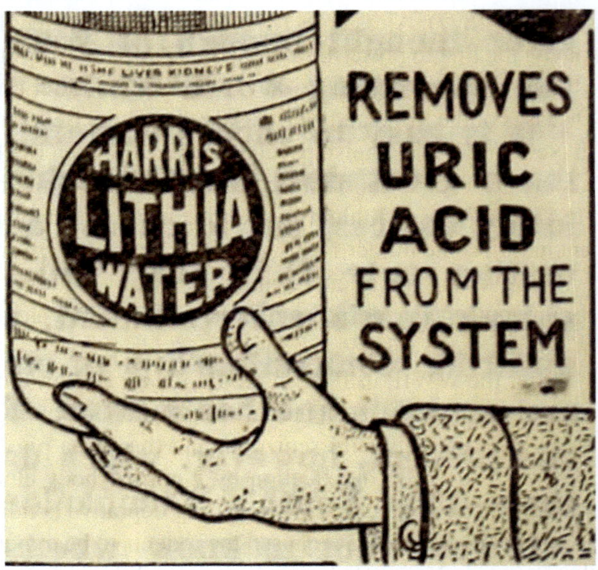

Fig. 16.4 Example of remedies with lithium which were marketed in the early twentieth century and were mostly indicated for the control of renal calculi and 'uric acid diathesis'

results from the treatment of ten acutely manic patients (Cade 1949, 2000); however, 2 years later he reported the first death because of lithium toxicity in a patient whose bipolar illness otherwise responded extremely well to treatment. Subsequent research with other ions (rubidium, cesium, lanthanum, neodymium and strontium) gave no positive results.

During the 1950s several researchers studied lithium and its usefulness in BD (Noack and Trautner 1951). However the important contribution that made the difference came from Denmark again in 1952, when Erik Stromgren (1909–1993), head of the Aarhus University psychiatric clinic in Risskov at that time, asked Mogens Schou (1918–2005) to undertake a randomized controlled trial of lithium in mania (Bech 2006). Mogens Schou was not a psychiatrist but a physician specialized in clinical chemistry and had observed a dramatic therapeutic effect of long-term lithium treatment in his younger brother. Schou randomized acutely manic patients with a flip of a coin to lithium or placebo, and in 1954 he published the results which made a significant impact (Schou et al. 1954). However lithium was still difficult to administer and blood levels a matter of guesswork. The situation changed with the introduction of the Coleman flame photometer in 1958 which made to monitor plasma lithium levels much more precisely in comparison to the previously used Beckman photometer.

It was, however, the Danish psychiatrist Poul Christian Baastrup (1918–2002) who demonstrated in 1964 the efficacy of lithium for the maintenance phase (Baastrup 1964). In the USA in 1960 Samuel Gershon joined the Schizophrenia and Psycho-pharmacology Joint Research Project of the University of Michigan at the mental hospital in Ypsilanti, Michigan, and the same year along with Arthur Yuwiler, also at Ypsilanti, they published the first North American paper on lithium (Gershon and Yuwiler 1960). For the next few years, there was significant academic opposition to the use of lithium as the standard treatment for BD, and much emphasis was given to its toxicity. Aubrey Lewis (1900–1975), professor of psychiatry and head of the Maudsley, considered lithium treatment 'dangerous nonsense', and Michael Shepherd (1923–1995) was also extremely negative towards it and suggested that lithium was toxic in mania and that claims of efficacy for it in preventing depression rested on 'dubious scientific methodology' (Blackwell and Shepherd 1968; Shepherd 1970; Blackwell 1969, 1970, 1971, 1972). However later studies established lithium and robustly linked it to the treatment of all phases of (Schou et al. 1970; Angst et al. 1969, 1970; Baastrup et al. 1970; Baastrup and Schou 1967; Bech 2006; Schioldann 1999, 2006, 2011; Johnstone et al. 1988; Mitchell and Hadzi-Pavlovic 2000). Later Fred Goodwin suggested that it could be also useful in the treatment of depression as add-on to antidepressants (Goodwin et al. 1969a, b, 1972, 2003; Goodwin 2002; Goodwin and Zis 1979). The recommended serum lithium levels were determined with certainty in 1976 (Bech et al. 1976). The term 'mood normalizer' was proposed by Mogens Schou for lithium (Schou 1963) after the term 'mood stabilizer, which was used during the 1950s to refer to a combination of amphetamine and a barbiturate to treat patients with neurotic instability but not patients with BD.

Lithium treatment for BD was approved in 1961 in France, in 1966 in the UK, in 1967 in Germany and in 1970 in Italy and the USA. In 1974, this application was extended to its use as a preventive agent for manic–depressive illness (Mitchell and Hadzi-Pavlovic 2000).

The specific biochemical mechanism of lithium action in mania is unknown. Interestingly unlike many other psychoactive drugs, it does not have any psychotropic effect in normal individuals at therapeutic concentrations. Treatment with lithium demands regular serum level tests and monitoring of thyroid and kidney function. Dehydration can result in increasing lithium levels. Serum lithium concentrations are recommended to be in the 0.4–1.2 mmol/l range (lower end of the range for maintenance therapy and the elderly, higher end for children) on samples taken 12 h after the preceding dose (Amdisen 1977; Chen et al. 2004; Solomon et al. 1996; Perlis et al. 2002).

The adverse effects of lithium include leukocytosis, polyuria and polydipsia, dry mouth, hand tremor, headache, neurocognitive problems, confusion, muscle weakness, ECG changes, nausea, vomiting, diarrhoea or constipation, muscle twitch, vertigo, EPS, euthyroid goitre, hypothyroidism, acne, hair loss and hair thinning, renal toxicity and renal interstitial fibrosis, seizures, coma, hallucinations, erythema multiforme, Brugada syndrome, sinus node dysfunction, pseudotumor cerebri, increased intracranial pressure and papilloedema and weight gain or loss. Lithium is also a teratogen, causing birth defects in a small number of newborn babies, including Ebstein's anomaly (Shepard et al. 2002). Most adverse effects are dose dependent. Dehydration in people taking lithium salts can be very hazardous, especially when combined with lithium-induced nephrogenic diabetes insipidus with polyuria. Lithium inhibits the action of the antidiuretic hormone causing an inability to concentrate urine, which leads to consequent loss of body water and thirst. Patients and therapists should be alert on heat and diarrhoea and other causes of dehydration. On the other hand, another danger is that rapid hydration may cause hyponatraemia with its danger of toxic sodium concentrations in plasma.

Lithium concentrations can be increased with concurrent use of diuretics especially loop diuretics and thiazides as well as with nonsteroidal anti-inflammatory drugs. Co-administration with antidepressants increases the risk of serotonin syndrome, and with antipsychotics it increases the risk for neuroleptic malignant syndrome.

Lithium toxicity manifestations include nausea, vomiting, diarrhoea, asthenia, ataxia, confusion, lethargy, polyuria, seizures and coma, coarse tremor, muscle twitching, convulsions and renal failure. Several authors have described a 'Syndrome of Irreversible Lithium-Effected Neurotoxicity' (SILENT), associated with episodes of acute lithium toxicity or long-term treatment within the appropriate dosage range. Symptoms are said to include cerebellar dysfunction (Ikeda et al. 2010; Porto et al. 2009; Adityanjee et al. 2005; Adityanjee 1989, 1987). Unfortunately, in long-term use, toxic effects might be induced even at therapeutic plasma levels (Fountoulakis et al. 2008c).

16.1.2 Antiepileptics

Although in much of the literature, the terms 'anticonvulsants' or 'antiepileptics' are used interchangeably with the term 'mood stabilizers', and only three antiepileptics (valproate, carbamazepine and lamotrigine) have proven efficacy in BD.

16.1.2.1 Valproate

Sodium valproate is the sodium salt of valproic acid. It is an anticonvulsant efficacious in the treatment of epilepsy (all partial and generalized seizures including absence seizures) as well as in the prevention of migraine headaches. It was first synthesized in 1882 by B.S. Burton as an analogue of valeric acid which can be found naturally in valerian and was used in the cosmetics industry. Valeric acid appears similar in structure to GABA but lacks the alcohol and amine functional groups that contribute to the biological activities of the GABA. Valproic acid was used for long in laboratories as a 'metabolically inert' solvent for organic compounds, and until in 1962 Pierre Eymard accidentally discovered its anticonvulsant properties while using it as a vehicle for other compounds that were being studied for antiepileptic properties (Meunier et al. 1963). Valproic acid was approved as an antiepileptic for the first time in 1967 in France.

Its mechanism of action includes weak blocking of sodium ion channels and weak inhibition of enzymes that deactivate GABA (e.g. GABA transaminase). It is unclear whether it also stimulates GABA synthesis.

Adverse effects include tiredness, tremor, nausea, vomiting, sedation and gastrointestinal symptoms as well as reversible hair loss in about 10 % of patients. Also some patients experience vision problems, endocrinological disorder (increased testosterone production in females and menstrual irregularities), memory problems, weight gain, infections, drowsiness and headache, liver damage, polycystic ovaries, movement disorders (even hallucinations, anxiety and confusion), swollen pancreas, low body temperature and potentially life-threatening blood abnormalities (e.g. low platelet count). Valproate has the highest risk of birth defects of any of the commonly used antiepileptic drugs during pregnancy (Cummings et al. 2011). Overdose results in tremor, respiratory depression, coma and metabolic acidosis and eventually can result to death. Serum or plasma levels of valproic acid concentrations should be in the range of 50–150 mg/l for the treatment of BD.

16.1.2.2 Carbamazepine

Carbamazepine is an antiepileptic efficacious against partial seizures, generalized tonic–clonic seizures and mixed seizures and also useful for the treatment of trigeminal neuralgia. It was discovered by chemist Walter Schindler at J.R. Geigy AG (today Novartis) in Basel, Switzerland, in 1953. It was first marketed as a drug to treat trigeminal neuralgia in 1962 and as an antiepileptic in the UK since 1965 and the USA since 1974. In 1971 the first studies concerning BD appeared in Japan (Okuma and Kishimoto 1998).

The mechanism of action of carbamazepine includes the stabilization of the inactivated state of sodium channels, making thus reducing the excitability of the neurons. It has also been shown to bind to GABA receptors (Granger et al. 1995).

The most common adverse effects with carbamazepine treatment may include drowsiness, dizziness, headaches and migraines, motor coordination impairment, nausea, vomiting, constipation, cardiac arrhythmias, blurry or double vision, aplastic anaemia or agranulocytosis and a dangerous or even fatal skin reaction (Stevens–Johnson syndrome and toxic epidermal necrolysis). It can also exacerbate pre-existing hypothyroidism. It can cause syndrome of inappropriate antidiuretic hormone, and it can aggravate juvenile myoclonic epilepsy and other types of epilepsy, especially absence seizures (Liu et al. 2006).

Among the agents used in the treatment of BD, carbamazepine is the drug most potent to interactions with other medication. It is a CYP450 inducer, and thus it might increase the metabolism and elimination of many agents, including warfarin, lamotrigine, phenytoin, theophylline, valproic acid, benzodiazepines and some antipsychotics. It also reduces the effectiveness of birth control pills thus leading to unexpected pregnancies. Other agents, like erythromycin, cimetidine, valproic acid, valnoctamide and calcium channel blockers as well as grapefruit juice, decrease carbamazepine metabolism and increase its serum availability often to toxic levels. As a drug that induces cytochrome P450 enzymes, it accelerates elimination of many benzodiazepines and decreases their action.

Carbamazepine is teratogenic and is associated among others with the development of spina bifida (Jentink et al. 2010), neurodevelopmental problems and delays (Cummings et al. 2011) craniofacial defects, cardiovascular malformations and hypospadias.

16.1.2.3 Lamotrigine

Lamotrigine is an antiepileptic efficacious in the treatment of focal seizures, primary and secondary tonic–clonic seizures and seizures associated with Lennox–Gastaut syndrome. It was marketed for the first time in 1994. It is chemically different to other antiepileptics.

Lamotrigine is a triazine derivate that inhibits voltage-sensitive sodium channels, leading to stabilization of neuronal membranes. It also blocks calcium channels and has a weak 5-HT3 receptor inhibition. Probably other actions also exist since lamotrigine exerts a variety of effects and adverse events which cannot be explained by its above pharmacodynamics properties alone (Rogawski and Loscher 2004a, b; Lees and Leach 1993). It is metabolized by hepatic glucuronidation.

Its adverse effects include life-threatening skin reactions, including Stevens–Johnson syndrome, DRESS syndrome and toxic epidermal necrolysis. Since December 2010, lamotrigine carries an FDA black box warning for aseptic meningitis. Other adverse events include loss of balance or coordination, double vision, blurred vision, dizziness, drowsiness, insomnia, anxiety, vivid dreams or nightmares, dry mouth, mouth ulcers, memory and cognitive problems, runny nose, cough, indigestion, abdominal pain, weight loss, missed or painful menstrual periods, vaginitis and leukopaenia.

Certain contraceptives decrease serum levels of lamotrigine (Reimers et al. 2005).

Lamotrigine has low teratogenic action; however, if used during the first trimester, it may increase the risk for cleft lip and palate malformation in newborns.

Lamotrigine has fewer drug interactions than other antiepileptics; however, caution is needed when co-administered with hepatic enzyme-inducing medications (Anderson 1998).

16.1.3 Antipsychotics

Antipsychotics or neuroleptics (also called previously major tranquilizers) were developed initially for the treatment of schizophrenia and psychotic symptoms.

Chlorpromazine was the first to be discovered in 1952 and initially was developed as an anaesthetic agent for general surgical use. The French Henri Laborit (1914–1995) reported that chlorpromazine was inducing indifference towards traumatic events in otherwise mentally healthy persons. Jean Delay (1907–1987) and Pierre Deniker (1917–1998) were the first to use it as monotherapy in agitated psychosis.

Antipsychotics are grouped into the first-generation antipsychotics (FGAs), also called typical antipsychotics, and the second-generation agents (SGAs), also called atypical antipsychotics. The common pharmacodynamics property of all antipsychotic agents is dopamine D2 receptor blockade. Most antipsychotics also affect a number of other neurotransmitters.

The most frequent adverse events for FGAs are extrapyramidal symptoms (EPS) and hyperprolactinaemia, while weight gain and metabolic abnormalities are caused mainly by SGAs. Other adverse effects include sedation, headaches, dizziness, diarrhoea, sexual dysfunction, osteoporosis, orthostatic hypotension, anticholinergic side effects, memory problems, angle-closure glaucoma, blurred vision, constipation, dry mouth or hypersalivation, agranulocytosis, leukopaenia, and neutropaenia and QT prolongation. Tardive dyskinesia and neuroleptic malignant syndrome are the most severe adverse events.

16.1.4 Antidepressants

Antidepressants are agents used for the treatment of depression but also of anxiety disorders, obsessive compulsive disorder, eating disorders, chronic pain, neuropathic pain and other neurological and psychiatric conditions.

In 1951, research on the two new anti-tuberculosis agents isoniazid and iproniazid developed by Hoffman–LaRoche, by Irving Selikoff (1915–1992) and Edward Robitzek (1912–1984) at Sea View Hospital on Staten Island suggested that the two agents also possessed some psychotropic properties (Selikoff and Robitzek 1952; Robitzek et al. 1952; Selifoff et al. 1952). Following these reports, in 1952 the Cincinnati psychiatrist Max Lurie (born 1920) treated some of his patients with these agents and together with Harry Salzer (born 1906) they reported that isoniazid improved depression in two-thirds of their patients. They also introduced the term antidepressant (Salzer and Lurie 1953). A year before, in France, Jean Delay with the resident Jean-Francois Buisson reported the positive effect of isoniazid on depressed patients, but they published these results years later (Delay and Buisson 1958). Roche has also produced iproniazid which showed a greater psychostimulant effect, but also more pronounced toxicity (Robitzek et al. 1953). Nathan Kline supported its use as an antidepressant, but eventually in 1961 it was withdrawn from the market because of lethal hepatotoxicity (Lopez-Munoz et al. 2007).

In 1957 the Swiss psychiatrist Roland Kuhn (1912–2005) discovered the first tricyclic antidepressant in the process of improvement of the efficacy of chlorpromazine in conjunction with the Geigy Pharmaceutical Company. He also coined the term 'thymoleptic' (Kuhn 1957, 1958). In 1988, fluoxetine, the first SSRI, was introduced. It was developed at Eli Lilly and Company in the early 1970s by Bryan Molloy, Klaus Schmiegel, David Wong and others. In spite of a long-lasting recent debate, the efficacy of antidepressants in the treatment of unipolar depression is no longer a matter of dispute (Fountoulakis et al. 2013b; Fountoulakis and Moller 2012; Sartorius et al. 2007).

Currently there are several classes of antidepressants including the selective serotonin reuptake inhibitors (SSRIs), the serotonin–norepinephrine reuptake inhibitors (SNRIs), the tricyclic antidepressants (TCAs) and the monoamine oxidase inhibitors (MAOIs).

The main neurotransmitter pathway through which antidepressants seem to exert their beneficial effect is that of serotonin. Pure noradrenergic action is unlikely to be sufficient to produce an antidepressant effect; however, double-acting agents (which affect both serotonin and noradrenaline pathways) might be more efficacious in comparison to purely serotonergic agents but also with more adverse effects.

The most common adverse effects include nausea, increased appetite and weight gain, loss of sexual desire and other sexual problems (e.g. erectile dysfunction and decreased ability to achieve orgasm), fatigue and drowsiness, insomnia, dry mouth, blurred vision, constipation, dizziness, agitation, irritability, anxiety, sexual problems and hyperprolactinaemia. Serotonergic syndrome is a potentially lethal event. Treatment with antidepressants also might induce suicidal thoughts, but no completed suicide has been attributed to treatment with antidepressants. Some agents after abrupt stop of treatment might cause withdrawal symptoms which persist for no more than 1–2 weeks.

Although the teratogenic risk is low with antidepressants, SSRI use in pregnancy has been associated with an increased risk of spontaneous abortion, preterm birth and low birth weight (Malm 2012; Rahimi et al. 2006).

The usefulness of antipsychotics in the treatment of bipolar depression is a matter of continuous debate (Pacchiarotti et al. 2013). It is interesting that some data suggest that norepinephrine activity is necessary for an antidepressant to act in bipolar depression; still this very activity increases the risk for the patients to switch to mania or hypomania (Fountoulakis et al. 2012c).

16.2 Evidence-Based Treatment

The literature was searched and the text that follows is updated through August 2014. The method which was followed in order to rank the agents according to the data is a modification of the PORT method, and it is shown in detail in Table 16.1. However the lack of data did not make this feasible for all facets and aspects of the disease. Thus, also a binomial classification was also made with agents being efficacious ('yes') or proven not to be ('neg'). It is disappointing that for the majority of agents vs. aspects, there are no data to refer to (–). All the evidence-based data are shown in Tables 16.2, 16.3, 16.4, 16.5, 16.6, 16.7, 16.8, and 16.9.

Table 16.1 Description of the method which was followed to rank the data in the present book chapter. Essentially it is a modified PORT method for the grading of data, on the basis of efficacy alone

Level A	Good research-based evidence, supported by at least 1 placebo-controlled study of sufficient magnitude. If there are non-placebo trials controlled with a comparator and with different results, the placebo controlled is the only taken into consideration
Level B	Fair research-based evidence, from at least one randomised, double-blind controlled trial which, however, fails to fulfil all the criteria above (e.g. very small sample size or no placebo control)
Eq	Equivocal data, that is, one positive and one negative RCT, only failed but not negative studies, positive meta-analysis, etc. Equivocal data as a level is superior to level C
Level C	At least one double-blind study with placebo or not, with a special design (e.g. ABA, discontinuation studies, etc.) or at least one open-label study with comparator or prospective open-label study or two prospective open-label studies with >10 participants
Level D	Recommendation based on prospective case studies with a minimum of 10 patients or large-scale retrospective chart analyses and support by expert opinion
Neg	Negative data

Table 16.2 Summary table of monotherapy data for the treatment of acute bipolar mania

Agent/modality (alphabetical order)	Effect start day	Overall	Core manic	Depressive	Psychotic	Agitation
Amisulpride	–	C	–	–	–	–
Aripiprazole	2–4	A	–	Yes	Yes	–
Asenapine	2	A	–	Eq	–	–
Carbamazepine	14	A	Yes	Yes	–	–
Cariprazine	4	A	Yes	No	–	–
Chlorpromazine	–	B	–	–	–	–
Clozapine	–	C	–	–	–	–
ECT	–	C	–	–	–	–
Eslicarbazepine	–	Neg	–	–	–	–
Gabapentin	–	Neg	–	–	–	–
Haloperidol	4	A	No	No	Yes	Yes
Lamotrigine	–	Neg	–	–	–	–
Licarbazepine	–	Neg	–	–	–	–
Lithium	7	A	Eq	No	No	–
Loxapine inhalant	–	–	–	–	–	Yes
Olanzapine	2–7	A	Yes	Yes	Yes	Yes
Oxcarbazepine	–	C	–	–	–	–
Paliperidone	2	A	–	–	–	–
Perphenazine	–	–	–	–	–	–
Quetiapine	4	A	–	Yes	Yes	–
Risperidone	3	A	–	Yes	Yes	–
Tamoxifen	5	A	Yes	No	Yes	–
TMS	–	C	–	–	–	–
Topiramate	–	Neg	–	–	–	–
Valproate	5–15	A	No	No	–	Yes
Verapamil	–	Neg	–	–	–	–
Ziprasidone	2	A	Yes	Eq	Yes	–

– no data, *Neg* negative data

Table 16.3 Summary table of data for the combination treatment of acute bipolar mania

Agent/modality (alphabetical order)	MS	Cbz	Lam	Li	Val	FGAs
Amisulpride	–	–	–	–	–	–
Aripiprazole	A	–	–	A	A	–
Asenapine	A	–	–	A	A	–
Carbamazepine	–	–	–	–	–	–
Cariprazine	–	–	–	–	–	–
Chlorpromazine	–	–	–	–	–	–
Clozapine	–	–	–	–	–	–
ECT	–	–	–	–	–	–
Eslicarbazepine	–	–	–	–	–	–
Gabapentin	Neg	–	–	–	–	–
Haloperidol	–	B	–	A	A	–
Lamotrigine	–	–	–	–	–	–
Licarbazepine	–	–	–	–	–	–
Lithium	–	B	–	–	–	–
Loxapine inhalant	–	–	–	–	–	–
Olanzapine	Yes	Neg	–	A	A	–
Oxcarbazepine	–	–	–	B	–	–
Paliperidone	Neg	–	–	Neg	Neg	–
Perphenazine	–	–	–	–	–	–
Quetiapine	A	–	–	A	A	–
Risperidone	–	A	–	A	A	–
Tamoxifen	–	–	–	–	–	–
TMS	–	–	–	–	–	–
Topiramate	Neg	–	–	–	–	–
Valproate	–	–	–	–	–	Yes
Verapamil	–	–	–	–	–	–
Ziprasidone	A	–	–	Neg	–	–

– no data, *Neg* negative data

16.2.1 Acute Mania

16.2.1.1 Monotherapy

A summary of monotherapy data for the treatment of acute mania is shown in Table 16.2.

16.2.1.1.1 Lithium

Although the first placebo-controlled study concerning the efficacy of lithium against acute mania was conducted in 1971 (Stokes et al. 1971), the first properly done study was in 179 hospitalized, acutely manic patients in academic settings across the USA, appeared as late as 1994, although lithium was available with a label for the treatment of BD already since decades. In that first 3-week study, the

Table 16.4 Summary table of monotherapy data for the treatment of acute bipolar depression overall and in BD-I and BD-II patients

Agent/modality (alphabetical order)	Monotherapy	BD-I	BD-II	Depressive core
Amisulpride	–	–	–	–
Aripiprazole	Eq	–	–	–
Asenapine	–	–	–	–
Bupropion	–	–	–	–
Carbamazepine	Eq	–	–	–
Chlorpromazine	–	–	–	–
Clozapine	–	–	–	–
Desipramine	–	–	–	–
Escitalopram	C	–	C	–
ECT	D	–	–	–
Fluoxetine	A	–	–	–
Gabapentin	Neg	–	–	–
Haloperidol	–	–	–	–
Imipramine	C	–	–	–
Ketamine	–	–	–	–
Lamotrigine	Eq	–	Eq	Yes
Levetiracetam	–	–	–	–
Lithium	Neg	–	Eq	–
Lurasidone	A	–	–	Yes
Olanzapine	Eq	Eq	–	Eq
OFC	A	Yes	–	Yes
Oxcarbazepine	–	–	–	–
Paliperidone	–	–	–	–
Paroxetine	Neg	No	No	–
Perphenazine	–	–	–	–
Quetiapine	A	Yes	Yes	Yes
Risperidone	–	–	–	–
Sleep deprivation	–	–	–	–
Tamoxifen	–	–	–	–
TMS	–	–	–	–
Topiramate	–	–	–	–
Valproate	Eq	Eq	–	Eq
Venlafaxine	–	–	–	–
Ziprasidone	Neg	–	–	–
CBT	–	–	–	–
Psychoeducation	–	–	–	–

– no data, *Neg* negative data

Table 16.5 Summary table of data for the combination treatment of acute bipolar depression

Agent/modality (alphabetical order)	MS	Cbz	Lam	Li	Val
Amisulpride	–	–	–	–	–
Aripiprazole	–	–	–	Neg	–
Asenapine	–	–	–	–	–
Bupropion	Neg	Neg	–	Neg	Neg
Carbamazepine	–	–	–	–	–
Chlorpromazine	–	–	–	–	–
Clozapine	–	–	–	–	–
Desipramine	–	–	–	–	–
Escitalopram	–	–	–	–	–
ECT	–	–	–	–	–
Fluoxetine	–	–	–	–	–
Gabapentin	–	–	–	–	–
Haloperidol	–	–	–	–	–
Imipramine	–	–	–	Neg	–
Ketamine	–	–	–	B	B
Lamotrigine	–	–	–	A	–
Levetiracetam	Neg	–	–	–	–
Lithium	–	–	A	–	–
Lurasidone	–	–	–	A	A
Olanzapine	–	–	–	–	–
OFC	–	–	–	–	–
Oxcarbazepine	–	–	–	B	–
Paliperidone	–	–	–	–	–
Paroxetine	Neg	Neg	–	Neg	Neg
Perphenazine	–	–	–	–	–
Quetiapine	–	–	–	–	–
Risperidone	–	–	–	–	–
Sleep deprivation	–	–	–	–	–
Tamoxifen	–	–	–	–	–
TMS	–	–	–	–	–
Topiramate	–	–	–	–	–
Valproate	–	–	–	–	–
Venlafaxine	–	–	–	–	–
Ziprasidone	Neg	–	Neg	Neg	Neg
CBT	–	–	–	–	–
Psychoeducation	–	–	–	–	–

– no data, *Neg* negative data

Table 16.6 Summary table of monotherapy data for the maintenance treatment phase

Agent/modality (alphabetical order)	Index episode	Enriched sample	Manic	Depressive	Mixed
Amisulpride	–	–	–	–	–
Aripiprazole	m[a]	Yes	Yes	No	–
Asenapine	–	–	–	–	–
Carbamazepine	–	–	–	–	–
Chlorpromazine	–	–	–	–	–
Clozapine	–	–	–	–	–
Electroconvulsive therapy	–	–	–	–	–
Fluoxetine	d	Yes	–	Eq	–
Gabapentin	–	–	–	–	–
Haloperidol	–	–	–	–	–
Imipramine	d	?	–	Eq	–
Lamotrigine	m/d	Yes	Yes	Yes	–
Lithium	m/d	No	Yes	Yes	–
N-acetyl cysteine	d	Yes		–	–
Olanzapine	m	Yes/no	Yes	Yes	Yes
Olanzapine–fluoxetine combination	–	–	–	Yes	–
Oxcarbazepine	–	–	–	–	–
Paliperidone	m	Yes	Yes	No	–
Paroxetine	–	–	–	–	–
Perphenazine	m	Yes	–	–	–
Phenytoin	euth	No	–	–	–
Pramipexole	euth	No	–	–	–
Quetiapine	m/d	Yes	Yes	Yes	–
Risperidone, long-acting injectable	m	Yes	Yes	No	–
Sertraline	–	–	–	–	–
Sleep deprivation	–	–	–	–	–
Tamoxifen	–	–	–	–	–
Transcranial magnetic stimulation	–	–	–	–	–
Topiramate	–	–	–	–	–
Valproate	m	Yes	Neg	Eq	–
Ziprasidone	m	Yes	–	–	–
CBT	d	No	–	–	–
Psychoeducation	m/d	No	–	–	–

Index episode also refers to data presented in Tables 16.7, 16.8, and 16.9
m mania/mixed, *d* depression, *m/d* both mania and depression, *UT* treatment as usual, *MS* mood stabilizers
[a]Aripiprazole is efficacious with a manic but not mixed index episode

Table 16.7 Summary table of combination data for the maintenance treatment phase and also concerning the maintenance treatment of rapid cycling patients and the risk for switching to the opposite pole

Agent/modality (alphabetical order)	TAU	Cbz	Lam	Li	Val	Rapid cycling	Switch
Amisulpride	–	–	–	–	–	–	–
Aripiprazole	–	–	Neg	Yes	Yes	Yes	No
Asenapine	–	–	–	–	–	–	No
Carbamazepine	–	–	–	Neg	–	Li + cbz	No
Chlorpromazine	–	–	–	–	–	–	–
Clozapine	–	–	–	–	–	–	–
Electroconvulsive therapy	–	–	–	–	–	–	–
Fluoxetine	–	–	–	–	–	–	No
Gabapentin	–	Yes	–	Yes	Yes	–	–
Haloperidol	–	–	–	–	–	–	Eq
Imipramine	–	–	–	Neg		–	Yes
Lamotrigine	–	–	–	Neg	Neg	Neg	No
Lithium	–	–	Neg	–	–	Li + cbz	No
N-acetyl cysteine	Neg	–	–	–	–	–	–
Olanzapine	–	–	–	Eq	Eq	–	No
Olanzapine–fluoxetine combination	–	–	–	–	–	–	No
Oxcarbazepine	–	–	–	Neg	–	–	–
Paliperidone	–	–	–	–	–	–	No
Paroxetine	–	–	–	–	Yes	–	No
Perphenazine	–	Neg	–	Neg	Neg	–	Yes
Phenytoin	Yes	–	–	–	–	–	–
Pramipexole	Neg	–	–	–	–	–	–
Quetiapine	–	–	–	m/d	m/d	Quet + val/li	No
Risperidone, long-acting injectable	m	–	–	–	–	RLAI + TAU	No
Sertraline	–	–	–	–	Yes	–	No
Sleep deprivation	–	–	–	–	–	–	–
Tamoxifen	–	–	–	–	–	–	–
Transcranial magnetic stimulation	–	–	–	–	–	–	–
Topiramate	–	–	–	–	–	–	–
Valproate	–	–	–	–	–	–	No
Ziprasidone	–	m	–	M	m	–	No
CBT	d	–	–	–	–	–	–
Psychoeducation	m/d	–	–	–	–	–	–

m mania/mixed, *d* depression, *m/d* both mania and depression, *TAU* treatment as usual, *MS* mood stabilizers

Table 16.8 Summary table of data for the treatment of acute mixed episodes and acute bipolar mania/mixed in rapid cycling patients

Agent/modality (alphabetical order)	Mixed episodes		
	Manic component	Depressive component	Rapid cycling
Amisulpride	–	–	–
Aripiprazole	Yes	Yes	Yes
Asenapine	Yes	–	–
Carbamazepine	Yes	Yes	–
Cariprazine	–	–	–
Chlorpromazine	–	–	–
Clozapine	–	–	–
ECT	–	–	–
Eslicarbazepine	–	–	–
Gabapentin	–	–	–
Haloperidol	–	–	–
Lamotrigine	–	–	–
Licarbazepine	–	–	–
Lithium	No	–	Neg[a]
Loxapine inhalant	–	–	–
Olanzapine	Yes	Eq	Yes
Oxcarbazepine	–	–	–
Paliperidone	Yes	No	–
Perphenazine	–	–	–
Quetiapine	Eq	–	No
Risperidone	Yes	–	–
Tamoxifen	–	–	–
TMS	–	–	–
Topiramate	–	–	–
Valproate	Yes	Eq	Neg[a]
Verapamil	–	–	–
Ziprasidone	Eq	Eq	–

– no data, *Neg* negative data
[a]For the combination lithium plus valproate

efficacy and safety of lithium (serum levels below 1.5 mmol/l; $N=36$) and divalproex (serum levels below 150 μg/ml; $N=69$) were compared to placebo ($N=74$). Half of them were previously nonresponsive to lithium, and none had previously received valproate; thus, the study sample was enriched in favour of divalproex. After 3 weeks, both treatment arms manifested a higher change in MRS in comparison to placebo, and this change was significant since day 15 for both agents. Unfortunately the results are reported only through a chart, and no exact means and standard deviations are available. Interestingly, the analysis of separate items of the MRS revealed that divalproex but not lithium had a beneficial effect on the core manic symptoms. The response rate was higher for lithium and divalproex in

Table 16.9 Summary table of data for the treatment of comorbid anxiety in bipolar depressed patient, the efficacy against acute bipolar depression in rapid cycling patients and the risk of switch to mania/hypomania

Agent/modality (alphabetical order)	Anxiety	Rapid cycling	Switch risk
Amisulpride	–	–	–
Aripiprazole	–	–	No
Asenapine	–	–	–
Bupropion	–	–	No
Carbamazepine	–	–	–
Chlorpromazine	–	–	–
Clozapine	–	–	–
Desipramine	–	–	Yes
Escitalopram	–	–	No
ECT	–	–	–
Fluoxetine	–	–	–
Gabapentin	–	–	–
Haloperidol	–	–	–
Imipramine	–	–	Yes
Ketamine	–	–	–
Lamotrigine	–	–	–
Levetiracetam	–	–	–
Lithium	Neg	Eq	–
Lurasidone	Yes	–	–
Olanzapine	–	–	No
OFC	–	–	No
Oxcarbazepine	–	–	–
Paliperidone	–	–	–
Paroxetine	Yes	No	No
Perphenazine	–	–	–
Quetiapine	Yes	Yes	No
Risperidone	No	–	–
Sleep deprivation	–	–	–
Tamoxifen	–	–	–
TMS	–	–	–
Topiramate	–	–	–
Valproate	Eq	Neg	–
Venlafaxine	–	–	Yes
Ziprasidone	–	–	–
CBT	–	–	–
Psychoeducation	–	–	–

– no data, *Neg* negative data

comparison to placebo (49 % vs. 48 % vs. 25 %; $p=0.025$). In spite of the fact that half of the patients were previously unresponsive to lithium, no inferiority of lithium in comparison to divalproex was observed. Fewer patients in the divalproex arm dropped out (61 % vs. 48 % vs. 64 %). Dropouts because of lack of efficacy were fewer in the two treatment arms in comparison to placebo (33 % vs. 30 % vs. 51 %), while dropouts because of adverse events were more frequent with lithium (11 % vs. 6 % vs. 3 %). The most frequent adverse events with lithium were asthenia, constipation, dizziness, nausea, fever, twitching and vomiting (Bowden et al. 1994). A post hoc analysis of the previous study confirmed the efficacy of lithium in classic manic but not mixed patients. All other effects were negative (Swann et al. 1997). An international multicentre 12-week RCT (3 weeks with placebo) in 302 acutely manic BD patients compared lithium (target serum levels 0.6–1.4 mEq/l; $N=98$) vs. quetiapine IR (flexibly dosed up to 800 mg/day; $N=107$) and vs. placebo ($N=97$). The improvement in YMRS score was significantly greater for lithium, and quetiapine IR in comparison to placebo at week 3 (−15.2 vs. −14.6 vs. −6.7; $p<0.001$) was present already during day 7 and persisted throughout the duration of the study. Significantly more lithium- and quetiapine IR-treated patients were responders in comparison with placebo patients at week 3 (53.1 % vs. 53.3 % vs. 27.4 %; $p<0.001$), and the picture was similar concerning the remission rates (49 % vs. 46.7 % vs. 22.1 %; $p<0.001$). The picture was similar concerning remission rates. While the quetiapine IR data concerning all individual YMRS items were reported, this was not reported also for lithium. Quetiapine IR but not lithium significantly improved the PANSS positive subscale, and both improved the activation and the aggression subscale. The effect on the negative subscale was not reported. Both medications significantly improved the MADRS score, but lithium achieved this only at endpoint while quetiapine IR already at day 21. Fewer patients in the lithium and quetiapine IR groups dropped out from the study compared with the placebo group (31.6 % vs. 32.7 % vs. 63.9 %). Also fewer of them dropped out because of lack of efficacy (12.2 % vs. 14.9 % vs. 39.2 %), while the dropout rate because of adverse events was similar among groups (6.1 % vs. 6.5 % vs. 4.1 %). The most common adverse events for lithium were tremor and insomnia (Bowden et al. 2005b). The third was an international multicentre study (PDMD-004), and it included 444 acutely manic or mixed BD patients and studied the efficacy and safety of lithium (1,500 mg/day; $N=113$) vs. topiramate (200 mg/day; $N=110$ or 400 mg/day; $N=110$) vs. placebo ($N=111$). At week 3, lithium-treated patients manifested significantly more reduction in their YMRS scores in comparison both to the topiramate arms and to placebo (−12.9 vs. −5.8 vs. −6.2 vs. −7.7; $p<0.001$). The withdrawal rate was similar among groups (26–29 %) with no difference concerning the cause. The fourth study was PDMD-008 which compared 1,500 mg of lithium daily ($N=114$) vs. 400 mg topiramate daily ($N=116$) vs. placebo ($N=112$) in 342 BD-I acutely manic or mixed patients. The withdrawal rate was 18 % for lithium and 13 % for placebo, with lithium-treated patients dropping out more frequently because of adverse effects and placebo-treated patients because of lack of efficacy. At week 3, lithium-treated patients manifested significantly more reduction in their YMRS scores in comparison to placebo (−13.8 vs, −8.4; $p<0.001$).

These two studies were not published independently but only together with the other two negative topiramate trials in an exploratory analysis in search of a potential efficacy signal. That analysis pooled all data from these four studies and reported that the percentage of responders at week 3 was 37 % for lithium vs. 22 % for placebo. Again there was no effect of lithium on the MADRS score. Nausea, diarrhoea, dizziness and weight gain were the more frequent side effects of lithium treatment (Kushner et al. 2006). A fourth 12-week (3 weeks with placebo) multicentre US study in 480 acutely manic or mixed patients (rapid cycling excluded) investigated lithium (900–1,500 mg/day; $N=160$) vs. aripiprazole (15–30 mg/day; $N=155$) vs. placebo ($N=165$). Both lithium and aripiprazole demonstrated significantly greater improvement than placebo in YMRS score at week 3 (−12.0 vs. −12.6 vs. −9.0; $p<0.005$), and the improvement was evident since week 1 for lithium and since day 2 for aripiprazole and continued for all the study period. The response rate was significantly higher in both the lithium and the aripiprazole groups in comparison to placebo at week 3 (45.8 % vs. 46.8 % vs. 34.4 %; $p<0.05$). A similar picture was evident concerning the remission rates (40 % vs. 40.3 % vs. 28.2 %). No effect on PANSS total or MADRS was observed for lithium. No results concerning the PANSS positive and negative subscales were reported. The dropout rate was similar between groups (51 % vs. 53 % vs. 53 %) at week 3. The dropout rate for lithium because of lack of efficacy was between that of aripiprazole and placebo (16 % vs. 6 % vs. 22 %), while more patients in the two medication arms dropped out because of adverse events in comparison to placebo (13 % vs. 15 % vs. 8 %). The most common adverse events with lithium were nausea, headache, constipation and tremor (Keck et al. 2009).

Overall, the literature suggests that lithium is effective for the treatment of acute manic episodes with or without mixed features. It has four positive studies (Bowden et al. 1994, 2005b; Kushner et al. 2006; Keck et al. 2009). The effect size for response has the magnitude of NNT equal to 5–6 at week 3, and the therapeutic effect appears after 7 days of treatment, that is, later in comparison to antipsychotics. There are limited data which dispute the effect of lithium on the core symptoms of mania. Its effect specifically on mixed episodes is unknown. Probably there is no therapeutic effect on concomitant depressive and psychotic symptoms. The most common adverse events with lithium were nausea, vomiting, dizziness headache, insomnia, asthenia, constipation, diarrhoea, tremor and weight gain.

16.2.1.1.2 Antiepileptics

Valproate

Limited data concerning the efficacy of valproate in acute mania exist from earlier studies which utilized very small study samples and a very different study design. Fourteen patients from these early studies were tested under double-blind conditions, and ten of them (71.4 %) were reported to have significantly improved (McElroy et al. 1989). Such an early study utilized an ABA design in five acutely ill manic patients who were treated with valproate 1.8–3.8 g/day (serum concentrations 50–100 μg/ml). These authors reported that in four cases a marked improvement (over 60 %) was observed within 3–15 days. They also reported that another seven patients with frequently recurrent episodes of a manic or maniform schizoaffective psychosis, previously unresponsive to lithium prophylaxis, were chronically treated with valproate in combination with low doses of lithium (one case only with valproate). Over an observation period of 1.5–3 years, none of the patients suffered from a relapse (Emrich et al. 1980, 1981).

As in the case of lithium, the first study with modern methodology on the efficacy and safety of valproate in the treatment of acute mania took place only in 1991. It was conducted in a small study sample which was enriched for lithium refractoriness and included 36 acutely manic patients (refractory or intolerant to lithium). Valproate serum concentrations were between 50 and 100 mg/l. The patients randomized to valproate ($N=17$) manifested a 54 % reduction in their YMRS in comparison to 5 % in patients of the placebo group ($N=19$). The treatment effect was present 1–4 days after achieving therapeutic serum concentrations (>50 mg/l). Fewer patients under valproate dropped out because of lack of efficacy (24 % vs. 63 %) but more because of adverse events (12 % vs. 5.3 %). There was no difference in the adverse effects profile between the treatment arms (Pope et al. 1991). Another 3-week study in 179 hospitalized, acutely manic patients in academic settings across the USA investigated the efficacy and safety of divalproex (serum levels below 150 μg/ml; $N=69$) and lithium (serum levels below 1.5 mmol/l; $N=36$) vs. placebo ($N=74$). Half of them were previously nonresponsive to lithium, and none had previously received valproate; thus, the study sample was enriched in favour of divalproex. After 3 weeks, both treatment arms manifested a higher change in MRS in comparison to placebo, and this change was significant since day 15 for both agents. Unfortunately the results were reported only through a chart, and no exact means and standard deviations are available. Interestingly, the analysis of separate items of the MRS revealed that divalproex but not lithium had a beneficial effect on the core manic symptoms. The response rate was higher for divalproex and lithium in comparison to placebo (48 % vs. 49 % vs. 25 %; $p=0.025$). In spite of the fact that half of patients were previously unresponsive to lithium, no superiority of divalproex was observed. Fewer patients in the divalproex arm dropped out (48 % vs. 61 % vs. 64 %). Dropouts because of lack of efficacy were fewer in the two treatment arms in comparison to placebo (30 % vs. 33 % vs. 51 %), while dropouts because of adverse events were more frequent with lithium (6 % vs. 11 % vs. 3 %). The most frequent adverse events for divalproex were asthenia, constipation, dizziness, nausea, twitching and vomiting (Bowden et al. 1994). A post hoc analysis of the previous study did not find any beneficial effect for divalproex either in classic or in mixed manic patients (Swann et al. 1997). Another multicentre study in 377 hospitalized patients suffering from an acute manic or mixed episode was conducted in the USA and investigated the efficacy and safety of divalproex sodium extended release (divalproex ER; $N=187$) against placebo ($N=177$). The target was serum valproate concentrations of 85–125 μg/ml. Patients receiving divalproex ER manifested more improvement in the MRS scores at week 3 (−11.5 vs.−9.0; $p=0.01$), and the difference was observable already at day 5. At week 3, 48 % of divalproex-treated patients were responders in comparison to 34 % in the placebo group

($p=0.01$). One problematic finding of this study is that divalproex ER did not differ from placebo in its effect on core manic symptoms like elevated mood, pressured speech and grandiosity. More patients in the divalproex ER group discontinued because of adverse events (10 % vs. 3 %), while less discontinued because of lack of efficacy (13 % vs. 26 %) in comparison to placebo. The overall discontinuation rates were comparable (58 % vs. 52 %). The most frequent side effects associated with treatment with divalproex ER were somnolence, dizziness and gastrointestinal complaints (Bowden et al. 2006). Another international multicentre study in 521 acutely manic or mixed patients evaluated the efficacy and safety of divalproex (500–2,500 mg/day; $N=201$) vs. olanzapine (5–20 mg/day; $N=215$) vs. placebo ($N=105$). At week 3, divalproex-treated patients were not better than placebo in contrast to olanzapine-treated patients in terms of change in their YMRS scores (−8.2 vs. −9.4 vs. −7.4). There was no difference in the MADRS score change between the medication arms and placebo. The response rates did not differ between the medication arms and placebo (40.3 % vs. 40.8 % vs. 31.3 %) and neither did the remission (40.3 % vs. 42.8 % vs. 35.4 %) nor the dropout rates (26 % vs. 24.9 % vs. 26.6 %). Overall, divalproex did not differ from placebo, and the negative findings persisted throughout the study. It is interesting that while 35.4 % (at 3 weeks) to 57.1 % (at 12 weeks) had valproate plasma concentrations lower than the recommended valproate therapeutic range, the YMRS scores of these patients were lower than those of patients with valproate concentrations above or within range. Patients treated with divalproex had significant decreases in leukocytes and platelets compared with olanzapine at week 12 (Tohen et al. 2008b). The next study was a small RCT which took place in a single academic setting in the USA and included a heterogeneous sample consisting of ambulatory bipolar spectrum disorder patients and patients with moderate-to-severe hypomanic or mild manic symptoms (hypomania/mild mania). Sixty patients were randomized to divalproex ER (15–30 mg/kg/day) or placebo. Probably due to the small study sample, no difference was detected in any of the outcome measures or the adverse effects between the treatment groups. There was no difference in the dropout rate between divalproex ER and placebo (57 % vs. 50 %) although in terms of reason, lack of efficacy was twofold higher in the placebo group (24 % vs. 47 %). There are a number of methodological and reporting issues pertaining to this study (McElroy et al. 2010a). The last was a failed multicentre study conducted in the USA and randomized 225 acutely manic or mixed patients to receive either divalproex ER ($N=147$) or placebo ($N=78$). The mean dose of divalproex ER was 2,211 mg/day, and the mean maximum serum valproic acid serum concentration was 77.9 μg/ml. At week 3, there was no difference in the outcome, the adverse effects or the dropout rate between the two treatment groups. The dropout rate was exceptionally high for a 3-week trial and similar for both groups (83 % vs. 80 %) (Hirschfeld et al. 2010).

Overall the data support the usefulness of valproate against acute mania. However it should be noted that a number of issues exist and future studies are needed to clarify them. Valproate has three positive (Pope et al. 1991; Bowden et al. 1994, 2006) and two failed (Tohen et al. 2008b; Hirschfeld et al. 2010) studies. Its effect on psychotic symptoms is unknown, and there seems to be no effect on concomitant depressive symptoms. It is problematic that the most recent and rigorously conducted studies on large samples either failed to support its overall efficacy or failed to find an effect on the core clinical features of acute mania. The NNT for response is probably around ten, and the therapeutic effect is present after 5–15 days. It is important to note that although the dosages utilized in these studies were somewhat higher than those usually used in everyday clinical practice (15–30 mg/kg/day which for a 75 k person correspond to 1,125–2,250 mg/day), they hardly achieved the target serum concentrations (50–100 μg/ml). On the other hand, the adverse effect profile was mild and without significant difference from the placebo group. The most frequent adverse events were somnolence, nausea, dizziness, asthenia, constipation, twitching and vomiting. Decreases in leukocytes and platelets have also been reported.

Carbamazepine

The first study on carbamazepine was published in 1980 and reported that 7 out of 9 manic and 5 out of 13 depressed patients had a partial to marked response when administered with carbamazepine (600–1,600 mg/day, blood levels 8–12 μg/ml). Also that several patients showed relapses when placebo was introduced and improvement when carbamazepine was reinstituted (Ballenger and Post 1980). Another study which utilized the ABAB design included 19 acutely manic patients and utilized carbamazepine in doses averaging 1,240 mg/day (blood levels 10.4 ± 2.2 μg/ml). These authors reported a rapid clinical improvement in 12 patients (63.2 %), and response was related to significantly more manic symptoms during the baseline placebo period, more dysphoric picture and rapid cycling. That study suggested that several predictors of poor response to lithium carbonate (manic severity, anxiety and dysphoria, rapid cycling and negative family history) may be associated with good response to carbamazepine (Post et al. 1987). The first multicentre US study on carbamazepine which conducted with a modern methodology utilized 204 acutely manic or mixed patients and was published in 2004. It was a 3-week RCT and compared carbamazepine extended release (carbamazepine ER; 400–1,600 mg/day; mean plasma level 8.9 μg/ml; $N=101$) vs. placebo ($N=103$). Half of the patients dropped out. Carbamazepine ER exhibited a significant reduction in YMRS scores ($p=0.032$), and this was evident since week 2. Unfortunately the results were published only in the form of charts, and thus precise mean and standard deviations of change scores are not available. More patients under carbamazepine ER were responders (41.5 % vs. 22.4 %; $p=0.007$). It is unclear whether it improved mixed patients also, and not only purely manic, because of a large placebo effect in the mixed group. There was no effect on the depressive score as measured by the HAM-D in the manic patients; however, there was a significant improvement in the mixed patients. The most frequent adverse events related to carbamazepine were dizziness, nausea and somnolence (Weisler et al. 2004). The second multicentre international study (USA and India) in 239 hospitalized acutely manic or mixed patients compared carbamazepine ER (400–1,600 mg/day; $N=122$) vs. placebo ($N=117$). Numerically fewer patients in the carbamazepine arm dropped out (34.4 % vs. 45.3 %) with more patients in the placebo arm discontinuing due to lack of efficacy (6.6 % vs. 23.1 %; $p<0.001$), while the dropout rate because of adverse events was similar in the two arms. Carbamazepine ER exhibited a significant reduction in YMRS scores since day 7 ($p<0.05$); however, again the publication of results is incomplete. The adverse events related to the carbamazepine ER arm included dizziness (39.3 %), somnolence (30.3 %) and nausea (23.8 %). Carbamazepine-treated patients also experienced a significant increase in total cholesterol, composed of increases in both high-density and low-density lipoproteins (Weisler et al. 2005). The pooled data of the 443 patients which took part in the two above-mentioned studies suggested that there was a trend less patients in the carbamazepine ER group to drop out in comparison to the placebo arm (42 % vs. 50 %; $p=0.087$). Significantly less patients under carbamazepine ER dropped out because of lack of efficacy (10 % vs. 22 %; $p<0.001$). At week 3 carbamazepine ER was related to significantly more reduction in the YMRS score in comparison to placebo (for manic episodes, $p<0.0001$; for mixed, $p<0.01$). There was also a significant reduction in the HAM-D scores of mixed patients (−4.8 vs. −2.3; $p<0.05$). More patients under carbamazepine ER patients experienced an adverse event (90 % vs. 64 %), and more of them dropped out because of adverse events (10.8 % vs. 5.5 %) (Weisler et al. 2006).

Finally, there is a 12-week double-blind, randomized, placebo-controlled study from China in 111 patients with acute mania which were randomized to carbamazepine (300–800 mg/day; $N=43$) vs. carbamazepine plus the herbal Free and Easy Wanderer Plus (FEWP; 36 g/day; $N=46$) vs. placebo ($N=22$). At endpoint both carbamazepine arms produced significantly greater improvement on YMRS score, and the improvement was present already at week 4, but they did not differ from each other (−22.9 vs. −25.4 vs. −17). In terms of response rates, more patients in the carbamazepine arms were superior to placebo (87.8 % vs. 93 % vs. 57.1 %, $p=0.012$). Interestingly, although there was no difference between the two carbamazepine groups concerning the carbamazepine dosage, fewer patients under the combination dropped out (25.6 % vs. 13 % vs. 40.9 %), and this was also true concerning dropout because of lack of efficacy (7 % vs. 4.3 % vs. 27.3 %). Depressed and manic patients were pooled for the analysis of adverse events, and the adverse events occurring in over 5 % of the patients in any treatment group were dizziness, laboratory testing abnormality, skin rash, headache, fatigue, blurred vision, somnolence and nausea. Compared to carbamazepine monotherapy, patients in the combination therapy had a lesser incidence of dizziness (18.2 % vs. 7.9 %; $p=0.069$) and fatigue (9.1 % vs. 1.1 %; $p=0.038$). No difference in the incidence of other adverse events was found between the combination therapy and CBZ monotherapy. Although this study supports the efficacy of carbamazepine during the acute manic phase, the low carbamazepine dosage, in combination with the possible dramatic reduction of carbamazepine levels when co-administered with FEWP, plus the unusually high response rate even in the placebo group and the unusually low dropout rate, makes conclusions difficult (Zhang et al. 2007).

Overall the data concerning the efficacy and safety of carbamazepine at dosages 400–1,600 mg/day and mean plasma level 8.9 μg/ml are robust, with three positive studies (Weisler et al. 2004, 2005; Zhang et al. 2007) and suggest an NNT of approximately 5 for response. Response starts since week 2. It is unknown whether carbamazepine has a beneficial effect on the core manic symptoms. There seems to be a beneficial effect on concomitant depressive symptoms only in mixed patients but not in purely manic, and the efficacy against psychotic symptoms is unknown. The most frequent adverse events related to carbamazepine treatment were dizziness, nausea, somnolence and an increase in total cholesterol which was composed of increases in both high-density and low-density lipoproteins.

Other Antiepileptics

Recently two 3-week multicentre, double-blind, randomized, placebo-controlled studies in acute mania were conducted concerning eslicarbazepine. The first one (BIA-2093-203) utilized a dose titrated by response (600–1,800 mg or 800–2,400 mg/day) and it was negative, while the second (BIA-2093-204) utilized fixed doses of 600, 1,200 and 1,800 mg/day, and it was a failed trial (Robertson et al. 2010). Three other also unpublished RCTs (NCT00107926, NCT00107939 and NCT00099229) concerning the racemic mixture licarbazepine were also negative.

There are two unpublished negative trials concerning lamotrigine against acute manic episodes (SCAA2008/GW609 and SCAA2009/GW610). The SCAA2008/GW609 study had 3-week duration and investigated the efficacy and safety of lamotrigine (50 mg/day; $N=84$) vs. lithium (titrated to a serum level of 0.8–1.3 mEq/l; $N=36$) vs. placebo ($N=95$). This study was generally underpowered. The SCAA2009/GW610 was a 6-week study and investigated lamotrigine (200 mg/day; $N=74$) vs. lithium (titrated to a serum level of 0.7–1.3 mEq/l; $N=77$) vs. placebo ($N=77$). In this later study the MRS scores were significantly reduced in patients receiving lithium vs. placebo ($p=0.05$). Lamotrigine was not associated with worsening manic symptoms in these trials (Goldsmith et al. 2003). One additional small RCT evaluated the efficacy and safety of lamotrigine (max 500 mg/day) and gabapentin (max 4,800 mg/day) monotherapy vs. placebo in 31 patients with refractory bipolar and unipolar mood disorders. At week 6, 52 % of patients under lamotrigine and 26 % under gabapentin were responders vs. 23 % in the placebo group. Lamotrigine differed significantly from placebo ($p=0.022$) but not gabapentin ($p=0.08$). Both agents were generally well tolerated (Frye et al. 2000). Four trials which tested the efficacy and safety of topiramate (target doses: 200, 400 or 600 mg/day) vs. placebo (two trials included lithium, 1,500 mg/day as an active comparator) in hospitalized BD-I acutely manic or mixed patients were negative concerning the YMRS score change at week 3 vs. placebo (−5.1 vs. −8.4), while lithium was related to a significant change vs. placebo and vs. topiramate. The same finding occurred at week 12. The most frequent adverse effects related to topiramate were paraesthesia, appetite decrease, dry mouth and weight loss. Topiramate was not associated with mood destabilization measured as mania exacerbation or treatment-emergent depression (Kushner et al. 2006).

Thus, the data concerning the efficacy of lamotrigine, gabapentin, topiramate, eslicarbazepine and licarbazepine against acute mania are negative. This suggests that there is no class effect concerning antiepileptics in the treatment of BD (Fountoulakis et al. 2011a; Rosa et al. 2011).

16.2.1.1.3 Antipsychotics

Antipsychotics were developed for the treatment of psychosis, and probably the first patients on whom they were used were manic–depressive in an excited state. However, eventually their primary indication was schizophrenia and related psychotic disorders. It is well known that there is a general efficacy–effectiveness gap, and only recently there were hard data available concerning their efficacy in BP. The first study was a small, placebo-controlled study supporting the efficacy of chlorpromazine (Klein 1967). Another one took place in 1975, and it utilized a problematic methodology especially concerning the psychometric scales; it compared lithium, haloperidol and chlorpromazine and suggested that antipsychotics acted more rapidly, but lithium was more globally effective (Shopsin et al. 1975).

Haloperidol

The efficacy and safety of haloperidol was studied in five RCTs and all were positive. All of them were of 12-week duration with the first 3 weeks as a double-blind placebo-controlled phase and the next 9 weeks as the extension phase without placebo. The primary outcome was positioned at week 3. The first one was an international multicentre study of 302 hospitalized patients with acute mania and compared haloperidol (up to 8 mg/day; $N=99$) vs. quetiapine IR (flexibly dosed up to 800 mg/day; $N=102$) and placebo ($N=101$). It showed that at week 3, haloperidol- and quetiapine IR-treated patients manifested significantly more reduction in the YMRS scores (−15.71 vs. −12.29 vs. −8.32; $p<0.01$), and this was evident as early as day 4. Quetiapine IR improved all individual items of the YMRS, while no such data are reported concerning haloperidol. Although both agents reduced the PANSS positive score at endpoint, only haloperidol had an effect at week 21, and only haloperidol differed from placebo concerning the reduction of YMRS score in psychotic patients, and this was true throughout the study. On the contrary, haloperidol had a favourable effect on the MADRS at week 3 which did not last until the end of the study in contrast to quetiapine which had a sustained effect. The response rate at day 21 was in favour of the haloperidol and quetiapine IR groups in comparison to placebo (56.1 % vs. 42.6 % vs. 35.0 %). Remission rates were not significant for either drug vs. placebo at day 21, but they were at week 12 (63.3 % vs. 61.4 % vs. 38.0 %). More patients under haloperidol withdrew from the study because of adverse events in comparison to quetiapine IR and placebo (10.1 % vs. 4.9 % vs. 5.9 %). The only frequent adverse events related to haloperidol treatment were EPS which occurred more often with haloperidol than with quetiapine IR or placebo (59.6 % vs. 12.7 % vs. 15.8 %) (McIntyre et al. 2005). Another international (outside the USA) 12-week multicentre trial in 438 hospitalized acutely manic BD patients (mixed and rapid cycling excluded) compared haloperidol (2–12 mg/day; $N=144$) vs. risperidone (1–6 mg/day; $N=154$) vs. placebo ($N=140$). At week 3 both agents exhibited higher change in YMRS scores (−13.9 vs. −15.1 vs. −9.4; $p<0.001$). The effect persisted throughout the study duration, and there were no differences between the two active drug arms. There was no difference between patients with vs. without psychotic features. Response rate at week 3 was also superior for the two active drugs vs. placebo (47 % vs. 48 % vs. 33 %). Response was stable during the whole study duration. Risperidone manifested a significant change also in the MADRS score at week 3 and at endpoint while haloperidol did only at endpoint. However in those patients who completed the study, the effect of haloperidol on the MADRS was larger than that of risperidone. EPS were more frequent in the haloperidol arm (40 % vs. 17 % vs. 9 %) at week 3, and a similar picture persisted throughout the study. There were similar rates of dropouts in the three arms at week 3 (10 % vs. 11 % vs. 15 %). Discontinuation because of adverse events was similar across arms (≤5 %), while there was some difference in the dropouts because of insufficient response (1 % vs. 3 % vs. 6 %) (Smulevich et al. 2005). The next study was again international and multicentre, included 485 acutely manic or mixed patients and assessed the efficacy and safety of aripiprazole (15 or 30 mg/day; $N=167$) vs. haloperidol (5–15 mg/day; $N=165$) vs. placebo ($N=153$). At week 3 both haloperidol and aripiprazole manifested significantly higher change in YMRS scores in comparison to placebo (−12.8 vs. −12.0 vs. −9.7; $p<0.01$), and this was maintained through week 12. Both medication arms significantly improved the positive but not the negative subscale of the PANSS. The response rates at week 3 were numerically greater with haloperidol and aripiprazole in comparison to placebo, but neither was significant (49.7 % vs. 47.0 % vs. 38.2 %; $p>0.05$). This was true also for the remission rates (45.3 % vs. 44 % vs. 36.8 %; $p>0.05$). The dropout rate was similar across the study arms at week 3 (27 % vs. 25 % vs. 29 %). Extrapyramidal adverse events were more frequent with haloperidol than aripiprazole (53.3 % vs. 23.5 %), but otherwise the adverse effects profile was similar (Young et al. 2009). Next was a 12-week international RCT on 438 acutely manic or mixed BD patients which compared haloperidol (8–30 mg/day; $N=172$) vs. ziprasidone (80–160 mg/day; $N=178$) and vs. placebo ($N=88$). At week 3, haloperidol produced greater change in MRS score in comparison to ziprasidone, but both arms did significantly better than placebo (−15.93 vs. −10.41 vs. −6.10; $p\leq0.01$). The positive subscale of the PANSS but not the other subscales was also significantly improved by the active drugs. At week 3, the response rate was significantly superior for haloperidol vs. both ziprasidone and placebo (54.7 % vs. 36.9 % vs. 20.5 %, respectively, $p<0.05$). Response was maintained until the end of the study (week 12) for both agents. At week 12, 31.9 % of haloperidol-treated patients were in remission vs. 22.7 % in the ziprasidone arm. Significantly more patients in the placebo group dropped out (59 % vs. 55 % vs. 72 %), and this was also true because of lack of efficacy (27 % vs. 12 % vs. 44 %) but not because of adverse events (9 % vs. 21 % vs. 5 %). More patients under haloperidol dropped out in comparison to patients under ziprasidone during the extension phase (weeks 4–12; 21.1 % vs. 9.6 %) and also had significantly higher rates of movement disorders as adverse events. At week 3, haloperidol-treated patients experienced more often adverse events in comparison to ziprasidone-treated patients and placebo (80.1 % vs. 64.6 % vs. 39.8 %). Throughout the study period more patients under haloperidol experienced adverse events in comparison to ziprasidone (87.1 % vs. 73.6 %). Through week 3, more patients under haloperidol had discontinued because of adverse events in comparison to ziprasidone and placebo (21 % vs. 9 % vs. 5 %) and at week 12 (21.1 % vs. 9.6 %). There was no significant difference in the cardiovascular adverse events between the three treatment arms and in the rate of switching to depression although numerically more patients under haloperidol switched during the entire 12-week duration of the study in comparison to ziprasidone (8.7 % vs. 4.5 %). This study was powered to detect weight gain since patients included should had had body weight ≥80 % of the lower weight limit and within 150 % of the upper weight limit of the ideal weight for sex, height and frame. It is interesting that there was a big difference in body weight between countries (Vieta et al. 2010c). Finally, a 3-week study from Japan randomized 224 manic or mixed BD patients to receive haloperidol (2.5–10 mg/day; $N=20$), olanzapine (5–20 mg/day; $N=105$) or placebo ($N=99$). The haloperidol arm included only 20 patients. At week 3 the haloperidol-treated patients had significant reduction in their YMRS score in comparison to placebo and similar to olanzapine (−14.3 vs. −12.6 vs. −6.8). Olanzapine had an effect on the core symptoms of mania, while a similar effect was not present for haloperidol. The response rates were similar in the three groups (65 % vs. 51 % vs. 44.3 %), while the remission rate was higher (but not significantly) in the haloperidol group (65 % vs. 47.1 % vs. 41.2 %). Haloperidol numerically increased the HAM-D score in, while olanzapine significantly decreased it in comparison to both haloperidol and placebo. More patients under haloperidol dropped out (60 % vs. 30.5 % vs. 45.5 %), fewer because of lack of efficacy (5 % vs. 14.3 % vs. 28.9 %) but more because of adverse events (25 % vs. 8.6 % vs. 7 %). More haloperidol-treated patients switched to symptomatic depression in comparison to olanzapine (16.7 % vs. 2.4 %, $p=0.014$). The adverse events rate related with haloperidol treatment were somnolence, EPS, weight gain and constipation. EPS in the haloperidol group were more severe than in the olanzapine group (Katagiri et al. 2012).

Overall, with five positive studies (McIntyre et al. 2005; Smulevich et al. 2005; Young et al. 2009; Vieta et al. 2010c; Katagiri et al. 2012), the data are strong in favour of haloperidol (up to 30 mg/day) in the treatment of acute mania with an NNT roughly equal to 5–8 for response, which is present already since day 4. There is signal for the induction of depression in the short term. One study reported no effect on the core symptoms of mania; however, it does have an effect on psychotic symptoms. It might be particularly efficacious in psychotic patients, but its effect on mixed patients is unknown. The adverse events rate related with haloperidol treatment were somnolence, EPS, weight gain and constipation.

Olanzapine

A multicentre US 3-week duration RCT on 139 acutely manic or mixed patients (half of them psychotic) from academic centres investigated the efficacy and safety of olanzapine (up to 10 mg/day; $N=70$) vs. placebo ($N=69$). The olanzapine group experienced significantly greater mean improvement in YMRS vs. the placebo group at week 3 (−10.26 vs. −4.88, $p=0.02$), and most of the improvement was observed already since week 1. However the analysis of separate YMRS items showed that only sleep and irritability differed between arms. There was also a significant effect of olanzapine on the positive subscale of the PANSS but not on the negative subscale. Olanzapine was equally effective in patients with and without psychotic features, mixed features and rapid cycling. There was no significant effect on the HAM-D. More patients in the olanzapine group responded in comparison to placebo (48.6 % vs. 24.2 %). More patients under placebo dropped out (65.2 % vs. 38.6 %) and also more dropped out because of lack of efficacy (47.8 % vs. 28.6 %). There was no difference in the dropout rate because of adverse effects. Somnolence, dizziness, dry mouth and weight gain but not EPS occurred significantly more often in the olanzapine-treated patients (Tohen et al. 1999). A multicentre 4-week RCT conducted in university-affiliated sites in the USA included 115 acutely manic or mixed patients (half of them psychotic) and studied the efficacy and safety of olanzapine (5–20 mg/day; $N=55$) vs. placebo ($N=60$). At week 4, olanzapine-treated patients had significantly greater reduction in the YMRS score (−14.78 vs. −8.13, $p<0.001$). This difference was evident since week 1. There was also a significant reduction in the PANSS positive subscale but not in the PANSS negative or the HAM-D. Olanzapine-treated patients demonstrated a higher rate of response (65 % vs. 43 %, $p=0.02$) than placebo-treated patients. Numerically fewer patients in the olanzapine arm dropped out (38.2 % vs. 58.3 %). Numerically more patients under olanzapine dropped out because of adverse effects (3.6 % vs. 1.7 %) and less because of lack of efficacy (27.3 % vs. 38.3 %). EPS were similar between arms; however, patients in the olanzapine arm manifested more weight gain and somnolence (Tohen et al. 2000). One study investigated the efficacy and safety of intramuscular olanzapine (10 mg, first two injections; 5 mg, third injection) vs. lorazepam (2 mg, first two injections; 1 mg, third injection) or placebo (placebo, first two injections; olanzapine, 10 mg, third injection) within a 24-h period in 201 agitated manic patients. At 2 h after the first injection, olanzapine-treated patients experienced a significantly greater reduction in agitation in comparison both to placebo and lorazepam, and the difference persisted throughout the study duration. On the contrary, lorazepam did not differ from placebo. There was no difference between groups concerning the adverse events rate, including EPS or QTc interval changes (Meehan et al. 2001). Another international multicentre study in 521 acutely manic or mixed patients evaluated the efficacy and safety of olanzapine (5–20 mg/day; $N=215$) vs. divalproex (500–2,500 mg/day; $N=201$) vs. placebo ($N=105$). At week 3, olanzapine but not divalproex-treated patients had significantly more reduction in their YMRS scores in comparison to the placebo arm (−9.4 vs. −8.2 vs. −7.4). The response rates did not differ between the medication arms and placebo (40.8 % vs. 40.3 % vs. 31.3 %) and neither did the remission rates (42.8 % vs. 40.3 % vs. 35.4 %). There was no difference in the MADRS score change between the medication arms and placebo. The dropout rate was not different between groups (26 % vs. 24.9 % vs. 26.6 %). Weight gain and somnolence were the most frequent adverse events associated with olanzapine treatment. It is interesting that while 35.4 % (at 3 weeks) to 57.1 % (at 12 weeks) had valproate plasma concentrations lower than the recommended valproate therapeutic range, the YMRS scores of these patients were lower than those of patients with valproate concentrations above or within range (Tohen et al. 2008b). Another international multicentre 3-week study in 488 acutely manic or mixed patients (rapid cycling excluded) compared olanzapine (5–20 mg/day; $N=190$) vs. asenapine (10–20 mg/day; $N=194$) vs. placebo ($N=104$). At day 21 both olanzapine and asenapine had superior changes from baseline in the YMRS scores (−12.6 vs. −10.8 vs. −5.5, $p<0.001$), and the change was evident since day 2. Olanzapine but not asenapine significantly improved the MADRS score in comparison to placebo. This improvement was evident since day 7. Olanzapine but not asenapine improved mixed patients also. More patients under olanzapine and asenapine responded in comparison to placebo (50 % vs. 42.3 % vs. 25.2 %, $p<0.01$). The picture was similar concerning the remission rates. The dropout rate was similar in the three treatment arms (30.9 % vs. 37.1 % vs. 38.5 %); however, fewer patients dropped out because of lack of efficacy in the olanzapine group (5.8 % vs. 8.2 % vs. 16.3 %). Also the fewer patients under olanzapine dropped out because of adverse events in comparison to asenapine and similar to placebo (4.2 % vs. 10.3 % vs. 6.7 %). EPS were reported in numerically more olanzapine- and asenapine-treated patients in comparison to placebo (7.9 % vs. 7.2 % vs. 2.9 %). The most frequent adverse effects of olanzapine included sedation, dry mouth, dizziness, somnolence and weight gain (McIntyre et al. 2009a). Another international multicentre RCT of 3-week duration included 488 acutely manic or mixed BD patients (rapid cycling excluded) and studied the efficacy and safety of olanzapine (5–20 mg/day; $N=205$) vs. asenapine (10–20 mg/day; $N=185$) vs. placebo ($N=98$). Olanzapine and asenapine were superior to placebo at day 21 (−14.6 vs. −11.5 vs. −7.8, $p<0.01$). For both medication arms the treatment effect was significant since day 2. Olanzapine but not asenapine significantly improved the MADRS score at endpoint. The response rate of olanzapine, but not of asenapine, was superior to that of placebo (54.7 % vs. 42.6 % vs. 34 %). This was true also for remission rates. The dropout rate was lower in the olanzapine arm (21.5 % vs. 33 % vs. 41.8 %). Fewer patients in the olanzapine arm discontinued because of lack of efficacy (6.3 % vs. 7.6 % vs. 14.3 %) or adverse events (3.4 % vs. 9.2 % vs. 4.1 %). Most frequent adverse events related with olanzapine treatment were somnolence, dizziness, sedation and EPS. More EPS in comparison to placebo were registered in the olanzapine group but lower in comparison to asenapine (6.8 % vs. 10.3 % vs. 3.1 %). Weight gain was significantly more frequent in the olanzapine arm (19.0 % vs. 7.2 % vs. 1.2 %) (McIntyre et al. 2010b). Finally, a 3-week study from Japan randomized 224 manic or mixed BD patients to receive haloperidol (2.5–10 mg/day; $N=20$), olanzapine (5–20 mg/day; $N=105$) or placebo ($N=99$). The haloperidol arm included only 20 patients. At week 3 the haloperidol-treated patients had significant reduction in their YMRS score in comparison to placebo and similar to olanzapine (−14.3 vs. −12.6 vs. −6.8). Olanzapine had an effect on the core symptoms of mania, while a similar effect was not present for haloperidol. The response rates were similar in the three groups (65 % vs. 51 % vs. 44.3 %), while the remission rate was higher (but not significantly) in the haloperidol group (47.1 % vs. 65 % vs. 41.2 %). Haloperidol numerically increased the HAM-D score, while olanzapine significantly decreased it in comparison to both haloperidol and placebo. More patients under haloperidol dropped out (60 % vs. 30.5 % vs. 45.5 %), fewer because of lack of efficacy (5 % vs. 14.3 % vs. 28.9 %) but more because of adverse events (25 % vs. 8.6 % vs. 7 %). More haloperidol-treated patients switched to symptomatic depression in comparison to olanzapine (16.7 % vs. 2.4 %, $p=0.014$). The adverse events related with olanzapine treatment were somnolence, dizziness, thirst and weight gain. EPS in olanzapine group were less severe than in the haloperidol group (Katagiri et al. 2012). The efficacy and safety of olanzapine has also been investigated in a study sample of 45 outpatients (24 BD-1, 22 BD-II and 4 BD-NOS) with HAM-D ≥10 and/or YMRS ≥10 and ≤24. This diverse group of patients was randomized to double-blind olanzapine (2.5–20 mg/day; $N=23$) vs. placebo ($N=22$) for 1 week. At endpoint, olanzapine did not differ from placebo in any outcome; however, there were trends towards a superiority of olanzapine, and the study was underpowered. On the other hand there was a significant weight gain and more EPS in the olanzapine group (Srivastava et al. 2012).

Taken together the above, the literature supports the efficacy of olanzapine 5–20 mg/day for the treatment of manic or mixed episodes and concomitant psychotic features. There are six positive trials supporting this efficacy (Tohen et al. 1999, 2000, 2008b; McIntyre et al. 2009a, 2010b; Katagiri et al. 2012). The NNT is approximately around 5 for response. Although the results are not satisfactorily consistent, olanzapine seems to have a beneficial effect on the core symptoms of mania, on psychotic symptoms, and treats mixed patients as well as rapid cycling, and the response is visible as early as days 2–7. Olanzapine does not seem to switch to depression and possibly improves the coexisting depressive symptoms. The adverse events related with olanzapine treatment were somnolence, dizziness, dry mouth, thirst and weight gain. There was also a low rate of EPS.

Quetiapine

An international multicentre 12-week RCT (3 weeks with placebo) in 302 acutely manic patients compared quetiapine IR (flexibly dosed up to 800 mg/day; $N=107$) vs. lithium (target serum levels 0.6–1.4 mEq/l; $N=98$) and vs. placebo ($N=97$). The improvement in YMRS score was significantly greater for quetiapine IR, and lithium in comparison to placebo at day 21 (−14.6 vs. −15.2 vs.−6.7; $p<0.001$) was present already during day 7 and persisted throughout the duration of the study. Significantly more quetiapine IR- and lithium-treated patients were responders in comparison with placebo patients at day 21 (53.3 % vs. 53.1 % vs. 27.4 %; $p<0.001$), and the picture was similar concerning the remission rates (46.7 % vs. 49 % vs. 22.1 %; $p<0.001$). The picture was similar concerning remission rates. Quetiapine IR improved all individual YMRS items, but the respected data for lithium were not reported. Quetiapine IR but not lithium significantly improved the PANSS positive subscale, and both improved the activation and the aggression subscale. The effect on the negative subscale was not reported. Both medications significantly improved the MADRS score, but quetiapine IR achieved this already at day 21 while lithium only at endpoint. Fewer patients in the quetiapine IR and lithium groups dropped out from the study compared with the placebo group (32.7 % vs. 31.6 % vs. 63.9 %). Also fewer of them dropped out because of lack of efficacy (14.9 % vs. 12.2 % vs. 39.2 %), while the dropout rate because of adverse events was similar among groups (6.5 % vs. 6.1 % vs. 4.1 %). The most common adverse events for quetiapine IR were dry mouth, somnolence, and weight gain. The quetiapine IR and placebo groups had similar, low levels of EPS (Bowden et al. 2005b). Another international multicentre study of 302 hospitalized BD patients with acute mania compared quetiapine IR (flexibly dosed up to 800 mg/day; $N=102$) vs. haloperidol (up to 8 mg/day; $N=99$) and placebo ($N=101$). It showed that at week 3, quetiapine IR- and haloperidol-treated patients manifested significantly more reduction in the YMRS scores (−12.29 vs. −15.71 vs. −8.32; $p<0.01$), and this was evident as early as day 4. Quetiapine IR improved all individual items of the YMRS, while no such data are reported concerning haloperidol. Although both agents reduced the PANSS positive score at endpoint, quetiapine had no effect at week 21 and did not differ from placebo concerning the reduction of YMRS score in psychotic patients, and this was true throughout the study. On the contrary, quetiapine IR had a sustained effect on the MADRS which started as early as week 3, while haloperidol had a favourable effect at week 3 which however did not last until the end of the study. The response rate at day 21 was in favour of the quetiapine IR and haloperidol groups in comparison to placebo (42.6 % vs. 56.1 % vs. 35.0 %). Remission rates were not significant for either drug vs. placebo at day 21, but they were at week 12 (61.4 % vs. 63.3 % vs. 38.0 %). Quetiapine IR had less frequent EPS in comparison to haloperidol and similar to placebo (12.7 % vs. 59.6 % vs. 15.8 %). Also fewer patients under quetiapine IR withdrew from the study because of adverse events in comparison to haloperidol and similar to placebo (4.9 % vs. 10.1 % vs. 5.9 %). The only frequent adverse events related to quetiapine were somnolence and postural hypotension (McIntyre et al. 2005). The NCT00309699 was an international multicentre 12-week (3 weeks with placebo) study which included 493 acutely manic or mixed patients and compared quetiapine IR (400–800 mg/day; $N=193$) vs. paliperidone ER (3–12 mg/day; $N=195$), vs. placebo ($N=105$). Both quetiapine IR and paliperidone ER significantly improved the YMRS at week 3 in comparison to placebo (−11.7 vs. −13.2 vs. −7.4; $p<0.001$). The treatment effect was evident as early as day 2 and lasted for the entire duration of the study, and it was similar for manic and mixed patients. Although a beneficial effect on total PANSS score was reported, no specific effects on the positive or negative subscales of the PANSS or on a depressive scale were included in the report. At week 3 more patients in the two treatment arms were responders in comparison to placebo (49 % vs. 55.8 % vs. 34.6 %). Similarly the remission rate was higher in both treatment arms in comparison to placebo at week 3 (47.4 % vs. 52.1 % vs. 28.8 %). This picture lasted for the entire duration of the study, and a similar picture was observed concerning the remission rates. The NNT for response or remission was 6–7 for quetiapine IR. At week 3 fewer patients under quetiapine IR or paliperidone ER dropped out in comparison to placebo (21.2 % vs. 20.5 % vs. 39 %). Fewer patients in the medication arms withdrew because of lack of efficacy in comparison to placebo, and these withdrawals were more in the quetiapine IR group in comparison to the paliperidone ER group (7.8 % vs. 3.1 % vs. 18.1 %). Dropout because of adverse events was similar in the three arms. The most common treatment-emergent adverse events related to quetiapine were somnolence, sedation, dry mouth, headache and dizziness. At week 12 the body weight increase was more frequent in the quetiapine IR group (17 % vs. 8 %), but more patients under paliperidone ER switched to depression (13.9 % vs. 7.5 %) (Vieta et al. 2010b). Another one, the NCT00422123, which was a US multicentre 3-week RCT, included 308 acutely manic or mixed BD patients and compared quetiapine XR (400–800 mg/day, $N=149$) with placebo ($N=159$). At week 3 quetiapine IR improved the YMRS in comparison to placebo (−14.3 vs. −10.5; $p<0.001$). The treatment effect was evident as early as day 4 and lasted for the entire duration of the study, and it was significant for manic but not for mixed or rapid cycling patients. Quetiapine XR improved 6 out of 11 YMRS items, including core items. There was also a beneficial effect on the MADRS score as early as day 4 for manic patients alone. No effect on psychotic symptoms was reported. At week 3 more patients in quetiapine XR arm were responders in comparison to placebo (55.0 % vs. 33.3 %). This picture lasted for the entire duration of the study, and a similar picture was observed concerning the remission rates. The NNT for response or remission was 6–7 for quetiapine IR. The dropout rate was similar in the two groups (29.1 % vs. 28.1 %). Fewer patients in the medication arm withdrew because of lack of efficacy in comparison to placebo (3.9 % vs. 9.4 %). The dropout because of adverse events was higher in the placebo group. The adverse events associated with quetiapine XR treatment were mild to moderate in intensity and included sedation, dry mouth and somnolence (Cutler et al. 2011). Finally a small 8-week RCT in two US sites in 41 bipolar spectrum disorder patients and moderate-to-severe hypomanic or mild manic symptoms (hypomania/mild mania) studied quetiapine IR (up to 800 mg/day; $N=21$) vs. placebo ($N=20$). Quetiapine IR-treated patients had a marginally but nonsignificant improvement in YMRS score in comparison to placebo ($p=0.06$). Some secondary outcomes were significant. Discontinuation rates were high and similar in the two groups (McElroy et al. 2010b).

Taken together the above, with four positive studies (Bowden et al. 2005b; McIntyre et al. 2005; Vieta et al. 2010b; Cutler et al. 2011), the literature supports the efficacy of quetiapine up to 800 mg/day for the treatment of acute mania. There is some doubt concerning its efficacy against mixed episodes and concomitant psychotic features, while it is not efficacious in rapid cycling patients. The NNT is approximately 2–6 for response. Quetiapine does not seem to switch to depression, and on the contrary there is a clear beneficial effect on concomitant depressive symptoms. The adverse events associated with quetiapine treatment included sedation, dry mouth, somnolence, headache, dizziness and postural hypotension.

Aripiprazole

Aripiprazole was studied in four studies. The first one was a 3-week multicentre US study in 262 acutely manic or mixed BD patients and tested aripiprazole (15–30 mg/day; $N=130$) vs. placebo ($N=132$). Aripiprazole significantly improved the YMRS score at week 3 in comparison to placebo (−8.2 vs. −3.4; $p=0.002$) and produced a significantly higher response rate (40 % vs. 19 %; $p<0.005$). Improvement was evident as early as day 4. This study did not report on the effect on psychotic and depressive symptoms. Fewer patients under aripiprazole dropped out (58 % vs. 79 %). Dropout due to adverse events or lack of efficacy was similar between groups. The most frequent aripiprazole-related adverse events were nausea, dyspepsia, somnolence, anxiety, vomiting, insomnia, light-headedness, constipation and akathisia. There were no significant changes in body weight, serum prolactin or QTc prolongation (Keck et al. 2003a). Another 3-week multicentre US study in 272 hospitalized acutely manic or mixed BD patients compared aripiprazole (15–30 mg/day; $N=137$), with placebo ($N=135$). Aripiprazole significantly improved the YMRS score at week 3 in comparison to placebo (−12.5 vs. −7.2; $p<0.001$), and this was evident as early as day 4. It also produced a significantly higher response rate (53 % vs. 32 %; $p<0.001$) which was present already at day 7. Aripiprazole produced significant change in the PANSS positive and hostility subscales but not in the PANSS negative subscale or the MADRS. The therapeutic effect was evident also in the rapid cycling and mixed patients subgroups. In the latter group, a significant effect on the MADRS was also present. Dropout rate was similar in the two groups (55 % vs. 52 %) and was also similar due to adverse events but due to lack of efficacy was double in the placebo group (9 % vs. 21 %). It was similar for aripiprazole (8.8 %) and placebo (7.5 %). Aripiprazole treatment resulted in no significant difference from placebo in change in mean body weight and was not associated with elevated serum prolactin or QTc prolongation. The most common adverse events with aripiprazole were nausea, somnolence, akathisia, dyspepsia, extremity pain and constipation (Sachs et al. 2006). Another one was a 12-week multicentre US study in 480 acutely manic or mixed patients (rapid cycling excluded) which investigated aripiprazole (15–30 mg/day; $N=155$) vs. lithium (900–1,500 mg/day; $N=160$) vs. placebo ($N=165$). Both aripiprazole and lithium demonstrated significantly greater improvement than placebo in YMRS score at week 3 (−12.6 vs. −12.0 vs. −9.0; $p<0.005$), and the improvement was evident since day 2 for aripiprazole and since week 1 for lithium and continued during all the study period. The response rate was significantly higher in both the aripiprazole and lithium groups in comparison to placebo at week 3 (46.8 % vs. 45.8 % vs. 34.4 %; $p<0.05$). A similar picture was concerning remission rates (40.3 % vs. 40 % vs. 28.2 %). Aripiprazole improved the PANSS cognitive and hostility subscales at week 3, but no effect on PANSS was observed for lithium. No results concerning the PANSS positive and negative subscales were reported. Neither agent had any effect on the MADRS scores. The dropout rate was similar between groups (53 % vs. 51 % vs. 53 %) at week 3. Fewer patients in the aripiprazole group dropped out because of lack of efficacy (6 % vs. 16 % vs. 22 %), while more patients in the two medication arms dropped out because of adverse events in comparison to placebo (15 % vs. 13 % vs. 8 %). The most common adverse events with aripiprazole were headache, nausea, akathisia, sedation and constipation (Keck et al. 2009). The next study was again international and multicentre, included 485 acutely manic or mixed patients and assessed the efficacy and safety of aripiprazole (15 or 30 mg/day; $N=167$) vs. haloperidol (5–15 mg/day; $N=165$) vs. placebo ($N=153$). At week 3 both aripiprazole and haloperidol manifested significantly higher change in YMRS scores in comparison to placebo (−12.0 vs. −12.8 vs. −9.7; $p<0.01$), and this was maintained through week 12. Both medication arms significantly improved the positive but not the negative subscale of the PANSS. The response rates at week 3 were numerically greater with haloperidol and aripiprazole in comparison to placebo, but neither was significant (47.0 % vs. 49.7 % vs. 38.2 %; $p>0.05$). This was true also for the remission rates (44 % vs. 45.3 % vs. 36.8 %; $p>0.05$). The dropout rate was similar across the study arms at week 3 (25 % vs. 27 % vs. 29 %). Extrapyramidal adverse events were less frequent with aripiprazole in comparison to haloperidol (23.5 % vs. 53.3 %), but otherwise the adverse effects profile was similar (Young et al. 2009). Finally, one international 3-week RCT on 401 hospitalized acutely manic or mixed BD patients evaluated the efficacy and safety of two fixed doses of aripiprazole (15 mg/day, $N=131$ and 30 mg/day, $N=136$) vs. placebo ($N=134$). Neither aripiprazole arm was better than placebo in any of the outcomes (YMRS, MADRS, PANSS total and hostility subscale and response rates), and overall withdrawal rates were similar also. Interestingly, the placebo response was generally higher than expected. The most frequent adverse events for either of the aripiprazole treatment groups were headache, nausea, dyspepsia, insomnia, agitation, constipation, akathisia, anxiety, lightheadedness, vomiting, diarrhoea, asthenia and extremity pain (El Mallakh et al. 2010). One study has not been completed and reported no results (A Multicentre, Randomized, Double-Blind, Placebo-Controlled Study of Aripiprazole in the Treatment of Acutely Manic Patients with Bipolar Disorder (Protocol CN138077)).

Taken together the above, with three positive (Keck et al. 2003a, 2009; Sachs et al. 2006) and one negative fixed dosage study (El Mallakh et al. 2010), the literature supports the efficacy of aripiprazole 15–30 mg/day for the treatment of acute manic and mixed episodes. The effect on the core symptoms of mania is unknown. There is a significant effect in mixed and rapid cycling patients, and it also treats concomitant positive psychotic features and agitation but not negative symptoms. It does not seem to have any effect on depressive symptoms. The NNT is approximately around 5–10 for response. Aripiprazole does not seem to switch to depression. Nausea, dyspepsia, somnolence, anxiety, vomiting, insomnia, light-headedness, constipation and akathisia were the most common adverse events. There were no significant effects on body weight, serum prolactin or QTc prolongation.

Risperidone

Another 3-week multicentre US study included 259 acutely manic BD patients (mixed excluded) and assessed the efficacy and safety of risperidone (1–6 mg/day; $N=134$) vs. placebo ($N=125$). Risperidone-treated patients manifested a significant change in the YMRS scores in comparison to placebo (−10.6 vs. −4.8; $p<0.001$), and the effect was evident since day 3. More patients under risperidone responded at week 3 (43 % vs. 24 %). The improvements in the MADRS score and four of the five PANSS factors (positive symptoms, disorganized thoughts, uncontrolled hostility/excitement and anxiety/depression) were also significant. The results were similar in patients with and without psychotic features. The most common risperidone-related adverse events were somnolence, dyspepsia, nausea and EPS (Hirschfeld et al. 2004). A second 3-week multicentre study from India included 290 acutely manic or mixed hospitalized BD patients (rapid cycling excluded) that assessed the efficacy and safety of risperidone (1–6 mg /day; $N=146$) vs. placebo ($N=144$). Risperidone-treated patients manifested significantly more change in the YMRS at week 3 (−23.2 vs. −10.8, $p<0.001$), and the improvement was evident since week 1. More patients under risperidone were responders at week 3 (73 % vs. 36 %; $p<0.001$). There was a significant effect also on the MADRS scores and the PANSS positive symptoms and uncontrolled excitement/hostility factors but not on the other PANSS subscales. The therapeutic effect was similar in manic vs. mixed and psychotic vs. nonpsychotic patients. Fewer patients under risperidone dropped out (10.9 % vs. 28.9 %). The dropout rate was similar because of adverse events, while fewer patients under risperidone dropped out because of lack of efficacy (4.8 % vs. 14.5 %). EPS were the most frequently reported adverse events in the risperidone group (Khanna et al. 2005). This study sparked a debate concerning the limits of the use of placebo in similar studies (Mudur 2006; Patel 2006). Another international (outside the USA) 12-week multicentre trial in 438 hospitalized acutely manic patients (mixed and rapid cycling excluded) compared risperidone (1–6 mg/day; $N=154$) vs. haloperidol (2–12 mg/day; $N=144$) vs. placebo ($N=140$). At week 3 both agents exhibited higher change in YMRS scores (−15.1 vs. −13.9 vs. −9.4; $p<0.001$). The effect persisted throughout the study duration, and there were no differences between the two active drug arms. There was no difference between patients with vs. without psychotic features. Response rate at week 3 was also superior for the two active drugs vs. placebo (48 % vs. 47 % vs. 33 %). Response was stable during the whole study duration. Risperidone manifested a significant change also in the MADRS score at week 3 and at endpoint, while haloperidol did only at endpoint. However in those patients who completed the study, the effect of haloperidol on the MADRS was larger than that of risperidone. EPS were more frequent in the haloperidol arm (17 % vs. 40 % vs. 9 %) at week 3, and a similar picture persisted throughout the study. There were similar rates of dropouts in the three arms at week 3 (11 % vs. 10 % vs. 15 %). Discontinuation because of adverse events was similar across arms (≤5 %), while there was some difference in the dropouts because of insufficient response (3 % vs. 1 % vs. 6 %) (Smulevich et al. 2005).

Thus, the literature with four positive studies (Gopal et al. 2005; Hirschfeld et al. 2004; Khanna et al. 2005; Smulevich et al. 2005) supports the efficacy of risperidone 1–6 mg/day for the treatment of acute manic and mixed episodes, which is evident since day 3. It seems also effective in the treatment of positive psychotic features and agitation and concomitant depressive but not negative symptoms. The NNT is approximately around 3–5 for response. It is unknown whether risperidone has an effect on the core symptoms of mania or whether it is beneficial for rapid cycling patients. It does not seem to switch to depression. Somnolence, dyspepsia, nausea and EPS were the most common adverse events.

Ziprasidone

An international (USA and Brazil) 3-week multicentre RCT in 210 acutely manic or mixed patients assessed the efficacy and safety of ziprasidone (80–160 mg/day; $N=140$) or placebo ($N=70$). At week 3, ziprasidone-treated patients achieved more reduction in the MRS score in comparison to placebo (12.4 vs. 7.8; $p<0.005$). The improvement was evident already since day 2, concerned also the core symptoms of mania and was similar in manic and mixed patients. There was a beneficial effect of ziprasidone on total PANSS score, but no effect on the subscales is reported. Significantly more patients under ziprasidone were responders (50 % vs. 35 %; $p<0.05$). Fewer patients under ziprasidone dropped out (46.4 % vs. 55.7 %), and this was also true because of lack of efficacy (19.3 % vs. 35.7 %) but not because of adverse events (3.6 % vs. 1.4 %). Ziprasidone was related to a low rate of EPS. There was no weight gain observed. The most frequent adverse events were somnolence, dizziness, akathisia and hypertonia (Keck et al. 2003b). Another 3-week international (USA, Brazil and Mexico) RCT included 206 acutely manic or mixed BD patients and studied the efficacy and safety of ziprasidone (80–160 mg/day; $N=140$) vs. placebo ($N=66$). Ziprasidone-treated patients manifested significantly greater reduction in the MRS scores at week 3 (−11.1 vs. −5.6; $p<0.01$). The improvement concerned also the core symptoms of mania and was evident as early as day 2. The responder rate at study endpoint was significantly higher in the ziprasidone group (46 % vs. 29 %; $p<0.05$). A significant improvement was also evident concerning the positive but not the negative subscale of the PANSS. There was an early improvement of HAM-D and MADRS scores; however, at endpoint ziprasidone did not differ from placebo. The discontinuation rate was similar in the two arms (39.3 % vs. 45.5 %). Fewer patients under ziprasidone dropped out because of lack of efficacy (12.9 % vs. 28.8 %) but more because of adverse events (5.7 % vs. 1.5 %). Ziprasidone treatment was related with EPS, somnolence and dizziness (Potkin et al. 2005). The next was a 12-week international RCT on 438 acutely manic or mixed BD patients which compared ziprasidone (80–160 mg/day; $N=178$) vs. haloperidol (8–30 mg/day; $N=172$) and vs. placebo ($N=88$). At week 3, ziprasidone produced smaller change in MRS score in comparison to haloperidol, but both arms did significantly better than placebo (−10.41 vs. −15.93 vs. −6.10, $p<0.01$), and the change concerned the core manic symptoms and was significant since day 2. Both medication arms improved the positive but not the negative subscale of the PANSS. There was no significant effect of either medication on the HAM-D or the MADRS. At week 3, the response rate was significantly superior for haloperidol vs. both ziprasidone and placebo (36.9 % vs. 54.7 % vs. 20.5 %; $p<0.05$). Response was maintained until the end of the study (week 12) for both agents. At week 12, 31.9 % of haloperidol-treated patients were in remission vs. 22.7 % in the ziprasidone arm. Significantly more patients in the placebo group dropped out (59 % vs. 55 % vs. 72 %), and this was also true because of lack of efficacy (27 % vs. 12 % vs. 44 %) but not because of adverse events (9 % vs. 21 % vs. 5 %). The adverse events related with ziprasidone treatment were EPS, akathisia, somnolence, dystonia/hypotonia, dizziness, tremor, anxiety and dyspepsia. There was no significant difference in the cardiovascular adverse events between the three treatment arms and in the rate of switching to depression although numerically more patients under haloperidol switched during the entire 12-week duration of the study in comparison to ziprasidone (8.7 % vs. 4.5 %). This study was powered to detect weight gain since patients included should had had body weight ≥80 % of the lower weight limit and within 150 % of the upper weight limit of the ideal weight for sex, height and frame. It is interesting that there was a big difference in body weight between countries (Vieta et al. 2010c).

Taken together the above, on the basis of three positive studies (Keck et al. 2003b; Potkin et al. 2005; Vieta et al. 2010c), the literature supports the efficacy of ziprasidone 80–160 mg/day for the treatment of acute manic and mixed episodes. It has a treatment effect on the core symptoms of mania, but the effect in rapid cycling patients is unknown. It is effective in the treatment of concomitant positive psychotic features but not negative symptoms. It does not seem to have any significant effect on depressive symptoms. The NNT is approximately 6 for response. Ziprasidone does not seem to switch to depression. The adverse events related with ziprasidone treatment were EPS, somnolence, dizziness, anxiety and dyspepsia. There were no significant effects on body weight or serum lipids. There was a small QTc prolongation.

Asenapine

Concerning asenapine, the first international multicentre RCT of 3-week duration (Ares 7501004; NCT00159744) included 488 acutely manic or mixed patients (rapid cycling excluded) and studied the efficacy and safety of asenapine (10–20 mg/day; $N=185$) vs. olanzapine (5–20 mg/day; $N=205$) vs. placebo ($N=98$). Asenapine and olanzapine were superior to placebo at day 21 (−11.5 vs. −14.6 vs. −7.8, $p<0.01$). For both medication arms the treatment effect was significant since day 2. Asenapine did not improve significantly the MADRS score at endpoint; however, olanzapine did. The response rate of asenapine was not superior to that of placebo, while that of olanzapine was 42.6 % vs. 54.7 % vs. 34 %. This was true also for remission rates. The dropout rate was lower in the olanzapine arm (33 % vs. 21.5 % vs. 41.8 %). Fewer patients in the treatment arms discontinued because of lack of efficacy (7.6 % vs. 6.3 % vs. 14.3 %) or adverse events (9.2 % vs. 3.4 % vs. 4.1 %). Most frequent adverse events related with asenapine treatment were somnolence, dizziness, sedation and EPS. The asenapine group experienced more EPS in comparison to placebo and to the olanzapine group (10.3 % vs. 6.8 % vs. 3.1 %). Weight gain was significantly more frequent in both treatment arms in comparison to placebo, but it was more pronounced in the olanzapine arm (19.0 % vs. 7.2 % vs. 1.2 %) (McIntyre et al. 2010b). The second was a 3-week duration (Ares 7501005; NCT00159796) in 488 BD patient suffering from an acute manic or mixed episode (rapid cycling excluded) and investigated the efficacy and safety of asenapine (10–20 mg/day; $N=194$) vs. olanzapine (5–20 mg/day; $N=190$) vs. placebo ($N=104$). At day 21 both asenapine and olanzapine had superior changes from baseline in the YMRS scores (−10.8 vs. −12.6 vs. −5.5, $p<0.001$), and the change was evident since day 2. Olanzapine but not asenapine improved mixed patients also. Asenapine did not improve the MADRS score in comparison to placebo; however, olanzapine did. More patients under asenapine and olanzapine responded in comparison to placebo (42.3 % vs. 50 %vs. 25.2 %, $p<0.01$). The picture was similar concerning the remission rates. The dropout rate was similar in the three treatment arms (37.1 % vs. 30.9 % vs. 38.5 %); however, fewer patients dropped out because of lack of efficacy in the asenapine group in comparison to placebo (8.2 % vs. 5.8 % vs. 16.3 %). However more patients under asenapine dropped out because of adverse events in comparison to olanzapine and placebo (10.3 % vs. 4.2 % vs. 6.7 %). EPS were reported in numerically more asenapine- and olanzapine-treated patients in comparison to placebo (7.2 % vs. 7.9 % vs. 2.9 %). The most frequent adverse effects of asenapine included sedation, dizziness, somnolence, fatigue, oral hypaesthesia, dry mouth, EPS and weight gain (McIntyre et al. 2009a).

Thus, on the basis of two positive trials (McIntyre et al. 2009a, 2010b), the literature supports the efficacy of asenapine 10–20 mg/day for the treatment of acute manic and mixed episodes and is effective as early as day 2. It is not reported whether it has a treatment effect on the core symptoms of mania, and the effect in rapid cycling patients is unknown. It is unknown whether it is effective in the treatment of concomitant positive or negative psychotic features, and it does not seem to have any significant effect on depressive symptoms. The NNT is between 6 and 12 for response. Asenapine does not seem to switch to depression. The adverse events related with asenapine treatment were EPS, somnolence, dizziness, sedation, fatigue, oral hypaesthesia, dry mouth, weight gain and EPS.

Paliperidone

Paliperidone was studied in two RCTs. The NCT00309699 was an international multicentre 12-week study which included 493 acutely manic or mixed patients and compared paliperidone ER (3–12 mg/day; $N=195$) vs. quetiapine IR (400–800 mg/day; $N=193$) vs. placebo ($N=105$). Both paliperidone ER and quetiapine IR significantly improved the YMRS at week 3 in comparison to placebo (−13.2 vs. −11.7 vs. −7.4; $p<0.001$). The treatment effect was evident as early as day 2 and lasted for the entire duration of the study, and it was similar for manic and mixed patients. Although a beneficial effect on total PANSS score was reported, no specific effects on the positive or negative subscales of the PANSS or on a depressive scale were included in the report. At week 3 more patients in the two treatment arms were responders in comparison to placebo (55.8 % vs. 49 % vs. 34.6 %). Similarly the remission rate was higher in both treatment arms in comparison to placebo at week 3 (52.1 % vs. 47.4 % vs. 28.8 %). This picture lasted for the entire duration of the study, and a similar picture was observed concerning the remission rates. The NNT for response or remission was 5 for paliperidone ER. At week 3 fewer patients under paliperidone ER or quetiapine IR dropped out in comparison to placebo (20.5 % vs. 21.2 % vs. 39 %). Fewer patients in the medication arms withdrew because of lack of efficacy in comparison to placebo, and these withdrawals were more in the quetiapine IR group in comparison to the paliperidone ER group (3.1 % vs. 7.8 % vs. 18.1 %). Dropout because of adverse events were similar in the three arms. The most common treatment-emergent adverse events were headache, somnolence and akathisia for paliperidone ER. At week 12 the body weight increase was more frequent in the quetiapine IR group (17 % vs. 8 %), but more patients under paliperidone ER switched to depression (13.9 % vs. 7.5 %) (Vieta et al. 2010b). The second paliperidone ER study was an international 3-week RCT in 469 BD patients in an acute manic or mixed episode and investigated the efficacy and safety of three fixed doses of once-daily paliperidone ER (3 mg/day; $N=112$, 6 mg/day; $N=120$, or 12 mg/day; $N=115$) or placebo ($n=122$). At week 3 the chance in YMRS was different in comparison to placebo only in the ER 12 mg group (−13.5 vs. −10.1; $p=0.025$), but not in the 6 mg or 3 mg groups compared with placebo. There was no effect on the MADRS or PANSS total score, and paliperidone ER did not shift patients to depression. There was no difference between any medication arm and placebo concerning response and remission rates. It was not reported whether the 12 mg dosage had an effect on the core manic symptoms. The dropout rate was similar in the 12 mg group and placebo (34.8 % vs. 41 %). Fewer patients in the 12 mg group dropped out because of lack of efficacy (6 % vs. 19.7 %) but more because of adverse events (7.8 % vs. 4.9 %) in comparison to placebo. Headache, EPS and prolactin elevation were the most common treatment-emergent adverse events. It is interesting to note that a significant treatment-by-country interaction occurred, which confounded interpretation of study results. There was no response observed in patients from the US sites (74 % of study sample), while on the contrary such an effect was observed in the rest countries. The efficacy for the overall study population was driven largely, but not exclusively, by patients from India (Berwaerts et al. 2012b).

These two studies (Vieta et al. 2010b; Berwaerts et al. 2012b) provide some support for the efficacy of paliperidone ER 3–12 mg/day for the treatment of acute manic and mixed episodes and is effective as early as day 2. It is not reported whether it has a treatment effect on the core symptoms of mania, positive psychotic symptoms and depression, and the effect in rapid cycling patients is unknown. The NNT is approximately around 5 for response. It is unclear whether paliperidone ER switches to depression. The adverse events related with paliperidone ER treatment were headache, somnolence and EPS, and prolactin elevation was the most common treatment-emergent adverse event.

Cariprazine

Three unpublished studies (NCT00488618, NCT01058096 and NCT01058668) confirmed the efficacy of cariprazine vs. placebo in the treatment of acute mania. The NCT00488618 was an international multicentre randomized, double-blind, placebo-controlled study which tested cariprazine (3–12 mg/day; $N=118$) vs. placebo ($N=120$) in acutely manic or mixed type, with or without psychotic features BD patients (rapid cycling excluded). The results suggested that cariprazine significantly reduced YMRS score at week 3 compared to placebo. The effect was present in all YMRS items separately. Cariprazine also improved the total PANSS but had no effect on the MADRS. More patients under cariprazine were responders (48 % vs. 25 %), and this was the picture concerning remission also. The most common adverse events were EPS, headache, constipation, nausea and dyspepsia. The NCT01058096 was an international multicentre randomized, double-blind, placebo-controlled study which tested cariprazine (3–12 mg/day; $N=158$) vs. placebo ($N=154$) in acutely manic or mixed type, with or without psychotic features BD patients (rapid cycling excluded), and suggested that cariprazine was superior to placebo already since day 4. Cariprazine also improved the total PANSS but had no effect on the MADRS. More patients under cariprazine were responders (59 % vs. 44 %), and this was the picture concerning remission also. The adverse effect profile included EPS but not weight gain, metabolic disturbances, prolactin increase or QTc prolongation. The dropout rate because of adverse events was similar with placebo (10 % vs. 7 %). The results of the NCT01058668 which tested cariprazine 3–6 mg/day ($N=167$) and 6–12 mg/day ($N=169$) vs. placebo ($N=161$) have not been fully publicized yet. However that study included acutely manic or mixed type, with or without psychotic features BD patients, and there was a statistically significant improvement in both cariprazine dose groups vs. placebo on the YMRS scores. The most common adverse events were akathisia (both cariprazine groups) and constipation (for the cariprazine 6–12 mg/day group). Discontinuations due to adverse events were similar (9 % in the 3–6 mg/day group; 15 % in the 6–12 mg/day group and 5 % in the placebo group) (Altinbas et al. 2013; Citrome 2013).

Overall these data support the efficacy of cariprazine against acute manic or mixed episodes. The NNT for response or remission is approximately 4–6. Cariprazine is reported to improve the core symptoms of mania but had no effect on the MADRS. It improves the total PANSS, but the specific effect on the PANSS positive subscale is unknown. Its efficacy in mixed and rapid cycling patients is unknown.

16.2.1.1.4 Other Agents and Treatment Modalities

Tamoxifen

A small pilot 3-week study on 16 manic or mixed patients with or without psychotic features subjects (treatment-naïve patients excluded) investigated the efficacy and safety of tamoxifen (20–140 mg/day; $N=8$) vs. placebo ($N=8$) for 3 weeks. Tamoxifen-treated patients showed significant improvement in the YMRS in comparison to placebo (−18.3 vs. +4.7) already since day 5, an effect that remained significant throughout the 3-week trial. Tamoxifen had a significant effect on the core symptoms of mania, and the overall effect size was very large ($d=1.08$; $p=0.001$). There was no significant effect on PANSS and MADRS scores. At study endpoint, response rates were 63 % for tamoxifen and 13 % for placebo. The small study sample precluded the detection of a significant outcome concerning response and remission rates; however, the study supported the notion that further research on tamoxifen was important. The most common adverse event related with tamoxifen was loss of appetite (Zarate et al. 2007). Two trials followed: An NIMH-sponsored clinical trial (NCT00026585) has not reported results yet, while a second one came from Turkey and was sponsored by the Stanley Medical Research Institute (NCT00411203). This was 3 weeks small in 66 manic or mixed patients with or without psychotic features which investigated the efficacy and safety of tamoxifen (40–160 mg/day; $N=35$) vs. placebo ($N=31$). At week 3 tamoxifen significantly reduced the YMRS score in comparison to placebo (−5.84 vs. +1.5; $p<0.01$) and had an effect in the core symptoms of mania. It also reduced significantly the PANSS positive and general psychopathology subscales but not the negative PANSS subscale or the MADRS. There was a superiority also concerning the response rate (48 % vs. 5 %; $p<0.002$) and a similar picture concerning the remission rate. Fewer patients under tamoxifen dropped out because of worsening (17 % vs. 32 %). The adverse events reported in the tamoxifen group were headache, worsening of acne, dry skin, urticaria, flushing and loss of appetite (Yildiz et al. 2008). Overall, the data for tamoxifen are positive; however, the total patient sample is still small.

Verapamil

One small 3-week study on 32 acutely manic patients investigated the efficacy and safety of verapamil ($N=17$) vs. placebo ($N=15$). The results suggested no benefit of verapamil over placebo in treating acute mania (Janicak et al. 1998).

Electroconvulsive Therapy (ECT)

There are no RCTs testing the efficacy and safety of monotherapy ECT vs. a placebo condition in acutely manic or mixed BD patients.

Transcranial Magnetic Stimulation (rTMS)

The data concerning rTMS are conflicting. There are two RCTs testing the efficacy and safety of rTMS vs. a placebo condition in acutely manic BD patients. The first utilized a right vs. sham prefrontal TMS of 20 Hz, 2-s duration per train, 20 trains per day for 10 treatment days, in 25 acutely manic patients. The results suggested there was no difference between treatment groups (Kaptsan et al. 2003). The second examined the efficacy of adjunctive right prefrontal high-frequency suprathreshold rTMS (20 Hz, 110 % of MT, 20 trains, 10 s intertrain interval for 10 days) vs. sham stimulation in 41 right-handed acutely manic patients. At endpoint there was a significant effect of treatment over time (Praharaj et al. 2009).

16.2.1.1.5 Summary of Monotherapy Trials for Acute Mania

Overall there are sufficient data in the literature to support the general efficacy of a number of agents in the treatment of acute mania; however, many details remain to be explored concerning many of the agents. Lithium, valproate, carbamazepine, haloperidol, olanzapine, quetiapine, aripiprazole, risperidone, ziprasidone, asenapine, paliperidone, cariprazine and probably tamoxifen are efficacious in the treatment of acute manic episodes. It is sad that there are no controlled data concerning the usefulness of ECT and rTMS.

A significant problem for the everyday clinical practice is that the average clinician often utilizes the so-called 'class effect' in order to easily navigate among therapeutic options. However, what needs to be stressed is that while antipsychotics seem to possess a 'class effect' restricted to the treatment of acute mania (possibly an antidopaminergic effect) (Brugue and Vieta 2007), there is no such an effect in anticonvulsants concerning any phase of BD (Fountoulakis et al. 2011a; Rosa et al. 2011).

16.2.1.2 Comparison of Agents

16.2.1.2.1 Lithium Versus Others

Lithium was used as the standard in order to compare the efficacy and safety of newer compounds. Therefore there is a wealth of data comparing it with other agents.

It has been compared with valproate in two studies. The first was a 3-week study in 27 manic patients that compared lithium (at serum levels 1.5 mmol/l) vs. valproate (1,500–3,000 mg/day). The response rate was higher in the lithium arm (92.3 % vs. 64.3 %). The favourable response to valproate was associated with high pretreatment depression scores, thus implying that treatment with valproate alone may be particularly efficacious in manic patients with mixed affective states (Freeman et al. 1992). The second was a 3-week study in 179 hospitalized, acutely manic patients in academic settings across the USA, which tested the efficacy and safety of lithium (serum levels below 1.5 mmol/l; $N=36$) vs. divalproex (serum levels below 150 μg/ml; $N=69$) and vs. placebo ($N=74$). Half of patients were previously nonresponsive to lithium, and none had previously received valproate; thus, the study sample was enriched in favour of divalproex. After 3 weeks, both treatment arms manifested a higher change in MRS in comparison to placebo, and this change was significant since day 15 for both agents. Unfortunately the results are reported only through a chart, and no exact means and standard deviations are available. Interestingly, the analysis of separate items of the MRS revealed that divalproex but not lithium had a beneficial effect on the core manic symptoms. The response rate was higher for lithium and divalproex in comparison to placebo (49 % vs. 48 % vs. 25 %; $p=0.025$). In spite of the fact that half of patients were previously unresponsive to lithium, no inferiority of lithium in comparison to divalproex was observed. Fewer patients in the divalproex arm dropped out (61 % vs. 48 % vs. 64 %). Dropouts because of lack of efficacy were fewer in the two treatment arms in comparison to placebo (33 % vs. 30 % vs. 51 %), while dropouts because of adverse events were more frequent with lithium (11 % vs. 6 % vs. 3 %). The most frequent adverse events with lithium were asthenia, constipation, dizziness, nausea, fever, twitching and vomiting, while with divalproex were asthenia, constipation, dizziness, nausea, twitching and vomiting (Bowden et al. 1994).

Lithium was compared with carbamazepine in three studies. The first one was a small 4-week study on 34 manic patients testing carbamazepine vs. lithium reported that the two treatment arms were similar in terms of efficacy. The dropout rate was similar too (17.6 %). There was a signal suggesting that while lithium was effective in a homogenous way in the total sample of patients which were included in the lithium arm, carbamazepine had a beneficial effect only in a minority of patients in the carbamazepine-treated group. The findings suggest that carbamazepine has antimanic potential in specific bipolar patients whose clinical characteristics remain to be clearly defined (Lerer et al. 1987). The second was a multicentre 4-week study from Japan in 105 patients (of which 80 % were also receiving antipsychotics and were somewhat refractory to them at dosages equivalent to 8 mg of haloperidol) with bipolar disorders. It compared carbamazepine ($N=51$) vs. lithium ($N=54$) both at 400–1,200 mg/day and showed that both agents had similar response rates (moderate to marked amelioration of manic symptoms in 62 and 59 %, respectively). Carbamazepine had a somewhat earlier onset of actin, but both agents needed at least 2 weeks for the majority of the responders to manifest the response. However the mean lithium serum levels were below the recommended therapeutic range (0.46 ± 0.22 mEq/l). The dropout rate was similar (15.7 % vs. 22.2 %), but more patients in the carbamazepine group dropped out because of adverse events while more in the lithium group because of lack of efficacy. The incidence of adverse events was higher in the carbamazepine group (60 % vs. 43 %). The main adverse events encountered in patients receiving carbamazepine were drowsiness, unsteadiness, lassitude, dizziness, weakness, thirst, constipation and cutaneous symptoms, while in the patients receiving lithium, they were unsteadiness, thirst, drowsiness, lassitude, dizziness, anorexia and polyuria. The incidence of cutaneous symptoms (exanthema) was significantly higher in the carbamazepine group (12 % vs. 0 %) (Okuma et al. 1990). The third study was on 52 hospitalized and rather refractory to treatment of manic patients, which were randomized to carbamazepine vs. lithium carbonate for 8 weeks, and reported that one-third were responders without any difference between arms (Small et al. 1991).

One small 4-week pilot study in 30 manic inpatients compared lamotrigine (25 mg once daily for 1 week, 50 mg once daily for the second week and 100 mg once daily for the last 2 weeks) vs. lithium (800 mg/day). Of course it should be noted that monotherapy data for lamotrigine in acute mania are clearly negative. There were no significant differences between groups at any time point, suggesting that the dose escalation required for lamotrigine did not adversely affect its onset of action. However both agents were probably administered at a too low dosage. Secondary outcome measures, including the use of lorazepam as rescue medication, did not differ between the groups. No significant adverse events were noted in either group. However since lamotrigine has negative placebo-controlled RCTs, this should be considered to be a failed study (Ichim et al. 2000).

Three studies compared lithium with chlorpromazine. The first study was small, included 23 manic patients and tested lithium carbonate ($N=13$) vs. chlorpromazine ($N=10$). It reported that lithium carbonate was superior to chlorpromazine on all six parameters selected from an objective rating scale (Platman 1970). The second one was a multicentre trial which included 18 hospitals and 255 newly admitted manic patients. It tested lithium carbonate vs. chlorpromazine for 3 weeks. Patients were classified as highly active or mildly active on the basis of degree of motor activity shown at admission. Chlorpromazine acted earlier and was superior to lithium in the more agitated patients, but lithium overall produced a better subjective mental state in patients. Chlorpromazine had fewer dropouts and had a lower incidence of severe side effects, but lithium had a lower incidence of overall side effects (Prien et al. 1972). Finally, a 3-week comparison, in 30 severely ill hospitalized manic patients, tested lithium carbonate (up to blood levels of 2.0 mEq/l; $N=10$) vs. haloperidol (up to 26 mg/day; $N=10$) vs. chlorpromazine (up to 2,500 mg/day; $N=10$). The results suggested the three agents were equal, although the scales used were not satisfactorily sensitive. Lithium produced a highly significant improvement of manic symptoms without sedation, while chlorpromazine produced considerable sedation but had little effect on the core manic symptoms per se. More patients under lithium remitted and met discharge criteria at study termination (Shopsin et al. 1975).

Another two studies compared lithium with haloperidol. In a 3-week comparison, 30 severely ill hospitalized manic patients were administered with lithium carbonate (up to blood levels of 2.0 mEq/l; $N=10$), haloperidol (up to 26 mg/day; $N=10$) or chlorpromazine (up to 2,500 mg/day; $N=10$). The results suggested the three agents were equal, although the scales used were not satisfactorily sensitive. Lithium and haloperidol produced a highly significant improvement of manic symptoms without sedation, while chlorpromazine produced considerable sedation but had little effect on the core manic symptoms per se. The comparison of haloperidol and lithium revealed some qualitative differences with haloperidol having a more rapid effect especially on behaviour and motor activity, while lithium acted more evenly and completely on the entire manic symptomatology. More patients under lithium remitted and met discharge criteria at study termination (Shopsin et al. 1975). The second was again a 3-week study in 21 severely ill manic inpatients and investigated the comparative efficacy of lithium (up to 900 mg/day; $N=7$) vs. haloperidol (up to 30 mg/day; $N=7$) vs. a combination of haloperidol–lithium ($N=7$). Subjects on haloperidol and the haloperidol–lithium combination were significantly improved after 7 days in comparison to the lithium-treated group. The haloperidol and the haloperidol–lithium combination groups did not differ from each other, either in degree of improvement or in side effects and were superior to lithium monotherapy (Garfinkel et al. 1980).

Lithium was compared with olanzapine in three studies. In the first, which was a small one, 30 acutely manic patients were randomly allocated to receive either olanzapine (10 mg/day; $N=15$) or lithium (800 mg/day; $N=15$) in a 4-week double-blind randomized controlled design. There were no significant differences between the two groups on any of the primary outcome measures and especially in the mania scale (10.2 vs. 13.2; $p=0.315$). There was no difference between arms concerning EPS (Berk et al. 1999). Another multicentre 4-week study in 140 acutely manic or mixed patients from China examined the efficacy and safety of olanzapine (5–20 mg/day, $N=69$) vs. lithium carbonate (600–1,800 mg/day, $N=71$). A significantly greater mean change was observed in the olanzapine arm concerning the YMRS score (−24.63 vs. −20.15; $p=0.013$). Both arms showed a significant reduction in the MADRS score, which did not differ between arms. More patients under olanzapine responded (87 % vs. 73.2 %; $p=0.035$), while the remission rate was similar in the two arms (82.6 % vs. 70.4 %; $p=0.073$). However 32.8 % of the lithium-treated patients did not achieve the target serum levels. Fewer (though not significantly) patients under olanzapine dropped out (8.7 % vs. 21.1 %; $p=0.07$), but more patients experienced at least one adverse event (36.2 % vs. 19.7 %; $p=0.038$). The most common adverse events related to olanzapine were weight gain, constipation, nausea, somnolence, nasopharyngitis, vomiting, diarrhoea, dizziness and restlessness, while those related with lithium were nausea and nasopharyngitis. More patients under olanzapine manifested a clinically significant weight increase (16.2 % vs. 2.9 %; $p=0.009$) (Niufan et al. 2008). A 3-week study from Iran included 40 female acutely manic inpatients (mixed excluded) and studied the efficacy and safety of olanzapine (20.52±4.37 mg/day; $N=20$) vs. lithium (1,156±249.32 mg/day and serum level 0.78±0.269 mEq/l; $N=20$). At the end of the trial, although lithium performed better than olanzapine in terms of the mania scale used, more patients under olanzapine manifested at least 50 % improvement (25 % vs. 15 %). The main reported side effects of olanzapine were weight gain, tremor and sedation, while for lithium it was tremor (Shafti 2010).

There are two studies comparing lithium with quetiapine. An international multicentre 12-week RCT (3 weeks with placebo) in 302 acutely manic BD patients compared lithium (target serum levels 0.6–1.4 mEq/l; $N=98$) vs. quetiapine IR (flexibly dosed up to 800 mg/day; $N = 107$) and vs. placebo ($N = 97$). The improvement in YMRS score was significantly greater for lithium, and quetiapine IR in comparison to placebo at week 3 (−15.2 vs. −14.6 vs. −6.7; $p < 0.001$) was present already during day 7 and persisted throughout the duration of the study. Significantly more lithium- and quetiapine IR-treated patients were responders in comparison with placebo patients at week 3 (53.1 % vs. 53.3 % vs. 27.4 %; $p < 0.001$), and the picture was similar concerning the remission rates (49 % vs. 46.7 % vs. 22.1 %; $p < 0.001$). While the quetiapine IR data concerning all individual YMRS items were reported, this was not done also for lithium. Quetiapine IR but not lithium significantly improved the PANSS positive subscale, and both improved the activation and the aggression subscale. The effect on the negative subscale was not reported. Both medications significantly improved the MADRS score, but lithium achieved this only at endpoint, while quetiapine IR already at day 21. Fewer patients in the lithium and quetiapine IR groups dropped out from the study compared with the placebo group (31.6 % vs. 32.7 % vs. 63.9 %). Also fewer of them dropped out because of lack of efficacy (12.2 % vs. 14.9 % vs. 39.2 %), while the dropout rate because of adverse events was similar among groups (6.1 % vs. 6.5 % vs. 4.1 %). The most common adverse events for lithium were tremor and insomnia, while for quetiapine they were dry mouth, somnolence and weight gain (Bowden et al. 2005b). The second study came from China and was a 4-week multicentre study in 154 manic patients (mixed excluded, more than 70 % without psychotic symptoms) that compared quetiapine (up to 800 mg/day; $N = 77$) vs. lithium (up to 2,000 mg/day with target serum concentration 0.6–1.2 mmol/l; $N = 77$). At week 4, a significant change in the YMRS scores was present in both treatment arms (−18.2 vs. −15.9). A similar significant change was present concerning the MADRS and the total PANSS scores also. The response rate was higher in the quetiapine group (77.9 % vs. 59.7 %; $p = 0.01$), and a similar picture was present concerning the remission rates (70.1 % vs. 48.1 %; $p < 0.01$). More patients under lithium dropped out (5.2 % vs. 19.5 %). For two consecutive visits, 20.8 % of lithium-treated patients had serum levels below 0.6 mmol/l. More patients under quetiapine experienced at least one adverse event (78.2 % vs. 68.8 %). The most common adverse events experienced by the quetiapine-treated group were constipation, dizziness, diarrhoea, alanine aminotransferase increase, palpitations, aspartate aminotransferase increase, pharyngolaryngeal pain, upper respiratory tract infection and dry mouth, while in the lithium-treated patients, they were nausea, constipation, vomiting, nasopharyngitis, dizziness, diarrhoea and upper respiratory tract infection. The proportion of patients with weight gain of >70 % at week 4 was higher in the quetiapine group (9.9 % vs. 6.5 %) (Li et al. 2008).

Finally, it has also been compared to aripiprazole in a 12-week (3 weeks with placebo) multicentre US study in 480 acutely manic or mixed patients (rapid cycling excluded). The study investigated lithium (900–1,500 mg/day; $N = 160$) vs. aripiprazole (15–30 mg/day; $N = 155$) vs. placebo ($N = 165$). Both lithium and aripiprazole demonstrated significantly greater improvement than placebo in YMRS score at week 3 (−12.0 vs. −12.6 vs. −9.0; $p < 0.005$), and the improvement was evident since week 1 for lithium and since day 2 for aripiprazole and continued for all the study period. The response rate was significantly higher in both the lithium and the aripiprazole groups in comparison to placebo at week 3 (45.8 % vs. 46.8 % vs. 34.4 %; $p<0.05$). A similar picture was evident concerning the remission rates (40 % vs. 40.3 % vs. 28.2 %). No effect on PANSS total or MADRS was observed for lithium. No results concerning the PANSS positive and negative subscales were reported. The dropout rate was similar between groups (51 % vs. 53 % vs. 53 %) at week 3. The dropout rate for lithium because of lack of efficacy was between that of aripiprazole and placebo (16 % vs. 6 % vs. 22 %), while more patients in the two medication arms dropped out because of adverse events in comparison to placebo (13 % vs. 15 % vs. 8 %). The most common adverse events with lithium were nausea, headache, constipation and tremor while with aripiprazole were headache, nausea, akathisia, sedation and constipation (Keck et al. 2009).

Conclusively, lithium was found superior or non-inferior to valproate (Freeman et al. 1992; Bowden et al. 1994) and equal to carbamazepine (Lerer et al. 1987; Okuma et al. 1990; Small et al. 1991), olanzapine (Berk et al. 1999; Niufan et al. 2008; Shafti 2010), quetiapine (Bowden et al. 2005b; Li et al. 2008) and aripiprazole (Keck et al. 2009), but inferior to haloperidol (Shopsin et al. 1975; Garfinkel et al. 1980). Overall lithium manifested a wider antimanic effect than valproate and carbamazepine but without an effect on psychotic symptoms and with slower onset of action in comparison to antipsychotics. Overall it manifested a more favourable adverse effect profile in comparison to all other agents except aripiprazole and valproate.

16.2.1.2.2 Valproate Versus Others

Valproate has also been used as kind of a standard for comparison with newer agents. Thus there is a significant number of studies involving it.

It has been compared to lithium in two studies (Freeman et al. 1992; Bowden et al. 1994). Both are discussed above in the 'lithium' section.

There is only one study comparing valproate with carbamazepine. That study came from India and was conducted in 30 manic inpatients (24 of them females; valproate $N=15$; carbamazepine $N=15$). It reported that the valproate group showed a significant fall in YMRS total scores already after week 1, while the carbamazepine group showed a significant fall only after week 2. At endpoint the difference was significant in favour of valproate (−32.8 vs. −20.8; $p=0.02$). The valproate group demonstrated a numerically greater mean improvement relative to the carbamazepine group on all YMRS items except sleep. More patients under valproate responded (73 % vs. 53 %). Only three patients in each group dropped out. Serum levels for carbamazepine did not correlate with clinical response, while on the contrary the levels of valproate correlated with clinical response. Significantly more patients in the carbamazepine group reported adverse events, including nausea, vomiting and dizziness, than valproate (17 % vs. 67 %) (Vasudev et al. 2000).

Another three papers compared valproate to olanzapine. One randomized, 12-week multicentre study included 120 patients hospitalized for acute mania or mixed episode and randomly assigned them to treatment with divalproex (750–3,250 mg/day; $N=63$) vs. olanzapine (5–25 mg/day; $N=57$). No significant differences between groups were found concerning the change in MRS scores from baseline to week 3 (−14.8 vs. −17.2; $p=0.210$). The two treatment arms produced similar changes in the BPRS and the HAM-D as well. The effect on psychotic symptoms was unclear. At week 3 numerically more patients under divalproex dropped out (38 % vs. 32 %). Similarly, numerically more patients under divalproex dropped out because of adverse events (11 % vs. 9 %) and because of lack of efficacy (22 % vs. 19 %) at the end of the study. More olanzapine-treated subjects experienced somnolence, weight gain, oedema, rhinitis and speech disorder (slurred speech), while no adverse events were significantly greater in the divalproex group (Zajecka et al. 2002). The second was a 3-week study in 148 hospitalized manic or mixed patients (approximately half of them mixed and half of them rapid cycling) that compared olanzapine (5–20 mg/day; $N=125$) vs. divalproex (500–2,500 mg/day in divided doses; targeted therapeutic range 50–125 μg/ml; $N=123$) and reported that there was a greater decrease in the YMRS score for the olanzapine group (−13.4 vs. −10.4; $p=0.03$), and the difference was present already at day 2. There was also a superiority concerning the response (54.4 % vs. 42.3 %; $p=0.06$) and remission rates (47.2 % vs. 34.1 %; $p=0.04$) which were also achieved faster in the olanzapine group. The change in the HAM-D was similar in the two treatment groups. In the subgroup without psychotic features, olanzapine was superior to divalproex, while in the psychotic group the two arms were equal. Also the overall dropout rate was similar (31.2 % vs. 35.7 %) also concerning because of adverse events (9.6 % vs. 7.1 %) and lack of efficacy (8.8 % vs. 9.5 %). The most common treatment-emergent adverse events related to olanzapine were dry mouth, increased appetite and somnolence, while for divalproex, nausea was more frequently observed. The average weight gain with olanzapine treatment was 2.5 kg, compared to 0.9 kg with divalproex treatment (Tohen et al. 2002a). Finally, an international multicentre study in 521 acutely manic or mixed patients evaluated the efficacy and safety of olanzapine (5–20 mg/day; $N=215$) vs. divalproex (500–2,500 mg/day; $N=201$) vs. placebo ($N=105$). At week 3, olanzapine- but not divalproex-treated patients had significantly more reduction in their YMRS scores in comparison to the placebo arm (−9.4 vs. −8.2 vs. −7.4). The response rates did not differ between the medication arms and placebo (40.8 % vs. 40.3 % vs. 31.3 %) and neither did the remission rates (42.8 % vs. 40.3 % vs. 35.4 %). There was no difference in the MADRS score change between the medications arms and placebo. The dropout rate was not different between groups (26 % vs. 24.9 % vs. 26.6 %). Weight gain and somnolence were the most frequent adverse events associated with olanzapine treatment. It is interesting that while 35.4 % (at 3 weeks) to 57.1 % (at 12 weeks) had valproate plasma concentrations lower than the recommended valproate therapeutic range, the YMRS scores of these patients were lower than those of patients with valproate concentrations above or within range (Tohen et al. 2008b).

One 12-week study from India in 60 patients with acute mania (mixed and rapid cycling excluded) assessed divalproex (750–2,000 mg/day; $N=30$) vs. oxcarbazepine (1,000–2,400 mg/day; $N=30$). At endpoint, the improvement in YMRS scores was comparable, and the remission rates were also similar (90 % vs. 80 %). A significantly greater number of patients in the divalproex group experienced one or more adverse events (66.7 % vs. 30 %, $p<0.01$). The most frequent adverse events related to divalproex were nausea, dizziness, vomiting, headache, pain in abdomen, sedation, weight gain, dyspepsia, increased appetite and constipations, while those related with oxcarbazepine were nausea, dizziness, vomiting, headache, sedation and dyspepsia (Kakkar et al. 2009).

Conclusively, in comparison to lithium, valproate was less efficacious and with a tendency to manifest fewer adverse events and dropouts, but its efficacy might be restricted to a specific minority of patients with mixed features (Freeman et al. 1992; Bowden et al. 1994). In one small study it was superior to carbamazepine and with faster action (Vasudev et al. 2000). In another it was superior to oxcarbazepine but with more frequent adverse events (Kakkar et al. 2009). It might be less efficacious in comparison to olanzapine and with a slower onset of action (although this could be a function of dosage), but also with fewer adverse events (Tohen et al. 2002a, 2008b; Zajecka et al. 2002).

16.2.1.2.3 Carbamazepine Versus Others

There are three studies comparing carbamazepine with lithium (Lerer et al. 1987; Okuma et al. 1990; Small et al. 1991) and one with valproate (Vasudev et al. 2000). All are discussed above in the respected sections.

One study in 17 manic patients tested carbamazepine (up to 1,600 mg/day; $N=8$) vs. haloperidol (up to 80 mg/day; $N=9$). The response to carbamazepine started between days 3–7, while that to haloperidol started within the first 3 days. However after day 7 the change in YMRS score was similar in both groups (−11.9 vs. −12.0) although more patients under carbamazepine manifested remission (75 % vs. 33 %) (Brown et al. 1989).

One more small 5-week study from Japan in 60 manic (only one mixed) patients assessed the efficacy and safety of carbamazepine (up to 900 mg/day; $N=30$) vs. chlorpromazine (up to 450 mg/day; $N=30$). Although there was a trend for carbamazepine to be more efficacious, the difference was not significant. More than one-third of patients responded by week 1, and almost all who responded had done so by week 2. At least one adverse event was present in 59 % of carbamazepine and 86 % of the chlorpromazine group. The main side effects encountered in patients receiving carbamazepine were drowsiness, headache, cutaneous symptoms (exanthema), dry mouth, lassitude and dizziness, while in the chlorpromazine group they were drowsiness, headache, dizziness, dry mouth, lassitude, orthostatic hypotension, feeling of weakness, hypersalivation and nasal stuffiness. Three patients in the carbamazepine and 5 in the chlorpromazine arm dropped out; two patients from each arm dropped out because of adverse events (Okuma et al. 1979).

Conclusively, carbamazepine was reported to be equally effective in comparison to lithium and with more frequent adverse events, but its efficacy was somewhat restricted to an undefined subgroup of patients in contrast to a wider efficacy of lithium (Lerer et al. 1987; Okuma et al. 1990; Small et al. 1991). In one other study carbamazepine was inferior to valproate and with slower onset of action (Vasudev et al. 2000). In two other studies carbamazepine was found equal to chlorpromazine but with fewer adverse events (Okuma et al. 1979) and equal to haloperidol but with slower onset of action (Brown et al. 1989).

16.2.1.2.4 Other Antiepileptics

Although except valproate and carbamazepine all other antiepileptics have negative data concerning the treatment of acute mania, it is interesting to see the comparison trials they are involved. Essentially these trials might be considered as including some kind of 'active placebo'.

There is probably one failed study on lamotrigine vs. lithium (Ichim et al. 2000) and another one on oxcarbazepine vs. divalproex (Kakkar et al. 2009). Both are discussed above in the respected sections of lithium and valproate.

16.2.1.2.5 Haloperidol Versus Others

Haloperidol has served as the golden standard in trials of any kind of psychotic states for long. It has also served as the golden standard for acute mania trials no matter whether psychotic features were present or not.

There is one study comparing haloperidol with carbamazepine (Brown et al. 1989) and two with lithium (Garfinkel et al. 1980; Shopsin et al. 1975). They are both discussed above in the respected carbamazepine and lithium sections.

Two studies compared haloperidol with olanzapine. A 12-week (2 successive, 6-week, double-blind periods) international study in 453 acutely manic or mixed patients compared the efficacy and safety of olanzapine (5–20 mg/day; $N=234$) vs. haloperidol (3–15 mg/day; $N=219$). At week 6 the change in YMRS scores was greater for the haloperidol group (−23.5 vs. −21.3; $p=0.03$), but olanzapine-treated patients covered the difference by week 12 (−26.5 vs. −26.8). Rates of response and remission at week 6 were similar (55 % vs. 62 % and 52.1 % vs. 46.1 %, respectively), and time to remission was also similar (median 34 vs. 29 days). For the subgroup of patients whose index episode did not include psychotic features, rates of remission were significantly greater for the olanzapine group compared with the haloperidol group (56.7 % vs. 41.6 %, $p=0.04$). A trend towards a higher efficacy of olanzapine in the more severely ill patients was also present. The dropout rate was lower for the olanzapine group (40.2 % vs. 47 %), but it was identical because of lack of efficacy (15 % vs. 15 %) and slightly different because of adverse events (8.1 % vs. 11.4 %). Both agents were equally effective in reducing the HAM-D score in mixed patients and in patients with higher depressive scores. Relapse rates into an affective episode (mania and/or depression) was similar in both groups (13.1 % vs. 14.8 %) but switch to depression occurred significantly more rapidly with haloperidol than with olanzapine. A trend for patients under haloperidol to switch more frequently to depression was also present (9.4 % vs. 16.8 %; $p=0.1$). Significantly more haloperidol-treated patients experienced worsening of EPS and increased salivation, while somnolence, sedation, weight gain, infection, dizziness and fever were significantly greater in the olanzapine group. It is important that 5 (2.3 %) haloperidol-treated patients developed tardive dyskinesia vs. none in the olanzapine group (Tohen et al. 2003a). A 3-week study from Japan randomized 224 manic or mixed BD patients to receive haloperidol (2.5–10 mg/day; $N=20$), olanzapine (5–20 mg/day; $N=105$) or placebo ($N=99$). The haloperidol arm included only 20 patients. At week 3 the haloperidol-treated patients had significant reduction in their YMRS score in comparison to placebo and similar to olanzapine (−14.3

vs. −12.6 vs. −6.8). Olanzapine had an effect on the core symptoms of mania, while a similar effect was not present for haloperidol. The response rates were similar in the three groups (65 % vs. 51 % vs. 44.3 %), while the remission rate was higher (but not significantly) in the haloperidol group (65 % vs. 47.1 % vs. 41.2 %). Haloperidol numerically increased the HAM-D score, while olanzapine significantly decreased it in comparison to both haloperidol and placebo. More patients under haloperidol dropped out (60 % vs. 30.5 % vs. 45.5 %), fewer because of lack of efficacy (5 % vs. 14.3 % vs. 28.9 %) but more because of adverse events (25 % vs. 8.6 % vs. 7 %). More haloperidol-treated patients switched to symptomatic depression in comparison to olanzapine (16.7 % vs. 2.4 %, $p=0.014$). The adverse events rate related with haloperidol treatment were somnolence, EPS, weight gain and constipation, while those related with olanzapine treatment were somnolence, dizziness, thirst and weight gain. EPS in olanzapine group were less severe than in the haloperidol group. EPS in the haloperidol group were more severe than in the olanzapine group (Katagiri et al. 2012).

One international multicentre study of 302 hospitalized patients with acute mania and compared haloperidol (up to 8 mg/day; $N=99$) vs. quetiapine IR (flexibly dosed up to 800 mg/day; $N=102$) and placebo ($N=101$). It showed that at week 3, haloperidol- and quetiapine IR-treated patients manifested significantly more reduction in the YMRS scores (−15.71 vs. −12.29 vs. −8.32; $p<0.01$), and this was evident as early as day 4. Haloperidol was superior to quetiapine ($p<0.05$). Quetiapine IR improved all individual items of the YMRS, while no such data are reported concerning haloperidol. Although both agents reduced the PANSS positive score at endpoint, only haloperidol had an effect at week 21, and only haloperidol differed from placebo concerning the reduction of YMRS score in psychotic patients, and this was true throughout the study. On the contrary, haloperidol had a favourable effect on the MADRS at week 3 which did not last until the end of the study in contrast to quetiapine which had a sustained effect. The response rate at day 21 was in favour of the haloperidol and quetiapine IR groups in comparison to placebo (56.1 % vs. 42.6 % vs. 35.0 %). Remission rates were not significant for either drug vs. placebo at day 21, but they were at week 12 (63.3 % vs. 61.4 % vs. 38.0 %). More patients under haloperidol withdrew from the study because of adverse events in comparison both to quetiapine IR and placebo (10.1 % vs. 4.9 % vs. 5.9 %). The only frequent adverse events related to haloperidol treatment were insomnia and EPS which occurred more often with haloperidol than with quetiapine IR or placebo (59.6 % vs. 12.7 % vs. 15.8 %). Insomnia, somnolence and EPS were the most frequent adverse events related with quetiapine IR treatment (McIntyre et al. 2005).

Two studies compared haloperidol with risperidone. A 4-week study in 45 inpatients with acute mania, of risperidone (6 mg/day; $N=15$) vs. haloperidol (10 mg/day; $N=15$) vs. lithium (800–1,200 mg/daily; $N=15$), reported no differences among groups. The extrapyramidal side effects of risperidone and haloperidol were not significantly different (Segal et al. 1998). Another international (outside the USA) 12-week multicentre trial in 438 hospitalized acutely manic BD patients (mixed and rapid cycling excluded) compared haloperidol (2–12 mg/day; $N=144$) vs. risperidone (1–6 mg/day; $N=154$) vs. placebo ($N=140$). At week 3 both agents exhibited higher change in YMRS scores (−13.9 vs. −15.1 vs. −9.4; $p<0.001$). The effect persisted throughout the study duration, and there were no differences between the two active drug arms. There was no difference between patients with vs. without psychotic features. Response rate at week 3 was also superior for the two active drugs vs. placebo (47 % vs. 48 % vs. 33 %). Response was stable during the whole study duration. Risperidone manifested a significant change also in the MADRS score at week 3 and at endpoint, while haloperidol did only at endpoint. However in those patients who completed the study, the effect of haloperidol on the MADRS was larger than that of risperidone. EPS were more frequent in the haloperidol arm (40 % vs. 17 % vs. 9 %) at week 3, and a similar picture persisted throughout the study. There were similar rates of dropouts in the three arms at week 3 (10 % vs. 11 % vs. 15 %). Discontinuation because of adverse events was similar across arms (≤5 %), while there was some difference in the dropouts because of insufficient response (1 % vs. 3 % vs. 6 %). Adverse events reported in more than 10 % of patients during the whole 12 weeks of double-blind treatment were EPS, somnolence and hyperkinesia in the risperidone group and EPS, hyperkinesia, tremor and hypertonia in the haloperidol group (Smulevich et al. 2005).

There are two studies comparing haloperidol with aripiprazole. An international 12-week multicentre study in 347 manic or mixed patients (only 11 % mixed, rapid cycling excluded) compared aripiprazole (15–30 mg/day; $N=175$) vs. haloperidol (10–15 mg/day; $N=172$). At week 12, the change in YMRS score was similar in the two treatment arms (−19.9 vs. −18.2), but significantly more patients taking aripiprazole were responders (49.7 % vs. 28.4 %; $p<0.001$) and remitters (50 % v. 27 %; $p<0.001$). Aripiprazole improved significantly more the MADRS score than haloperidol, and more haloperidol-treated patients switched to depression (11 % vs. 17.7 %; $p=0.08$). Fewer patients under aripiprazole dropped out (49.1 % vs. 70.1 %), and this was true also due to adverse events (18.3 % vs. 48.8 %) but not due to lack of efficacy (17.1 % vs. 5.8 %). In both groups the most frequent adverse events were EPS, insomnia and headache. EPS were more frequent with haloperidol than aripiprazole (24.0 % vs. 62.7 %) (Vieta et al. 2005a). The next study was again international and multicentre, included 485 acutely manic or mixed patients and assessed the efficacy and safety of aripiprazole (15 or 30 mg/day; $N=167$) vs. haloperidol (5–15 mg/day; $N=165$) vs. placebo ($N=153$). At week 3 both haloperidol and aripiprazole manifested significantly higher change in YMRS scores in comparison to placebo (−12.8 vs. −12.0 vs. −9.7; $p<0.01$), and this was maintained through week 12. Both medication arms significantly improved the positive but not the negative subscale of the PANSS. The response rates at week 3 were numerically greater with haloperidol and aripiprazole in comparison to placebo, but neither was significant (49.7 % vs. 47.0 % vs. 38.2 %; $p>0.05$). This was true also for the remission rates (45.3 % vs. 44 % vs. 36.8 %; $p>0.05$). The dropout rate was similar across the study arms at week 3 (27 % vs. 25 % vs. 29 %). Extrapyramidal adverse events were more frequent with haloperidol than aripiprazole (53.3 % vs. 23.5 %), but otherwise the adverse effects profile was similar (Young et al. 2009).

One study compared haloperidol with ziprasidone. It was a 12-week international RCT on 438 acutely manic or mixed BD patients which compared haloperidol (8–30 mg/day; $N=172$) vs. ziprasidone (80–160 mg/day; $N=178$) and vs. placebo ($N=88$). At week 3, haloperidol produced greater change in MRS score in comparison to ziprasidone, but both arms did significantly better than placebo (−15.93 vs. −10.41 vs. −6.10; $p \leq 0.01$). The positive subscale of the PANSS but not the other subscales was also significantly improved by the active drugs. At week 3, the response rate was significantly superior for haloperidol vs. both ziprasidone and placebo (54.7 % vs. 36.9 % vs. 20.5 %, respectively; $p<0.05$). Response was maintained until the end of the study (week 12) for both agents. At week 12, 31.9 % of haloperidol-treated patients were in remission vs. 22.7 % in the ziprasidone arm. Significantly more patients in the placebo group dropped out (59 % vs. 55 % vs. 72 %), and this was also true because of lack of efficacy (27 % vs. 12 % vs. 44 %) but not because of adverse events (9 % vs. 21 % vs. 5 %). More patients under haloperidol dropped out in comparison to patients under ziprasidone during the extension phase (weeks 4–12; 21.1 % vs. 9.6 %) and also had significantly higher rates of movement disorders as adverse events. At week 3, haloperidol-treated patients experienced more often adverse events in comparison to ziprasidone-treated patients and placebo (80.1 % vs. 64.6 % vs. 39.8 %). Throughout the study period more patients under haloperidol experienced adverse events in comparison to ziprasidone (87.1 % vs. 73.6 %). Through week 3, more patients under haloperidol had discontinued because of adverse events in comparison to ziprasidone and placebo (21 % vs. 9 % vs. 5 %) and at week 12 (21.1 % vs. 9.6 %). There was no significant difference in the cardiovascular adverse events between the three treatment arms and in the rate of switching to depression although numerically more patients under haloperidol switched during the entire 12-week duration of the study in comparison to ziprasidone (8.7 % vs. 4.5 %). This study was powered to detect weight gain since patients included should had had body weight ≥80 % of the lower weight limit and within 150 % of the upper weight limit of the ideal weight for sex, height and frame. It is interesting that there was a big difference in body weight between countries (Vieta et al. 2010c).

Finally two different dosages of haloperidol were compared. That study tested 25 mg/day vs. 5 mg/day of haloperidol as add-on lithium, placebo or lorazepam for 21 days in 63 acutely psychotic bipolar manic inpatients reported that the high haloperidol dose produced greater improvement (response rate 41 % vs. 24 % at day 4; 78 % vs. 48 % at day 21) and more side effects than did the low dose but with more side effects (Chou et al. 1999).

Overall haloperidol was found comparable in efficacy with carbamazepine (Brown et al. 1989), olanzapine (Tohen et al. 2003a; Katagiri et al. 2012), quetiapine (McIntyre et al. 2005), risperidone (Segal et al. 1998; Smulevich et al. 2005) and aripiprazole (Vieta et al. 2005a; Young et al. 2009). It was found superior to lithium (Shopsin et al. 1975; Garfinkel et al. 1980) and ziprasidone (Vieta et al. 2010c). It acted faster in comparison to lithium (Shopsin et al. 1975; Garfinkel et al. 1980), carbamazepine (Brown et al. 1989) and olanzapine (Tohen et al. 2003a; Katagiri et al. 2012). Overall it manifested superior efficacy on psychotic patients but less effect (if any) on depressive symptoms. It also manifested more adverse events (especially EPS), switching to depression and dropouts than the comparison agents.

16.2.1.2.6 Olanzapine Versus Others

Three studies comparing olanzapine with lithium (Berk et al. 1999; Shafti 2010; Niufan et al. 2008), three with valproate (Zajecka et al. 2002; Tohen et al. 2002a, 2008b) and two with haloperidol (Tohen et al. 2003a; Katagiri et al. 2012) have been discussed above in the respected sections.

There are two studies comparing olanzapine with asenapine. The first was an international multicentre 3-week study in 488 acutely manic or mixed patients (rapid cycling excluded) which compared olanzapine (5–20 mg/day; $N=190$) vs. asenapine (10–20 mg/day; $N=194$) vs. placebo ($N=104$). At day 21 both olanzapine and asenapine had superior changes from baseline in the YMRS scores (−12.6 vs. −10.8 vs. −5.5, $p<0.001$), and the change was evident since day 2. Olanzapine but not asenapine significantly improved the MADRS score in comparison to placebo. This improvement was evident since day 7. Olanzapine but not asenapine improved mixed patients also. More patients under olanzapine and asenapine responded in comparison to placebo (50 % vs. 42.3 % vs. 25.2 %, $p<0.01$). The picture was similar concerning the remission rates. The dropout rate was similar in the three treatment arms (30.9 % vs. 37.1 % vs. 38.5 %); however, fewer patients dropped out because of lack of efficacy in the olanzapine group (5.8 % vs. 8.2 % vs. 16.3 %). Also the fewer patients under olanzapine dropped out because of adverse events in comparison to asenapine and similar to placebo (4.2 % vs. 10.3 % vs. 6.7 %). EPS were reported in numerically more olanzapine- and asenapine-treated patients in comparison to placebo (7.9 % vs. 7.2 % vs. 2.9 %). The most frequent adverse effects of olanzapine included sedation, dry mouth, dizziness, somnolence and weight gain (McIntyre et al. 2009a). The second one was again an international multicentre RCT of 3-week duration which included 488 acutely manic or mixed BD patients (rapid cycling excluded) and studied the efficacy and safety of olanzapine (5–20 mg/day; $N=205$) vs. asenapine (10–20 mg/day; $N=185$) vs. placebo ($N=98$). Olanzapine and asenapine were superior to placebo at day 21 (−14.6 vs. −11.5 vs. −7.8, $p<0.01$). For both medication arms the treatment effect was significant since day 2. Olanzapine but not asenapine significantly improved the MADRS score at endpoint. The response rate of olanzapine, but not of asenapine, was superior to that of placebo (54.7 % vs. 42.6 % vs. 34 %). This was true also for remission rates. The dropout rate was lower in the olanzapine arm (21.5 % vs. 33 % vs. 41.8 %). Fewer patients in the olanzapine arm discontinued because of lack of efficacy (6.3 % vs. 7.6 % vs. 14.3 %) or adverse events (3.4 % vs. 9.2 % vs. 4.1 %). Most frequent adverse events related with olanzapine treatment were somnolence, dizziness, sedation and EPS, while with asenapine they were somnolence dizziness, sedation and EPS. More EPS in comparison to placebo were registered in the olanzapine group but lower in comparison to asenapine (6.8 % vs. 10.3 % vs. 3.1 %). Weight gain was significantly more frequent in both treatment arms in comparison to placebo, but it was more pronounced in the olanzapine arm (19.0 % vs. 7.2 % vs. 1.2 %) (McIntyre et al. 2010b).

One 3-week US multicentre study in 329 manic or mixed hospitalized patients without psychotic features compared olanzapine (5–20 mg/day; $N=165$) vs. risperidone (1–6 mg/day; $N=164$). The authors reported only MMRM analysis (not

LOCF), and according to it, there was no difference between the two treatment arms in terms of YMRS, HAM-D and MADRS change. The response rate was also similar (62.1 % vs. 59.5 %), while there was a tendency more for olanzapine-treated patients to remit (38.5 % vs. 28.5 %; $p=0.07$). The effect on rapid cycling patients was similar to the rest of patients. Significantly less olanzapine-treated patients dropped out (21.3 % vs. 33 %; $p=0.019$), but the dropout rates because of adverse events and lack of efficacy were similar (5.4 % vs. 8.5 % and 4.2 % vs. 4.2 %, respectively). Olanzapine-treated patients experienced greater elevations in liver function enzymes, dry mouth and increase in weight, while risperidone-treated patients were more likely to experience prolactin elevation and sexual dysfunction (Perlis et al. 2006a).

Finally the NCT00329108 unpublished study of olanzapine (15–20 mg/day) vs. ziprasidone (120–160 mg/day) was stopped prematurely, after recruiting only 29 patients, and did not report any efficacy results (NCT00329108 study results 2009).

Olanzapine was found to have similar efficacy with risperidone in patients without psychotic features, in terms of YMRS, HAM-D and MADRS change. The two agents were also equal in the subgroup of rapid cycling patients. Fewer olanzapine-treated patients dropped out, but there was more weight gain in the olanzapine group (Perlis et al. 2006a). Finally the NCT00329108 unpublished study of olanzapine vs. ziprasidone was stopped prematurely (NCT00329108 study results 2009).

16.2.1.2.7 Quetiapine Versus Others

There are two studies comparing quetiapine with lithium (Bowden et al. 2005b; Li et al. 2008) and one with haloperidol (McIntyre et al. 2005) which were discussed above in the respected sections.

There is one study comparing quetiapine with paliperidone. That was an international multicentre 12-week (3 weeks with placebo) study which included 493 acutely manic or mixed patients and compared quetiapine IR (400–800 mg/day; $N=193$) vs. paliperidone ER (3–12 mg/day; $N=195$) vs. placebo ($N=105$). Both quetiapine IR and paliperidone ER significantly improved the YMRS at week 3 in comparison to placebo (−11.7 vs. −13.2 vs. −7.4; $p<0.001$). The treatment effect was evident as early as day 2 and lasted for the entire duration of the study, and it was similar for manic and mixed patients. Although a beneficial effect on total PANSS score was reported, no specific effects on the positive or negative subscales of the PANSS or on a depressive scale were included in the report. At week 3 more patients in the two treatment arms were responders in comparison to placebo (49 % vs. 55.8 % vs. 34.6 %). Similarly the remission rate was higher in both treatment arms in comparison to placebo at week 3 (47.4 % vs. 52.1 % vs. 28.8 %). This picture lasted for the entire duration of the study, and a similar picture was observed concerning the remission rates. The NNT for response or remission was 6–7 for quetiapine IR. At week 3 fewer patients under quetiapine IR or paliperidone ER dropped out in comparison to placebo (21.2 % vs. 20.5 % vs. 39 %). Fewer patients in the medication arms withdrew because of lack of efficacy in comparison to placebo, and these withdrawals were more in the quetiapine IR group in comparison to the paliperidone ER group (7.8 % vs. 3.1 % vs. 18.1 %). Dropout because of adverse events was similar in the three arms. The most common treatment-emergent adverse events related to quetiapine were somnolence, sedation, dry mouth, headache and dizziness, and for paliperidone ER they were headache, somnolence and akathisia. At week 12 the body weight increase was more frequent in the quetiapine IR group (17 % vs. 8 %), but more patients under paliperidone ER switched to depression (13.9 % vs. 7.5 %) (Vieta et al. 2010b).

Conclusively, quetiapine is reported to be equal to lithium but with more dropouts and adverse events (Bowden et al. 2005b; Li et al. 2008). Also it is reported to be equal to haloperidol, with fewer dropouts and less frequent EPS, but less efficacious in psychotic patients. In contrast to haloperidol it had an effect on depressive symptoms (McIntyre et al. 2005). Quetiapine is reported to be equal to paliperidone, and both agents had a similar effect in manic and mixed patients. Body weight increase was more frequent in the quetiapine group, but more patients under paliperidone switched to depression (Vieta et al. 2010b).

16.2.1.2.8 Other Antipsychotics

There is also a one old 2-week study in 23 acutely manic inpatients (one admitted twice during two discrete episodes) that compared pimozide (6–32 mg/day; $N=12$) vs. chlorpromazine (200–1,600 mg/day; $N=12$). It reported that both agents led to clinical improvement, with a significant effect being noted within 24 h. Maybe chlorpromazine acted faster probably due to its greater sedative effect, but by 7 both drugs were equally effective. Sedation was the side effect most frequent with chlorpromazine, and EPS were more frequent with pimozide (Cookson et al. 1981).

All the studies concerning the rest of agents have been reported and discussed above; however, it is important to cite them again from a reverse angle. There are two studies which compared risperidone with haloperidol (Segal et al. 1998; Smulevich et al. 2005) and one vs. olanzapine (Perlis et al. 2006a). There is one study comparing aripiprazole with lithium (Keck et al. 2009) and two with haloperidol (Vieta et al. 2005a; Young et al. 2009), two studies comparing asenapine with olanzapine (McIntyre et al. 2009a, 2010b), one study comparing paliperidone with quetiapine (Vieta et al. 2010b), one unpublished study comparing ziprasidone with olanzapine (NCT00329108 study results 2009) and another one with haloperidol (Vieta et al. 2010c). Finally there are two studies comparing chlorpromazine with lithium (Platman 1970; Prien et al. 1972) and one with carbamazepine (Okuma et al. 1979).

16.2.1.2.9 Comparison of ECT Methods

In one 3-week study, 36 inpatients suffering from acute mania and referred for ECT were randomized to receive bifrontal (BFECT; $N=17$) or bitemporal (BTECT; $N=19$) ECT. None of the subjects were on mood stabilizers during the course of ECT. The YMRS scores showed faster decline in the BFECT than in the BTECT group. More patients in the BFECT group responded, and this happened significantly earlier than in the BTECT group. There were no significant differences between the groups in performance on cognitive function tests (Hiremani et al. 2008).

16.2.1.2.10 Conclusion of Comparison Studies

Overall, comparison studies suggest that the higher the efficacy, the more frequent the adverse events are. Although there are no sufficient data to support a big difference between agents, it seems that antipsychotics and lithium are more efficacious than valproate and carbamazepine unless you apply a loading strategy. Also it seems clear that antipsychotics act earlier in comparison to the other compounds. The effect on depressive symptoms is unclear, but it seems that haloperidol-treated patients might switch more often to depression. An effect of dosing on the above-mentioned differences cannot be ruled out.

Earlier studies suggested that lithium could be specifically useful against the more 'classic' cases of euphoric mania, while antiepileptics might have a better efficacy in the rest of cases. This is not supported by more recent data (Fountoulakis et al. 2012d). A factor which could have affected the results is the well-known lithium discontinuation-related refractoriness (present probably in up to 15 % of patients) (Post et al. 1992). Because of this, patients enrolled in RCTs could constitute a sample more refractory to lithium treatment than expected. However even when samples enriched for lithium refractoriness were used, no inferiority of lithium to the other agent was documented (Bowden et al. 1994).

16.2.1.3 Combination and Add-On Treatment

A number of studies examine the efficacy and safety of agents given not as monotherapy but combined. This simultaneous administration of agents is given under a variety of conditions concerning the study sample, ranging from patients being refractory to a baseline treatment to absolutely usual patients. In the first instance, an agent is used as adjunct or add-on therapy on a pre-existing treatment to which the patient has shown unsatisfactory response. The definition of this unsatisfactory response varies widely, from explicitly recruiting some sort of refractory patients to simply demand pretreatment with the baseline therapy for at least 1–2 weeks, and still the patients fulfil the inclusion criteria. In the second instance, both the baseline agent and the second one which is compared with placebo are started simultaneously with the initiation of the trial. In this case the study tests a combination treatment against monotherapy. Although essentially both designs provide information on how to treat patients with unsatisfactory response to monotherapy, the conclusions and the generalizability differ, since studies on samples which include only refractory or partial responders (add-on studies) are more sensitive to the effect of the joint treatment in comparison to combination studies.

16.2.1.3.1 Combination Treatment

A summary of combination treatment data for the treatment of acute mania is shown in Table 16.3.

Carbamazepine Combinations

A 6-week international trial of olanzapine (10–30 mg/day; $N=58$) vs. placebo ($n=60$) on carbamazepine (400–1,200 mg/day) followed by open-label, 20-week olanzapine plus carbamazepine ($N=86$) reported no significant differences in efficacy measures between treatment groups, but at 6 weeks triglyceride levels were significantly higher ($p=0.008$), and potentially clinically significant weight gain (≥7 %) occurred more frequently in the combined olanzapine and carbamazepine group (24.6 % vs. 3.4 %, $p=0.002$). Carbamazepine reduced olanzapine concentrations, but olanzapine had no effect on carbamazepine concentrations. Both agents were started simultaneously, and the results do not support the utility of such a treatment strategy (Tohen et al. 2008a). It should be noted that carbamazepine significantly reduces the serum concentration levels of many other agents.

A second 12-week double-blind, randomized, placebo-controlled study from China in 111 patients with acute mania randomized them to carbamazepine (300–800 mg/day; $N=43$) vs. carbamazepine plus the herbal Free and Easy Wanderer Plus (FEWP; 36 g/day; $N=46$) vs. placebo ($N=22$). At endpoint both carbamazepine arms produced significantly greater improvement on YMRS score, and the improvement was present already at week 4, but they did not differ from each other (−22.9 vs. −25.4 vs. −17). In terms of response rates, more patients in the carbamazepine arms were superior to placebo (87.8 % vs. 93 % vs. 57.1 %, $p=0.012$). Interestingly, although there was no difference between the two carbamazepine groups concerning the carbamazepine dosage, fewer patient under the combination dropped out (25.6 % vs. 13 % vs. 40.9 %), and this was also true concerning dropout because of lack of efficacy (7 % vs. 4.3 % vs. 27.3 %). Depressed and manic patients were pooled for the analysis of adverse events, and the adverse events occurring in over 5 % of the patients in any treatment group were dizziness, laboratory testing abnormality, skin rash, headache, fatigue, blurred vision, somnolence and nausea. Compared to carbamazepine monotherapy, patients in the combination therapy had a lesser incidence of dizziness (18.2 % vs. 7.9 %; $p=0.069$) and fatigue (9.1 % vs. 1.1 %; $p=0.038$). No difference in the incidence of other adverse events was found between the combination therapy and carbamazepine monotherapy. Although this study supports the efficacy of carbamazepine during the acute manic phase, the low carbamazepine dosage, in combination with the possible dramatic reduction of carbamazepine levels when co-administered with FEWP, plus the unusually high response rate even in the placebo group and the unusually low dropout rate, makes conclusions difficult. Technically it does not support the use of FEWP in acute mania, but a number of other interpretations also exist, for example, that adding FEWP compensates for the drop in carbamazepine levels (Zhang et al. 2007).

FGAs Combinations

One 3-week study in 136 hospitalized patients with acute mania utilized the adding of valproate (20 mg/kg; $N=69$) vs. placebo ($N=69$) on FGAs (preferably haloperidol and/or perazine). The valproate group had a higher response rate (70 % vs. 46 %; $p=0.005$). The mean neuroleptic dose declined continuously in the valproate group, whereas only slight variations were observed in the placebo group, and the difference was statistically significant ($p=0.0007$) for study weeks 2 and 3. Premature discontinuations occurred in only 13 % of the patients (Muller-Oerlinghausen et al. 2000).

Haloperidol Combinations

A 5-week study on 23 patients with carbamazepine ($N=23$) vs. placebo ($n=20$) on haloperidol suggested a superior performance in the combination group in terms of change in the Brief Psychiatric Rating Scale ratings (Klein et al. 1984). Another 3-week study in 21 severely ill manic inpatients investigated the comparative efficacy of lithium (up to 900 mg/day; $N=7$) vs. haloperidol (up to 30 mg/day; $N=7$) vs. a combination of haloperidol–lithium ($N=7$). All medications were initiated simultaneously. Subjects on haloperidol and the haloperidol–lithium combination were significantly improved after 7 days in comparison to the lithium-treated group. The haloperidol and the haloperidol–lithium combination groups did not differ from each other, either in degree of improvement or in side effects, and were superior to lithium monotherapy. Conclusively, that study suggested that combining haloperidol with lithium was not superior to haloperidol alone (Garfinkel et al. 1980). However, a more recent study reported that the combination of lithium with haloperidol at low dosage (5 mg/daily) but not the combination with haloperidol at high dosage (25 mg/daily) increased the efficacy against acute mania. In contrast, the combination of haloperidol with lorazepam had no added effect neither on the low nor on the high dosage (Chou et al. 1999).

Overall the data on combinations of agents with haloperidol vs. haloperidol monotherapy are equivocal, and the results might depend on the haloperidol dosage.

Lithium Combinations

As mentioned above, a 3-week study in 21 severely ill manic inpatients investigated the comparative efficacy of lithium (up to 900 mg/day; $N=7$) vs. haloperidol (up to 30 mg/day; $N=7$) vs. a combination of haloperidol–lithium ($N=7$). Subjects on haloperidol and the haloperidol–lithium combination were significantly improved after 7 days in comparison to the lithium-treated group. Conclusively, that study suggested that the combination of haloperidol plus lithium is superior to lithium alone (Garfinkel et al. 1980). The lithium plus haloperidol combination was tested vs. lithium plus lorazepam in 20 hospitalized patients. There was no evidence for a significant difference between the two treatment groups in the magnitude of or time to response (5.0 ± 0.82 days for haloperidol; 6.5 ± 0.93 days for lorazepam). Of the patients who were terminated from the protocol early, nonresponse was the primary reason in the lorazepam group, while side effects were the reason in the haloperidol group (Lenox et al. 1992). It was also tested vs. carbamazepine plus lithium in 33 hospitalized manic patients which were withdrawn from psychoactive medications for 2 weeks after which they were randomized to double-blind treatment. Again the two groups were similar. However the haloperidol group had more EPS that were major reasons for dropout, whereas carbamazepine group patients were more often noncompliant and initially required more rescue medications (Small et al. 1995). Overall the haloperidol plus lithium combination seems to be somewhat more effective than lithium monotherapy and other combinations with lithium but with more adverse effects.

A 3-week trial on with a manic or mixed episode was randomized to receive ziprasidone (80–160 mg/day; $N=101$) vs. placebo ($N=103$) on top of lithium (serum levels 0.8–1.2 mEq/l). All medications were initiated since the beginning of the study. There was no superiority of the ziprasidone group over placebo at endpoint concerning the MRS (Weisler et al. 2003; Bowden 2005).

A 4-week study from Brazil in 180 inpatients in a manic episode with or without psychotic features (mixed and rapid cycling excluded) compared fixed oral doses of allopurinol (600 mg/day; $N=60$) vs. dipyridamole (200 mg/day; $N=60$) vs. placebo ($N=60$) as adjunct treatment on lithium. All medications started together in all the study arms. Allopurinol resulted in greater mean reductions in YMRS scores from baseline to day 21 ($p<0.001$) and day 28 ($p=0.003$) compared with placebo. Remission rates were significantly higher for allopurinol compared with dipyridamole and placebo ($p=0.008$). The dipyridamole group did not differ from placebo. The presence of psychotic symptoms did not influence the results. The dropout rate was similar in the three groups. Decrease in plasma uric acid levels showed a significant positive association with antimanic effects in the allopurinol group ($p<0.001$) (Machado-Vieira et al. 2008).

Finally, a 6-week study on 40 manic inpatients allocated to tamoxifen (80 mg/day; $N=$) vs. placebo on top of lithium (1–1.2 mEq/l) B) reported significant difference in favour of the tamoxifen group ($p=0.02$) concerning the YMRS and the total PANSS without any difference on adverse events except for fatigue that occurred more often in the tamoxifen group simultaneously (Amrollahi et al. 2010).

Overall the combination data support the conclusion that all the combinations which included lithium (haloperidol, lorazepam, carbamazepine, ziprasidone, tamoxifen, allopurinol) were proven superior to lithium alone, with the exception of the dipyridamole plus lithium. Most of these combinations had more adverse events in comparison to monotherapy, and there was a trend that the more effective the combination, the more adverse events it showed.

Lithium or Valproate Combinations

A number of trials investigate the addition of an agent on top of lithium or valproate, since these two constituted the backbone of the treatment of bipolar disorder for decades.

A multicentre trial from the USA on 117 patients on mania, hypomania or mixed episodes of gabapentin (900–3,600 mg/day; $N=58$) vs. placebo ($N=59$) on lithium or valproate or both (it included a 2 weeks placebo lead-in) was negative (Pande et al. 2000). Similarly negative was a 3-week multicentre trial on 156 patients with manic or mixed episode which tested the administration of risperidone (1–6 mg/day; $N=52$) vs. haloperidol (2–12 mg/day; $N=53$) vs. placebo (N=51) as combination therapy with lithium (29 %) or divalproex (71 %). For the whole sample a significantly greater reduction in the YMRS score was observed in both combination medication groups in comparison to placebo (−14.3 vs. −13.4 vs. 8.2); however, the small subsample of patients which did not receive mood stabilizers until the start of the trial precluded any conclusion for this specific subgroup ($N=17$, −11.3 vs. $N=17$, −10.1 vs. $N=19$, −9.4). The trial was discontinued by 49 % of the placebo group patients, 35 % of the risperidone group patients and 53 % of the haloperidol group patients (Sachs et al. 2002).

A small 4-week study on 13 women with acute mania/hypomania which were given tamoxifen (40 mg/day; $N=5$) or medroxyprogesterone acetate (MPA; 20 mg/

day; $N=4$) or placebo ($N=4$) as add-on to lithium and/or valproate reported that at endpoint only the tamoxifen group manifested a significant change from baseline in the CARS-M score (−22.2 vs. −13 vs. −8.5). No effect on the PANSS positive subscale was evident in any group. Although it is not reported specifically, the study sample was not constituted of refractory patients, and all medications were started simultaneously. The small study sample precludes any strong conclusions (Kulkarni et al. 2006).

Finally, a 12-week study in 324 manic or mixed episodes with asenapine (5–10 mg; $N=158$) vs. placebo (N=166) on lithium or valproate reported that adjunctive asenapine significantly improved the YMRS score at week 3 and the response and remission rates at week 12 (Szegedi et al. 2012).

Conclusively, the data are in support of combining lithium or valproate with asenapine or tamoxifen.

Valproate Combinations

One 3-week study on 88 manic patients evaluated folic acid (3 mg/day; $N=44$) vs. placebo ($N=44$) on top of valproate. There was a statistically significant difference in the YMRS results between the case and control groups after 3 weeks of treatment ($p=0.005$), although the analysis of the results was not the standard. Only four patients dropped out (Behzadi et al. 2009). Also, one small study on 15 manic patients which investigated the use of omega-3 fatty acids as combination therapy with valproate was negative (Chiu et al. 2005).

Risperidone Combinations

A 3-week study on 81 partially responding acutely manic patients which were receiving a mood stabilizer for at least 2 weeks prior to study entry allocated them to risperidone ($n=42$) vs. placebo ($n=39$) on top of lithium, valproate or carbamazepine. The results suggested that there was no difference between arms in terms of change in the YMRS score (−14.9 vs. 13.2). It should be noted that in carbamazepine-treated patients the risperidone plasma levels were 40 % lower. The incidence of adverse events was similar in both groups (Yatham et al. 2003).

Conclusively, there are few but still important data suggesting that specific combinations are superior to monotherapy in non-refractory or otherwise selected samples, although it is difficult to assess the quality of many study samples. In spite of the very small number of trials and the problems with the data quality, one could generalize that the combination of an antipsychotic plus lithium or valproate is superior to lithium or valproate alone. Tamoxifen and probably allopurinol are also valuable agents to use in combination with other treatment modalities.

16.2.1.3.2 Add-On Treatment

Add-On to Haloperidol

A small 5-week study on 12 refractory patients with acute mania of phenytoin ($N=6$) vs. placebo ($N=6$) on haloperidol reported that there was more improvement in the patients receiving phenytoin (Mishory et al. 2000).

Add-On to Lithium

An 8-week trial on 52 incomplete responders to lithium utilized the addition of 600–1,200 mg/day carbamazepine ($N=26$) or oxcarbazepine ($N=26$) during maintenance treatment. All patients completed the study. Although this trial was on patients in the 'maintenance' phase the design and the results are more relevant to the acute manic phase. The study sample constituted of manic, mixed and depressed patients. Both groups improved with the addition of either drug, but those receiving oxcarbazepine improved significantly more on the YMRS score at endpoint. Oxcarbazepine improved also the HAM-D and the MADRS score and exhibited better tolerability in comparison to carbamazepine (Juruena et al. 2009).

Add-On to Lithium or Valproate

A 3-week multicentre trial on 156 patients with manic or mixed episode tested the administration of risperidone (1–6 mg/day; $N=52$) vs. haloperidol (2–12 mg/day; $N=53$) vs. placebo (N=51) as add-on therapy on lithium (29 %) or divalproex (71 %). The results suggested a significantly greater reduction in the YMRS score in both add-on medication groups in comparison to placebo (−14.3 vs. −13.4 vs. 8.2). Especially among patients who were receiving mood stabilizers at the start of the trial ('breakthrough' patients), the mean total score on the YMRS decreased more in the medication add-on groups in comparison to placebo ($N=34$, −15.7 vs. $N=33$, −14.9; $N=28$, −7.4). The trial was discontinued by 49 % of the placebo group patients, 35 % of the risperidone group patients and 53 % of the haloperidol group patients (Sachs et al. 2002).

In another 6-week trial on 344 partially responsive manic or mixed patients, olanzapine (5–20 mg/day) vs. placebo as add-on treatment on valproate or lithium was tested, and the results suggested that that olanzapine co-therapy improved the patients' YMRS total scores significantly more than monotherapy (−13.11 vs. −9.10; $p=0.003$). A similar picture was there concerning the response rate (67.7 % vs. 44.7 %; $p<0.001$). Olanzapine co-therapy improved also the HAM-D. Treatment-emergent symptoms that were significantly higher for the olanzapine co-therapy group included somnolence, dry mouth, weight gain, increased appetite, tremor and slurred speech (Tohen et al. 2002b).

In a 3-week combination treatment study, patients under lithium (0.7–1.0 mEq/l) or valproate (50–100 μg/ml) were randomized to receive quetiapine IR (up to 800 mg/day; $N=91$) or placebo ($N=100$). Patients should have been treated with li/val at 7 days prior to randomization. More patients in the quetiapine group completed the study (61.5 % vs. 49 %). A significantly greater mean reduction in the YMRS score was observed at endpoint in the quetiapine group (−13.76 vs. −9.93; $p=0.021$). Also the response rate was significantly higher in the quetiapine group (54.3 % vs. 32.6 %; $p=0.005$), as was the remission rate (45.7 % vs. 25.8 %; $p=0.007$). Common adverse events in the quetiapine group included somnolence, dry mouth, asthenia and postural hypotension (Sachs et al. 2004). Another 3-week study on 402 partial responders with acute mania tested the adding of quetiapine IR up to 800 mg/day ($N=197$) vs. placebo ($N=205$) on lithium (serum concentration 0.7–1.0 mEq/l) or valproate (serum concentration 50–100 μg/ml). The improvement in the YMRS in the quetiapine group was significant at day 21 (−15.29 vs. −2.19; $p<0.05$). Similarly, the quetiapine group was superior concerning the response rate (55.7 % vs. 41.6 %; $p<0.01$). More patients in the quetiapine group completed the trial, and there was no difference in discontinuation rates due to adverse events between the two groups. Common adverse events in the quetiapine group were somnolence, dry mouth and asthenia (Yatham et al. 2004). A third study utilizing quetiapine was a 6-week study on 200 partial responders with acute mania which tested the adding of quetiapine IR up to 800 mg/day ($N=104$) vs. placebo ($n=96$) on lithium (serum concentration 0.7–1.0 mEq/l) or valproate (serum concentration 50–100 μg/ml). There was no difference in the YMRS change between groups (Yatham et al. 2007).

A 6-week multicentre study included 384 partial responders experiencing a manic or mixed episode (with or without psychotic features) and utilized the addition of aripiprazole (15–30 mg/day; $N=253$) vs. placebo ($N=131$) on lithium (0.6–1.0 mmol/l) or valproate (50–125 μg/ml). The mean improvement from baseline in YMRS total score at week 6 was significantly greater with aripiprazole (−13.3 vs. −10.7), and the difference was present already since week 1. There was also a superiority concerning the response rate at week 6 (62.8 % vs. 48.5 % for both the lithium and valproate groups). Discontinuation rates due to adverse events were higher with aripiprazole than with placebo (9 % vs. 5 %). Akathisia was the most frequently reported extrapyramidal symptom-related adverse event and occurred significantly more frequently among those receiving aripiprazole (18.6 % vs. 5.4 %). There were no significant differences between treatments in weight change from baseline to week 6 (+0.55 kg vs. +0.23 kg) (Vieta et al. 2008c).

A 3-week multicentre US study on 448 patients with acute manic or mixed episode utilized ziprasidone (40–80 mg/day; $N=226$ or 80–160 mg/day; $N=232$) vs. placebo ($N=222$) on top of lithium or divalproex. There was no difference at endpoint in the change in the YMRS scores from baseline (−11.0 vs. −10.2 vs, −9.5), and similarly there was no difference in any of the outcomes (Sachs et al. 2012a, b).

A 12-week study in 287 patients in a manic or mixed episode to investigate the efficacy and safety of topiramate (50–400 mg/day; $N=143$) vs. placebo ($N=144$) as adjunctive therapy on valproate (serum levels 45–100 mg/l) or lithium (serum levels 0.5–1.2 mEq/l) reported that at endpoint there was no difference in the YMRS score change in the two groups (−10.1 vs. −9.6). Similarly there was no difference concerning the response rates (39 % vs. 38 %) and the secondary outcomes. Topiramate did not worsen mania or induce depression. Paraesthesia, diarrhoea and anorexia were more common in the topiramate group. However the topiramate group achieved greater reductions than the placebo group in body weight (−2.5 vs. 0.2 kg, $p<0.001$) and body mass index (−0.84 vs. 0.07 kg/m(2), $p<0.001$) (Roy Chengappa et al. 2006).

A 6-week study on 300 patients with acute mania or mixed episode (33 % mixed; with or without psychotic features) which were allocated to paliperidone ER (3–12 mg/day; $N=150$) vs. placebo ($N=150$) in addition to lithium (38 %) or valproate (62 %) reported that there was no significant difference between groups in terms of YMRS change (−14.3 vs. −13.2; $p=0.16$) or in any of the secondary outcomes. More patients under the combination treatment manifested an adverse event (70 % vs. 54 %) (Berwaerts et al. 2011).

Finally, a 12-week international multicentre study in 324 patients experiencing manic (60 %) or mixed (40 %) episodes evaluated the efficacy and safety of asenapine (10–20 mg/day; $N=158$) vs. placebo ($N=166$) as adjunctive treatment on lithium or valproate. Adjunctive asenapine significantly improved the YMRS score at week 3 (−10.3 vs. −7.9; $p=0.026$). The response rates were similar at week 3 (32 % vs. 27 %) but significantly better with asenapine at week 12 (47.7 % vs. 34.4 %; $p=0.0152$). The remission rates were significantly greater with asenapine at weeks 3 (33.5 % vs. 21.5 %; $p=0.0158$) and 12 (43.2 % vs. 30.1 %; $p=0.0148$). Some but not all of the secondary outcomes were significantly better with asenapine at weeks 3 and 12. Overall discontinuation rates were higher with adjunctive placebo than with adjunctive asenapine. Treatment-emergent adverse events related with asenapine treatment were sedation, somnolence, depressive symptoms, oral hypoesthesia and increased weight (Szegedi et al. 2012).

Overall, the data suggest that in patients who are refractory or partial responders to lithium or valproate, it is beneficial to add risperidone, haloperidol, olanzapine, quetiapine, aripiprazole and asenapine but not ziprasidone, topiramate or paliperidone.

Add-On to Lithium, Valproate or Carbamazepine

A 3-week study on 60 partially responding acutely manic patients which were receiving a mood stabilizer for at least 2 weeks prior to study entry allocated them to risperidone ($n=26$) vs. placebo ($n=34$) on top of lithium, valproate or carbamazepine. The results suggested that there was no difference between arms in terms of change in the YMRS score (−13.8 vs. 7.1); however, there was a numerical difference, and the small study subsample precluded significance. Again it should be noted that in carbamazepine-treated patients the risperidone plasma levels were 40 % lower. The incidence of adverse events was similar in both groups (Yatham et al. 2003).

Add-On to Lithium, Valproate or Carbamazepine or Atypical Antipsychotics

A 6-week study randomized 27 manic or mixed subjects to allopurinol (600 mg/day; $N=15$) vs. placebo ($N=12$) on top of lithium, valproic acid, carbamazepine or atypical antipsychotic medications. Allopurinol augmentation did not show a statistically significant improvement over placebo. Subjects with restricted caffeine use showed a greater effect size compared to caffeine users (Fan et al. 2012).

Add-On ECT

There is only one sham-controlled trial of ECT as adjunctive treatment on chlorpromazine (600 mg/day) in 30 acutely manic patients. That study supported the efficacy of ECT with a faster rate of improvement (Sikdar et al. 1994).

Add-On to Treatment as Usual

One small 8-week study in 21 ambulatory mild-to-moderate manic patients with insomnia evaluated the efficacy and tolerability of ramelteon (fixed-dose 8 mg/day;

$N=10$) vs. placebo ($N=11$). There was no difference between groups in terms of outcome concerning the manic symptoms. However, ramelteon was associated with improvement in a global rating of depressive symptoms and was also well tolerated and associated with no serious adverse events (McElroy et al. 2010d).

Overall, the data on partial responders or refractory patients support the addition of specific antipsychotics on top of lithium or valproate and also the use of allopurinol and the combination of lithium with carbamazepine or oxcarbazepine.

Other Add-On Options

A recent placebo-controlled 4-week RCT in 180 acutely manic patients supported the efficacy and safety of the purinergic agents allopurinol (600 mg/day) and dipyridamole (200 mg/day) as adjunctive to lithium in acute bipolar mania (Machado-Vieira et al. 2008). Folic acid was also found to be useful as an adjunct to valproate against acute mania (Behzadi et al. 2009). There is one 5-week trial from Israel on 32 recently admitted manic inpatients which compared valnoctamide (600–1,200 mg/day; $N=15$) vs. placebo ($N=17$) on top of risperidone (1–6 mg/day). All medications were started at day 1. In all efficacy measures the valnoctamide plus risperidone combination was more effective than risperidone plus placebo from week 3 to week 5. Valnoctamide is an anticonvulsant analogue of valproate that does not undergo biotransformation to the corresponding free acid and in mice has been shown to be distinctly less teratogenic than valproate (Bersudsky et al. 2010). A pilot 8-week study in 21 acutely manic outpatients on the usefulness of adjunctive ramelteon against acute mania/mixed failed to produce a positive result for the agent (McElroy et al. 2010d).

16.2.1.4 Post Hoc Analyses and Meta-analytic Studies

16.2.1.4.1 Post Hoc Analyses

Olanzapine

A secondary analysis of a trial on olanzapine (Tohen et al. 2000) reported that olanzapine is effective in acutely manic or mixed patients irrespective of whether or not they have failed to respond to another treatment in the past (Baker et al. 2002). The data of two trials of olanzapine in acute mania (Tohen et al. 1999, 2000) were pooled and analysed in combination. The sample was stratified in terms of gender, age, episode type, psychotic features, substance abuse and specific clinical features. The results showed significant antimanic efficacy in all subgroups. There was somewhat superior efficacy of olanzapine in patients who were younger at illness onset, without prior substance abuse and had not previously received antipsychotic treatment (Baldessarini et al. 2003). Another reanalysis of the pooled data of these two specific trials (Tohen et al. 1999, 2000) reported that olanzapine monotherapy resulted in significant clinical improvement in over half of the patients, and just under 20 % of them achieved a near complete remission of both manic and accompanying depressive symptoms (Chengappa et al. 2003). A post hoc analysis of a study which compared olanzapine (5–20 mg/day) to divalproex sodium (500–2,500 mg/day) for bipolar manic or mixed episodes ($N=251$) (Tohen et al. 2003c) classified patients at study entry as 'rapid cyclers' if they experienced at least four episodes within the last year. Olanzapine was proven superior in non-rapid cyclers, while both agents were equal in rapid cycling patients. Under olanzapine, non-rapid cycling patients improved more than rapid cycling, while under divalproex both groups improved to a similar extent. Overall rapid cycling patients did less well over long-term treatment than non-rapid cycling patients. Conclusively this post hoc analysis suggests that olanzapine has a broader efficacy in the treatment of acutely manic or mixed patients, while divalproex matches the efficacy of olanzapine only in rapid cycling patients (Suppes et al. 2005).

Quetiapine

An a priori-defined combined analysis of data from two placebo-controlled studies (McIntyre et al. 2005; Bowden et al. 2005b) reported that a significant improvement in the quetiapine group (both psychotic and nonpsychotic patients) vs. placebo concerning the change in YMRS score was observed already since day 4 ($p=0.021$), and the improvement continued until the end of the trials and concerned all YMRS individual items. The response and remission rates were also higher for the quetiapine group. Quetiapine significantly improved the PANSS total and the positive subscale as well as the MADRS score ($p<0.001$). Treatment with quetiapine was related with the emergence of somnolence, dry mouth, weight gain and dizziness (Vieta et al. 2005b).

Risperidone

A post hoc analysis of one multicentre risperidone study from India (Khanna et al. 2005) of 3-week duration which included 291 acutely manic or mixed BD patients (rapid cycling excluded) and assessed the efficacy and safety of risperidone (1–6 mg/day, $N=146$) vs. placebo ($N=145$) reported that more patients under risperidone achieved remission (42 % vs. 13 %), and fewer dropped out (11 % vs. 29 %) especially because of lack of efficacy (5 % vs. 15 %). The dropout because of adverse events was similar in the two patient groups. This analysis did not report adverse events or the effect of the intervention in any other scale except YRMS in terms of remission alone (Gopal et al. 2005).

Asenapine

Exploratory pooled post hoc analyses from two trials of asenapine in acute mania (McIntyre et al. 2009a, 2010b) evaluated the efficacy of asenapine and olanzapine on depressive symptoms, in those patients with significant baseline depressive symptoms. In the original trials, 977 patients were randomized to flexible-dose sublingual asenapine (10–20 mg/day), oral olanzapine (5–20 mg/day) or placebo. The pooled analysis identified three populations by using baseline depressive symptoms: a. MADRS score ≥20 ($N=132$), b. CGI for Bipolar Disorder-Depression (CGI-BP-D) scale severity score ≥4 ($N=170$) and c. diagnosis of mixed episodes ($N=302$). The results suggested that the decreases in MADRS total score were statistically greater with asenapine vs. placebo at days 7 and 21 in all populations, while the differences between olanzapine and placebo were not significant. Olanzapine manifested some efficacy on the basis of the decreases in CGI-BP-D scores, but its results appeared to be less consistent (Szegedi et al. 2011). A second analysis confirmed its efficacy in mixed episodes (Azorin et al. 2013). Another meta-analyses suggested that asenapine had an effect on every individual YMRS item, and thus it has an effect on the core of mania (Cazorla et al. 2013).

Aripiprazole

Another analysis was designed to assess the efficacy and safety of aripiprazole in subpopulations of patients with acute manic or mixed episodes. The 516 patients from two trials (Sachs et al. 2006; Keck et al. 2003a) were stratified by severity, episode type, presence or absence of psychotic features, episode frequency, age, gender, and baseline severity of depressive symptoms. Analyses concerning safety and adverse event analyses were also performed. The results suggested that aripiprazole significantly improved the YMRS total scores in comparison to placebo in all subpopulations except the >55 years age group. The treatment-emergent adverse events profile differed between genders and age groups (Suppes et al. 2008a).

Ziprasidone

A pooled data analysis from two similarly designed trials on ziprasidone in acute bipolar mania (Keck et al. 2003b; Potkin et al. 2005) selected all patients with scoring ≥2 on at least two items of the extracted HAM-D. These 179 patients (ziprasidone, $N=124$; placebo, $N=55$) were considered to meet criteria for dysphoric mania and were included in the post hoc analysis. Patients treated with ziprasidone manifested a significant reduction in their HAM-D scores beginning at day 4 in comparison to placebo ($p<0.05$). They had also significant improvements on the MRS score and all secondary efficacy measures, and had significantly higher response and remission rates compared with placebo (Stahl et al. 2010). Another pooled analysis of the same two trials of ziprasidone (Keck et al. 2003b; Potkin et al. 2005) reported that significantly greater antipsychotic effects were observed with ziprasidone already by day 4, and the magnitude of improvement increased significantly with time, and it concerned all patients and predicted subsequent acute manic episode remission (Ketter et al. 2010).

Lithium

A post hoc analysis of a lithium trial (Bowden et al. 1994) confirmed the efficacy of lithium in classic manic but not mixed patients. All other effects were negative (Swann et al. 1997).

16.2.1.4.2 Meta-analyses

The first meta-analysis included only randomized controlled clinical trials with a double-blind assessment of outcomes, and lithium levels were required to be within the therapeutic range of 0.4–1.5 mmol/l. It compared lithium vs. valproate and carbamazepine and reported that there is no significant difference between them; however, there was a general tendency in favour of the antiepileptics with regard to adverse events and treatment tolerance. These results questioned the widely accepted opinion that lithium is the first choice and antiepileptics follow (Emilien et al. 1996).

More recent meta-analytic studies suggest that the efficacy of second-generation antipsychotics is established both as monotherapy and as add-on therapy to mood stabilizers. An early comparison of second-generation antipsychotics found aripiprazole, olanzapine, quetiapine, risperidone and ziprasidone superior to placebo as monotherapy but failed to detect any differences between them (Perlis et al. 2006b). Another study compared second-generation antipsychotics with placebo, first-generation antipsychotics or mood stabilizers in the treatment of acute mania and reported that the second-generation antipsychotics were significantly more efficacious than placebo both as monotherapy and also as adjunct treatment on mood-stabilizing agents. They were associated with EPS and somnolence (Scherk et al. 2007). Another one tested whether combination treatment is superior to monotherapy and reported that significant reductions in YMRS scores were shown with haloperidol, olanzapine, risperidone and quetiapine as adjunctive treatment on a mood stabilizer vs. a mood stabilizer alone. Also significantly more patients under co-therapy responded. However, the combination treatment manifested more adverse events (especially weight gain) and lower tolerability (Smith et al. 2007). One meta-analysis suggested that that antimanic agents are roughly equal in efficacy against acute mania (Tamayo et al. 2010); however, two others reported that second-generation antipsychotics are superior to antiepileptics, but this should be balanced against increased adverse events (EPS, somnolence and weight gain) especially in youth (Correll et al. 2010; Tarr et al. 2010), while a more recent one reported that haloperidol shows a faster onset of antimanic action in comparison to second-generation antipsychotics (Goikolea et al. 2013a) but also the most likely to switch patients to depression (Goikolea et al. 2013b). Olanzapine and aripiprazole are confirmed to be efficacious against psychotic features (Baldessarini et al. 2003; Fountoulakis et al. 2009; Suppes et al. 2008a). One meta-analysis reported that combination treatment was more effective than monotherapy, studies outside the USA had higher effect size and the baseline YMRS predicted the outcome (Tarr et al. 2011) probably because of a structural coupling effect (Fountoulakis and Kontis 2012). Year of study publication was not associated with YMRS score change. Also the study size, number of study sites, YMRS score required for study entry, inclusion of patients with mixed mania or treatment resistance and inclusion of inpatients vs. outpatients had no significant influence on the outcome.

The review and meta-analysis of data available for oxcarbazepine suggests that although there are some positive data (Hirschfeld and Kasper 2004) the level of evidence is insufficient (Vasudev et al. 2011).

Two recent meta-analyses attempted to rank antimanic agents according to efficacy. The first one utilized the method of multiple treatments meta-analysis and reported that the ranking in terms of efficacy was haloperidol, risperidone, olanzapine, lithium, quetiapine, aripiprazole, carbamazepine, asenapine, valproate and ziprasidone. According to that meta-analysis, overall, antipsychotics were significantly more effective than mood stabilizers (Cipriani et al. 2011). However this meta-analysis has been criticized both concerning the overall methodology but also concerning the incomplete list of RCTs which was utilized (Fountoulakis and Siamouli 2012). A more balanced meta-analysis confirmed that the response to antipsychotics was greater and more rapid in comparison to lithium, valproate or carbamazepine, but it did not confirm any difference between haloperidol and second-generation antipsychotics (Yildiz et al. 2010).

A meta-analysis which pooled data from nine randomized, double-blind, placebo-controlled, acute studies of ziprasidone reported that the discontinuation rate due to adverse events or 7 % or greater weight gain between ziprasidone and placebo was not significant in all psychiatric conditions. In acute mania the risk for akathisia with ziprasidone had a NNTH = 12, the risk for overall EPS had a NNTH = 12 and the reported somnolence had NNTH = 7 (Gao et al. 2013).

The number needed to treat to harm (NNTH) of ziprasidone relative to placebo was estimated when an RD was statistically significant. Results: The RD in discontinuation due to adverse events or 7 % or greater weight gain between ziprasidone and placebo was not significant in all three psychiatric conditions. The risk for akathisia with ziprasidone was significantly higher in BPD with an RD of 2.3 % (NNTH = 44) and in BPM with an RD of 8.4 % (NNTH = 12). Risk for overall EPS with ziprasidone was significantly higher in BPM with an RD of 8.7 % (NNTH = 12) and schizophrenia with an RD of 3.3 % (NNTH = 30). Risk of reported somnolence with ziprasidone was also significantly higher in BPD with an RD of 11.8 % (NNTH = 8), BPM with an RD of 14.3 % (NNTH = 7) and schizophrenia with an RD of 7 % (NNTH = 14). Dose-dependent increase in the risk for reported somnolence with ziprasidone was observed in BPD and schizophrenia. Conclusions: Ziprasidone was associated with significant differential adverse effects relative to placebo in BPM, BPD and schizophrenia with no significant difference in weight gain in all three groups. Self-reported somnolence was increased across the three conditions. Subjects with BPM were more vulnerable to EPS than those with BPD or schizophrenia.

Finally, a recent network meta-analysis reported that there is no superiority of any antimanic agent vs. another except for risperidone vs. aripiprazole and valproate. Aripiprazole, olanzapine, quetiapine, risperidone and valproate had less all-cause discontinuation rates than placebo. Sensitivity analysis by drug class indicated similar efficacy profiles for haloperidol, second-generation antipsychotics and mood stabilizers (Yildiz et al. 2014).

Overall, post hoc and meta-analytic studies confirm the superiority of antipsychotics vs. lithium, valproate and carbamazepine both in terms of faster onset of action but also in terms of the overall outcome in the treatment of acute mania. However they also confirmed that this higher efficacy comes with the cost of more frequent adverse events, mainly EPS, weight gain and somnolence. Olanzapine was proven efficacious against mixed episodes, depressive symptoms and psychotic features as well as in rapid cycling patients. Quetiapine was proven efficacious for all YMRS individual items, depressive symptoms and also against psychotic features. Asenapine was confirmed to be efficacious against depressive symptoms. Aripiprazole was found to have no effect in patients aged >55 years but is effective against psychotic symptoms. Ziprasidone was reported to be effective against dysphoric mania. Meta-analytic studies also suggest that combination treatment is superior to monotherapy; however, they did not distinguish between add-on and combination studies and populations. The data of oxcarbazepine were found to be insufficient.

16.2.2 Acute Bipolar Depression

Bipolar depression is not well studied, in spite of the fact that it is the facet of BD responsible for most of the burden of the disease. Until not many years ago, it was mostly considered to be similar in clinical and neurobiological terms with 'endogenous' or 'melancholic' unipolar depression and was treated accordingly. The only reservation was that antidepressants might switch to the manic pole. Therefore, only a limited number of RCTs exist, and the common practice among clinicians is to carry the clinical data and wisdom from the treatment of unipolar to bipolar depression. However the data clearly suggest such an approach to be wrong.

The agents are listed below in a 'historical' sequence with lithium and anticonvulsants first, then antidepressants and finally with antipsychotics on the basis of the year of the first study they were investigated.

16.2.2.1 Monotherapy

A summary of monotherapy data for the treatment of acute bipolar depression is shown in Table 16.4.

16.2.2.1.1 Lithium

In spite of the widely spread belief that lithium is an effective treatment option against bipolar depression, there are no data in support of it. The earlier studies provided some positive data but are difficult to interpret (Mendels 1976; Stokes et al. 1971; Goodwin et al. 1969b, 1972; Greenspan et al. 1970; Noyes and Dempsey 1974; Noyes et al. 1974; Baron et al. 1975; Donnelly et al. 1978; Srisurapanont et al. 1995). There is only one rigorously conducted 8-week RCT (EMBOLDEN I) in 802 bipolar depressed patients (499 BD-I, 303 BD-II) which investigated the efficacy and tolerability of lithium (600–1,800 mg/day; $N=136$) vs. quetiapine (300 mg/day; $N=265$ or 600 mg/day; $N=268$) vs. placebo ($N=133$). The change in the mean MADRS total score at endpoint was not significant for lithium ($p=0.123$), while it was significant concerning both quetiapine groups ($p<0.001$) vs. placebo (−13.6 vs. −15.4 vs. −16.1 vs. −11.8). Quetiapine improved most of the MADRS individual items suggesting an effect on the core depressive symptoms, while lithium improved only 'inner tension' and 'reduced sleep'. A similar picture emerged with the HAM-D and the Hamilton Anxiety Scale. At endpoint, the response rate was not significant for lithium ($p=0.279$), but it was significant for the two quetiapine groups ($p<0.001$) in comparison to placebo (62.5 % vs. 68.6 % vs. 69.6 % vs. 55.8 %) and so were the remission rates (62.5 % vs. 69.8 % vs. 70.3 % vs. 55.0 %). The overall dropout rate was lower in the lithium group (14.4 % vs. 24.5 % vs. 23.5 % vs. 27.8 %), and this was in part due to a lower dropout rate in the lithium group because of adverse events (5.1 % vs. 9.8 % vs. 13.1 % vs. 8.3 %). Concerning the dropout rate due to lack of efficacy, the lithium group had a rate similar to placebo, while the 600 mg quetiapine group had the lowest rate (4.2 % vs. 4.2 % vs. 0.7 % vs. 5.3 %). The most common adverse event with lithium treatment was nausea with lithium. A problem is that in this particular study the mean lithium serum levels were 0.61 mEq/l, with 34.9 % of patients having levels below 0.6 mEq/l, which are lower than the generally recommended. However a further post hoc analysis which included only patients with lithium levels >0.8 mEq/l ($N=34$) reported again no significant difference between lithium and placebo, and the numerical difference (−2.5 point of the MADRS scale) was similar to that of the whole lithium group vs. placebo (−1.8). The difference was not significant in patients who completed the study either. Quetiapine was significantly effective in BD-I but not in BD-II patients. It is unclear whether quetiapine or lithium are effective in rapid cycling patients although there is some signal for lithium (Young et al. 2010). It seems that in spite of these negative findings, it is reasonable to keep lithium in mind as a therapeutic option, and the authors believe the data are inconclusive.

16.2.2.1.2 Valproate

The efficacy and safety of divalproex was tested in an 8-week clinical trial in 25 outpatients with BD-I depression. These patients were randomized to receive either divalproex (rapidly titrated up to 2,500 mg/day, as tolerated, to a target serum level of 50–100 mg/dl; $N=13$) or placebo ($N=12$). Although the sample size was small and the analysis was not the standard, the results suggested that divalproex-treated patients had significant improvement in their depression as this was reflected in the change in HAM-D scores from baseline (−11.5 vs. −6.5; $p=0.002$) and anxiety ratings in comparison to placebo. More patients under divalproex remitted (46 % vs. 25 %). Apart from the small study sample, another limitation of this study was that most patients were male (Davis et al. 2005). Another 6-week small study on 18 acute non-refractory bipolar depressed patients investigated divalproex ER (target dose level 70–90 ng/dl; $N=9$) vs. placebo ($N=9$). The results suggested that the divalproex ER treatment group showed significantly greater reduction in the MADRS scores compared to placebo (−13.6 vs. −1.4; $p=0.003$), and the analysis of individual MADRS items supported an effect of divalproex ER on the core symptoms of depression (Ghaemi et al. 2007).

An exploratory evaluation of the efficacy and safety of divalproex ER with a 6-week trial on 54 mood stabilizer-naïve patients with BD-I ($N=20$) or BD-II ($N=34$), of whom 36 (67 %) were rapid cyclers, randomized them to receive divalproex ER (1,000–2,000 mg/day, serum levels 50–100 mg/ml; $N=26$) or placebo ($N=28$). Divalproex treatment produced statistically significant improvement in MADRS scores compared with placebo from week 1 onward, but this concerned only BD-I patients (−16 vs. −2). The divalproex ER group had significantly higher response (38.5 % vs. 10.7 %) and remission rates (23.1 % vs. 10.7 %). Response and remission appeared at day 38. Treatment effect concerned only BD-I patients. The dropout rate was similar between the two groups (50 % vs. 46.4 %), numerically higher for the divalproex ER group because of adverse events (7.7 % vs. 0 %)

and similar because of lack of efficacy (26.9 % vs. 28.6 %). The most common adverse events related with divalproex ER treatment were nausea, increased appetite, diarrhoea, dry mouth and cramps (Muzina et al. 2010).

A fourth study (Sachs et al. 2001) is not published and can be assessed only through two meta-analyses papers (Bond et al. 2010; Smith et al. 2010). This was an 8-week small study on 43 patients with BD-I ($N=24$) or BD-II ($N=19$), of whom 13 (29 %) were rapid cyclers. These patients were randomized to receive divalproex ER (titrated up to achieve serum levels of 45–95 μg/ml, $N=21$) or placebo ($N=22$). The two groups were similar concerning the improvement in MADRS scores (−9.7 vs. −8.1). The divalproex ER group had significantly higher response (42.9 % vs. 27.3 %) and remission rates (66.6 % vs. 45.5 %). The overall dropout rate was similar between the two groups (30.4 % vs. 36.4 %) and numerically higher for the placebo group because of adverse events (0 % vs. 9.1 %). The authors reported no difference in adverse events between the treatment groups.

Taken together the above, it seems that there are some (though somewhat inconsistent and not sufficient) data, coming from small trials supporting the efficacy of valproate in bipolar depression especially in BD-I patients and on the core symptoms of depression. There is possibly some efficacy against concomitant anxiety and in rapid cycling patients.

16.2.2.1.3 Carbamazepine

Although carbamazepine is considered to be one of the traditional 'mood stabilizers', and a cornerstone for the treatment strategy for many clinicians worldwide, there are only two studies. The first is an old positive small withdrawal study concerning its efficacy against bipolar depression. These authors evaluated carbamazepine (600–1,600 mg/day at blood levels of 8–12 μg/ml) on 13 bipolar depressed patients and reported that 5 of them (38.5 %) had a good to marked response. Three manifested a relapse when placebo substituted carbamazepine. Dizziness, ataxia, clumsiness, drowsiness, slurred speech and diplopia were the most frequent carbamazepine-related adverse events (Ballenger and Post 1980). The second was a 12-week double-blind, randomized, placebo-controlled study from China in 124 patients with acute bipolar depression which were randomized to carbamazepine (300–800 mg/day; $N=49$) vs. carbamazepine plus the herbal Free and Easy Wanderer Plus (FEWP; 36 g/day; $N=50$) vs. placebo ($N=25$). At endpoint patients under carbamazepine plus FEWP showed a significantly greater improvement on HAM-D score vs. both carbamazepine monotherapy and placebo, and the improvement was present already at week 4 (−13.5 vs. −16 vs. −10.6). A similar picture was there concerning the MADRS results. Carbamazepine monotherapy was similar with placebo in terms of HAM-D, and MADRS total score change from baseline and superior to placebo in terms of CGI change. In terms of response rates, carbamazepine plus FEWP was superior to carbamazepine alone, and both were superior to placebo (63.88 % vs. 84.8 % vs. 34.8 %, $p<0.001$). There was a similar dropout rate between the two carbamazepine groups and lower in comparison to placebo (26.5 % vs. 20 % vs. 40 %), and this was also true concerning dropout because of lack of efficacy (6.1 % vs. 6 % vs. 24 %). Depressed and manic patients were pooled for the analysis of adverse events, and the adverse events occurring in over 5 % of the patients in any treatment group were dizziness, laboratory testing abnormality, skin rash, headache, fatigue, blurred vision, somnolence and nausea. Compared to carbamazepine monotherapy, patients in the combination therapy had a lesser incidence of dizziness (18.2 % vs. 7.9 %; $p=0.069$) and fatigue (9.1 % vs. 1.1 %; $p=0.038$). No difference in the incidence of other adverse events was found between the combination therapy and CBZ monotherapy. This study does not support the use of carbamazepine monotherapy against bipolar depression, but it leaves significant doubt (Zhang et al. 2007).

16.2.2.1.4 Lamotrigine

There are five trials which investigate the efficacy and safety of lamotrigine in the treatment of acute bipolar depression (SCA100223/NCT00274677, SCA30924/NCT00056277, SCA40910, SCAA2010 and SCAB2001). One included BD-II patients alone and one a mixed population of BD-I and BD-II patients. All were negative concerning the primary outcome. They showed some benefit on some of the secondary outcomes (Goldsmith et al. 2003; Calabrese et al. 2008).

In one of these studies, 195 outpatients with BD-I depression received fixed dosages of lamotrigine (50 mg/day; $N=66$ or 200 mg/day; $N=63$) or placebo ($N=66$) for 7 weeks. At endpoint there was no difference between groups in terms of change in HAM-D or MADRS scores, but there was a significant improvement for the 200 mg lamotrigine group in several secondary outcomes, and these improvements were seen as early as week 3. The response rate for lamotrigine 200 mg was 51 %, and it was higher than the reported 26 % for placebo. There was no difference in the overall dropout rate between the three groups (35 % vs. 29 % vs. 29 %), in the dropout rate because of adverse events (18 % vs. 16 % vs. 15 %) or because of lack of efficacy (0 % vs. 2 % vs. 3 %). The adverse events and other safety results were similar across treatment groups, with the exception of a higher rate of headache in the lamotrigine groups (Calabrese et al. 1999). In the other studies a flexible dose of 100–400 mg daily was used in one of them and a fixed dose of 200 mg/day in the three others. The trial duration for these studies varied from 7 to 10 weeks. In all of them lamotrigine was well tolerated but did not differ significantly from placebo at endpoint on the primary outcomes (HAM-D or MADRS), and seldom it differed on secondary outcomes (Calabrese et al. 2008). Finally, a small double-blind, randomized study with crossover series of three 6-week monotherapy evaluations compared lamotrigine (500 mg/day) vs. gabapentin (4,800 mg/day) vs. placebo in a mixed unipolar–bipolar population of 31 refractory depressed patients. The response rate according to CGI improvement was 52 % vs. 26 % vs. 23 %; $p=0.031$ (Frye et al. 2000).

Overall the data are negative concerning the efficacy of lamotrigine in bipolar depression although the presence of a weak signal cannot be ruled out.

16.2.2.1.5 Antidepressants

In spite of the fact that antidepressants have an established efficacy against unipolar depression, and this defines them as a class of drugs which includes different kinds of molecules, such a 'class effect' is not present also for bipolar depression (Fountoulakis et al. 2011a). Although the data are problematic, the use of antidepressants is neither encouraged nor prohibited by all treatment algorithms which, however, consistently advise the concomitant use of an antimanic agent. Older placebo-controlled studies were mostly positive but difficult to judge on the basis of modern criteria and needs.

The first was a 6-week study on 59 refractory anergically depressed patients which were randomly assigned to tranylcypromine vs. placebo. At endpoint tranylcypromine was superior to placebo, and the effect was evident since week 1. The authors suggest that these results support the efficacy of tranylcypromine against bipolar depression since anergic depression most typically occurs in primary bipolar and in pseudounipolar affective illnesses (Himmelhoch et al. 1982).

However the first trial was properly conducted, and investigating the acute phase of bipolar depression took part only in 1989. It was a 6-week, double-blind study on 89 patients and compared fluoxetine (20–80 mg/day; $N=30$, of which 11 were receiving also lithium), imipramine (75–300 mg/day; $N=30$, which 5 were receiving also lithium) and placebo ($N=29$, which 6 were receiving also lithium) with bipolar depression. At endpoint there was a significant change in both treatment arms in comparison with placebo in terms of HAM-D score change (−13.9 vs. −9.7 vs. −3.9), and the response rate was 86 % for fluoxetine vs. 57 % for imipramine and 38 % for placebo. Fewer patients under fluoxetine dropped out (43 % vs. 53 % vs. 66 %), and this was also true because of lack of efficacy (7 % vs. 7 % vs. 38 %) and adverse events (7 % vs. 30 % vs. 10 %). The most frequent adverse events were insomnia, nervousness and excessive sweating for fluoxetine and dry mouth for imipramine. The interpretation of the results of this study is complicated by the concomitant use of lithium, especially in the fluoxetine group. Half of the patients on fluoxetine were receiving 80 mg daily, while 65 % under imipramine were receiving 150–300 mg daily (Cohn et al. 1989).

Another 8-week study on 34 depressed patients (32 BP-I and 2 BP-II) utilized fluoxetine monotherapy (10–60 mg/day; $N=8$) vs. olanzapine monotherapy (5–20 mg/day; $N=8$) vs. OFC, that is, olanzapine–fluoxetine combination (10–40 mg/day fluoxetine plus 2.5–15 mg/day olanzapine; $N=9$) and vs. placebo ($N=9$). There were significant reductions over time in mean HAM-D and MADRS ratings for all treatment groups (including the placebo group), but no difference between them. Interestingly, while there was no significant increase in YMRS scores over time in any treatment group, there was a significant reduction in the mean YMRS score in the fluoxetine group ($p=0.008$). This study was underpowered to detect any treatment effect (Amsterdam and Shults 2005a).

A small placebo-controlled crossover study lasting 9 months (on 10 BD-II depressed patients without any previous treatment with any antidepressant, antipsychotic or mood stabilizer drug) suggested that escitalopram (10 mg/day) might be better than placebo as monotherapy for depression. The results suggested that treatment with escitalopram led to a significant improvement in depression severity, lower percentage of days depressed or high and lower percentage of days impaired, in comparison with placebo. There was no indication that escitalopram led to a worsening of illness course. Interestingly there was some signal that escitalopram was beneficial even concerning hypomania (Parker et al. 2006).

The only properly conducted study on a sample of adequate size was an international trial on 740 patients with bipolar depression (478 BD-I and 262 BD-II) which randomized them to receive quetiapine 300 mg/day ($N=245$), quetiapine 600 mg/day ($N=247$), paroxetine 20 mg/day ($N=122$) or placebo ($N=126$) for 8 weeks. The results suggested that both quetiapine groups demonstrated statistically significant improvement in the MADRS score vs. placebo at endpoint, but paroxetine did not (−16.9 vs. −16 vs. −11.9). Also, both quetiapine groups but not the paroxetine group manifested significantly higher response rates (66.8 % vs. 67.2 % vs. 51.1 % vs. 52.9 %); however, only the 600 mg/day quetiapine group manifested a significantly higher remission rate in comparison to placebo (64.6 % vs. 68.5 % vs. 56.8 % vs. 55.4 %). The overall dropout rate was similar in the four groups (34.7 % vs. 35.6 % vs. 37.7 % vs. 39.7 %), and it was numerically higher in the quetiapine and paroxetine groups due to adverse events (8.6 % vs. 12.1 % vs. 12.3 % vs. 7.9 %) and lower in both the quetiapine groups because of lack of efficacy (1.2 % vs. 2 % vs. 4.1 % vs. 4.8 %). Both quetiapine dosages and paroxetine produced a significant improvement in anxiety in terms of change of HAM-A scale score from baseline. Paroxetine had no significant effect on any MADRS item. A sub-analysis suggested that quetiapine was efficacious both in BD-I and in BD-II patients, while paroxetine was not efficacious in any subgroup of patients, not even in non-rapid cycling. The incidence of treatment-emergent mania/hypomania was numerically lower in the quetiapine groups compared with paroxetine and placebo (2.1 % vs. 4.1 % vs. 10.7 % vs. 8.9 %). The most frequent adverse events were dry mouth, sedation, headache, insomnia and nausea with paroxetine treatment (McElroy et al. 2010c).

16.2.2.1.6 Olanzapine

As mentioned above, an 8-week study on 34 bipolar depressed patients which utilized olanzapine monotherapy vs. fluoxetine monotherapy vs. OFC and vs. placebo was underpowered and negative (Amsterdam and Shults 2005a). Also another international 8-week trial (also mentioned above in detail) on 833 BD-I depressed patients which utilized olanzapine vs. OFC or placebo reported a superiority of both treatment groups in comparison to placebo in terms of MADRS score reduction as well as a longer time to treatment discontinuation. However, the analysis of individual MADRS items suggested that the OFC had an effect on the core symptoms of depression, while this was not the case for olanzapine monotherapy (Tohen et al. 2003c). It is widely accepted that when attempting to demonstrate a purely antidepressive effect, the total HAM-D or MADRS scores are not appropriate; instead subscales which include only the 'core items' of depression should be used, like the HAM-D depression factor (Bech 2001; Lecrubier and Bech 2007). To answer this question, another trial was conducted, on 514 patients with bipolar depression which were allocated to receive olanzapine (5–20 mg/day, $N=343$) or placebo ($N=171$) for 6 weeks. The results suggested that olanzapine demonstrated a significantly greater improvement on the MADRS (−13.8 vs. −11.67; $p=0.018$), the HAM-D and the YMRS scores. There was significantly higher response (52.5 % vs.

43.3 %; $p=0.049$) and remission rates (38.5 % vs. 29.2 %; $p=0.038$) for the olanzapine group in comparison to placebo. The response was evident since week 2. The analysis of individual MADRS items and the MADRS-6 subscale did not show an effect of olanzapine on the 'core' of depressive symptoms according to LOCF analysis, but on the contrary MMRM analysis showed a significant effect. The overall dropout rate was similar in the two groups (22.2 % vs. 28.7 %), and this was also true concerning dropout because of adverse events (8.7 % vs. 7.6 %) but not because of lack of efficacy (1.7 % vs. 7.6 %). Olanzapine caused significantly greater mean increases in weight, fasting cholesterol and triglycerides ($p<0.01$), and significantly more patients gained at least 7 % in body weight ($p<0.001$) (Tohen et al. 2012).

16.2.2.1.7 Quetiapine

The first trial on quetiapine in bipolar depression included 542 outpatients (BD-I, $N=360$; BD-II, $N=182$; 20 % rapid cycling) which were randomly assigned to 8 weeks of quetiapine (300 mg/day; $N=181$ or 600 mg/day; $N=180$) or placebo ($N=181$). Both quetiapine groups demonstrated statistically significant improvement in the MADRS score vs. placebo at endpoint (−16.4 vs. −16.7 vs. −10.3; $p<0.001$), and this was evident since week 1. The response rate was in favour of the quetiapine groups (57.6 % vs. 58.2 % vs. 36.1 %; $p<0.001$) and so was the remission rate (52.9 % in the quetiapine groups vs. 28.4 % for placebo; $p<0.001$). The overall dropout rate was similar in the three groups (33.3 % vs. 45.5 % vs. 40.9 %), numerically higher in the quetiapine groups due to adverse events (16 % vs. 26.1 % vs. 8.8 %) and lower because of lack of efficacy (2.2 % vs. 1.7 % vs. 13.3 %). Both quetiapine dosages produced a significant improvement in anxiety in terms of change of HAM-A scale from baseline. Both quetiapine dosages improved the core symptoms of depression; however, sub-analysis suggested that quetiapine was efficacious only in BD-I and not in BD-II patients but both in rapid and non-rapid cycling patients. Treatment-emergent mania rates were low and similar for all groups (3.2 % vs. 3.9 %). The most common quetiapine related adverse events were dry mouth, somnolence, dizziness and sedation (Calabrese et al. 2005a). A second study included 509 bipolar depressed outpatients (BD-I, $N=338$; BD-II, $N=171$; 30 % rapid cycling) which were randomly assigned to 8 weeks of quetiapine (300 mg/day; $N=172$ or 600 mg/day; $N=169$) or placebo ($N=162$). Both quetiapine groups demonstrated statistically significant improvement in the MADRS score vs. placebo at endpoint (−16.9 vs. −16 vs. −11.9; $p<0.001$), and this was evident since week 1. The response rate was in favour of the quetiapine groups (60 % vs. 58.3 % vs. 44.7 %; $p<0.05$) and so was the remission rates (51.6 % vs. 52.35 vs. 37.3 %, $p<0.05$). The overall dropout rate was similar in the three groups (41.3 % vs. 46.7 % vs. 34.5 %), numerically higher in the quetiapine groups due to adverse events (8.1 % vs. 11.2 % vs. 1.2 %) and lower because of and lack of efficacy (1.7 % vs. 2.9 % vs. 7.7 %). Both quetiapine dosages produced a significant improvement in anxiety in terms of change of HAM-A scale. Both quetiapine dosages improved the core symptoms of depression, and sub-analysis suggested that quetiapine was efficacious both in BD-I and in BD-II patients and also in rapid and non-rapid cycling patients. Treatment-emergent mania rates were low and similar for all groups (2–4 % vs. 7 %). The most common quetiapine-related adverse events were dry mouth, somnolence, dizziness, sedation and constipation (Thase et al. 2006). A third international study on 740 patients with bipolar depression (478 BD-I and 262 BD-II) randomized them to receive quetiapine 300 mg/day (*N*=245), quetiapine 600 mg/day (*N*=247), paroxetine 20 mg/day (*N*=122) or placebo (*N*=126) for 8 weeks. Both quetiapine groups demonstrated statistically significant improvement in the MADRS score vs. placebo at endpoint, but paroxetine did not (−16.9 vs. −16 vs. −11.9). The improvement was evident since week 2. Both quetiapine groups but not the paroxetine group manifested significantly higher response rates in comparison to placebo (66.8 % vs. 67.2 % vs. 51.1 % vs. 52.9 %); however, only the 600 mg/day quetiapine group manifested a significantly higher remission rate (64.6 % vs. 68.5 % vs. 56.8 % vs. 55.4 %). The overall dropout rate was similar in the four groups (34.7 % vs. 35.6 % vs. 37.7 % vs. 39.7 %), numerically higher in the quetiapine and paroxetine groups due to adverse events (8.6 % vs. 12.1 % vs. 12.3 % vs. 7.9 %) and lower in the quetiapine groups because of lack of efficacy (1.2 % vs. 2 % vs. 4.1 % vs. 4.8 %). Both quetiapine dosages and paroxetine produced a significant improvement in anxiety in terms of change of HAM-A scale from baseline. Quetiapine 600 mg/day improved the core symptoms of depression, while this was equivocal for the 300 mg/day dosage. Paroxetine had no significant effect on any MADRS item. A sub-analysis suggested that quetiapine was efficacious both in BD-I and in BD-II patients, while paroxetine was not efficacious in any subgroup of patients, not even in non-rapid cycling. The incidence of treatment-emergent mania/hypomania was numerically lower with quetiapine compared with paroxetine and placebo (2.1 % vs. 4.1 % vs. 10.7 % vs. 8.9 %). The most frequent adverse events with both dosages of quetiapine treatment were dry mouth, somnolence, sedation and dizziness (McElroy et al. 2010c). Another 8-week study in 802 bipolar depressive patients (499 BD-I, 303 BD-II) investigated the efficacy and tolerability of quetiapine (300 mg/day; *N*=265 or 600 mg/day; *N*=268) vs. lithium (600–1,800 mg/day; *N*=136) and vs. placebo (*N*=133). The change in the mean MADRS total score at endpoint (−15.4 vs. −16.1 vs. −13.6 vs. −11.8) was significant concerning both quetiapine groups ($p<0.001$) vs. placebo, but it was not significant for lithium ($p=0.123$). Quetiapine improved most of the MADRS individual items suggesting the presence of an effect on the core depressive symptoms. A similar picture emerged with the HAM-D and the HAM-A. At endpoint, the response rate (68.6 % vs. 69.6 % vs. 62.5 % vs. 55.8 %) was significant for the two quetiapine groups ($p<0.05$ and <0.01) but not for lithium ($p=0.279$) in comparison to placebo and so were the remission rates (69.8 % vs. 70.3 % vs. 62.5 % vs. 55.0 %). The overall dropout rate in the quetiapine groups was similar to placebo but numerically higher of the dropout of the lithium group (24.5 % vs. 23.5 % vs. 14.4 % vs. 27.8 %), and this was in part due to a lower dropout rate in the lithium group because of adverse events (9.8 % vs. 13.1 % vs. 5.1 % vs. 8.3 %). The 600 mg quetiapine group had the lowest rate of dropout rate due to lack of efficacy (4.2 % vs. 0.7 % vs. 4.2 % vs. 5.3 %). The most common adverse events for both quetiapine groups were somnolence, dry mouth and dizziness. Quetiapine was significantly effective in BD-I but not in BD-II patients. It is unclear whether quetiapine or lithium was effective in rapid cycling patients although there is some signal for lithium (Young et al. 2010). Finally, another study utilized 277 bipolar depressed outpatients (80 % BD-I; 27.4 % rapid cycling) which were randomly assigned to 8 weeks of quetiapine XR (300 mg/day, $N=139$) or placebo ($N=138$). The quetiapine XR group demonstrated statistically significant improvement in the MADRS score vs. placebo at endpoint (−17.4 vs. −11.9; $p<0.001$). The response rate was in favour of the quetiapine XR group (65.4 % vs. 43.1 %; $p<0.001$), and this was evident since week 2. Also significantly different was the remission rate (54.1 % vs. 39.4 %, $p=0.02$). The overall dropout rate was similar in the two groups (37.4 % vs. 30.4 %), numerically higher in the quetiapine XR group due to adverse events (12.2 % vs. 1.4 %) and lower because of and lack of efficacy (1.4 % vs. 7.2 %). Quetiapine XR improved the core symptoms of depression, and MMRM sub-analysis suggested that quetiapine XR was efficacious both in BD-I and in BD-II patients and also in rapid and non-rapid cycling patients. Treatment-emergent mania rates were low and similar in the two groups (4.4 % vs. 6.4 %). The most common quetiapine XR-related adverse events were dry mouth, somnolence, sedation and increased appetite (Suppes et al. 2010).

Overall, in five studies, all of whom were positive, quetiapine IR or XR is reported to be efficacious at dosages of 300 and 600 mg/day and produced response and remission rates approximately 20 % higher than placebo. It is important that quetiapine had a similar efficacy in BD-I and BD-II patients as well as in rapid cycling, and it significantly improved all the MADRS items corresponding to the core symptoms of depression and also improved concomitant anxiety.

16.2.2.1.8 Aripiprazole

Two identically designed, 8-week, multicentre, randomized, double-blind, placebo-controlled studies (CN138-096 and CN138-146) to evaluate the efficacy and safety of aripiprazole monotherapy in depressed BD-I outpatients without psychotic features were both negative for aripiprazole. Patients were randomized to receive aripiprazole (5–30 mg/day; $N=186$ and $N=187$) or placebo ($N=188$ and $N=188$). In both studies, although statistically significant differences were observed concerning the change in the MADRS score during weeks 1–6, aripiprazole did not achieve statistical significance vs. placebo at endpoint in either study (−11.9 and −12.3 vs. −10.6 and −11.5). The dropout rate was higher in the aripiprazole group in comparison to placebo (46.8 % and 41.2 % vs. 35.1 % and 29.8 %), and this was also the case due to adverse events (16.7 % and 10.2 % vs. 7.4 % and 5.3 %) but not because of lack of efficacy (3.2 % and 5.3 % vs. 8.5 % and 5.9 %). Treatment-emergent mania was similar in the two groups (3.9 % and 2.2 % vs. 2.2 % and 1.1 %). Treatment with aripiprazole was associated with a higher incidence of akathisia, insomnia, nausea, fatigue, restlessness and dry mouth vs. placebo (Thase et al. 2008). It has been argued that the failure of these two trials was due to the 'catching up' of the placebo group after week 6 rather than because of a lack of efficacy of aripiprazole. The fact is that at endpoint the placebo response in terms of MADRS score change in the aripiprazole studies (−10.6 and −11.5) is similar to what was observed also in the quetiapine studies (from −10.3 to −11.9), while the aripiprazole response (−11.9 and −12.3) is clearly lower to the response observed with quetiapine (from −15.4 to −17.4).

16.2.2.1.9 Ziprasidone

There are two negative unpublished trials concerning ziprasidone (Lombardo et al. 2012). The first was a 6-week, multicentre US study which utilized a fixed-flexible dose and evaluated the efficacy and safety of ziprasidone in 504 depressed outpatients with BD-I. Patients were randomized to ziprasidone (40–80 mg/day; $N=165$ or 120–160 mg/day; $N=171$) or placebo ($N=168$). The results suggested no difference between study groups in terms of change in MADRS score from baseline (−14.8 vs. −13.8 vs. −13.3) or in the response rates (53 % vs. 46 % vs. 49 %). The dropout rate was similar between groups (35.8 % vs. 43 % vs. 32.8 %), numerically higher for the ziprasidone groups due to adverse events (9.78 % vs. 14 % vs. 5.4 %) and also due to lack of efficacy (4.2 % vs. 4.1 % vs. 1.8 %) (NCT00141271). The second was also a 6-week, multicentre US study which again utilized a fixed-flexible dose and evaluated the efficacy and safety of ziprasidone in 392 depressed outpatients with BD-I. Patients were randomized to ziprasidone (40–160 mg/day; $N=192$) or placebo ($N=200$). Again the results suggested no difference between study groups in terms of change in MADRS score (−14.9 vs. −13.2) from baseline or response rates (53 % vs. 51 %). The dropout rate was similar between groups (38 % vs. 31 %) (NCT00282464).

16.2.2.1.10 Lurasidone

One 6-week trial on 335 bipolar depressed patients without psychotic features which were randomly assigned to receive lurasidone (20–60 mg/day; $N=166$ or 80–120 mg/day; $N=169$) or placebo ($N=170$) reported that both lurasidone dosages significantly reduced the MADRS total scores at endpoint (−15.4 and −15.4 vs. −10.7). Lurasidone had an effect on the core symptoms of depression. Both lurasidone groups also experienced significant improvements compared with placebo in anxiety symptoms and in patient-reported measures of quality of life and functional impairment. Discontinuation rates were similar in the three groups (25.9 % vs. 26.6 % vs. 25.3 %), and this was true also due to adverse events (6.6 % vs. 5.9 % vs. 6.5 %). Dropout because of lack of efficacy was lower in the 80–120 mg/day lurasidone group (7.2 % vs. 3 % vs. 7.6 %). More patients in the lurasidone groups were experiencing response (53 % vs. 51 % vs. 30 %; $p<0.001$) and remission (42 % vs. 40 % vs. 25 %; $p<0.01$) at endpoint. The most frequent adverse events associated with lurasidone were nausea, headache, akathisia and somnolence. Minimal changes in weight, lipids and measures of glycaemic control were observed with lurasidone (Loebel et al. 2013). Although this was a 6-week study and given the negative findings at endpoint (week 8) for aripiprazole while the data was positive at week 6, one should be cautions concerning the interpretation of the lurasidone data. However the magnitude of improvement and the absolute values of lurasidone- and placebo-induced change in the MADRS score argue in favour of lurasidone.

16.2.2.1.11 Other Agents and Therapeutic Modalities

There is a small number of early studies on very small samples (Jimerson et al. 1980; Osman et al. 1989; Kastin et al. 1972). A prospective, randomized controlled, multicentre 6-week trial involving 132 bipolar depressive patients resistant to treatment compared ECT vs. algorithm-based pharmacological treatment as usual has been announced (Kessler et al. 2010). No results have been publicized until now. One uncontrolled trial on 220 patients suggested that bipolar depressives respond to ECT in a similar magnitude unipolar depressives do. The study included 170 unipolar and 50 bipolar depressive patients. The response and remission rates and numbers of ECT for both groups were equivalent (Bailine et al. 2010). However another uncontrolled study suggested that BD-I depressed patients respond less well in comparison to BD-II, and in turn BD-II respond less well in comparison to unipolar depressives (Medda et al. 2009).

There is one study on repetitive transcranial magnetic stimulation (rTMS) which included 23 depressed BD patients (12 BP-I, 9 BP-II and 2 BP-I in a mixed state). Patients were randomly assigned to daily left prefrontal rTMS (5 Hz, 110 % motor threshold, 8 s on, 22 s off, over 20 min) vs. placebo each weekday morning for 2 weeks. The results suggested that the two treatment groups were similar in terms of response and mean HAM-D change from baseline over the 2 weeks (Nahas et al. 2003).

16.2.2.1.12 Conclusion of Monotherapy Trials for the Treatment of Acute Bipolar Depression

The data are clearly negative for lithium even at high serum concentration levels and also for lamotrigine, while there are some (though somewhat inconsistent and not sufficient) positive data concerning valproate. They are equivocal for carbamazepine. Antidepressants as a class do not have an established efficacy against bipolar depression. Older placebo-controlled studies were somewhat positive but difficult to judge on the basis of modern criteria and needs. There are some inconclusive data concerning escitalopram and fluoxetine monotherapy, while the data are clearly negative for paroxetine. Quetiapine and lurasidone have positive data with a clear beneficial effect on the core depressive symptoms, while the evidence is negative concerning aripiprazole and ziprasidone. Olanzapine monotherapy might work against bipolar depression but probably without an effect on the 'core' of depressive symptoms.

Quetiapine, lurasidone and maybe valproate have some positive efficacy against concomitant anxiety as well. This is true also for paroxetine which seems to improve concomitant anxiety independently of its lack of effect on depression.

16.2.2.2 Comparison of Treatment Options

Since only a limited number of options for the treatment of bipolar depression exist, comparison studies are limited, and often they compare agents with unproven efficacy.

Some early studies were too small and with problems in methodology (Kessell and Holt 1975; Coppen et al. 1972; Aberg-Wistedt 1982).

The first properly conducted comparison trial was a 6-week, double-blind study on 89 patients with bipolar depression and compared fluoxetine (20–80 mg/day; $N=30$, 11 receiving also lithium), imipramine (75–300 mg/day; $N=30$, 5 receiving also lithium) and placebo ($N=29$, 6 receiving also lithium). At endpoint there was a significant change in both treatment arms in comparison to placebo in terms of HAM-D score change from baseline (−13.9 vs. −9.7 vs. −3.9), and the response rate was 86 % for fluoxetine vs. 57 % for imipramine and 38 % for placebo. Fewer patients under fluoxetine dropped out (43 % vs. 53 % vs. 66 %), and this was also true because of lack of efficacy (7 % vs. 7 % vs. 38 %) and adverse events (7 % vs. 30 % vs. 10 %). The most frequent adverse events were insomnia, nervousness and excessive sweating for fluoxetine and dry mouth for imipramine. The interpretation of the results of this study is complicated by the concomitant use of lithium especially in the fluoxetine group. Half of the patients on fluoxetine were receiving 80 mg daily, while 65 % under imipramine were receiving 150–300 mg daily (Cohn et al. 1989).

A 4-week multicentre trial compared moclobemide (400–600 mg/day; $N=18$) vs. imipramine (133–200 mg/day; $N=15$) in 33 patients (some receiving also lithium) and reported similar efficacy in both treatment arms with response rates of 53 and 60 %, respectively. Dropout rates were comparable. The number of patients presenting with adverse events, as well as the total number of adverse events, was greater with imipramine (Baumhackl et al. 1989). A small 6-week study on 56 BD-I ($N=24$) and BD-II ($N=32$) (rapid cycling excluded) patients suffering from 'anergic depression' compared the efficacy of tranylcypromine (30–60 mg/day; $N=28$) with that of imipramine (150–300 mg/day; $N=28$). The results suggested that tranylcypromine produced statistically significant superior outcome in terms of greater symptomatic improvement. More patients under tranylcypromine who completed the study responded (81 % vs. 48 %; $p=0.02$), while fewer dropped out (7 % vs. 25 %; $p=0.03$), and the proportion of patients which switched to mania/hypomania was numerically higher in the imipramine group (12 % vs. 24 %). The authors proposed that tranylcypromine had a specific effect on anergia and reversed neurovegetative symptoms. BD-I and BD-II patients had comparable outcomes, but BD-I patients had a significantly greater risk of treatment-emergent mood swings (38 % vs. 13 %; $p=0.03$) (Himmelhoch et al. 1991). A crossover study of nonresponders of the previous study reported that 9 out of 12 patients which were crossed over from imipramine to tranylcypromine responded, but in comparison only 1 out of 4 patients which were switched from tranylcypromine to imipramine responded (Thase et al. 1992).

Another small 6-week study included 16 BD-I depressed patients that were randomly assigned in this double-blind outpatient study to receive either idazoxan (up to 240 mg/day; $N=7$) or bupropion (up to 450 mg/day; $N=9$). The small study sample did not allow the detection of any differences between treatment arms (Grossman et al. 1999). A study compared 15 depressed women with BP-II with 17 women with unipolar depression which were randomized to receive once vs. twice daily venlafaxine monotherapy up to 225 mg for 6 weeks. The results suggested a similar efficacy for venlafaxine in the two diagnostic groups without any episodes of drug-induced hypomania or rapid cycling (Amsterdam and Garcia-Espana 2000).

An 8-week international multicentre study in 156 bipolar depressed patients randomized them to moclobemide (450–750 mg/day; $N=81$) or imipramine (150–250 mg/day; $N=75$). There were no statistically significant differences between the two groups on any efficacy measures or on the dropout rate for any reason. Anticholinergic side effects were three times more common with imipramine than moclobemide, and weight gain was also greater on imipramine. More patients under imipramine switched to mania (3.7 % vs. 11 %) (Silverstone 2001).

As already mentioned above, olanzapine and the OFC were compared vs. placebo in one international 8-week trial on 833 BD-I depressed patients (one-third rapid cycling). These patients were assigned to receive olanzapine (5–20 mg/day; $N=370$) or OFC (6 and 25, 6 and 50 or 12 and 50 mg/day, $N=86$) or placebo ($N=377$). Both treatment groups showed statistically significant improvement in depressive symptoms (MADRS score) vs. the placebo group (−15 vs. −18.5 vs. −11.9; $p<0.001$). The response rate was higher in the two treatment groups in comparison to placebo (39 % vs. 56.1 % vs. 30.4 %), and this was true also for remission rates (32.8 % vs. 48.8 % vs. 24.5 %). Treatment-emergent mania did not differ among groups (5.7 % vs. 6.4 % vs. 6.7 %). The overall dropout rate was in favour of the OFC (51.6 % vs. 36 % vs. 61.5 %), and this was also true concerning the dropout rate due to adverse events (9.2 % vs. 2.3 % vs. 5 %) and due to lack of efficacy (19.7 % vs. 9.3 % vs. 32.1 %). Also the time to discontinuation was significantly longer in the olanzapine and the OFC group. Conclusively the OFC was superior to olanzapine monotherapy, and both were superior to placebo in the treatment of acute bipolar depression. The OFC arm was relatively small (only 86 patients). The analysis of individual MADRS items suggested that the OFC had an effect on the core symptoms of depression, while this was not the case for olanzapine monotherapy (Tohen et al. 2003c). One 7-week trial compared OFC (6/25, 6/50, 12/25 or 12/50 mg/day; $N=205$) vs. lamotrigine (titrated to 150–200 mg/day; $N=205$) in 410 BD-I depressed patients (one-third rapid cyclers). The OFC-treated patients had significantly greater improvement than lamotrigine-treated patients in MADRS score change from baseline (−18.5 vs. −16.4; $p=0.02$). The response rates did not significantly differ between groups (68.8 % vs. 59.7 %; $p=0.073$) and neither did remission rates (56.4 % vs. 49.2 %; $p=0.16$). Time to response was significantly shorter for OFC-treated patients (17 vs. 23 days; $p=0.010$), but not time to remission or time to discontinuation. There was a significantly higher incidence of 'suicidal and self-injurious behaviour' adverse events in the lamotrigine group (0.5 % vs. 3.4 %; $p=0.037$). The dropout rate was similar between treatment groups (33.2 % vs. 34.6 %). Somnolence, increased appetite, dry mouth, sedation, weight gain and tremor occurred more frequently in the OFC group ($p<0.05$), and also weight and total cholesterol and triglyceride levels were significantly elevated in the OFC group ($p<0.001$) (Brown et al. 2006).

The single-blind 6-week comparison of paroxetine ($N=28$) vs. venlafaxine ($N=27$) in 55 bipolar depressed patients which were already receiving mood stabilizers reported no significant differences in either efficacy or safety between the two treatment groups. The change in the HAM-D total score from baseline (−6.9 vs. −9), the response (43 % vs. 48 %) and the remission rates (42 % vs. 43 %) were similar in the two groups. Also the dropout rate was similar (43 % vs. 50 %), but more patients under paroxetine dropped out because of lack of efficacy (7 % vs. 0 %), while more under venlafaxine dropped out because of switching to mania (3 % vs. 13 %). The adverse effect profile was similar between groups. There was no difference between BD-I and BD-II patients or between those taking lithium and those taking anticonvulsants (Vieta et al. 2002). The relatively higher risk of treatment-emergent affective switches with venlafaxine compared to sertraline or bupropion has also been confirmed in an add-on trial (Post et al. 2006).

Overall the comparison data are sparse. They suggest that antidepressants are equal in efficacy but with a different adverse events profile. However the efficacy of antidepressants should be considered in combination with the negative monotherapy data. The frequent use of concomitant mood stabilizers as 'background' medication complicates the interpretation of results. The OFC is superior to olanzapine alone and to lamotrigine and with an effect on the core symptoms of depression. The comparison of paroxetine with venlafaxine suggests a higher switching risk for patients treated with venlafaxine.

16.2.2.3 Combination and Add-On Treatment

A summary of combination treatment data for the treatment of acute bipolar depression is shown in Table 16.5.

16.2.2.3.1 Combination Treatment

There are only three studies of proper methodology and size utilizing a combination treatment. The first was one international 8-week trial on 833 BD-I depressed patients (one-third rapid cycling) which were assigned to receive olanzapine (5–20 mg/day; $N=370$) or OFC (6 and 25, 6 and 50 or 12 and 50 mg/day, $N=86$) or placebo ($N=377$). Both treatment groups showed statistically significant improvement in the depressive symptoms (MADRS score) vs. the placebo group (−15 vs. −18.5 vs. −11.9; $p<0.001$). The response rate was higher in the two treatment groups in comparison to placebo (39 % vs. 56.1 % vs. 30.4 %), and this was true also for remission rates (32.8 % vs. 48.8 % vs. 24.5 %). Treatment-emergent mania did not differ among groups (5.7 % vs. 6.4 % vs. 6.7 %). The dropout rate was in favour of the OFC. This was true concerning the overall dropout rate (51.6 % vs. 36 % vs. 61.5 %), as well as dropout due to adverse events (9.2 % vs. 2.3 % vs. 5 %) and due to lack of efficacy (19.7 % vs. 9.3 % vs. 32.1 %). The time to discontinuation was significantly longer in the olanzapine and the OFC group. That study concluded that the OFC was superior to olanzapine monotherapy, and both were superior to placebo in the treatment of acute bipolar depression. The OFC arm was relatively small (only 86 patients), and this was one of the limitations of the study. Other limitations were that in comparison to placebo and olanzapine, the OFC arm had a lower number of inpatients, less frequent psychotic features, more rapid cycling (possibly higher rates of 'spontaneous remission') and lower number of centres. The analysis of individual MADRS items suggested that the OFC had an effect on the core symptoms of depression, while this was not the case for olanzapine monotherapy (Tohen et al. 2003c).

A second recent double-blind 26-week placebo-controlled study from the USA (STEP-BD) compared the adding of paroxetine (10–40 mg/day; $N=93$) or bupropion (150–375 mg/day; $N=86$) vs. placebo ($N=187$) on a mood stabilizer in 366 bipolar depressed patients (two-thirds BD-I, 29.4 % rapid cycling). The results suggested that the two antidepressant arms did not perform significantly better than placebo after 26 weeks of treatment in terms of recovery rates (23.5 % vs. 27.3 %)

or transient remission (17.9 % vs. 21.4 %). Switch rates were similar (10.1 % vs. 10.7 %) as was the dropout rate (34.1 % vs. 33.7 %) and adverse events (9.5 % vs. 7 %). Modest nonsignificant trends favouring the placebo group were observed across the secondary outcomes. There was no difference between BD-I and BD-II patients (Sachs et al. 2007).

The third was a 12-week double-blind, randomized, placebo-controlled study from China in 124 patients with acute bipolar depression which were randomized to carbamazepine (300–800 mg/day; $N=49$) vs. carbamazepine plus the herbal Free and Easy Wanderer Plus (FEWP; 36 g/day; $N=50$) vs. placebo ($N=25$). At endpoint patients under carbamazepine plus FEWP showed a significantly greater improvement on HAM-D score vs. both carbamazepine monotherapy and placebo, and the improvement was present already at week 4 (−13.5 vs. −16 vs. −10.6). A similar picture was there concerning the MADRS results. In terms of response rates, more patients in the carbamazepine plus FEWP responded both in comparison to carbamazepine monotherapy and in comparison to placebo (63.88 % vs. 84.8 % vs. 34.8 %, $p<0.001$). There was a similar dropout rate between the two carbamazepine groups and lower in comparison to placebo (26.5 % vs. 20 % vs. 40 %), and this was also true concerning the dropout because of lack of efficacy (6.1 % vs. 6 % vs. 24 %). Depressed and manic patients were pooled for the analysis of adverse events, and the adverse events occurring in over 5 % of the patients in any treatment group were dizziness, laboratory testing abnormality, skin rash, headache, fatigue, blurred vision, somnolence and nausea. Compared to carbamazepine monotherapy, patients in the combination therapy had a lesser incidence of dizziness (18.2 % vs. 7.9 %; $p=0.069$) and fatigue (9.1 % vs. 1.1 %; $p=0.038$). No difference in the incidence of other adverse events was found between the combination therapy and CBZ monotherapy. This study supports the use of carbamazepine plus FEWP against bipolar depression. The negative results concerning carbamazepine monotherapy, in combination with the possible dramatic reduction of carbamazepine levels when co-administered with FEWP, plus the unusually high response rate even in the placebo group and the unusually low dropout rate, make conclusions difficult (Zhang et al. 2007).

A small study in 21 patients with BD-II in an acute depressive phase on therapeutic levels of lithium or valproate was randomly assigned to treatment with pramipexole ($N=10$) or placebo ($n=11$) for 6 weeks. All subjects except for one in each group completed the study. There was a superiority of pramipexole in terms of response (60 % vs. 9 %; $p=0.02$). One subject on pramipexole and two on placebo developed hypomanic symptoms (Zarate et al. 2004). Another small study randomized 17 BD depressed patients to receive adjunctive inositol or placebo for 6 weeks on lithium or valproate. The results were numerically in favour of inositol in terms of response rates (44 % vs. 0 %; $p=0.053$) (Eden Evins et al. 2006).

16.2.2.3.2 Add-On Treatment

Add-On Treatment on Lithium

There are a few studies which investigate the efficacy and safety of adding various agents on top of ongoing lithium treatment which was proven inadequate either to treat the acute depressive episode or to prevent its development.

The first properly conducted trial took place only in 1993, and it was a 4-week trial in 30 BD outpatients on maintenance treatment with lithium, suffering from a major depressive recurrence. They were randomized to L-sulpiride (50–75 mg/day; $N=15$) or amitriptyline (50–75 mg/day; $N=15$). L-sulpiride showed equivalent antidepressant activity to amitriptyline at endpoint in terms of HAM-D score change from baseline and in terms of response rate (93 % vs. 86 %). The onset of action was faster in the L-sulpiride group. The adverse events rate was similar in the two groups. Two patients in the amitriptyline group dropped out, and one patient from each group switched to mania or hypomania. The lack of a placebo arm in this trial makes conclusions difficult (Bocchetta et al. 1993).

Another multicentre 10-week study in 117 BD depressed outpatients (rapid cyclers excluded) investigated paroxetine (20–50 mg/day; $N=35$) vs. imipramine (50–300 mg/day; $N=39$) vs. placebo ($N=43$) as add-on to lithium (at least 7 weeks of lithium treatment before entering the study). In addition to lithium monotherapy, patients may have received either carbamazepine or valproate (but not both) in combination with lithium for the control of manic symptoms. The authors stratified patients on the basis of trough serum lithium levels determined at the screening visit (cut-off 0.8 meq/l). At endpoint there was no difference in terms of HAM-D score change in the three groups (−10.2 vs. −11.1 vs. −8.6), and the authors reported that antidepressants were beneficial for patients with low (−10.4 vs. −10.7 vs. 5.8) but not for high levels of lithium. A similar picture was present concerning the response (45.5 % vs. 38.9 % vs. 34.9 %) and remission rates (56.0 % vs. 47.8 % vs. 53.8 %). Compared to imipramine, paroxetine resulted in a lower incidence of adverse events, most notably emergence of manic symptoms (Nemeroff et al. 2001). This particular study has been criticized concerning the way it presented the data and because it puts too much emphasis on a post hoc analysis of the subgroup of patients with low lithium levels (Amsterdam and McHenry 2012).

Another 8-week study from the Netherlands in 124 depressed outpatients with BD (two-thirds BD-I, without psychotic features, severe rapid cycling excluded, 12.9 % rapid cycling) reported that adding lamotrigine (titrated to 200 mg/day; $N=64$) to ongoing lithium treatment (serum levels 0.6–1.2 mmol/l) was better than placebo ($N=60$). At endpoint, the lamotrigine group manifested significantly greater mean change from baseline in the MADRS total score (−15.38 vs. −11.03; $p=0.024$). Also, lamotrigine was effective in the core symptoms of depression. Significantly more patients responded to lamotrigine than to placebo (51.6 % vs. 31.7 %, $p=0.030$). The overall dropout rate was similar in the two groups (18.7 % vs. 15 %), and this was also true because of lack of efficacy (3.1 % vs. 5 %) and adverse events (6.3 % vs. 3.3 %). Switch to mania or hypomania occurred more often in the lamotrigine group, but this was not significant (7.8 % vs. 3.3 %; $p=0.441$) (van der Loos et al. 2009). In the second phase of the previous study, paroxetine 20 mg was added to ongoing treatment in those who were nonresponders after 8 weeks of treatment. After an additional 8-week treatment, the improvement in the two groups (lamotrigine plus lithium plus paroxetine vs. lithium plus paroxetine) was similar, and the difference was not significant. The disappearance of the difference was not due to a further improvement in the group of patients treated previously with lithium plus lamotrigine but in an improvement in the lithium plus placebo group. Thus, the conclusion from this complex series of studies could be that lithium plus paroxetine is effective at least in a subgroup of BD patients which were refractory to lithium monotherapy. Since lithium monotherapy is not efficacious in the treatment of bipolar depression (as shown above in the monotherapy section), it could be assumed (although not entirely supported by the data) that both lamotrigine and paroxetine are effective in the treatment of bipolar depression as add-on to ongoing lithium treatment (van der Loos et al. 2010). However a careful analysis of the results of this series of studies questions whether the therapeutic effect persists beyond week 12 (van der Loos et al. 2010, 2011).

Another 8-week trial on 52 incomplete responders (two-thirds female; 27 BD-I, 25 BD-II) utilized the adding of carbamazepine (600–1,200 mg/day; $N=26$) or oxcarbazepine (600–1,200 mg/day; $N=26$) during maintenance treatment with lithium. Although this trial was on patients in the 'maintenance' phase, the design and the results are more relevant to the acute depressive phase since the study sample included depressed patients. All patients completed the trial. Both groups improved with the addition of either drug, but those receiving oxcarbazepine improved significantly more on their MADRS (−6.1 vs. −12.2; $p<0.001$) and HAM-D scores at endpoint (Juruena et al. 2009).

Finally, a 6-week double-blind study investigated the efficacy and safety of antidepressant augmentation in 42 bipolar patients under lithium maintenance treatment who were suffering from a breakthrough episode of major depression. These patients were randomly assigned to receive paroxetine (20–40 mg/day; $N=19$) or amitriptyline (75–150 mg/day; $N=23$). At the end of the study, there was no difference between study groups in terms of HAM-D score change from baseline (−14.9 vs. −15.5 $p=0.798$) or in response, remission or dropout rates. No effect of lithium levels on antidepressant efficacy was found (Bauer et al. 1999; Pilhatsch et al. 2010).

Overall, the data suggest that in bipolar depressed patients who experience depression while under lithium treatment, it is appropriate to add lamotrigine or oxcarbazepine but not imipramine. The data on adding paroxetine are equivocal.

Add-On Treatment on Lithium or Valproate

A 6-week study in 27 depressed outpatients (9 men and 18 women) with bipolar disorder (BD-I, $N=11$; BD-II, $N=16$) without psychotic features, being treated with lithium or divalproex, tried to clarify the appropriate treatment strategy by comparing the addition of paroxetine ($N=11$) vs. a second mood stabilizer ($N=16$). Although there was a numerically greater improvement in the combined mood stabilizers group concerning the change in the HAM-D score (−14 vs. −9), this was not significant. There were significantly more dropouts in the combined mood stabilizers group (Young et al. 2000).

One of the most interesting recent trials was single centred and utilized a randomized, placebo-controlled, double-blind, crossover design. It included 18 refractory bipolar depressed patients (44 % BD-I) without psychotic features who were maintained at therapeutic levels of lithium or valproate. These patients received an intravenous infusion of either ketamine hydrochloride (0.5 mg/kg) or placebo on 2 test days 2 weeks apart. The MADRS was applied at baseline and at 40, 80, 110 and 230 min and on days 1, 2, 3, 7, 10 and 14 post-infusion. The results suggested that within 40 min, depressive symptoms significantly improved in the ketamine group in comparison to the placebo group (effect size $d = 0.52$). The improvement remained significant through day 3. There was also a significant difference concerning the response rate (71 % vs. 6 %). One patient from each group developed manic symptoms. The most common adverse effect related to ketamine treatment was dissociative symptoms, only at the 40-min point (Diazgranados et al. 2010). A second small double-blind, randomized, crossover, placebo-controlled study on 15 refractory bipolar depressed patients (60 % BD-I, no rapid cycling during the past year) without psychotic features, maintained on therapeutic levels of lithium or valproate, randomized them to receive a single intravenous infusion of either ketamine hydrochloride (0.5 mg/kg) or placebo with a protocol identical to that of the previous study. The results suggested again that within 40 min, depressive symptoms, as well as suicidal ideation, significantly improved in the ketamine group vs. placebo ($d = 0.89$). The improvement remained significant through day 3. More patients in the ketamine group responded in comparison to placebo (79 % vs. 0 %) at some point during the trial. The most common side effect was dissociative symptoms, which occurred only at the 40-min time point. These results were similar to a previous study and replicated previous findings. In addition, this study reported an effect of ketamine on the suicidal ideation in these patients (Zarate et al. 2012).

The most recent international study was of 6-week duration in 348 BD-I depressed patients without psychotic features and investigated the efficacy of lurasidone (20–120 mg/day; $N = 183$) vs. placebo ($N = 165$) as adjunctive therapy on lithium or valproate. At endpoint, lurasidone was superior to placebo in terms of MADRS score reduction from baseline (−17.1 vs. −13.5; $p = 0.005$). Significantly more patients in the lurasidone group were responders (57 % vs. 42 %; $p = 0.005$), and significantly more achieved remission (50 % vs. 35 %; $p = 0.008$) at endpoint. Adjunctive lurasidone had an effect on the core depressive symptoms, and the overall effect was unrelated to whether the patient was receiving lithium or valproate. Lurasidone exerted a significantly greater improvement in anxiety symptoms and in patient-reported measures of quality of life and functional impairment. The overall dropout rates were similar in the two groups (21.9 % vs. 17.6 %), and this was also true concerning the dropouts because of adverse events (6 % vs. 7.9 %) and lack of efficacy (4.9 % vs. 3 %). The most frequent adverse events related to lurasidone treatment were nausea, somnolence, tremor, akathisia and insomnia. Minimal changes in weight, lipids and measures of glycaemic control were observed during treatment with lurasidone (Loebel et al. 2014).

Overall the data suggest that in BD patients experiencing depression during treatment with lithium or valproate, it would be appropriate to add ketamine or lurasidone. Lurasidone also improves anxiety, and ketamine improves suicidality in these patients. Response to a single ketamine infusion appears within minutes and does not last more than 3 days.

Add-On Treatment on Lithium Plus Other Agents

A small placebo-controlled adjunctive study on 23 BD patients (rapid cycling excluded) of aripiprazole on lithium and citalopram was negative. Before randomization, patients had to be on a constant mood stabilizer treatment with lithium or valproate for at least 1 week. After inclusion, all patients were openly treated with additional citalopram (20–40 mg/day) and with additional aripiprazole (10–30 mg/day; $N=12$) or placebo ($N=11$) for 6 weeks. At endpoint there was no significant difference between the two groups with respect to the HAM-D change or response or dropout rates. However the study was underpowered, and the study sample was too small to detect any differences (Quante et al. 2010).

Add-On Treatment on a Mood Stabilizer

A small 8-week trial on 15 bipolar depressed patients to assess efficacy and rate of treatment-emergent mood elevation in depressed BD patients when bupropion (358 ± 62 mg/day; $N=7$) or desipramine (140 ± 46 mg/day; $N=8$) was added to an ongoing therapeutic regimen of lithium, valproate or carbamazepine reported that there was no difference concerning the acute efficacy between the two drugs. The response rate was similar (63 % vs. 71 %). Switching to mania/hypomania was more frequent in the desipramine group (11 % vs. 50 %; $p=0.01$) (Sachs et al. 1994).

Sixty-four BD patients (one-third BD-II, almost half rapid cycling) with a breakthrough major depressive episode despite ongoing adequately dosed mood stabilizer medication were randomized in a double-blind manner to bupropion (up to 450 mg/day), sertraline (up to 200 mg/day) or venlafaxine (up to 375 mg/day) for 10 weeks. Nonresponders were re-randomized such that there were 95 acute treatment phases. The results suggested that 37 % of the acute treatment phases were associated with a much or very much improved rating in depression, and 14 % were associated with switches. No comparisons between agents were reported by this study (Post et al. 2001).

A 12-week small study on 30 BD nonpsychotic depressed patients who were receiving a stable dose of a mood stabilizer investigated the efficacy and safety of add-on risperidone (1–4 mg/day; $N=10$) vs. paroxetine (20–40 mg/day; $N=10$) vs. the combination of risperidone and paroxetine ($N=10$). There was no difference in the HAM-D score change between the three groups (–5.2 vs. −5.6 vs. −6.3), and this was true also concerning the MADRS score change. There was a significant improvement of the combination group in comparison to the paroxetine group in terms of YMRS score change, but the switch rate into mania or hypomania was very low, with only one patient in the paroxetine plus placebo condition experiencing mild hypomania. More patients in the risperidone groups dropped out in comparison to the paroxetine group (Shelton and Stahl 2004).

Another 10-week trial in 174 BD (26 % BD-II; 27 % rapid cycling) depressed patients (stratified for rapid cycling) examined the relative acute effects of bupropion (75–450 mg/day; $N=51$), sertraline (50–200 mg/day; $N=58$) and venlafaxine (37.5–375 mg/day; $N=65$) as adjuncts to ongoing mood stabilizers. The response (49 % vs. 53 % vs. 51 %) and the remission rate (41 % vs. 36 % vs. 34 %) were similar in the three groups, and the specific combination with lithium vs. other mood stabilizers did not alter the results. The dropout rate was numerically higher in the venlafaxine group (31 % vs. 41 % vs. 45 %), and this was also true for reasons of lack of efficacy or worsening of mood (29 % vs. 28 % vs. 38 %). There was a significantly increased risk of switches into hypomania or mania in the venlafaxine group (10 % vs. 9 % vs. 29 %; $p=0.002$). This was true for rapid cycling (0 % vs. 8 % vs. 29 %; $p<0.01$) but not non-rapid cycling patients (7 % vs. 6 % vs. 12 %; $p=0.55$) (Post et al. 2006).

A 12-week pilot trial in 20 BD depressed patients (85 % females, 60 % BD-I, 20 % rapid cycling) without psychotic features investigated the addition of lamotrigine (50–200 mg/day; $N=10$) vs. citalopram (10–30 mg/day; $N=10$) on ongoing treatment with a mood stabilizer. At endpoint there was no difference between the treatment groups in the MADRS score change from baseline (−13.3 vs. −14.2; $p=0.78$). There was a numerical but not significant difference in both the response (45 % vs. 60 %) and the remission (35 % vs. 60 %) rates at endpoint in favour of citalopram. Switching to hypomania occurred in 10 % of patients in each group (Schaffer et al. 2006).

A 10-week trial with three treatment cycles on 174 bipolar depressed patients randomized them to receive bupropion, sertraline or venlafaxine on top of their ongoing mood stabilizer. Each cycle included shift to treatment with another one from the three antidepressants. Half of the patients responded at the endpoint of the first treatment cycle, but only a few additional responded during the subsequent treatment cycles (Altshuler et al. 2009).

The small 6-week study in 32 BD depressed patients (71.9 % BD-I, 21.9 % rapid cycling) compared levetiracetam (up to 2,500 mg/day; $N=17$) vs. placebo ($N=15$) as adjunctive treatment to their ongoing medication. There was no significant difference between the two treatment groups in terms of MADRS score change from baseline; however, there was a numerical superiority of the placebo group. Also significantly more patients in the placebo group remitted (0 % vs. 23 %; $p=0.02$). More patients in the levetiracetam group dropped out (41.2 % vs. 26.6 %). This is the only study showing some kind of superiority of placebo vs. the active drug, thus suggesting that levetiracetam might in fact worsen depression in BD patients (Saricicek et al. 2010).

Finally, an international study included 298 depressed BD-I patients without psychotic features and assessed the efficacy and safety of ziprasidone (40–160 mg/day; $N=147$) vs. placebo ($N=147$) as adjunct therapy to an ongoing treatment with lithium, lamotrigine or valproate. At endpoint there was no difference between groups in terms of MADRS total score change for baseline (−13.2 vs. −12.9; $p=0.792$). More patients under ziprasidone dropped out (40.1 % vs. 29.3 %), and this was also true concerning dropout because of adverse events (17 % vs. 9.5 %) but not because of lack of efficacy (2.7 % vs. 5.4 %). A quality analysis suggested that although poor quality data might confuse the results, this was not a causal factor for the negative findings of the study. More patients under ziprasidone reported the emergence of adverse events (72.8 % vs. 46.9 %). The presence of mixed features and the specific co-administered mood stabilizer had no effect on the results (Sachs et al. 2011).

Overall the data on the options to treat BD patients who experience a depressed episode during treatment with mood stabilizers in general suggest that it is not appropriate to add ziprasidone, and levetiracetam should be avoided because there is a risk to worsen depression. Imipramine and venlafaxine might pose the patients at an increased risk of switching to the opposite pole without any visible therapeutic benefits in comparison to other antidepressants.

Add-On Treatment on Lamotrigine

An 8-week study in 29 BD depressed outpatients (62 % BD-I) on a stable dose of lamotrigine (100 mg or more) randomized them to receive either memantine (20 mg/day; *N*=14) or placebo (*N*=15). The results revealed no difference between the two treatment groups at endpoint (Anand et al. 2012).

Add-On Treatment on ECT

A pilot study on 16 BD refractory depressed patients referred for ECT treatment randomized them to thiopental alone (*N*=8) or thiopental plus ketamine (0.5 mg/kg; *N*=8) for anaesthesia before each ECT session. The results of this pilot suggest that ketamine, at a dose of 0.5 mg/kg, given just before ECT, did not enhance the antidepressant effect of ECT (Abdallah et al. 2012).

Other Add-On Options

Another placebo-controlled study on 85 bipolar depressive patients of adjunctive modafinil (177 mg/day) has been shown to improve the outcome of bipolar depression without switching to mania or hypomania. Both the response and remission rates were significantly higher in the modafinil group (44 and 39 %) compared with the placebo group (23 and 18 %) (Frye et al. 2007). Although that study did not report a higher risk for manic switches, it has been reported that modafinil could cause subclinical switches (Fountoulakis et al. 2008b). Also the proof of concept study for the treatment of acute BD-I depression for adjunct armodafinil (the longer-lasting isomer of modafinil; dosage 150 mg/day; *N*=128) on lithium, valproate or olanzapine was positive (Calabrese et al. 2010). The investigation of celecoxib (400 mg/day) did not support its efficacy as an adjunct in the treatment of depressive or mixed episodes (Nery et al. 2008).

Some data support the usefulness of omega-3 fatty acids as adjunctive therapy in bipolar depression but not mania, but the data are conflicting and inconclusive (Sarris et al. 2012; Frangou et al. 2006, 2007; Keck et al. 2006b; Chiu et al. 2005; Stoll et al. 1999; Murphy et al. 2012; Sylvia et al. 2013).

Although there is a wide consensus on the usefulness of ECT both against acute mania and acute bipolar depression and in refractory cases, controlled hard data are lacking (Loo et al. 2010). Another useful tool could be transcranial magnetic stimulation (TMS); however, it has been poorly investigated in bipolar depression (Dell'Osso et al. 2009). Sleep deprivation and other noninvasive circadian-related interventions could be useful add-on treatment in order to accelerate and sustain the antidepressant response (Wu et al. 2009). One study on bright light therapy in bipolar depression was negative (Dauphinais et al. 2012).

16.2.2.3.3 Conclusions Concerning Combination Treatment and Add-On Treatment

Taken together, the above-mentioned trials suggest that only the OFC has solid scientific support concerning its efficacy against acute bipolar depression. Combination treatment with paroxetine or bupropion with a mood stabilizer does not improve the outcome. In BD depressed patients who experience depression while under lithium treatment, it is appropriate to add lamotrigine, oxcarbazepine, ketamine or lurasidone but not imipramine. The data on adding paroxetine are equivocal. In BD patients experiencing depression during treatment with valproate, it would be appropriate to add ketamine or lurasidone. In these patients, lurasidone improves also anxiety and ketamine improves suicidality. The data are also negative concerning the adding of memantine on lamotrigine and ketamine simultaneously with ECT.

Overall the data on the options to treat BD patients who experience a depressed episode during treatment with mood stabilizers in general suggest that it is not appropriate to add ziprasidone. Levetiracetam should be avoided because there is a risk to worsen depression. Imipramine and venlafaxine might pose the patients at an increased risk of switching to the opposite pole without any visible therapeutic benefit in comparison to other antidepressants.

16.2.2.4 Post Hoc Review and Meta-analytic Studies

16.2.2.4.1 Post Hoc Studies

Olanzapine and OFC

A post hoc analysis of the OFC and olanzapine data (Tohen et al. 2003c) reported that in comparison to placebo, the olanzapine-treated patients exhibited statistically significant greater improvements on SF-36 mental component summary (MCS) score and on 3 out of 8 SF-36 dimension scores (mental health, role-emotional and social functioning). The OFC-treated patients exhibited statistically greater improvements on MCS score and on 5 out of 8 SF-36 dimension scores (general health perception, mental health, role-emotional, social functioning and vitality), as well as on QLDS total score vs. both placebo and olanzapine. These results suggest that patients with bipolar depression receiving olanzapine or OFC for 8 weeks had greater improvement in health-related quality of life than those receiving placebo, and additionally OFC treatment is superior to olanzapine alone (Shi et al. 2004a). A second post hoc analysis of the same data set data (Tohen et al. 2003c) reported that the beneficial effect was already present since day 7. A number of alternative methods of analysis of the data (pattern analysis, survival analysis and mixed-effects regression analysis) confirmed the superiority of both olanzapine and OFC vs. placebo (Dube et al. 2007). A sub-analysis of Japanese subpopulation from the second olanzapine study (Tohen et al. 2012) further supported the efficacy of olanzapine in the treatment of bipolar depression (Katagiri et al. 2013). A pooled analysis of the two olanzapine studies (Tohen et al. 2003c, 2012) which utilized LOCF data supported the efficacy of olanzapine on the core depressive items (Tohen et al. 2013).

Quetiapine

There are a number of post hoc analyses which utilize data from two individual quetiapine trials. The first one included both of them (Calabrese et al. 2005a; Thase et al. 2006) and confirmed the efficacy of quetiapine as monotherapy, in comparison to placebo, for the treatment of acute depressive episodes in BD-II disorder (Suppes et al. 2008b). Another post hoc analysis of only one of these trials (Calabrese et al.

2005a) concluded that quetiapine significantly improved quality of life in comparison with placebo, which was evident since week 4. Quetiapine treatment also effected a significant improvement in quality of sleep (Endicott et al. 2007). A further post hoc analysis of the same study (Calabrese et al. 2005a) calculated the number needed to treat (NNT) and reported that the NNT was 5 for both response and remission for quetiapine (600 and 300 mg/day) compared with placebo. It also reported that the median time to response and remission were significantly shorter with quetiapine 600 and 300 mg/day than placebo. There was no difference between the treatment groups in the incidence of treatment-emergent mania or hypomania (quetiapine 600 mg/day: 2.2 %, quetiapine 300 mg/day: 3.9 % and placebo: 3.9 %) (Cookson et al. 2007). Another post hoc analysis of both trials (Calabrese et al. 2005a; Thase et al. 2006) which utilized the data only concerning BD-I patients reported that quetiapine was effective in this subset of patients already since week 1 (MADRS score change at endpoint: quetiapine 300 mg/day = −19.4; 600 mg/day = −19.6; placebo = −12.6; $p<0.001$), and the effect sizes were 0.78 and 0.80, respectively. Changes in MADRS were unrelated to reports of sedation and somnolence (Weisler et al. 2008).

Aripiprazole

One post hoc analysis of pooled data from two similarly designed trials who assessed the impact of aripiprazole monotherapy (Thase et al. 2008) classified patients as severely depressed (Bech-6 total score >15) or less severely depressed (Bech-6 total score <15) and reported that at endpoint the mean reduction in the MADRS total score was not significant in the group of severely depressed patients (aripiprazole: −19.4 vs. placebo: −15.4; $p=0.14$) and neither was in the less severely depressed group (−13.8 vs. −10.3; $p=0.07$). The adverse event profiles were similar between the two severity groups (Thase et al. 2012).

Ziprasidone

The post hoc analysis of the two negative unpublished ziprasidone monotherapy trials confirmed that ziprasidone 40–160 mg/day did not show superiority over placebo at week 6 in the treatment of bipolar depression and detected serious inconsistencies in subject rating that may have limited the ability to detect a difference between drug and placebo response. It also reported that ziprasidone was not efficacious in the more or less severely depressed patients (Lombardo et al. 2012).

Antidepressants

A post hoc analysis of a 6-week trial of imipramine, phenelzine or placebo reported that BD-II depressive patients respond in a similar way unipolars do (Agosti and Stewart 2007).

16.2.2.4.2 Review and Meta-analytic Studies

Lamotrigine which was investigated in five RCTs had a disappointingly negative performance, and all of the studies were negative concerning the primary outcome (Amann et al. 2010). However the fact that there was a kind of positive signal in some of the secondary outcomes justified the meta-analysis of the data. According to it, the data from 1,072 patients suggested that lamotrigine was superior to placebo in terms of response (on the basis of HAM-D score change: relative risk (RR) = 1.27, 95 % CI: 1.09–1.47, $p=0.002$). The NNT was 11 (95 % CI: 7–25) on HAM-D and 13 (95 % CI: 7–33) on the MADRS. The remission rates were not statistically significantly higher for lamotrigine on HAM-D (pooled RR = 1.10, 95 % CI: 0.90–1.36, $p=0.060$) but were on MADRS (pooled RR = 1.21, 95 % CI: 1.03–1.42, $p=0.021$). There was a significant change in the MADRS total score from baseline ($p=0.04$) but not in the HAM-D ($p=0.08$). There was no difference in the discontinuation rates either ($p=0.292$). Baseline severity of depression seemed to play a significant role, and lamotrigine was superior to placebo in patients with HAM-D score >24 (RR = 1.47, $p=0.001$) but not in those with HAM-D score < or =24 (RR = 1.07, $p=0.445$). In the severe group, the response rate to lamotrigine was 45.5 % vs. 30.1 % in the placebo group, while in the moderate severity group, the response rate to lamotrigine was 47.5 % vs. 44.6 % in the placebo group. According to these data, the interaction by severity was because of a higher response rate in the placebo group in the moderately ill patients, while the response rate to lamotrigine was independent of severity (Geddes et al. 2009).

Three meta-analyses which were published a later reported that only quetiapine and to a lesser extent olanzapine monotherapy exert efficacy in the treatment of bipolar depression. It also reported negative results for lamotrigine and aripiprazole. Both quetiapine and olanzapine analyses suffered from substantial heterogeneity. These authors also comment that although some early lithium RCTs were positive for bipolar depression, they utilized a small study sample and suffered from a number of methodological shortcomings which limit their usefulness (Tamayo et al. 2010; Cruz et al. 2010; De Fruyt et al. 2011). For aripiprazole, the mean Number Needed to Harm (NNTH) for discontinuation due to adverse events during the treatment of acute bipolar depression was 14 and for olanzapine it was 24, while with quetiapine XR treatment the NNTH appeared to be associated with dose, and it was 9 for the 300 mg/day dosage (Gao et al. 2011). A systematic review of the efficacy and safety of SGAs identified seven published papers on the use of aripiprazole, olanzapine and quetiapine. While the internal validity of the trials was fairly good, the external validity was only moderate. Both clinical heterogeneity of the included trials and statistical heterogeneity of the meta-analytic data were considerable. The data were in favour of quetiapine and to a lesser extent of olanzapine, but they were not in favour of aripiprazole. These authors concluded that the adverse events are a major problem of the use of SGAs with weight gain, akathisia and somnolence/sedation being the most frequent and problematic (De Fruyt et al. 2012).

The stringent criteria used by the previous meta-analyses precluded the inclusion of the valproate trials. These four randomized placebo-controlled trials (6- and 8-week duration) were analysed in two meta-analytical studies. The total study sample was small and included only 142 patients, but the quality of the trials was good. The results suggested that divalproex is efficacious vs. placebo both in terms of response rates (39.3 % vs. 17.5 %) as well as remission rates (40.6 % vs. 24.3 %). The relative risks of response (RR = 2.10, $p=0.02$) and remission (RR = 1.61,

$p = 0.04$) were significantly greater for divalproex in comparison to placebo (Bond et al. 2010). The standardized effect size concerning the change from baseline in the depressive scales was statistically significant (–0.35), but the effect on anxiety symptoms was not. There was no evidence of induction of manic symptoms, and there was no difference in the adverse events rate (Smith et al. 2010). Similarly, the meta-analysis of the two negative aripiprazole studies produced positive results with a standardized effect size equal to 0.17 (Fountoulakis et al. 2011b).

Another meta-analysis focused on depressed patients with BD-II. The authors included studies with different methodology (monotherapy and add-on, with or without placebo, double-blind as well as open and acute together with maintenance studies) and reported that according to their results, quetiapine was judged as having compelling evidence supporting its efficacy, while there was some support for the efficacy of lithium, antidepressants and pramipexole. The data for lamotrigine were equivocal (Swartz and Thase 2011).

The first meta-analysis concerning antidepressants included 12 studies with variable designs and suggested that antidepressants are both effective and safe for bipolar depression (Gijsman et al. 2004). However subsequent analyses on 15 antidepressant trials suggested that antidepressants as a class are no more efficacious than placebo, and they do not increase the risk of switching to the opposite pole (Sidor and Macqueen 2010, 2012). The opposite conclusion has been reported by another more recent analysis which reported that overall there is a positive signal for antidepressants and that the risk for switching to mania is overestimated (Vazquez et al. 2013).

Another meta-analysis on 18 RCTs compared the efficacy, acceptability and safety of mood stabilizer monotherapy with combination and antidepressant treatment. The results suggested that mood stabilizer monotherapy was associated with increased rates of response (RR = 1.30, NNT = 10) and remission (RR = 1.51, NNT = 8) in comparison to placebo. Combination therapy was not statistically superior to monotherapy, and there were no differences between individual medications or drug classes (Van Lieshout and MacQueen 2010). However it is clear that a class effect is not present concerning antidepressants in bipolar depression (Fountoulakis et al. 2011a). Moreover, the utilization of the 'class effect' concept in meta-analytic studies produces erroneous results like 'Mood stabilisers are moderately efficacious' (Van Lieshout and MacQueen 2010).

A recent meta-analysis of data concerning BD-I and BD-II depression suggested that patients who do not respond in the first 2 weeks of treatment are unlikely to respond eventually and would benefit from a change in treatment. It analysed the data from 1,913 patients which had been randomized to aripiprazole, lamotrigine, olanzapine, OFC or quetiapine and from 1,456 which had received placebo. Early improvement predicted response and remission with high sensitivity (86 and 88 %, respectively), but rates of false positives were high (53 and 59 %, respectively). The pooled negative predictive values for response/remission were 74 and 82 %, respectively, with low rates of false negatives (14 and 12 %, respectively). These results suggest that although early improvement does not predict eventual response or remission its absence predicts of eventual nonresponse. Thus clinicians can have an idea when to change treatment because of lack of efficacy during short-term treatment, and 2 weeks seem to be a reasonable time point to consider a change in therapy (Kemp et al. 2010).

Another recent meta-analysis on the efficacy of quetiapine, lamotrigine, paroxetine, lithium, olanzapine, aripiprazole, phenelzine and divalproex included 19 trials and reported that not all medications were associated with symptomatic improvement, with lamotrigine, paroxetine, aripiprazole and lithium not being different from placebo. The highest reductions in MADRS scores vs. placebo were reported for the OFC (–6.6; $p=0.000$) and quetiapine monotherapy (for 300 mg/day, –4.8; $p=0.000$; for 600 mg/day, –4.8; $p=0.000$), with quetiapine monotherapy also showing the highest reduction in HAM-D scores (–4.0; $p=0.000$) (Vieta et al. 2010a). A meta-analysis confirmed the superiority of OFC vs. olanzapine monotherapy (RR = 1.58; 95 % CI: 1.27–1.97) and vs. placebo (RR = 1.99; 95 % CI: 1.49–2.65) but not to lamotrigine; however, the authors noted that these data were of low quality. Similar results were found for remission and relapse rates. No differences were identified for levels of depression and mania symptoms (low-quality evidence) and incidence of mania (moderate-quality evidence). Adverse effects were more common in patients treated with OFC than in those treated with lamotrigine, but no difference was found relative to the patients treated with olanzapine monotherapy (Silva et al. 2013). A systematic review from all antiepileptics supported the use only of divalproex and lamotrigine in the treatment of acute bipolar depression (Reinares et al. 2013).

A meta-analysis which pooled data from nine randomized, double-blind, placebo-controlled, acute studies of ziprasidone including the two unpublished in bipolar depression reported that the discontinuation rate due to adverse events or 7 % or greater weight gain between ziprasidone and placebo was not significant in all psychiatric conditions. In bipolar depression the risk for akathisia with ziprasidone had an NNTH = 44, and reported somnolence had NNTH = 8 which seemed to be dose dependent (Gao et al. 2013).

Two reviews investigated the issue of the treatment of refractory bipolar depression and identified several open but only seven RCTs, of whom two with (ar) modafinil and ECT and one with each ketamine, lamotrigine, pramipexole, inositol and risperidone. Therefore these authors concluded that the available hard data for treatment strategies in resistant bipolar depression is extremely scarce, and most of the strategies remain essentially experimental; however, they seem to be efficacious and promising (Sienaert et al. 2013; Aan Het Rot et al. 2012).

One meta-analysis compared the efficacy of ECT in unipolar vs. bipolar depression and identified six relevant studies. It reported a similar rate of response (50.9 % vs. 53.2 %) (Dierckx et al. 2012).

16.2.3 Maintenance Treatment

16.2.3.1 Monotherapy

A summary of monotherapy data for maintenance treatment is shown in Table 16.6.

16.2.3.1.1 Lithium

There is a number of old small studies which investigated the usefulness of lithium in the maintenance treatment of BD, and all of them reported positive findings concerning the efficacy of lithium. However these studies are problematic not only because the study samples were often mixed and as small as with only 15 (Melia 1970), 18 (Fyro and Petterson 1977), 53 (Fieve et al. 1976) and 24 patients (Cundall et al. 1972) but also because they followed a methodological approach which is no longer considered adequate in psychopharmacology research. Thus, although there are several studies with mixed and small samples and inadequate design (Hullin et al. 1972; Klein et al. 1981; Prien et al. 1973b; Fieve et al. 1976), small non-randomized case-control studies with placebo (Margo and McMahon 1982; Persson 1972), small crossover studies (Mander and Loudon 1988) and discontinuation studies (Post et al. 1992; Baastrup et al. 1970; Small et al. 1971; Christodoulou and Lykouras 1982; Melia 1970; Cundall et al. 1972; Hullin et al. 1972), conclusions are impossible since these trials are difficult to interpret.

Most of these early studies suggested that lithium is efficacious for the prophylaxis against both manic and depressive episodes in both BD-I and BD-II patients (Dunner et al. 1976; Prien et al. 1973a, b; Kane et al. 1982). However in one of them, the efficacy of lithium in the prevention of bipolar depression has been questioned. That study was in 205 BD patients who were hospitalized because of acute mania. It reported that lithium was superior to placebo in preventing relapses, and this was due mainly to the lower incidence of manic relapses in the lithium group (Prien et al. 1973a). Interestingly, in another study a discontinuation-induced refractoriness phenomenon was described for the first time (Post et al. 1992).

The first properly conducted randomized, double-blind, parallel-group multicentre study concerning lithium took part in 2000 and included 372 BD patients who met the inclusion criteria within 3 months of the onset of an index manic episode. These patients were randomized to maintenance treatment with lithium (0.8–1.2 mmol/l; $N=91$), divalproex (75–125 μg/ml; $N=372$) or placebo ($N=94$) for a period of 52 weeks. The patients should have been randomized within 3 months from the onset of the index episode, and they were required to be manic, partially recovered or remitted but not depressed at randomization. They were required to fulfil the inclusion criteria for two subsequent assessments, 6 days apart from each other. The three treatment groups did not differ concerning the time to manifestation of any mood episode, and this was also the case concerning manic or depressive episodes alone. The median times to 50 % survival without a mood episode were 24, 40 and 28 weeks, respectively. The lithium group had higher rates of tremor, thirst and polyuria (Bowden et al. 2000).

Another study utilized an 8–16-week open-label lamotrigine treatment of 349 BD-I patients (rapid cycling excluded, polarity was balanced) with acute mania/hypomania. Other psychotropic drug regimens were discontinued, and 175 patients who responded and maintained a CGI score of 3 or less for 4 consecutive weeks were randomized to lithium (0.8–1.1 mEq/l; $N=46$) or lamotrigine (100–400 mg/day; $N=59$) or placebo ($N=70$) as double-blind maintenance treatment for 18 months. The results suggested that both lithium ($p=0.006$) and lamotrigine ($p=0.02$) were superior to placebo at prolonging the time to intervention for any mood episode. The median survival times were 292, 140 and 85 days, respectively. Lamotrigine was superior to placebo at prolonging the time to a depressive episode, while lithium was superior to placebo at prolonging the time to a manic, hypomanic or mixed episode. The most common adverse event reported for lithium was diarrhoea. The interpretation of this study is complex, because the study sample was enriched for response to lamotrigine, although lamotrigine is not efficacious against acute manic or mixed episodes. Thus, one interpretation could be that the study sample comprised of patients which manifested spontaneous remission (Bowden et al. 2003). A study with a similar design but on 966 BD-I depressed patients (rapid cycling excluded) utilized open-label lamotrigine (titrated to 200 mg/day) for 8–16 weeks during which period concomitant drugs were gradually withdrawn. Those patients who responded and maintained a CGI score of 3 or less for 4 consecutive weeks ($N=463$) were then randomly assigned to lithium (0.8–1.1 mEq/l; $N=121$), lamotrigine (50, 200, or 400 mg/day; $N=221$) or placebo ($N=121$) monotherapy for up to 18 months. The results suggested that the time to intervention for any mood episode was statistically superior ($p=0.029$) for both lithium and lamotrigine vs. placebo. The median survival times were 170, 200 and 93 days, respectively. Lamotrigine was significantly superior to placebo at prolonging the time to intervention for a depressive episode ($p=0.047$) while lithium at prolonging the time to intervention for a manic or hypomanic episode ($p=0.026$). There was no difference in the proportion of patients who were intervention-free for depression (46 % vs. 57 % vs. 45 %) or mania (86 % vs. 77 % vs. 72 %) at 1 year. Headache was the most frequent adverse event for all three treatment groups (Calabrese et al. 2003a).

Also there is one short-term placebo-controlled discontinuation study which assessed the efficacy and safety of lithium for the maintenance treatment of BD in adolescents. Participants with acute mania ($N=100$) received open treatment with lithium at therapeutic serum levels (mean 0.99 mEq/l) for at least 4 weeks. The patients who responded ($N=40$) were randomly assigned to continue ($N=19$) or discontinue lithium ($N=21$) during a 2-week double-blind, placebo-controlled phase. There was no significant difference between the two groups in terms of experiencing a clinically significant symptom exacerbation during the 2-week double-blind phase (52.6 % under lithium vs. 61.9 % under placebo) (Kafantaris et al. 2004).

Finally there is also one recent study (NCT00314184 or trial 144, also named 'SPARCLE') which investigated the efficacy and safety of lithium vs. quetiapine (300–800 mg/day) vs. placebo as maintenance treatment in BD-I. During the open-label phase, 2,438 BD-I patients with a current or recent manic, depressive or mixed episode received open-label quetiapine, and those achieving stabilization ($N=1{,}226$; 50.3 %) were randomized to continue quetiapine or to switch to placebo or lithium (0.6–1.2 mEq/l) for up to 104 weeks in a double-blind trial. The study was terminated early after planned interim analysis provided positive results. The results suggested that the time to recurrence of any mood event was significantly longer for lithium and for quetiapine vs. placebo ($p<0.0001$). Both lithium and quetiapine significantly increased time to recurrence of both manic events and depressive events compared with placebo. Overall rates of adverse events were generally similar between treatment groups (Weisler et al. 2011).

Overall there are four large randomized placebo-controlled studies (plus one small) concerning the efficacy of lithium in the maintenance treatment of BD. One is negative and three are positive. Two positive studies support the usefulness of lithium in the prevention of manic but not depressive episodes irrespective of the polarity of the index episodes. The third study supports its usefulness in the prevention of depressive episodes also. There are some data concerning index mixed episodes, but there are no data supporting the efficacy in the prevention of mixed episodes. There are no specific data concerning rapid cycling patients. The study samples were not enriched for response to lithium and probably contained a significant proportion of patients in spontaneous improvement since lamotrigine is neither active in acute mania nor in acute depression. One study had a sample enriched for response to quetiapine. The design of the studies was somewhat problematic, especially concerning the magnitude of improvement during the acute treatment phase and the duration the patients were stable before entering the double-blind phase.

16.2.3.1.2 Valproate

As mentioned above, there is one properly conducted randomized, double-blind, parallel-group multicentre study concerning valproate. That study included 372 BD patients who met the recovery criteria within 3 months of the onset of an index manic episode. These patients were randomized to maintenance treatment with divalproex (75–125 μg/ml; $N=372$) or lithium (0.8–1.2 mmol/l; $N=91$) or placebo ($N=94$) for a period of 52 weeks. The patients should have been randomized within 3 months from the onset of the index episode, and they were required to be manic, partially recovered or remitted but not depressed at randomization. They were required to fulfil the inclusion criteria for two subsequent assessments, 6 days apart from each other. The three treatment groups did not differ concerning the time to manifestation of any mood episode, and this was also the case concerning manic or depressive episodes alone. The divalproex group had higher rates of tremor, sedation, weight gain and reduction in platelet blood count (Bowden et al. 2000).

This study is the only one available so far concerning the efficacy of valproate. Valproate was the agent under investigation, while lithium served as active control. Taking into consideration the fact that lithium has proven efficacy in the prevention of mood episodes, this should be considered to be a failed study and not negative for valproate.

16.2.3.1.3 Carbamazepine

Similarly, the data are essentially absent for carbamazepine. There is only a small old study with an inadequate design, which applied carbamazepine 200–600 mg/day for 1 year in 32 patients (22 on agent and 10 on placebo). The results suggested that more patients under carbamazepine had a good response in comparison to placebo (60 % vs. 22.2 %), but the difference was not significant because of the small study sample (Okuma et al. 1981).

16.2.3.1.4 Lamotrigine

There are three trials which investigate the efficacy and safety of lamotrigine in the maintenance treatment of BD. In the first study, open-label lamotrigine was added to current treatment of 324 BD patients with rapid cycling bipolar disorder. From those patients, 182 were stabilized. Psychotropics were tapered off, and these patients were randomly assigned to lamotrigine or placebo monotherapy for 6 months. The results suggested that the two treatment groups were similar in terms of time to additional pharmacotherapy, which was the primary outcome. However, survival in the study was statistically different between the treatment groups ($p=0.036$) and also was the median survival time ($p=0.03$), both in favour of the lamotrigine group. More patients under lamotrigine were stable without relapse for 6 months of monotherapy (41 % vs. 26 %; $p=0.03$). There were no treatment-related changes in laboratory parameters, vital signs or body weight, and no serious rashes occurred (Calabrese et al. 2000).

The next two studies both utilized a similar design. The first of them utilized an 8–16-week open-label lamotrigine treatment of 349 patients (rapid cycling excluded) with acute mania/hypomania. Other psychotropic drug regimens were discontinued, and the 175 patients who responded and maintained a CGI score of 3 or less for 4 consecutive weeks were randomized to lamotrigine (100–400 mg/day; $N=59$) or lithium (0.8–1.1 mEq/l; $N=46$) or placebo ($N=70$) as double-blind maintenance treatment for 18 months. The results suggested that both lamotrigine ($p=0.02$) and lithium ($p=0.006$) were superior to placebo at prolonging the time to intervention for any mood episode. Lamotrigine was superior to placebo at prolonging the time to a depressive episode, while lithium was superior to placebo at prolonging the time to a manic, hypomanic or mixed episode. The most common adverse event reported for lamotrigine was headache and diarrhoea for lithium (Bowden et al. 2003). A study with a similar design but on 966 BD-I depressed patients (rapid cycling excluded) utilized open-label lamotrigine (titrated to 200 mg/day) for 8–16 weeks during which period concomitant drugs were gradually withdrawn. Those patients who responded and maintained a CGI score of 3 or less for 4 consecutive weeks ($N=463$) were then randomly assigned to monotherapy with lamotrigine (50, 200 or 400 mg/day; $N=221$), lithium (0.8–1.1 mEq/l; $N=121$) or placebo ($N=121$) for up to 18 months. The results suggested that the time to intervention for any mood episode was statistically superior ($p=0.029$) for both lamotrigine and lithium vs. placebo. The median survival times were 200, 170 and 93 days, respectively. Lamotrigine was statistically superior to placebo at prolonging the time to intervention for a depressive episode ($p=0.047$) while lithium at prolonging the time to intervention for a manic or hypomanic episode ($p=0.026$). There was no difference in the proportion of patients who were intervention-free for depression (46 % vs. 57 % vs. 45 %) or mania (86 % vs. 77 % vs. 72 %) at 1 year. Headache was the most frequent adverse event for all 3 treatment groups (Calabrese et al. 2003a).

Overall there are three randomized placebo-controlled studies concerning the efficacy of lamotrigine in the maintenance treatment of BD and specifically in the prevention of depressive but not of manic episodes. This efficacy was present irrespective of the polarity of the index episodes. There are no data concerning index mixed episodes or features. Although the only study on rapid cycling patients was negative concerning the primary outcome, it provided some positive data concerning the secondary outcomes. Although technically the study samples were enriched for response to lamotrigine, probably they contained a significant proportion of patients in spontaneous improvement since lamotrigine is not efficacious neither in acute mania nor in acute bipolar depression. The design of the studies was somewhat problematic, especially concerning the magnitude of improvement during the acute treatment phase and the duration the patients were stable before entering the double-blind phase.

16.2.3.1.5 Antidepressants

In the first published study, 44 BD patients with an index episode of depression, after remission, were randomly assigned to lithium carbonate, imipramine or placebo for 2 years. The results suggested that imipramine was similar to placebo and inferior to lithium. The difference between treatments was due primarily to depressive episodes; manic episodes occurred infrequently (Prien et al. 1973b). Another early small study on 22 BD-II patients in remission for at least 6 months, which were treated openly with imipramine 150 mg/day, randomly assigned them on a double-blind basis to treatment with lithium, imipramine, lithium carbonate plus imipramine or placebo. Lithium was found to prevent any type of relapse among patients BD-II; however, imipramine was no better than placebo (Kane et al. 1982).

A placebo-controlled study in 839 depressed patients, which investigated the efficacy and safety of short- and long-term fluoxetine treatment, compared in a retrospective way the results concerning patients with BD-II ($n=89$) with those concerning patients with unipolar depression (UP; $N=661$ unmatched and 89 matched). All patients received 12 weeks of open-label 20 mg/day fluoxetine therapy. Complete remission was defined as a total HAM-D score ≤ 7 by week 9 that was then maintained for 3 additional weeks. Remitted patients were then randomly assigned to receive double-blind treatment with one of the following: (1) fluoxetine 20 mg daily for 52 weeks; (2) fluoxetine for 38 weeks, then placebo for 14 weeks; (3) fluoxetine for 14 weeks, then placebo for 38 weeks; or (4) placebo for 52 weeks. The results suggested that fluoxetine had similar efficacy in the two groups during the long-term relapse prevention therapy. More BD-II patients experienced a manic switch, but this was not statistically significant (Amsterdam et al. 1998).

In another trial, 37 BD-II and BD-NOS patients in a depressive episode received open-label fluoxetine monotherapy 20 mg/day for up to 8 weeks. The 12 patients who responded (HAM-D ≤ 9) were randomized to receive continuation therapy with fluoxetine 20 mg/day or placebo for up to 6 months. During the continuation phase, 43 % of fluoxetine-treated patients and 100 % of placebo-treated patients relapsed ($p=0.08$). Fluoxetine-treated patients had a small but significant increase in YMRS score in comparison to placebo (3.0 vs. 0.2; $p=0.01$), but no hypomanic switch episodes were observed. Overall the study sample was too small to permit valid conclusions (Amsterdam and Shults 2005b). Finally, one trial examined the safety and efficacy of long-term (50 weeks) fluoxetine monotherapy (10–40 mg/day; $N=28$) vs. lithium monotherapy (300–1,200 mg/day; $N=26$) and vs. placebo ($N=27$) in the preventing of relapse and recurrence of depressive episodes in BD-II patients. There was a significantly prolonged mean time to relapse in the fluoxetine group in comparison to the others (249.9 days vs. 156.4 days vs. 186.9; $p=0.03$). There were no statistically significant differences in hypomanic symptoms among treatment groups over time (Amsterdam and Shults 2010).

Overall two small old studies were negative concerning the value of imipramine in the prevention of depressive episodes in BD. Three other small studies provide some support for the usefulness of fluoxetine monotherapy in the prevention of depressive episodes in BD-II patients. All studies suffer from methodological problems and are essentially continuation studies.

16.2.3.1.6 Olanzapine

The first trial included 361 BD-I patients with an index manic or mixed episode in at least partial remission for 2 consecutive weekly visits after olanzapine 5–20 mg/day open-label treatment of the acute phase. These patients were randomized to receive olanzapine ($N=225$) or placebo ($N=136$) for up to 48 weeks. The results suggested that the median time to symptomatic relapse into any mood episode was significantly longer among patients receiving olanzapine vs. placebo (174 days vs. 22). The times to symptomatic relapse into manic, depressive and mixed episodes were all significantly longer among patients receiving olanzapine than among patients receiving placebo. The relapse rate to any mood episode was significantly lower in the olanzapine group (46.7 % vs. 80.1 %), and this was also true concerning any type of episode. During olanzapine treatment, the most common emergent event was weight gain. Placebo patients lost a mean of 2.0 kg while in contrast patients in the olanzapine group gained 1.0 kg (Tohen et al. 2006).

A second study on 766 BD-I patients with current manic or mixed episodes (rapid cycling excluded) which were initially randomized to flexibly dosed paliperidone ER (3–12 mg/day; $N=617$) or olanzapine (5–20 mg/day; $N=149$) for a duration of 3-week acute treatment phase. The responders continued the same treatment (12-week continuation phase). Those patients on paliperidone ER who achieved remission during this phase were randomized to fixed-dose paliperidone ER ($N=152$) or placebo ($N=148$), while those on olanzapine continued to receive that at a fixed dose ($N=83$). This maintenance phase continued until at least 140 recurrences occurred among patients originally assigned to paliperidone ER in the acute treatment phase. The median time to recurrence of any mood symptoms was significantly longer for paliperidone vs. placebo (558 vs. 283 days; $p=0.017$) and not observed with olanzapine (<50 % of patients experienced recurrence). Olanzapine-treated patients had significantly longer time to recurrence for any mood symptoms in comparison to either group ($p<0.001$). For paliperidone the difference was significant for preventing recurrence of manic, but not depressive symptoms. This clarification is not reported concerning olanzapine. Treatment-emergent adverse events occurred more often in olanzapine group (64 %) than placebo (59 %) or paliperidone ER groups (55 %) (Berwaerts et al. 2012a).

Finally, one trial utilized a 12-week open-label period with risperidone long-acting injection (RLAI) in 560 patients with manic or mixed episode (rapid cycling excluded). Those who did not experience a recurrence entered an 18-month randomized, double-blind period with oral olanzapine (10 mg/day; $N=131$), RLAI ($N=132$) or placebo ($N=135$). Time to recurrence of any mood episode was significantly longer with olanzapine and RLAI vs. placebo ($p = p<0.001$ and 0.031). Again the difference concerning the time to recurrence was significant for both mania and depression concerning olanzapine ($p<0.001$ and $p=0.01$) and for mania ($p=0.005$) but not depression ($p=0.655$) concerning RLAI. Fewer patients in the olanzapine and RLAI groups relapsed into any mood episode in comparison to placebo (23.8 % vs. 38.9 % vs. 56.4 %). Both medication arms manifested lower relapses into mania (14.6 % vs. 19.8 % vs. 39.1 %), but only olanzapine manifested fewer relapses also concerning depression (9.2 % vs. 19.1 % vs. 17.3 %) (Vieta et al. 2012).

These results provide support for the efficacy of olanzapine in the prevention of any kind of mood relapse after an index manic or mixed episode which responded to olanzapine treatment during the acute phase. However the efficacy of olanzapine does not seem to be restricted to those patients who responded to olanzapine during the acute phase. Its effect on rapid cycling patients is unknown.

16.2.3.1.7 Aripiprazole

There are two trials supporting the efficacy of aripiprazole during the maintenance phase of BD. In the first one, which took place in 76 centres in 3 countries, 161 recently manic- or mixed-episode BD-I patients stabilized on aripiprazole (15 or 30 mg/day, 6–18 weeks) and maintained on aripiprazole treatment for 6 weeks were randomized to aripiprazole ($N=78$) or placebo ($N=83$) for 26 weeks. The results suggested that aripiprazole was superior to placebo in delaying the time to relapse ($p=0.020$), and this was specifically due to a significant delay in the development of manic ($p=0.01$) but not depressive ($p=0.68$) relapses. Aripiprazole-treated patients had significantly fewer relapses than placebo patients (25 % vs. 43 %; $p=0.013$). The adverse events related with aripiprazole treatment were weight gain (13 % vs. 0 %) and akathisia, pain in the extremities, tremor and vaginitis (Keck et al. 2006a). A second study included a 26-week, double-blind, placebo-controlled relapse prevention with a prospective, 74-week, double-blind, placebo-controlled extension phase (100 weeks in total) in 567 BD-I patients with a recent manic or mixed episode who had received open-label aripiprazole 15 or 30 mg/day (started at 30 mg/day) for 6–18 weeks. Those patients who achieved stabilization ($N=161$; YMRS ≤ 10 and MADRS ≤ 13 for 6 consecutive weeks) were randomly assigned to double-blind treatment with aripiprazole ($N=78$) or placebo ($N=83$) for 26 weeks. Patients who completed the 26-week stabilization continued in a double-blind fashion with aripiprazole ($N=39$) or placebo ($N=27$) for an additional 74 weeks and were monitored for relapse, efficacy and tolerability. At 100 weeks, time to relapse was significantly longer with aripiprazole than placebo ($p=0.01$). The rate of relapse was 33 % in the aripiprazole group vs. 52 % in the placebo group at endpoint. Aripiprazole was superior to placebo in delaying time to manic relapse ($p=0.005$) but not to depressive relapse ($p=0.602$). Eventually only seven patients in the aripiprazole group and five in the placebo group completed the 100 weeks of the study, and this should be considered vs. the 567 who entered the 6–18 weeks of the stabilization phase. The adverse events reported during 100 weeks of treatment with aripiprazole vs. placebo were tremor, akathisia, dry mouth, hypertension, weight gain, vaginitis, abnormal thinking, pharyngitis and flu syndrome. Mean weight change from baseline to 100 weeks (LOCF) was +0.4 kg with aripiprazole and −1.9 kg with placebo (Keck et al. 2007).

Overall these two trials support the efficacy of aripiprazole in the maintenance treatment of BD but only concerning the prevention of manic but not depressive episodes in patients after an index manic or mixed episode who responded to aripiprazole during the acute phase. These two correspond to stringent criteria concerning the definition of 'maintenance' treatment.

16.2.3.1.8 Quetiapine

There is one published positive study that used quetiapine IR (NCT00314184 or trial 144, also named 'SPARCLE') which investigated the efficacy and safety of quetiapine monotherapy (300–800 mg/day) as maintenance treatment in BD-I patients compared with switching to placebo or lithium. During the open-label phase, 2,438 BD-I patients with a current or recent manic, depressive or mixed episode received open-label quetiapine, and those achieving stabilization ($N=1{,}226$; 50.3 %) were randomized to continue quetiapine or to switch to placebo or lithium (0.6–1.2 mEq/l) for up to 104 weeks in a double-blind fashion. The study was terminated early after planned interim analysis provided positive results. The results suggested that the time to recurrence of any mood event was significantly longer for quetiapine vs. placebo ($p<0.0001$) and for lithium vs. placebo ($p<0.0001$). Both quetiapine and lithium significantly increased time to recurrence of both manic events and depressive events compared with placebo. Overall rates of adverse events were generally similar between treatment groups, and safety findings for quetiapine were consistent with its known profile (Weisler et al. 2011).

16.2.3.1.9 Paliperidone

There is one study on 766 BD-I patients with current manic or mixed episodes (rapid cycling excluded) which were initially randomized to flexibly dosed paliperidone ER (3–12 mg/day; $N=617$) or olanzapine (5–20 mg/day; $N=149$) for a duration of 3-week acute treatment phase. The responders continued the same treatment (12-week continuation phase). Those patients on paliperidone ER who achieved remission during this phase were randomized to fixed-dose paliperidone ER ($N=152$) or placebo ($N=148$), while those on olanzapine continued to receive that at fixed dose ($N=83$). This maintenance phase continued until at least 140 recurrences occurred among patients originally assigned to paliperidone ER in the acute treatment phase. The median time to recurrence of any mood symptoms was significantly longer for paliperidone vs. placebo (558 vs. 283 days; $p=0.017$) and not observed with olanzapine (<50 % of patients experienced recurrence). Olanzapine-treated patients had significantly longer time to recurrence for any mood symptoms in comparison to either group ($p<0.001$). For paliperidone the difference was significant for preventing recurrence of manic, but not depressive symptoms. Treatment-emergent adverse events occurred more often in olanzapine group (64 %) than placebo (59 %) or paliperidone ER groups (55 %) (Berwaerts et al. 2012a). Overall this trial supports the usefulness of paliperidone maintenance treatment for the prevention of manic recurrences in patients with index manic or mixed episodes who responded to paliperidone during the acute phase.

16.2.3.1.10 Risperidone Long-Acting Injectable (RLAI)

The first study on the efficacy of RLAI in the maintenance treatment of BD-I was conducted in 559 BD-I patients with current or recent manic or mixed episode (rapid cycling excluded). The patients were treated with open-label oral risperidone for 3 weeks and open-label RLAI for 26 weeks. Those patients who maintained response ($N=303$) were randomly allocated to continue RLAI ($N=154$) or to placebo injections ($N=149$) for up to 24 months. Most patients (77 %) on RLAI received a dose of 25 mg every 2 weeks. The results suggested that the time to recurrence for any mood episode was significantly longer in the RLAI group vs. placebo ($p<0.001$); the difference was significant for time to recurrence of mania ($p<0.001$) but not time to recurrence of depression ($p=0.805$). Fewer patients in the RLAI group experienced recurrence in comparison to placebo (30 % vs. 56 %). Weight gain was more in the risperidone group (Quiroz et al. 2010). The second trial utilized a 12-week open-label period with RLAI in 560 patients with manic or mixed episode (rapid cycling excluded). Those who did not experience a recurrence entered an 18-month randomized, double-blind period with RLAI ($N=132$) or placebo ($N=135$) or oral olanzapine (10 mg/day; $N=131$). Of patients under RLAI, 25 mg were received by 66 % of patients, 37.5 mg by 31 % and 50 mg by 4 %. The results demonstrated a median time to mood episode recurrence of 198 days in the placebo arm, whereas the median was not reached in the RLAI arm ($p=0.057$). Time to recurrence of any mood episode was significantly longer with RLAI and olanzapine vs. placebo ($p=0.031$ and $p<0.001$). Again the difference was significant for time to recurrence of mania ($p=0.005$) but not depression ($p=0.655$) concerning RLAI but for both concerning olanzapine ($p<0.001$ and $p=0.01$). Fewer patients in the RLAI and olanzapine groups relapsed into any mood episode in comparison to placebo (38.9 % vs. 23.8 % vs. 56.4 %). Both medication arms manifested lower relapses into mania (19.8 % vs. 14.6 % vs. 39.1 %), but only olanzapine manifested fewer relapses also concerning depression (19.1 % vs. 9.2 % vs. 17.3 %). There was no evidence of worsening of depression in the RLAI arm (Vieta et al. 2012).

Overall the data suggest that RLAI is efficacious in the prevention of manic but not depressive episodes in BD-I patients with a manic or mixed index episode who responded to oral risperidone or RLAI during the acute phase. No data concerning the efficacy in rapid cycling patients exist.

16.2.3.1.11 Conclusions of Monotherapy Trials

The data that come from placebo-controlled monotherapy trials suggest that lithium, aripiprazole, paliperidone and RLAI are efficacious in the prevention of manic episodes in patients who recovered from an index manic or mixed episode. Olanzapine and quetiapine were efficacious in the prevention of both manic and depressive episodes. Quetiapine was efficacious irrespective of index episode, while olanzapine was proven efficacious in the prevention of mixed episodes also. There are no data for carbamazepine or valproate (failed study).

Irrespective of index episode, lamotrigine is efficacious in the prevention of depressive but not manic episodes and was not efficacious in the prevention of mixed episodes or in rapid cycling patients. The data were negative for imipramine, while there was some support for the efficacy of fluoxetine in BD-II patients.

All except lithium and maybe olanzapine were proven efficacious in samples enriched for response during the acute phase. Except from the negative data concerning lamotrigine, there are no data concerning rapid cycling patients. Also except from the data concerning olanzapine, there are no data concerning specifically the prevention of mixed episodes or the response of patients at an index mixed episode.

16.2.3.2 Comparison of Treatments

16.2.3.2.1 Lithium Versus Others

Lithium Versus Carbamazepine

There are a number of studies comparing lithium with carbamazepine. The first study included 83 in- and outpatients suffering from major affective, schizoaffective or schizophreniform psychoses. The duration was 3 years, and it was a prospective double-blind randomized trial. There was no difference between lithium and carbamazepine with two-thirds of patients responding well to either agent. There was a significantly higher dropout rate for patients with mood-incongruent psychotic features in the lithium group. Both drugs appeared more effective in preventing excited rather than depressive symptoms (Placidi et al. 1986). Another trial reported some superiority for lithium (Watkins et al. 1987), while two others reported that the two agents had comparative efficacy (Lusznat et al. 1988; Stoll et al. 1989).

A study on 52 hospitalized acutely manic patients randomized them to treatment with either lithium or carbamazepine after a 2-week drug withdrawal period for up to 2 years. Double-blind assessments revealed no significant differences between the two treatment groups (Small et al. 1991). Another 12-month double-blind trial in 31 BD patients who were previously stabilized on lithium randomized them to receive either lithium ($N=16$) or carbamazepine ($N=15$) and reported that the overall relapse rate was similar in the two treatment groups (Coxhead et al. 1992). A 2-year duration open trial suggested that there was no significant difference between the two medication arms (Simhandl et al. 1993). An interesting study randomized 52 outpatients with BD to receive lithium or carbamazepine, a crossover to the opposite drug in the second year and then a third year on the combination. There was no difference between the treatment groups in terms of marked or moderate improvement (33.3 % vs. 31.4 % vs. 55.2 %). Lithium was superior to carbamazepine in the prophylaxis of mania. Patients with a past history of rapid cycling did poorly on monotherapy and better on combination treatment (28.0 % vs. 19.0 % vs. 56.3 %; $p<0.05$) (Denicoff et al. 1997).

One of the most important is the MAP study which took place in nine university hospitals in Germany. It included 144 BD patients which were randomized to open treatment with lithium ($N=74$; mean serum level 0.63 mmol/l) vs. carbamazepine ($N=70$; mean dosage 621 mg/day) for 2.5 years. There was no difference between the two drugs in terms of number of recurrences. There was some superiority of lithium when comedication ($p=0.041$) or adverse effects ($p=0.007$) was taken into consideration. More patients in the carbamazepine group dropped out (5.4 % vs. 12.9 %) although more patients in the lithium group reported any adverse event

(61 % vs. 21 %; $p<0.001$). In those patients who completed the 2.5 years of the study, there was a higher but not significant number of recurrences in the carbamazepine group (47 % vs. 28 %; $p=0.06$). Overall there was no difference between the two agents although there was a trend for lithium to perform better concerning some secondary outcomes (Greil et al. 1997). A further analysis of the study sample separated BD-I ($N=114$) vs. BD-II and BD NOS ($N=57$). Lithium was superior in BD-I patients, while there was no difference between the two agents in the second subsample. A second sub-analysis contrasted a 'classical subgroup' (BD-I without mood-incongruent delusions and without comorbidity; $N=67$) and a 'nonclassical subgroup' (all other patients $N=104$). Lithium was superior in the 'classical' group with a significantly lower hospitalization rate (26 vs. 62 %; $p=0.012$), while there was no difference between the two agents in the 'nonclassical' group, although a tendency in favour of carbamazepine was found. The results did not find any effect concerning the episode sequence prior to the index episode although there was a tendency of the pattern mania–depression-free interval to respond better to lithium. There was also a trend for suicidal behaviour to respond better to lithium, but the data on patients' satisfaction were significantly in favour of carbamazepine. Overall the results of this sub-analysis suggest that lithium has a global efficacy in BD, while the effect of carbamazepine might be restricted to the 'nonclassical' patients (Kleindienst and Greil 2000; Greil and Kleindienst 1999a, b). A further analysis of the data suggested that after taking a variety of outcomes into consideration (inter-episodic morbidity, dropout and rehospitalization), lithium had superior performance in comparison to carbamazepine (Kleindienst and Greil 2002).

A 2-year duration double-blind study in 94 BD patients with at least two mood episodes during the previous 3 years who were in remission at entry into the study compared lithium ($N=44$) vs. carbamazepine ($N=50$). These patients were not treated with lithium or carbamazepine for more than a total of 6 months during their lifetime. No concurrent antipsychotics or antidepressants were allowed. Fewer patients under lithium relapsed into any mood episode (27.3 % vs. 42 %). Lithium was superior to carbamazepine in those patients with an index manic or hypomanic episode that had not been treated with study drug during the index episode ($p<0.01$) and also in patients with prior hypomanic but no manic episodes ($p<0.05$). Their dropout rate was similar in the two groups (36.4 % vs. 26 %). There was no difference between treatment arms in terms concerning the relapse into a mood episode when only completers were considered (36 % vs. 32 %). Overall the data suggested that lithium was found to be superior in prophylactic efficacy to carbamazepine in BD patients not previously treated with mood stabilizers (Hartong et al. 2003).

Overall the data suggest that there are no significant differences between lithium and carbamazepine. There might be some superiority of lithium in the treatment of more 'classic' patients, but in the rest of patients, the two agents were comparable.

Lithium Versus Valproate

The first comparison trial included 372 BD patients who met the recovery criteria within 3 months of the onset of an index manic episode. These patients were randomized to maintenance treatment with lithium (0.8–1.2 mmol/l; $N=91$), divalproex (75–125 μg/ml; $N=372$) or placebo ($N=94$) for a period of 52 weeks. The patients should have been randomized within 3 months from the onset of the index episode, and they were required to be manic, partially recovered or remitted but not depressed at randomization. They were required to fulfil the inclusion criteria for two subsequent assessments, 6 days apart from each other. The three treatment groups did not differ concerning the time to manifestation of any mood episode, and this was also the case concerning manic or depressive episodes alone. Thus this is considered to be a failed study. The lithium group had higher rates of tremor, thirst and polyuria, while the divalproex group had higher rates of tremor, sedation, weight gain and reduction in platelet blood count (Bowden et al. 2000).

A second study investigated the efficacy of lithium vs. valproate in rapid cycling patients. That trial lasted 20 months and included 254 recently hypomanic/manic patients who had experienced a persistent bimodal response to combined treatment with lithium and divalproex. Only 60 patients remained after the open-label phase and were randomly assigned to lithium or divalproex monotherapy. The two agents had comparable efficacy in terms of relapse into any mood episode (56 % vs. 50 %), and this was also true both for depressive (34 % vs. 29 %) as well as for hypomanic/manic relapses (19 % vs. 22 %). There were no significant differences in time to relapse. More patients in the lithium group dropped out because of adverse events (16 % vs. 4 %) (Calabrese et al. 2005b).

Finally one study recruited 98 BD patients with a history of suicide attempts and assigned them to receive in a double-blind way lithium ($N=49$) or valproate ($N=49$) plus adjunctive medications as indicated for 2.5 years. Overall there were 45 suicide events in 35 participants (35.7 %), but no suicides. There were no differences between treatment groups in time to suicide attempt or to suicide event (Oquendo et al. 2011).

Again lithium was comparable to valproate in terms of prevention of mood episodes and suicidality.

Lithium Versus Lamotrigine

As mentioned before, three placebo-controlled RCTs suggested that at dosages of 50–400 mg daily, lamotrigine was comparable to lithium and superior to placebo at prolonging the time to intervention for any mood episode in BD-I patients who had recently experienced a manic or hypomanic episode. Lamotrigine was more efficacious in the prevention of depressive episodes and lithium in the prevention of manic, hypomanic and mixed episodes. It is important that in these two RCTs patients received lamotrigine during the acute phase, thus suggesting that the study sample was not really enriched in favour of either compound, since lamotrigine is not efficacious during the acute phase (Bowden et al. 2003; Calabrese et al. 2003a).

Lithium Versus Antidepressants

There are three studies comparing lithium and antidepressants during the maintenance phase. In the first one, 122 patients with recurrent affective illness were randomly assigned to lithium, imipramine or placebo therapy for 2 years following discharge from hospitalization for acute depression. In bipolar patients lithium was significantly more effective than imipramine or placebo in preventing any mood episode. Both treatments were significantly more effective than placebo. It is interesting that the difference between medication arms was due primarily to depressive episodes (Prien et al. 1973b). In the second one, 117 BD patients which received lithium carbonate or imipramine hydrochloride or both reported that lithium carbonate and the combination treatment were superior to imipramine in the prevention of manic recurrences and were as effective as imipramine in the preventing of depressive episodes. This was the first study to document that the efficacy of lithium might not include all phases of BD (Prien et al. 1984). The third one included 81 BD-II patients who recovered from their major depressive episode during initial open-label fluoxetine monotherapy that was randomly assigned to receive 50 weeks of double-blind monotherapy with fluoxetine (10–40 mg/day; $N=28$) or lithium (300–1,200 mg/day; $N=26$) or placebo ($N=27$). The mean time to relapse was significantly longer for fluoxetine (249.9 vs. 156.4 vs. 186.9 days). The estimated hazard of relapse was 2.5 times greater with lithium than with fluoxetine (Amsterdam and Shults 2010).

Thus the above studies suggest that lithium was superior to imipramine concerning the prevention of depression in BD-I patients but inferior to fluoxetine in BD-II patients.

Lithium Versus SGAs

There are two trials which compare lithium with an SGA. In the first one, acutely manic or mixed BD-I patients entered the study and received open-label co-treatment with olanzapine and lithium for 6–12 weeks. Those who remitted were randomly assigned to 52 weeks of double-blind monotherapy with olanzapine (5–20 mg/day; $N=217$) or lithium (target blood level: 0.6–1.2 meq/l; $N=214$). The two treatment groups had similar relapse rates (30 % vs. 38.8 %). There was some superiority of olanzapine in the prevention of manic or mixed episodes. The two agents did not differ concerning the prevention of depressive episodes. There was a significantly greater weight gain olanzapine than with lithium (1.8 kg vs. −1.4 kg) (Tohen et al. 2005). That study sample included patients in a manic/mixed episode and was possibly biased towards a manic/mixed predominant polarity. During the acute phase patients received a combination of lithium plus olanzapine, and no duration of response/remission was required in order to continue to the 'maintenance' phase.

The second study randomized manic or mixed BD-I patients to 12 weeks of lithium vs. aripiprazole monotherapy and those who responded to an additional 40-week maintenance (52 weeks total treatment). During this phase, patients continued receiving either aripiprazole (15 or 30 mg/day) or lithium (900, 1,200 or 1,500 mg/day). Of the 66 patients who entered the extension phase, only 20 patients (30.3 %) completed the entire phase (aripiprazole $N=7$; lithium $N=13$). The two agents appeared to be comparable. The most common treatment-emergent adverse events in the extension phase for aripiprazole were akathisia, headache, somnolence, anxiety and nasopharyngitis (all 8 %) and for lithium were insomnia (15.8 %), headache (13.2 %), diarrhoea (13.2 %) and vomiting (10.5 %) (El-Mallakh et al. 2012).

According to the above data, lithium was comparable to olanzapine and aripiprazole for the maintenance treatment of BD.

16.2.3.2.2 Valproate Versus Others

The studies concerning the comparison of valproate with lithium have already been discussed above (Bowden et al. 2000; Calabrese et al. 2005b; Oquendo et al. 2011).

Two trials compare valproate vs. olanzapine. The first one was a 47-week, randomized, double-blind study and compared olanzapine (5–20 mg/day) to divalproex (500–2,500 mg/day) in 251 BD-I patients in a manic or mixed episode. At endpoint there was no difference between the treatment groups in terms of mean improvement in YMRS score. The median time to symptomatic mania remission was significantly shorter for olanzapine (14 days vs. 62 days), but there were no significant differences between groups in the rates of symptomatic mania remission (56.8 % vs. 45.5 %) and subsequent relapse into mania or depression (42.3 % vs. 56.5 %). Treatment-emergent adverse events occurring significantly more frequently during olanzapine treatment were somnolence, dry mouth, increased appetite, weight gain, akathisia and high alanine aminotransferase levels; those for divalproex were nausea and nervousness (Tohen et al. 2003b). The cost analysis of the results of the previous study suggested that the overall per-patient treatment costs were similar for olanzapine and divalproex (Zhu et al. 2005).

16.2.3.2.3 Carbamazepine Versus Others

Carbamazepine has been studied only in comparison to lithium, and these studies have been discussed previously in the paragraph concerning lithium (Greil et al. 1997; Small et al. 1991; Kleindienst and Greil 2000, 2002; Hartong et al. 2003; Coxhead et al. 1992; Denicoff et al. 1997; Greil and Kleindienst 1999a; Placidi et al. 1986; Watkins et al. 1987; Lusznat et al. 1988; Simhandl et al. 1993).

16.2.3.2.4 Olanzapine Versus Others

The comparisons of olanzapine with lithium (Tohen et al. 2005) and valproate (Tohen et al. 2003b; Zhu et al. 2005) have been discussed above.

There is one study which compared olanzapine with asenapine, and it was an extension of the acute phase of an asenapine vs. olanzapine trial (McIntyre et al. 2009b). The extension phase included a 9-week double-blind extension followed by a 40-week double-blind extension. Patients entering the extension phase maintained their pre-established treatment, but those originally randomized to placebo received flexible-dose asenapine. Eventually all were receiving either flexible-dose asenapine (10–20 mg/day; $N=111$) or olanzapine (5–20 mg/day; $N=107$). At endpoint the change in the mean YMRS score was similar in the two groups (–28.2 vs. −28.6). Also the adverse events rate was similar between groups. The most frequent treatment-emergent AEs were insomnia, sedation and depression with asenapine and weight gain, somnolence and sedation with olanzapine (McIntyre et al. 2010a).

There is also only one study which compared olanzapine with paliperidone. It included 766 BD-I patients with current manic or mixed episodes (rapid cycling excluded) which were initially randomized to olanzapine (5–20 mg/day; $N=149$) or paliperidone ER (3–12 mg/day; $N=617$) for an acute treatment phase of 3-week duration. The responders continued the same treatment during a 12-week continuation phase, and those patients on paliperidone ER who achieved remission during this phase were randomized to fixed-dose paliperidone ER ($N=152$) or placebo ($N=148$), while those on olanzapine continued to receive that at fixed dose ($N=83$). This maintenance phase continued until at least 140 recurrences occurred among patients originally assigned to paliperidone ER in the acute treatment phase. The median time to recurrence of any mood symptoms was not observed with olanzapine (<50 % of patients experienced recurrence) and was significantly longer for paliperidone vs. placebo (558 vs. 283 days; $p=0.017$). Olanzapine-treated patients had significantly longer time to recurrence for any mood symptoms in comparison to either group ($p<0.001$). For paliperidone the difference was significant for preventing recurrence of manic, but not depressive symptoms. This clarification is not reported concerning olanzapine. Treatment-emergent adverse events occurred more often in olanzapine group (64 %) than placebo (59 %) or paliperidone ER groups (55 %) (Berwaerts et al. 2012a).

16.2.3.2.5 Other Comparisons

The comparison of aripiprazole (El-Mallakh et al. 2012), fluoxetine (Amsterdam and Shults 2010) imipramine (Prien et al. 1984) and lamotrigine (Bowden et al. 2003; Calabrese et al. 2003a) with lithium and of asenapine (McIntyre et al. 2010a) and paliperidone with olanzapine (Berwaerts et al. 2012a) has been discussed previously.

One 25-week RCT (expansion of an acute phase study (Brown et al. 2006) compared the olanzapine–fluoxetine combination (OFC 6/25, 6/50, 12/25 or 12/50 mg/day) vs. lamotrigine (titrated to 200 mg/day) in the prevention of bipolar depression in patients who responded to either the OFC or lamotrigine during the acute phase (note: the acute data are negative for lamotrigine vs. placebo). The results suggested that at endpoint patients with BD-I depression had significantly greater symptom improvement in terms of YMRS and MADRS scores on OFC compared with lamotrigine, but there was no treatment difference in the incidence of relapse. OFC-treated patients had more treatment-emergent adverse events and greater incidence of weight gain and hypercholesterolaemia. Thus, bipolar depressive patients who responded to OFC do better on long-term OFC in comparison to spontaneously improved patients on long-term lamotrigine (Brown et al. 2009).

Finally, there is one 6-week study which compared the efficacy of venlafaxine monotherapy (37.5–225 mg/day) in 15 women with BD-II vs. 17 women with unipolar (UP) depression years). The results suggested that the efficacy of venlafaxine was similar in the two treatment groups. No episodes of drug-induced hypomania or rapid cycling were observed (Amsterdam and Garcia-Espana 2000).

16.2.3.2.6 Summary of Comparison Studies

Overall the literature suggests that lithium is comparable with carbamazepine, valproate, olanzapine and aripiprazole. It might be more efficacious than carbamazepine in more 'classic' patients, but not less efficacious in the rest. Lamotrigine is more efficacious in the prevention of depressive episodes and lithium in the prevention of manic, hypomanic and mixed episodes. In the prevention of depressive episodes, lithium was shown to be superior to imipramine but inferior to fluoxetine in BD-II patients, while OFC has shown some superiority in comparison to lamotrigine. Valproate and olanzapine were shown to be comparable, which is in accord with their comparison with lithium separately. Olanzapine was shown to be comparable with asenapine but superior to paliperidone ER.

16.2.3.3 Combination and Add-On Treatment

A summary of combination and add-on treatment data for the maintenance phase is shown in Table 16.7.

16.2.3.3.1 Combination Treatment

There are three early studies which investigated the combination of lithium with another agent. All were negative, but the problems in their design limit the interpretation of the results. In the first combination treatment trial, 22 BD-II patients in remission for at least 6 months were randomly assigned to lithium, imipramine, lithium plus imipramine or placebo. The results suggested that lithium was efficacious in the prevention of relapse of any type, but imipramine was not efficacious either as monotherapy or in the combination group (Kane et al. 1982). In the second one, 117 BD patients received lithium, imipramine or both and reported that lithium and the combination treatment were superior to imipramine in the prevention of manic recurrences and were as effective as imipramine in the preventing of depressive episodes (Prien et al. 1984). In the third study, 52 outpatients with BD were randomized to receive lithium or carbamazepine, a crossover to the opposite drug in the second year, and then a third year on the combination. There was no difference between the treatment groups in terms of marked or moderate improvement (33.3 % vs. 31.4 % vs. 55.2 %). Lithium was superior to carbamazepine in the prophylaxis of mania. Patients with a past history of rapid cycling did poorly on monotherapy and better on combination treatment (28.0 % vs. 19.0 % vs. 56.3 %; $p<0.05$) (Denicoff et al. 1997).

The first study with a modern methodology took part in 2004 and was a 6-month maintenance study of lithium, carbamazepine or valproate plus perphenazine (4–64 mg/day; $N=18$) or placebo ($N=19$) in patients who had just remitted from an acute manic or mixed episode with or without psychotic features and retained remission for at least 2 weeks. The results suggested that patients receiving perphenazine had not had a better course in comparison to those receiving placebo, but on the contrary they had a shorter time to depressive relapse, more dropouts and have increased rates of dysphoria and depressive symptoms (Zarate and Tohen 2004).

One 18-month discontinuation placebo-controlled study included 99 BD-I patients who had achieved syndromic remission after 6 weeks of treatment with combination of olanzapine 5–20 mg/day plus lithium (0.6–1.2 mmol/l) or valproate (50–125 μg/ml). During the double-blind phase, patients were randomized to lithium or valproate plus olanzapine ($N=51$) or placebo ($N=48$). The results suggested that there was no difference between study groups in terms of syndromic relapse but was significant for symptomatic relapse (163 days vs. 42 days; $p=0.023$) (Tohen et al. 2004).

Another international study examined the efficacy and safety of quetiapine on lithium or divalproex in the prevention of mood episodes in BD-I patients with most recent episode manic/mixed or depressive. All patients received open-label quetiapine plus lithium or divalproex for up to 36 weeks to achieve at least 12 weeks of clinical stability. Then they were subsequently randomized to lithium (target serum concentrations 0.5–1.2 mEq/l) or divalproex (target serum concentrations 50–125 μg/ml) plus quetiapine (400–800 mg/day; $N=336$) or placebo ($N=367$) for up to 104 weeks. The results suggested that the combination significantly increased the time to recurrence of any mood event in comparison to placebo, and the relapse rate was lower in the combination group (18.5 % vs. 49.0 %). This beneficial effect concerned both manic and depressive episodes and corresponded to risk reductions >70 %. The combination was more efficacious than a mood stabilizer alone irrespective of index episode, mood stabilizer and rapid cycling status. During the randomization phase, there was an increase in weight of 0.5 kg in the quetiapine group and a reduction of 1.9 kg in the placebo group. More patients in the combination group manifested an elevation of serum glucose levels (Vieta et al. 2008b). There was a North American study with a similar design as the previous one (combination group $N=310$; placebo group $N=313$) and reported the same results with the international study (Suppes et al. 2009). These combination studies appear to be the first to report prevention on both depression and mania regardless of the type of index episode and rapid cycling status.

The OFC is a standard combination with proven efficacy against acute bipolar depression (Brown et al. 2006). There is one 25-week RCT (expansion of the acute phase study) which compared the OFC (6/25, 6/50, 12/25 or 12/50 mg/day) vs. lamotrigine (titrated to 200 mg/day) in the prevention of bipolar depression in patients who responded to either the OFC or lamotrigine during the acute phase (note: the acute data are negative for lamotrigine vs. placebo). The results suggested that at endpoint patients with BD-I depression had significantly greater symptom improvement in terms of YMRS and MADRS scores on OFC compared with lamotrigine, but there was no treatment difference in terms of incidence of relapse. OFC-treated patients had more treatment-emergent adverse events and greater incidence of weight gain and hypercholesterolaemia. Thus, bipolar depressive patients who responded to OFC do better on long-term OFC in comparison to spontaneously improved patients on long-term lamotrigine (Brown et al. 2009).

Another discontinuation 6-month RCT included 240 BD-I patients in an acute manic episode who responded to open-label ziprasidone plus a mood stabilizer and maintained response for at least eight consecutive weeks. These patients were randomized to receive either the combination of lithium or valproate plus ziprasidone (80–160 mg/day; $N=127$) or lithium or valproate alone ($N=113$). The results suggested that the combination was superior to mood stabilizer alone (relapse rate 19.7 % vs. 32.4 %; longer median time to intervention for the combination: 43.0 days vs. 26.5 days; $p=0.01$). Also the time to discontinuation for any reason was significantly longer for the combination arm ($p=0.0047$). Only tremor occurred more frequently in the combination arm (6.3 % vs. 3.6 %) (Bowden et al. 2010).

One open-label 24-month study (BALANCE trial) included 330 BD-I patients from 41 sites in the UK, France, USA and Italy and randomized them to lithium monotherapy (plasma concentration 0.4–1.0 mmol/l, $N=110$), valproate monotherapy (750–1,250 mg, $N=110$) or both agents in combination ($N=110$), after an active run-in of 4–8 weeks on the combination. The results revealed that the combination group had less outcome events (59 % vs. 69 % vs. 54 %). The hazard ratios for the primary outcome were 0.59 ($p=0.0023$) for combination therapy vs. valproate, 0.82 ($p=0.27$) for combination therapy vs. lithium and 0.71 ($p=0.0472$) for lithium vs. valproate. It is important to note that 16 participants had serious adverse events after randomization. Of them seven were receiving valproate monotherapy (three deaths), five lithium monotherapy (two deaths) and four combination therapy (one death). Overall the results neither reliably confirm nor refute a benefit of combination therapy compared with lithium monotherapy, but clearly suggest that it is superior to valproate alone (Geddes et al. 2010). There are some methodological issues that might be responsible for these results at least partially (Fountoulakis 2010a).

A 24-week discontinuation trial of aripiprazole from Korea included 175 BD-I patients in a manic or mixed episode who were treated for 6 weeks with open-label divalproex plus aripiprazole. Stabilized patients for at least 2 weeks were randomized to 24 weeks of divalproex (50–125 μg/ml) plus aripiprazole (10–30 mg/day; $N=40$) or placebo ($N=43$). The results suggested that the time to relapse of any mood episode was similar in the two treatment groups ($p=0.098$). Weight gain was similar in the two groups and so were other adverse events (Woo et al. 2011).

One study included 787 BD-I patients with a recent manic or mixed episode (rapid cycling included) and applied a 9–24-week stabilization phase to them with single-blind aripiprazole (10–30 mg/day) plus open-label lamotrigine (100 or 200 mg/day). Of them 351 were stabilized for eight consecutive weeks and were randomized to aripiprazole plus lamotrigine ($N=178$) or placebo plus lamotrigine ($N=173$) and were followed-up for 52 weeks. At endpoint the two groups were not different in terms of time to any relapse, and this was also true concerning manic, mixed or depressive relapses although the combination group had a numerically longer time to relapse. Fewer patients in the combination group had relapsed at endpoint (11 % vs. 23 %) yielding a NNT of 9 (95 % CI: 5–121). The three most common adverse events in the combination group were akathisia, insomnia and anxiety (Carlson et al. 2012).

Another study included 164 recently depressed BD-I or BD-II patients, treated them with a combination of lamotrigine (up to 200 mg/day) plus divalproex (45–120 μg/ml or maximum daily dosage of 2,500 mg) and randomized those who were stabilized to 8 months of double-blind treatment with lamotrigine plus placebo ($N=45$) vs. lamotrigine plus divalproex ($N=41$). At endpoint the time to depressive episode did not differ significantly between groups (Bowden et al. 2012).

Overall, there is no compelling data that combination treatment in general does better than monotherapy. Most of the combination trials are negative and suggest that starting with monotherapy could be the best option for most patients. However for those patients stabilized on combination treatment, shifting them to monotherapy is the wrong choice. The exception is combination treatment with quetiapine or ziprasidone plus a mood stabilizer which according to the data might do better than a mood stabilizer alone, and thus they might constitute the only combinations worth to start with from the beginning.

16.2.3.3.2 Add-On Treatment

The first add-on study was a randomized, open study of clozapine ($N=19$) as add-on therapy vs. treatment as usual ($N=19$) in patients with treatment-resistant BD or schizoaffective disorder who were followed up for 1 year. The results suggested the presence of significant clinical improvement in the clozapine group in comparison to treatment as usual (Suppes et al. 1999).

Another add-on study investigated the efficacy of phenytoin in 23 BD patients who had at least one episode per year in the previous 2 years despite ongoing prophylaxis but were stable for a mean of 4 months (range 1–13) before entering the study. Phenytoin or placebo was added to their current therapy in a double-blind crossover design for 6 months in each phase, leading to 30 observation periods of 6 months each. At the end of the study three patients on phenytoin and nine on placebo experienced a relapse, suggesting the presence of a significant prophylactic effect for phenytoin ($p=0.02$) (Mishory et al. 2003).

One small 1-year, double-blind, randomized, comparative, placebo-controlled, parallel-group, multicentre study investigated the efficacy of gabapentin ($N=13$) or placebo ($N=12$) added to the current treatment (lithium, valproate, carbamazepine or any combination but not antipsychotics or antidepressants) in euthymic BD-I or BD-II patients with at least two mood episodes during the last year. The results suggested that the combination was superior to placebo at endpoint in terms of change in the CGI-BP-Mania score (−2.1 vs. −0.6; $p=0.0046$). No emerging manic or depressive symptoms were seen in either group. The combination group manifested also a significant reduction in the use of sleeping medication (Vieta et al. 2006).

A 52-week, double-blind, randomized, placebo-controlled, parallel-group, multicentre, clinical trial included 55 BD-I and BD-II outpatients which had had two or more episodes during the last year, but currently being in remission and assigned them to oxcarbazepine ($N=26$) or placebo ($N=29$) as adjunctive treatment to ongoing therapy with lithium. Overall there was no difference between the treatment groups either in time to recurrence for any mood episode (19.2 vs. 18.6; $p=0.315$) or in the recurrence rates (38.46 % vs. 58.62 %; $p=0.135$). There was a trend for depressive episodes being less likely in the oxcarbazepine group (11.54 % vs. 31.03 %; $p=0.085$) and for better functionality with the GAF ($p=0.074$). The only significant finding concerned impulsivity was significantly better prevented by oxcarbazepine ($p=0.044$) (Vieta et al. 2008a).

One trial included 83 outpatients with bipolar depression and unsatisfactory response to treatment with lithium, valproate or carbamazepine and treated them for 10 weeks with the same mood stabilizer plus one of three double-blind randomly assigned antidepressants. Both the 61 patients who showed response as well as the 22 patients who showed partial response entered the 1-year double-blind continuation trial of their medication. At study endpoint, 42 (69 %) of the 61 acute positive responders maintained positive response and 32 (53 %) achieved remission. Only 6 (27 %) of the 22 acute partial responders had achieved positive treatment response at study endpoint.

Eight acute positive responders (13 %) and five acute partial responders (22 %) developed mania. These results suggest that patients who respond to treatment with mood stabilizers plus antidepressants maintain response with the same continued treatment; however, those patients who manifest only a partial acute response are unlikely to further improve when the same treatment is sustained (Altshuler et al. 2009).

The only large controlled trial which evaluated adjunctive maintenance treatment with a long-acting injectable antipsychotic in BD included 240 BD-I patients with at least four mood episodes in the 12 months prior to study entry. These patients entered a 16-week, open-label stabilization phase with RLAI plus TAU. Those who remitted ($N=124$) entered a 52-week, double-blind, placebo-controlled phase and were randomized to continued treatment with adjunctive RLAI (25–50 mg every 2 weeks) plus TAU ($N=65$) or to adjunctive placebo injection plus TAU ($N=59$). The time to relapse was longer ($p=0.010$), and the relapse rates were lower in patients receiving adjunctive RLAI (23.1 % vs. 45.8 % $p=0.011$). More patients under RLAI discontinued because of adverse events (4.6 % vs. 1.7 %). The most frequent adverse events related to RLAI treatment in comparison to placebo were tremor (24.6 % vs. 10.2 %), insomnia (20.0 % vs. 18.6 %), muscle rigidity (12.3 % vs. 5.1 %), increased weight (6.2 % vs. 1.7 %) and hypokinesia (7.7 % vs. 0.0 %) (Macfadden et al. 2009).

A recent complex trial included 124 bipolar depressed patients refractory to lithium. As previously discussed, these patients were randomized to addition of lamotrigine ($N=64$) or placebo ($n=60$) (van der Loos et al. 2009), and after 8 weeks, paroxetine was added to nonresponders for another 8 weeks ($N=27$) (van der Loos et al. 2010). The patients who responded ($N=65$, of them 25 under lithium plus lamotrigine, 5 under lithium plus lamotrigine plus paroxetine, 6 under paroxetine plus lithium and 19 under lithium monotherapy) continued medication and were followed for up to 68 weeks or until a relapse or recurrence of a depressive or manic episode. These authors compared the two groups defined by the presence of lamotrigine or not. The results suggested that although a numerical superiority in the time to relapse or recurrence was observed for the lamotrigine group vs. the other group (median time 10.0 vs. 3.5 months), this difference was not significant, and therefore these results do not support the authors' conclusion that the maintenance treatment with combination of lamotrigine plus lithium is superior to lithium alone. Furthermore, at study endpoint a similar percentage of patients was still in the study (28.1 % vs. 23.3 %) (van der Loos et al. 2011).

Another trial included 1,270 BD-I patients with a current manic or mixed episode and treated them with lithium or valproate for 2 weeks. Those with inadequate response ($N=686$) received adjunctive single-blind aripiprazole or placebo, and those patients who achieved stability for 12 consecutive weeks ($N=337$) were randomized to double-blind aripiprazole (10–30 mg/day; $N=168$) or placebo ($N=169$) on top of lithium or valproate for 52 weeks. Fewer patients in the aripiprazole group relapsed (17 % vs. 29 %; $p=0.014$). Also the aripiprazole group manifested significantly delayed time to any relapse compared to the placebo group. The significant difference concerned manic and mixed but not depressive relapses. The most common adverse events with adjunctive aripiprazole treatment were headache (13.2 %

vs. 10.8 %), weight increase (9.0 % vs. 6.6 %), tremor (6.0 % vs. 2.4 %) and insomnia (5.4 % vs. 9.6 %) (Marcus et al. 2011).

One study on 50 stable outpatients with BD-I or BD-II added pramipexole ($N=21$) or placebo ($N=24$) on TAU for 8 weeks. Although this is a short duration study, it could be considered to belong to the maintenance phase since it included stabilized patients. The primary cognitive analyses indicated no compelling cognitive benefit of pramipexole vs. placebo, although several methodological problems were present. The major issue was the presence of subsyndromal mood symptoms. In strictly euthymic patients pramipexole might had exerted a beneficial effect ($p=0.03$) (Burdick et al. 2012)

A 12-week study in 324 manic or mixed episodes with asenapine (5–10 mg; $N=158$) vs. placebo ($N=166$) on lithium or valproate reported that adjunctive asenapine significantly improved the YMRS score at week 3 and the response and remission rates at week 12. Those patients who completed this core study were eligible for a 40-week double-blind extension which however assessed only safety and tolerability, because only a small number of patients entered the extension. Treatment-emergent adverse events reported by 5 % or more of asenapine patients and at twice the incidence of placebo were sedation, somnolence, depressive symptoms, oral hypoesthesia and increased weight. Overall adjunctive asenapine to lithium or valproate was well tolerated for up to 52 weeks (Szegedi et al. 2012).

The efficacy of 2 g/day N-acetyl cysteine (NAC) which is a glutathione precursor as adjunct maintenance treatment for BD was examined in 149 BD patients with MADRS score ≥12 at trial entry. After 8 weeks of open-label NAC treatment, they were randomized to adjunctive NAC or placebo, in addition to treatment as usual. Overall there were no significant between-group differences in recurrence or symptomatic outcomes during the maintenance phase of the trial (Berk et al. 2012).

Two trials investigated the efficacy of adjunctive N-acetyl cysteine (NAC). The first one randomized 75 BD patients during the maintenance phase and reported that NAC treatment caused a significant improvement on the MADRS score in comparison to placebo ($p=0.002$). Improvements were lost after washout. There was no effect of NAC on time to a mood episode and no significant between-group differences in adverse events (Berk et al. 2008). The second randomized 14 patients (not all of them with high depression scores) and reported a superiority of the NAC group vs. placebo in terms of remission ($p=0.031$) (Magalhaes et al. 2011). One maintenance study supported the usefulness of ramelteon in the prevention of relapse in BD patients (Norris et al. 2013).

There are some studies suggesting that there is a role for various nutritional supplements such as n-3 fatty acids, chromium, choline, magnesium and tryptophan alone or in combination with pharmacotherapies for the treatment of BD, but the data are of low quality (Sylvia et al. 2013).

16.2.3.4 Post Hoc Reviews and Meta-analytic Studies

16.2.3.4.1 Post Hoc Analyses

There are a number of post hoc analyses which shed some light on a number of questions. They are mentioned below in chronological order of publication.

A sub-analysis of the MAP study which subdivided the patients into 'classical' BD-I without mood-incongruent delusions and without comorbidity ($N=67$) and a nonclassical subgroup including all other patients ($N=104$) reported that the 'classical' group had a lower rehospitalization rate with lithium than with carbamazepine prophylaxis ($p=0.005$), while in the nonclassical group there was no difference between agents although a trend in favour of carbamazepine was found. An additional sub-analysis included mixed states as an additional nonclassical feature and confirmed the results (Greil et al. 1998).

Breakthrough depression is a common problem in the treatment of bipolar disorder. Only one, recently published, double-blind, placebo-controlled trial has examined the efficacy of divalproex in the prevention of depressive episodes in bipolar patients in the frame of an additional analysis of a previously mentioned trial (Bowden et al. 2000). That study lasted for 52 weeks after an index manic episode and randomized patients to maintenance treatment with divalproex ($N=187$), lithium ($N=91$) or placebo ($N=94$) plus adjunctive paroxetine or sertraline for breakthrough depression. The results of the additional analysis suggested that the discontinuation rate for any reason was lower among patients in the divalproex group taking an SSRI than among patients in the placebo group taking an SSRI (56 % vs. 85 %; $p=0.043$) (Gyulai et al. 2003b).

The post hoc analysis of a 24-week, double-blind, placebo-controlled study of ziprasidone or placebo plus lithium or valproate (Bowden et al. 2010) with the utilization of four different remission criteria suggested that the application of different definitions of remission does not make any significant difference concerning the results (Pae et al. 2012).

Another post hoc analysis investigated the response of symptoms associated with suicidality in BD-I patients and assessed the suicide risk during treatment with olanzapine in combination with lithium or divalproex. It utilized data from a previously published trial (Tohen et al. 2004), in which manic or mixed-episode patients who were partially responsive to at least 2 weeks of lithium or divalproex monotherapy prior to study entry were randomly assigned to augmentation therapy with olanzapine (5–20 mg/day) or placebo. That study reported that patients taking olanzapine added to lithium or valproate experienced sustained symptomatic remission, but not syndromic remission, for longer than those receiving lithium or valproate monotherapy. The results of the post hoc analysis suggested that suicidality in adult, mixed-episode, BD-I disorder patients was associated with somatic discomfort, agitated depression and psychosis and that the addition of an atypical antipsychotic–antimanic agent in some BD patients might help to reduce suicidal ideation (Houston et al. 2006).

Another analysis suggested that using olanzapine early in the course of the disorder is possibly more beneficial than lithium during the maintenance phase. This study was a post hoc analysis of data from a multicentre, double-blind, 12-month maintenance trial in 431 BD-I initially euthymic patients with at least two prior manic/mixed episodes which were randomly assigned to olanzapine (5–20 mg/day) or lithium (serum concentration 0.6–1.2 mEq/l) (Tohen et al. 2005). The post hoc analysis subcategorized the patients by illness stage according to number of prior manic/mixed episodes, early stage, 2 prior episodes ($N=53$, lithium; $N=48$, olanzapine); intermediate stage, 3–5 prior episodes ($N=80$, lithium; $N=98$, olanzapine); and later stage, more than 5 prior episodes ($N=81$, lithium; $N=71$, olanzapine), and reported that there were significant effects for treatment ($p<0.001$) and illness stage ($p=0.006$) but no significant interaction ($p=0.107$) on rate of manic/mixed relapse/recurrence. The rates for a manic or mixed relapse or recurrence for olanzapine vs. lithium were 2.1 % vs. 26.4 % ($p=0.008$), 13.3 % vs. 23.8 % ($p=0.073$) and 23.9 % vs. 33.3 % ($p=0.204$) for early-, intermediate- and later-stage groups, respectively. There was no significant effect for treatment ($p=0.096$) or illness stage ($p=0.731$) for depressive relapse or recurrence. These authors concluded that olanzapine maintenance therapy may be particularly effective early in the course of BD (Ketter et al. 2006).

Post hoc analyses were conducted on data from patients presenting with a mixed index episode who were enrolled in a larger maintenance trial of olanzapine vs. placebo for 48 weeks (Tohen et al. 2006). The original study included 731 BD patients, and of them 304 were suffering from an acute mixed episode (41.6 %). Of them, a total of 121 (39.8 %) remitted after the open-label phase and were randomized to olanzapine ($N=76$) or placebo ($N=45$). Compared to the placebo group, the olanzapine group had a lower incidence of 59.2 % vs. 91.1 %; $p<0.001$ and a longer time (46 vs. 15 days; $p<0.001$) to symptomatic relapse of any kind. This was true both for depressive symptomatic relapse (85 vs. 22 days; $p=0.001$) and manic symptomatic relapse (too few relapses to calculate vs. 42 days; $p<0.001$) (Tohen et al. 2009).

A post hoc analysis of a double-blind trial in which BD-I patients who had achieved stabilization from a manic, depressive or mixed episode during open-label treatment with quetiapine were randomized to continue quetiapine or to switch to lithium or placebo for up to 104 weeks (Weisler et al. 2011) reported that of patients randomized to lithium, 201 (59.5 %) obtained lithium levels between 0.6 and 1.2 mEq/l, and 137 (40.5 %) obtained lithium levels <0.6 mEq/l. Their outcomes were compared with those of patients receiving placebo ($N=404$), and the results suggested that the times to recurrence of any mood episode as well as a manic or depressive episode separately were significantly longer for the lithium 0.6–1.2 mEq/l group vs. placebo and vs. lithium <0.6 mEq/l, with no differences between lithium <0.6 mEq/l and placebo (Nolen and Weisler 2013).

Two clinical trials, prospectively designed for combined analysis, compared lithium and lamotrigine vs. placebo for the treatment of BD-I disorder in recently depressed or manic patients (Bowden et al. 2003; Calabrese et al. 2003a). Together they included 1,315 BD-I patients of which 638 were stabilized during the open-label phase and randomly assigned to double-blind monotherapy with lamotrigine (50–400 mg/day fixed dose or 100–400 mg/day flexible dose; $N=280$;), lithium (serum level of 0.8–1.1 mEq/l; $N=167$) or placebo ($N=191$) for 18 months. The results suggested that both lamotrigine and lithium were superior to placebo for time to intervention for any mood episode (197 vs. 184 vs. 86 days). Lamotrigine was superior to placebo for time to intervention for both mania and depression, and lithium was superior to placebo only concerning the time to intervention for mania.

Additional analyses adjusted for index mood did not change the results (Goodwin et al. 2004; Calabrese et al. 2003b). Both lamotrigine and lithium were more effective than placebo in delaying the time to intervention for any mood episode when relapses that occurred in the first 90 or 180 days were excluded from the analyses (Calabrese et al. 2006). A fourth post hoc analysis suggested that the lithium-induced thyroid function abnormalities could be partially responsible for its failure to prevent depression. The analysis showed that patients for whom lithium was ineffective in the prevention of depressive episodes had a significantly higher adjusted mean TSH level in comparison to those for whom lithium was successful (4.4 microIU/ml vs. 2.4 microIU/ml) (Frye et al. 2009). A fifth post hoc analysis of the same two trials focused on subsyndromal symptoms. It reported that significantly more patients under lamotrigine but not under lithium were in remission in comparison to placebo (63 % vs. 60 % vs. 53 %; $p=0.02$ and $p=0.165$, respectively). The median time to onset of subsyndromal symptoms was significantly longer in both treatment groups in comparison to placebo (15 vs. 15 vs. 9 days; $p<0.05$), and this was also true concerning the duration from onset of subsyndromal symptoms to subsequent mood episode (Frye et al. 2006). Finally, aripiprazole maintenance treatment as adjunctive on lithium or valproate is efficacious for a manic but not for a mixed index episode (Yatham et al. 2013).

16.2.3.4.2 Review and Meta-analyses

One review confirmed the efficacy of lithium but reported that there is no definitive evidence as to whether or not lithium has an anti-suicidal effect (Burgess et al. 2001). Two others supported the usefulness of RLAI (Bobo and Shelton 2010) and that of ziprasidone for the maintenance treatment of BD-I disorder in adults as an adjunct to lithium or valproate (Citrome 2010). One review on the usefulness of aripiprazole in the maintenance phase of BD identified two publications, both describing the results of a single trial. It also identified four issues that the authors suggested they limit the interpretation of that trial (insufficient duration, enriched sample, possible conflation of iatrogenic adverse effects of abrupt medication discontinuation with beneficial effects of treatment and a low overall completion rate). They also stressed that the literature rarely mentions these limitations (Tsai et al. 2011). It should be mentioned however that these limitations are present in most maintenance trials and are valid for almost all agents. A number of papers discussed the place of aripiprazole in the treatment of BD (Goodwin et al. 2011; Sayyaparaju et al. 2014).

Concerning meta-analysis, the first one included four RCTs and failed to prove the prophylactic efficacy of carbamazepine (Dardennes et al. 1995). A second one on the usefulness of oxcarbazepine in the maintenance treatment of BD concluded that the data are of low quality and the evidence base is not sufficiently rigorous in terms of methodology to provide guidance on the use of oxcarbazepine in the maintenance treatment of BD (Vasudev et al. 2008).

A number of meta-analyses had focused on lithium. One of them analysed 19 lithium trials (865 patients) and found lithium highly efficacious in terms or recurrence prevention in comparison to placebo (29 % vs. 74 %). However it failed to find sufficient evidence to prove that the lithium-withdrawal relapse phenomenon really exists (Davis et al. 1999). A more recent study included 22 lithium studies (5,647 patients; 33,473 patient-years of risk) and showed that suicide was 82 % less frequent during periods of treatment with lithium (Tondo et al. 2001). The presumed selectivity of lithium against mania was suggested to be a biased result caused by the discontinuation design of many studies, since discontinuation seems to predispose more to mania than depression (Burgess et al. 2001), but a more recent meta-analysis of 5 RCTs (with 770 participants) reported that lithium is especially strong concerning manic relapse prevention, while in the prevention of depressive relapses, it was found to be less potent, but still efficacious (Geddes et al. 2004).

A number of meta-analytic studies confirmed the antimanic efficacy of specific agents and the antidepressant of others. A systematic review and meta-analysis of 34 randomized and quasi-randomized controlled trials suggested that there is evidence for the efficacy of lithium, valproate and lamotrigine as maintenance therapy for the prevention of relapse in BD. Three drugs have a significant effect in the prevention of manic relapses (lithium, olanzapine and aripiprazole) and three in the prevention of depressive symptoms (valproate, lamotrigine and imipramine) (Beynon et al. 2009). Another one confirmed the efficacy of olanzapine in the prevention of mania but questioned its efficacy in the preventing of depressive relapses. It also pointed out that this efficacy was restricted to patients who have responded to olanzapine during the acute manic or mixed episode and who have not previously had a satisfactory response to lithium or valproate (Cipriani et al. 2010). Finally, the analysis of maintenance data from 15 studies reported that quetiapine, lithium, RLAI, aripiprazole and olanzapine were proven effective in manic recurrence prevention, while lamotrigine, quetiapine and lithium were proven effective also for the prevention of depressive relapses (Popovic et al. 2010).

Two analyses investigated combination treatment and both questioned its efficacy. The first reported that there is little evidence to support the efficacy of combination therapy (Beynon et al. 2009), while the second utilized data from 7 trials with a total of 350 BD patients. It reported that those long-term treatments that included antidepressants yielded 27 % lower risk of a depressive relapse in comparison to mood stabilizer alone or to no treatment. However the presence of an antidepressant was related with a 72 % greater risk for a manic relapse. The risk ratio was not significant in either case; therefore, these authors suggested that long-term adjunctive antidepressant treatment was not superior to a mood stabilizer alone (Ghaemi et al. 2008).

One final meta-analysis included 20 trials (5,364 patients). It confirmed that the majority of studies included samples enriched for response to a specific agent during the acute phase. The results suggested that no monotherapy was associated with a significantly reduced risk for both manic/mixed and depressed relapse. Of the combination treatments, only quetiapine + lithium/divalproex was associated with a significantly reduced risk vs. comparator (placebo + lithium/valproate) for relapse at both the manic/mixed and depressed poles of bipolar illness. Other limitations for the analysis and interpretation include differences in study durations and definitions of relapse (Vieta et al. 2011).

16.2.4 Treatment of Mixed Episodes

Mixed episodes are no longer accepted as a diagnostic entity by DSM-5; instead 'mixed features' is included as a specifier. The two concepts are significantly different, and the results concerning mixed episodes from the clinical trials so far cannot be applied directly in patients with this specifier. It is important to note that in clinical trials, mixed episodes are treated together with manic episodes. Some studies report the results concerning mixed episodes separately; however, they always concern trials of acute mania. No data on mixed episodes are reported in clinical trials of bipolar depression. An important limitation is the fact that in most studies, even when results are reported separately for mixed patients, they usually concern the manic but not the depressive component of the clinical picture (Fountoulakis et al. 2012d).

A summary of the data for the treatment of mixed episodes is shown in Table 16.8.

16.2.4.1 Treatment of Acute Mixed Episodes

Aripiprazole was reported to be efficacious in the treatment of acute mixed episodes, and this efficacy concerned both the manic and the depressive component. Additionally, the efficacy against the manic component was independent from the severity of the depressive component (Suppes et al. 2008a; Sachs et al. 2006; Keck et al. 2003b).

Asenapine is reported not to be efficacious against the manic component, but no data exist concerning the depressive component (McIntyre et al. 2009c). Olanzapine was reported to be efficacious against the manic, but the data are inconclusive concerning the depressive component (there might be some efficacy in the most severe cases and in specific subgroups) (McIntyre et al. 2009c; Tohen et al. 1999, 2000; Baldessarini et al. 2003; Baker et al. 2003; Shi et al. 2004b). Paliperidone is efficacious against the manic but not against the depressive component (Berwaerts et al. 2010; Vieta et al. 2010a). Risperidone is reported to be efficacious against the manic component, but it is unknown whether this is also true for the depressive component (Khanna et al. 2005). Ziprasidone is reported to be efficacious against both the manic and the depressive component, but this was reported in mixed states not similar to the DSM definition (Keck et al. 2003b; Potkin et al. 2005; Stahl et al. 2010; McElroy et al. 1992). Carbamazepine is efficacious both against the manic and against the depressive component (Weisler et al. 2004, 2005, 2006). Valproate is efficacious against the manic component, but the data concerning the depressive component are inconclusive (Bowden et al. 2006; Ghaemi et al. 2007).

In mixed depression, the OFC was comparable to olanzapine, and both were superior to placebo, but the report does not permit to derive conclusions (Benazzi et al. 2009; Tohen et al. 2003c).

The data concerning the combination of haloperidol or risperidone plus lithium or valproate were negative (Sachs et al. 2002), while the combinations of olanzapine plus lithium or valproate have positive data concerning both components (Tohen et al. 2002b; Baker et al. 2004; Houston et al. 2006, 2009, 2011). Overall it seems that SGAs are effective in the treatment of acute mixed episodes of BD, with predominant manic symptoms. Their efficacy in treating depressed mixed episodes remains unclear (Muralidharan et al. 2013).

16.2.4.2 Maintenance Treatment of Mixed Bipolar Episodes

The data so far suggest that olanzapine prolongs relapse into any episode in patients with an index mixed episode (Tohen et al. 2006, 2009), while lithium and valproate had negative results in patients with a dysphoric manic index episode (Bowden et al. 2005a). The data are in support of the combination of quetiapine plus lithium or valproate (Vieta et al. 2008b; Suppes et al. 2009) but are negative concerning aripiprazole in patients with an index mixed episode (Yatham et al. 2013).

16.2.5 Treatment of Rapid Cycling Patients

The treatment of rapid cycling patients constitutes a challenge. Often their course frustrates the therapist, and the evaluation of treatment is difficult because of the rapid switching from one pole to another. Careful registration and evaluation of the long-term course is necessary in order to verify whether the overall frequency and/or severity of episodes improved (Fountoulakis et al. 2013a).

A summary of the data for the treatment of rapid cycling patients specifically for acute mania is shown in Table 16.8 and for acute bipolar depression is shown in Table 16.9.

16.2.5.1 Treatment of Acute Episodes in Rapid Cycling Patients

The secondary analysis of the data from a trial of olanzapine in acute mania suggested that olanzapine was effective in the reducing of the symptoms of mania and was well tolerated in rapid cycling BD-I patients (Sanger et al. 2003). The pooling of data from two RCTs reported that improvement of mania with olanzapine was similar in rapid cyclers and non-rapid cyclers. However, rapid cyclers showed an earlier response (Vieta et al. 2004). One trial was also positive concerning aripiprazole in acutely manic patients (Sachs et al. 2006).

Although one study on acute mania in rapid cycling patients was negative (Cutler et al. 2011), one a priori planned sub-analysis of data from rapid cycling patients with acute BD-I or BD-II depression suggested that quetiapine monotherapy (300–600 mg/day) was effective and well tolerated (Vieta et al. 2007). This was also confirmed by the post hoc analysis of the rapid cycling subsample of bipolar depressives from the BOLDER study (Cookson et al. 2007). Finally the sub-analysis of the data from a small number of depressed rapid cycling BD patients again suggested that 300 mg of quetiapine monotherapy was superior to placebo (Suppes et al. 2010).

Additionally there is some weak but positive signal for lithium (Young et al. 2010) and some positive but equivocal data for valproate (Muzina et al. 2010); however, the results are clearly negative for paroxetine (McElroy et al. 2010c).

The combination of lithium and divalproex is probably not effective, and the further addition of lamotrigine does not seem to add anything in terms of efficacy (Kemp et al. 2012a).

16.2.5.2 Relapse Prevention in Rapid Cycling Patients

The treatment during the maintenance phase and the relapse prevention is the most challenging aspect of the treatment of rapid cycling BD patients.

The data so far suggest that divalproex was not more effective than lithium (Calabrese et al. 2005b) and also the combination of lithium plus divalproex was not better than lithium alone (Kemp et al. 2009). However the combination of lithium plus carbamazepine did better than either agent alone, but the study sample of that trial was very small (Denicoff et al. 1997). The data are negative for lamotrigine although in some secondary outcomes there was a beneficial signal especially in BD-II patients (Calabrese et al. 2000). It is interesting to note that the popular concept among clinicians that divalproex is more effective than lithium in the long-term management of rapid cycling bipolar disorder was not supported by a trial on 139 patients (Findling et al. 2005).

In patients who continued open-label olanzapine therapy for 1 year after 3 weeks of double-blind therapy for acute mania, non-rapid cyclers were more likely to experience a symptomatic remission and were less likely to experience a recurrence, especially into a depressive phase. They also were less likely to be hospitalized and to make a suicide attempt (Vieta et al. 2004).

One post hoc analysis suggested that aripiprazole was efficacious (Muzina et al. 2008). There are no data on monotherapy with other antipsychotics concerning the maintenance phase. Another post hoc analysis reported that rapid cycling patients did less well during the extended observation period than non-rapid cycling patients, regardless of treatment, and that overall olanzapine and divalproex appeared comparable (Suppes et al. 2005).

An international study confirmed the efficacy and safety of quetiapine on lithium or divalproex in the prevention of mood episodes in rapid cycling BD-I patients with most recent episode being manic/mixed or depressive (Vieta et al. 2008b). There was a North American study with a similar design as the previous one and reported the same results (Suppes et al. 2009). A large controlled trial which evaluated adjunctive maintenance treatment with RLAI on TAU in 240 BD-I patients with at least four mood episodes in the 12 months prior to study entry returned positive results. These patients did not correspond exactly to the 'rapid cycling' definition; however, the results of the study are relevant for consideration in the treatment of rapid cycling patients (Macfadden et al. 2009).

Data from the STEP-BD support the role of antidepressants in the development of rapid cycling. A rapid cycling course predicted three times more depressive episodes in spite of continuation treatment with antidepressants. However, the study sample was very small (Ghaemi et al. 2010). Again according to the STEP-BD data, during follow-up, antidepressant use was associated with more frequent mood episodes (Schneck et al. 2008). A similar conclusion came from an earlier randomized controlled study of rapid cycling patients which utilized a double-blind on-off-on-off design with the use of tricyclic antidepressants (Wehr et al. 1988).

Finally, the data are negative concerning the administration of ethyl-eicosapentaenoate (EPA) 6 g/day as augmentation on ongoing treatment with mood stabilizers in rapid cycling patients with acute bipolar depression (Keck et al. 2006b).

One meta analysis suggested that lithium was at least partially efficacious in rapid cycling patients (Kupka et al. 2003), and another one suggested there is no clear advantage of any treatment option vs. the others (Tondo et al. 2003), while a third one found that some atypical antipsychotics (especially quetiapine and olanzapine) could be considered as the first-line treatment option (Cruz et al. 2010). The meta-analysis of 20 studies published from 1974 to 2002 comparing subjects with rapid and non-rapid cycling BD reported that in contrast to common beliefs, lithium prophylaxis had at least partial efficacy in a considerable number of rapid cyclers, especially when antidepressants were avoided. It should be mentioned however that hypothyroidism, which is a frequent adverse effect of lithium, might be associated with mood destabilization in vulnerable patients (Kupka et al. 2003).

16.2.6 Treatment of Special Conditions

16.2.6.1 Treatment of Comorbid Conditions

Comorbidity is a significant issue in bipolar patients and often needs specific therapeutic intervention. Simply adding medication might not be the correct strategy, at least not always.

16.2.6.1.1 Treatment of Comorbid Substance Abuse Disorder (SUD)

As shown in Chap. 9 of the current book, substance use, abuse and dependence is not uncommon in BD patients. Their coexistence perplexes the treatment for both conditions. Unfortunately, the data concerning the pharmacological treatment of substance use in patients with BD are limited.

There are two placebo-controlled trials suggesting that the combination of valproate and lithium in BD patients with co-occurring alcohol dependence improves both mood and alcohol use symptoms and that lithium treatment in BD adolescents improves both mood and substance use symptoms (Cerullo and Strakowski 2007). Lithium can be used for the treatment of concomitant substance and polysubstance abuse (Geller et al. 1992, 1998), and quetiapine and risperidone can reduce drug craving (Nejtek et al. 2008). However, the data concerning quetiapine for alcohol abuse are negative (Brown et al. 2008). For bipolar patients with alcohol dependence, naltrexone could be useful (Sherwood Brown et al. 2009), and a preliminary report is positive for acamprosate (Tolliver et al. 2012).

There are open-label medication trials which provide limited support to quetiapine, aripiprazole and lamotrigine for the treatment of BD patients with cocaine dependence. Also, aripiprazole might be helpful in patients with alcohol use disorders (Cerullo and Strakowski 2007).

It is important to mention that during treatment with antidepressants, the presence of substance use might increase the risk of switching (Goldberg and Whiteside 2002).

In spite of the magnitude of the problem and the resulting disability, burden and cost, the existing data are insufficient to support an informed design of pharmaceutical treatment strategy in BD patients with SUD. Some data are available for alcohol, cannabis and cocaine use comorbid with BD, but the literature is poor concerning heroin, amphetamine, methamphetamine and poly-SUD comorbid with BD (Beaulieu et al. 2012).

16.2.6.1.2 Treatment of Comorbid Anxiety and Anxiety Disorders

A post hoc analysis of anxiety symptoms with data from two RCTs (Calabrese et al. 2005a; Thase et al. 2006) of 8-week duration concerning quetiapine (300 or 600 mg/day) reported that at endpoint there was no difference between treatment groups and placebo concerning the total HAM-A score, but there was concerning both the psychic and somatic anxiety subscale scores in comparison with placebo ($p<0.001$). The baseline severity of anxiety did not impact the improvement in depressive symptoms (Lydiard et al. 2009). Also, quetiapine XR (50–300 mg/day) was superior both to divalproex ER (500–3,000 mg/day) and to placebo in the improvement of anxiety in BD patients with comorbid panic attack or GAD (Sheehan et al. 2013). In another study, again quetiapine (300 or 600 mg/day) and paroxetine (20 mg/day) produced a significant improvement in anxiety in terms of change of HAM-A scale score from baseline in acutely depressed BD patients (McElroy et al. 2010c). Finally, quetiapine (300–600 mg/day) significantly improved the HAM-A score from baseline, while this was not the case with lithium (600–1,800 mg/day; $p=0.279$) (Young et al. 2010).

Also lurasidone (20–60 mg/day; $N=166$ or 80–120 mg/day) significantly improved anxiety symptoms in comparison to placebo (Loebel et al. 2013).

On the contrary, risperidone monotherapy was not an effective anxiolytic for BD patients with comorbid panic disorder or GAD in doses of 0.5–4 mg/day over 8 weeks of treatment (Sheehan et al. 2009). As mentioned previously, negative were also the data concerning lithium (600–1,800 mg/day; $p=0.279$) (Young et al. 2010).

The data concerning divalproex (rapidly titrated up to 2,500 mg/day, as tolerated, to a target serum level of 50–100 mg/dl) are equivocal because the only positive study was based on a small study sample (25 outpatients with BD-I depression) (Davis et al. 2005).

It is reasonable to suggest that also benzodiazepines can be used as adjunctive medication for sedation or for the treatment of anxiety, although abuse, tolerance and dependence constitute important problems. Although approved for the treatment of GAD, pregabalin has no data on BD. However, again it is reasonable to suggest it might be a useful agent for the treatment of anxiety disorders that commonly accompany BD and could substitute for benzodiazepines, according to the clinical judgement of the therapist. A significant advantage is that it is not metabolized in the liver.

A summary of the data for the treatment of anxiety mostly during a bipolar depressive episode is shown in Table 16.9.

16.2.6.1.3 Weight Gain

Weight gain and the metabolic syndrome in general constitute a significant public health problem which is especially important in psychiatric patients.

Although the general approach is that lifestyle modifications are the main tool to control and even avoid weight gain, such approaches are of limited value in psychiatric populations, who find it difficult to discipline concerning food intake and lack motivation to exercise. Therefore, besides the psychoeducation to push a change in lifestyle, a number of medications have been proposed as useful to tackle this problem.

Topiramate is not effective in the treatment of BD per se; however, it is unique because of its ability to cause weight loss at dosages of 50–200 mg/day. A review reported that more than 70 % of patients taking topiramate for a mean duration of 5 months lost a mean of 5–6 kg (Arnone 2005). The problem is that most agents with proven efficacy in weight loss might cause depression de novo, and topiramate itself could induce suicidality in some patients although no completed suicides related to topiramate have been reported (Fountoulakis et al. 2012a).

16.2.6.1.4 Treatment of Agitation

Agitation constitutes an important clinical problem which perplexes treatment. It is mostly present during the acute phase, both manic and depressive, but milder forms could be present during all phases of the illness. When severe, it often affects insight and interferes with proper treatment, and it usually demands specialized treatment itself.

A number of treatments have been proposed, but most are not studied adequately due to a number of methodological issues, including the obtaining of informed consent from the side of the patient. Probably most clinicians choose antipsychotics in their everyday clinical practice, and this option is supported by a double-blind clinical trial which reported that intramuscular haloperidol (5–10 mg) was equal in efficacy but faster acting in comparison to intramuscular clonazepam (1–2 mg) in agitated mania at 0, 30 and 60 min (Chouinard et al. 1993). Similarly, intramuscular olanzapine (10 mg, first two injections; 5 mg, third injection) was reported to be superior to lorazepam (2 mg, first two injections; 1 mg, third injection), for the controlling of agitation in manic patients. Already 2 h after the first injection, patients treated with olanzapine showed a significantly greater reduction in scores on all agitation scales compared with patients treated with either placebo or lorazepam (Meehan et al. 2001).

Valproate oral loading of 20 mg/kg/day was reported to be comparable to haloperidol 0.2 mg/kg/day for the treatment of excited manic patients in a single-blind study, and the effect was evident within 3 days from starting (McElroy et al. 1996). Overall, valproate loading up to 30 mg/kg/day was reported to be safe and well tolerated (Hirschfeld et al. 1999).

The most recent addition in the armamentarium for the treatment of acute agitation concerned the development of inhaled loxapine which could be considered as not as invasive as injections but still faster acting in comparison to oral formulas. One clinical trial was conducted in BD-I patients with agitation associated with manic or mixed episodes. The anti-agitation effect was observed at 10 min (first time point measured) for both the 5 mg and 10 mg doses. Loxapine remained superior to placebo throughout the remainder of the study at all time points measured. The effect size was comparable to what has been previously reported for intramuscular antipsychotics and benzodiazepines. For safety reasons it has been recommended that inhaled loxapine be restricted to a single dose in 24 h and be subject to a Risk Evaluation and Mitigation Strategy programme (Citrome 2012; Kwentus et al. 2012).

16.2.6.1.5 Treatment of the Neurocognitive Deficit

One study compared pramipexole ($N=21$) vs. placebo ($N=24$) for the treatment of the neurocognitive deficit in stable BD-I or BD-II outpatients. Overall the two groups showed similar effect on neurocognitive function, but there was some efficacy for pramipexole in euthymic patients only (Burdick et al. 2012). Similarly, a trial which utilized N-acetyl cysteine (NAC) failed to support its efficacy for the improvement of neurocognitive function in BD patients (Dean et al. 2012).

On the contrary there are some data supporting the usefulness of insulin and mifepristone. In one study, euthymic BD patients were randomized to receive adjunctive intranasal insulin (40 IU q.i.d.; $N=34$) or placebo ($N=28$) for 8 weeks. A significant improvement vs. placebo was noted with intranasal insulin therapy on executive function but not on the other neurocognitive measures (McIntyre et al. 2012). The data were more robust concerning the effect of 600 mg/day of mifepristone (a synthetic steroid compound with both antiprogesterone and antiglucocorticoid properties) vs. placebo as an adjunctive treatment, for 1 week, in 60 patients with bipolar depression. Mifepristone improved the primary outcome which was spatial working memory, and this was evident 7 weeks after the cessation of treatment. The magnitude of this neuropsychological response was predicted by the magnitude of the cortisol response to mifepristone, but it was unrelated with the change in depressed mood (Watson et al. 2012).

16.2.6.1.6 Suicide

Suicide is not an uncommon outcome in the course of BD (see Chap. 19), and there is much discussion concerning the potential anti-suicidal efficacy of specific drugs and especially of lithium. However almost all the data come from studies of naturalistic and epidemiological nature, and no controlled studies exist.

There is only one post hoc analysis which investigated suicidality in BD-I patients during treatment with olanzapine in combination with lithium or divalproex. In mixed patients with residual suicidality, suicidal thoughts were associated with somatic discomfort, agitated depression and psychosis. It seems that combination therapy with olanzapine plus lithium ($N=36$) vs. lithium alone ($N=22$) differentially reduced the score in the suicidal item of the HAM-D by 58 % vs. 29 % ($p<0.05$) within 1 week and all associated symptoms within 2 weeks by averages of 31 % vs. 12 % ($p<0.05$) (Houston et al. 2006).

16.2.7 Cautions for Pharmaceutical Treatment in BD Patients

There are a number of issues that need attention during the treatment of BD with medication. It is well known that lithium has a narrow therapeutic window concerning its dosage and plasma levels (recommended plasma level 0.6–1.2 mmol/l).

Although the research data suggest it is well accepted with a good tolerability profile, often in clinical practice patients are dissatisfied because of sedation and tremor, and sometimes a decline in creative thinking is reported (see Chap. 20), although in patients under long-term lithium treatment, no further decline of neurocognitive function was observed (Engelsmann et al. 1988). Adverse events are more frequent with higher doses, while 'rebound mania' has been described on withdrawal. Additional drawbacks with lithium therapy also include laboratory testing and thorough investigation before starting treatment (ECG, kidney function, etc.), which often delay the initiation of treatment and disappoint the patient. It seems that overall fewer than 20 % of patients have no adverse effects at all, but also only about 30 % have more than minor complaints. The most frequent adverse events include neurological, endocrinological (more often from the thyroid), cardiovascular, renal, gastrointestinal, haematological and dermatological manifestations, while also lithium intoxication is not rare. It seems there is a complex relationship between lithium treatment, female gender, hypothyroidism and rapid cycling (Bauer and Whybrow 1990; Cowdry et al. 1983; Fountoulakis et al. 2008c; Bauer et al. 1990; Gyulai et al. 2003a). While most authors argue that lithium is neuroprotective, a neurotoxic effect is also possible in the long term, even at therapeutic levels, especially in combination with antipsychotics (Fountoulakis et al. 2008c). It is reported also that lithium plasma levels peak during the summer (Cusin et al. 2002; Wilting et al. 2007), especially in males (D'Mello et al. 1995), and this difference could be up to 25 % (Medhi et al. 2008).

As mentioned above, it is very interesting and well known that many patients under lithium complain that treatment inhibits their creativity and productivity (Shaw et al. 1986). It is important to note that this loss of creativity might be specifically related to lithium and not divalproex (Stoll et al. 1996) although there are studies rejecting this (Schou 1979). Overall it seems that patients are more creative when well stabilized and their symptoms are under good control (see Chap. 20). At any case, fortunately, cognitive complaints do not seem to be significant predictors of discontinuation of lithium treatment (Connelly et al. 1982; Maarbjerg et al. 1988). Apart from reduced creativity, a general negative impact of lithium on neurocognitive function has been reported, especially on memory and psychomotor functioning (Squire et al. 1980; Kocsis et al. 1993; Honig et al. 1999; Lund et al. 1982; Kessing 1998), but fortunately the insult does not seem to be cumulative (Engelsmann et al. 1988). More specifically, lithium impairs both mental and motor speed, short-term memory and verbal or associative fluency, but the deficit is reversible when lithium is withdrawn and re-establishes when lithium is re-administered (Goldberg 2008; Shaw et al. 1987; Kocsis et al. 1993). Lithium also causes a deficit in the long-term recall (retrieval) without having an effect on attention or encoding (Shaw et al. 1987; Squire et al. 1980; Reus et al. 1979; Karniol et al. 1978; Kropf and Muller-Oerlinghausen 1979). This deficit might especially concern verbal memory (Bora et al. 2007; Senturk et al. 2007). The overall effect size related to the negative impact of lithium treatment on neurocognition is small (Arts et al. 2008), but could be significant concerning specific domains (Wingo et al. 2009). Precise guidelines concerning lithium treatment and its optimal therapeutic levels are available (Malhi et al. 2011).

The recommended valproate therapeutic serum concentration is 50–150 mg/ml. It needs caution when used in women of childbearing age, due to the high frequency of unplanned pregnancies in bipolar females and the relatively high teratogenicity of valproate. Other potential acute side effects are weight gain and hair loss. It is unclear whether it induces polycystic ovarian syndrome.

The typical dosage of carbamazepine in the treatment of acute mania is 600–1,800 mg/day (serum concentration 4–12 mg/ml). However, after several weeks under carbamazepine, an induction of hepatic enzymes (CYP 3A4) occurs. Consequently the drug levels drop and may require additional upward dose titration (Bertilsson and Tomson 1986). The dosage-related adverse effects include double or blurred vision, dizziness, sedation, ataxia, vertigo, gastrointestinal disturbances, cognitive impairment, haematological effects and Stevens–Johnson syndrome and its related dermatological effects (Tohen et al. 1991, 1995; Blackburn et al. 1998).

The most significant drawback of lamotrigine treatment is the need to initiate it slowly with a rate of 25 mg at 2-week intervals in order to avoid a moderately high incidence of dangerous rash (Seo et al. 2010).

Carbamazepine decreases lamotrigine concentrations by approximately 50 %, and during combination therapy, lamotrigine can be started with higher dosages and faster titration. It exerts similar effects on other agents as well, e.g. risperidone (Ono et al. 2002).

It is also important to note the adverse effects of topiramate because although it is not used in the treatment of BD per se, it is often administered in BD patients in order to lose weight or to treat a comorbid substance abuse disorder. It is reported that topiramate impairs attention, verbal memory, psychomotor slowing, and word finding even at very low dosages (25–50 mg/day). This impairment is reversible after discontinuation of the drug (Goldberg 2008; Salinsky et al. 2005).

The adverse effects of FGAs and especially of haloperidol include extrapyramidal signs and symptoms (EPS), tardive dyskinesia and hyperprolactinaemia, while the most frequent side effects of chlorpromazine are EPS, tardive dyskinesia, postural hypotension and hepatotoxicity. On the other hand, the most significant problem with some of the SGAs is weight gain, hyperlipidaemia and diabetes mellitus in a significant percentage of the patients. The treatment of these somatic conditions is difficult, and the methods proposed have produced rather unsatisfactory results so far. Hyperprolactinaemia and EPS are the most frequent adverse effects with amisulpride. Akathisia and EPS are the adverse effects most often reported with aripiprazole.

Concerning olanzapine, the most frequent adverse effects include dry mouth, weight gain, increased appetite, diabetes mellitus and metabolic syndrome and somnolence. The main adverse effects of quetiapine are persistent sedation and weight gain, however, to a lower extent than olanzapine. Maybe the XR formulation of quetiapine induces less sedation in comparison to the IR formulation (Riesenberg et al. 2012). The main side effects of risperidone are dose-related EPS, weight gain, sedation and hyperprolactinaemia. Somnolence, akathisia and EPS, as well as a potential QTc prolongation, are the main adverse effects of ziprasidone treatment; however, ziprasidone is not associated with the metabolic syndrome (Kemp et al. 2012b).

Reports on antipsychotics concerning their adverse effect on neurocognition are rare and conflicting (Holmes et al. 2008; Pan et al. 2011; Goldberg and Chengappa 2009). There are data suggesting that the executive function deficit was correlated with years of exposure to antipsychotic drugs (Zubieta et al. 2001). This latter finding could reflect the toxic effect of chronic psychosis, the toxic effect of long-term medication or both. In general, neuroleptics have been associated with sustained attention and visuomotor speed deficits (King 1994). Current antipsychotic treatment in BD patients is reported to relate to worse performance across all executive function tests as well as in semantic fluency, verbal learning and recognition memory, even when clinical features were controlled for (Frangou et al. 2005; Jamrozinski et al. 2009; Altshuler et al. 2004).

16.2.8 Switching to the Opposite Pole

There were several reports in the 1970s suggesting that the use of antidepressants might induce mania, mixed episodes and rapid cycling. On the other hand, there is a wide belief among clinicians that antipsychotics induce depression. Often these two suggestions are not limited to BD but are considered to be true for all mental disorders. Overall, it is widely accepted among psychiatrists that both antidepressants and FGAs can induce the opposite pole, a chronic, dysphoric, mixed or irritable state in BD patients, and may accelerate episode frequency and/or may cause other forms of course destabilization in patients with BD. However, hard data are rare, and the bulk of evidence comes from chart reviews and retrospective and open studies.

The earlier studies utilized the medical records of patients in a retrospective way and suggested that without the concomitant use of an antimanic agent, the switch rate to mania or hypomania is around 25 % (Bottlender et al. 2001). Additionally they suggested that the concomitant use of an antimanic agent reduces the switch rate to 14 % but does not eliminate the risk (Post et al. 2001, 2006). It seems also that the switch rate depends on lithium levels (5.9 % for high and 10.5 % for low lithium levels) (Nemeroff et al. 2001). The review of the medical records of 158 depressed BD-I patients suggested that pharmacological intervention and the number of mixed depressive symptoms at admission acted as risk factors for the development of manic-like symptomatology (Bottlender et al. 2004).

The analysis of the results of the STEP-BD patients is of particular interest. The results from the first 500 patients reported that from the 338 subjects with prior antidepressant treatment and complete data on switch event outcomes, 44 % reported at least 1 switching. Shorter duration of illness and history of multiple antidepressant trials seemed to act as risk factors. Also switch was less common during treatment with electroconvulsive therapy or monoamine oxidase inhibitors than other antidepressants (Truman et al. 2007). The results from the first 1,500 patients suggested a 10 times higher risk for the presence of dysphoria, irritability and middle insomnia for those patients with current antidepressant treatment although this could be predicted also by past antidepressant-related manic switch and gender (El-Mallakh et al. 2008).

The data from double-blind RCTs concerning the switch rates of paroxetine and bupropion suggest that they are similar to placebo (Sachs et al. 2007). A problem is that since paroxetine is not efficacious in the treatment of acute bipolar depression (McElroy et al. 2010c), no real conclusions can be made. The data are also negative for fluoxetine even as monotherapy in BD-II patients (Amsterdam et al. 2004) and for citalopram whose rates are similar to those of lamotrigine when added on a mood stabilizer (Schaffer et al. 2006).

However there are some data suggesting that venlafaxine might have higher rates of switching in comparison to the other antidepressants or placebo. The results from a 10-week RCT, on 174 patients which were randomly treated with a flexible dose of bupropion, sertraline and venlafaxine or placebo as adjuncts to mood stabilizers, suggested that while the three antidepressants were comparable in terms of efficacy, there was a significantly increased risk of switches into hypomania or mania in those patients treated with venlafaxine in comparison to bupropion or sertraline (Post et al. 2006). The comparison of venlafaxine with bupropion after 1 year found higher rates of switch into hypomania and mania in the venlafaxine group (21.8 % vs. 14.9 %) (Leverich et al. 2006). A small study which compared 15 BD-II depressed women with 17 women with unipolar depression which were randomized to receive once vs. twice daily venlafaxine monotherapy up to 225 mg for 6 weeks reported similar efficacy for venlafaxine in the two diagnostic groups without any episodes of drug-induced hypomania or rapid cycling (Amsterdam and Garcia-Espana 2000). A single-blind 6-week comparison of paroxetine vs. venlafaxine in 55 bipolar depressed patients which were already receiving mood stabilizers reported no significant differences in either efficacy or safety between the two treatment groups; however, although the dropout rate was similar (43 % vs. 50 %), more patients under paroxetine dropped out because of lack of efficacy (7 % vs. 0 %), while more under venlafaxine dropped out because of switching to mania (3 % vs. 13 %) (Vieta et al. 2002). Two more recent publications from the same research group reported conflicting results concerning venlafaxine (Altshuler et al. 2006, 2009). The interpretation of the data concerning venlafaxine is difficult, but one of the available interpretations could be that venlafaxine is efficacious in the treatment of bipolar depression but at the same time puts patients at a higher risk to switch to mania or hypomania. This switch causes dropouts and could mask the therapeutic effect.

Similarly, there are data suggesting that treatment with imipramine increases the risk for an affective switch. A small 6-week study on BD patients suffering from 'anergic depression' compared the efficacy of tranylcypromine (30–60 mg/day; $N=28$) with that of imipramine (150–300 mg/day; $N=28$), and the results suggested that tranylcypromine produced statistically significant superior outcome in terms of greater symptomatic improvement, while the proportion of patients which switched to mania/hypomania was numerically higher in the imipramine group (12 % vs. 24 %). BD-I patients had a significantly greater risk of treatment-emergent mood swings (38 % vs. 13 %; $p=0.03$) (Himmelhoch et al. 1991). Another 8-week international multicentre study in 156 bipolar depressed patients randomized them to moclobemide (450–750 mg/day; $N=81$) or imipramine (150–250 mg/day; $N=75$). There were no statistically significant differences between the two groups on any efficacy measures or on the dropout rate for any reason; however, more patients under imipramine switched to mania (3.7 % vs. 11 %) (Silverstone 2001). Finally, a multicentre 10-week study in 117 BD depressed outpatients compared paroxetine (20–50 mg/day; *N*=35) vs. imipramine (50–300 mg/day; *N*=39) vs. placebo (*N*=43) as add-on to lithium and reported that the three groups were comparable in terms of efficacy; however, in comparison to imipramine, paroxetine resulted in a lower incidence of the emergence of manic symptoms (Nemeroff et al. 2001).

It is important to mention that switching to mania or hypomania has been reported during treatment with antidepressants of comorbid OCD (White et al. 1986; Steiner 1991; Vieta and Bernardo 1992; Rihmer et al. 1996; Perugi et al. 2002) or panic disorder (Pecknold and Fleury 1986; Sholomskas 1990).

There are a number of reviews which suggest a possible connection between switching and antidepressant treatment; however, they also stress that all available studies suffer from various forms of bias. The switch rate has been calculated to be as high as 18.2 % in the short term and 35.6 % during the continuation phase; however, it has also been pointed out that antidepressant discontinuation is associated with a substantially increased risk of depression relapse over the subsequent year with no reduced risk of switching into mania (Post et al. 2003). The risk is higher in BD-I patients in comparison to BD-II (14.2 % vs. 7.1 % in acute trials and 23.4 % vs. 13.9 % in maintenance studies). The rates of switching in unipolar patients are lower than those in bipolar (1.5 % in acute trials and 6.0 % in maintenance studies) (Bond et al. 2008). Another review suggested that all classes of antidepressants have been reported to relate to affective switches in a subgroup of about 20–40 % of BD patients. The patients at the highest risk seem to be those whose initial illness begun in adolescence or young adulthood (Goldberg and Truman 2003). Furthermore, it is reported that when combined with a mood stabilizer, antidepressants given for acute bipolar depression do not induce a switch into hypomania or mania (Licht et al. 2008; Harel and Levkovitz 2008). The most recent systematic review of 73 reports (109 trials, 114 521 adult patients), 35 of which were suitable for meta-analysis, suggested that the overall risk of mania with vs. without antidepressants averaged 12.5 % vs. 7.5 %, with antidepressant-associated mania being more frequent in bipolar than unipolar patients. TCAs were riskier than SSRIs, while data for other types of ADs were inconclusive. Mood stabilizers had minor effects probably confounded by their preferential use in mania-prone patients (Tondo et al. 2010). A genetic study of BD-I (*N*=103) and BD-II (*N*=66) patients during antidepressant therapy, who manifested an affective switch that occurred within a period of 3 weeks in comparison to 247 patients which never showed switches concerning the functional polymorphism in the upstream regulatory region of the serotonin transporter (SERTPR), tryptophan hydroxylase (TPH), G-protein beta 3 subunit (Gbeta3), monoamine oxidase A (MAO-A), catechol-O-methyltransferase (COMT), serotonin receptor 2A (5-HT2A), dopamine receptor D2 (DRD2) and dopamine receptor D4 (DRD4) gene variants, produced no significant results (Serretti et al. 2004).

FGAs are also considered to induce the opposite pole and cause dysphoria and depression. Although one study in acutely manic patients suggested that haloperidol-treated patients relapsed earlier than olanzapine-treated patients into a depressive episode, this could simply mean that haloperidol is less effective than olanzapine in the prevention of depressive episodes (Tohen et al. 2003a). On the contrary, one trial which compared continuation treatment of perphenazine vs. discontinuation (placebo) as adjunct on lithium, carbamazepine or valproate for 6 months reported that those patients randomly assigned to continue perphenazine treatment, relative to those who discontinued it, were more likely to have a shorter time to depressive relapse, discontinue the study and have increased rates of dysphoria, depressive symptoms and extrapyramidal symptoms (Zarate and Tohen 2004).

On the contrary, in most studies SGAs do not appear to switch patients into depression, while some authors suggest they possess a mild protective property against switching. Both SGAs and the OFC seem to be efficacious without posing the patients at an increased risk for an affective switch (Tohen et al. 2003c; Amsterdam and Shults 2005a; Keck et al. 2005; Benazzi et al. 2009; Calabrese et al. 2005a; Thase et al. 2006). A recent meta-analysis reported that treating acute mania with SGAs is associated with 42 % less risk of switch to depression than with haloperidol. Nevertheless, caution should be taken when considering this a class effect, as only olanzapine, quetiapine and ziprasidone may show a better profile (Goikolea et al. 2013b).

Overall there are no data to suggest a generalized and class effect for antidepressants or FGAs concerning the induction of an affective switch. There are negative data concerning all SSRIs and SGAs studied and some positive data only concerning venlafaxine, imipramine and perphenazine. Some authors believe that at least the switch risk and perhaps also the risk for rapid cycling and new-onset suicidality have been over-interpreted (Grunze 2008).

Conclusively, the issue of switching is still open and further research is needed. No solid conclusions can be made so far. A summary of the data concerning the switch risk is shown in Table 16.9.

References

A Multicenter, Randomized, Double-Blind, Placebo-Controlled Study of Aripiprazole in the Treatment of Acutely Manic Patients with Bipolar Disorder (Protocol CN138077). Unpublished

Aan Het Rot M, Zarate CA Jr, Charney DS, Mathew SJ (2012) Ketamine for depression: where do we go from here? Biol Psychiatry 72(7):537–547. doi:10.1016/j.biopsych.2012.05.003, S0006-3223(12)00417-9 [pii]

Abdallah CG, Fasula M, Kelmendi B, Sanacora G, Ostroff R (2012) Rapid antidepressant effect of ketamine in the electroconvulsive therapy setting. J ECT 28(3):157–161. doi:10.1097/YCT.0b013e31824f8296

Aberg-Wistedt A (1982) Comparison between zimelidine and desipramine in endogenous depression. A cross-over study. Acta Psychiatr Scand 66(2):129–138

Adityanjee (1987) The syndrome of irreversible lithium effectuated neurotoxicity. J Neurol Neurosurg Psychiatry 50(9):1246–1247

Adityanjee (1989) The syndrome of irreversible lithium-effectuated neurotoxicity (SILENT). Pharmacopsychiatry 22(2):81–83. doi:10.1055/s-2007-1014583

Adityanjee, Munshi KR, Thampy A (2005) The syndrome of irreversible lithium-effectuated neurotoxicity. Clin Neuropharmacol 28(1):38–49

Agosti V, Stewart JW (2007) Efficacy and safety of antidepressant monotherapy in the treatment of bipolar-II depression. Int Clin Psychopharmacol 22(5):309–311. doi:10.1097/YIC.0b013e3280c28410

Altinbas K, Guloksuz S, Oral ET (2013) Clinical potential of cariprazine in the treatment of acute mania. Psychiatr Danub 25(3):207–213

Altshuler LL, Ventura J, van Gorp WG, Green MF, Theberge DC, Mintz J (2004) Neurocognitive function in clinically stable men with bipolar I disorder or schizophrenia and normal control subjects. Biol Psychiatry 56(8):560–569. doi:10.1016/j.biopsych.2004.08.002, S0006-3223(04)00853-4 [pii]

Altshuler LL, Suppes T, Black DO, Nolen WA, Leverich G, Keck PE Jr, Frye MA, Kupka R, McElroy SL, Grunze H, Kitchen CM, Post R (2006) Lower switch rate in depressed patients with bipolar II than bipolar I disorder treated adjunctively with second-generation antidepressants. Am J Psychiatry 163(2):313–315. doi:10.1176/appi.ajp.163.2.313, 163/2/313 [pii]

Altshuler LL, Post RM, Hellemann G, Leverich GS, Nolen WA, Frye MA, Keck PE Jr, Kupka RW, Grunze H, McElroy SL, Sugar CA, Suppes T (2009) Impact of antidepressant continuation after acute positive or partial treatment response for bipolar depression: a blinded, randomized study. J Clin Psychiatry 70(4):450–457, ej08m04191 [pii]

Amann B, Born C, Crespo JM, Pomarol-Clotet E, McKenna P (2010) Lamotrigine: when and where does it act in affective disorders? A systematic review. J Psychopharmacol 10:1289–1294. doi:10.1177/0269881110376695, 0269881110376695 [pii]

Amdisen A (1977) Serum level monitoring and clinical pharmacokinetics of lithium. Clin Pharmacokinet 2(2):73–92

Amrollahi Z, Rezaei F, Salehi B, Modabbernia AH, Maroufi A, Esfandiari GR, Naderi M, Ghebleh F, Ahmadi-Abhari SA, Sadeghi M, Tabrizi M, Akhondzadeh S (2010) Double-blind, randomized, placebo-controlled 6-week study on the efficacy and safety of the tamoxifen adjunctive to lithium in acute bipolar mania. J Affect Disord 129(1–3):327–331. doi:10.1016/j.jad.2010.08.015, S0165-0327(10)00549-5 [pii]

Amsterdam JD, Garcia-Espana F (2000) Venlafaxine monotherapy in women with bipolar II and unipolar major depression. J Affect Disord 59(3):225–229

Amsterdam JD, McHenry LB (2012) The paroxetine 352 bipolar trial: a study in medical ghostwriting. Int J Risk Saf Med 24(4):221–231. doi:10.3233/JRS-2012-0571

Amsterdam JD, Shults J (2005a) Comparison of fluoxetine, olanzapine, and combined fluoxetine plus olanzapine initial therapy of bipolar type I and type II major depression–lack of manic induction. J Affect Disord 87(1):121–130

Amsterdam JD, Shults J (2005b) Fluoxetine monotherapy of bipolar type II and bipolar NOS major depression: a double-blind, placebo-substitution, continuation study. Int Clin Psychopharmacol 20(5):257–264

Amsterdam JD, Shults J (2010) Efficacy and safety of long-term fluoxetine versus lithium monotherapy of bipolar II disorder: a randomized, double-blind, placebo-substitution study. Am J Psychiatry 167(7):792–800. doi:10.1176/appi.ajp.2009.09020284, appi.ajp.2009.09020284 [pii]

Amsterdam JD, Garcia-Espana F, Fawcett J, Quitkin FM, Reimherr FW, Rosenbaum JF, Schweizer E, Beasley C (1998) Efficacy and safety of fluoxetine in treating bipolar II major depressive episode. J Clin Psychopharmacol 18(6):435–440

Amsterdam JD, Shults J, Brunswick DJ, Hundert M (2004) Short-term fluoxetine monotherapy for bipolar type II or bipolar NOS major depression - low manic switch rate. Bipolar Disord 6(1):75–81

Anand A, Gunn AD, Barkay G, Karne HS, Nurnberger JI, Mathew SJ, Ghosh S (2012) Early antidepressant effect of memantine during augmentation of lamotrigine inadequate response in bipolar depression: a double-blind, randomized, placebo-controlled trial. Bipolar Disord 14(1):64–70. doi:10.1111/j.1399-5618.2011.00971.x

Anderson GD (1998) A mechanistic approach to antiepileptic drug interactions. Ann Pharmacother 32(5):554–563

Angst J, Grof P, Schou M (1969) Lithium. Lancet 1(7605):1097

Angst J, Weis P, Grof P, Baastrup PC, Schou M (1970) Lithium prophylaxis in recurrent affective disorders. Br J Psychiatry 116(535):604–614

Arnone D (2005) Review of the use of topiramate for treatment of psychiatric disorders. Ann Gen Psychiatry 4(1):5

Arts B, Jabben N, Krabbendam L, van Os J (2008) Meta-analyses of cognitive functioning in euthymic bipolar patients and their first-degree relatives. Psychol Med 38(6):771–785. doi:10.1017/S0033291707001675, S0033291707001675 [pii]

Azorin JM, Sapin C, Weiller E (2013) Effect of asenapine on manic and depressive symptoms in bipolar I patients with mixed episodes: results from post hoc analyses. J Affect Disord 145(1):62–69. doi:10.1016/j.jad.2012.07.013, S0165-0327(12)00532-0 [pii]

Baastrup PC (1964) The use of lithium in manic-depressive psychosis. Compr Psychiatry 5(6):396–408

Baastrup PC, Schou M (1967) Lithium as a prophylactic agents. Its effect against recurrent depressions and manic-depressive psychosis. Arch Gen Psychiatry 16(2):162–172

Baastrup PC, Poulsen JC, Schou M, Thomsen K, Amdisen A (1970) Prophylactic lithium: double blind discontinuation in manic-depressive and recurrent-depressive disorders. Lancet 2(7668):326–330

Bailine S, Fink M, Knapp R, Petrides G, Husain MM, Rasmussen K, Sampson S, Mueller M, McClintock SM, Tobias KG, Kellner CH (2010) Electroconvulsive therapy is equally effective in unipolar and bipolar depression. Acta Psychiatr Scand 121(6):431–436. doi:10.1111/j.1600-0447.2009.01493.x, ACP1493 [pii]

Baker RW, Goldberg JF, Tohen M, Milton DR, Stauffer VL, Schuh LM (2002) The impact of response to previous mood stabilizer therapy on response to olanzapine versus placebo for acute mania. Bipolar Disord 4(1):43–49

Baker RW, Tohen M, Fawcett J, Risser RC, Schuh LM, Brown E, Stauffer VL, Shao L, Tollefson GD (2003) Acute dysphoric mania: treatment response to olanzapine versus placebo. J Clin Psychopharmacol 23(2):132–137

Baker RW, Brown E, Akiskal HS, Calabrese JR, Ketter TA, Schuh LM, Trzepacz PT, Watkin JG, Tohen M (2004) Efficacy of olanzapine combined with valproate or lithium in the treatment of dysphoric mania. Br J Psychiatry 185:472–478. doi:10.1192/bjp.185.6.472, 185/6/472 [pii]

Baldessarini RJ, Hennen J, Wilson M, Calabrese J, Chengappa R, Keck PE Jr, McElroy SL, Sachs G, Vieta E, Welge JA, Yatham LN, Zarate CA Jr, Baker RW, Tohen M (2003) Olanzapine versus placebo in acute mania: treatment responses in subgroups. J Clin Psychopharmacol 23(4):370–376

Ballenger JC, Post RM (1980) Carbamazepine in manic-depressive illness: a new treatment. Am J Psychiatry 137(7):782–790

Baron M, Gershon ES, Rudy V, Jonas WZ, Buchsbaum M (1975) Lithium carbonate response in depression. Prediction by unipolar/bipolar illness, average-evoked response, catechol-O-methyl transferase, and family history. Arch Gen Psychiatry 32(9):1107–1111

Bauer MS, Whybrow PC (1990) Rapid cycling bipolar affective disorder. II. Treatment of refractory rapid cycling with high-dose levothyroxine: a preliminary study. Arch Gen Psychiatry 47(5):435–440

Bauer MS, Whybrow PC, Winokur A (1990) Rapid cycling bipolar affective disorder. I. Association with grade I hypothyroidism. Arch Gen Psychiatry 47(5):427–432

Bauer M, Zaninelli R, Muller-Oerlinghausen B, Meister W (1999) Paroxetine and amitriptyline augmentation of lithium in the treatment of major depression: a double-blind study. J Clin Psychopharmacol 19(2):164–171

Baumhackl U, Biziere K, Fischbach R, Geretsegger C, Hebenstreit G, Radmayr E, Stabl M (1989) Efficacy and tolerability of moclobemide compared with imipramine in depressive disorder (DSM-III): an Austrian double-blind, multicentre study. Br J Psychiatry Suppl 6:78–83

Beaulieu S, Saury S, Sareen J, Tremblay J, Schutz CG, McIntyre RS, Schaffer A (2012) The Canadian Network for Mood and Anxiety Treatments (CANMAT) task force recommendations for the management of patients with mood disorders and comorbid substance use disorders. Ann Clin Psychiatry 24(1):38–55, acp_2401e [pii]

Bech P (2001) Meta-analysis of placebo-controlled trials with mirtazapine using the core items of the Hamilton Depression Scale as evidence of a pure antidepressive effect in the short-term treatment of major depression. Int J Neuropsychopharmacol 4(4):337–345

Bech P (2006) The full story of lithium. A tribute to Mogens Schou (1918–2005). Psychother Psychosom 75(5):265–269. doi:10.1159/000093947

Bech P, Vendsborg PB, Rafaelsen OJ (1976) Lithium maintenance treatment of manic-melancholic patients: its role in the daily routine. Acta Psychiatr Scand 53(1):70–81

Behzadi AH, Omrani Z, Chalian M, Asadi S, Ghadiri M (2009) Folic acid efficacy as an alternative drug added to sodium valproate in the treatment of acute phase of mania in bipolar disorder: a double-blind randomized controlled trial. Acta Psychiatr Scand 120(6):441–445. doi:10.1111/j.1600-0447.2009.01368.x, ACP1368 [pii]

Benazzi F, Berk M, Frye MA, Wang W, Barraco A, Tohen M (2009) Olanzapine/fluoxetine combination for the treatment of mixed depression in bipolar I disorder: a post hoc analysis. J Clin Psychiatry 70(10):1424–1431. doi:10.4088/JCP.08m04772gre

Berk M, Ichim L, Brook S (1999) Olanzapine compared to lithium in mania: a double-blind randomized controlled trial. Int Clin Psychopharmacol 14(6):339–343

Berk M, Copolov DL, Dean O, Lu K, Jeavons S, Schapkaitz I, Anderson-Hunt M, Bush AI (2008) N-acetyl cysteine for depressive symptoms in bipolar disorder–a double-blind randomized placebo-controlled trial. Biol Psychiatry 64(6):468–475. doi:10.1016/j.biopsych.2008.04.022, S0006-3223(08)00500-3 [pii]

Berk M, Dean OM, Cotton SM, Gama CS, Kapczinski F, Fernandes B, Kohlmann K, Jeavons S, Hewitt K, Moss K, Allwang C, Schapkaitz I, Cobb H, Bush AI, Dodd S, Malhi GS (2012) Maintenance N-acetyl cysteine treatment for bipolar disorder: a double-blind randomized placebo controlled trial. BMC Med 10:91. doi:10.1186/1741-7015-10-91, 1741-7015-10-91 [pii]

Bersudsky Y, Applebaum J, Gaiduk Y, Sharony L, Mishory A, Podberezsky A, Agam G, Belmaker RH (2010) Valnoctamide as a valproate substitute with low teratogenic potential in mania: a double-blind, controlled, add-on clinical trial. Bipolar Disord 12(4):376–382. doi:10.1111/j.1399-5618.2010.00828.x, BDI828 [pii]

Bertilsson L, Tomson T (1986) Clinical pharmacokinetics and pharmacological effects of carbamazepine and carbamazepine-10,11-epoxide. An update. Clin Pharmacokinet 11(3):177–198

Berwaerts J, Xu H, Nuamah I, Lim P, Hough D (2010) Evaluation of the efficacy and safety of paliperidone extended-release in the treatment of acute mania: a randomized, double-blind, dose-response study. J Affect Disord. doi:10.1016/j.jad.2010.06.030, S0165-0327(10)00458-1 [pii]

Berwaerts J, Lane R, Nuamah IF, Lim P, Remmerie B, Hough DW (2011) Paliperidone extended-release as adjunctive therapy to lithium or valproate in the treatment of acute mania: a randomized, placebo-controlled study. J Affect Disord 129:252–260. doi:10.1016/j.jad.2010.09.011, S0165-0327(10)00579-3 [pii]

Berwaerts J, Melkote R, Nuamah I, Lim P (2012a) A randomized, placebo- and active-controlled study of paliperidone extended-release as maintenance treatment in patients with bipolar I disorder after an acute manic or mixed episode. J Affect Disord 138(3):247–258. doi:10.1016/j.jad.2012.01.047, S0165-0327(12)00094-8 [pii]

Berwaerts J, Xu H, Nuamah I, Lim P, Hough D (2012b) Evaluation of the efficacy and safety of paliperidone extended-release in the treatment of acute mania: a randomized, double-blind, dose-response study. J Affect Disord 136(1–2):e51–e60. doi:10.1016/j.jad.2010.06.030, S0165-0327(10)00458-1 [pii]

Beynon S, Soares-Weiser K, Woolacott N, Duffy S, Geddes JR (2009) Pharmacological interventions for the prevention of relapse in bipolar disorder: a systematic review of controlled trials. J Psychopharmacol 23(5):574–591. doi:10.1177/0269881108093885

Blackburn S, Oliart A, Garcia Rodriguez L, Perez Gutthann S (1998) Antiepileptics and blood dyscrasias: a cohort study. Pharmacotherapy 18:1277

Blackwell B (1969) Need for careful evaluation of lithium. Am J Psychiatry 125(8):1131

Blackwell B (1970) Lithium. Lancet 2(7678):875–876

Blackwell B (1971) Lithium prophylaxis in recurrent affective disorders. Br J Psychiatry 118(542):131–132

Blackwell B (1972) Prophylactic lithium: science or science fiction? Am Heart J 83(1):139–141

Blackwell B, Shepherd M (1968) Prophylactic lithium: another therapeutic myth? An examination of the evidence to date. Lancet 1(7549):968–971

Bobo WV, Shelton RC (2010) Risperidone long-acting injectable (Risperdal Consta(R)) for maintenance treatment in patients with bipolar disorder. Expert Rev Neurother 10(11):1637–1658. doi:10.1586/ern.10.143

Bocchetta A, Bernardi F, Burrai C, Pedditzi M, Del Zompo M (1993) A double-blind study of L-sulpiride versus amitriptyline in lithium-maintained bipolar depressives. Acta Psychiatr Scand 88(6):434–439

Bond DJ, Noronha MM, Kauer-Sant'Anna M, Lam RW, Yatham LN (2008) Antidepressant-associated mood elevations in bipolar II disorder compared with bipolar I disorder and major depressive disorder: a systematic review and meta-analysis. J Clin Psychiatry 69(10):1589–1601

Bond DJ, Lam RW, Yatham LN (2010) Divalproex sodium versus placebo in the treatment of acute bipolar depression: a systematic review and meta-analysis. J Affect Disord 124(3):228–234. doi:10.1016/j.jad.2009.11.008

Bora E, Vahip S, Akdeniz F, Gonul AS, Eryavuz A, Ogut M, Alkan M (2007) The effect of previous psychotic mood episodes on cognitive impairment in euthymic bipolar patients. Bipolar Disord 9:468–477. doi:10.1111/j.1399-5618.2007.00469.x

Bottlender R, Rudolf D, Strauss A, Moller HJ (2001) Mood-stabilisers reduce the risk of developing antidepressant-induced maniform states in acute treatment of bipolar I depressed patients. J Affect Disord 63(1–3):79–83

Bottlender R, Sato T, Kleindienst N, Strauss A, Moller HJ (2004) Mixed depressive features predict maniform switch during treatment of depression in bipolar I disorder. J Affect Disord 78(2):149–152

Bowden CL (2005) Atypical antipsychotic augmentation of mood stabilizer therapy in bipolar disorder. J Clin Psychiatry 66(Suppl 3):12–19

Bowden CL, Brugger AM, Swann AC, Calabrese JR, Janicak PG, Petty F, Dilsaver SC, Davis JM, Rush AJ, Small JG et al (1994) Efficacy of divalproex vs lithium and placebo in the treatment of mania. The Depakote Mania Study Group. JAMA 271(12):918–924

Bowden CL, Calabrese JR, McElroy SL, Gyulai L, Wassef A, Petty F, Pope HG Jr, Chou JC, Keck PE Jr, Rhodes LJ, Swann AC, Hirschfeld RM, Wozniak PJ (2000) A randomized, placebo-controlled 12-month trial of divalproex and lithium in treatment of outpatients with bipolar I disorder. Divalproex Maintenance Study Group. Arch Gen Psychiatry 57(5):481–489

Bowden CL, Calabrese JR, Sachs G, Yatham LN, Asghar SA, Hompland M, Montgomery P, Earl N, Smoot TM, DeVeaugh-Geiss J (2003) A placebo-controlled 18-month trial of lamotrigine and lithium maintenance treatment in recently manic or hypomanic patients with bipolar I disorder. Arch Gen Psychiatry 60(4):392–400

Bowden CL, Collins MA, McElroy SL, Calabrese JR, Swann AC, Weisler RH, Wozniak PJ (2005a) Relationship of mania symptomatology to maintenance treatment response with divalproex, lithium, or placebo. Neuropsychopharmacology 30(10):1932–1939. doi:10.1038/sj.npp.1300788, 1300788 [pii]

Bowden CL, Grunze H, Mullen J, Brecher M, Paulsson B, Jones M, Vagero M, Svensson K (2005b) A randomized, double-blind, placebo-controlled efficacy and safety study of quetiapine or lithium as monotherapy for mania in bipolar disorder. J Clin Psychiatry 66(1):111–121

Bowden CL, Swann AC, Calabrese JR, Rubenfaer LM, Wozniak PJ, Collins MA, Abi-Saab W, Saltarelli M (2006) A randomized, placebo-controlled, multicenter study of divalproex sodium extended release in the treatment of acute mania. J Clin Psychiatry 67(10):1501–1510

Bowden CL, Vieta E, Ice KS, Schwartz JH, Wang PP, Versavel M (2010) Ziprasidone plus a mood stabilizer in subjects with bipolar I disorder: a 6-month, randomized, placebo-controlled, double-blind trial. J Clin Psychiatry 71(2):130–137. doi:10.4088/JCP.09m05482yel

Bowden CL, Singh V, Weisler R, Thompson P, Chang X, Quinones M, Mintz J (2012) Lamotrigine vs. lamotrigine plus divalproex in randomized, placebo-controlled maintenance treatment for bipolar depression. Acta Psychiatr Scand 126(5):342–350. doi:10.1111/j.1600-0447.2012.01890.x

Brown D, Silverstone T, Cookson J (1989) Carbamazepine compared to haloperidol in acute mania. Int Clin Psychopharmacol 4(3):229–238

Brown EB, McElroy SL, Keck PE Jr, Deldar A, Adams DH, Tohen M, Williamson DJ (2006) A 7-week, randomized, double-blind trial of olanzapine/fluoxetine combination versus lamotrigine in the treatment of bipolar I depression. J Clin Psychiatry 67(7):1025–1033

Brown ES, Garza M, Carmody TJ (2008) A randomized, double-blind, placebo-controlled add-on trial of quetiapine in outpatients with bipolar disorder and alcohol use disorders. J Clin Psychiatry 69(5):701–705, ej07m03431 [pii]

Brown E, Dunner DL, McElroy SL, Keck PE, Adams DH, Degenhardt E, Tohen M, Houston JP (2009) Olanzapine/fluoxetine combination vs. lamotrigine in the 6-month treatment of bipolar I depression. Int J Neuropsychopharmacol 12(6):773–782. doi:10.1017/S1461145708009735, S1461145708009735 [pii]

Brugue E, Vieta E (2007) Atypical antipsychotics in bipolar depression: neurobiological basis and clinical implications. Prog Neuropsychopharmacol Biol Psychiatry 31(1):275–282

Burdick KE, Braga RJ, Nnadi CU, Shaya Y, Stearns WH, Malhotra AK (2012) Placebo-controlled adjunctive trial of pramipexole in patients with bipolar disorder: targeting cognitive dysfunction. J Clin Psychiatry 73(1):103–112. doi:10.4088/JCP.11m07299

Burgess S, Geddes J, Hawton K, Townsend E, Jamison K, Goodwin G (2001) Lithium for maintenance treatment of mood disorders. Cochrane Database Syst Rev (3):CD003013

Cade J (1949) Lithium salts in the treatment of psychotic excitement. Med J Aust 36:349–352

Cade JF (2000) Lithium salts in the treatment of psychotic excitement. 1949. Bull World Health Organ 78(4):518–520

Calabrese JR, Bowden CL, Sachs GS, Ascher JA, Monaghan E, Rudd GD (1999) A double-blind placebo-controlled study of lamotrigine monotherapy in outpatients with bipolar I depression. Lamictal 602 Study Group. J Clin Psychiatry 60(2):79–88

Calabrese JR, Suppes T, Bowden CL, Sachs GS, Swann AC, McElroy SL, Kusumakar V, Ascher JA, Earl NL, Greene PL, Monaghan ET (2000) A double-blind, placebo-controlled, prophylaxis study of lamotrigine in rapid-cycling bipolar disorder. Lamictal 614 Study Group. J Clin Psychiatry 61(11):841–850

Calabrese JR, Bowden CL, Sachs G, Yatham LN, Behnke K, Mehtonen OP, Montgomery P, Ascher J, Paska W, Earl N, DeVeaugh-Geiss J (2003a) A placebo-controlled 18-month trial of lamotrigine and lithium maintenance treatment in recently depressed patients with bipolar I disorder. J Clin Psychiatry 64(9):1013–1024

Calabrese JR, Vieta E, Shelton MD (2003b) Latest maintenance data on lamotrigine in bipolar disorder. Eur Neuropsychopharmacol 13(Suppl 2):S57–S66

Calabrese JR, Keck PE Jr, Macfadden W, Minkwitz M, Ketter TA, Weisler RH, Cutler AJ, McCoy R, Wilson E, Mullen J (2005a) A randomized, double-blind, placebo-controlled trial of quetiapine in the treatment of bipolar I or II depression. Am J Psychiatry 162(7):1351–1360

Calabrese JR, Shelton MD, Rapport DJ, Youngstrom EA, Jackson K, Bilali S, Ganocy SJ, Findling RL (2005b) A 20-month, double-blind, maintenance trial of lithium versus divalproex in rapid-cycling bipolar disorder. Am J Psychiatry 162(11):2152–2161

Calabrese JR, Goldberg JF, Ketter TA, Suppes T, Frye M, White R, DeVeaugh-Geiss A, Thompson TR (2006) Recurrence in bipolar I disorder: a post hoc analysis excluding relapses in two double-blind maintenance studies. Biol Psychiatry 59(11):1061–1064

Calabrese JR, Huffman RF, White RL, Edwards S, Thompson TR, Ascher JA, Monaghan ET, Leadbetter RA (2008) Lamotrigine in the acute treatment of bipolar depression: results of five double-blind, placebo-controlled clinical trials. Bipolar Disord 10(2):323–333. doi:10.1111/j.1399-5618.2007.00500.x, BDI500 [pii]

Calabrese JR, Ketter TA, Youakim JM, Tiller JM, Yang R, Frye MA (2010) Adjunctive armodafinil for major depressive episodes associated with bipolar I disorder: a randomized, multicenter, double-blind, placebo-controlled, proof-of-concept study. J Clin Psychiatry 71(10):1363–1370. doi:10.4088/JCP.09m05900gry

Carlson BX, Ketter TA, Sun W, Timko K, McQuade RD, Sanchez R, Vester-Blokland E, Marcus R (2012) Aripiprazole in combination with lamotrigine for the long-term treatment of patients with bipolar I disorder (manic or mixed): a randomized, multicenter, double-blind study (CN138-392). Bipolar Disord 14(1):41–53. doi:10.1111/j.1399-5618.2011.00974.x

Cazorla P, Zhao J, Mackle M, Szegedi A (2013) Asenapine effects on individual Young Mania Rating Scale items in bipolar disorder patients with acute manic or mixed episodes: a pooled analysis. Neuropsychiatr Dis Treat 9:409–413. doi:10.2147/NDT.S38390

Cerullo MA, Strakowski SM (2007) The prevalence and significance of substance use disorders in bipolar type I and II disorder. Subst Abus Treat Prev Policy 2:29. doi:10.1186/1747-597X-2-29, 1747-597X-2-29 [pii]

Chen KP, Shen WW, Lu ML (2004) Implication of serum concentration monitoring in patients with lithium intoxication. Psychiatry Clin Neurosci 58(1):25–29

Chengappa KN, Baker RW, Shao L, Yatham LN, Tohen M, Gershon S, Kupfer DJ (2003) Rates of response, euthymia and remission in two placebo-controlled olanzapine trials for bipolar mania. Bipolar Disord 5(1):1–5

Chiu CC, Huang SY, Chen CC, Su KP (2005) Omega-3 fatty acids are more beneficial in the depressive phase than in the manic phase in patients with bipolar I disorder. J Clin Psychiatry 66(12):1613–1614

Chou JC, Czobor P, Charles O, Tuma I, Winsberg B, Allen MH, Trujillo M, Volavka J (1999) Acute mania: haloperidol dose and augmentation with lithium or lorazepam. J Clin Psychopharmacol 19(6):500–505

Chouinard G, Annable L, Turnier L, Holobow N, Szkrumelak N (1993) A double-blind randomized clinical trial of rapid tranquilization with I.M. clonazepam and I.M. haloperidol in agitated psychotic patients with manic symptoms. Can J Psychiatr 38(Suppl 4):S114–S121

Christodoulou GN, Lykouras EP (1982) Abrupt lithium discontinuation in manic-depressive patients. Acta Psychiatr Scand 65(5):310–314

Cipriani A, Rendell J, Geddes JR (2010) Olanzapine in the long-term treatment of bipolar disorder: a systematic review and meta-analysis. J Psychopharmacol 24(12):1729–1738. doi:10.1177/0269881109106900

Cipriani A, Barbui C, Salanti G, Rendell J, Brown R, Stockton S, Purgato M, Spineli LM, Goodwin GM, Geddes JR (2011) Comparative efficacy and acceptability of antimanic drugs in acute mania: a multiple-treatments meta-analysis. Lancet 378(9799):1306–1315. doi:10.1016/S0140-6736(11)60873-8, S0140-6736(11)60873-8 [pii]

Citrome L (2010) Ziprasidone HCl capsules for the adjunctive maintenance treatment of bipolar disorder in adults. Expert Rev Neurother 10(7):1031–1037. doi:10.1586/ern.10.66

Citrome L (2012) Inhaled loxapine for agitation revisited: focus on effect sizes from 2 Phase III randomised controlled trials in persons with schizophrenia or bipolar disorder. Int J Clin Pract 66(3):318–325. doi:10.1111/j.1742-1241.2011.02890.x

Citrome L (2013) Cariprazine in bipolar disorder: clinical efficacy, tolerability, and place in therapy. Adv Ther 30(2):102–113. doi:10.1007/s12325-013-0004-9

Cohn JB, Collins G, Ashbrook E, Wernicke JF (1989) A comparison of fluoxetine imipramine and placebo in patients with bipolar depressive disorder. Int Clin Psychopharmacol 4(4):313–322

Connelly CE, Davenport YB, Nurnberger JI Jr (1982) Adherence to treatment regimen in a lithium carbonate clinic. Arch Gen Psychiatry 39(5):585–588

Cookson J, Silverstone T, Wells B (1981) Double-blind comparative clinical trial of pimozide and chlorpromazine in mania. A test of the dopamine hypothesis. Acta Psychiatr Scand 64(5):381–397

Cookson J, Keck PE Jr, Ketter TA, Macfadden W (2007) Number needed to treat and time to response/remission for quetiapine monotherapy efficacy in acute bipolar depression: evidence from a large, randomized, placebo-controlled study. Int Clin Psychopharmacol 22(2):93–100

Coppen A, Whybrow PC, Noguera R, Maggs R, Prange AJ Jr (1972) The comparative antidepressant value of L-tryptophan and imipramine with and without attempted potentiation by liothyronine. Arch Gen Psychiatry 26(3):234–241

Correll CU, Sheridan EM, DelBello MP (2010) Antipsychotic and mood stabilizer efficacy and tolerability in pediatric and adult patients with bipolar I mania: a comparative analysis of acute, randomized, placebo-controlled trials. Bipolar Disord 12(2):116–141. doi:10.1111/j.1399-5618.2010.00798.x, BDI798 [pii]

Cowdry RW, Wehr TA, Zis AP, Goodwin FK (1983) Thyroid abnormalities associated with rapid-cycling bipolar illness. Arch Gen Psychiatry 40(4):414–420

Coxhead N, Silverstone T, Cookson J (1992) Carbamazepine versus lithium in the prophylaxis of bipolar affective disorder. Acta Psychiatr Scand 85(2):114–118

Cruz N, Sanchez-Moreno J, Torres F, Goikolea JM, Valenti M, Vieta E (2010) Efficacy of modern antipsychotics in placebo-controlled trials in bipolar depression: a meta-analysis. Int J Neuropsychopharmacol 13(1):5–14. doi:10.1017/S1461145709990344, S1461145709990344 [pii]

Cummings C, Stewart M, Stevenson M, Morrow J, Nelson J (2011) Neurodevelopment of children exposed in utero to lamotrigine, sodium valproate and carbamazepine. Arch Dis Child 96(7):643–647. doi:10.1136/adc.2009.176990

Cundall RL, Brooks PW, Murray LG (1972) A controlled evaluation of lithium prophylaxis in affective disorders. Psychol Med 2(3):308–311

Cusin C, Serretti A, Mandelli L, Lucca A, Smeraldi E (2002) Seasonal variations of lithium plasma levels. Psychiatry Res 111(1):35–41, S0165178102001300 [pii]

Cutler AJ, Datto C, Nordenhem A, Minkwitz M, Acevedo L, Darko D (2011) Extended-release quetiapine as monotherapy for the treatment of adults with acute mania: a randomized, double-blind, 3-week trial. Clin Ther 33(11):1643–1658. doi:10.1016/j.clinthera.2011.10.002, S0149-2918(11)00673-4 [pii]

D'Mello DA, McNeil JA, Msibi B (1995) Seasons and bipolar disorder. Ann Clin Psychiatry 7(1):11–18

Dardennes R, Even C, Bange F, Heim A (1995) Comparison of carbamazepine and lithium in the prophylaxis of bipolar disorders. A meta-analysis. Br J Psychiatry 166(3):378–381

Dauphinais DR, Rosenthal JZ, Terman M, DiFebo HM, Tuggle C, Rosenthal NE (2012) Controlled trial of safety and efficacy of bright light therapy vs. negative air ions in patients with bipolar depression. Psychiatry Res 196(1):57–61. doi:10.1016/j.psychres.2012.01.015, S0165-1781(12)00045-5 [pii]

Davis JM, Janicak PG, Hogan DM (1999) Mood stabilizers in the prevention of recurrent affective disorders: a meta-analysis. Acta Psychiatr Scand 100(6):406–417

Davis LL, Bartolucci A, Petty F (2005) Divalproex in the treatment of bipolar depression: a placebo-controlled study. J Affect Disord 85(3):259–266

De Fruyt J, Deschepper E, Audenaert K, Constant E, Floris M, Pitchot W, Sienaert P, Souery D, Claes S (2011) Second generation antipsychotics in the treatment of bipolar depression: a systematic review and meta-analysis. J Psychopharmacol. doi:10.1177/0269881111408461, 0269881111408461 [pii]

De Fruyt J, Deschepper E, Audenaert K, Constant E, Floris M, Pitchot W, Sienaert P, Souery D, Claes S (2012) Second generation antipsychotics in the treatment of bipolar depression: a systematic review and meta-analysis. J Psychopharmacol 26(5):603–617. doi:10.1177/0269881111408461, 0269881111408461 [pii]

Dean OM, Bush AI, Copolov DL, Kohlmann K, Jeavons S, Schapkaitz I, Anderson-Hunt M, Berk M (2012) Effects of N-acetyl cysteine on cognitive function in bipolar disorder. Psychiatry Clin Neurosci 66(6):514–517. doi:10.1111/j.1440-1819.2012.02392.x

Delay J, Buisson JF (1958) Psychic action of isoniazid in the treatment of depressive states. J Clin Exp Psychopathol 19(2 Suppl 1):51–55

Dell'Osso B, Mundo E, D'Urso N, Pozzoli S, Buoli M, Ciabatti M, Rosanova M, Massimini M, Bellina V, Mariotti M, Altamura AC (2009) Augmentative repetitive navigated transcranial magnetic stimulation (rTMS) in drug-resistant bipolar depression. Bipolar Disord 11(1):76–81. doi:10.1111/j.1399-5618.2008.00651.x, BDI651 [pii]

Denicoff KD, Smith-Jackson EE, Disney ER, Ali SO, Leverich GS, Post RM (1997) Comparative prophylactic efficacy of lithium, carbamazepine, and the combination in bipolar disorder. J Clin Psychiatry 58(11):470–478

Diazgranados N, Ibrahim L, Brutsche NE, Newberg A, Kronstein P, Khalife S, Kammerer WA, Quezado Z, Luckenbaugh DA, Salvadore G, Machado-Vieira R, Manji HK, Zarate CA Jr (2010) A randomized add-on trial of an N-methyl-D-aspartate antagonist in treatment-resistant bipolar depression. Arch Gen Psychiatry 67(8):793–802. doi:10.1001/archgenpsychiatry.2010.90, 67/8/793 [pii]

Dierckx B, Heijnen WT, van den Broek WW, Birkenhager TK (2012) Efficacy of electroconvulsive therapy in bipolar versus unipolar major depression: a meta-analysis. Bipolar Disord 14(2):146–150. doi:10.1111/j.1399-5618.2012.00997.x

Donnelly EF, Goodwin FK, Waldman IN, Murphy DL (1978) Prediction of antidepressant responses to lithium. Am J Psychiatry 135(5):552–556

Dube S, Tollefson GD, Thase ME, Briggs SD, Van Campen LE, Case M, Tohen M (2007) Onset of antidepressant effect of olanzapine and olanzapine/fluoxetine combination in bipolar depression. Bipolar Disord 9(6):618–627

Dunner DL, Stallone F, Fieve RR (1976) Lithium carbonate and affective disorders. V: a double-blind study of prophylaxis of depression in bipolar illness. Arch Gen Psychiatry 33(1):117–120

Eden Evins A, Demopulos C, Yovel I, Culhane M, Ogutha J, Grandin LD, Nierenberg AA, Sachs GS (2006) Inositol augmentation of lithium or valproate for bipolar depression. Bipolar Disord 8(2):168–174

El Mallakh RS, Vieta E, Rollin L, Marcus R, Carson WH, McQuade R (2010) A comparison of two fixed doses of aripiprazole with placebo in acutely relapsed, hospitalized patients with bipolar disorder I (manic or mixed) in subpopulations (CN138-007). Eur Neuropsychopharmacol 20(11):776–783. doi:10.1016/j.euroneuro.2010.07.003, S0924-977X(10)00159-8 [pii]

El-Mallakh RS, Ghaemi SN, Sagduyu K, Thase ME, Wisniewski SR, Nierenberg AA, Zhang HW, Pardo TA, Sachs G (2008) Antidepressant-associated chronic irritable dysphoria (ACID) in STEP-BD patients. J Affect Disord 111(2-3):372–377. doi:10.1016/j.jad.2008.03.025, S0165-0327(08)00136-5 [pii]

El-Mallakh RS, Marcus R, Baudelet C, McQuade R, Carson WH, Owen R (2012) A 40-week double-blind aripiprazole versus lithium follow-up of a 12-week acute phase study (total 52 weeks) in bipolar I disorder. J Affect Disord 136(3):258–266. doi:10.1016/j.jad.2011.11.043, S0165-0327(11)00760-9 [pii]

Emilien G, Maloteaux JM, Seghers A, Charles G (1996) Lithium compared to valproic acid and carbamazepine in the treatment of mania: a statistical meta-analysis. Eur Neuropsychopharmacol 6(3):245–252, 0924-977X(96)00029-6 [pii]

Emrich HM, von Zerssen D, Kissling W, Moller HJ, Windorfer A (1980) Effect of sodium valproate on mania. The GABA-hypothesis of affective disorders. Archiv fur Psychiatrie und Nervenkrankheiten 229(1):1–16

Emrich HM, von Zerssen D, Kissling W, Moller HJ (1981) Therapeutic effect of valproate in mania. Am J Psychiatry 138(2):256

Endicott J, Rajagopalan K, Minkwitz M, Macfadden W (2007) A randomized, double-blind, placebo-controlled study of quetiapine in the treatment of bipolar I and II depression: improvements in quality of life. Int Clin Psychopharmacol 22(1):29–37

Engelsmann F, Katz J, Ghadirian AM, Schachter D (1988) Lithium and memory: a long-term follow-up study. J Clin Psychopharmacol 8(3):207–212

Fan A, Berg A, Bresee C, Glassman LH, Rapaport MH (2012) Allopurinol augmentation in the outpatient treatment of bipolar mania: a pilot study. Bipolar Disord 14(2):206–210. doi:10.1111/j.1399-5618.2012.01001.x

Fieve RR, Kumbaraci T, Dunner DL (1976) Lithium prophylaxis of depression in bipolar I, bipolar II, and unipolar patients. Am J Psychiatry 133(8):925–929

Findling RL, McNamara NK, Youngstrom EA, Stansbrey R, Gracious BL, Reed MD, Calabrese JR (2005) Double-blind 18-month trial of lithium versus divalproex maintenance treatment in pediatric bipolar disorder. J Am Acad Child Adolesc Psychiatry 44(5):409–417

Fountoulakis KN (2008) The contemporary face of bipolar illness: complex diagnostic and therapeutic challenges. CNS Spectr 13(9):763–774, 777–769
Fountoulakis KN (2010a) The BALANCE trial. Lancet 375(9723):1343–1344; author reply 1344. doi:10.1016/S0140-6736(10)60569-7, S0140-6736(10)60569-7 [pii]
Fountoulakis KN (2010b) Pharmaceutical treatment of acute bipolar depression. F1000 Med Rep 2:47. doi:10.3410/M2-47
Fountoulakis KN (2012a) Introduction–bipolar illness: current understanding and future perspectives. CNS Neurosci Ther 18(3):193. doi:10.1111/j.1755-5949.2012.00298.x
Fountoulakis KN (2012b) Refractoriness in bipolar disorder: definitions and evidence-based treatment. CNS Neurosci Ther 18(3):227–237. doi:10.1111/j.1755-5949.2011.00259.x
Fountoulakis KN, Kontis D (2012) Mathematical coupling and the true role of baseline severity in acute mania trials. Neuropsychopharmacology 37(3):850. doi:10.1038/npp.2011.234
Fountoulakis KN, Moller HJ (2012) Antidepressant drugs and the response in the placebo group: the real problem lies in our understanding of the issue. J Psychopharmacol 26(5):744–750. doi:10.1177/0269881111421969
Fountoulakis KN, Siamouli M (2012) Comparative efficacy of anti-manic drugs in acute mania. Lancet 379(9819):893–894. doi:10.1016/S0140-6736(12)60391-2, author reply 894. S0140-6736(12)60391-2 [pii]
Fountoulakis KN, Vieta E (2008) Treatment of bipolar disorder: a systematic review of available data and clinical perspectives. Int J Neuropsychopharmacol 11(7):999–1029. doi:10.1017/S1461145708009231
Fountoulakis KN, Nimatoudis I, Iacovides A, Kaprinis G (2004a) Off-label indications for atypical antipsychotics: a systematic review. Ann Gen Hosp Psychiatry 3(1):4. doi:10.1186/1475-2832-3-4
Fountoulakis KN, Nimatoudis I, Iacovides A, Kaprinis G (2004b) Report of three cases that received maintenance treatment with risperidone as a mood stabilizer. Ann Gen Hosp Psychiatry 3(1):10. doi:10.1186/1475-2832-3-10
Fountoulakis KN, Vieta E, Sanchez-Moreno J, Kaprinis SG, Goikolea JM, Kaprinis GS (2005) Treatment guidelines for bipolar disorder: a critical review. J Affect Disord 86(1):1–10. doi:10.1016/j.jad.2005.01.004
Fountoulakis KN, Magiria S, Siamouli M, Panagiotidis P, Nimatoudis I, Iacovides A, Kaprinis GS (2007a) A seven- year follow-up of an extremely refractory bipolar I patient. CNS Spectr 12(10):733–734
Fountoulakis KN, Vieta E, Siamouli M, Valenti M, Magiria S, Oral T, Fresno D, Giannakopoulos P, Kaprinis GS (2007b) Treatment of bipolar disorder: a complex treatment for a multi-faceted disorder. Ann Gen Psychiatry 6:27. doi:10.1186/1744-859X-6-27
Fountoulakis KN, Grunze H, Panagiotidis P, Kaprinis G (2008a) Treatment of bipolar depression: an update. J Affect Disord 109(1–2):21–34. doi:10.1016/j.jad.2007.10.016
Fountoulakis KN, Siamouli M, Panagiotidis P, Magiria S, Kantartzis S, Iacovides A, Kaprinis GS (2008b) Ultra short manic-like episodes after antidepressant augmentation with modafinil. Prog Neuropsychopharmacol Biol Psychiatry 32(3):891–892. doi:10.1016/j.pnpbp.2007.11.006, S0278-5846(07)00396-X [pii]
Fountoulakis KN, Vieta E, Bouras C, Notaridis G, Giannakopoulos P, Kaprinis G, Akiskal H (2008c) A systematic review of existing data on long-term lithium therapy: neuroprotective or neurotoxic? Int J Neuropsychopharmacol 11(2):269–287. doi:10.1017/S1461145707007821
Fountoulakis KN, Gonda X, Vieta E, Schmidt F (2009) Treatment of psychotic symptoms in bipolar disorder with aripiprazole monotherapy: a meta-analysis. Ann Gen Psychiatry 8:27. doi:10.1186/1744-859X-8-27, 1744-859X-8-27 [pii]
Fountoulakis KN, Gonda X, Vieta E, Rihmer Z (2011a) Class effect of pharmacotherapy in bipolar disorder: fact or misbelief? Ann Gen Psychiatry 10(1):8, 1744-859X-10-8 [pii]
Fountoulakis KN, Vieta E, Schmidt F (2011b) Aripiprazole monotherapy in the treatment of bipolar disorder: a meta-analysis. J Affect Disord 133(3):361–370. doi:10.1016/j.jad.2010.10.018, S0165-0327(10)00632-4 [pii]
Fountoulakis KN, Gonda X, Samara M, Siapera M, Karavelas V, Ristic DI, Iacovides A (2012a) Antiepileptic drugs and suicidality. J Psychopharmacol 26(11):1401–1407. doi:10.1177/0269881112440514

Fountoulakis KN, Kasper S, Andreassen O, Blier P, Okasha A, Severus E, Versiani M, Tandon R, Moller HJ, Vieta E (2012b) Efficacy of pharmacotherapy in bipolar disorder: a report by the WPA section on pharmacopsychiatry. Eur Arch Psychiatry Clin Neurosci 262(Suppl 1):1–48. doi:10.1007/s00406-012-0323-x

Fountoulakis KN, Kelsoe JR, Akiskal H (2012c) Receptor targets for antidepressant therapy in bipolar disorder: an overview. J Affect Disord 138(3):222–238. doi:10.1016/j.jad.2011.04.043

Fountoulakis KN, Kontis D, Gonda X, Siamouli M, Yatham LN (2012d) Treatment of mixed bipolar states. Int J Neuropsychopharmacol 15(7):1015–1026. doi:10.1017/S1461145711001817

Fountoulakis KN, Kontis D, Gonda X, Yatham LN (2013a) A systematic review of the evidence on the treatment of rapid cycling bipolar disorder. Bipolar Disord 15(2):115–137. doi:10.1111/bdi.12045

Fountoulakis KN, Veroniki AA, Siamouli M, Moller HJ (2013b) No role for initial severity on the efficacy of antidepressants: results of a multi-meta-analysis. Ann Gen Psychiatry 12(1):26. doi:10.1186/1744-859X-12-26

Frangou S, Donaldson S, Hadjulis M, Landau S, Goldstein LH (2005) The Maudsley Bipolar Disorder Project: executive dysfunction in bipolar disorder I and its clinical correlates. Biol Psychiatry 58(11):859–864. doi:10.1016/j.biopsych.2005.04.056, S0006-3223(05)00579-2 [pii]

Frangou S, Lewis M, McCrone P (2006) Efficacy of ethyl-eicosapentaenoic acid in bipolar depression: randomised double-blind placebo-controlled study. Br J Psychiatry 188:46–50. doi:10.1192/bjp.188.1.46, 188/1/46 [pii]

Frangou S, Lewis M, Wollard J, Simmons A (2007) Preliminary in vivo evidence of increased N-acetyl-aspartate following eicosapentanoic acid treatment in patients with bipolar disorder. J Psychopharmacol 21(4):435–439. doi:10.1177/0269881106067787, 0269881106067787 [pii]

Freeman TW, Clothier JL, Pazzaglia P, Lesem MD, Swann AC (1992) A double-blind comparison of valproate and lithium in the treatment of acute mania. Am J Psychiatry 149(1):108–111

Frye MA, Ketter TA, Kimbrell TA, Dunn RT, Speer AM, Osuch EA, Luckenbaugh DA, Cora-Ocatelli G, Leverich GS, Post RM (2000) A placebo-controlled study of lamotrigine and gabapentin monotherapy in refractory mood disorders. J Clin Psychopharmacol 20(6):607–614

Frye MA, Yatham LN, Calabrese JR, Bowden CL, Ketter TA, Suppes T, Adams BE, Thompson TR (2006) Incidence and time course of subsyndromal symptoms in patients with bipolar I disorder: an evaluation of 2 placebo-controlled maintenance trials. J Clin Psychiatry 67(11):1721–1728

Frye MA, Grunze H, Suppes T, McElroy SL, Keck PE Jr, Walden J, Leverich GS, Altshuler LL, Nakelsky S, Hwang S, Mintz J, Post RM (2007) A placebo-controlled evaluation of adjunctive modafinil in the treatment of bipolar depression. Am J Psychiatry 164(8):1242–1249

Frye MA, Yatham L, Ketter TA, Goldberg J, Suppes T, Calabrese JR, Bowden CL, Bourne E, Bahn RS, Adams B (2009) Depressive relapse during lithium treatment associated with increased serum thyroid-stimulating hormone: results from two placebo-controlled bipolar I maintenance studies. Acta Psychiatr Scand 120(1):10–13. doi:10.1111/j.1600-0447.2008.01343.x, ACP1343 [pii]

Fyro B, Petterson U (1977) A double-blind study of the prophylactic effect of lithium in manic-depressive disease. Acta Psychiatr Scand 269(Suppl):17–22

Gao K, Kemp DE, Fein E, Wang Z, Fang Y, Ganocy SJ, Calabrese JR (2011) Number needed to treat to harm for discontinuation due to adverse events in the treatment of bipolar depression, major depressive disorder, and generalized anxiety disorder with atypical antipsychotics. J Clin Psychiatry 72(8):1063–1071. doi:10.4088/JCP.09r05535gre

Gao K, Pappadopulos E, Karayal ON, Kolluri S, Calabrese JR (2013) Risk for adverse events and discontinuation due to adverse events of ziprasidone monotherapy relative to placebo in the acute treatment of bipolar depression, mania, and schizophrenia. J Clin Psychopharmacol 33(3):425–431. doi:10.1097/JCP.0b013e3182917f3f

Garfinkel PE, Stancer HC, Persad E (1980) A comparison of haloperidol, lithium carbonate and their combination in the treatment of mania. J Affect Disord 2(4):279–288

Geddes JR, Burgess S, Hawton K, Jamison K, Goodwin GM (2004) Long-term lithium therapy for bipolar disorder: systematic review and meta-analysis of randomized controlled trials. Am J Psychiatry 161(2):217–222

Geddes JR, Calabrese JR, Goodwin GM (2009) Lamotrigine for treatment of bipolar depression: independent meta-analysis and meta-regression of individual patient data from five randomised trials. Br J Psychiatry 194(1):4–9. doi:10.1192/bjp.bp.107.048504, 194/1/4 [pii]

Geddes JR, Goodwin GM, Rendell J, Azorin JM, Cipriani A, Ostacher MJ, Morriss R, Alder N, Juszczak E (2010) Lithium plus valproate combination therapy versus monotherapy for relapse prevention in bipolar I disorder (BALANCE): a randomised open-label trial. Lancet 375(9712):385–395. doi:10.1016/S0140-6736(09)61828-6, S0140-6736(09)61828-6 [pii]

Geller B, Cooper TB, Watts HE, Cosby CM, Fox LW (1992) Early findings from a pharmacokinetically designed double-blind and placebo-controlled study of lithium for adolescents comorbid with bipolar and substance dependency disorders. Prog Neuropsychopharmacol Biol Psychiatry 16(3):281–299

Geller B, Cooper TB, Sun K, Zimerman B, Frazier J, Williams M, Heath J (1998) Double-blind and placebo-controlled study of lithium for adolescent bipolar disorders with secondary substance dependency. J Am Acad Child Adolesc Psychiatry 37(2):171–178

Gershon S, Yuwiler A (1960) Lithium ion: a specific psychopharmacological approach to the treatment of mania. J Neuropsychiatry 1:229–241

Ghaemi SN, Gilmer WS, Goldberg JF, Zablotsky B, Kemp DE, Kelley ME, Bauer AD, Fleck J, Filkowski MM, Stan VA, Dunn RT (2007) Divalproex in the treatment of acute bipolar depression: a preliminary double-blind, randomized, placebo-controlled pilot study. J Clin Psychiatry 68(12):1840–1844

Ghaemi SN, Wingo AP, Filkowski MA, Baldessarini RJ (2008) Long-term antidepressant treatment in bipolar disorder: meta-analyses of benefits and risks. Acta Psychiatr Scand 118(5):347–356. doi:10.1111/j.1600-0447.2008.01257.x, ACP1257 [pii]

Ghaemi SN, Ostacher MM, El-Mallakh RS, Borrelli D, Baldassano CF, Kelley ME, Filkowski MM, Hennen J, Sachs GS, Goodwin FK, Baldessarini RJ (2010) Antidepressant discontinuation in bipolar depression: a Systematic Treatment Enhancement Program for Bipolar Disorder (STEP-BD) randomized clinical trial of long-term effectiveness and safety. J Clin Psychiatry 71(4):372–380. doi:10.4088/JCP.08m04909gre

Gijsman HJ, Geddes JR, Rendell JM, Nolen WA, Goodwin GM (2004) Antidepressants for bipolar depression: a systematic review of randomized, controlled trials. Am J Psychiatry 161(9):1537–1547. doi:10.1176/appi.ajp.161.9.1537

Goikolea JM, Colom F, Capapey J, Torres I, Valenti M, Grande I, Undurraga J, Vieta E (2013a) Faster onset of antimanic action with haloperidol compared to second-generation antipsychotics. A meta-analysis of randomized clinical trials in acute mania. Eur Neuropsychopharmacol 23(4):305–316. doi:10.1016/j.euroneuro.2012.05.017, S0924-977X(12)00152-6 [pii]

Goikolea JM, Colom F, Torres I, Capapey J, Valenti M, Undurraga J, Grande I, Sanchez-Moreno J, Vieta E (2013b) Lower rate of depressive switch following antimanic treatment with second-generation antipsychotics versus haloperidol. J Affect Disord 144(3):191–198. doi:10.1016/j.jad.2012.07.038, S0165-0327(12)00569-1 [pii]

Goldberg J (2008) Adverse cognitive effects of psychotropic medications. In: Goldberg J, Burdick K (eds) Cognitive dysfunction in bipolar disorder: a guide for clinicians. American Psychiatric Press, Washington, DC, pp 137–158

Goldberg JF, Chengappa KN (2009) Identifying and treating cognitive impairment in bipolar disorder. Bipolar Disord 11(Suppl 2):123–137. doi:10.1111/j.1399-5618.2009.00716.x, BDI716 [pii]

Goldberg JF, Truman CJ (2003) Antidepressant-induced mania: an overview of current controversies. Bipolar Disord 5(6):407–420, 067 [pii]

Goldberg JF, Whiteside JE (2002) The association between substance abuse and antidepressant-induced mania in bipolar disorder: a preliminary study. J Clin Psychiatry 63(9):791–795

Goldsmith DR, Wagstaff AJ, Ibbotson T, Perry CM (2003) Lamotrigine: a review of its use in bipolar disorder. Drugs 63(19):2029–2050

Goodwin FK (2002) Rationale for long-term treatment of bipolar disorder and evidence for long-term lithium treatment. J Clin Psychiatry 63(Suppl 10):5–12

Goodwin FK, Zis AP (1979) Lithium in the treatment of mania: comparisons with neuroleptics. Arch Gen Psychiatry 36(8 Spec No):840–844

Goodwin FK, Murphy DL, Bunney WE Jr (1969a) Lithium. Lancet 2(7613):212–213

Goodwin FK, Murphy DL, Bunney WE Jr (1969b) Lithium-carbonate treatment in depression and mania. A longitudinal double-blind study. Arch Gen Psychiatry 21(4):486–496

Goodwin FK, Murphy DL, Dunner DL, Bunney WE Jr (1972) Lithium response in unipolar versus bipolar depression. Am J Psychiatry 129(1):44–47

Goodwin FK, Fireman B, Simon GE, Hunkeler EM, Lee J, Revicki D (2003) Suicide risk in bipolar disorder during treatment with lithium and divalproex. JAMA 290(11):1467–1473. doi:10.1001/jama.290.11.1467, 290/11/1467 [pii]

Goodwin GM, Bowden CL, Calabrese JR, Grunze H, Kasper S, White R, Greene P, Leadbetter R (2004) A pooled analysis of 2 placebo-controlled 18-month trials of lamotrigine and lithium maintenance in bipolar I disorder. J Clin Psychiatry 65(3):432–441

Goodwin GM, Abbar M, Schlaepfer TE, Grunze H, Licht RW, Bellivier F, Fountoulakis KN, Altamura AC, Pitchot W, Agren H, Holsboer-Trachsler E, Vieta E (2011) Aripiprazole in patients with bipolar mania and beyond: an update of practical guidance. Curr Med Res Opin 27(12):2285–2299. doi:10.1185/03007995.2011.628380

Gopal S, Steffens DC, Kramer ML, Olsen MK (2005) Symptomatic remission in patients with bipolar mania: results from a double-blind, placebo-controlled trial of risperidone monotherapy. J Clin Psychiatry 66(8):1016–1020

Granger P, Biton B, Faure C, Vige X, Depoortere H, Graham D, Langer SZ, Scatton B, Avenet P (1995) Modulation of the gamma-aminobutyric acid type A receptor by the antiepileptic drugs carbamazepine and phenytoin. Mol Pharmacol 47(6):1189–1196

Greenspan K, Schildkraut JJ, Gordon EK, Baer L, Aronoff MS, Durell J (1970) Catecholamine metabolism in affective disorders. 3. MHPG and other catecholamine metabolites in patients treated with lithium carbonate. J Psychiatr Res 7(3):171–183

Greil W, Kleindienst N (1999a) The comparative prophylactic efficacy of lithium and carbamazepine in patients with bipolar I disorder. Int Clin Psychopharmacol 14(5):277–281

Greil W, Kleindienst N (1999b) Lithium versus carbamazepine in the maintenance treatment of bipolar II disorder and bipolar disorder not otherwise specified. Int Clin Psychopharmacol 14(5):283–285

Greil W, Ludwig-Mayerhofer W, Erazo N, Schochlin C, Schmidt S, Engel RR, Czernik A, Giedke H, Muller-Oerlinghausen B, Osterheider M, Rudolf GA, Sauer H, Tegeler J, Wetterling T (1997) Lithium versus carbamazepine in the maintenance treatment of bipolar disorders–a randomised study. J Affect Disord 43(2):151–161

Greil W, Kleindienst N, Erazo N, Muller-Oerlinghausen B (1998) Differential response to lithium and carbamazepine in the prophylaxis of bipolar disorder. J Clin Psychopharmacol 18:455

Grossman F, Potter WZ, Brown EA, Maislin G (1999) A double-blind study comparing idazoxan and bupropion in bipolar depressed patients. J Affect Disord 56(2–3):237–243

Grunze HC (2008) Switching, induction of rapid cycling, and increased suicidality with antidepressants in bipolar patients: fact or overinterpretation? CNS Spectr 13(9):790–795

Gyulai L, Bauer M, Bauer MS, Garcia-Espana F, Cnaan A, Whybrow PC (2003a) Thyroid hypofunction in patients with rapid-cycling bipolar disorder after lithium challenge. Biol Psychiatry 53(10):899–905, S0006322302015731 [pii]

Gyulai L, Bowden CL, McElroy SL, Calabrese JR, Petty F, Swann AC, Chou JC, Wassef A, Risch CS, Hirschfeld RM, Nemeroff CB, Keck PE Jr, Evans DL, Wozniak PJ (2003b) Maintenance efficacy of divalproex in the prevention of bipolar depression. Neuropsychopharmacology 28(7):1374–1382

Harel EV, Levkovitz Y (2008) Effectiveness and safety of adjunctive antidepressants in the treatment of bipolar depression: a review. Isr J Psychiatry Relat Sci 45(2):121–128

Hartong EG, Moleman P, Hoogduin CA, Broekman TG, Nolen WA (2003) Prophylactic efficacy of lithium versus carbamazepine in treatment-naive bipolar patients. J Clin Psychiatry 64(2):144–151

Himmelhoch JM, Fuchs CZ, Symons BJ (1982) A double-blind study of tranylcypromine treatment of major anergic depression. J Nerv Ment Dis 170(10):628–634

Himmelhoch JM, Thase ME, Mallinger AG, Houck P (1991) Tranylcypromine versus imipramine in anergic bipolar depression. Am J Psychiatry 148(7):910–916

Hiremani RM, Thirthalli J, Tharayil BS, Gangadhar BN (2008) Double-blind randomized controlled study comparing short-term efficacy of bifrontal and bitemporal electroconvulsive therapy in acute mania. Bipolar Disord 10(6):701–707. doi:10.1111/j.1399-5618.2008.00608.x, BDI608 [pii]

Hirschfeld RM, Kasper S (2004) A review of the evidence for carbamazepine and oxcarbazepine in the treatment of bipolar disorder. Int J Neuropsychopharmacol 7(4):507–522. doi:10.1017/S1461145704004651, S1461145704004651 [pii]

Hirschfeld RM, Allen MH, McEvoy JP, Keck PE Jr, Russell JM (1999) Safety and tolerability of oral loading divalproex sodium in acutely manic bipolar patients. J Clin Psychiatry 60(12):815–818

Hirschfeld RM, Keck PE Jr, Kramer M, Karcher K, Canuso C, Eerdekens M, Grossman F (2004) Rapid antimanic effect of risperidone monotherapy: a 3-week multicenter, double-blind, placebo-controlled trial. Am J Psychiatry 161(6):1057–1065

Hirschfeld RM, Bowden CL, Vigna NV, Wozniak P, Collins M (2010) A randomized, placebo-controlled, multicenter study of divalproex sodium extended-release in the acute treatment of mania. J Clin Psychiatry 71(4):426–432. doi:10.4088/JCP.08m04960yel

Holmes MK, Erickson K, Luckenbaugh DA, Drevets WC, Bain EE, Cannon DM, Snow J, Sahakian BJ, Manji HK, Zarate CA Jr (2008) A comparison of cognitive functioning in medicated and unmedicated subjects with bipolar depression. Bipolar Disord 10(7):806–815. doi:10.1111/j.1399-5618.2008.00628.x, BDI628 [pii]

Honig A, Arts BM, Ponds RW, Riedel WJ (1999) Lithium induced cognitive side-effects in bipolar disorder: a qualitative analysis and implications for daily practice. Int Clin Psychopharmacol 14(3):167–171

Houston JP, Ahl J, Meyers AL, Kaiser CJ, Tohen M, Baldessarini RJ (2006) Reduced suicidal ideation in bipolar I disorder mixed-episode patients in a placebo-controlled trial of olanzapine combined with lithium or divalproex. J Clin Psychiatry 67(8):1246–1252

Houston JP, Tohen M, Degenhardt EK, Jamal HH, Liu LL, Ketter TA (2009) Olanzapine-divalproex combination versus divalproex monotherapy in the treatment of bipolar mixed episodes: a double-blind, placebo-controlled study. J Clin Psychiatry 70(11):1540–1547. doi:10.4088/JCP.08m04895yel

Houston JP, Ketter TA, Case M, Bowden C, Degenhardt EK, Jamal HH, Tohen M (2011) Early symptom change and prediction of subsequent remission with olanzapine augmentation in divalproex-resistant bipolar mixed episodes. J Psychiatr Res 45(2):169–173. doi:10.1016/j.jpsychires.2010.05.016, S0022-3956(10)00176-7 [pii]

Hullin RP, McDonald R, Allsopp MN (1972) Prophylactic lithium in recurrent affective disorders. Lancet 1(7759):1044–1046

Ichim L, Berk M, Brook S (2000) Lamotrigine compared with lithium in mania: a double-blind randomized controlled trial. Ann Clin Psychiatry 12(1):5–10

Ikeda Y, Kameyama M, Narita K, Takei Y, Suda M, Aoyama Y, Yuuki N, Sakurai N, Fukuda M, Mikuni M, Amanuma M (2010) Total and regional brain volume reductions due to the Syndrome of Irreversible Lithium-Effectuated Neurotoxicity (SILENT): a voxel-based morphometric study. Prog Neuropsychopharmacol Biol Psychiatry 34(1):244–246. doi:10.1016/j.pnpbp.2009.10.010

Jamrozinski K, Gruber O, Kemmer C, Falkai P, Scherk H (2009) Neurocognitive functions in euthymic bipolar patients. Acta Psychiatr Scand 119(5):365–374. doi:10.1111/j.1600-0447.2008.01320.x, ACP1320 [pii]

Janicak PG, Sharma RP, Pandey G, Davis JM (1998) Verapamil for the treatment of acute mania: a double-blind, placebo-controlled trial. Am J Psychiatry 155(7):972–973

Jentink J, Dolk H, Loane MA, Morris JK, Wellesley D, Garne E, de Jong-van den Berg L, Group EASW (2010) Intrauterine exposure to carbamazepine and specific congenital malformations: systematic review and case-control study. BMJ 341:c6581. doi:10.1136/bmj.c6581

Jimerson DC, Post RM, Stoddard FJ, Gillin JC, Bunney WE Jr (1980) Preliminary trial of the noradrenergic agonist clonidine in psychiatric patients. Biol Psychiatry 15(1):45–57

Johnson FN, Amdisen A (1983) The first era of lithium in medicine. An historical note. Pharmacopsychiatria 16(2):61–63. doi:10.1055/s-2007-1017450

Johnstone EC, Crow TJ, Frith CD, Owens DG (1988) The Northwick Park "functional" psychosis study: diagnosis and treatment response. Lancet 2(8603):119–125

Juruena MF, Ottoni GL, Machado-Vieira R, Carneiro RM, Weingarthner N, Marquardt AR, Fleig SS, Broilo L, Busnello EA (2009) Bipolar I and II disorder residual symptoms: oxcarbazepine and carbamazepine as add-on treatment to lithium in a double-blind, randomized trial. Prog Neuropsychopharmacol Biol Psychiatry 33(1):94–99. doi:10.1016/j.pnpbp.2008.10.012, S0278-5846(08)00318-7 [pii]

Kafantaris V, Coletti DJ, Dicker R, Padula G, Pleak RR, Alvir JM (2004) Lithium treatment of acute mania in adolescents: a placebo-controlled discontinuation study. J Am Acad Child Adolesc Psychiatry 43(8):984–993

Kakkar AK, Rehan HS, Unni KE, Gupta NK, Chopra D, Kataria D (2009) Comparative efficacy and safety of oxcarbazepine versus divalproex sodium in the treatment of acute mania: a pilot study. Eur Psychiatry 24(3):178–182. doi:10.1016/j.eurpsy.2008.12.014, S0924-9338(09)00011-X [pii]

Kane JM, Quitkin FM, Rifkin A, Ramos-Lorenzi JR, Nayak DD, Howard A (1982) Lithium carbonate and imipramine in the prophylaxis of unipolar and bipolar II illness: a prospective, placebo-controlled comparison. Arch Gen Psychiatry 39(9):1065–1069

Kaptsan A, Yaroslavsky Y, Applebaum J, Belmaker RH, Grisaru N (2003) Right prefrontal TMS versus sham treatment of mania: a controlled study. Bipolar Disord 5(1):36–39

Karniol IG, Dalton J, Lader MH (1978) Acute and chronic effects of lithium chloride on physiological and psychological measures in normals. Psychopharmacology (Berl) 57(3):289–294

Kastin AJ, Ehrensing RH, Schalch DS, Anderson MS (1972) Improvement in mental depression with decreased thyrotropin response after administration of thyrotropin-releasing hormone. Lancet 2(7780):740–742

Katagiri H, Takita Y, Tohen M, Higuchi T, Kanba S, Takahashi M (2012) Efficacy and safety of olanzapine in the treatment of Japanese patients with bipolar I disorder in a current manic or mixed episode: a randomized, double-blind, placebo- and haloperidol-controlled study. J Affect Disord 136(3):476–484. doi:10.1016/j.jad.2011.10.045, S0165-0327(11)00712-9 [pii]

Katagiri H, Tohen M, McDonnell DP, Fujikoshi S, Case M, Kanba S, Takahashi M, Gomez JC (2013) Efficacy and safety of olanzapine for treatment of patients with bipolar depression: Japanese subpopulation analysis of a randomized, double-blind, placebo-controlled study. BMC Psychiatry 13:138. doi:10.1186/1471-244X-13-138

Keck PE Jr, Marcus R, Tourkodimitris S, Ali M, Liebeskind A, Saha A, Ingenito G (2003a) A placebo-controlled, double-blind study of the efficacy and safety of aripiprazole in patients with acute bipolar mania. Am J Psychiatry 160(9):1651–1658

Keck PE Jr, Versiani M, Potkin S, West SA, Giller E, Ice K (2003b) Ziprasidone in the treatment of acute bipolar mania: a three-week, placebo-controlled, double-blind, randomized trial. Am J Psychiatry 160(4):741–748

Keck PE Jr, Corya SA, Altshuler LL, Ketter TA, McElroy SL, Case M, Briggs SD, Tohen M (2005) Analyses of treatment-emergent mania with olanzapine/fluoxetine combination in the treatment of bipolar depression. J Clin Psychiatry 66(5):611–616

Keck PE Jr, Calabrese JR, McQuade RD, Carson WH, Carlson BX, Rollin LM, Marcus RN, Sanchez R (2006a) A randomized, double-blind, placebo-controlled 26-week trial of aripiprazole in recently manic patients with bipolar I disorder. J Clin Psychiatry 67(4):626–637

Keck PE Jr, Mintz J, McElroy SL, Freeman MP, Suppes T, Frye MA, Altshuler LL, Kupka R, Nolen WA, Leverich GS, Denicoff KD, Grunze H, Duan N, Post RM (2006b) Double-blind, randomized, placebo-controlled trials of ethyl-eicosapentanoate in the treatment of bipolar depression and rapid cycling bipolar disorder. Biol Psychiatry 60(9):1020–1022. doi:10.1016/j.biopsych.2006.03.056, S0006-3223(06)00537-3 [pii]

Keck PE Jr, Calabrese JR, McIntyre RS, McQuade RD, Carson WH, Eudicone JM, Carlson BX, Marcus RN, Sanchez R (2007) Aripiprazole monotherapy for maintenance therapy in bipolar I disorder: a 100-week, double-blind study versus placebo. J Clin Psychiatry 68(10):1480–1491

Keck PE, Orsulak PJ, Cutler AJ, Sanchez R, Torbeyns A, Marcus RN, McQuade RD, Carson WH (2009) Aripiprazole monotherapy in the treatment of acute bipolar I mania: a randomized, double-blind, placebo- and lithium-controlled study. J Affect Disord 112(1–3):36–49. doi:10.1016/j.jad.2008.05.014, S0165-0327(08)00230-9 [pii]

Kemp DE, Gao K, Ganocy SJ, Elhaj O, Bilali SR, Conroy C, Findling RL, Calabrese JR (2009) A 6-month, double-blind, maintenance trial of lithium monotherapy versus the combination of lithium and divalproex for rapid-cycling bipolar disorder and Co-occurring substance abuse or dependence. J Clin Psychiatry 70(1):113–121, ej07m04022 [pii]

Kemp DE, Ganocy SJ, Brecher M, Carlson BX, Edwards S, Eudicone JM, Evoniuk G, Jansen W, Leon AC, Minkwitz M, Pikalov A, Stassen HH, Szegedi A, Tohen M, Van Willigenburg AP, Calabrese JR (2010) Clinical value of early partial symptomatic improvement in the prediction of response and remission during short-term treatment trials in 3369 subjects with bipolar I or II depression. J Affect Disord 130(1–2):171–179. doi:10.1016/j.jad.2010.10.026, S0165-0327(10)00640-3 [pii]

Kemp DE, Gao K, Fein EB, Chan PK, Conroy C, Obral S, Ganocy SJ, Calabrese JR (2012a) Lamotrigine as add-on treatment to lithium and divalproex: lessons learned from a double-blind, placebo-controlled trial in rapid-cycling bipolar disorder. Bipolar Disord 14(7):780–789. doi:10.1111/bdi.12013

Kemp DE, Karayal ON, Calabrese JR, Sachs GS, Pappadopulos E, Ice KS, Siu CO, Vieta E (2012b) Ziprasidone with adjunctive mood stabilizer in the maintenance treatment of bipolar I disorder: Long-term changes in weight and metabolic profiles. Eur Neuropsychopharmacol 22(2):123–131. doi:10.1016/j.euroneuro.2011.06.005, S0924-977X(11)00152-0 [pii]

Kessell A, Holt NF (1975) A controlled study of a tetracyclic antidepressant–maprotiline (Ludiomil). Med J Aust 1(25):773–776

Kessing LV (1998) Cognitive impairment in the euthymic phase of affective disorder. Psychol Med 28(5):1027–1038

Kessler U, Vaaler AE, Schoyen H, Oedegaard KJ, Bergsholm P, Andreassen OA, Malt UF, Morken G (2010) The study protocol of the Norwegian randomized controlled trial of electroconvulsive therapy in treatment resistant depression in bipolar disorder. BMC Psychiatry 10(1):16. doi:10.1186/1471-244X-10-16, 1471-244X-10-16 [pii]

Ketter TA, Houston JP, Adams DH, Risser RC, Meyers AL, Williamson DJ, Tohen M (2006) Differential efficacy of olanzapine and lithium in preventing manic or mixed recurrence in patients with bipolar I disorder based on number of previous manic or mixed episodes. J Clin Psychiatry 67(1):95–101

Ketter TA, Agid O, Kapur S, Loebel A, Siu CO, Romano SJ (2010) Rapid antipsychotic response with ziprasidone predicts subsequent acute manic/mixed episode remission. J Psychiatr Res 44(1):8–14. doi:10.1016/j.jpsychires.2009.07.006, S0022-3956(09)00170-8 [pii]

Khanna S, Vieta E, Lyons B, Grossman F, Eerdekens M, Kramer M (2005) Risperidone in the treatment of acute mania: double-blind, placebo-controlled study. Br J Psychiatry 187:229–234

King DJ (1994) Psychomotor impairment and cognitive disturbances induced by neuroleptics. Acta Psychiatr Scand Suppl 380:53–58

Klein DF (1967) Importance of psychiatric diagnosis in prediction of clinical drug effects. Arch Gen Psychiatry 16(1):118–126

Klein HE, Broucek B, Greil W (1981) Lithium withdrawal triggers psychotic states. Br J Psychiatry 139:255–256

Klein E, Bental E, Lerer B, Belmaker RH (1984) Carbamazepine and haloperidol v placebo and haloperidol in excited psychoses. A controlled study. Arch Gen Psychiatry 41(2):165–170

Kleindienst N, Greil W (2000) Differential efficacy of lithium and carbamazepine in the prophylaxis of bipolar disorder: results of the MAP study. Neuropsychobiology 42(Suppl 1):2–10

Kleindienst N, Greil W (2002) Inter-episodic morbidity and drop-out under carbamazepine and lithium in the maintenance treatment of bipolar disorder. Psychol Med 32(3):493–501

Kocsis JH, Shaw ED, Stokes PE, Wilner P, Elliot AS, Sikes C, Myers B, Manevitz A, Parides M (1993) Neuropsychologic effects of lithium discontinuation. J Clin Psychopharmacol 13(4):268–275

Kropf D, Muller-Oerlinghausen B (1979) Changes in learning, memory, and mood during lithium treatment. Approach to a research strategy. Acta Psychiatr Scand 59(1):97–124

Kuhn R (1957) Treatment of depressive states with an iminodibenzyl derivative (G 22355). Schweizerische medizinische Wochenschrift 87(35–36):1135–1140

Kuhn R (1958) The treatment of depressive states with G 22355 (imipramine hydrochloride). Am J Psychiatry 115(5):459–464

Kulkarni J, Garland KA, Scaffidi A, Headey B, Anderson R, de Castella A, Fitzgerald P, Davis SR (2006) A pilot study of hormone modulation as a new treatment for mania in women with bipolar affective disorder. Psychoneuroendocrinology 31(4):543–547

Kupka RW, Luckenbaugh DA, Post RM, Leverich GS, Nolen WA (2003) Rapid and non-rapid cycling bipolar disorder: a meta-analysis of clinical studies. J Clin Psychiatry 64(12):1483–1494

Kushner SF, Khan A, Lane R, Olson WH (2006) Topiramate monotherapy in the management of acute mania: results of four double-blind placebo-controlled trials. Bipolar Disord 8(1):15–27

Kwentus J, Riesenberg RA, Marandi M, Manning RA, Allen MH, Fishman RS, Spyker DA, Kehne JH, Cassella JV (2012) Rapid acute treatment of agitation in patients with bipolar I disorder: a multicenter, randomized, placebo-controlled clinical trial with inhaled loxapine. Bipolar Disord 14(1):31–40. doi:10.1111/j.1399-5618.2011.00975.x

Lecrubier Y, Bech P (2007) The Ham D(6) is more homogenous and as sensitive as the Ham D(17). Eur Psychiatry 22(4):252–255

Lees G, Leach MJ (1993) Studies on the mechanism of action of the novel anticonvulsant lamotrigine (Lamictal) using primary neurological cultures from rat cortex. Brain Res 612(1–2):190–199

Lenox RH, Watson DG (1994) Lithium and the brain: a psychopharmacological strategy to a molecular basis for manic depressive illness. Clin Chem 40(2):309–314

Lenox RH, Newhouse PA, Creelman WL, Whitaker TM (1992) Adjunctive treatment of manic agitation with lorazepam versus haloperidol: a double-blind study. J Clin Psychiatry 53(2):47–52

Lerer B, Moore N, Meyendorff E, Cho SR, Gershon S (1987) Carbamazepine versus lithium in mania: a double-blind study. J Clin Psychiatry 48(3):89–93

Leverich GS, Altshuler LL, Frye MA, Suppes T, McElroy SL, Keck PE Jr, Kupka RW, Denicoff KD, Nolen WA, Grunze H, Martinez MI, Post RM (2006) Risk of switch in mood polarity to hypomania or mania in patients with bipolar depression during acute and continuation trials of venlafaxine, sertraline, and bupropion as adjuncts to mood stabilizers. Am J Psychiatry 163(2):232–239

Li H, Ma C, Wang G, Zhu X, Peng M, Gu N (2008) Response and remission rates in Chinese patients with bipolar mania treated for 4 weeks with either quetiapine or lithium: a randomized and double-blind study. Curr Med Res Opin 24(1):1–10. doi:10.1185/030079908X253933

Licht RW, Gijsman H, Nolen WA, Angst J (2008) Are antidepressants safe in the treatment of bipolar depression? A critical evaluation of their potential risk to induce switch into mania or cycle acceleration. Acta Psychiatr Scand 118(5):337–346. doi:10.1111/j.1600-0447.2008.01237.x, ACP1237 [pii]

Liu L, Zheng T, Morris MJ, Wallengren C, Clarke AL, Reid CA, Petrou S, O'Brien TJ (2006) The mechanism of carbamazepine aggravation of absence seizures. J Pharmacol Exp Ther 319(2):790–798. doi:10.1124/jpet.106.104968

Loebel A, Cucchiaro J, Silva R, Kroger H, Hsu J, Sarma K, Sachs G (2013) Lurasidone monotherapy in the treatment of bipolar I depression: a randomized, double-blind. Placebo-controlled study. Am J Psychiatry. doi:10.1176/appi.ajp.2013.13070984, 1763708 [pii]

Loebel A, Cucchiaro J, Silva R, Kroger H, Sarma K, Xu J, Calabrese JR (2014) Lurasidone as adjunctive therapy with lithium or valproate for the treatment of bipolar I depression: a randomized, double-blind, placebo-controlled study. Am J Psychiatry 171(2):169–177. doi:10.1176/appi.ajp.2013.13070985

Lombardo I, Sachs G, Kolluri S, Kremer C, Yang R (2012) Two 6-week, randomized, double-blind, placebo-controlled studies of ziprasidone in outpatients with bipolar I depression: did baseline characteristics impact trial outcome? J Clin Psychopharmacol 32(4):470–478. doi:10.1097/JCP.0b013e31825ccde5

Loo C, Katalinic N, Mitchell PB, Greenberg B (2010) Physical treatments for bipolar disorder: a review of electroconvulsive therapy, stereotactic surgery and other brain stimulation techniques. J Affect Disord 132(1–2):1–13. doi:10.1016/j.jad.2010.08.017, S0165-0327(10)00552-5 [pii]

Lopez-Munoz F, Alamo C, Juckel G, Assion HJ (2007) Half a century of antidepressant drugs: on the clinical introduction of monoamine oxidase inhibitors, tricyclics, and tetracyclics. Part I: monoamine oxidase inhibitors. J Clin Psychopharmacol 27(6):555–559. doi:10.1097/jcp.0b013e3181bb617

Lund Y, Nissen M, Rafaelsen OJ (1982) Long-term lithium treatment and psychological functions. Acta Psychiatr Scand 65(3):233–244

Lusznat RM, Murphy DP, Nunn CM (1988) Carbamazepine vs lithium in the treatment and prophylaxis of mania. Br J Psychiatry 153:198–204

Lydiard RB, Culpepper L, Schioler H, Gustafsson U, Paulsson B (2009) Quetiapine monotherapy as treatment for anxiety symptoms in patients with bipolar depression: a pooled analysis of results from 2 double-blind, randomized, placebo-controlled studies. Prim Care Companion J Clin Psychiatry 11(5):215–225. doi:10.4088/PCC.08m00659

Maarbjerg K, Aagaard J, Vestergaard P (1988) Adherence to lithium prophylaxis: I. Clinical predictors and patient's reasons for nonadherence. Pharmacopsychiatry 21(3):121–125. doi:10.1055/s-2007-1014662

Macfadden W, Alphs L, Haskins JT, Turner N, Turkoz I, Bossie C, Kujawa M, Mahmoud R (2009) A randomized, double-blind, placebo-controlled study of maintenance treatment with adjunctive risperidone long-acting therapy in patients with bipolar I disorder who relapse frequently. Bipolar Disord 11(8):827–839. doi:10.1111/j.1399-5618.2009.00761.x, BDI761 [pii]

Machado-Vieira R, Soares JC, Lara DR, Luckenbaugh DA, Busnello JV, Marca G, Cunha A, Souza DO, Zarate CA Jr, Kapczinski F (2008) A double-blind, randomized, placebo-controlled 4-week study on the efficacy and safety of the purinergic agents allopurinol and dipyridamole adjunctive to lithium in acute bipolar mania. J Clin Psychiatry 69(8):1237–1245, ej07m03858 [pii]

Magalhaes PV, Dean OM, Bush AI, Copolov DL, Malhi GS, Kohlmann K, Jeavons S, Schapkaitz I, Anderson-Hunt M, Berk M (2011) N-acetyl cysteine add-on treatment for bipolar II disorder: a subgroup analysis of a randomized placebo-controlled trial. J Affect Disord 129(1-3):317–320. doi:10.1016/j.jad.2010.08.001, S0165-0327(10)00520-3 [pii]

Malhi GS, Tanious M, Gershon S (2011) The lithiumeter: a measured approach. Bipolar Disord 13(3):219–226. doi:10.1111/j.1399-5618.2011.00918.x

Malm H (2012) Prenatal exposure to selective serotonin reuptake inhibitors and infant outcome. Ther Drug Monit 34(6):607–614. doi:10.1097/FTD.0b013e31826d07ea

Mander AJ, Loudon JB (1988) Rapid recurrence of mania following abrupt discontinuation of lithium. Lancet 2(8601):15–17

Marcus R, Khan A, Rollin L, Morris B, Timko K, Carson W, Sanchez R (2011) Efficacy of aripiprazole adjunctive to lithium or valproate in the long-term treatment of patients with bipolar I disorder with an inadequate response to lithium or valproate monotherapy: a multicenter, double-blind, randomized study. Bipolar Disord 13(2):133–144. doi:10.1111/j.1399-5618.2011.00898.x

Margo A, McMahon P (1982) Lithium withdrawal triggers psychosis. Br J Psychiatry 141:407–410

Marmol F (2008) Lithium: bipolar disorder and neurodegenerative diseases Possible cellular mechanisms of the therapeutic effects of lithium. Prog Neuropsychopharmacol Biol Psychiatry 32(8):1761–1771. doi:10.1016/j.pnpbp.2008.08.012

McElroy SL, Keck PE Jr, Pope HG Jr, Hudson JI (1989) Valproate in psychiatric disorders: literature review and clinical guidelines. J Clin Psychiatry 50(Suppl):23–29

McElroy SL, Keck PE Jr, Pope HG Jr, Hudson JI, Faedda GL, Swann AC (1992) Clinical and research implications of the diagnosis of dysphoric or mixed mania or hypomania. Am J Psychiatry 149(12):1633–1644

McElroy SL, Keck PE, Stanton SP, Tugrul KC, Bennett JA, Strakowski SM (1996) A randomized comparison of divalproex oral loading versus haloperidol in the initial treatment of acute psychotic mania. J Clin Psychiatry 57(4):142–146

McElroy SL, Martens BE, Creech RS, Welge JA, Jefferson L, Guerdjikova AI, Keck PE Jr (2010a) Randomized, double-blind, placebo-controlled study of divalproex extended release loading monotherapy in ambulatory bipolar spectrum disorder patients with moderate-to-severe hypomania or mild mania. J Clin Psychiatry 71(5):557–565. doi:10.4088/JCP.08m04854yel

McElroy SL, Martens BE, Winstanley EL, Creech R, Malhotra S, Keck PE Jr (2010b) Placebo-controlled study of quetiapine monotherapy in ambulatory bipolar spectrum disorder with moderate-to-severe hypomania or mild mania. J Affect Disord 124(1–2):157–163. doi:10.1016/j.jad.2009.11.014, S0165-0327(09)00507-2 [pii]

McElroy SL, Weisler RH, Chang W, Olausson B, Paulsson B, Brecher M, Agambaram V, Merideth C, Nordenhem A, Young AH (2010c) A double-blind, placebo-controlled study of quetiapine and paroxetine as monotherapy in adults with bipolar depression (EMBOLDEN II). J Clin Psychiatry 71(2):163–174. doi:10.4088/JCP.08m04942gre

McElroy SL, Winstanley EL, Martens B, Patel NC, Mori N, Moeller D, McCoy J, Keck PE Jr (2010d) A randomized, placebo-controlled study of adjunctive ramelteon in ambulatory bipolar I disorder with manic symptoms and sleep disturbance. Int Clin Psychopharmacol 26(1):48–53. doi:10.1097/YIC.0b013e3283400d35

McIntyre RS, Brecher M, Paulsson B, Huizar K, Mullen J (2005) Quetiapine or haloperidol as monotherapy for bipolar mania–a 12-week, double-blind, randomised, parallel-group, placebo-controlled trial. Eur Neuropsychopharmacol 15(5):573–585

McIntyre RS, Cohen M, Zhao J, Alphs L, Macek TA, Panagides J (2009a) A 3-week, randomized, placebo-controlled trial of asenapine in the treatment of acute mania in bipolar mania and mixed states. Bipolar Disord 11(7):673–686. doi:10.1111/j.1399-5618.2009.00748.x, BDI748 [pii]

McIntyre RS, Cohen M, Zhao J, Alphs L, Macek TA, Panagides J (2009b) Asenapine versus olanzapine in acute mania: a double-blind extension study. Bipolar Disord 11(8):815–826. doi:10.1111/j.1399-5618.2009.00749.x, BDI749 [pii]

McIntyre RS, Muzina DJ, Adams A, Lourenco MT, Law CW, Soczynska JK, Woldeyohannes HO, Nathanson J, Kennedy SH (2009c) Quetiapine XR efficacy and tolerability as monotherapy and as adjunctive treatment to conventional antidepressants in the acute and maintenance treatment of major depressive disorder: a review of registration trials. Expert Opin Pharmacother 10(18):3061–3075. doi:10.1517/14656560903448837

McIntyre RS, Cohen M, Zhao J, Alphs L, Macek TA, Panagides J (2010a) Asenapine for long-term treatment of bipolar disorder: a double-blind 40-week extension study. J Affect Disord 126(3):358–365. doi:10.1016/j.jad.2010.04.005, S0165-0327(10)00341-1 [pii]

McIntyre RS, Cohen M, Zhao J, Alphs L, Macek TA, Panagides J (2010b) Asenapine in the treatment of acute mania in bipolar I disorder: a randomized, double-blind, placebo-controlled trial. J Affect Disord 122(1–2):27–38. doi:10.1016/j.jad.2009.12.028, S0165-0327(10)00007-8 [pii]

McIntyre RS, Soczynska JK, Woldeyohannes HO, Miranda A, Vaccarino A, Macqueen G, Lewis GF, Kennedy SH (2012) A randomized, double-blind, controlled trial evaluating the effect of intranasal insulin on neurocognitive function in euthymic patients with bipolar disorder. Bipolar Disord 14(7):697–706. doi:10.1111/bdi.12006

Medda P, Perugi G, Zanello S, Ciuffa M, Cassano GB (2009) Response to ECT in bipolar I, bipolar II and unipolar depression. J Affect Disord 118(1–3):55–59. doi:10.1016/j.jad.2009.01.014

Medhi B, Prakash O, Jose VM, Pradhan B, Chakrabarty S, Pandhi P (2008) Seasonal variation in plasma levels of lithium in the Indian population: is there a need to modify the dose? Singapore Med J 49(9):724–727

Meehan K, Zhang F, David S, Tohen M, Janicak P, Small J, Koch M, Rizk R, Walker D, Tran P, Breier A (2001) A double-blind, randomized comparison of the efficacy and safety of intramuscular injections of olanzapine, lorazepam, or placebo in treating acutely agitated patients diagnosed with bipolar mania. J Clin Psychopharmacol 21(4):389–397

Melia PI (1970) Prophylactic lithium: a double-blind trial in recurrent affective disorders. Br J Psychiatry 116(535):621–624

Mendels J (1976) Lithium in the treatment of depression. Am J Psychiatry 133(4):373–378

Meunier H, Carraz G, Neunier Y, Eymard P, Aimard M (1963) Pharmacodynamic properties of N-dipropylacetic acid. Therapie 18:435–438
Mishory A, Yaroslavsky Y, Bersudsky Y, Belmaker RH (2000) Phenytoin as an antimanic anticonvulsant: a controlled study. Am J Psychiatry 157(3):463–465
Mishory A, Winokur M, Bersudsky Y (2003) Prophylactic effect of phenytoin in bipolar disorder: a controlled study. Bipolar Disord 5(6):464–467, 070 [pii]
Mitchell S (1870) On the use of bromide of lithium. Am J Med Sci 60:443–445
Mitchell S (1877) Clinical lecture on nervousness in the male. Med News 35:177–184
Mitchell PB, Hadzi-Pavlovic D (2000) Lithium treatment for bipolar disorder. Bull World Health Organ 78(4):515–517
Mudur G (2006) Indian study sparks debate on the use of placebo in psychiatry trials. BMJ 332(7541):566
Muller-Oerlinghausen B, Retzow A, Henn FA, Giedke H, Walden J (2000) Valproate as an adjunct to neuroleptic medication for the treatment of acute episodes of mania: a prospective, randomized, double-blind, placebo-controlled, multicenter study. European Valproate Mania Study Group. J Clin Psychopharmacol 20(2):195–203
Muralidharan K, Ali M, Silveira LE, Bond DJ, Fountoulakis KN, Lam RW, Yatham LN (2013) Efficacy of second generation antipsychotics in treating acute mixed episodes in bipolar disorder: a meta-analysis of placebo-controlled trials. J Affect Disord 150(2):408–414. doi:10.1016/j.jad.2013.04.032
Murphy BL, Stoll AL, Harris PQ, Ravichandran C, Babb SM, Carlezon WA Jr, Cohen BM (2012) Omega-3 fatty acid treatment, with or without cytidine, fails to show therapeutic properties in bipolar disorder: a double-blind, randomized add-on clinical trial. J Clin Psychopharmacol 32(5):699–703. doi:10.1097/JCP.0b013e318266854c
Muzina DJ, Momah C, Eudicone JM, Pikalov A, McQuade RD, Marcus RN, Sanchez R, Carlson BX (2008) Aripiprazole monotherapy in patients with rapid-cycling bipolar I disorder: an analysis from a long-term, double-blind, placebo-controlled study. Int J Clin Pract 62(5):679–687. doi:10.1111/j.1742-1241.2008.01735.x, IJCP1735 [pii]
Muzina DJ, Gao K, Kemp DE, Khalife S, Ganocy SJ, Chan PK, Serrano MB, Conroy CM, Calabrese JR (2010) Acute efficacy of divalproex sodium versus placebo in mood stabilizer-naive bipolar I or II depression: a double-blind, randomized, placebo-controlled trial. J Clin Psychiatry 72:813–819. doi:10.4088/JCP.09m05570gre
Nahas Z, Kozel FA, Li X, Anderson B, George MS (2003) Left prefrontal transcranial magnetic stimulation (TMS) treatment of depression in bipolar affective disorder: a pilot study of acute safety and efficacy. Bipolar Disord 5(1):40–47
NCT00141271 A six-week, randomized, double-blind, multicenter, fixed-flexible dose, placebo-controlled study evaluating the efficacy and safety of oral ziprasidone in outpatients with bipolar I depression. Unpublished
NCT00282464 A six-week flexible dose study evaluating the efficacy and safety of geodon in patients with bipolar I depression
NCT00329108 study results (2009) http://165.112.8.96/ct2/show/results/NCT00329108
Nejtek VA, Avila M, Chen LA, Zielinski T, Djokovic M, Podawiltz A, Kaiser K, Bae S, Rush AJ (2008) Do atypical antipsychotics effectively treat co-occurring bipolar disorder and stimulant dependence? A randomized, double-blind trial. J Clin Psychiatry 69(8):1257–1266, ej07m03385 [pii]
Nemeroff CB, Evans DL, Gyulai L, Sachs GS, Bowden CL, Gergel IP, Oakes R, Pitts CD (2001) Double-blind, placebo-controlled comparison of imipramine and paroxetine in the treatment of bipolar depression. Am J Psychiatry 158(6):906–912
Nery FG, Monkul ES, Hatch JP, Fonseca M, Zunta-Soares GB, Frey BN, Bowden CL, Soares JC (2008) Celecoxib as an adjunct in the treatment of depressive or mixed episodes of bipolar disorder: a double-blind, randomized, placebo-controlled study. Hum Psychopharmacol 23(2):87–94. doi:10.1002/hup.912
Niufan G, Tohen M, Qiuqing A, Fude Y, Pope E, McElroy H, Ming L, Gaohua W, Xinbao Z, Huichun L, Liang S (2008) Olanzapine versus lithium in the acute treatment of bipolar mania: a double-blind, randomized, controlled trial. J Affect Disord 105(1–3):101–108

Nivoli AM, Colom F, Murru A, Pacchiarotti I, Castro-Loli P, Gonzalez-Pinto A, Fountoulakis KN, Vieta E (2011) New treatment guidelines for acute bipolar depression: a systematic review. J Affect Disord 129(1–3):14–26. doi:10.1016/j.jad.2010.05.018

Noack CH, Trautner EM (1951) The lithium treatment of maniacal psychosis. Med J Aust 2(7):219–222

Nolen WA, Weisler RH (2013) The association of the effect of lithium in the maintenance treatment of bipolar disorder with lithium plasma levels: a post hoc analysis of a double-blind study comparing switching to lithium or placebo in patients who responded to quetiapine (Trial 144). Bipolar Disord 15(1):100–109. doi:10.1111/bdi.12027

Norris ER, Karen B, Correll JR, Zemanek KJ, Lerman J, Primelo RA, Kaufmann MW (2013) A double-blind, randomized, placebo-controlled trial of adjunctive ramelteon for the treatment of insomnia and mood stability in patients with euthymic bipolar disorder. J Affect Disord 144(1–2):141–147. doi:10.1016/j.jad.2012.06.023, S0165-0327(12)00472-7 [pii]

Noyes R Jr, Dempsey GM (1974) Lithium treatment of depression. Dis Nerv Syst 35(12):573–576

Noyes R Jr, Dempsey GM, Blum A, Cavanaugh GL (1974) Lithium treatment of depression. Compr Psychiatry 15(3):187–193

Okuma T, Kishimoto A (1998) A history of investigation on the mood stabilizing effect of carbamazepine in Japan. Psychiatry Clin Neurosci 52(1):3–12. doi:10.1111/j.1440-1819.1998.tb00966.x

Okuma T, Inanaga K, Otsuki S, Sarai K, Takahashi R, Hazama H, Mori A, Watanabe M (1979) Comparison of the antimanic efficacy of carbamazepine and chlorpromazine: a double-blind controlled study. Psychopharmacology (Berl) 66(3):211–217

Okuma T, Inanaga K, Otsuki S, Sarai K, Takahashi R, Hazama H, Mori A, Watanabe S (1981) A preliminary double-blind study on the efficacy of carbamazepine in prophylaxis of manic-depressive illness. Psychopharmacology (Berl) 73(1):95–96

Okuma T, Yamashita I, Takahashi R, Itoh H, Otsuki S, Watanabe S, Sarai K, Hazama H, Inanaga K (1990) Comparison of the antimanic efficacy of carbamazepine and lithium carbonate by double-blind controlled study. Pharmacopsychiatry 23(3):143–150

Ono S, Mihara K, Suzuki A, Kondo T, Yasui-Furukori N, Furukori H, de Vries R, Kaneko S (2002) Significant pharmacokinetic interaction between risperidone and carbamazepine: its relationship with CYP2D6 genotypes. Psychopharmacology (Berl) 162(1):50–54. doi:10.1007/s00213-002-1056-8

Oquendo MA, Galfalvy HC, Currier D, Grunebaum MF, Sher L, Sullivan GM, Burke AK, Harkavy-Friedman J, Sublette ME, Parsey RV, Mann JJ (2011) Treatment of suicide attempters with bipolar disorder: a randomized clinical trial comparing lithium and valproate in the prevention of suicidal behavior. Am J Psychiatry 168(10):1050–1056. doi:10.1176/appi.ajp.2011.11010163, appi.ajp.2011.11010163 [pii]

Osman OT, Rudorfer MV, Potter WZ (1989) Idazoxan: a selective alpha 2-antagonist and effective sustained antidepressant in two bipolar depressed patients. Arch Gen Psychiatry 46(10):958–959

Pacchiarotti I, Bond DJ, Baldessarini RJ, Nolen WA, Grunze H, Licht RW, Post RM, Berk M, Goodwin GM, Sachs GS, Tondo L, Findling RL, Youngstrom EA, Tohen M, Undurraga J, Gonzalez-Pinto A, Goldberg JF, Yildiz A, Altshuler LL, Calabrese JR, Mitchell PB, Thase ME, Koukopoulos A, Colom F, Frye MA, Malhi GS, Fountoulakis KN, Vazquez G, Perlis RH, Ketter TA, Cassidy F, Akiskal H, Azorin JM, Valenti M, Mazzei DH, Lafer B, Kato T, Mazzarini L, Martinez-Aran A, Parker G, Souery D, Ozerdem A, McElroy SL, Girardi P, Bauer M, Yatham LN, Zarate CA, Nierenberg AA, Birmaher B, Kanba S, El-Mallakh RS, Serretti A, Rihmer Z, Young AH, Kotzalidis GD, MacQueen GM, Bowden CL, Ghaemi SN, Lopez-Jaramillo C, Rybakowski J, Ha K, Perugi G, Kasper S, Amsterdam JD, Hirschfeld RM, Kapczinski F, Vieta E (2013) The International Society for Bipolar Disorders (ISBD) task force report on antidepressant use in bipolar disorders. Am J Psychiatry 170(11):1249–1262. doi:10.1176/appi.ajp.2013.13020185

Pae CU, Masand PS, Mandel FS, O'Gorman C (2012) Achieving and sustaining remission in bipolar I disorder with ziprasidone : a post hoc analysis of a 24-week, double-blind, placebo-controlled study. Clin Drug Investig 32(11):747–754. doi:10.1007/s40261-012-0009-1

Pan YJ, Hsieh MH, Liu SK (2011) Visuospatial working memory deficits in remitted patients with bipolar disorder: susceptibility to the effects of GABAergic agonists. Bipolar Disord 13(4):365–376. doi:10.1111/j.1399-5618.2011.00931.x
Pande AC, Crockatt JG, Janney CA, Werth JL, Tsaroucha G (2000) Gabapentin in bipolar disorder: a placebo-controlled trial of adjunctive therapy. Gabapentin Bipolar Disorder Study Group. Bipolar Disord 2(3 Pt 2):249–255
Parker G, Tully L, Olley A, Hadzi-Pavlovic D (2006) SSRIs as mood stabilizers for bipolar II disorder? A proof of concept study. J Affect Disord 92(2–3):205–214
Patel V (2006) Ethics of placebo-controlled trial in severe mania. Indian J Med Ethics 3(1):11–12
Pecknold JC, Fleury D (1986) Alprazolam-induced manic episode in two patients with panic disorder. Am J Psychiatry 143(5):652–653
Perlis RH, Sachs GS, Lafer B, Otto MW, Faraone SV, Kane JM, Rosenbaum JF (2002) Effect of abrupt change from standard to low serum levels of lithium: a reanalysis of double-blind lithium maintenance data. Am J Psychiatry 159(7):1155–1159
Perlis RH, Baker RW, Zarate CA Jr, Brown EB, Schuh LM, Jamal HH, Tohen M (2006a) Olanzapine versus risperidone in the treatment of manic or mixed States in bipolar I disorder: a randomized, double-blind trial. J Clin Psychiatry 67(11):1747–1753
Perlis RH, Welge JA, Vornik LA, Hirschfeld RM, Keck PE Jr (2006b) Atypical antipsychotics in the treatment of mania: a meta-analysis of randomized, placebo-controlled trials. J Clin Psychiatry 67(4):509–516
Persson G (1972) Lithium prophylaxis in affective disorders. Acta Psychiatr Scand 48:462–479
Perugi G, Toni C, Frare F, Travierso MC, Hantouche E, Akiskal HS (2002) Obsessive-compulsive-bipolar comorbidity: a systematic exploration of clinical features and treatment outcome. J Clin Psychiatry 63(12):1129–1134
Pilhatsch M, Wolf R, Winter C, Lewitzka U, Bauer M (2010) Comparison of paroxetine and amitriptyline as adjunct to lithium maintenance therapy in bipolar depression: a reanalysis of a randomized, double-blind study. J Affect Disord 126(3):453–457. doi:10.1016/j.jad.2010.04.025, S0165-0327(10)00361-7 [pii]
Placidi GF, Lenzi A, Lazzerini F, Cassano GB, Akiskal HS (1986) The comparative efficacy and safety of carbamazepine versus lithium: a randomized, double-blind 3-year trial in 83 patients. J Clin Psychiatry 47(10):490–494
Platman SR (1970) A comparison of lithium carbonate and chlorpromazine in mania. Am J Psychiatry 127(3):351–353
Pope HG Jr, McElroy SL, Keck PE Jr, Hudson JI (1991) Valproate in the treatment of acute mania. A placebo-controlled study. Arch Gen Psychiatry 48(1):62–68
Popovic D, Reinares M, Amann B, Salamero M, Vieta E (2010) Number needed to treat analyses of drugs used for maintenance treatment of bipolar disorder. Psychopharmacology (Berl) 213(4):657–667. doi:10.1007/s00213-010-2056-8
Porto FH, Leite MA, Fontenelle LF, Marrocos RP, Szczerback NF, de Freitas MR (2009) The Syndrome of Irreversible Lithium-Effectuated Neurotoxicity (SILENT): one-year follow-up of a single case. J Neurol Sci 277(1–2):172–173. doi:10.1016/j.jns.2008.10.010
Post RM, Uhde TW, Roy-Byrne PP, Joffe RT (1987) Correlates of antimanic response to carbamazepine. Psychiatry Res 21(1):71–83
Post R, Leverich G, Altshuler L, Mikalauskas K (1992) Lithium-discontinuation-induced refractoriness: preliminary observations. Am J Psychiatry 149:1727
Post RM, Altshuler LL, Frye MA, Suppes T, Rush AJ, Keck PE Jr, McElroy SL, Denicoff KD, Leverich GS, Kupka R, Nolen WA (2001) Rate of switch in bipolar patients prospectively treated with second-generation antidepressants as augmentation to mood stabilizers. Bipolar Disord 3(5):259–265
Post RM, Leverich GS, Nolen WA, Kupka RW, Altshuler LL, Frye MA, Suppes T, McElroy S, Keck P, Grunze H, Walden J (2003) A re-evaluation of the role of antidepressants in the treatment of bipolar depression: data from the Stanley Foundation Bipolar Network. Bipolar Disord 5(6):396–406, 065 [pii]

Post RM, Altshuler LL, Leverich GS, Frye MA, Nolen WA, Kupka RW, Suppes T, McElroy S, Keck PE, Denicoff KD, Grunze H, Walden J, Kitchen CM, Mintz J (2006) Mood switch in bipolar depression: comparison of adjunctive venlafaxine, bupropion and sertraline. Br J Psychiatry 189:124–131

Potkin SG, Keck PE Jr, Segal S, Ice K, English P (2005) Ziprasidone in acute bipolar mania: a 21-day randomized, double-blind, placebo-controlled replication trial. J Clin Psychopharmacol 25(4):301–310

Praharaj SK, Ram D, Arora M (2009) Efficacy of high frequency (rapid) suprathreshold repetitive transcranial magnetic stimulation of right prefrontal cortex in bipolar mania: a randomized sham controlled study. J Affect Disord 117(3):146–150. doi:10.1016/j.jad.2008.12.020, S0165-0327(09)00004-4 [pii]

Prien RF, Caffey EM Jr, Klett CJ (1972) Comparison of lithium carbonate and chlorpromazine in the treatment of mania. Report of the Veterans Administration and National Institute of Mental Health Collaborative Study Group. Arch Gen Psychiatry 26(2):146–153

Prien RF, Caffey EM Jr, Klett CJ (1973a) Prophylactic efficacy of lithium carbonate in manic-depressive illness. Report of the Veterans Administration and National Institute of Mental Health collaborative study group. Arch Gen Psychiatry 28(3):337–341

Prien RF, Klett CJ, Caffey EM Jr (1973b) Lithium carbonate and imipramine in prevention of affective episodes. A comparison in recurrent affective illness. Arch Gen Psychiatry 29(3):420–425

Prien RF, Kupfer DJ, Mansky PA, Small JG, Tuason VB, Voss CB, Johnson WE (1984) Drug therapy in the prevention of recurrences in unipolar and bipolar affective disorders. Report of the NIMH Collaborative Study Group comparing lithium carbonate, imipramine, and a lithium carbonate-imipramine combination. Arch Gen Psychiatry 41(11):1096–1104

Quante A, Zeugmann S, Luborzewski A, Schommer N, Langosch J, Born C, Anghelescu I, Wolf J (2010) Aripiprazole as adjunct to a mood stabilizer and citalopram in bipolar depression: a randomized placebo-controlled pilot study. Hum Psychopharmacol 25(2):126–132. doi:10.1002/hup.1096

Quiroz JA, Yatham LN, Palumbo JM, Karcher K, Kushner S, Kusumakar V (2010) Risperidone long-acting injectable monotherapy in the maintenance treatment of bipolar I disorder. Biol Psychiatry 68(2):156–162. doi:10.1016/j.biopsych.2010.01.015, S0006-3223(10)00057-0 [pii]

Rahimi R, Nikfar S, Abdollahi M (2006) Pregnancy outcomes following exposure to serotonin reuptake inhibitors: a meta-analysis of clinical trials. Reprod Toxicol 22(4):571–575. doi:10.1016/j.reprotox.2006.03.019

Reimers A, Helde G, Brodtkorb E (2005) Ethinyl estradiol, not progestogens, reduces lamotrigine serum concentrations. Epilepsia 46(9):1414–1417. doi:10.1111/j.1528-1167.2005.10105.x

Reinares M, Rosa AR, Franco C, Goikolea JM, Fountoulakis K, Siamouli M, Gonda X, Frangou S, Vieta E (2013) A systematic review on the role of anticonvulsants in the treatment of acute bipolar depression. Int J Neuropsychopharmacol 16(2):485–496. doi:10.1017/S1461145712000491, S1461145712000491 [pii]

Reus VI, Targum SD, Weingarter H, Post RM (1979) Effect of lithium carbonate on memory processes of bipolar affectively ill patients. Psychopharmacology (Berl) 63(1):39–42

Riesenberg RA, Baldytcheva I, Datto C (2012) Self-reported sedation profile of quetiapine extended-release and quetiapine immediate-release during 6-day initial dose escalation in bipolar depression: a multicenter, randomized, double-blind, phase IV study. Clin Ther 34(11):2202–2211. doi:10.1016/j.clinthera.2012.09.002, S0149-2918(12)00524-3 [pii]

Rihmer Z, Barsi J, Belso N, Pestality P, Gyorgy S (1996) Antidepressant-induced hypomania in obsessive-compulsive disorder. Int Clin Psychopharmacol 11(3):203–205

Robertson B, Grunze H, Versavel M, Costa R, Almeida L, Soares-da-Silva P (2010) Results of a double-blind, randomized, dose-titration, placebo controlled multicenter trial (SCO/BIA-2093-203 study) on safety and efficacy of eslicarbazepine acetate (BIA 2-093) for acute manic episodes associated with biopolar I disorder. Bipolar Disord 12(Suppl 12):46

Robitzek EH, Selikoff IJ, Ornstein GG (1952) Chemotherapy of human tuberculosis with hydrazine derivatives of isonicotinic acid; preliminary report of representative cases. Q Bull Sea View Hosp N Y Sea View Hosp Staten Island Clin Soc 13(1):27–51

Robitzek EH, Selikoff IJ, Mamlok E, Tendlau A (1953) Isoniazid and its isopropyl derivative in the therapy of tuberculosis in humans: comparative therapeutic and toxicologic properties. Dis Chest 23(1):1–15

Rogawski MA, Loscher W (2004a) The neurobiology of antiepileptic drugs. Nat Rev Neurosci 5(7):553–564. doi:10.1038/nrn1430

Rogawski MA, Loscher W (2004b) The neurobiology of antiepileptic drugs for the treatment of nonepileptic conditions. Nat Med 10(7):685–692. doi:10.1038/nm1074

Rosa AR, Fountoulakis K, Siamouli M, Gonda X, Vieta E (2011) Is anticonvulsant treatment of mania a class effect? Data from randomized clinical trials. CNS Neurosci Ther 17(3):167–177. doi:10.1111/j.1755-5949.2009.00089.x, CNS89 [pii]

Roy Chengappa KN, Schwarzman LK, Hulihan JF, Xiang J, Rosenthal NR (2006) Adjunctive topiramate therapy in patients receiving a mood stabilizer for bipolar I disorder: a randomized, placebo-controlled trial. J Clin Psychiatry 67(11):1698–1706

Sachs GS, Lafer B, Stoll AL, Banov M, Thibault AB, Tohen M, Rosenbaum JF (1994) A double-blind trial of bupropion versus desipramine for bipolar depression. J Clin Psychiatry 55(9):391–393

Sachs GS, Collins MA, Altshuler LL, Ketter TA, Suppes T, Rasgon NL, Frye MA, Wozniak P (2001) Divalproex sodium versus placebo in the treatment of bipolar depression. In: 40th Annual Meeting of the American College of Neuropsychopharmacology, San Juan, 8th Dec 2001

Sachs GS, Grossman F, Ghaemi SN, Okamoto A, Bowden CL (2002) Combination of a mood stabilizer with risperidone or haloperidol for treatment of acute mania: a double-blind, placebo-controlled comparison of efficacy and safety. Am J Psychiatry 159(7):1146–1154

Sachs G, Chengappa KN, Suppes T, Mullen JA, Brecher M, Devine NA, Sweitzer DE (2004) Quetiapine with lithium or divalproex for the treatment of bipolar mania: a randomized, double-blind, placebo-controlled study. Bipolar Disord 6(3):213–223

Sachs G, Sanchez R, Marcus R, Stock E, McQuade R, Carson W, Abou-Gharbia N, Impellizzeri C, Kaplita S, Rollin L, Iwamoto T (2006) Aripiprazole in the treatment of acute manic or mixed episodes in patients with bipolar I disorder: a 3-week placebo-controlled study. J Psychopharmacol 20(4):536–546

Sachs GS, Nierenberg AA, Calabrese JR, Marangell LB, Wisniewski SR, Gyulai L, Friedman ES, Bowden CL, Fossey MD, Ostacher MJ, Ketter TA, Patel J, Hauser P, Rapport D, Martinez JM, Allen MH, Miklowitz DJ, Otto MW, Dennehy EB, Thase ME (2007) Effectiveness of adjunctive antidepressant treatment for bipolar depression. N Engl J Med 356(17):1711–1722. doi:10.1056/NEJMoa064135, NEJMoa064135 [pii]

Sachs GS, Ice KS, Chappell PB, Schwartz JH, Gurtovaya O, Vanderburg DG, Kasuba B (2011) Efficacy and safety of adjunctive oral ziprasidone for acute treatment of depression in patients with bipolar I disorder: a randomized, double-blind, placebo-controlled trial. J Clin Psychiatry 72:1413–1422. doi:10.4088/JCP.09m05934

Sachs GS, Vanderburg DG, Edman S, Karayal ON, Kolluri S, Bachinsky M, Cavus I (2012a) Adjunctive oral ziprasidone in patients with acute mania treated with lithium or divalproex, part 1: results of a randomized, double-blind, placebo-controlled trial. J Clin Psychiatry 73(11):1412–1419. doi:10.4088/JCP.11m07388

Sachs GS, Vanderburg DG, Edman S, Karayal ON, Kolluri S, Bachinsky M, Cavus I (2012b) Adjunctive oral ziprasidone in patients with acute mania treated with lithium or divalproex, part 2: influence of protocol-specific eligibility criteria on signal detection. J Clin Psychiatry 73(11):1420–1425. doi:10.4088/JCP.11m07389

Salinsky MC, Storzbach D, Spencer DC, Oken BS, Landry T, Dodrill CB (2005) Effects of topiramate and gabapentin on cognitive abilities in healthy volunteers. Neurology 64(5):792–798. doi:10.1212/01.WNL.0000152877.08088.87, 64/5/792 [pii]

Salzer HM, Lurie ML (1953) Anxiety and depressive states treated with isonicotinyl hydrazide (isoniazid). AMA Arch Neurol Psychiatry 70(3):317–324

Sanger TM, Tohen M, Vieta E, Dunner DL, Bowden CL, Calabrese JR, Feldman PD, Jacobs TG, Breier A (2003) Olanzapine in the acute treatment of bipolar I disorder with a history of rapid cycling. J Affect Disord 73(1–2):155–161, S0165032702003348 [pii]

Saricicek A, Maloney K, Muralidharan A, Ruf B, Blumberg HP, Sanacora G, Lorberg B, Pittman B, Bhagwagar Z (2010) Levetiracetam in the management of bipolar depression: a randomized, double-blind, placebo-controlled trial. J Clin Psychiatry 72(6):744–750. doi:10.4088/JCP.09m05659gre

Sarris J, Mischoulon D, Schweitzer I (2012) Omega-3 for bipolar disorder: meta-analyses of use in mania and bipolar depression. J Clin Psychiatry 73(1):81–86. doi:10.4088/JCP.10r06710

Sartorius N, Baghai TC, Baldwin DS, Barrett B, Brand U, Fleischhacker W, Goodwin G, Grunze H, Knapp M, Leonard BE, Lieberman J, Nakane Y, Pinder RM, Schatzberg AF, Svestka J, Baumann P, Ghalib K, Markowitz JC, Padberg F, Fink M, Furukawa T, Fountoulakis KN, Jensen P, Kanba S, Riecher-Rossler A (2007) Antidepressant medications and other treatments of depressive disorders: a CINP Task Force report based on a review of evidence. Int J Neuropsychopharmacol 10(Suppl 1):S1–S207. doi:10.1017/S1461145707008255

Sayyaparaju KK, Grunze H, Fountoulakis KN (2014) When to start aripiprazole therapy in patients with bipolar mania. Neuropsychiatr Dis Treat 10:459–470. doi:10.2147/NDT.S40066

Schaffer A, Zuker P, Levitt A (2006) Randomized, double-blind pilot trial comparing lamotrigine versus citalopram for the treatment of bipolar depression. J Affect Disord 96(1–2):95–99

Scherk H, Pajonk FG, Leucht S (2007) Second-generation antipsychotic agents in the treatment of acute mania: a systematic review and meta-analysis of randomized controlled trials. Arch Gen Psychiatry 64(4):442–455. doi:10.1001/archpsyc.64.4.442, 64/4/442 [pii]

Schioldann J (1999) John Cade's seminal lithium paper turns fifty. Acta Psychiatr Scand 100(6):403–405

Schioldann J (2006) Obituary: Mogens Abelin Schou (1918-2005) – half a century with lithium. Hist Psychiatry 17(2):247–252

Schioldann J (2011) 'On periodical depressions and their pathogenesis' by Carl Lange (1886). Hist Psychiatry 22(85 Pt 1):108–130

Schneck CD, Miklowitz DJ, Miyahara S, Araga M, Wisniewski S, Gyulai L, Allen MH, Thase ME, Sachs GS (2008) The prospective course of rapid-cycling bipolar disorder: findings from the STEP-BD. Am J Psychiatry 165:370–377

Schou M (1963) Normothymotics, "mood-normalizers": are lithium and the imipramine drugs specific for affective disorders? Br J Psychiatry 109:803–809

Schou M (1979) Artistic productivity and lithium prophylaxis in manic-depressive illness. Br J Psychiatry 135:97–103

Schou M, Juel-Nielsen N, Stromgren E, Voldby H (1954) The treatment of manic psychoses by the administration of lithium salts. J Neurol Neurosurg Psychiatry 17(4):250–260

Schou M, Baastrup PC, Grof P, Weis P, Angst J (1970) Pharmacological and clinical problems of lithium prophylaxis. Br J Psychiatry 116(535):615–619

Segal J, Berk M, Brook S (1998) Risperidone compared with both lithium and haloperidol in mania: a double-blind randomized controlled trial. Clin Neuropharmacol 21(3):176–180

Selifoff IJ, Robitzek EH, Ornstein GG (1952) Toxicity of hydrazine derivatives of isonicotinic acid in the chemotherapy of human tuberculosis; a preliminary report. Q Bull Sea View Hosp N Y Sea View Hosp Staten Island Clin Soc 13(1):17–26

Selikoff IJ, Robitzek EH (1952) Tuberculosis chemotherapy with hydrazine derivatives of isonicotinic acid. Dis Chest 21(4):385–438

Senturk V, Goker C, Bilgic A, Olmez S, Tugcu H, Oncu B, Atbasoglu EC (2007) Impaired verbal memory and otherwise spared cognition in remitted bipolar patients on monotherapy with lithium or valproate. Bipolar Disord 9(Suppl 1):136–144. doi:10.1111/j.1399-5618.2007.00481.x, BDI481 [pii]

Seo HJ, Chiesa A, Lee SJ, Patkar AA, Han C, Masand PS, Serretti A, Pae CU (2010) Safety and tolerability of lamotrigine: results from 12 placebo-controlled clinical trials and clinical implications. Clin Neuropharmacol 34(1):39–47. doi:10.1097/WNF.0b013e3182055c07, 00002826-201101000-00009 [pii]

Serretti A, Artioli P, Zanardi R, Lorenzi C, Rossini D, Cusin C, Arnoldi A, Catalano M (2004) Genetic features of antidepressant induced mania and hypo-mania in bipolar disorder. Psychopharmacology (Berl) 174(4):504–511. doi:10.1007/s00213-004-1948-x

Shafti SS (2010) Olanzapine vs. lithium in management of acute mania. J Affect Disord 122(3):273–276. doi:10.1016/j.jad.2009.08.013, S0165-0327(09)00396-6 [pii]

Shaw ED, Mann JJ, Stokes PE, Manevitz AZ (1986) Effects of lithium carbonate on associative productivity and idiosyncrasy in bipolar outpatients. Am J Psychiatry 143(9):1166–1169

Shaw ED, Stokes PE, Mann JJ, Manevitz AZ (1987) Effects of lithium carbonate on the memory and motor speed of bipolar outpatients. J Abnorm Psychol 96(1):64–69

Sheehan DV, McElroy SL, Harnett-Sheehan K, Keck PE Jr, Janavs J, Rogers J, Gonzalez R, Shivakumar G, Suppes T (2009) Randomized, placebo-controlled trial of risperidone for acute treatment of bipolar anxiety. J Affect Disord 115(3):376–385. doi:10.1016/j.jad.2008.10.005, S0165-0327(08)00401-1 [pii]

Sheehan DV, Harnett-Sheehan K, Hidalgo RB, Janavs J, McElroy SL, Amado D, Suppes T (2013) Randomized, placebo-controlled trial of quetiapine XR and divalproex ER monotherapies in the treatment of the anxious bipolar patient. J Affect Disord 145(1):83–94. doi:10.1016/j.jad.2012.07.016, S0165-0327(12)00535-6 [pii]

Shelton RC, Stahl SM (2004) Risperidone and paroxetine given singly and in combination for bipolar depression. J Clin Psychiatry 65(12):1715–1719

Shepard TH, Brent RL, Friedman JM, Jones KL, Miller RK, Moore CA, Polifka JE (2002) Update on new developments in the study of human teratogens. Teratology 65(4):153–161. doi:10.1002/tera.10032

Shepherd M (1970) A prophylactic myth. Int J Psychiatry 9:423–425

Sherwood Brown E, Carmody TJ, Schmitz JM, Caetano R, Adinoff B, Swann AC, John Rush A (2009) A randomized, double-blind, placebo-controlled pilot study of naltrexone in outpatients with bipolar disorder and alcohol dependence. Alcohol Clin Exp Res 33(11):1863–1869. doi:10.1111/j.1530-0277.2009.01024.x, ACER1024 [pii]

Shi L, Namjoshi MA, Swindle R, Yu X, Risser R, Baker RW, Tohen M (2004a) Effects of olanzapine alone and olanzapine/fluoxetine combination on health-related quality of life in patients with bipolar depression: secondary analyses of a double-blind, placebo-controlled, randomized clinical trial. Clin Ther 26(1):125–134

Shi L, Schuh LM, Trzepacz PT, Huang LX, Namjoshi MA, Tohen M (2004b) Improvement of positive and negative syndrome scale cognitive score associated with olanzapine treatment of acute mania. Curr Med Res Opin 20(9):1371–1376. doi:10.1185/030079904125004493

Sholomskas AJ (1990) Mania in a panic disorder patient treated with fluoxetine. Am J Psychiatry 147(8):1090–1091

Shopsin B, Gershon S, Thompson H, Collins P (1975) Psychoactive drugs in mania. A controlled comparison of lithium carbonate, chlorpromazine, and haloperidol. Arch Gen Psychiatry 32(1):34–42

Shorter E (2009) The history of lithium therapy. Bipolar Disord 11(Suppl 2):4–9. doi:10.1111/j.1399-5618.2009.00706.x

Sidor MM, Macqueen GM (2010) Antidepressants for the acute treatment of bipolar depression: a systematic review and meta-analysis. J Clin Psychiatry 72:156–167. doi:10.4088/JCP.09r05385gre

Sidor MM, MacQueen GM (2012) An update on antidepressant use in bipolar depression. Curr Psychiatry Rep 14(6):696–704. doi:10.1007/s11920-012-0323-6

Sienaert P, Lambrichts L, Dols A, De Fruyt J (2013) Evidence-based treatment strategies for treatment-resistant bipolar depression: a systematic review. Bipolar Disord 15(1):61–69. doi:10.1111/bdi.12026

Sikdar S, Kulhara P, Avasthi A, Singh H (1994) Combined chlorpromazine and electroconvulsive therapy in mania. Br J Psychiatry 164(6):806–810

Silva MT, Zimmermann IR, Galvao TF, Pereira MG (2013) Olanzapine plus fluoxetine for bipolar disorder: a systematic review and meta-analysis. J Affect Disord 146(3):310–318. doi:10.1016/j.jad.2012.11.001, S0165-0327(12)00735-5 [pii]

Silverstone T (2001) Moclobemide vs. imipramine in bipolar depression: a multicentre double-blind clinical trial. Acta Psychiatr Scand 104(2):104–109, acp240 [pii]

Simhandl C, Denk E, Thau K (1993) The comparative efficacy of carbamazepine low and high serum level and lithium carbonate in the prophylaxis of affective disorders. J Affect Disord 28(4):221–231

Small JG, Small IF, Moore DF (1971) Experimental withdrawal of lithium in recovered manic-depressive patients: a report of five cases. Am J Psychiatry 127(11):1555–1558

Small JG, Klapper MH, Milstein V, Kellams JJ, Miller MJ, Marhenke JD, Small IF (1991) Carbamazepine compared with lithium in the treatment of mania. Arch Gen Psychiatry 48(10):915–921

Small JG, Klapper MH, Marhenke JD, Milstein V, Woodham GC, Kellams JJ (1995) Lithium combined with carbamazepine or haloperidol in the treatment of mania. Psychopharmacol Bull 31(2):265–272

Smith LA, Cornelius V, Warnock A, Tacchi MJ, Taylor D (2007) Acute bipolar mania: a systematic review and meta-analysis of co-therapy vs. monotherapy. Acta Psychiatr Scand 115(1):12–20. doi:10.1111/j.1600-0447.2006.00912.x, ACP912 [pii]

Smith LA, Cornelius VR, Azorin JM, Perugi G, Vieta E, Young AH, Bowden CL (2010) Valproate for the treatment of acute bipolar depression: systematic review and meta-analysis. J Affect Disord 122(1–2):1–9. doi:10.1016/j.jad.2009.10.033, S0165-0327(09)00495-9 [pii]

Smulevich AB, Khanna S, Eerdekens M, Karcher K, Kramer M, Grossman F (2005) Acute and continuation risperidone monotherapy in bipolar mania: a 3-week placebo-controlled trial followed by a 9-week double-blind trial of risperidone and haloperidol. Eur Neuropsychopharmacol 15(1):75–84

Solomon DA, Ristow WR, Keller MB, Kane JM, Gelenberg AJ, Rosenbaum JF, Warshaw MG (1996) Serum lithium levels and psychosocial function in patients with bipolar I disorder. Am J Psychiatry 153(10):1301–1307

Squire LR, Judd LL, Janowsky DS, Huey LY (1980) Effects of lithium carbonate on memory and other cognitive functions. Am J Psychiatry 137(9):1042–1046

Srisurapanont M, Yatham LN, Zis AP (1995) Treatment of acute bipolar depression: a review of the literature. Can J Psychiatr 40(9):533–544

Srivastava S, Wang PW, Hill SJ, Childers ME, Keller KL, Ketter TA (2012) Pilot study of the efficacy of double-blind, placebo-controlled one-week olanzapine stabilization therapy in heterogeneous symptomatic bipolar disorder patients. J Psychiatr Res 46(7):920–926. doi:10.1016/j.jpsychires.2012.04.004, S0022-3956(12)00110-0 [pii]

Stahl S, Lombardo I, Loebel A, Mandel FS (2010) Efficacy of ziprasidone in dysphoric mania: pooled analysis of two double-blind studies. J Affect Disord 122(1–2):39–45. doi:10.1016/j.jad.2009.06.023, S0165-0327(09)00280-8 [pii]

Steiner W (1991) Fluoxetine-induced mania in a patient with obsessive-compulsive disorder. Am J Psychiatry 148(10):1403–1404

Stokes PE, Shamoian CA, Stoll PM, Patton MJ (1971) Efficacy of lithium as acute treatment of manic-depressive illness. Lancet 1(7713):1319–1325

Stoll K, Goncalves N, Krober H, Demisch K, Bellaire W (1989) Use of carbamazepine in affective illness. In: Lerer G, Gershon S (eds) New directions in affective disorders. Springer, New York, pp 540–544

Stoll AL, Locke CA, Vuckovic A, Mayer PV (1996) Lithium-associated cognitive and functional deficits reduced by a switch to divalproex sodium: a case series. J Clin Psychiatry 57(8):356–359

Stoll AL, Severus WE, Freeman MP, Rueter S, Zboyan HA, Diamond E, Cress KK, Marangell LB (1999) Omega 3 fatty acids in bipolar disorder: a preliminary double-blind, placebo-controlled trial. Arch Gen Psychiatry 56(5):407–412

Strobusch AD, Jefferson JW (1980) The checkered history of lithium in medicine. Pharm Hist 22(2):72–76

Suppes T, Webb A, Paul B, Carmody T, Kraemer H, Rush AJ (1999) Clinical outcome in a randomized 1-year trial of clozapine versus treatment as usual for patients with treatment-resistant illness and a history of mania. Am J Psychiatry 156(8):1164–1169

Suppes T, Brown E, Schuh LM, Baker RW, Tohen M (2005) Rapid versus non-rapid cycling as a predictor of response to olanzapine and divalproex sodium for bipolar mania and maintenance of remission: post hoc analyses of 47-week data. J Affect Disord 89(1–3):69–77

Suppes T, Eudicone J, McQuade R, Pikalov A 3rd, Carlson B (2008a) Efficacy and safety of aripiprazole in subpopulations with acute manic or mixed episodes of bipolar I disorder. J Affect Disord 107(1–3):145–154. doi:10.1016/j.jad.2007.08.015, S0165-0327(07)00299-6 [pii]

Suppes T, Hirschfeld RM, Vieta E, Raines S, Paulsson B (2008b) Quetiapine for the treatment of bipolar II depression: analysis of data from two randomized, double-blind, placebo-controlled studies. World J Biol Psychiatry 9(3):198–211. doi:10.1080/15622970701317265, 778576702 [pii]

Suppes T, Vieta E, Liu S, Brecher M, Paulsson B (2009) Maintenance treatment for patients with bipolar I disorder: results from a north american study of quetiapine in combination with lithium or divalproex (trial 127). Am J Psychiatry 166(4):476–488. doi:10.1176/appi.ajp.2008.08020189, appi.ajp.2008.08020189 [pii]

Suppes T, Datto C, Minkwitz M, Nordenhem A, Walker C, Darko D (2010) Effectiveness of the extended release formulation of quetiapine as monotherapy for the treatment of acute bipolar depression. J Affect Disord 121(1–2):106–115. doi:10.1016/j.jad.2009.10.007, S0165-0327(09)00467-4 [pii]

Swann AC, Bowden CL, Morris D, Calabrese JR, Petty F, Small J, Dilsaver SC, Davis JM (1997) Depression during mania. Treatment response to lithium or divalproex. Arch Gen Psychiatry 54(1):37–42

Swartz HA, Thase ME (2011) Pharmacotherapy for the treatment of acute bipolar II depression: current evidence. J Clin Psychiatry 72(3):356–366. doi:10.4088/JCP.09r05192gre

Sylvia LG, Peters AT, Deckersbach T, Nierenberg AA (2013) Nutrient-based therapies for bipolar disorder: a systematic review. Psychother Psychosom 82(1):10–19. doi:10.1159/000341309, 000341309 [pii]

Szegedi A, Zhao J, van Willigenburg A, Nations KR, Mackle M, Panagides J (2011) Effects of asenapine on depressive symptoms in patients with bipolar I disorder experiencing acute manic or mixed episodes: a post hoc analysis of two 3-week clinical trials. BMC Psychiatry 11:101. doi:10.1186/1471-244X-11-101, 1471-244X-11-101 [pii]

Szegedi A, Calabrese JR, Stet L, Mackle M, Zhao J, Panagides J (2012) Asenapine as adjunctive treatment for acute mania associated with bipolar disorder: results of a 12-week core study and 40-week extension. J Clin Psychopharmacol 32(1):46–55. doi:10.1097/JCP.0b013e31823f872f

Tamayo JM, Zarate CA, Vieta E, Vazquez G, Tohen M (2010) Level of response and safety of pharmacological monotherapy in the treatment of acute bipolar I disorder phases: a systematic review and meta-analysis. Int J Neuropsychopharmacol 13(6):1–20. doi:10.1017/S1461145709991246, S1461145709991246 [pii]

Tarr GP, Glue P, Herbison P (2010) Comparative efficacy and acceptability of mood stabilizer and second generation antipsychotic monotherapy for acute mania–a systematic review and meta-analysis. J Affect Disord 134(1–3):14–19. doi:10.1016/j.jad.2010.11.009, S0165-0327(10)00691-9 [pii]

Tarr GP, Herbison P, de la Barra SL, Glue P (2011) Study design and patient characteristics and outcome in acute mania clinical trials. Bipolar Disord 13(2):125–132. doi:10.1111/j.1399-5618.2011.00904.x

Thase ME, Mallinger AG, McKnight D, Himmelhoch JM (1992) Treatment of imipramine-resistant recurrent depression, IV: a double-blind crossover study of tranylcypromine for anergic bipolar depression. Am J Psychiatry 149(2):195–198

Thase ME, Macfadden W, Weisler RH, Chang W, Paulsson B, Khan A, Calabrese JR (2006) Efficacy of quetiapine monotherapy in bipolar I and II depression: a double-blind, placebo-controlled study (the BOLDER II study). J Clin Psychopharmacol 26(6):600–609

Thase ME, Jonas A, Khan A, Bowden CL, Wu X, McQuade RD, Carson WH, Marcus RN, Owen R (2008) Aripiprazole monotherapy in nonpsychotic bipolar I depression: results of 2 randomized, placebo-controlled studies. J Clin Psychopharmacol 28(1):13–20

Thase ME, Bowden CL, Nashat M, Eudicone JM, Marcus R, McQuade RD, Carlson BX (2012) Aripiprazole in bipolar depression: a pooled, post-hoc analysis by severity of core depressive symptoms. Int J Psychiatry Clin Pract 16(2):121–131. doi:10.3109/13651501.2011.632680

Tohen M, Castillo J, Cole JO, Miller MG, de los Heros R, Farrer RJ (1991) Thrombocytopenia associated with carbamazepine: a case series. J Clin Psychiatry 52(12):496–498

Tohen M, Castillo J, Baldessarini RJ, Zarate C Jr, Kando JC (1995) Blood dyscrasias with carbamazepine and valproate: a pharmacoepidemiological study of 2,228 patients at risk. Am J Psychiatry 152(3):413–418

Tohen M, Sanger TM, McElroy SL, Tollefson GD, Chengappa KN, Daniel DG, Petty F, Centorrino F, Wang R, Grundy SL, Greaney MG, Jacobs TG, David SR, Toma V (1999) Olanzapine versus placebo in the treatment of acute mania. Olanzapine HGEH Study Group. Am J Psychiatry 156(5):702–709

Tohen M, Jacobs TG, Grundy SL, McElroy SL, Banov MC, Janicak PG, Sanger T, Risser R, Zhang F, Toma V, Francis J, Tollefson GD, Breier A (2000) Efficacy of olanzapine in acute bipolar mania: a double-blind, placebo-controlled study. The Olanzipine HGGW Study Group. Arch Gen Psychiatry 57(9):841–849

Tohen M, Baker RW, Altshuler LL, Zarate CA, Suppes T, Ketter TA, Milton DR, Risser R, Gilmore JA, Breier A, Tollefson GA (2002a) Olanzapine versus divalproex in the treatment of acute mania. Am J Psychiatry 159(6):1011–1017

Tohen M, Chengappa KN, Suppes T, Zarate CA Jr, Calabrese JR, Bowden CL, Sachs GS, Kupfer DJ, Baker RW, Risser RC, Keeter EL, Feldman PD, Tollefson GD, Breier A (2002b) Efficacy of olanzapine in combination with valproate or lithium in the treatment of mania in patients partially nonresponsive to valproate or lithium monotherapy. Arch Gen Psychiatry 59(1):62–69

Tohen M, Goldberg JF, Gonzalez-Pinto Arrillaga AM, Azorin JM, Vieta E, Hardy-Bayle MC, Lawson WB, Emsley RA, Zhang F, Baker RW, Risser RC, Namjoshi MA, Evans AR, Breier A (2003a) A 12-week, double-blind comparison of olanzapine vs haloperidol in the treatment of acute mania. Arch Gen Psychiatry 60(12):1218–1226

Tohen M, Ketter TA, Zarate CA, Suppes T, Frye M, Altshuler L, Zajecka J, Schuh LM, Risser RC, Brown E, Baker RW (2003b) Olanzapine versus divalproex sodium for the treatment of acute mania and maintenance of remission: a 47-week study. Am J Psychiatry 160(7):1263–1271

Tohen M, Vieta E, Calabrese J, Ketter TA, Sachs G, Bowden C, Mitchell PB, Centorrino F, Risser R, Baker RW, Evans AR, Beymer K, Dube S, Tollefson GD, Breier A (2003c) Efficacy of olanzapine and olanzapine-fluoxetine combination in the treatment of bipolar I depression. Arch Gen Psychiatry 60(11):1079–1088

Tohen M, Chengappa KN, Suppes T, Baker RW, Zarate CA, Bowden CL, Sachs GS, Kupfer DJ, Ghaemi SN, Feldman PD, Risser RC, Evans AR, Calabrese JR (2004) Relapse prevention in bipolar I disorder: 18-month comparison of olanzapine plus mood stabiliser v. mood stabiliser alone. Br J Psychiatry 184:337–345

Tohen M, Greil W, Calabrese JR, Sachs GS, Yatham LN, Oerlinghausen BM, Koukopoulos A, Cassano GB, Grunze H, Licht RW, Dell'Osso L, Evans AR, Risser R, Baker RW, Crane H, Dossenbach MR, Bowden CL (2005) Olanzapine versus lithium in the maintenance treatment of bipolar disorder: a 12-month, randomized, double-blind, controlled clinical trial. Am J Psychiatry 162(7):1281–1290

Tohen M, Calabrese JR, Sachs GS, Banov MD, Detke HC, Risser R, Baker RW, Chou JC, Bowden CL (2006) Randomized, placebo-controlled trial of olanzapine as maintenance therapy in patients with bipolar I disorder responding to acute treatment with olanzapine. Am J Psychiatry 163(2):247–256

Tohen M, Bowden CL, Smulevich AB, Bergstrom R, Quinlan T, Osuntokun O, Wang WV, Oliff HS, Martenyi F, Kryzhanovskaya LA, Greil W (2008a) Olanzapine plus carbamazepine v. carbamazepine alone in treating manic episodes. Br J Psychiatry 192(2):135–143. doi:10.1192/bjp.bp.107.041301, 192/2/135 [pii]

Tohen M, Vieta E, Goodwin GM, Sun B, Amsterdam JD, Banov M, Shekhar A, Aaronson ST, Bardenstein L, Grecu-Gabos I, Tochilov V, Prelipceanu D, Oliff HS, Kryzhanovskaya L, Bowden C (2008b) Olanzapine versus divalproex versus placebo in the treatment of mild to moderate mania: a randomized, 12-week, double-blind study. J Clin Psychiatry 69(11):1776–1789, ej07m03788 [pii]

Tohen M, Sutton VK, Calabrese JR, Sachs GS, Bowden CL (2009) Maintenance of response following stabilization of mixed index episodes with olanzapine monotherapy in a randomized, double-blind, placebo-controlled study of bipolar 1 disorder. J Affect Disord 116(1–2):43–50. doi:10.1016/j.jad.2008.11.003, S0165-0327(08)00442-4 [pii]

Tohen M, McDonnell DP, Case M, Kanba S, Ha K, Fang YR, Katagiri H, Gomez JC (2012) Randomised, double-blind, placebo-controlled study of olanzapine in patients with bipolar I depression. Br J Psychiatry 201(5):376–382. doi:10.1192/bjp.bp.112.108357, bjp.bp.112.108357 [pii]

Tohen M, Katagiri H, Fujikoshi S, Kanba S (2013) Efficacy of olanzapine monotherapy in acute bipolar depression: a pooled analysis of controlled studies. J Affect Disord 149(1–3):196–201. doi:10.1016/j.jad.2013.01.022

Tolliver BK, Desantis SM, Brown DG, Prisciandaro JJ, Brady KT (2012) A randomized, double-blind, placebo-controlled clinical trial of acamprosate in alcohol-dependent individuals with bipolar disorder: a preliminary report. Bipolar Disord 14(1):54–63. doi:10.1111/j.1399-5618.2011.00973.x

Tondo L, Hennen J, Baldessarini RJ (2001) Lower suicide risk with long-term lithium treatment in major affective illness: a meta-analysis. Acta Psychiatr Scand 104(3):163–172, acp464 [pii]

Tondo L, Hennen J, Baldessarini RJ (2003) Rapid-cycling bipolar disorder: effects of long-term treatments. Acta Psychiatr Scand 108(1):4–14, 126 [pii]

Tondo L, Vazquez G, Baldessarini RJ (2010) Mania associated with antidepressant treatment: comprehensive meta-analytic review. Acta Psychiatr Scand 121(6):404–414. doi:10.1111/j.1600-0447.2009.01514.x, ACP1514 [pii]

Truman CJ, Goldberg JF, Ghaemi SN, Baldassano CF, Wisniewski SR, Dennehy EB, Thase ME, Sachs GS (2007) Self-reported history of manic/hypomanic switch associated with antidepressant use: data from the Systematic Treatment Enhancement Program for Bipolar Disorder (STEP-BD). J Clin Psychiatry 68(10):1472–1479

Tsai AC, Rosenlicht NZ, Jureidini JN, Parry PI, Spielmans GI, Healy D (2011) Aripiprazole in the maintenance treatment of bipolar disorder: a critical review of the evidence and its dissemination into the scientific literature. PLoS Med 8(5):e1000434. doi:10.1371/journal.pmed.1000434, 10-PLME-RA-5815R3 [pii]

van der Loos ML, Mulder PG, Hartong EG, Blom MB, Vergouwen AC, de Keyzer HJ, Notten PJ, Luteijn ML, Timmermans MA, Vieta E, Nolen WA (2009) Efficacy and safety of lamotrigine as add-on treatment to lithium in bipolar depression: a multicenter, double-blind, placebo-controlled trial. J Clin Psychiatry 70(2):223–231, ej08m04152 [pii]

van der Loos ML, Mulder P, Hartong EG, Blom MB, Vergouwen AC, van Noorden MS, Timmermans MA, Vieta E, Nolen WA (2010) Efficacy and safety of two treatment algorithms in bipolar depression consisting of a combination of lithium, lamotrigine or placebo and paroxetine. Acta Psychiatr Scand 122(3):246–254. doi:10.1111/j.1600-0447.2009.01537.x, ACP1537 [pii]

van der Loos ML, Mulder P, Hartong EG, Blom MB, Vergouwen AC, van Noorden MS, Timmermans MA, Vieta E, Nolen WA (2011) Long-term outcome of bipolar depressed patients receiving lamotrigine as add-on to lithium with the possibility of the addition of paroxetine in nonresponders: a randomized, placebo-controlled trial with a novel design. Bipolar Disord 13(1):111–117. doi:10.1111/j.1399-5618.2011.00887.x

Van Lieshout RJ, MacQueen GM (2010) Efficacy and acceptability of mood stabilisers in the treatment of acute bipolar depression: systematic review. Br J Psychiatry 196:266–273. doi:10.1192/bjp.bp.108.057612, 196/4/266 [pii]

Vasudev K, Goswami U, Kohli K (2000) Carbamazepine and valproate monotherapy: feasibility, relative safety and efficacy, and therapeutic drug monitoring in manic disorder. Psychopharmacology (Berl) 150(1):15–23

Vasudev A, Macritchie K, Watson S, Geddes JR, Young AH (2008) Oxcarbazepine in the maintenance treatment of bipolar disorder. Cochrane Database Syst Rev (1):CD005171. doi:10.1002/14651858.CD005171.pub2

Vasudev A, Macritchie K, Vasudev K, Watson S, Geddes J, Young AH (2011) Oxcarbazepine for acute affective episodes in bipolar disorder. Cochrane Database Syst Rev (12):CD004857. doi:10.1002/14651858.CD004857.pub2

Vazquez GH, Tondo L, Undurraga J, Baldessarini RJ (2013) Overview of antidepressant treatment of bipolar depression. Int J Neuropsychopharmacol 16(7):1673–1685. doi:10.1017/S1461145713000023

Vieta E, Bernardo M (1992) Antidepressant-induced mania in obsessive-compulsive disorder. Am J Psychiatry 149(9):1282–1283

Vieta E, Martinez-Aran A, Goikolea JM, Torrent C, Colom F, Benabarre A, Reinares M (2002) A randomized trial comparing paroxetine and venlafaxine in the treatment of bipolar depressed patients taking mood stabilizers. J Clin Psychiatry 63(6):508–512

Vieta E, Calabrese JR, Hennen J, Colom F, Martinez-Aran A, Sanchez-Moreno J, Yatham LN, Tohen M, Baldessarini RJ (2004) Comparison of rapid-cycling and non-rapid-cycling bipolar I manic patients during treatment with olanzapine: analysis of pooled data. J Clin Psychiatry 65(10):1420–1428

Vieta E, Bourin M, Sanchez R, Marcus R, Stock E, McQuade R, Carson W, Abou-Gharbia N, Swanink R, Iwamoto T (2005a) Effectiveness of aripiprazole v. haloperidol in acute bipolar mania: double-blind, randomised, comparative 12-week trial. Br J Psychiatry 187:235–242

Vieta E, Mullen J, Brecher M, Paulsson B, Jones M (2005b) Quetiapine monotherapy for mania associated with bipolar disorder: combined analysis of two international, double-blind, randomised, placebo-controlled studies. Curr Med Res Opin 21(6):923–934

Vieta E, Manuel Goikolea J, Martinez-Aran A, Comes M, Verger K, Masramon X, Sanchez-Moreno J, Colom F (2006) A double-blind, randomized, placebo-controlled, prophylaxis study of adjunctive gabapentin for bipolar disorder. J Clin Psychiatry 67(3):473–477

Vieta E, Calabrese JR, Goikolea JM, Raines S, Macfadden W (2007) Quetiapine monotherapy in the treatment of patients with bipolar I or II depression and a rapid-cycling disease course: a randomized, double-blind, placebo-controlled study. Bipolar Disord 9(4):413–425

Vieta E, Cruz N, Garcia-Campayo J, de Arce R, Manuel Crespo J, Valles V, Perez-Blanco J, Roca E, Manuel Olivares J, Morinigo A, Fernandez-Villamor R, Comes M (2008a) A double-blind, randomized, placebo-controlled prophylaxis trial of oxcarbazepine as adjunctive treatment to lithium in the long-term treatment of bipolar I and II disorder. Int J Neuropsychopharmacol 11(4):445–452. doi:10.1017/S1461145708008596, S1461145708008596 [pii]

Vieta E, Suppes T, Eggens I, Persson I, Paulsson B, Brecher M (2008b) Efficacy and safety of quetiapine in combination with lithium or divalproex for maintenance of patients with bipolar I disorder (international trial 126). J Affect Disord 109(3):251–263. doi:10.1016/j.jad.2008.06.001, S0165-0327(08)00238-3 [pii]

Vieta E, T'Joen C, McQuade RD, Carson WH Jr, Marcus RN, Sanchez R, Owen R, Nameche L (2008c) Efficacy of adjunctive aripiprazole to either valproate or lithium in bipolar mania patients partially nonresponsive to valproate/lithium monotherapy: a placebo-controlled study. Am J Psychiatry 165(10):1316–1325. doi:10.1176/appi.ajp.2008.07101560, appi.ajp.2008.07101560 [pii]

Vieta E, Locklear J, Gunther O, Ekman M, Miltenburger C, Chatterton ML, Astrom M, Paulsson B (2010a) Treatment options for bipolar depression: a systematic review of randomized, controlled trials. J Clin Psychopharmacol 30(5):579–590. doi:10.1097/JCP.0b013e3181f15849

Vieta E, Nuamah IF, Lim P, Yuen EC, Palumbo JM, Hough DW, Berwaerts J (2010b) A randomized, placebo- and active-controlled study of paliperidone extended release for the treatment of acute manic and mixed episodes of bipolar I disorder. Bipolar Disord 12(3):230–243. doi:10.1111/j.1399-5618.2010.00815.x, BDI815 [pii]

Vieta E, Ramey T, Keller D, English PA, Loebel AD, Miceli J (2010c) Ziprasidone in the treatment of acute mania: a 12-week, placebo-controlled, haloperidol-referenced study. J Psychopharmacol 24(4):547–558. doi:10.1177/0269881108099418, 0269881108099418 [pii]

Vieta E, Gunther O, Locklear J, Ekman M, Miltenburger C, Chatterton ML, Astrom M, Paulsson B (2011) Effectiveness of psychotropic medications in the maintenance phase of bipolar disorder: a meta-analysis of randomized controlled trials. Int J Neuropsychopharmacol 14(8):1029–1049. doi:10.1017/S1461145711000885, S1461145711000885 [pii]

Vieta E, Montgomery S, Sulaiman AH, Cordoba R, Huberlant B, Martinez L, Schreiner A (2012) A randomized, double-blind, placebo-controlled trial to assess prevention of mood episodes with risperidone long-acting injectable in patients with bipolar I disorder. Eur Neuropsychopharmacol 22(11):825–835. doi:10.1016/j.euroneuro.2012.03.004, S0924-977X(12)00060-0 [pii]

Watkins SE, Callender K, Thomas DR, Tidmarsh SF, Shaw DM (1987) The effect of carbamazepine and lithium on remission from affective illness. Br J Psychiatry 150:180–182

Watson S, Gallagher P, Porter RJ, Smith MS, Herron LJ, Bulmer S, Young AH, Ferrier IN (2012) A randomized trial to examine the effect of mifepristone on neuropsychological performance and mood in patients with bipolar depression. Biol Psychiatry 72(11):943–949. doi:10.1016/j.biopsych.2012.05.029, S0006-3223(12)00507-0 [pii]

Wehr TA, Sack DA, Rosenthal NE, Cowdry RW (1988) Rapid cycling affective disorder: contributing factors and treatment responses in 51 patients. Am J Psychiatry 145(2):179–184

Weisler R, Dunn J, English P (2003) Adjunctive Ziprasidone for acute bipolar mania: randomized, placebo-controlled trial. Paper presented at the 4th International Forum on Mood and Anxiety Disorders, Monte Carlo, 19–21 Nov

Weisler RH, Kalali AH, Ketter TA (2004) A multicenter, randomized, double-blind, placebo-controlled trial of extended-release carbamazepine capsules as monotherapy for bipolar disorder patients with manic or mixed episodes. J Clin Psychiatry 65(4):478–484

Weisler RH, Keck PE Jr, Swann AC, Cutler AJ, Ketter TA, Kalali AH (2005) Extended-release carbamazepine capsules as monotherapy for acute mania in bipolar disorder: a multicenter, randomized, double-blind, placebo-controlled trial. J Clin Psychiatry 66(3):323–330

Weisler RH, Hirschfeld R, Cutler AJ, Gazda T, Ketter TA, Keck PE, Swann A, Kalali A (2006) Extended-release carbamazepine capsules as monotherapy in bipolar disorder : pooled results from two randomised, double-blind, placebo-controlled trials. CNS Drugs 20(3):219–231

Weisler RH, Calabrese JR, Thase ME, Arvekvist R, Stening G, Paulsson B, Suppes T (2008) Efficacy of quetiapine monotherapy for the treatment of depressive episodes in bipolar I disorder: a post hoc analysis of combined results from 2 double-blind, randomized, placebo-controlled studies. J Clin Psychiatry 69(5):769–782, ej07m03676 [pii]

Weisler RH, Nolen WA, Neijber A, Hellqvist A, Paulsson B (2011) Continuation of quetiapine versus switching to placebo or lithium for maintenance treatment of bipolar I disorder (Trial 144: a randomized controlled study). J Clin Psychiatry 72(11):1452–1464. doi:10.4088/JCP.11m06878

White K, Keck PE Jr, Lipinski J (1986) Serotonin-uptake inhibitors in obsessive-compulsive disorder: a case report. Compr Psychiatry 27(3):211–214

Wilting I, Fase S, Martens EP, Heerdink ER, Nolen WA, Egberts AC (2007) The impact of environmental temperature on lithium serum levels. Bipolar Disord 9(6):603–608. doi:10.1111/j.1399-5618.2007.00438.x, BDI438 [pii]

Wingo AP, Wingo TS, Harvey PD, Baldessarini RJ (2009) Effects of lithium on cognitive performance: a meta-analysis. J Clin Psychiatry 70(11):1588–1597. doi:10.4088/JCP.08r04972

Woo YS, Bahk WM, Chung MY, Kim DH, Yoon BH, Lee JH, Ahn YM, Chung SK, Kim JG, Lee KH, Paik KC (2011) Aripiprazole plus divalproex for recently manic or mixed patients with bipolar I disorder: a 6-month, randomized, placebo-controlled, double-blind maintenance trial. Hum Psychopharmacol 26(8):543–553. doi:10.1002/hup.1240

Wu JC, Kelsoe JR, Schachat C, Bunney BG, DeModena A, Golshan S, Gillin JC, Potkin SG, Bunney WE (2009) Rapid and sustained antidepressant response with sleep deprivation and chronotherapy in bipolar disorder. Biol Psychiatry 66(3):298–301. doi:10.1016/j.biopsych.2009.02.018, S0006-3223(09)00231-5 [pii]

Yatham LN, Grossman F, Augustyns I, Vieta E, Ravindran A (2003) Mood stabilisers plus risperidone or placebo in the treatment of acute mania. International, double-blind, randomised controlled trial. Br J Psychiatry 182:141–147

Yatham LN, Paulsson B, Mullen J, Vagero AM (2004) Quetiapine versus placebo in combination with lithium or divalproex for the treatment of bipolar mania. J Clin Psychopharmacol 24(6):599–606

Yatham LN, Vieta E, Young AH, Moller HJ, Paulsson B, Vagero M (2007) A double blind, randomized, placebo-controlled trial of quetiapine as an add-on therapy to lithium or divalproex for the treatment of bipolar mania. Int Clin Psychopharmacol 22(4):212–220

Yatham LN, Fountoulakis KN, Rahman Z, Ammerman D, Fyans P, Marler SV, Baker RA, Carlson BX (2013) Efficacy of aripiprazole versus placebo as adjuncts to lithium or valproate in relapse prevention of manic or mixed episodes in bipolar I patients stratified by index manic or mixed episode. J Affect Disord 147(1–3):365–372. doi:10.1016/j.jad.2012.11.042

Yildiz A, Guleryuz S, Ankerst DP, Ongur D, Renshaw PF (2008) Protein kinase C inhibition in the treatment of mania: a double-blind, placebo-controlled trial of tamoxifen. Arch Gen Psychiatry 65(3):255–263

Yildiz A, Vieta E, Leucht S, Baldessarini RJ (2010) Efficacy of antimanic treatments: meta-analysis of randomized, controlled trials. Neuropsychopharmacology 36(2):375–389. doi:10.1038/npp.2010.192, npp2010192 [pii]

Yildiz A, Nikodem M, Vieta E, Correll CU, Baldessarini RJ (2014) A network meta-analysis on comparative efficacy and all-cause discontinuation of antimanic treatments in acute bipolar mania. Psychol Med :1–19. doi:10.1017/S0033291714001305

Young LT, Joffe RT, Robb JC, MacQueen GM, Marriott M, Patelis-Siotis I (2000) Double-blind comparison of addition of a second mood stabilizer versus an antidepressant to an initial mood stabilizer for treatment of patients with bipolar depression. Am J Psychiatry 157(1):124–126

Young AH, Oren DA, Lowy A, McQuade RD, Marcus RN, Carson WH, Spiller NH, Torbeyns AF, Sanchez R (2009) Aripiprazole monotherapy in acute mania: 12-week randomised placebo- and haloperidol-controlled study. Br J Psychiatry 194(1):40–48. doi:10.1192/bjp.bp.108.049965, 194/1/40 [pii]

Young AH, McElroy SL, Bauer M, Philips N, Chang W, Olausson B, Paulsson B, Brecher M (2010) A double-blind, placebo-controlled study of quetiapine and lithium monotherapy in adults in the acute phase of bipolar depression (EMBOLDEN I). J Clin Psychiatry 71(2):150–162. doi:10.4088/JCP.08m04995gre

Zajecka JM, Weisler R, Sachs G, Swann AC, Wozniak P, Sommerville KW (2002) A comparison of the efficacy, safety, and tolerability of divalproex sodium and olanzapine in the treatment of bipolar disorder. J Clin Psychiatry 63(12):1148–1155

Zarate CA Jr, Tohen M (2004) Double-blind comparison of the continued use of antipsychotic treatment versus its discontinuation in remitted manic patients. Am J Psychiatry 161(1):169–171

Zarate CA Jr, Payne JL, Singh J, Quiroz JA, Luckenbaugh DA, Denicoff KD, Charney DS, Manji HK (2004) Pramipexole for bipolar II depression: a placebo-controlled proof of concept study. Biol Psychiatry 56(1):54–60

Zarate CA Jr, Singh JB, Carlson PJ, Quiroz J, Jolkovsky L, Luckenbaugh DA, Manji HK (2007) Efficacy of a protein kinase C inhibitor (tamoxifen) in the treatment of acute mania: a pilot study. Bipolar Disord 9(6):561–570

Zarate CA Jr, Brutsche NE, Ibrahim L, Franco-Chaves J, Diazgranados N, Cravchik A, Selter J, Marquardt CA, Liberty V, Luckenbaugh DA (2012) Replication of ketamine's antidepressant efficacy in bipolar depression: a randomized controlled add-on trial. Biol Psychiatry. doi:10.1016/j.biopsych.2011.12.010, S0006-3223(11)01210-8 [pii]

Zhang ZJ, Kang WH, Tan QR, Li Q, Gao CG, Zhang FG, Wang HH, Ma XC, Chen C, Wang W, Guo L, Zhang YH, Yang XB, Yang GD (2007) Adjunctive herbal medicine with carbamazepine for bipolar disorders: a double-blind, randomized, placebo-controlled study. J Psychiatr Res 41(3–4):360–369. doi:10.1016/j.jpsychires.2005.06.002

Zhu B, Tunis SL, Zhao Z, Baker RW, Lage MJ, Shi L, Tohen M (2005) Service utilization and costs of olanzapine versus divalproex treatment for acute mania: results from a randomized, 47-week clinical trial. Curr Med Res Opin 21(4):555–564

Zubieta JK, Huguelet P, O'Neil RL, Giordani BJ (2001) Cognitive function in euthymic bipolar I disorder. Psychiatry Res 102(1):9–20, S0165-1781(01)00242-6 [pii]

17 Psychosocial Treatment and Interventions

17.1 General Background

It has been solidly shown that BD has an unfavourable outcome in a considerable number of patients, in spite of the recent advances in its pharmacological treatment (Fountoulakis et al. 2012; Grunze et al. 2013). Many BD patients eventually suffer from chronic mood symptoms with significant global disability and burden, not only for themselves but also for their family and the society (Murray et al. 2012; Rosa et al. 2010). The overall functional outcome can be captured mainly by two dimensions representing clinical severity and cognitive dysfunction (Reinares et al. 2013). Unfortunately, symptomatic remission does not imply functional recovery which is absent in a significant number of clinically and symptomatically remitted patients (Tohen et al. 2000; Rosa et al. 2011).

Pharmacological treatment often fails to address all the patients' needs and there is a growing need for the development and implementation of effective and affordable interventions, tailored to the individual patient (Catala-Lopez et al. 2013). Early successful treatment, with full recovery if possible, is of prime importance for the long-term outcome. It has been clearly shown that subsyndromal symptoms together with psychosocial stress at baseline are factors predicting earlier relapse (De et al. 2012). Longitudinal studies show that poor adherence is also predictive of a poorer long-term outcome (Berk et al. 2010).

There are several specific adjunctive psychotherapies which have been developed with the aim to fill the above gaps and eventually to improve the illness outcome (Geddes and Miklowitz 2013). It is still unclear which psychotherapies truly work and which patients are eligible. The time of intervention is also an open question (Scott et al. 2006; Miller et al. 2004; Meyer and Hautzinger 2012; de Barros et al. 2013; Gomes et al. 2011; Reinares et al. 2014; Fountoulakis and Siamouli 2009a). Acute depression and the maintenance phase but not acute mania are at the centre of research.

Concerning the quality of the data available, the studies in BD patients suffer from the same limitations and methodological problems all psychotherapy

K.N. Fountoulakis, *Bipolar Disorder: An Evidence-Based Guide to Manic Depression*, DOI 10.1007/978-3-642-37216-2_17

trials do. There is no universally accepted standardized method to conduct this kind of studies and blindness and the nature of the control intervention are unresolved limitations.

17.2 Specific Psychotherapies and Psychosocial Interventions

17.2.1 Cognitive-Behavioural Therapy (CBT)

CBT for BD includes education about BD as a diathesis–stress illness, enhances the cognitive-behavioural skills to cope with prodromes, stresses the importance of routine and sleep, deals with cognitive and behavioural barriers to treatment adherence and guides the patient towards the identification of triggering factors and the dealing with long-term vulnerabilities. It also challenges dysfunctional thoughts and underlying maladaptive assumptions.

There are a small number of studies which investigate the usefulness of CBT in BD. All of them utilize CBT as adjunct treatment on pharmacotherapy and all have inadequate placebo conditions as control.

The first study on CBT in bipolar depression included 103 BD-I patients and randomized them to 14 sessions of CBT or a control group which however did not include any placebo condition. During a 12-month period, fewer patients in the CBT group relapsed in comparison to controls (44 % vs. 75 %). Also, patients in the control group had shorter duration in an episode, less admissions and mood symptoms and higher social functioning (Lam et al. 2003). However, the report of an extension (18-month follow-up) reported no effect of CBT on the relapse rate (Lam et al. 2005b).

Another study on 52 BD patients confirmed this loss of efficacy during the follow-up in a study which compared CBT plus additional emotive techniques vs. treatment as usual (TAU) (Ball et al. 2006). The comparison of CBT plus psychoeducation vs. TAU in 40 BD patients reported a beneficial effect even after 5 years in terms of symptoms and social–occupational functioning, but rate of recurrences and time to recurrence were not reported (Gonzalez-Isasi et al. 2012). CBT plus psychoeducation has been proven superior to psychoeducation alone in a study of 79 BD patients (52 BD-I and 27 BD-II). In that study, the combined treatment group had 50 % fewer depressed days per month, while at the same time the psychoeducation-alone group had more antidepressant use (Zaretsky et al. 2008). Similar results were reported from a study in 41 BD patients randomized to CBT vs. TAU. The results suggested an improvement in symptoms, frequency and duration of episodes (Costa et al. 2011).

A study which compared CBT vs. TAU in 253 BD patients reported that after 18 months more than half of the patients had a recurrence and there was no difference between groups. The post hoc analysis demonstrated that CBT was significantly more effective than TAU in those patients with fewer than 12 previous episodes, but less effective in those with more episodes (Scott et al. 2006). Similarly, no differences were reported at 12 months concerning the number of episodes and time to relapse by another study in 50 BD patients in remission which compared CBT vs. TAU (Gomes et al. 2011). Finally a 2-year study on 76 BD patients which were randomized to receive 20 sessions of CBT vs. support therapy reported negative findings concerning the relapse rate (Meyer and Hautzinger 2012).

Overall, the data so far give limited support for the usefulness of CBT during the acute phase of bipolar depression but definitely not for the maintenance for which booster sessions might be necessary and further research on the issue is needed. Probably patients at earlier stages of the illness might benefit more by this specific intervention, while those patients with a high chronicity and severity may have a worse response to the treatment. Unfortunately the type of patients which are more likely to benefit from CBT constitutes a minority in usual clinical practice.

17.3 Psychoeducation

Psychoeducation for BD includes training of patients regarding the overall awareness of the disorder, the treatment adherence, the avoiding of substance abuse as well as the early detection of new episodes. It also focuses on regular habits and stress management.

One of the first studies concerning the teaching of patients to recognize and identify the components of their disease and especially early symptoms of relapse and recurrence and to seek professional help as early as possible followed 69 patients for 18 months and compared psychoeducation to TAU and reported significant prolongation of the time to first manic relapse ($p=0.008$) and significant reductions in the number of manic relapses over 18 months (30 % vs. 52 %; $p=0.013$). The experimental treatment had no effect on time to first relapse or number of relapses with depression, but it significantly improved overall social functioning. It is important to note that the psychoeducation method included a limited number of sessions (7–12) (Perry et al. 1999).

The efficacy of adjunctive group psychoeducation was tested by the Barcelona group. Their trial included 120 euthymic BD patients who were randomly assigned to 21 sessions of group psychoeducation vs. non-specific group meetings. In this specific trial, psychoeducation involved improvement of illness awareness, detection of prodromes, adherence enhancement, substance use avoidance, encouragement of regular habits and stress management. The study included a follow-up with a duration of 2 years and reported that psychoeducation exerted a beneficial effect on the rate of and the time to recurrence as well as concerning hospitalizations per patient. This beneficial effect was high and was not reduced after 5 years (any episode 0.79 vs. 0.87; mania 0.40 vs. 0.57; hypomania 0.27 vs. 0.42 and mixed episodes 0.34 vs. 0.61), except for depressive episodes (0.91 vs. 0.80). Subjects in the psychoeducation group were acutely ill much less time (Colom et al. 2003, 2009).

Enhanced relapse prevention alone does not seem to work since another study with a different design reported that only occupational functioning but not time to recurrence improved with an intervention consisting of training community mental health teams to deliver enhanced relapse prevention (Lobban et al. 2010). Also a study with a 12-month follow-up and with a similar design to the first study of the Barcelona group but with 16 sessions found no differences between groups in mood symptoms, psychosocial functioning and quality of life, except for a subjectively perceived overall clinical improvement by subjects who received psychoeducation. The authors suggested that characteristics of the sample could explain this discrepancy, as patients with a more advanced stage of disease might have a worse response to psychoeducation (de Barros et al. 2013). In accord with the above, a post hoc analysis of the original Barcelona data revealed that patients with more than seven episodes did not show significant improvement with group psychoeducation in time to recurrence, and those with more than 14 episodes did not benefit from the treatment in terms of time spent ill (Colom et al. 2010).

The cost for the treatment of BD might be reduced with group psychoeducation (Scott et al. 2009). One trial in 204 BD patients applied 20 sessions of CBT or 6 sessions of group psychoeducation and found that overall the outcome was similar in the two groups in terms of reduction of symptoms and likelihood of relapse, but psychoeducation was associated with a decrease of costs ($180 per subject vs. $1,200 per subject for CBT) (Parikh et al. 2012) Currently there are some proposals of online psychoeducation programmes, but results are still inconclusive or pending (Smith et al. 2011; Proudfoot et al. 2012).

More complex multimodal approaches and multicomponent care packages have been developed and usually psychoeducation is a core element. One of these packages also included CBT and elements of dialectical behaviour therapy and social rhythms and has shown a beneficial effect after 1-year follow-up in comparison to TAU (Castle et al. 2010). The beneficial effect seems to be present concerning manic but not depressive episodes (Bauer et al. 2006; Simon et al. 2006), while a benefit on social role function and quality of life seems also to be present (Bauer et al. 2006).

Overall, the data so far suggest that interventions of a 6-month group psychoeducation seem to exert a long-lasting prophylactic effect, but this is probably restricted to manic episodes and to patients at the earlier stages of the disease who have achieved remission before the intervention has started. Although the mechanism of action of psychoeducation remains unknown, it is highly likely that the beneficial effect is mediated by the enhancement of treatment adherence, the promoting of lifestyle regularity and healthy habits and the teaching of early detection of prodromal signs.

17.4 Interpersonal and Social Rhythm Therapy (IPSRT)

IPSRT is based on the hypothesis that stressful life events and unstable or disrupted daily routines can lead to circadian rhythm instability and, in vulnerable individuals, to affective episodes (Reinares et al. 2014). It includes the management of affective symptoms through improvement of adherence to medication and stabilizing social rhythms and the resolution of interpersonal problems (unresolved grief, social role transitions, interpersonal role disputes, interpersonal deficits, grief for the lost healthy self).

There are only limited data concerning its usefulness. The first study included 175 acutely ill BD patients and followed them for 2 years. The trial involved four treatment groups depending on the combination of treatment and phase, that is, IPSRT vs. intensive clinical management during the acute and the maintenance phase. Overall, the data suggested there was no difference between IPSRT and intensive clinical management in terms of time to remission and in the proportion of patients achieving remission (70 % vs. 72 %). A positive finding was that those patients who received IPSRT during the acute treatment phase survived longer without an episode and showed higher regularity of social rhythms (Frank et al. 2005). Regarding psychosocial functioning, the results suggested that especially women who initially received IPSRT showed faster improvement in occupational functioning, but again there were no differences between groups at the end of the follow-up (Frank et al. 2008). More recently, a 12-week study in which unmedicated depressed BD-II patients were randomized to IPSRT ($N = 14$) vs. treatment with quetiapine (up to 300 mg/day; $N = 11$) showed that both groups experienced significant reduction in symptoms over time, but there were no group-by-time interactions. Response and dropout rates were similar (Swartz et al. 2012).

Overall, there are no convincing data on the usefulness of IPSRT during the maintenance phase of BD; however, there are some data suggesting that if applied early and particularly already during the acute phase, it might prolong the time to relapse.

17.5 Family Intervention

Family intervention for BD includes psychoeducation, communication enhancement and problem-solving skills training, as well as support and self-care training for caregivers. Family intervention targets the whole family and not only the patient.

There are significantly more studies on the possible usefulness of family intervention in BD patients. The importance of involving the whole family in the treatment intervention was highlighted in a study of 81 BD patients and 33 family dyads, which reported that the odds ratio for hospitalization at 1-year follow-up was related with high perceived criticism (by the patients from their relatives), poor adherence and the relatives' lack of knowledge concerning BD (OR 3.3; 95 % CI: 1.3–8.6) (Scott et al. 2012).

Several studies support the use of adjunctive family-focused treatment. One intervention design consists of 21 one-hour sessions which combine psychoeducation, communication skills training and problem-solving training. The sessions take place at home and include both the patient and his/her family during the post-episode period. The treatment has shown its efficacy vs. crisis management in 101 BD patients in reducing relapses (35 % vs. 54 %) and increasing time to relapse (53 vs. 73 weeks, respectively) (Miklowitz et al. 2000, 2003) and to reduce hospitalization risk compared with individual treatment (12 % vs. 60 %) (Rea et al. 2003).

The benefits extended to a 2-year follow-up and were particularly useful for depressive symptoms, in families with high expressed emotion and for the improvement of medication adherence (Miklowitz et al. 2003). Another format of intervention included 12 sessions of group psychoeducation for the patients and their families, and in comparison to TAU in 58 BD patients, it was reported to have a beneficial effect in the prevention of relapses, the decreasing of manic symptoms and the improvement of medication adherence (D'Souza et al. 2010).

Improvement in a variety of peripheral problems that accompany BD has been reported with several types of family intervention. Adjunctive psychoeducational marital intervention in acutely ill patients was reported to have a beneficial effect concerning medication adherence and global functioning but not for symptoms (Clarkin et al. 1998). It is almost certain that neither adjunctive family therapy nor adjunctive multifamily group therapy improves the recovery rate from acute bipolar episodes when compared with pharmacotherapy alone (Miller et al. 2004); however, it seems that these interventions could be beneficial for patients from families with high levels of impairment and could result in a reduction of both the number of depressive episodes and the time spent in depression (Cohen $d=0.7$–1.0) (Miller et al. 2008). In this frame, in those patients who recovered from the intake episode, multifamily group therapy was associated with the lowest hospitalization risk (Solomon et al. 2008).

A 15-month RCT showed the benefits in the prevention of recurrences of 12 group sessions of psychoeducation with a 90-min duration, delivered to caregivers of euthymic BD patients. This intervention was reported to have both reduced the risk of recurrence in comparison to a control group (42 % vs. 66 %; NNT: 4.1 with 95 % CI: 2.4–19.1) and also to have delayed recurrence (Reinares et al. 2008). It seemed that this intervention was particularly efficacious in the prevention of hypomanic/manic episodes and also in the reduction of the overall family burden (Reinares et al. 2004). It seems reasonable and also it is supported by research that carer-focused interventions improve the knowledge of the illness (van Gent and Zwart 1991), reduce burden (Madigan et al. 2012) and also reduce the general and mental health risk of caregivers (Perlick et al. 2010).

Overall, the literature supports the idea that interventions which focus on families and caregivers exert a beneficial impact especially on family members. The effect includes issues ranging from subjective well-being to general health. The effect on the patients themselves is controversial, but it is almost certain that there is a beneficial effect on issues like treatment adherence.

17.6 Intensive Psychosocial Intervention

'Intensive' psychotherapy is another option, but it is of unknown general efficacy. In BD patients it has been tested on 293 acutely depressive outpatients in multi-site study. These patients were randomized to 3 sessions of psychoeducation or up to 30 sessions of intensive psychotherapy (family-focused therapy, IPSRT or CBT). The methodology suffered from a number of drawbacks and the two groups were not well matched. The intensive psychotherapy group showed higher recovery rates, shorter times to recovery and greater likelihood of being clinically well in comparison to patients on the short intervention (Miklowitz et al. 2007b). The functional outcome was also reported to be better after 1 year (Miklowitz et al. 2007a).

17.7 Cognitive Remediation and Functional Remediation

As mentioned in the relevant chapter of the current book, BD patients suffer from severe and persistent neurocognitive dysfunction. There are already developed psychotherapeutic and other non-pharmacological methods to address this problem in patients with schizophrenia, but the experience from their application is rather disappointing in spite of favourable meta-analytic reports (Anaya et al. 2012).

Functional remediation tailored for the needs of BD patients includes education on neurocognitive deficits, communication, autonomy and stress management.

So far a similar picture seems to be in place concerning BD as well, with the limited research data that exist, failing to provide solid support to this kind of intervention.

One uncontrolled study in 15 BD patients applied a type of cognitive rehabilitation intervention and focused on mood monitoring and residual depressive symptoms, organization, planning and time management, attention and memory. An improvement of residual depressive symptoms, executive functions and general functioning was described. Patients with greater neurocognitive impairment had less benefit from the intervention (Deckersbach et al. 2010). The combination of neurocognitive techniques with psychoeducation and problem-solving within an ecological framework was tested in a multicentre trial in 239 euthymic BD patients with a moderate–severe degree of functional impairment ($N=77$) vs. psychoeducation ($N=82$) and vs. TAU ($N=80$). At endpoint the combined programme was superior to TAU but not to psychoeducation alone (Martinez-Aran et al. 2011; Torrent et al. 2013). A small study in 37 BD and schizoaffective patients tested Social Cognition and Interaction Training (SCIT) as adjunctive to TAU ($N=21$) vs. TAU alone ($N=16$). There was no difference between groups concerning social functioning, but there was a superiority of the combination group in the improvement of emotion perception, theory of mind, hostile attribution bias and depressive symptoms (Lahera et al. 2013).

17.8 Mindfulness-Based Interventions

The basic concept of mindfulness-based training is to enhance the ability to keep one's attention on purpose in the present moment and non-judgmentally. For BD patients it includes education about the illness and relapse prevention, combination of cognitive therapy and training in mindfulness meditation to increase the awareness of the patterns of thoughts, feelings and bodily sensations and the development of a different way (non-judgmentally) of relating to thoughts, feelings and bodily sensations. It also promotes the ability of the patients to choose the most skilful response to thoughts, feelings or situations.

The first study concerning the application of mindfulness-based cognitive therapy (MBCT) in BD tested it in comparison to waiting list and included only 8 patients in each group. The results suggested a beneficial effect with a reduction in anxiety and depressive symptoms (Williams et al. 2008).

Another study included 23 BD patients and 10 healthy controls and also utilized brain fMRI. Sixteen of these patients were tested before and after an 8-week MBCT intervention, and seven were wait-listed for training and tested at the same intervals. The results were compared with those of 10healthy controls. Following MBCT, there were significant improvements in BD patients concerning mindfulness, anxiety and emotion regulation, working memory, spatial memory and verbal fluency compared to the bipolar wait-list group (Ives-Deliperi et al. 2013).

The biggest study so far concerning MBCT included 95 BD patients and tested MBCT as adjunctive to TAU ($N=48$) vs. TAU alone ($N=47$) and followed the patients for 12 months. The results showed no difference between treatment groups in terms of relapse and recurrent rates of any mood episodes. There was some beneficial effect of MBCT on anxiety symptoms (Perich et al. 2013a, b).

Recently, the focus has expanded to analyse the impact of MBCT on brain activity and cognitive functioning in BD, but the findings are difficult to interpret (Howells et al. 2012; Stange et al. 2011; Ives-Deliperi et al. 2013).

A study which applied dialectical behaviour therapy in which mindfulness represented a large component also reported some positive outcomes (Van et al. 2013).

Overall, the data do not support a beneficial effect of MBCT on the core issues of BD but also suggest that MBCT could be useful in the reduction of anxiety in BD patients. So far there are no data supporting its efficacy in the prevention of recurrences.

Conclusions

Reviewing the data on the usefulness of psychosocial intervention in BD is rather disappointing. It seems that only psychoeducation is efficacious for the relapse prevention of mood episodes but only in a selected subgroup of patients at an early stage of the disease who have very good if not complete remission of the acute episode. CBT and IPSRT could have some beneficial effect during the acute phase, but more data are needed. Mindfulness interventions could only decrease anxiety, while interventions to improve neurocognition seem to be rather ineffective. Family intervention seems to have benefits mainly for caregivers, but it is uncertain whether they have an effect on patient outcomes. A summary of the specific areas of efficacy for each of the above-mentioned interventions is shown in Table 17.1.

The mechanisms responsible for the efficacy of the psychosocial treatments are unknown and poorly studied. Opinions suggest that the effect could be mediated through enhancement of treatment adherence (Colom et al. 2005); improving the lifestyle and especially biological rhythms, food intake and social zeitgebers (Frank et al. 2005); the changing of dysfunctional attitudes

Table 17.1 Specific psychosocial interventions and their targeted therapeutic effect in BD

Intervention	Efficacy					
	Relapse/recurrence	Manic symptoms	Depressive symptoms	Anxiety	Neurocognition	Overall functioning
CBT	No	–	Yes	–	–	–
Psychoeducation	Yes	No	No	–	–	Yes
IPSRT	E	E	E	–	–	–
Family intervention	No	No	No	–	–	No
Intensive psychosocial intervention	–	–	–	–	–	–
Cognitive remediation	No	No	No	–	No	No
Mindfulness-based interventions	No	No	No	Yes	–	–

(Ball et al. 2006); but also through the improvement of family interactions (Simoneau et al. 1999a, b). The enhanced ability for the early identification of signs of relapse may play an important role too (Perry et al. 1999).

As in any trial concerning any psychological intervention, the methodological issues hampering research are cardinal. The blindness problem together with the impossible task to have a valid placebo group limits the value of the data. Because of these methodological drawbacks, often small studies of this kind have an unexpectedly high effect size, while at the same time there is a lack of replication of the same treatment by different research groups under the same conditions. Psychosocial interventions suffer from an additional drawback themselves. The training of the therapist and the setting itself might play an important role and it is quite different to apply the same intervention in specialized centres than in real-world settings in the everyday clinical practice. Furthermore, the gathering of the data is far from systematic; adverse events are not routinely registered, outcomes are not hierarchically stated a priori and too many post hoc analyses are published without being stated as such.

The best timing for the implementation of psychological interventions is still uncertain, but it seems that they function better in subjects which are at an early stage of the disease and who were euthymic when recruited (Scott et al. 2007; Miller et al. 2004). It is highly possible that a higher number of previous episodes (Colom et al. 2010; Scott et al. 2006) as well as a higher psychiatric morbidity and more severe functional impairment (Reinares et al. 2010) might reduce treatment response although the data are not conclusive (Lam et al. 2009). In addition, it has been suggested that in the early phases, the intervention should be simpler, with a focus on neuroprotective strategies (Kapczinski et al. 2009). At later stages, the emphasis could focus more on rehabilitative interventions dealing with the specific disabilities of the patients (Berk et al. 2007).

IPSRT and CBT might be also efficacious during the acute episodes, but this is far from clear (Miklowitz et al. 2007b; Frank et al. 2005; Scott et al. 2006). Specific characteristics of the family environment have also been shown to influence the response to treatment (Miller et al. 2008; Miklowitz et al. 2009). Probably there were subpopulations who will especially benefit from these treatments (Scott et al. 2006; Miller et al. 2008), but these assumptions are based on post hoc analyses alone.

It should be mentioned that most of research concerns pure and classic BD-I patients although there are some rare data concerning special populations like BD-II (Colom et al. 2009; Swartz et al. 2012), schizoaffective disorder (Vieta 2010; Murru et al. 2012), patients with high suicide risk (Fountoulakis et al. 2009; Fountoulakis and Siamouli 2009b; Williams et al. 2008) and patients with comorbid substance abuse (Weiss et al. 2007, 2009).

The literature includes reports which suggest that the benefits of psychosocial interventions if achieved can last for up to 5 years (Gonzalez-Isasi et al. 2010; Colom et al. 2009) although some patients might need booster sessions (Lam et al. 2005a; Ball et al. 2006). The complete range of the effect these interventions have is still uncharted. It is reasonable to expect a beneficial effect in a number of problems, including suicidality, but research data on these issues are virtually non-existent (Fountoulakis et al. 2009; Fountoulakis and Siamouli 2009b).

Overall, there are some data in the literature supporting the notion that adjunctive specific psychological treatments can improve specific illness outcomes. It seems reasonable that any such intervention should be applied as early as possible and should always be tailored to the specific needs of the patient in the context of personalized patient care, since it is accepted that both the patients and their relatives have different needs and problems depending on the stage of the illness.

References

Anaya C, Martinez AA, yuso-Mateos JL, Wykes T, Vieta E, Scott J (2012) A systematic review of cognitive remediation for schizo-affective and affective disorders. J Affect Disord 142:13–21

Ball JR, Mitchell PB, Corry JC, Skillecorn A, Smith M, Malhi GS (2006) A randomized controlled trial of cognitive therapy for bipolar disorder: focus on long-term change. J Clin Psychiatry 67:277–286

Bauer MS, McBride L, Williford WO, Glick H, Kinosian B, Altshuler L, Beresford T, Kilbourne AM, Sajatovic M (2006) Collaborative care for bipolar disorder: part II. Impact on clinical outcome, function, and costs. Psychiatr Serv 57:937–945

Berk M, Conus P, Lucas N, Hallam K, Malhi GS, Dodd S, Yatham LN, Yung A, McGorry P (2007) Setting the stage: from prodrome to treatment resistance in bipolar disorder. Bipolar Disord 9:671–678

Berk L, Hallam KT, Colom F, Vieta E, Hasty M, Macneil C, Berk M (2010) Enhancing medication adherence in patients with bipolar disorder. Hum Psychopharmacol 25:1–16

Castle D, White C, Chamberlain J, Berk M, Berk L, Lauder S, Murray G, Schweitzer I, Piterman L, Gilbert M (2010) Group-based psychosocial intervention for bipolar disorder: randomised controlled trial. Br J Psychiatry 196:383–388

Catala-Lopez F, Genova-Maleras R, Vieta E, Tabares-Seisdedos R (2013) The increasing burden of mental and neurological disorders. Eur Neuropsychopharmacol 23:1337–1339

Clarkin JF, Carpenter D, Hull J, Wilner P, Glick I (1998) Effects of psychoeducational intervention for married patients with bipolar disorder and their spouses. Psychiatr Serv 49:531–533

Colom F, Vieta E, Martinez-Aran A, Reinares M, Goikolea JM, Benabarre A, Torrent C, Comes M, Corbella B, Parramon G, Corominas J (2003) A randomized trial on the efficacy of group psychoeducation in the prophylaxis of recurrences in bipolar patients whose disease is in remission. Arch Gen Psychiatry 60:402–407

Colom F, Vieta E, Sanchez-Moreno J, Martinez-Aran A, Reinares M, Goikolea JM, Scott J (2005) Stabilizing the stabilizer: group psychoeducation enhances the stability of serum lithium levels. Bipolar Disord 7(Suppl 5):32–36

Colom F, Vieta E, Sanchez-Moreno J, Palomino-Otiniano R, Reinares M, Goikolea JM, Benabarre A, Martinez-Aran A (2009) Group psychoeducation for stabilised bipolar disorders: 5-year outcome of a randomised clinical trial. Br J Psychiatry 194:260–265

Colom F, Reinares M, Pacchiarotti I, Popovic D, Mazzarini L, Martinez AA, Torrent C, Rosa AR, Palomino-Otiniano R, Franco C, Bonnin CM, Vieta E (2010) Has number of previous episodes any effect on response to group psychoeducation in bipolar patients? Acta Neuropsychiatrica 22:50–53

Costa RT, Cheniaux E, Rosaes PA, Carvalho MR, Freire RC, Versiani M, Range BP, Nardi AE (2011) The effectiveness of cognitive behavioral group therapy in treating bipolar disorder: a randomized controlled study. Rev Bras Psiquiatr 33:144–149

D'Souza R, Piskulic D, Sundram S (2010) A brief dyadic group based psychoeducation program improves relapse rates in recently remitted bipolar disorder: a pilot randomised controlled trial. J Affect Disord 120:272–276

de Barros PK, de O Costa LF, Silval KI, Dias VV, Roso MC, Bandeira M, Colom F, Moreno RA (2013) Efficacy of psychoeducation on symptomatic and functional recovery in bipolar disorder. Acta Psychiatr Scand 127:153–158

De DC, Ezquiaga E, Agud JL, Vieta E, Soler B, Garcia-Lopez A (2012) Subthreshold symptoms and time to relapse/recurrence in a community cohort of bipolar disorder outpatients. J Affect Disord 143:160–165

Deckersbach T, Nierenberg AA, Kessler R, Lund HG, Ametrano RM, Sachs G, Rauch SL, Dougherty D (2010) RESEARCH: cognitive rehabilitation for bipolar disorder: an open trial for employed patients with residual depressive symptoms. CNS Neurosci Ther 16:298–307

Fountoulakis KN, Siamouli M (2009) Re: How well do psychosocial interventions work in bipolar disorder? Can J Psychiatry 54:578

Fountoulakis KN, Gonda X, Siamouli M, Rihmer Z (2009) Psychotherapeutic intervention and suicide risk reduction in bipolar disorder: a review of the evidence. J Affect Disord 113:21–29

Fountoulakis KN, Kasper S, Andreassen O, Blier P, Okasha A, Severus E, Versiani M, Tandon R, Moller HJ, Vieta E (2012) Efficacy of pharmacotherapy in bipolar disorder: a report by the WPA section on pharmacopsychiatry. Eur Arch Psychiatry Clin Neurosci 262(Suppl 1):1–48

Frank E, Kupfer DJ, Thase ME, Mallinger AG, Swartz HA, Fagiolini AM, Grochocinski V, Houck P, Scott J, Thompson W, Monk T (2005) Two-year outcomes for interpersonal and social rhythm therapy in individuals with bipolar I disorder. Arch Gen Psychiatry 62:996–1004

Frank E, Soreca I, Swartz HA, Fagiolini AM, Mallinger AG, Thase ME, Grochocinski VJ, Houck PR, Kupfer DJ (2008) The role of interpersonal and social rhythm therapy in improving occupational functioning in patients with bipolar I disorder. Am J Psychiatry 165:1559–1565

Geddes JR, Miklowitz DJ (2013) Treatment of bipolar disorder. Lancet 381:1672–1682

Gomes BC, Abreu LN, Brietzke E, Caetano SC, Kleinman A, Nery FG, Lafer B (2011) A randomized controlled trial of cognitive behavioral group therapy for bipolar disorder. Psychother Psychosom 80:144–150

Gonzalez-Isasi A, Echeburua E, Mosquera F, Ibanez B, Aizpuru F, Gonzalez-Pinto A (2010) Long-term efficacy of a psychological intervention program for patients with refractory bipolar disorder: a pilot study. Psychiatry Res 176:161–165

Gonzalez-Isasi A, Echeburua E, Liminana JM, Gonzalez-Pinto A (2012) Psychoeducation and cognitive-behavioral therapy for patients with refractory bipolar disorder: a 5-year controlled clinical trial. Eur Psychiatry 29:134–141

Grunze H, Vieta E, Goodwin GM, Bowden C, Licht RW, Moller HJ, Kasper S (2013) The World Federation of Societies of Biological Psychiatry (WFSBP) guidelines for the biological treatment of bipolar disorders: update 2012 on the long-term treatment of bipolar disorder. World J Biol Psychiatry 14:154–219

Howells FM, Ives-Deliperi VL, Horn NR, Stein DJ (2012) Mindfulness based cognitive therapy improves frontal control in bipolar disorder: a pilot EEG study. BMC Psychiatry 12:15

Ives-Deliperi VL, Howells F, Stein DJ, Meintjes EM, Horn N (2013) The effects of mindfulness-based cognitive therapy in patients with bipolar disorder: a controlled functional MRI investigation. J Affect Disord 150:1152–1157

Kapczinski F, Dias VV, Kauer-Sant'Anna M, Frey BN, Grassi-Oliveira R, Colom F, Berk M (2009) Clinical implications of a staging model for bipolar disorders. Expert Rev Neurother 9:957–966

Lahera G, Benito A, Montes JM, Fernandez-Liria A, Olbert CM, Penn DL (2013) Social cognition and interaction training (SCIT) for outpatients with bipolar disorder. J Affect Disord 146:132–136

Lam DH, Watkins ER, Hayward P, Bright J, Wright K, Kerr N, Parr-Davis G, Sham P (2003) A randomized controlled study of cognitive therapy for relapse prevention for bipolar affective disorder: outcome of the first year. Arch Gen Psychiatry 60:145–152

Lam DH, McCrone P, Wright K, Kerr N (2005a) Cost-effectiveness of relapse-prevention cognitive therapy for bipolar disorder: 30-month study. Br J Psychiatry 186:500–506

Lam D, Donaldson C, Brown Y, Malliaris Y (2005b) Burden and marital and sexual satisfaction in the partners of bipolar patients. Bipolar Disord 7(5):431–440

Lam DH, Burbeck R, Wright K, Pilling S (2009) Psychological therapies in bipolar disorder: the effect of illness history on relapse prevention – a systematic review. Bipolar Disord 11:474–482

Lobban F, Taylor L, Chandler C, Tyler E, Kinderman P, Kolamunnage-Dona R, Gamble C, Peters S, Pontin E, Sellwood W, Morriss RK (2010) Enhanced relapse prevention for bipolar disorder by community mental health teams: cluster feasibility randomised trial. Br J Psychiatry 196:59–63

Madigan K, Egan P, Brennan D, Hill S, Maguire B, Horgan F, Flood C, Kinsella A, O'Callaghan E (2012) A randomised controlled trial of carer-focussed multi-family group psychoeducation in bipolar disorder. Eur Psychiatry 27:281–284

Martinez-Aran A, Torrent C, Sole B, Bonnin CM, Rosa AR, Sanchez-Moreno J, Vieta E (2011) Functional remediation for bipolar disorder. Clin Pract Epidemiol Ment Health 7:112–116

Meyer TD, Hautzinger M (2012) Cognitive behaviour therapy and supportive therapy for bipolar disorders: relapse rates for treatment period and 2-year follow-up. Psychol Med 42:1429–1439

Miklowitz DJ, Simoneau TL, George EL, Richards JA, Kalbag A, Sachs-Ericsson N, Suddath R (2000) Family-focused treatment of bipolar disorder: 1-year effects of a psychoeducational program in conjunction with pharmacotherapy. Biol Psychiatry 48:582–592

Miklowitz DJ, George EL, Richards JA, Simoneau TL, Suddath RL (2003) A randomized study of family-focused psychoeducation and pharmacotherapy in the outpatient management of bipolar disorder. Arch Gen Psychiatry 60:904–912

Miklowitz DJ, Otto MW, Frank E, Reilly-Harrington NA, Kogan JN, Sachs GS, Thase ME, Calabrese JR, Marangell LB, Ostacher MJ, Patel J, Thomas MR, Araga M, Gonzalez JM, Wisniewski SR (2007a) Intensive psychosocial intervention enhances functioning in patients with bipolar depression: results from a 9-month randomized controlled trial. Am J Psychiatry 164:1340–1347

Miklowitz DJ, Otto MW, Frank E, Reilly-Harrington NA, Wisniewski SR, Kogan JN, Nierenberg AA, Calabrese JR, Marangell LB, Gyulai L, Araga M, Gonzalez JM, Shirley ER, Thase ME, Sachs GS (2007b) Psychosocial treatments for bipolar depression: a 1-year randomized trial from the Systematic Treatment Enhancement Program. Arch Gen Psychiatry 64:419–426

Miklowitz DJ, Axelson DA, George EL, Taylor DO, Schneck CD, Sullivan AE, Dickinson LM, Birmaher B (2009) Expressed emotion moderates the effects of family-focused treatment for bipolar adolescents. J Am Acad Child Adolesc Psychiatry 48:643–651

Miller IW, Solomon DA, Ryan CE, Keitner GI (2004) Does adjunctive family therapy enhance recovery from bipolar I mood episodes? J Affect Disord 82:431–436

Miller IW, Keitner GI, Ryan CE, Uebelacker LA, Johnson SL, Solomon DA (2008) Family treatment for bipolar disorder: family impairment by treatment interactions. J Clin Psychiatry 69:732–740

Murray CJ, Vos T, Lozano R, Naghavi M, Flaxman AD, Michaud C, Ezzati M, Shibuya K, Salomon JA, Abdalla S, Aboyans V, Abraham J, Ackerman I, Aggarwal R, Ahn SY, Ali MK, Alvarado M, Anderson HR, Anderson LM, Andrews KG, Atkinson C, Baddour LM, Bahalim AN, Barker-Collo S, Barrero LH, Bartels DH, Basanez MG, Baxter A, Bell ML, Benjamin EJ, Bennett D, Bernabe E, Bhalla K, Bhandari B, Bikbov B, Bin AA, Birbeck G, Black JA, Blencowe H, Blore JD, Blyth F, Bolliger I, Bonaventure A, Boufous S, Bourne R, Boussinesq M, Braithwaite T, Brayne C, Bridgett L, Brooker S, Brooks P, Brugha TS, Bryan-Hancock C, Bucello C, Buchbinder R, Buckle G, Budke CM, Burch M, Burney P, Burstein R, Calabria B, Campbell B, Canter CE, Carabin H, Carapetis J, Carmona L, Cella C, Charlson F, Chen H, Cheng AT, Chou D, Chugh SS, Coffeng LE, Colan SD, Colquhoun S, Colson KE, Condon J, Connor MD, Cooper LT, Corriere M, Cortinovis M, de Vaccaro KC, Couser W, Cowie BC, Criqui MH, Cross M, Dabhadkar KC, Dahiya M, Dahodwala N, msere-Derry J, Danaei G,

Davis A, De Leo D, Degenhardt L, Dellavalle R, Delossantos A, Denenberg J, Derrett S, Des J, Dharmaratne SD, Dherani M, az-Torne C, Dolk H, Dorsey ER, Driscoll T, Duber H, Ebel B, Edmond K, Elbaz A, Ali SE, Erskine H, Erwin PJ, Espindola P, Ewoigbokhan SE, Farzadfar F, Feigin V, Felson DT, Ferrari A, Ferri CP, Fevre EM, Finucane MM, Flaxman S, Flood L, Foreman K, Forouzanfar MH, Fowkes FG, Fransen M, Freeman MK, Gabbe BJ, Gabriel SE, Gakidou E, Ganatra HA, Garcia B, Gaspari F, Gillum RF, Gmel G, Gonzalez-Medina D, Gosselin R, Grainger R, Grant B, Groeger J, Guillemin F, Gunnell D, Gupta R, Haagsma J, Hagan H, Halasa YA, Hall W, Haring D, Haro JM, Harrison JE, Havmoeller R, Hay RJ, Higashi H, Hill C, Hoen B, Hoffman H, Hotez PJ, Hoy D, Huang JJ, Ibeanusi SE, Jacobsen KH, James SL, Jarvis D, Jasrasaria R, Jayaraman S, Johns N, Jonas JB, Karthikeyan G, Kassebaum N, Kawakami N, Keren A, Khoo JP, King CH, Knowlton LM, Kobusingye O, Koranteng A, Krishnamurthi R, Laden F, Lalloo R, Laslett LL, Lathlean T, Leasher JL, Lee YY, Leigh J, Levinson D, Lim SS, Limb E, Lin JK, Lipnick M, Lipshultz SE, Liu W, Loane M, Ohno SL, Lyons R, Mabweijano J, MacIntyre MF, Malekzadeh R, Mallinger L, Manivannan S, Marcenes W, March L, Margolis DJ, Marks GB, Marks R, Matsumori A, Matzopoulos R, Mayosi BM, McAnulty JH, McDermott MM, McGill N, McGrath J, Medina-Mora ME, Meltzer M, Mensah GA, Merriman TR, Meyer AC, Miglioli V, Miller M, Miller TR, Mitchell PB, Mock C, Mocumbi AO, Moffitt TE, Mokdad AA, Monasta L, Montico M, Moradi-Lakeh M, Moran A, Morawska L, Mori R, Murdoch ME, Mwaniki MK, Naidoo K, Nair MN, Naldi L, Narayan KM, Nelson PK, Nelson RG, Nevitt MC, Newton CR, Nolte S, Norman P, Norman R, O'Donnell M, O'Hanlon S, Olives C, Omer SB, Ortblad K, Osborne R, Ozgediz D, Page A, Pahari B, Pandian JD, Rivero AP (2012) Disability-adjusted life years (DALYs) for 291 diseases and injuries in 21 regions, 1990–2010: a systematic analysis for the global burden of disease study 2010. Lancet 380:2197–2223

Murru A, Pacchiarotti I, Nivoli AM, Colom F, Vieta E (2012) Is schizoaffective disorder still a neglected condition in the scientific literature? Psychother Psychosom 81:389–390

Parikh SV, Zaretsky A, Beaulieu S, Yatham LN, Young LT, Patelis-Siotis I, Macqueen GM, Levitt A, Arenovich T, Cervantes P, Velyvis V, Kennedy SH, Streiner DL (2012) A randomized controlled trial of psychoeducation or cognitive-behavioral therapy in bipolar disorder: a Canadian Network for Mood and Anxiety treatments (CANMAT) study [CME]. J Clin Psychiatry 73:803–810

Perich T, Manicavasagar V, Mitchell PB, Ball JR (2013a) The association between meditation practice and treatment outcome in Mindfulness-based Cognitive Therapy for bipolar disorder. Behav Res Ther 51:338–343

Perich T, Manicavasagar V, Mitchell PB, Ball JR, Hadzi-Pavlovic D (2013b) A randomized controlled trial of mindfulness-based cognitive therapy for bipolar disorder. Acta Psychiatr Scand 127:333–343

Perlick DA, Miklowitz DJ, Lopez N, Chou J, Kalvin C, Adzhiashvili V, Aronson A (2010) Family-focused treatment for caregivers of patients with bipolar disorder. Bipolar Disord 12:627–637

Perry A, Tarrier N, Morriss R, McCarthy E, Limb K (1999) Randomised controlled trial of efficacy of teaching patients with bipolar disorder to identify early symptoms of relapse and obtain treatment. BMJ 318:149–153

Proudfoot J, Parker G, Manicavasagar V, Hadzi-Pavlovic D, Whitton A, Nicholas J, Smith M, Burckhardt R (2012) Effects of adjunctive peer support on perceptions of illness control and understanding in an online psychoeducation program for bipolar disorder: a randomised controlled trial. J Affect Disord 142:98–105

Rea MM, Tompson MC, Miklowitz DJ, Goldstein MJ, Hwang S, Mintz J (2003) Family-focused treatment versus individual treatment for bipolar disorder: results of a randomized clinical trial. J Consult Clin Psychol 71:482–492

Reinares M, Vieta E, Colom F, Martinez-Aran A, Torrent C, Comes M, Goikolea JM, Benabarre A, Sanchez-Moreno J (2004) Impact of a psychoeducational family intervention on caregivers of stabilized bipolar patients. Psychother Psychosom 73:312–319

Reinares M, Colom F, Sanchez-Moreno J, Torrent C, Martinez-Aran A, Comes M, Goikolea JM, Benabarre A, Salamero M, Vieta E (2008) Impact of caregiver group psychoeducation on the course and outcome of bipolar patients in remission: a randomized controlled trial. Bipolar Disord 10:511–519

Reinares M, Colom F, Rosa AR, Bonnin CM, Franco C, Sole B, Kapczinski F, Vieta E (2010) The impact of staging bipolar disorder on treatment outcome of family psychoeducation. J Affect Disord 123:81–86

Reinares M, Papachristou E, Harvey P, Mar BC, Sanchez-Moreno J, Torrent C, yuso-Mateos JL, Ploubidis GB, Vieta E, Frangou S (2013) Towards a clinical staging for bipolar disorder: defining patient subtypes based on functional outcome. J Affect Disord 144:65–71

Reinares M, Sanchez-Moreno J, Fountoulakis KN (2014) Psychosocial interventions in bipolar disorder: what, for whom, and when. J Affect Disord 156:46–55. doi:10.1016/j.jad.2013.12.017

Rosa AR, Reinares M, Michalak EE, Bonnin CM, Sole B, Franco C, Comes M, Torrent C, Kapczinski F, Vieta E (2010) Functional impairment and disability across mood states in bipolar disorder. Value Health 13:984–988

Rosa AR, Reinares M, Amann B, Popovic D, Franco C, Comes M, Torrent C, Bonnin CM, Sole B, Valenti M, Salamero M, Kapczinski F, Vieta E (2011) Six-month functional outcome of a bipolar disorder cohort in the context of a specialized-care program. Bipolar Disord 13:679–686

Scott J, Paykel E, Morriss R, Bentall R, Kinderman P, Johnson T, Abbott R, Hayhurst H (2006) Cognitive-behavioural therapy for severe and recurrent bipolar disorders: randomised controlled trial. Br J Psychiatry 188:313–320

Scott J, Colom F, Vieta E (2007) A meta-analysis of relapse rates with adjunctive psychological therapies compared to usual psychiatric treatment for bipolar disorders. Int J Neuropsychopharmacol 10:123–129

Scott J, Colom F, Popova E, Benabarre A, Cruz N, Valenti M, Goikolea JM, Sanchez-Moreno J, Asenjo MA, Vieta E (2009) Long-term mental health resource utilization and cost of care following group psychoeducation or unstructured group support for bipolar disorders: a cost-benefit analysis. J Clin Psychiatry 70:378–386

Scott J, Colom F, Pope M, Reinares M, Vieta E (2012) The prognostic role of perceived criticism, medication adherence and family knowledge in bipolar disorders. J Affect Disord 142:72–76

Simon GE, Ludman EJ, Bauer MS, Unutzer J, Operskalski B (2006) Long-term effectiveness and cost of a systematic care program for bipolar disorder. Arch Gen Psychiatry 63:500–508

Simoneau TL, Miklowitz DJ, Richards JA, Saleem R, George EL (1999a) Bipolar disorder and family communication: effects of a psychoeducational treatment program. J Abnorm Psychol 108:588–597

Simoneau B, Lavallee P, Anderson PC, Bailey M, Bantle G, Berthiaume S, Chabot C, Fazal G, Halmos T, Ogilvie WW, Poupart MA, Thavonekham B, Xin Z, Thibeault D, Bolger G, Panzenbeck M, Winquist R, Jung GL (1999b) Discovery of non-peptidic P2-P3 butanediamide renin inhibitors with high oral efficacy. Bioorg Med Chem 7(3):489–508

Smith DJ, Griffiths E, Poole R, di Florio A, Barnes E, Kelly MJ, Craddock N, Hood K, Simpson S (2011) Beating bipolar: exploratory trial of a novel Internet-based psychoeducational treatment for bipolar disorder. Bipolar Disord 13:571–577

Solomon DA, Keitner GI, Ryan CE, Kelley J, Miller IW (2008) Preventing recurrence of bipolar I mood episodes and hospitalizations: family psychotherapy plus pharmacotherapy versus pharmacotherapy alone. Bipolar Disord 10:798–805

Stange JP, Eisner LR, Holzel BK, Peckham AD, Dougherty DD, Rauch SL, Nierenberg AA, Lazar S, Deckersbach T (2011) Mindfulness-based cognitive therapy for bipolar disorder: effects on cognitive functioning. J Psychiatr Pract 17:410–419

Swartz HA, Frank E, Cheng Y (2012) A randomized pilot study of psychotherapy and quetiapine for the acute treatment of bipolar II depression. Bipolar Disord 14:211–216

Tohen M, Hennen J, Zarate CM Jr, Baldessarini RJ, Strakowski SM, Stoll AL, Faedda GL, Suppes T, Gebre-Medhin P, Cohen BM (2000) Two-year syndromal and functional recovery in 219 cases of first-episode major affective disorder with psychotic features. Am J Psychiatry 157:220–228

Torrent C, Bonnin CM, Martinez-Aran A, Valle J, Amann BL, Gonzalez-Pinto A, Crespo JM, Ibanez A, Garcia-Portilla MP, Tabares-Seisdedos R, Arango C, Colom F, Sole B, Pacchiarotti I, Rosa AR, yuso-Mateos JL, Anaya C, Fernandez P, Landin-Romero R, onso-Lana S, Ortiz-Gil J, Segura B, Barbeito S, Vega P, Fernandez M, Ugarte A, Subira M, Cerrillo E, Custal N, Menchon JM, Saiz-Ruiz J, Rodao JM, Isella S, Alegria A, Al-Halabi S, Bobes J, Galvan G, Saiz PA, Balanza-Martinez V, Selva G, Fuentes-Dura I, Correa P, Mayoral M, Chiclana G, Merchan-Naranjo J, Rapado-Castro M, Salamero M, Vieta E (2013) Efficacy of functional remediation in bipolar disorder: a multicenter randomized controlled study. Am J Psychiatry 170:852–859

van Gent EM, Zwart FM (1991) Psychoeducation of partners of bipolar-manic patients. J Affect Disord 21:15–18

Van Dijk S, Jeffrey J, Katz MR (2013) A randomized, controlled, pilot study of dialectical behavior therapy skills in a psychoeducational group for individuals with bipolar disorder. J Affect Disord 145:386–393

Vieta E (2010) Individualizing treatment for patients with schizoaffective disorder. J Clin Psychiatry 71:e26

Weiss RD, Griffin ML, Kolodziej ME, Greenfield SF, Najavits LM, Daley DC, Doreau HR, Hennen JA (2007) A randomized trial of integrated group therapy versus group drug counseling for patients with bipolar disorder and substance dependence. Am J Psychiatry 164:100–107

Weiss RD, Griffin ML, Jaffee WB, Bender RE, Graff FS, Gallop RJ, Fitzmaurice GM (2009) A "community-friendly" version of integrated group therapy for patients with bipolar disorder and substance dependence: a randomized controlled trial. Drug Alcohol Depend 104:212–219

Williams JM, Alatiq Y, Crane C, Barnhofer T, Fennell MJ, Duggan DS, Hepburn S, Goodwin GM (2008) Mindfulness-based cognitive therapy (MBCT) in bipolar disorder: preliminary evaluation of immediate effects on between-episode functioning. J Affect Disord 107:275–279

Zaretsky A, Lancee W, Miller C, Harris A, Parikh SV (2008) Is cognitive-behavioural therapy more effective than psychoeducation in bipolar disorder? Can J Psychiatry 53:441–448

Treatment Guidelines 18

18.1 Background

Treatment guidelines constitute one of the important developments in the field of psychiatry, after the introduction of the operationalized diagnostic criteria in the frame of modern classification systems and the advancing of evidence-based medicine (EBM) also in psychiatry. They emerged as an important element in order to summarize and clarify the research data and to the extent this is possible, to standardize treatment on the basis of evidence. They also emerged as a response to the need of many clinicians for algorithms, which would be able to carry research findings to the everyday clinical practice by organizing information from diverse sources into an easily accessible and reliable format.

To fulfil the above goals and satisfy these needs, in principle, the development of algorithms obeys the rules of EBM and is based primarily on research data from studies conducted in a rigorous way. However, these data cannot always support the decision-making, and often in the real-world clinical practice, the recommendations fail to satisfy the needs of the individual patient. Therefore, a supplementary method is to utilize expert opinion or clinical consensus. In the last few years, the consumer opinion as well as economic issues have an increasing strength and importance and may play a significant role in the shaping of steps. The standard approach in the development of algorithms as this has been shaped in the last 20 years is to utilize EBM standards for the earlier steps; however, as algorithms move from earlier to later steps, the evidence become more and more insufficient, and expert opinion or clinical consensus gradually take over. Socioeconomic forces from patient advocates, the industry and the economic interest of the government and insurance companies exert pressure already since the beginning and the first step and up to the end of the procedure.

Eventually, the use of algorithms and guidelines is supposed to bring benefits for the patients in terms of a more favourable overall outcome as a combination of better efficacy and safety/tolerability. It is also supposed to bring benefits for the health system in general, since the use of algorithms and guidelines facilitates

K.N. Fountoulakis, *Bipolar Disorder: An Evidence-Based Guide to Manic Depression*, DOI 10.1007/978-3-642-37216-2_18

clinical decision-making, reduces clinically inappropriate or cost-inefficient clinical practice decisions, provides similar treatment across different installations and provides a metric to assess patient response and a framework to estimate the cost of treatment (Fountoulakis et al. 2005).

However, on the other hand, there are several potential risks associated with the use of algorithms and guidelines (Rush et al. 1999). The biggest problem is that often the evidence might be insufficient to lead to the development of an algorithm and the consensus panels whose decisions will cover the gap often express biased opinions. The use of algorithms may increase the costs disproportionally in comparison to benefits, and this poses important ethical dilemmas, especially when efficacy collides with safety and cost. It is important to have in mind that rigid algorithms may be difficult to follow or to keep, especially when they demand much time and sophisticated skills to gather the necessary clinical information. They may thus lead to poorer standard of care because of fast and inappropriate application, and what is of prime importance is that rigid algorithms might be subject to inappropriate use by the administration with important legal and ethical implications. Deviation from algorithms may constitute an excuse for legal action by malpractice lawyers.

18.2 List of Existing Guidelines

A list of guidelines has been created after systematic search of the literature (Fountoulakis et al. 2005, 2012; Fountoulakis and Vieta 2008). So far, the search for treatment guidelines for BD resulted in 52 papers concerning published structured treatment algorithms proposed by official panels (Expert consensus guidelines are released for the treatment of bipolar disorder. Consensus Development Conferences 1997; AACAP 1997; Allen et al. 2001; APA 1994, 1995, 2002; Barreira et al. 1999; Dennehy 2000; Gilbert et al. 1998; Goldberg 2000; Goodwin et al. 1997; Goodwin 2003, 2009; Grunze et al. 2002, 2003, 2004, 2009, 2010, 2013; Jobson 1997; Kusumakar et al. 1997; Licht et al. 2003; McClellan and Werry 1997; Montgomery 2001; Rush et al. 1999, 2003; Sachs et al. 2000; Suppes et al. 1995, 2001, 2002, 2003; O'Dowd 2006; Frances et al. 1996; Bauer et al. 1999; Yatham et al. 2005, 2006, 2009, 2013a, b; Ng et al. 2009; Hirschfeld 2005; International Consensus Group on the evidence-based pharmacologic treatment of bipolar I and II depression 2008; International consensus group on depression prevention in bipolar disorder 2011; Australian and New Zealand clinical practice guidelines for the treatment of bipolar disorder 2004; NCCfMH 2006; Jon et al. 2009; Nolen et al. 2008; Beaulieu et al. 2012; Bond et al. 2012; McIntyre et al. 2012; Rosenbluth et al. 2012; Schaffer et al. 2012). An additional source is the National Institute of Clinical Excellence (NICE) whose guidelines concerning BD are available in draft format and will be finalized by the end of 2014 (NICE 2014). A number of other national and international guidelines and algorithms exist in the internet. The most important sources and bodies concerning the development of guidelines for the treatment of BD are shown in Table 18.1. In the text that follows, only the most recent

Table 18.1 Major sources of guidelines (in alphabetical order)

Body	Country	Comments
American Psychiatric Association (APA)	USA	Stopped in 2008
British Association for Psychopharmacology	UK	
Canadian Network for Mood and Anxiety group (CANMAT)	Canada	
Collegium International NeuroPsychopharmacologicum (CINP)	International	To be published in 2015
European College of NeuroPsychopharmacology (ECNP)	Europe	Last in 2000
National Institute of Clinical Excellence (NICE)	UK	To be published in 2014
Texas Medication Algorithm Project.	USA	Stopped in 2002
World Federation of Societies of Biological Psychiatry (WFSBP)	International	

guidelines will be analyzed in depth concerning their specific recommendations, and this because the author wishes to avoid confusing the reader with obsolete information.

18.3 Critical Review of the Most Important Guidelines

18.3.1 American Psychiatric Association Treatment Guidelines for BD

Historically, the first detailed operational treatment guidelines concerning BD were those of the American Psychiatric Association in 1994 (APA 1994, 1995). Their development was under the auspices of the Steering Committee on Practice Guidelines and was based on expert opinion and reviewers which evaluated all available evidence. A second and last version was published in 2002 (APA 2002), while a third version in 2010 never made it to publication because of unresolved issues concerning conflict of interest.

A characteristic of the 1994 version was that it identified five types of medications: Mood stabilizers (lithium, valproate and carbamazepine), antimanic agents, antidepressant agents, adjunctive medication and new or atypical medications. It was also giving priority to lithium and considered it as first choice for all phases of BD. Interestingly, lithium was considered to be superior to neuroleptics even during the acute manic phase. Valproate and carbamazepine were considered to be a second choice of treatment, while benzodiazepines and neuroleptics were considered effective in the rapid control of agitation during the acute mania phase, but lithium was considered more effective specifically concerning the normalization of mood. At that time, it is important to note that most data which were utilized concerned chlorpromazine. Antidepressants were considered to be efficacious in the treatment of bipolar depression but were also considered to worsen the overall course of

BD. ECT was reserved as the last resort, and the possibility to induce mania was stressed. Psychosocial interventions were recommended but without specific targets for them.

These guidelines were revised in 2002 (APA 2002). This new version was much advanced, and the work group classified the guidelines into three categories reflecting the support from clinical data: (I) recommended with substantial clinical confidence, (II) recommended with moderate clinical confidence, and (III) may be recommended on the basis of individual circumstances.

Overall the APA 2002 guidelines coded the generally accepted treatment of BD without any radical suggestions. They did not suggest any detailed algorithms but rather they attempted to evaluate treatment options by reviewing the existing data. The term 'mood stabilizer' was omitted, because of the absence of a consensus definition on what exactly this term should mean; however, in essence, those agents previously considered as being 'stabilizers' (e.g. lithium, valproex) were treated by the guidelines as such. There was a clear suggestion that psychosocial therapies should be used only in combination with pharmacotherapy. The work group was reserved concerning the usefulness of atypical antipsychotics and considered them an adjunct treatment option. Olanzapine was clearly stated as a valid alternative at dosages over 15 mg/day, but it was also stressed that except from the acute manic phase, data were inconclusive, although olanzapine monotherapy or in combination with fluoxetine might be effective in the treatment of bipolar depression. The work group also clearly stated that higher doses of lithium so as to keep serum levels at 0.8–1.0 meq/l may be more effective during the maintenance phase.

In 2008 the APA developed a draft of new guidelines after a thorough review of the literature; however, eventually they were never published because of unresolved issues pertaining to the conflict of interest. Since then, the development of guidelines by the APA has stopped.

18.3.2 The Canadian Network for Mood and Anxiety Treatments and International Society on Bipolar Disorder Guidelines (CANMAT/ISBD)

The Canadian Network for Mood and Anxiety Treatments (CANMAT) (Yatham et al. 2013a) published guidelines for the first time in 1997 (Kusumakar et al. 1997) and revised editions followed in 2005, 2007 and 2009 (Yatham et al. 2005, 2006, 2009). In 2013 the most recent version appeared as a collaboration of the CANMAT with the International Society on Bipolar Disorders (ISBD) (Yatham et al. 2013b).

The CANMAT/ISBD guidelines were based on an extensive review of the literature and data from clinical trials. Also the support for use from the experience coming from the clinical practice and the safety and tolerability of the intervention were considered in formulating the clinical recommendations. Eventually every intervention was categorized into a first, second, or third line, or as 'not recommended'.

The CANMAT/ISBD guidelines concern a range of populations (e.g. children, women and the elderly) and also provide specific recommendations on how to manage BD-II. They tried to incorporate an international perspective and to reflect international variations in practice. A number of additional guidelines were issued by CANMAT to treat special cases of mood disorder patients with psychiatric and somatic comorbidity (McIntyre et al. 2012; Rosenbluth et al. 2012; Beaulieu et al. 2012; Bond et al. 2012; Schaffer et al. 2012).

The most recent 2013 version of the CANMAT/ISBD guidelines (Yatham et al. 2013b) suggest that for the treatment of acute manic episodes, the first-line recommendation is monotherapy with lithium, divalproex, divalproex ER, olanzapine, risperidone, quetiapine, quetiapine XR, aripiprazole, ziprasidone, asenapine or paliperidone ER and adjunctive therapy with risperidone, quetiapine, olanzapine, aripiprazole, asenapine on lithium or divalproex. The second line includes monotherapy with carbamazepine, carbamazepine ER, ECT or haloperidol and combination therapy with lithium plus divalproex. The third line of treatment includes monotherapy with chlorpromazine, clozapine, oxcarbazepine, tamoxifen or cariprazine and combination therapy with lithium or divalproex plus haloperidol, lithium plus carbamazepine or adjunctive tamoxifen. They do not recommend monotherapy with gabapentin, topiramate, lamotrigine, verapamil, tiagabine and combination therapy with risperidone or olanzapine plus carbamazepine.

For the treatment of acute BD-I depression as first-line option, they recommend monotherapy with lithium, lamotrigine, quetiapine or quetiapine XR and combination therapy with lithium or divalproex or olanzapine plus an SSRI, lithium plus divalproex and lithium or divalproex plus bupropion. The second line includes monotherapy with divalproex or lurasidone and combination therapy with quetiapine plus an SSRI, adjunctive modafinil and lithium or divalproex plus lamotrigine or lurasidone. The third line includes monotherapy with carbamazepine, olanzapine or ECT or combination therapy with lithium plus carbamazepine or pramipexole, lithium or divalproex plus venlafaxine, lithium plus MAOI, lithium or divalproex or atypical antipsychotic plus a tricyclic antidepressant, lithium or divalproex or carbamazepine plus an SSRI plus lamotrigine and quetiapine plus lamotrigine. They do not recommend monotherapy with gabapentin, aripiprazole or ziprasidone and combination therapy with adjunctive ziprasidone or levetiracetam.

For the maintenance treatment, the first-line recommendation includes monotherapy with lithium, lamotrigine, divalproex, olanzapine, quetiapine, risperidone LAI and aripiprazole and adjunctive therapy with quetiapine, risperidone LAI, aripiprazole or ziprasidone on lithium or divalproex. The second-line monotherapy includes carbamazepine and paliperidone ER and combination therapy with lithium plus divalproex or carbamazepine, lithium or divalproex plus olanzapine, risperidone or lamotrigine and olanzapine plus fluoxetine. The third-line monotherapy includes asenapine, and the adjunctive therapy includes phenytoin, clozapine, ECT, topiramate, omega-3-fatty acids, oxcarbazepine, gabapentin and asenapine. They do not recommend monotherapy with gabapentin, topiramate or antidepressants and adjunctive therapy with flupenthixol.

Overall the CANMAT/ISBD guidelines reflect a clinically oriented mentality in their development. They are close to the practice of the average clinician; they organize it and protect the clinician from known caveats. However, they are not always in accord with the hard data available, especially concerning bipolar depression.

18.3.3 The Texas Medication Algorithm Project (TMAP) for the Treatment of BD

These guidelines were started developing in 1995, and the first publication came in 1999 (Rush et al. 1999; Gilbert et al. 1998), and their most recent and last version was published in 2002 (Suppes et al. 2002). There were efforts to empirically validate and assess the earlier versions of the algorithm (Suppes et al. 2003), and the areas of outcome which were expected to improve were defined (better quality of life, increased productive activity, less reliance on treatment system, fewer negative social outcomes like arrest, prison time, etc., decreased cost) (Rush et al. 2003).

At that time, there was little evidence to support the development of algorithms for BD-II and rapid cycling disorder, so the algorithm was focused only on BD-I and the panel suggested the use of the guidelines in BD-II also.

The TMAP was revolutionary for a number of reasons. These guidelines were developed by a panel of academic clinicians and researchers, practicing clinicians in the TDMHMR system, administrators, advocates and consumers. It was the first to involve as many stakeholders as possible in BD. Another breakthrough issue was the core proposal that all bipolar patients should receive continuous treatment with an antimanic agent and thus follow the algorithm concerning the treatment of mania/hypomania with an intermittent use of the depression algorithm. This constituted a shift in the way we understand and practice the treatment of BD, and it is the basis of our current concept and practice. Finally it was the first algorithm to put an atypical antipsychotic (olanzapine) as first-choice treatment and equal to lithium and divalproex. Two important recommendations were made concerning the maintenance phase. The first was that maintenance treatment is considered to be necessary only for patients with two manic episodes or with one which was severe or for those patients with a positive family history of affective disorder. For the rest of patients (first manic episode without family history), it is recommended to gradually discontinue treatment usually after the completion of 6 months in full remission. In terms of nomenclature, an important element was that they consider mania and antimanic medication as the core of BD and its treatment, putting depression at a somewhat lower level. Antidepressant medication was considered as an adjunctive therapy to the antimanic. Lithium, anticonvulsants and atypical antipsychotics were grouped under the label 'antimanic agents' in the mania/hypomania algorithm. However, at the stage 1 of the depression algorithm, their label changes to 'mood stabilizers' without any explanation for this change. In an earlier paper from this panel, the term 'mood stabilizer' includes lithium, carbamazepine and divalproex, but not atypical antipsychotics (Suppes et al. 2001). However, the most recent paper put lithium and divalproex at a similar position with atypical antipsychotics.

The validation of the early versions of these guidelines was attempted by their use in 69 acutely ill BD patients with satisfactory results (Suppes et al. 2001), but further testing of the algorithms (but not of the final version) (Suppes et al. 2002) was unimpressive (Suppes et al. 2003).

Overall the TMAP was a breakthrough effort and was the first to adopt a number of innovations which today are considered the standard in our conceptualizing of the treatment of BD. It was short-lived, however, and it stopped producing algorithms after 2002.

18.3.4 The World Federation of Societies of Biological Psychiatry (WFSBP) Guidelines for the Biological Treatment of BD

This work group published guidelines for bipolar depression in 2002 (Grunze et al. 2002), mania in 2003 (Grunze et al. 2003) and maintenance treatment in 2004 (Grunze et al. 2004). A second 'wave' of guidelines was published during 2009–2013 (Grunze et al. 2009, 2010, 2013).

The latest WFSBP guidelines utilized a modified version of the PORT method to grade the data concerning efficacy and afterwards utilized a secondary classification to include also safety and tolerability.

For the treatment of acute mania, as first-choice agents are ranked aripiprazole, valproate, risperidone and ziprasidone. As second choice, olanzapine, quetiapine, asenapine, carbamazepine, haloperidol and lithium were recommended. The third choice includes chlorpromazine, paliperidone, phenytoin, pimozide and tamoxifen. The fourth includes amisulpride, clonazepam, clozapine, levetiracetam, lorazepam, nimodipine, oxcarbazepine, retigabine, zonisamide, zotepine and ECT. The fifth and final choice includes verapamil.

With the utilization of this classification, the WFSBP suggests that concerning the treatment of acute mania, the first step includes monotherapy with first-choice agents. The second step would be the switching to another first-choice agent or combine two first-choice agents. Similarly the third step includes combination of two first-choice agents. The fourth and fifth steps include combinations of agents essentially according to the judgement of the therapist.

For the treatment of acute bipolar depression, the WFSBP guidelines suggest that first-choice agent is only quetiapine, while their next best option includes olanzapine, fluoxetine, lamotrigine, valproate, OFC, lithium plus lamotrigine, adjunctive modafinil, N-acetylcysteine on lithium or valproate and FEWP plus carbamazepine. A variety of combinations are proposed as next steps.

For the treatment during the maintenance phase, the guidance is more complex, and on the basis of the available data, the WFSBP guidelines suggest the use of aripiprazole, lamotrigine, lithium, quetiapine, olanzapine and risperidone, but they note that not all of them prevent both mania and depression. They also note the problems because of the metabolic syndrome induced by some of these agents when used for prolonged periods of time. They also suggest the avoiding of typical antipsychotics because of the risk to induce tardive dyskinesia.

Overall the WFSBP guidelines are based on the existing research evidence and try to avoid suggestions which are not evidence based, but at the same time, they try to provide the clinician with solutions. They constitute a step forward towards the evidence-based pharmacotherapy and evidence-based psychiatry.

18.3.5 British Association for Psychopharmacology (BAP)

The BAP issued guidelines for the treatment of BD for the first time in 2003 (Goodwin 2003) and revised them in 2009 (Goodwin 2009). Both versions were based on a consensus panel after extensive review of the literature

The 2009 guidelines cover the assessment and treatment of BD in a global way and strongly suggest a multidisciplinary approach in the frame of enhanced care.

For acute mania, they recommend antipsychotics or valproate for the more severe cases and antipsychotics, lithium, valproate or carbamazepine for the milder ones. In case of refractoriness, they recommend combination treatment or ECT.

For acute bipolar depression, they recommend ECT for the more severe cases and quetiapine or lithium for the milder ones, plus an SSRI if needed.

It is interesting that for the maintenance phase, it is the first guidelines, the only one so far, that suggest the choice of treatment on the basis of predominant polarity. Thus, they recommend maintenance treatment with lithium, aripiprazole, quetiapine, valproate or olanzapine if the predominant polarity is manic and lamotrigine or quetiapine if the predominant polarity is depressive.

18.3.6 The UK National Institute of Clinical Excellence (NICE) Treatment Guidelines for BD

The NICE issued the first version of guidelines for the treatment of BD in 2006, and the revised version is expected to be published officially in September 2014; however, a draft version was available online at the time of the writing of the current chapter and it is discussed here (NICE 2014).

Concerning acute mania, the draft of the 2014 NICE guidelines recommends the use of olanzapine, risperidone, quetiapine or haloperidol. If the patient does not respond, it is recommended to change to another antipsychotic, and the choice should be made also on the basis of previous response if it exists. If the patient is already under treatment with lithium or valproate, then the recommendation is to increase dosage to the highest permitted and reassessment should follow before the changing of medication. If an antidepressant is in place, it should be discontinued. The second step includes combination of lithium or valproate plus an antipsychotic, and the third step demands hospitalization. The NICE warns against the use of gabapentin, lamotrigine and topiramate in acute mania.

Concerning acute bipolar depression, the NICE recommends olanzapine, OFC, quetiapine, lamotrigine, lithium and valproate. If the patient is already under treatment with lithium or valproate, then the recommendation is to increase the dosage to the highest permitted, and reassessment should follow before the changing of medication. The next step includes combination of lithium or valproate plus quetiapine or OFC. The third step includes lithium plus lamotrigine or olanzapine and valproate plus lamotrigine. The NICE warns against the use of gabapentin and topiramate.

During the maintenance phase, the NICE guidelines recommend as first-line treatment the continuation of the treatment the patient received during the acute phase and led to the resolution of the symptoms. Irrespective of polarity, the continuation of this treatment should be done for at least 3–6 months. In case the patient does not wish to follow this, it is recommended to change treatment to lithium, olanzapine, quetiapine, valproate or lithium plus valproate. Again the NICE warns against the use of gabapentin and topiramate.

18.4 Critical View of Treatment Guidelines for BD

As discussed in previous chapters, BD has a complex clinical picture and an even more complex treatment. Only recently hard data became available concerning the efficacy and safety of various treatment options and many beliefs have been discredited. Still we know little concerning the treatment of many aspects of the disorder.

It is almost impossible for the research findings to make it to the everyday clinical practice rapidly and in a proper way by themselves. Clinicians do not have the time to dig into primary research papers and might not have the background to read them critically. Treatment guidelines serve the purpose of gathering and evaluating the research data and synthesize them into a comprehensive and operational treatment algorithm. If this is not possible, because the data are often not sufficient, the classification of treatment options according to efficacy and safety/tolerability is also an important task for guidelines.

In the past, the difference in the treatment views between the academic authorities in Europe and the USA was prominent. The European view was in favour of the use of antipsychotics and antidepressants, while the US approach was in favour of 'mood stabilizers'. This difference no longer exists at least concerning antipsychotics. However, the reality is that in spite of previous algorithms, the use of antipsychotics to treat acute mania was widespread both in Europe (Licht et al. 1994) and in the USA (Chou et al. 1996) often as monotherapy. This practice was based on evidence that antimanic properties of antipsychotics are different from their sedative ones and might relate to dopamine receptor blockade (Cookson 2001).

The various treatment guidelines generally seem to have a common starting point, best described by the 1994 APA guidelines (APA 1994), which interestingly seem to reflect the opinion of many clinicians still today. Some guidelines try to keep up with the evidence; others rely more on expert opinion. The greatest problem guidelines face is from the second-line recommendation and beyond. At this level, after monotherapy with first-line agents fails, data are sparse. Guidelines insist in suggesting monotherapy as the first option, although data suggest that such an approach is effective in less than half of patients and is likely to leave residual symptoms. It is rather true that guidelines sacrifice much effectiveness in favour of safety and fewer adverse effects. However, the reality is that suboptimally treated BD is a potentially disabling and lethal disease.

The three most recent guidelines (NICE, CANMAT/ISBD and WFSBP) agree in that first-choice treatment for acute mania should be olanzapine, quetiapine, risperidone, lithium and valproate. The guidelines of CANMAT/ISBD and of WFSBP agree that the second-line treatment includes haloperidol and lithium plus valproate. The combination of lithium or valproate plus an antipsychotic is proposed as second-line treatment by NICE and WFSBP, while the CANMAT/ISBD consider it as first-line option. There is no agreement concerning the third-line option. ECT is considered as second line by the CANMAT/ISBD and as third-line option by the WFSBP. It should be noted that the NICE excludes from recommendations aripiprazole and asenapine due to high cost without a corresponding higher efficacy. It also excludes paliperidone because it considers it to be an active metabolite of risperidone which should not be considered separately. It did not consider cariprazine because the pharmaceutical company which markets it refused to provide the NICE with the data required, while ziprasidone is not marketed in the UK.

Concerning acute bipolar depression, these guidelines agree that the first-line option is lamotrigine, lithium, quetiapine, olanzapine (the CANMAT/ISBD suggest in combination with an SSRI) and valproate (again the CANMAT/ISBD suggest in combination with an SSRI). The combination of olanzapine with fluoxetine (OFC) is suggested by the NICE specifically, while the CANMAT/ISBD suggests the combination of olanzapine with any SSRI except paroxetine. According to the WFSBP, the OFC is the second-line recommendation. The second- and third-line options have little in common. The combination of lithium plus lamotrigine is the second-line option for WFSBP and CANMAT/ISBD and third line according to NICE. The combination of venlafaxine plus lithium or valproate is the third-line option according to CANMAT/ISBD and second line according to WFSBP. The NICE guidelines suggest the use of lithium and valproate monotherapy as first-line option and their combination with another agent as second- and third-line option. They also do not recommend gabapentin or topiramate at any phase of the disorder.

The CANMAT/ISBD guidelines suggest a greater variety of treatment options and include ECT also as first- or second-line treatment depending on the severity of the clinical picture and the clinical judgement of the therapist. The WFSBP guidelines are reserved towards the efficacy of lithium at least as monotherapy, and they seem to be more open to novel suggestions (e.g. FEWP). Eventually they strongly recommend quetiapine, the OFC, the combination of an antimanic agent plus an SSRI, lamotrigine as monotherapy but also in combination with lithium and adjunctive treatment with modafinil.

For the maintenance phase, the three guidelines agree concerning the use of lithium, olanzapine and quetiapine as first-line treatment options in the maintenance treatment for the prevention of any mood episode. Valproate is also recommended as the first-line treatment option but second line according to the WFSBP due to equivocal research data. Lamotrigine is recommended by the WFSBP and the CANMAT/ISBD mainly for the prevention of depressive episodes, while the NICE prefers to recommend lithium but not lamotrigine. The CANMAT/ISBD guidelines recommend the use of atypical antipsychotics as prophylactic therapy but only concerning the prevention of manic episodes, with the exception of quetiapine which is recommended also for the prevention of depressive episodes. The WFSBP and the CANMAT/ISBD agree almost perfectly concerning the third-line treatment options.

It is evident that there are many issues that need further study, data are rare and insufficient and many questions remain unanswered. Overall it seems that disagreements are more than agreements even though all treatment guidelines claim to be 'evidence based'. Probably this is because of the different way to approach and utilize the data. A point of relative consensus is that antidepressants do not have a major role in the treatment of bipolar depression at least as monotherapy with the exception of fluoxetine, especially in combination with olanzapine.

Furthermore, the NICE takes under serious consideration the financial cost, and because of this, it significantly narrows its suggestions. The WFSBP takes special consideration of adverse events, while the CANMAT/ISBD provide with a greater variety of options while leaving the consideration of the adverse events to the therapist.

There is a nonspecific consensus among guidelines that the second line of treatment should include various combinations of first-line agents although often this is not supported by the data.

Guidelines also agree that there is lack of hard data concerning the treatment of mixed episodes and rapid cycling. On the contrary, they agree that although there is also a lack of hard data, hypomania should be treated the same way as mania. All agents are somewhat considered to be more effective towards one pole of the illness in comparison to the other. More specifically, lithium, valproate, carbamazepine and antipsychotics are all more effective for the treatment and prevention of mania and to a lesser degree for depression, while on the contrary, lamotrigine is more effective for the treatment and prevention of depression and to a lesser degree for mania.

It is important to note that in spite of the publication of various treatment guidelines, clinicians do not seem to widely adopt any of them. Their impact on clinical practice is quite limited even in the USA. After the publication of the first APA 1994 guidelines, only about 16 % of manic patients without psychotic features, 38 % with mania with psychotic features, 31 % of bipolar depressed with psychotic features and 17 % of bipolar depressed without psychotic features were reported to be treated according to treatment guidelines (Lim et al. 2001).

Several studies registered the prescribing patterns in Europe and the USA and their results are most interesting. They reported at the dawn of the twenty-first century, up to 23 % of diagnosed bipolar patients did not receive any medication at all, half were under antidepressants, half under a 'mood stabilizer' (lithium or anticonvulsant) and one-third was receiving antipsychotics. According to the same authors, only 20 % of patients were on monotherapy, and half of them were receiving at least three agents, while 18 % did not receive any 'mood stabilizer' (lithium or anticonvulsant) at all. Discontinuation rates for lithium were between 50 and 60 % (Levine et al. 2000; Frangou et al. 2002).

The pressure to develop guidelines for the treatment of severe and disabling mental disorders becomes stronger and stronger because of the need to provide better treatment in combination with a lower cost. However, sufficient empirical data are not always sufficient and the evaluation of guidelines in the real-world environment does not always support their use, as many times they lead to an increased cost without an impressive improvement in the treatment outcome. To complicate things more, the installations where the algorithms were tested are not representative of the average treatment setting.

It is almost certain that the generalization of the use of evidence-based guidelines for the treatment of bipolar disorders will improve treatment outcome and at the same time lower the cost of bipolar illness even though they may increase the short-term cost for medication and rehabilitation programs. But the least these algorithms may achieve is to ensure a minimum quality of treatment and care and the minimum necessary discipline from the side of the therapist.

However, the psychiatric community should guard the right of the therapist to make independent decisions concerning treatment, on the basis of the individual patient and available scientific data; that means algorithms cannot replace education and training and may not be considered a 'golden standard of treatment' the deviation from which should be justified. Such an extreme situation may lead to unnecessary legal complications.

On the technical field, there are several issues that need to be clarified. These include the term 'mood stabilizer', the usefulness of newer antipsychotics, the treatment of the acute phase of bipolar depression, the true value of combination therapy, whether antimanic properties of medication are distinct from sedation effects, the treatment of mixed features and rapid cycling, the role of psychosocial interventions and the assessment and treatment of the neurocognitive deficit, the functional impairment and disability which often burden the patients and their families during symptom-free intervals.

References

AACAP (1997) AACAP official action. Practice parameters for the assessment and treatment of children and adolescents with bipolar disorder. J Am Acad Child Adolesc Psychiatry 36(1):138–157

Allen MH, Currier GW, Hughes DH, Reyes-Harde M, Docherty JP (2001) The expert consensus guideline series. Treatment of behavioral emergencies. Postgrad Med (Spec no):1–88; quiz 89–90

APA (1994) Practice guideline for the treatment of patients with bipolar disorder. Am J Psychiatry 151(12 Suppl):1–36

APA (1995) American Psychiatric Association releases treatment guideline for bipolar disease. Am Fam Physician 51(6):1605–1606

APA (2002) Practice guideline for the treatment of patients with bipolar disorder (revision). Am J Psychiatry 159(4 Suppl):1–50

Australian and New Zealand clinical practice guidelines for the treatment of bipolar disorder (2004) Aust N Z J Psychiatry 38(5):280–305. doi:10.1111/j.1440-1614.2004.01356.x, ANP1356 [pii]

Barreira P, Duckworth K, Goff D, Flannery RB Jr (1999) Clinical practice guidelines: the Massachusetts experience in psychiatry. Harv Rev Psychiatry 7(4):230–232

Bauer MS, Callahan AM, Jampala C, Petty F, Sajatovic M, Schaefer V, Wittlin B, Powell BJ (1999) Clinical practice guidelines for bipolar disorder from the department of veterans affairs. J Clin Psychiatry 60(1):9–21

Beaulieu S, Saury S, Sareen J, Tremblay J, Schutz CG, McIntyre RS, Schaffer A, Canadian Network for M, Anxiety Treatments Task F (2012) The Canadian Network for Mood and Anxiety Treatments (CANMAT) task force recommendations for the management of patients with mood disorders and comorbid substance use disorders. Ann Clin Psychiatry 24(1):38–55

Bond DJ, Hadjipavlou G, Lam RW, McIntyre RS, Beaulieu S, Schaffer A, Weiss M, Canadian Network for M, Anxiety Treatments Task F (2012) The Canadian Network for Mood and Anxiety Treatments (CANMAT) task force recommendations for the management of patients with mood disorders and comorbid attention-deficit/hyperactivity disorder. Ann Clin Psychiatry 24(1):23–37

Chou J, Zito J, Vitrai J, Craig T, Allingham B, Czobor P (1996) Neuroleptics in acute mania: a pharmacoepidemiologic study. Ann Pharmacother 30:1396–1398

Cookson J (2001) Use of antipsychotic drugs and lithium in mania. Br J Psychiatry Suppl 41:s148–s156

Dennehy EB (2000) Guidelines for treatment of bipolar disorder. Curr Psychiatry Rep 2(4):316–321

Expert consensus guidelines are released for the treatment of bipolar disorder. Consensus Development Conferences (1997) Am Fam Physician 55(4):1447–1449

Fountoulakis KN, Kasper S, Andreassen O, Blier P, Okasha A, Severus E, Versiani M, Tandon R, Moller HJ, Vieta E (2012) Efficacy of pharmacotherapy in bipolar disorder: a report by the WPA section on pharmacopsychiatry. Eur Arch Psychiatry Clin Neurosci 262(Suppl 1):1–48. doi:10.1007/s00406-012-0323-x

Fountoulakis KN, Vieta E (2008) Treatment of bipolar disorder: a systematic review of available data and clinical perspectives. Int J Neuropsychopharm 11(7):999–1029. doi:10.1017/S1461145708009231

Fountoulakis KN, Vieta E, Sanchez-Moreno J, Kaprinis SG, Goikolea JM, Kaprinis GS (2005) Treatment guidelines for bipolar disorder: a critical review. J Affect Disord 86(1):1–10. doi:10.1016/j.jad.2005.01.004

Frances A, Docherty J, Kahn D (1996) The expert consensus guideline series: treatment of bipolar disorder. J Clin Psychiatry 57(Suppl 12A):1–88

Frangou S, Raymont V, Bettany D (2002) The Maudsley bipolar disorder project. A survey of psychotropic prescribing patterns in bipolar I disorder. Bipolar Disord 4(6):378–385

Gilbert DA, Altshuler KZ, Rago WV, Shon SP, Crismon ML, Toprac MG, Rush AJ (1998) Texas medication algorithm project: definitions, rationale, and methods to develop medication algorithms. J Clin Psychiatry 59(7):345–351

Goldberg JF (2000) Treatment guidelines: current and future management of bipolar disorder. J Clin Psychiatry 61(Supp 13):12–18

Goodwin G, Bourgeois M, Conti L (1997) Treatment of bipolar depressive mood disorders: algorithms for pharmacotherapy. Int J Psychiatry Clin Pract 1:S9–S12

Goodwin GM (2003) Evidence-based guidelines for treating bipolar disorder: recommendations from the British Association for Psychopharmacology. J Psychopharmacol 17(2):149–173; discussion 147

Goodwin GM (2009) Evidence-based guidelines for treating bipolar disorder: revised second edition – recommendations from the British Association for Psychopharmacology. J Psychopharmacol 23(4):346–388. doi:10.1177/0269881109102919, 0269881109102919 [pii]

Grunze H, Kasper S, Goodwin G, Bowden C, Baldwin D, Licht R, Vieta E, Moller HJ (2002) World Federation of Societies of Biological Psychiatry (WFSBP) guidelines for biological treatment of bipolar disorders. Part I: treatment of bipolar depression. World J Biol Psychiatry 3(3):115–124

Grunze H, Kasper S, Goodwin G, Bowden C, Baldwin D, Licht RW, Vieta E, Moller HJ (2003) The World Federation of Societies of Biological Psychiatry (WFSBP) guidelines for the biological treatment of bipolar disorders, part II: treatment of mania. World J Biol Psychiatry 4(1):5–13

Grunze H, Kasper S, Goodwin G, Bowden C, Moller H (2004) WFSBP task force on treatment guidelines for bipolar disorders: the World Federation of Societies of Biological Psychiatry (WFSBP) guidelines for the biological treatment of bipolar disorders, part III: maintenance treatment. World J Biol Psychiatry 5(3):120–135

Grunze H, Vieta E, Goodwin GM, Bowden C, Licht RW, Moller HJ, Kasper S (2009) The World Federation of Societies of Biological Psychiatry (WFSBP) guidelines for the biological treatment of bipolar disorders: update 2009 on the treatment of acute mania. World J Biol Psychiatry 10(2):85–116. doi:10.1080/15622970902823202, 910249156 [pii]

Grunze H, Vieta E, Goodwin GM, Bowden C, Licht RW, Moller HJ, Kasper S, Disorders WTFOTGFB (2010) The World Federation of Societies of Biological Psychiatry (WFSBP) guidelines for the biological treatment of bipolar disorders: update 2010 on the treatment of acute bipolar depression. World J Biol Psychiatry 11(2):81–109. doi:10.3109/15622970903555881

Grunze H, Vieta E, Goodwin GM, Bowden C, Licht RW, Moller HJ, Kasper S, Disorders WTFoTGfB (2013) The World Federation of Societies of Biological Psychiatry (WFSBP) guidelines for the biological treatment of bipolar disorders: update 2012 on the long-term treatment of bipolar disorder. World J Biol Psychiatry 14(3):154–219. doi:10.3109/15622975.2013.770551

Hirschfeld R (2005) Guideline watch for the practice guideline for the treatment of patients with bipolar disorder. http://www.psych.org/psych_pract/treatg/pg/prac_guide.cfm

International consensus group on depression prevention in bipolar disorder (2011) J Clin Psychiatry 72(10):1295–1310. doi:10.4088/JCP.10123co1c

International Consensus Group on the evidence-based pharmacologic treatment of bipolar I and II depression (2008) J Clin Psychiatry 69(10):1632–1646, eaz7127 [pii]

Jobson K (1997) International psychopharmacology algorithm project: algorithms in psychopharmacology. Int J Psychiatry Clin Pract 1:S3–S8

Jon DI, Bahk WM, Yoon BH, Shin YC, Cho HS, Lee E, Ha K, Kim W, Chung SK, Seo JS, Min KJ (2009) Revised Korean medication algorithm for bipolar disorder. World J Biol Psychiatry 10(4 Pt 3):846–855. doi:10.1080/15622970802144865, 794876687 [pii]

Kusumakar V, Yatham L, Parikh S (1997) Bipolar disorder: a summary of clinical issues and treatment options. CANMAT Monograph, Halifax/Nova Scotia

Levine J, Chengappa KN, Brar JS, Gershon S, Yablonsky E, Stapf D, Kupfer DJ (2000) Psychotropic drug prescription patterns among patients with bipolar I disorder. Bipolar Disord 2(2):120–130

Licht R, Gouliaev G, Vestergaard P, Dybbro J, Lund H, Merinder L (1994) Treatment of manic episodes in Scandinavia: the use of neuroleptic drugs in a clinical routine setting. J Affect Disord 32:179–185

Licht RW, Vestergaard P, Kessing LV, Larsen JK, Thomsen PH (2003) Psychopharmacological treatment with lithium and antiepileptic drugs: suggested guidelines from the Danish Psychiatric Association and the Child and Adolescent Psychiatric Association in Denmark. Acta Psychiatr Scand 108(Suppl 419):1–22

Lim PZ, Tunis SL, Edell WS, Jensik SE, Tohen M (2001) Medication prescribing patterns for patients with bipolar I disorder in hospital settings: adherence to published practice guidelines. Bipolar Disord 3(4):165–173

McClellan J, Werry J (1997) Practice parameters for the assessment and treatment of children and adolescents with bipolar disorder. American Academy of Child and Adolescent Psychiatry. J Am Acad Child Adolesc Psychiatry 36(10 Suppl):157S–176S

McIntyre RS, Alsuwaidan M, Goldstein BI, Taylor VH, Schaffer A, Beaulieu S, Kemp DE, Canadian Network for M, Anxiety Treatments Task F (2012) The Canadian Network for Mood and Anxiety Treatments (CANMAT) task force recommendations for the management of patients with mood disorders and comorbid metabolic disorders. Ann Clin Psychiatry 24(1):69–81

Montgomery DB (2001) ECNP Consensus Meeting March 2000 Nice: guidelines for investigating efficacy in bipolar disorder. European College of Neuropsychopharmacology. Eur Neuropsychopharmacol 11(1):79–88

NCCfMH (2006) Bipolar disorder. The management of bipolar disorder in adults, children and adolescents, in primary and secondary care. CG38 NICE guideline. http://www.kenniscentrumbipolairestoornissen.nl/wp-content/uploads/NHS-guideline-bipolar-disorder.pdf

Ng F, Mammen OK, Wilting I, Sachs GS, Ferrier IN, Cassidy F, Beaulieu S, Yatham LN, Berk M (2009) The International Society for Bipolar Disorders (ISBD) consensus guidelines for the safety monitoring of bipolar disorder treatments. Bipolar Disord 11(6):559–595. doi:10.1111/j.1399-5618.2009.00737.x, BDI737 [pii]

NICE (2014) Bipolar disorder. https://www.nice.org.uk/Guidance/Conditions-and-diseases/Mental-health-and-behavioural-conditions/Bipolar-disorder

Nolen W, Kupka R, Schulte P, Knoppert-van der Klein E, Honig A, Reichart C (2008) Richtlijn bipolaire stoornissen, 2nd edn. De Tijdstrom Uitgerverij BV, Utrecht

O'Dowd A (2006) NICE issues new guidance to improve the treatment of bipolar disorder. BMJ 333(7561):220

Rosenbluth M, Macqueen G, McIntyre RS, Beaulieu S, Schaffer A, Canadian Network for M, Anxiety Treatments Task F (2012) The Canadian Network for Mood and Anxiety Treatments (CANMAT) task force recommendations for the management of patients with mood disorders and comorbid personality disorders. Ann Clin Psychiatry 24(1):56–68

Rush AJ, Crismon ML, Kashner TM, Toprac MG, Carmody TJ, Trivedi MH, Suppes T, Miller AL, Biggs MM, Shores-Wilson K, Witte BP, Shon SP, Rago WV, Altshuler KZ (2003) Texas Medication Algorithm Project, phase 3 (TMAP-3): rationale and study design. J Clin Psychiatry 64(4):357–369

Rush AJ, Rago WV, Crismon ML, Toprac MG, Shon SP, Suppes T, Miller AL, Trivedi MH, Swann AC, Biggs MM, Shores-Wilson K, Kashner TM, Pigott T, Chiles JA, Gilbert DA, Altshuler KZ (1999) Medication treatment for the severely and persistently mentally ill: the Texas Medication Algorithm Project. J Clin Psychiatry 60(5):284–291

Sachs GS, Printz DJ, Kahn DA, Carpenter D, Docherty JP (2000) The expert consensus guideline series: medication treatment of bipolar disorder 2000. Postgrad Med Spec No:1–104

Schaffer A, McIntosh D, Goldstein BI, Rector NA, McIntyre RS, Beaulieu S, Swinson R, Yatham LN, Canadian Network for M, Anxiety Treatments Task F (2012) The CANMAT task force recommendations for the management of patients with mood disorders and comorbid anxiety disorders. Ann Clin Psychiatry 24(1):6–22

Suppes T, Calabrese J, Mitchell P, Pazzaglia P, Potter W, Zarin D (1995) Algorithms for the treatment of bipolar manic-depressive illness. Psychopharmacol Bull 31(3):469–474

Suppes T, Dennehy EB, Swann AC, Bowden CL, Calabrese JR, Hirschfeld RM, Keck PE Jr, Sachs GS, Crismon ML, Toprac MG, Shon SP (2002) Report of the Texas Consensus Conference Panel on medication treatment of bipolar disorder 2000. J Clin Psychiatry 63(4):288–299

Suppes T, Rush AJ, Dennehy EB, Crismon ML, Kashner TM, Toprac MG, Carmody TJ, Brown ES, Biggs MM, Shores-Wilson K, Witte BP, Trivedi MH, Miller AL, Altshuler KZ, Shon SP (2003) Texas Medication Algorithm Project, phase 3 (TMAP-3): clinical results for patients with a history of mania. J Clin Psychiatry 64(4):370–382

Suppes T, Swann AC, Dennehy EB, Habermacher ED, Mason M, Crismon ML, Toprac MG, Rush AJ, Shon SP, Altshuler KZ (2001) Texas Medication Algorithm Project: development and feasibility testing of a treatment algorithm for patients with bipolar disorder. J Clin Psychiatry 62(6):439–447

Yatham LN, Kennedy SH, O'Donovan C, Parikh S, MacQueen G, McIntyre R, Sharma V, Silverstone P, Alda M, Baruch P, Beaulieu S, Daigneault A, Milev R, Young LT, Ravindran A, Schaffer A, Connolly M, Gorman CP, Canadian Network for M, Anxiety T (2005) Canadian Network for Mood and Anxiety Treatments (CANMAT) guidelines for the management of patients with bipolar disorder: consensus and controversies. Bipolar Disord 7(Suppl 3):5–69. doi:10.1111/j.1399-5618.2005.00219.x

Yatham LN, Kennedy SH, O'Donovan C, Parikh SV, MacQueen G, McIntyre RS, Sharma V, Beaulieu S, Guidelines Group C (2006) Canadian Network for Mood and Anxiety Treatments (CANMAT) guidelines for the management of patients with bipolar disorder: update 2007. Bipolar Disord 8(6):721–739. doi:10.1111/j.1399-5618.2006.00432.x

Yatham LN, Kennedy SH, Parikh SV, Schaffer A, Beaulieu S, Alda M, O'Donovan C, Macqueen G, McIntyre RS, Sharma V, Ravindran A, Young LT, Milev R, Bond DJ, Frey BN, Goldstein BI (2013a) The evolution of CANMAT Bipolar Disorder Guidelines: past, present, and future. Bipolar Disord 15(1):58–60. doi:10.1111/bdi.12038

Yatham LN, Kennedy SH, Parikh SV, Schaffer A, Beaulieu S, Alda M, O'Donovan C, Macqueen G, McIntyre RS, Sharma V, Ravindran A, Young LT, Milev R, Bond DJ, Frey BN, Goldstein BI, Lafer B, Birmaher B, Ha K, Nolen WA, Berk M (2013b) Canadian Network for Mood and Anxiety Treatments (CANMAT) and International Society for Bipolar Disorders (ISBD) collaborative update of CANMAT guidelines for the management of patients with bipolar disorder: update 2013. Bipolar Disord 15(1):1–44. doi:10.1111/bdi.12025

Yatham LN, Kennedy SH, Schaffer A, Parikh SV, Beaulieu S, O'Donovan C, MacQueen G, McIntyre RS, Sharma V, Ravindran A, Young LT, Young AH, Alda M, Milev R, Vieta E, Calabrese JR, Berk M, Ha K, Kapczinski F (2009) Canadian Network for Mood and Anxiety Treatments (CANMAT) and International Society for Bipolar Disorders (ISBD) collaborative update of CANMAT guidelines for the management of patients with bipolar disorder: update 2009. Bipolar Disord 11(3):225–255. doi:10.1111/j.1399-5618.2009.00672.x, BDI672 [pii]

19 Special Issues

19.1 Gender

It is well known that concerning the prevalence of unipolar depression, females have almost double rates in comparison to males (Lloyd and Miller 1997; Blazer et al. 1994). However, this does not hold true concerning BD, for which similar rates between males and females are reported. There are some data suggesting that males might be over-represented in those diagnosed with a BD-I and females over-represented in those diagnosed with a BD-II disorder (Parker et al. 2014).

Some authors suggest that females with less social support and experiencing social stressors might be at the greatest risk to develop depression, but this concerns unipolar and not bipolar cases. It has been documented that women are more likely to experience stressful and even threatening life events and are at a higher risk of early sexual abuse and current spousal abuse (Roesler and McKenzie 1994; Finkelhor et al. 1990). Women also might use oral contraceptive and often experience mood disorders temporally related to their gender identity (e.g. premenstrual- or postpartum-onset mood disorders) which might have an impact on the course of BD (Meinhard et al. 2014). A number of adverse experiences related to sexual life and determined by gender seem to happen in the lives of bipolar women. In comparison to healthy women, bipolar women might be more likely to have been forced by their partners to have sex, raped or suffering from sexually transmitted diseases. The use of contraceptives is usually sporadic and their rates of pregnancy and abortion are high (Ozcan et al. 2014).

Also, in almost all societies, unequal roles for women are in place, and additionally there is a gender difference in copying styles; men might react to emotional distress by trying not to think about it, while women are more likely to ruminate over their problems (Nolen-Hoeksema and Girgus 1994; Nolen-Hoeksema et al. 1999, 2007). In this frame, women are more likely to report depressive symptoms due to marital problems than men (Joiner et al. 1992; Hammen and Peters 1978) and are more likely to be diagnosed with depression because they seek professional help more often for their depressive symptoms and maybe because they are more

K.N. Fountoulakis, *Bipolar Disorder: An Evidence-Based Guide to Manic Depression*, DOI 10.1007/978-3-642-37216-2_19

sensitive to negative relationships (Phillips and Segal 1969). Concerning the neurocognitive function, the data are inconsistent (Bucker et al. 2014; Suwalska and Lojko 2014).

Overall there does not seem to be any significant gender difference concerning the risk of recurrence, thus suggesting that gender is among the risk factors for initiating depressive symptoms in unipolar depression but not among those determining the course and outcome either in unipolar or in bipolar cases (Nazroo et al. 1997; Philibert et al. 1997).

There are a number of comorbid conditions which seem to be more frequent in bipolar women, including abdominal obesity. This happens possibly because of a higher frequency of predominant depressive polarity in women and more seasonal variations in mood disturbance and reproductive life events and related treatments (Baskaran et al. 2014). Another condition concerns subclinical hypothyroidism which seems to be more frequent in bipolar females and increases with age. It occurs in up to 20 % of postmenopausal women, and if present, it might induce some kind of treatment refractoriness and it complicates treatment especially with lithium (Bauer et al. 2014; Ozerdem et al. 2014). Migraine is also a common comorbidity of BD-II and is more prevalent in women than men (Saunders et al. 2014).

19.2 Suicidality

Suicide is a complex and multi-causal behaviour and thus it demands a complex and sophisticated approach (Rihmer et al. 2010). One of the first issues that should be clarified is the difference between suicidal ideation, suicide attempts and death by suicide. The difference is not only in the quality of behaviour but also it is reflected in the numbers. Although a significant percent of the population experiences thoughts of death, especially transient ones (Fountoulakis et al. 2012b), only a few persons attempt and those who die from suicide are so few that they constitute suicide a rare phenomenon. The rate of attempted to completed suicide is about 5 to 1 in patients with any mood disorder (Tondo et al. 2003).

The latest statistics point to an increase in suicides worldwide after a substantial decline during the past two decades. The decline as well as the rise are of unknown aetiology; however, the major reason for the decline is believed to be the better recognition of mood disorders and the wider availability of treatment (Isometsa et al. 1994b; Rihmer and Akiskal 2006; Akiskal et al. 2005; Cipriani et al. 2005; Rihmer et al. 2002), while the relationship of the rise in suicides with the economic crisis which begun in 2008 is vague (Fountoulakis et al. 2013, 2014).

The average rate of suicide in the general population is approximately 11.4 per 100,000 persons worldwide, while in the USA and Europe, it is around 12 per 100,000. Across countries and cultures, a robust finding is that males have double rates in comparison to females (Saxena and Fleischmann 2014; WHO 2014). Studies in BD patients suggest that the rate of suicide in this population is 0.4 % per year with equal rates between males and females. These rates are 40 times higher in comparison to those of the general population (Tondo et al. 2003). Suicide attempts in BD patients have a lifetime prevalence from 9 to 19 % with no significant difference between BD-I (10–38 %) and BD-II (18–56 %) (Dunner et al. 1976; Endicott et al. 1985; Coryell et al. 1987; Cassano et al. 1992; Rihmer and Pestality 1999; Vieta et al. 1997; Tondo et al. 1999). Again these rates are approximately 10–20 times higher than those observed in the general population.

It is important to understanding suicidality because it is likely that this could lead to its prevention which is one of the most challenging tasks for psychiatry today. It has been solidly confirmed by psychological autopsy studies that the majority of suicidal victims were suffering from a mood disorder, often untreated, with frequent comorbidity of anxiety and substance-use disorders (Rihmer et al. 2002; Henriksson et al. 1993; Rihmer 2007; Barraclough et al. 1974; Monkman 1987; Badawi et al. 1999). In spite of the robustness of these findings, the specific prevalence and incidence of suicide in BD and vice versa is vague. Reports are conflicting. Although around 60–80 % of all suicide victims are reported to be suffering from depression and on the other hand, an estimated 15 % of patients with severe major depression eventually die from suicide, only 15 % of suicidal victims are reported to suffer from BD (Gomez-Duran et al. 2014). On the contrary, a meta-review reported that BD has one of the highest suicide risks (Chesney et al. 2014) and other studies reported that the percentage of BD patients who attempt suicide after 1.5 year is double in comparison with unipolar depression (19.9 % vs. 9.5 %) (Holma et al. 2014). Probably the heterogeneity of results has its source in the quality of the study samples. BD patients during manic episodes rarely attempt suicide; however, they suffer more from chronic depression and subthreshold depressive symptoms in comparison to unipolar depression (Holma et al. 2014).

Prevention is based to a significant extend to the successful prediction of suicide. Important risk factors are male gender, recent hospitalization because of bipolar depression or suicide attempt and presence of mixed features (Isometsa et al. 2014). Especially the presence of a mixed features during a depressive episode as well as agitation substantially increase the risk of both attempted and committed suicide (Balazs et al. 2006; Isometsa et al. 1994b; Rihmer and Akiskal 2006; Akiskal et al. 2005; Rihmer 2007). However, other studies suggest that female gender is a risk factor (Schaffer et al. 2014). Probably there is a complex interplay of a number of factors including age, gender, family history of suicide, marital status, living circumstances, higher number of prior depressive episodes, history of psychotic features, comorbid anxiety, personality disorders (especially borderline), past and recent suicide attempts, substance and alcohol abuse, recent hospitalization and interpersonal, employment/financial and legal/police stressors (Tidemalm et al. 2014; Umamaheswari et al. 2014; Zimmerman et al. 2014; Bernal et al. 2006; Rihmer et al. 2002; Rihmer 2007; Balazs et al. 2006; Rihmer and Akiskal 2006; Henriksson et al. 1993; Carra et al. 2014; Schaffer et al. 2014). Patients with severe suicide attempts were reported to manifest lower affective intensity and lability and higher neurocognitive function in comparison to patients with less severe attempts and normal controls (Olie et al. 2014).

Although biological research has so far identified several biological correlates of suicide today, there is no biological marker found yet to distinguish explicitly between suicidal and non-suicidal depressives (Samuelsson et al. 2006; Nordstrom et al. 1994), but there are at least some data concerning the contribution of biological factors to the development of various stages of suicidality (Fountoulakis et al. 2004).

Especially important risk factors with clinical significance are the presence of mixed features or agitated depression (Isometsa et al. 1994b, 2014; Balazs et al. 2006; Rihmer and Akiskal 2006; Akiskal et al. 2005; Rihmer 2007), borderline personality (Zimmerman et al. 2014) and substance abuse (Carra et al. 2014).

Since prevention is believed to be possible, common reason would expect to be far more efficacious; it is an impressive fact that in spite of frequent medical contact before committing suicide, only a small minority of victims had received appropriate treatment. This is particularly a problem in primary care, where most patients seek help (Luoma et al. 2002; Rihmer et al. 1990, 2002; Henriksson et al. 1993; Isometsa et al. 1994a). Thus, not only early identification of suicidal behaviour is possible but also early intervention is possible and could make a difference. The patient should hospitalized or be put on a plan of regular psychiatric visits on an interval ranging from once to twice weekly. Latter visits could be planned on a month interval or even less frequently. The main factors determining hospitalization and frequency of visits include the clinical picture, social and family support, history of adherence, insight into the illness and the risk and medication adverse effects. However, one should have in mind that no feature in the clinical picture is in fact a reliable index of the true risk and of the danger for the patient's life and health.

The pharmacological treatment of BD patients at risk to commit suicide is complex and with a lot of caveats. It is of outmost importance that the US Food and Drug Administration (FDA) has issued a warning concerning the use of antidepressants in children and adolescents and possibly in all age groups because of possible induction of suicidality (thinking and behaviour but not completed suicide) by antidepressants in juvenile depressives (FDA 2009). Antidepressants are the only formally approved treatment for major depression (Akiskal et al. 2005; Rihmer and Akiskal 2006; Yerevanian et al. 2004) and there are no data supporting the effectiveness of any other approach (Fountoulakis et al. 2008); however, this holds true for unipolar but not for bipolar depression (see Chap. 16).

The warning was based on data from RCTs but there is doubt whether the design of these studies permits this kind of conclusions, mainly because suicidal patients are not included in studies of this kind due of ethical reasons. A recent study reported that after the warning (between 2003 and 2005), the SSRIs prescriptions for children and adolescents in the USA and the Netherlands decreased by about 22 %, but simultaneously there was a 49 % youth suicide rate increase in the Netherlands (between 2003 and 2005) and a 14 % in the USA (between 2003 and 2004) (Gibbons et al. 2007).

Thus, it is highly possible that the 'natural' population of mood disorder patients does not respond to treatment concerning their suicidal symptoms the way randomized trials imply. On the contrary it seems that proper and 'aggressive' treatment of mental disorders and especially of depression aiming at achieving full remission should always be the target and determines to a large extent whether suicidal behaviour is expressed or not (Tiihonen et al. 2006; Sondergard et al. 2007; Moller 2006; Angst et al. 2005). In this frame it is interesting to mention that one study reported that antidepressants reduced by half the risk for manifesting suicidal behaviour in BD-I and by one-third in BD-II patients but not at all in unipolar depressives (Leon et al. 2014).

A similar warning is in place by the FDA now concerning anticonvulsants. This is very important also, since specific anticonvulsants are typically used in the treatment of BD. Of these, lamotrigine was found to increase the risk for suicidal behaviour and this is an oxymoron since lamotrigine is efficacious in the treatment of bipolar depression. A number of methodological issues and problems are in place again and further research is necessary (Ferrer et al. 2014; Fountoulakis et al. 2012a).

On the other hand, lithium is believed to exert a robust anti-suicidal effect. This conclusion is based on uncontrolled observational data (Rihmer and Akiskal 2006; Cipriani et al. 2005; Angst et al. 2005; Isometsa et al. 2014; Curran and Ravindran 2014) and probably reflects an inherent bias in the study samples. A number of strategies have been proposed for the treatment of refractory BD patients and the rapid alleviation of suicidal symptoms, including the combination of total sleep deprivation, light therapy and lithium (Benedetti et al. 2014) and also the use of a single sub-anaesthetic infusion of ketamine (0.5 mg/kg over 40 min) (Ballard et al. 2014). Unfortunately the data concerning psychosocial interventions are weak and mostly essentially negative (Gonda et al. 2007; Rihmer et al. 2009; Fountoulakis et al. 2009). The only and probably best way to prevent suicide is the development of social support networks which can act as buffers and also as networks continuously tracking for patients with subtle suicidal symptoms. Such networks have been proved to be particularly effective in the prevention of any suicidal behaviours including completed suicides in the elderly in Japan (Fountoulakis et al. 2011).

19.3 Paediatric BD

The focus of the current book is adult BD; thus, it will include only a short description of BD in children and adolescents. BD in these age groups constitutes an important field of both clinical and research interest because it represents a very early stage and proper diagnosis and treatment is expected to alter the long-term course of the illness to the better.

Although the core features of mood disorders are essentially the same across the life span, traditionally children are considered somewhat separately. This happens because of the special features their phase of life includes and the way these special features might influence the overall manifestation and treatment of mental disorders. Additionally, an early age at onset of any disorder probably implies a more severe and chronic disease and also poor response to treatment.

19.3.1 Epidemiology of Paediatric BD

The incidence of mood disorders in general, among children and adolescents, is reported to increase during the last few decades. These reports are rather consistent and they also suggest there is a decrease of the age at onset of mood disorders. The general picture suggests that the prevalence of BD in the general population aged below 21 years is 0.2–0.4 % in children and 1 % in adolescents but rates close to 2 % have been reported worldwide (Van Meter et al. 2011; McClellan et al. 2007). In hospitals, it seems that up to 20 % of youth referred to mental health services suffer from BD (Weller et al. 1986; Wozniak et al. 1995).

Concerning suicide and related behaviours, the prevalence of attempted suicide is 1 % in children and 1.7–5.9 % in adolescents, while the annual completed suicide rate ranges from nearly zero in children below the age of 10 to a peak of above 18/100,000 in boys 15–19 years old. The data suggest that among 15–19-year-olds, the suicide rates have quadrupled over the last four decades, and the reason for this is not known. Unfortunately, suicide is currently the fourth leading cause of death in children aged 10–15 years and the third leading cause of death among adolescents and young adults aged 15–25 years. The great majority of attempts among children and adolescents have little lethal potential partially because of restricted access to lethal material and inadequate cognitive potential to plan a successful attempt. What is unique in this age group is suicide imitation and contagion. This means that the suicidal behaviour increases in adolescents following exposure to well-publicized news stories of suicide or a film involving a teen suicide, but this seems to concern vulnerable individuals and not the age group as a whole (Brent et al. 1993; Cheng et al. 2007; Gould and Shaffer 1986).

19.3.2 Clinical Features of Paediatric BD

It is highly unlikely that the true epidemiology of paediatric BD has changed. Rather the criteria used and the better training of mental health professionals as well as the increasing awareness of the disease have led to this increase in the figures (Dickstein and Leibenluft 2012). The true role of the pharmaceutical industry in this procedure is unknown and should be closely monitored in the future (Mitchell et al. 2010). Some authors have expressed concerns about an overdiagnosis of BD in children and adolescents (Carlson and Meyer 2006; Harris 2005; McClellan 2005). There are significant differences between countries in the way the diagnosis is put and this in turn returns different rates. For example, there has been reported a 12.5 times higher discharge rate with the diagnosis of paediatric BD in the USA in comparison to the UK (James et al. 2014). A comparison of Italian and US bipolar children revealed that Italian children had more elevated mood whereas US children presented more flight of ideas and productivity. Also there was a difference in the comorbidity rates (Donfrancesco et al. 2014b).

Recently it has been reported that the number of American children and adolescents diagnosed with BD in community hospitals increased fourfold in

10 years with the rates reaching 40 %, while in outpatient clinics it doubled reaching the 6 % (Leibenluft and Rich 2008). For the same period, the outpatient office visits for children and adolescents with BD in the USA increased 40-fold (Mitchell et al. 2010). In contrast, in Germany only 8 % of child and adolescent psychiatrists had ever diagnosed BD (Meyer et al. 2004).

Overall, clinically, mood disorders in this age group present with the same core features manifested in adults and they can be diagnosed on the basis of operationalized criteria (Leibenluft 2008). However, the presence of some age-specific features should be noted. It seems that the developmental phase might influence the expression of certain mood symptoms and that's why, e.g. pervasive anhedonia or significant psychomotor retardation are rare among depressive children and auditory hallucinations and somatic complaints are seen more often in prepubertal children. The mood seems to be more often irritable rather than euphoric or depressed mood, and failure to attain expected weight gain is present instead of weight loss. Among preschool children often lack of smiling, apathy towards play, lack of involvement in all activities, physical complaints and physical aggression while among school-aged children, deteriorating school performance, increased irritability, fighting or argumentativeness and avoidance of peers may signal a mood disorder (Leibenluft 2011). Also, it is reported that in children, mania might present with a chronic instead of an episodic pattern, with mixed and rapid cycling features instead of classic manifestations (Geller and Luby 1997). All these should be considered in the frame that approximately 40–70 % of children and adolescents with a mood disorder have also at least one additional comorbid psychiatric disorder.

Children are often difficult to diagnose because abnormal thought content is masked by the normal vivid imagination characteristic of the age, and behavioural disorders can often be considered in the frame of normal development or of antisocial traits rather than in the frame of bipolarity. In adolescents, symptomatology could be hidden under the otherwise normal intense behavioural patterns of the age and perplexed by substance use.

However, there is a special consideration concerning generalized anxiety. Exacerbation of anxiety symptoms and school refusal are not uncommon among children who are depressed, and in the presence of family history of BD, this should be considered to be a possible prodrome of BD. The mania prodrome was reported to start gradually in most youth (88.5 %), with either slow (59.6 %) or rapid (28.8 %) deterioration. A rapid onset with rapid deterioration prodrome was rather rare (11.5 %) (Correll et al. 2014). Once BD is fully manifested, the presence of comorbid anxiety disorders is common and adversely affects the course of BD, as it relates to more frequent mood recurrences, longer time to recovery, less time euthymic, and more time spend in mixed and depressive episodes and rapid cycling (Sala et al. 2014; Castilla-Puentes et al. 2013).

It is frequent that depressive episodes appear first and the diagnosis of BD is not made until manic symptoms appear also. This switching of diagnosis from unipolar depression to BD is up to more than 30 % within a 5-year period, and it is significantly higher in children in comparison to adults (Geller and Luby 1997). It is also higher for youths with attention deficit hyperactivity disorder (ADHD) with subthreshold bipolar features at baseline (57 % vs. 21 %) as well as in those with deficient emotional self-regulation (Biederman et al. 2014). ADHD is frequently comorbid with BD and both disorder share many clinical and neurobiological features (Galanter and Leibenluft 2008). However, ADHD seems to be an independent nosological entity than BD, but when comorbid with BD in children, it is related with higher severity of ADHD symptoms, higher family load and more severe behavioural disorder (Donfrancesco et al. 2014a).

In children and adolescents with BD, there are data suggesting that a number of neurocognitive functions are impaired. These include verbal and visuospatial memory, processing speed, working memory, overall cognitive flexibility and social cognition and theory of mind and are more pronounced in BD-I patients and in those with comorbid ADHD (Frias et al. 2014; Schenkel et al. 2014; Dickstein et al. 2007; McClure et al. 2005a, b).

19.3.3 Aetiopathogenesis of Paediatric BD

The aetiopathogenesis of mood disorders in children and adolescents is not well understood. This is an age group which combines developmental vulnerability and high potency for neuroplasticity and compensation for any insults. It is generally believed that genetic factors play a significant role; however, there are vague data in support of this and no clear conclusions can be made. Non-shared environmental factors might also play an important role (Pike and Plomin 1996). At the cognitive level, the theoretical approach suggests the presence of cognitive distortions similar to those seen in adults but again data are inconsistent and scarce.

The traditional approach puts much emphasis on the family interactions and their relationship to the development of depression, but the conditions are usually complicated and difficult to interpret. The most difficult problem to deal with is that in the family genetic, epigenetic and psychosocial factors are combined and interplay and it is impossible to clarify the true cause or causes. When the family environment is problematic, then there is a high probability of a genetic vulnerability in the family and sometimes in both parents (assortative mating). However, this does not exclude the possibility of an emotional vulnerability induced upon the child by the environment by shaping the early experiences. Depressed parents may model negative cognitive styles and poor self-esteem, leading to a deficit of social problem-solving skills and in coping with stressful life events. Marital conflict and lack of an adequate family support system, especially when a mental illness of the parent(s) is present, disrupt parental functioning and put the child at a high risk for any mental disorder but especially for a mood disorder. In this frame, it is understandable why family conflict is the most frequent event adolescents report that they experienced the period before they manifest suicidal behaviour. There are several studies suggesting that depressed children and adolescents might experience more stressful life events like interpersonal losses, problems in relationships, parental divorce, bereavement, physical abuse and suicide in the environment (Gould et al. 1998; Kaplan et al. 1997; Williamson et al. 1995; Beautrais et al. 1997).

From a neurobiological point of view, obstetric complications seem to be specific to schizophrenia and are not found in bipolar children and adolescents (Arango et al. 2014). On the other hand, it is certain that genetics clearly play at least a moderate role while both shared and non-shared environmental influences appear to be also important. It is interesting that one study did not find any significant differences in white matter microstructure between BD patients, healthy offspring and healthy controls (Teixeira et al. 2014). To note, white matter findings are an early finding in adult BD.

It is also interesting that in sharp contrast with adult onset BD, there are data suggesting that in very early-onset psychotic bipolar patients there is a low premorbid IQ, more neurological signs, reduced frontal grey matter at the time of their first psychotic episode and greater brain changes than healthy controls. The overall pattern is similar to early-onset schizophrenia, but it seems that the findings are related more to the specific phenotypic features (e.g. early-onset psychotic symptoms) than to diagnosis per se (Arango et al. 2014).

19.3.4 Treatment of Paediatric BD

There have been important efforts to develop guidelines for the treatment of paediatric BD in spite of the lack of supporting evidence (Carlson et al. 2009; McClellan et al. 2007). The standard treatment of mental disorders during childhood and adolescence is some type of psychosocial treatment. The characteristics of the psychological treatments suitable for children and adolescents with mood disorders are similar to those of the treatments for adults. They aim to provide families with an understanding of symptoms, course and treatment, to teach both the youth and parents methods for coping with symptoms and prevent relapse. However, there is an almost complete lack of evidence concerning their efficacy (Fristad and MacPherson 2014).

On the contrary there is a significant controversy concerning pharmacotherapy. Double-blind studies are few and it seems that these age groups are particularly vulnerable for the induction of suicidality by antidepressants. The few controlled data suggest that aripiprazole has shown efficacy for relapse prevention in BD children 4–9 years of age in one placebo-controlled RCT, but the results were not robust in a second study on children 10–17 years of age (Diaz-Caneja et al. 2014; Findling et al. 2012, 2013). Olanzapine was found superior to placebo in the treatment of acute mania (Tohen et al. 2007) and so was quetiapine (Pathak et al. 2013). There is one negative placebo-controlled trial concerning quetiapine in paediatric bipolar depression (Findling et al. 2014) and another negative trial of divalproex in the treatment of acute mania (Wagner et al. 2009).

There are many reports in the literature on the efficacy and safety of a variety of medication in these age groups (Azorin and Findling 2007; Barzman et al. 2006; Chang 2008; DelBello et al. 2006, 2007; Jensen et al. 2007; Marchand et al. 2004; Andrade et al. 2006; Dudley et al. 2008; Tsapakis et al. 2008; Usala et al. 2008; Fraguas et al. 2011; Kryzhanovskaya et al. 2009; McCormack 2010; Seida et al. 2012;

Gentile 2011). However, the fact is that there are no hard data concerning lithium, carbamazepine, lamotrigine and the rest of antipsychotics (except those mentioned before). ECT and TMS might be reasonable alternatives if initial therapeutic attempts fail (Morales et al. 2005).

19.4 Geriatric BD

The elderly population is increasing both as absolute numbers as well as in percentage in the total population and this is a worldwide trend. This of course leads to an increase in the numbers of geriatric psychiatric patients and to a shift in the focus of health care services. At the same time, geriatric mental patients present with multiple challenges both at the diagnostic as well as the therapeutic level. Again, the focus of the current book is not geriatric populations; thus, only a short discussion of the issue is included.

19.4.1 Epidemiology of Geriatric BD

One needs to separate two distinct issues in geriatric BD. The overall prevalence of BD in old age includes all patients with BD who survived to become old, no matter their age at onset, and also the prevalence of those patients with BD whose illness appeared at a latter age, probably after the age of 65. It is generally unknown whether these are distinct forms of the disease; however, there are some data linking the late-onset BD with organic mental disorder, most often vascular encephalopathy.

There are some data including large-scale epidemiological data, suggesting that the prevalence of BD decreases with age and falls to 0.1–0.4 % in subjects aged 65 years or older (Young and Klerman 1992; Young 1992, 1997; Shulman et al. 1992; Snowdon 1991; Brieger and Marneros 2005; Sajatovic and Blow 2007; Berrios and Bakshi 1991). Since BD is a life-long disorder, this decreasing rates probably reflect the higher mortality of these patients but also probably some kind of 'masking' of the more benign cases because other somatic disorders become more prominent or the fact that the mental health of BD patients is perplexed by organic factors, which subsequently alters the current diagnosis. The concept that mania is burned out by increasing age is probably mistaken (Mirchandani and Young 1993).

Among psychiatric inpatients aged 55 year or older, the prevalence of BD is approximately 10 % while for outpatients it is estimated to be lower and equal to 6.1 % (Depp and Jeste 2004). In long-term care institutions, the reported prevalence ranges from 3 to 9.7 % (Koenig and Blazer 1992; Tariot et al. 1993). Concerning hypomania the percentage is as low as 1.6 % but it comes from only one study (Cravello et al. 2011).

It is important to know the prevalence of acute mania in the elderly for a number of reasons including the differences in the treatment and the dangers for the general health, even for the life itself of the geriatric manic patients. The overall prevalence of acute episodes of late-life mania is reported to be 6 % in psychiatric inpatients aged 50 or older. In this particular sample, the mean prevalence of late-onset mania was reported to be 44.2 % (Dols et al. 2014a). Other authors reported that late-onset mania (after the age of 50) exists in at least 10 % of all BD patients (Yassa et al. 1988; Van Gerpen et al. 1999), while only in 8 % of geriatric BD patients mania appeared before the age of 40 (Shulman and Post 1980). The prevalence reported for acute mania in outpatient settings ranges between 5 and 20 % (Prakash et al. 2009; Young and Klerman 1992; Young 1992).

As mentioned above, hypomania is rare; however, only half of patients are diagnosed as BD-I and only one-fourth experiences the onset of mood symptoms after the age of 50 (Dols et al. 2014b).

Depression is more prevalent than mania, and this is also a consequence of the fact that by passing the years in most BD patients, a depressive predominant polarity is in place. The prevalence of major depression (both unipolar and bipolar) is estimated to be 2 % in the general population over 65 years of age (Vaillant et al. 1996; Blazer et al. 1991; Reynolds 1992), with up to 15 % having some kind of other mood disorder (Branconnierm et al. 1983). Approximately 25–40 % of patients in the general hospital setting have some kind of subthreshold depression (Rapp et al. 1988). In residential homes, the accepted figure for patients with major depression is approximately 12 %, with an additional 30 % manifesting a milder form of depressive-like symptomatology (Katz et al. 1989; Foster et al. 1991; Parmelee et al. 1991; NIH 1992; Katz and Parmelee 1994; Weyerer et al. 1995).

The recognition of patients with a late-onset mood disorder is poor; less than half of hospitalised patients with depression in general medical practice are referred to a psychiatrist, and less than 20 % receive adequate treatment (Shah and De 1998). At the same time, geriatric patients with depression have up to 1.5–3 times higher morbidity (Parmelee et al. 1992), with the lifetime risk of suicide being as high as 15 %; almost 10 % of them die annually (Murphy 1994).

19.4.2 Clinical Features of Geriatric BD

It is not uncommon that geriatric BD patients spend most of their lives with episodes of depression and diagnosed as unipolar. The first manic episode could emerge only during their 50s or 60s (Shulman and Post 1980; Shulman et al. 1992; Snowdon 1991; Young 1992, 1997; Young and Klerman 1992; Stone 1989), and it has been reported that in one-quarter of them, the first manic episode occurs after the age of 65 (Stone 1989). Although a depressive predominant polarity seems to prevail with increasing age (Nivoli et al. 2014), it is clear that mania as a clinical entity does not disappear (Mirchandani and Young 1993).

Although a difference in the frequency of family history (Yassa et al. 1988; Young 1992; Dhingra and Rabins 1991), the presence of brain organic disease (Shulman and Post 1980; Snowdon 1991; Stone 1989; Tohen et al. 1994; McDonald et al. 1991) or somatic triggering factors (Krauthammer and Klerman 1978;

Young 1992; Young and Klerman 1992; Mirchandani and Young 1993) seem to exist between early- and late-onset mania, there is an ongoing debate whether BD differs between younger and older patients and in special consideration of the age at onset. Some differences have been confirmed concerning unipolar depression but the picture concerning BD is vague. Concerning unipolar depression a number of studies in the elderly reported that mood is more often irritable than depressive (Monfort 1995), and also several symptoms like loss of weight, feelings of guilt, suicidal ideation, melancholic features, hypochondriasis as well as associated symptoms of psychosis could be more frequent (Lader 1982; Nelson et al. 1989; Musetti et al. 1989; Brown et al. 1984; Lyness et al. 1992). However, these findings vary across studies. Many of these patients manifest a type of behaviour that can be characterized as 'passive–aggressive' or 'self-aggressive' because they often refuse to get up from bed, eat, wash themselves or talk. Also, they often hide important information concerning severe somatic disease and in this way they let it go untreated. Geriatric mania is considered to differ from mania in younger patients in terms of increased confusion and agitation, paranoid and mixed features (dysphoria and irritability) but recent studies tend to reject this assumption (Yassa et al. 1988; Kellner and Neher 1991; Khouzam et al. 1994; Tohen et al. 1994; Van Gerpen et al. 1999).

As discussed in more detail in Chaps. 4, 12, and 15, the neurocognitive impairment correlates with mania and psychotic features. This holds true both for younger and elderly BD patients (Mirchandani and Young 1993; Young 1992), but it seems that neurocognitive impairment is more frequent and more severe in elderly patients in comparison with younger ones (Aprahamian et al. 2014; Young 1992, 1997; Young and Klerman 1992), but this might simply reflect the accumulated burden of the disease and the progression into later stages (see Chap. 15). Eventually, a significant percentage of elderly BD patients obtain neuropsychological scores indicative of the presence of dementia (Aprahamian et al. 2014; Bartels et al. 2002; Gerson et al. 1999; Pampallona et al. 2004) although it is clear that BD is not correlated and does not constitute a risk factor for the development of dementia in the elderly (Shulman and Post 1980; Stone 1989). On the other hand, acute manic-like episodes are often seen in dementia patients (Lyketsos et al. 1995). In elderly individuals there is an increased possibility of the coexistence of depression and dementia or some other type of 'organic' decline of neurocognitive function. The syndrome of 'pseudodementia' has also been described (Kiloh 1961). This term refers to the manifestation of dementia symptomatology, which in fact is due to depression and disappears after successful antidepressant therapy. It is also described as the emergence of late-onset bipolarity in the frame of an ongoing dementing pathology (Akiskal and Pinto 1999; Ng et al. 2008; Akiskal and Benazzi 2005).

It is interesting to note that although psychiatric comorbidity is rather uncommon, medical comorbidity is high and this is of course a consequence of advanced age (Dols et al. 2014b). The assessment and diagnosis of somatic symptoms is a difficult task in mood disorders. As a general rule, physicians should avoid assigning this symptomatology to an underlying mental disorder, especially in the elderly, since in this age group it is highly likely the patient indeed suffers from a true 'somatic' disorder even in cases the physician is unable to diagnose it. On the other hand, it is generally believed that the elderly depressives manifest more somatoform symptomatology, in comparison to younger depressives. In this frame, the concept of 'masked depression' (Modai et al. 1982) used to be popular in the past, but today it is not accepted by either classification system although it is accepted that the onset of health concerns in old age is more likely to be either realistic or to reflect a mood disorder. Percentages of comorbidity between depression and physical illness vary from 6 to 45 % (Kok et al. 1995; Kitchell et al. 1982), and this large discrepancy reflects the difficulty in the application of operationalized criteria for the diagnosis of mood disorders in patients with general health problems. Greater overall severity of medical illness, cognitive impairment, physical disability and symptoms of pain or other somatic complaints seem to be a more important predictor of depression than specific medical diagnoses (Williamson and Schulz 1992).

Suicide constitutes an important health problem for the elderly. Elderly men are at a higher risk for completing suicide than elderly women. The coexistence of a serious somatic disease, like renal failure or cancer, represents a major risk factor for a well-planned suicide attempt (Heikkinen and Lonnqvist 1995). Other risk factors include loneliness and social isolation, usually as a consequence of bereavement. The failure to follow medical advice in serious general medical conditions could be considered to be a form of 'passive suicide'. On the other hand, 'rational' suicide plans are not common even in severely ill patients. There is a possibility of acute-onset suicidal plans (after an acute incidence concerning general health, e.g. stroke or heart attack) (Kishi et al. 1996). In the frame of BD, patients are unlikely to attempt while in mania; however, since depression is predominant in this age group, suicide constitutes an important problem.

19.4.3 Neurobiology of Geriatric BD

The neurobiology of geriatric BD is complex since a number of pathologies coexist. It is reasonable to accept that the physiological and pathological changes which happen in the human brain at advanced age are superimposed to those induced by BD, but the real question concerns late-onset cases and whether they are related to different neurobiological characteristics.

It has been proposed as a distinct type of BD within the bipolar spectrum (see Chap. 6) the emergence of late-onset bipolarity in the frame of an ongoing dementing pathology most frequently of vascular origin (Steffens and Krishnan 1998; Akiskal and Pinto 1999; Akiskal and Benazzi 2005; Ng et al. 2008). This directly implies a different neurobiological substrate and aetiopathogenetic mechanism for late-onset cases. It is well known that a large number of medications, metabolic disturbances as well as neurological conditions can cause secondary mania (Van Gerpen et al. 1999). Although the clinical data do not suggest the presence of clinical differences, it has been reported that late-onset mood patients are less likely to have a positive family history for mood disorders (Shulman and Post 1980; Stone 1989; Charron et al. 1991; Hopkinson 1964; Mendlewicz 1976; Yassa et al. 1988; Young 1992; Dhingra and Rabins 1991). Also, while overall the rate of positive family history for mood disorders is between 26.5 and 48 % in elderly BD patients (Snowdon 1991; Stone 1989; Tohen et al. 1994), when neurological disorders are present, the rate drops to 9–33 % (McDonald et al. 1991; Shulman et al. 1992; Snowdon 1991; Stone 1989). On the contrary late-onset patients have brain pathologies more frequent, which are detectable with routine neuroimaging (Shulman and Post 1980; Snowdon 1991; Stone 1989; Tohen et al. 1994; McDonald et al. 1991; Jacoby and Levy 1980; Burvill et al. 1989; Rabins et al. 1991; Jakoby et al. 1980, 1981; Greenwald et al. 1996; Uradhyaya et al. 1990; Sackheim et al. 1993; Steffens and Krishnan 1998). Additionally, geriatric mania is more likely to be secondary in comparison to mania in younger patients (Krauthammer and Klerman 1978; Young 1992; Young and Klerman 1992; Mirchandani and Young 1993). Some authors consider this secondary mania to be an equivalent of delirium (Shulman 1997) since it is related to the presence of stroke, traumatic brain injury, space-occupying lesions and other neurological disorders .(Tohen et al. 1994; Shulman and Post 1980; Shulman et al. 1992; Stone 1989; Young 1992; Cummings and Mendez 1984).

The literature suggests that 17–43 % of geriatric mania patients have demonstrable cerebral organic disorders (Shulman and Post 1980; Shulman et al. 1992; Stone 1989; Young and Klerman 1992), but it is doubtful that this is significantly higher in comparison to the general elderly population (Van Gerpen et al. 1999).

The data concerning the presence of neurocognitive dysfunction in late-life BD and its relationship with white matter pathologies are controversial (Rej et al. 2014; Salloway et al. 1996).

19.4.4 Treatment of Geriatric BD

The treatment of geriatric BD pays much attention to the comorbid medical disorders as well as the general physical condition of the patient which could be naturally compensated because of age. It also pays much attention to the possible causal relationship between mood symptoms and medical or even iatrogenic conditions. In these cases, treatment of the causal condition could alleviate or greatly improve mood symptoms.

The pharmacotherapy of geriatric BD includes lithium, valproate, carbamazepine and lamotrigine as well as antipsychotics (mostly atypicals) although they are not well studied in elderly patients (Fountoulakis et al. 2003; Sajatovic and Chen 2011). Some antipsychotics are under a warning for use in vascular patients because they are related to higher mortality. ECT is another option with many studies reporting better outcomes in older than in younger patients. However, by far the most troubling side effect of ECT, especially in the elderly, is the neurocognitive impairment.

In patients with dementia it is important to have in mind that treatment could induce manic-like symptomatology (Leung 2014).

Psychosocial interventions are also important since in geriatric BD patients, close social interactions and support are important even in the management of acute episodes (Beyer et al. 2014). Psychotherapy is always an option especially for depression (Gum and Arean 2004; Gerson et al. 1999). The presence and severity of medical illnesses, physical disability, cognitive impairment and psychomotor retardation make psychotherapeutic intervention difficult and affect its efficacy and success. The form of psychotherapy should be adjusted to the patient's personality, behaviour patterns as well as his/her cultural and educational level. Behavioural therapy, cognitive-behavioural therapy and problem-solving therapy have been extensively studied for their effectiveness in the treatment of depression in elderly. Fewer studies have been carried out for the efficacy of interpersonal psychotherapy. Non-standardized psychotherapies — as psychodynamic psychotherapy and reminiscence therapy — are also proposed as appropriate treatments for geriatric depression. The major problem is that all these options have been studied in unipolar samples.

Eventually, however, most studies support the opinion that geriatric BD carries a poorer prognosis than BD in younger patients for a number of reasons including medical comorbidities and advanced stage of the disease. However, many authors attribute this to factors like failure to make an early diagnosis and improper or insufficient treatment.

References

Akiskal HS, Benazzi F (2005) Atypical depression: a variant of bipolar II or a bridge between unipolar and bipolar II? J Affect Disord 84(2–3):209–217

Akiskal HS, Pinto O (1999) The evolving bipolar spectrum. Prototypes I, II, III, and IV. Psychiatr Clin North Am 22(3):517–534, vii

Akiskal HS, Benazzi F, Perugi G, Rihmer Z (2005) Agitated "unipolar" depression re-conceptualized as a depressive mixed state: implications for the antidepressant-suicide controversy. J Affect Disord 85(3):245–258

Andrade C, Bhakta SG, Singh NM (2006) Controversy revisited: selective serotonin reuptake inhibitors in paediatric depression. World J Biol Psychiatry 7(4):251–260. doi:10.1080/15622970600702690, J271045WTR587355 [pii]

Angst J, Angst F, Gerber-Werder R, Gamma A (2005) Suicide in 406 mood-disorder patients with and without long-term medication: a 40 to 44 years' follow-up. Arch Suicide Res 9(3): 279–300

Aprahamian I, Ladeira RB, Diniz BS, Forlenza OV, Nunes PV (2014) Cognitive impairment in euthymic older adults with bipolar disorder: a controlled study using cognitive screening tests. Am J Geriatr Psychiatry 22(4):389–397. doi:10.1016/j.jagp.2012.08.013

Arango C, Fraguas D, Parellada M (2014) Differential neurodevelopmental trajectories in patients with early-onset bipolar and schizophrenia disorders. Schizophr Bull 40(Suppl 2):S138–S146. doi:10.1093/schbul/sbt198

Azorin JM, Findling RL (2007) Valproate use in children and adolescents with bipolar disorder. CNS Drugs 21(12):1019–1033, 21125 [pii]

Badawi MA, Eaton WW, Myllyluoma J, Weimer LG, Gallo J (1999) Psychopathology and attrition in the Baltimore ECA 15-year follow-up 1981–1996. Soc Psychiatry Psychiatr Epidemiol 34(2):91–98

Balazs J, Benazzi F, Rihmer Z, Rihmer A, Akiskal KK, Akiskal HS (2006) The close link between suicide attempts and mixed (bipolar) depression: implications for suicide prevention. J Affect Disord 91(2–3):133–138

Ballard ED, Ionescu DF, Vande Voort JL, Niciu MJ, Richards EM, Luckenbaugh DA, Brutsche NE, Ameli R, Furey ML, Zarate CA Jr (2014) Improvement in suicidal ideation after ketamine infusion: relationship to reductions in depression and anxiety. J Psychiatr Res. doi:10.1016/j.jpsychires.2014.07.027

Barraclough B, Bunch J, Nelson B, Sainsbury P (1974) A hundred cases of suicide: clinical aspects. Br J Psychiatry 125:355–373

Bartels SJ, Dums AR, Oxman TE, Schneider LS, Arean PA, Alexopoulos GS, Jeste DV (2002) Evidence-based practices in geriatric mental health care. Psychiatr Serv 53(11):1419–1431

Barzman DH, DelBello MP, Adler CM, Stanford KE, Strakowski SM (2006) The efficacy and tolerability of quetiapine versus divalproex for the treatment of impulsivity and reactive aggression in adolescents with co-occurring bipolar disorder and disruptive behavior disorder(s). J Child Adolesc Psychopharmacol 16(6):665–670. doi:10.1089/cap.2006.16.665

Baskaran A, Cha DS, Powell AM, Jalil D, McIntyre RS (2014) Sex differences in rates of obesity in bipolar disorder: postulated mechanisms. Bipolar Disord 16(1):83–92. doi:10.1111/bdi.12141

Bauer M, Glenn T, Pilhatsch M, Pfennig A, Whybrow PC (2014) Gender differences in thyroid system function: relevance to bipolar disorder and its treatment. Bipolar Disord 16(1):58–71. doi:10.1111/bdi.12150

Beautrais AL, Joyce PR, Mulder RT (1997) Precipitating factors and life events in serious suicide attempts among youths aged 13 through 24 years. J Am Acad Child Adolesc Psychiatry 36(11):1543–1551

Benedetti F, Riccaboni R, Locatelli C, Poletti S, Dallaspezia S, Colombo C (2014) Rapid treatment response of suicidal symptoms to lithium, sleep deprivation, and light therapy (chronotherapeutics) in drug-resistant bipolar depression. J Clin Psychiatry 75(2):133–140. doi:10.4088/JCP.13m08455

Bernal M, Haro JM, Bernert S, Brugha T, de Graaf R, Bruffaerts R, Lepine JP, de Girolamo G, Vilagut G, Gasquet I, Torres JV, Kovess V, Heider D, Neeleman J, Kessler R, Alonso J (2006) Risk factors for suicidality in Europe: results from the ESEMED study. J Affect Disord 101:27–34

Berrios GE, Bakshi N (1991) Manic and depressive symptoms in the elderly: their relationships to treatment outcome, cognition and motor symptoms. Psychopathology 24(1):31–38

Beyer JL, Greenberg RL, Marino P, Bruce ML, Al Jurdi RK, Sajatovic M, Gyulai L, Mulsant BH, Gildengers A, Young RC (2014) Social support in late life mania: GERI-BD. Int J Geriatr Psychiatry. doi:10.1002/gps.4093

Biederman J, Wozniak J, Tarko L, Serra G, Hernandez M, McDermott K, Woodsworth KY, Uchida M, Faraone SV (2014) Re-examining the risk for switch from unipolar to bipolar major depressive disorder in youth with ADHD: a long term prospective longitudinal controlled study. J Affect Disord 152–154:347–351. doi:10.1016/j.jad.2013.09.036

Blazer D, Burchetti B, Service C et al (1991) The association of age in depression among the elderly: an epidemiologic exploration. J Gerontol 46:M210–M215

Blazer DG, Kessler RC, McGonagle KA, Swartz MS (1994) The prevalence and distribution of major depression in a national community sample: the National Comorbidity Survey. Am J Psychiatry 151(7):979–986

Branconnierm R, Cole J, Ghazvinian D, Spera K, Oxenkrug G, Bass J (1983) Clinical pharmacology of bupropion and imipramine in elderly depressives. J Clin Psychiatry 44:130–133

Brent DA, Perper JA, Moritz G, Allman C, Schweers J, Roth C, Balach L, Canobbio R, Liotus L (1993) Psychiatric sequelae to the loss of an adolescent peer to suicide. J Am Acad Child Adolesc Psychiatry 32(3):509–517

Brieger P, Marneros A (2005) Bipolar disorders in late life. In: Kasper S, Hirschfeld R (eds) Handbook of bipolar disorder: diagnosis and therapeutic approaches. Taylor & Francis Group, LLC, New York, pp 83–93

Brown R, Sweeney J, Loutsch E, Kocsis J, Frances A (1984) Involutional melancholia revisited. Am J Psychiatry 141:24–28

Bucker J, Popuri S, Muralidharan K, Kozicky JM, Baitz HA, Honer WG, Torres IJ, Yatham LN (2014) Sex differences in cognitive functioning in patients with bipolar disorder who recently recovered from a first episode of mania: data from the Systematic Treatment Optimization

Program for Early Mania (STOP-EM). J Affect Disord 155:162–168. doi:10.1016/j.jad.2013.10.044

Burvill P, Hall W, Stampfer H, Emmerson J (1989) A comparison of early onset and late onset depressive illness in the elderly. Br J Psychiatry 155:673–679

Carlson GA, Meyer SE (2006) Phenomenology and diagnosis of bipolar disorder in children, adolescents, and adults: complexities and developmental issues. Dev Psychopathol 18(4):939–969. doi:10.1017/S0954579406060470

Carlson GA, Findling RL, Post RM, Birmaher B, Blumberg HP, Correll C, DelBello MP, Fristad M, Frazier J, Hammen C, Hinshaw SP, Kowatch R, Leibenluft E, Meyer SE, Pavuluri MN, Wagner KD, Tohen M (2009) AACAP 2006 research forum–advancing research in early-onset bipolar disorder: barriers and suggestions. J Child Adolesc Psychopharmacol 19(1):3–12. doi:10.1089/cap.2008.100

Carra G, Bartoli F, Crocamo C, Brady KT, Clerici M (2014) Attempted suicide in people with co-occurring bipolar and substance use disorders: systematic review and meta-analysis. J Affect Disord 167C:125–135. doi:10.1016/j.jad.2014.05.066

Cassano GB, Akiskal HS, Savino M, Musetti L, Perugi G (1992) Proposed subtypes of bipolar II and related disorders: with hypomanic episodes (or cyclothymia) and with hyperthymic temperament. J Affect Disord 26(2):127–140

Castilla-Puentes R, Sala R, Ng B, Galvez J, Camacho A (2013) Anxiety disorders and rapid cycling: data from a cohort of 8129 youths with bipolar disorder. J Nerv Ment Dis 201(12):1060–1065. doi:10.1097/NMD.0000000000000052

Chang KD (2008) The use of atypical antipsychotics in pediatric bipolar disorder. J Clin Psychiatry 69(Suppl 4):4–8

Charron M, Fortin L, Paquette I (1991) De novo mania among elderly people. Acta Psychiatr Scand 84(6):503–507

Cheng AT, Hawton K, Lee CT, Chen TH (2007) The influence of media reporting of the suicide of a celebrity on suicide rates: a population-based study. Int J Epidemiol 36(6):1229–1234. doi:10.1093/ije/dym196, dym196 [pii]

Chesney E, Goodwin GM, Fazel S (2014) Risks of all-cause and suicide mortality in mental disorders: a meta-review. World Psychiatry 13(2):153–160. doi:10.1002/wps.20128

Cipriani A, Pretty H, Hawton K, Geddes JR (2005) Lithium in the prevention of suicidal behavior and all-cause mortality in patients with mood disorders: a systematic review of randomized trials. Am J Psychiatry 162(10):1805–1819

Correll CU, Hauser M, Penzner JB, Auther AM, Kafantaris V, Saito E, Olvet D, Carrion RE, Birmaher B, Chang KD, DelBello MP, Singh MK, Pavuluri M, Cornblatt BA (2014) Type and duration of subsyndromal symptoms in youth with bipolar I disorder prior to their first manic episode. Bipolar Disord 16(5):478–492. doi:10.1111/bdi.12194

Coryell W, Andreasen NC, Endicott J, Keller M (1987) The significance of past mania or hypomania in the course and outcome of major depression. Am J Psychiatry 144(3): 309–315

Cravello L, Palmer K, de Girolamo G, Caltagirone C, Spalletta G (2011) Neuropsychiatric symptoms and syndromes in institutionalized elderly people without dementia. Int Psychogeriatr 23(3):425–434. doi:10.1017/S1041610210001304

Cummings JL, Mendez MF (1984) Secondary mania with focal cerebrovascular lesions. Am J Psychiatry 141(9):1084–1087

Curran G, Ravindran A (2014) Lithium for bipolar disorder: a review of the recent literature. Expert Rev Neurother 14(9):1079–1098. doi:10.1586/14737175.2014.947965

DelBello MP, Kowatch RA, Adler CM, Stanford KE, Welge JA, Barzman DH, Nelson E, Strakowski SM (2006) A double-blind randomized pilot study comparing quetiapine and divalproex for adolescent mania. J Am Acad Child Adolesc Psychiatry 45(3):305–313. doi:10.1097/01.chi.0000194567.63289.97, 00004583-200603000-00006 [pii]

DelBello MP, Adler CM, Whitsel RM, Stanford KE, Strakowski SM (2007) A 12-week single-blind trial of quetiapine for the treatment of mood symptoms in adolescents at high risk for developing bipolar I disorder. J Clin Psychiatry 68(5):789–795

Depp CA, Jeste DV (2004) Bipolar disorder in older adults: a critical review. Bipolar Disord 6(5):343–367. doi:10.1111/j.1399-5618.2004.00139.x

Dhingra U, Rabins PV (1991) Mania in the elderly: a 5–7 year follow-up. J Am Geriatr Soc 39(6):581–583

Diaz-Caneja CM, Moreno C, Llorente C, Espliego A, Arango C, Moreno D (2014) Practitioner review: long-term pharmacological treatment of pediatric bipolar disorder. J Child Psychol Psychiatry 55(9):959–980. doi:10.1111/jcpp.12271

Dickstein DP, Leibenluft E (2012) Beyond dogma: from diagnostic controversies to data about pediatric bipolar disorder and children with chronic irritability and mood dysregulation. Isr J Psychiatry Relat Sci 49(1):52–61

Dickstein DP, Nelson EE, McClure EB, Grimley ME, Knopf L, Brotman MA, Rich BA, Pine DS, Leibenluft E (2007) Cognitive flexibility in phenotypes of pediatric bipolar disorder. J Am Acad Child Adolesc Psychiatry 46(3):341–355. doi:10.1097/chi.0b013e31802d0b3d

Dols A, Kupka RW, van Lammeren A, Beekman AT, Sajatovic M, Stek ML (2014a) The prevalence of late-life mania: a review. Bipolar Disord 16(2):113–118. doi:10.1111/bdi.12104

Dols A, Rhebergen D, Beekman A, Kupka R, Sajatovic M, Stek ML (2014b) Psychiatric and medical comorbidities: results from a Bipolar Elderly Cohort Study. Am J Geriatr Psychiatry. doi:10.1016/j.jagp.2013.12.176

Donfrancesco R, Di Trani M, Andriola E, Leone D, Torrioli MG, Passarelli F, DelBello MP (2014a) Bipolar disorder in children with ADHD: a Clinical Sample Study. J Atten Disord. doi:10.1177/1087054714539999

Donfrancesco R, Marano A, Innocenzi M, Toni L, Di Lelio A, Milone A, Sposato M, Mazzotta G, Valenti V, Melegari MG, DelBello MP (2014b) A comparison of bipolar disorders in children in Italy and the United States. J Affect Disord 159:53–55. doi:10.1016/j.jad.2014.01.003

Dudley M, Hadzi-Pavlovic D, Andrews D, Perich T (2008) New-generation antidepressants, suicide and depressed adolescents: how should clinicians respond to changing evidence? Aust N Z J Psychiatry 42(6):456–466. doi:10.1080/00048670802050538, 792988748 [pii]

Dunner DL, Gershon ES, Goodwin FK (1976) Heritable factors in the severity of affective illness. Biol Psychiatry 11(1):31–42

Endicott J, Nee J, Andreasen N, Clayton P, Keller M, Coryell W (1985) Bipolar II. Combine or keep separate? J Affect Disord 8(1):17–28

FDA (2009) Antidepressant use in children, adolescents, and adults. http://www.fda.gov/CDER/Drug/antidepressants/default.htm. Accessed 1 Jan 2009

Ferrer P, Ballarin E, Sabate M, Vidal X, Rottenkolber M, Amelio J, Hasford J, Schmiedl S, Ibanez L (2014) Antiepileptic drugs and suicide: a systematic review of adverse effects. Neuroepidemiology 42(2):107–120. doi:10.1159/000356807

Findling RL, Youngstrom EA, McNamara NK, Stansbrey RJ, Wynbrandt JL, Adegbite C, Rowles BM, Demeter CA, Frazier TW, Calabrese JR (2012) Double-blind, randomized, placebo-controlled long-term maintenance study of aripiprazole in children with bipolar disorder. J Clin Psychiatry 73(1):57–63. doi:10.4088/JCP.11m07104

Findling RL, Correll CU, Nyilas M, Forbes RA, McQuade RD, Jin N, Ivanova S, Mankoski R, Carson WH, Carlson GA (2013) Aripiprazole for the treatment of pediatric bipolar I disorder: a 30-week, randomized, placebo-controlled study. Bipolar Disord 15(2):138–149. doi:10.1111/bdi.12042

Findling RL, Pathak S, Earley WR, Liu S, DelBello MP (2014) Efficacy and safety of extended-release quetiapine fumarate in youth with bipolar depression: an 8 week, double-blind, placebo-controlled trial. J Child Adolesc Psychopharmacol 24(6):325–335. doi:10.1089/cap.2013.0105

Finkelhor D, Hotaling G, Lewis IA, Smith C (1990) Sexual abuse in a national survey of adult men and women: prevalence, characteristics, and risk factors. Child Abuse Negl 14(1):19–28

Foster J, Cataldo J, Boksay I (1991) Incidence of depression in a medical long-term facility: findings from a restricted sample of new admissions. Int J Geriatr Psychiatry 6:13–20

Fountoulakis KN, O' Hara R, Iacovides A, Camilleri CP, Kaprinis S, Kaprinis G, Yesavage J (2003) Unipolar late-onset depression: a comprehensive review. Ann Gen Hosp Psychiatry 2:11

Fountoulakis KN, Iacovides A, Fotiou F, Nimatoudis J, Bascialla F, Ioannidou C, Kaprinis G, Bech P (2004) Neurobiological and psychological correlates of suicidal attempts and thoughts of death in patients with major depression. Neuropsychobiology 49(1):42–52. doi:10.1159/000075338

Fountoulakis KN, Gonda X, Siamouli M, Rihmer Z (2008) Psychotherapeutic intervention and suicide risk reduction in bipolar disorder: a review of the evidence. J Affect Disord. doi:10.1016/j.jad.2008.06.014, S0165-0327(08)00268-1 [pii]

Fountoulakis KN, Gonda X, Siamouli M, Rihmer Z (2009) Psychotherapeutic intervention and suicide risk reduction in bipolar disorder: a review of the evidence. J Affect Disord 113(1–2):21–29. doi:10.1016/j.jad.2008.06.014

Fountoulakis KN, Gonda X, Rihmer Z (2011) Suicide prevention programs through community intervention. J Affect Disord 130(1–2):10–16. doi:10.1016/j.jad.2010.06.009

Fountoulakis KN, Gonda X, Samara M, Siapera M, Karavelas V, Ristic DI, Iacovides A (2012a) Antiepileptic drugs and suicidality. J Psychopharmacol 26(11):1401–1407. doi:10.1177/0269881112440514

Fountoulakis KN, Pantoula E, Siamouli M, Moutou K, Gonda X, Rihmer Z, Iacovides A, Akiskal H (2012b) Development of the Risk Assessment Suicidality Scale (RASS): a population-based study. J Affect Disord 138(3):449–457. doi:10.1016/j.jad.2011.12.045

Fountoulakis KN, Koupidis SA, Siamouli M, Grammatikopoulos IA, Theodorakis PN (2013) Suicide, recession, and unemployment. Lancet 381(9868):721–722. doi:10.1016/S0140-6736(13)60573-5

Fountoulakis KN, Gonda X, Dome P, Theodorakis PN, Rihmer Z (2014) Possible delayed effect of unemployment on suicidal rates: the case of Hungary. Ann Gen Psychiatry 13:12. doi:10.1186/1744-859X-13-12

Fraguas D, Correll CU, Merchan-Naranjo J, Rapado-Castro M, Parellada M, Moreno C, Arango C (2011) Efficacy and safety of second-generation antipsychotics in children and adolescents with psychotic and bipolar spectrum disorders: comprehensive review of prospective head-to-head and placebo-controlled comparisons. Eur Neuropsychopharmacol 21(8):621–645. doi:10.1016/j.euroneuro.2010.07.002

Frias A, Palma C, Farriols N (2014) Neurocognitive impairments among youth with pediatric bipolar disorder: a systematic review of neuropsychological research. J Affect Disord 166:297–306. doi:10.1016/j.jad.2014.05.025

Fristad MA, MacPherson HA (2014) Evidence-based psychosocial treatments for child and adolescent bipolar spectrum disorders. J Clin Child Adolesc Psychol 43(3):339–355. doi:10.1080/15374416.2013.822309

Galanter CA, Leibenluft E (2008) Frontiers between attention deficit hyperactivity disorder and bipolar disorder. Child Adolesc Psychiatr Clin N Am 17(2):325–346, viii–ix. doi:10.1016/j.chc.2007.11.001

Geller B, Luby J (1997) Child and adolescent bipolar disorder: a review of the past 10 years. J Am Acad Child Adolesc Psychiatry 36(9):1168–1176

Gentile S (2011) Clinical usefulness of second-generation antipsychotics in treating children and adolescents diagnosed with bipolar or schizophrenic disorders. Paediatr Drugs 13(5):291–302. doi:10.2165/11591250-000000000-00000

Gerson S, Belin TR, Kaufman A, Mintz J, Jarvik L (1999) Pharmacological and psychological treatments for depressed older patients: a meta-analysis and overview of recent findings. Harv Rev Psychiatry 7(1):1–28

Gibbons RD, Brown CH, Hur K, Marcus SM, Bhaumik DK, Erkens JA, Herings RM, Mann JJ (2007) Early evidence on the effects of regulators' suicidality warnings on SSRI prescriptions and suicide in children and adolescents. Am J Psychiatry 164(9):1356–1363

Gomez-Duran EL, Forti-Buratti MA, Gutierrez-Lopez B, Belmonte-Ibanez A, Martin-Fumado C (2014) Psychiatric disorders in cases of completed suicide in a hospital area in Spain between 2007 and 2010. Revista de psiquiatria y salud mental. doi:10.1016/j.rpsm.2014.02.001

Gonda X, Fountoulakis KN, Kaprinis G, Rihmer Z (2007) Prediction and prevention of suicide in patients with unipolar depression and anxiety. Ann Gen Psychiatry 6:23. doi:10.1186/1744-859X-6-23

Gould MS, Shaffer D (1986) The impact of suicide in television movies. Evidence of imitation. N Engl J Med 315(11):690–694

Gould MS, Shaffer D, Fisher P, Garfinkel R (1998) Separation/divorce and child and adolescent completed suicide. J Am Acad Child Adolesc Psychiatry 37(2):155–162

Greenwald B, Kramer-Ginsberg E, Krishnan R, Ashtari M, Aupperle P, Patel M (1996) MRI signal hyperintensities in geriatric depression. Am J Psychiatry 153(9):1212–1215

Gum A, Arean PA (2004) Current status of psychotherapy for mental disorders in the elderly. Curr Psychiatry Rep 6(1):32–38

Hammen CL, Peters SD (1978) Interpersonal consequences of depression: responses to men and women enacting a depressed role. J Abnorm Psychol 87(3):322–332

Harris J (2005) The increased diagnosis of "juvenile bipolar disorder": what are we treating? Psychiatr Serv 56(5):529–531. doi:10.1176/appi.ps.56.5.529

Heikkinen M, Lonnqvist J (1995) Recent life events in elderly suicide: a Nationwide Study in Finland. Int Psychogeriatr 7:287–300

Henriksson MM, Aro HM, Marttunen MJ, Heikkinen ME, Isometsa ET, Kuoppasalmi KI, Lonnqvist JK (1993) Mental disorders and comorbidity in suicide. Am J Psychiatry 150(6):935–940

Holma KM, Haukka J, Suominen K, Valtonen HM, Mantere O, Melartin TK, Sokero TP, Oquendo MA, Isometsa ET (2014) Differences in incidence of suicide attempts between bipolar I and II disorders and major depressive disorder. Bipolar Disord 16(6):652–661. doi:10.1111/bdi.12195

Hopkinson G (1964) A genetic study of affective illness in patients over 50. Br J Psychiatry 110:244–254

Isometsa ET, Aro HM, Henriksson MM, Heikkinen ME, Lonnqvist JK (1994a) Suicide in major depression in different treatment settings. J Clin Psychiatry 55(12):523–527

Isometsa ET, Henriksson MM, Aro HM, Heikkinen ME, Kuoppasalmi KI, Lonnqvist JK (1994b) Suicide in major depression. Am J Psychiatry 151(4):530–536

Isometsa E, Sund R, Pirkola S (2014) Post-discharge suicides of inpatients with bipolar disorder in Finland. Bipolar Disord. doi:10.1111/bdi.12237

Jacoby R, Levy R (1980) Computed tomography in the elderly-3: affective disorder. Br J Psychiatry 136:270–275

Jakoby R, Lewy R, Bird J (1980) Computed tomography in the elderly: affective disorders. Br J Psychiatry 136:270–275

Jakoby R, Lewy R, Bird J (1981) Computed tomography and the outcome of affective disorders: a follow-up study of elderly patients. Br J Psychiatry 139:288–292

James A, Hoang U, Seagroatt V, Clacey J, Goldacre M, Leibenluft E (2014) A comparison of American and English hospital discharge rates for pediatric bipolar disorder, 2000 to 2010. J Am Acad Child Adolesc Psychiatry 53(6):614–624. doi:10.1016/j.jaac.2014.02.008

Jensen PS, Buitelaar J, Pandina GJ, Binder C, Haas M (2007) Management of psychiatric disorders in children and adolescents with atypical antipsychotics: a systematic review of published clinical trials. Eur Child Adolesc Psychiatry 16(2):104–120. doi:10.1007/s00787-006-0580-1

Joiner TE Jr, Alfano MS, Metalsky GI (1992) When depression breeds contempt: reassurance seeking, self-esteem, and rejection of depressed college students by their roommates. J Abnorm Psychol 101(1):165–173

Kaplan SJ, Pelcovitz D, Salzinger S, Mandel F, Weiner M (1997) Adolescent physical abuse and suicide attempts. J Am Acad Child Adolesc Psychiatry 36(6):799–808

Katz I, Parmelee P (1994) Depression in elderly patients residential care settings. In: Schneider L, Reynolds C, Lebowitz B, Fiedhoff A (eds) Diagnosis and treatment of depression in late life: results of the NIH Consensus Development Conference. American Psychiatric Press, Washington, DC, pp 437–442

Katz I, Lesher E, Kleban M, Jethanandani V, Parmelee P (1989) Clinical features of depression in the nursing home. Int Psychogeriatr 1:5–15

Kellner MB, Neher F (1991) A first episode of mania after age 80. Can J Psychiatry Rev Can Psychiatry 36(8):607–608
Khouzam HR, Emery PE, Reaves B (1994) Secondary mania in late life. J Am Geriatr Soc 42(1):85–87
Kiloh L (1961) Pseudodementia. Acta Psychiatr Scand 37:336–351
Kishi Y, Robinson R, Kosier J (1996) Suicidal plans in patients with stroke: comparison between acute-onset and delayed-onset suicidal plans. Int Psychogeriatr 8(4):623–634
Kitchell M, Barnes R, Veith R et al (1982) Screening for depression in hospitalized geriatric medical patients. J Am Geriatr Soc 30:174–177
Koenig HG, Blazer DG (1992) Epidemiology of geriatric affective disorders. Clin Geriatr Med 8(2):235–251
Kok R, Heeren T, Hooijer C et al (1995) The prevalence of depression in elderly medical inpatients. J Affect Disord 33:77–82
Krauthammer C, Klerman GL (1978) Secondary mania: manic syndromes associated with antecedent physical illness or drugs. Arch Gen Psychiatry 35(11):1333–1339
Kryzhanovskaya LA, Robertson-Plouch CK, Xu W, Carlson JL, Merida KM, Dittmann RW (2009) The safety of olanzapine in adolescents with schizophrenia or bipolar I disorder: a pooled analysis of 4 clinical trials. J Clin Psychiatry 70(2):247–258
Lader M (1982) Differential diagnosis of anxiety in the elderly. J Clin Psychiatry 43:4–7
Leibenluft E (2008) Pediatric bipolar disorder comes of age. Arch Gen Psychiatry 65(10): 1122–1124. doi:10.1001/archpsyc.65.10.1122
Leibenluft E (2011) Severe mood dysregulation, irritability, and the diagnostic boundaries of bipolar disorder in youths. Am J Psychiatry 168(2):129–142. doi:10.1176/appi.ajp.2010.10050766
Leibenluft E, Rich BA (2008) Pediatric bipolar disorder. Annu Rev Clin Psychol 4:163–187. doi:10.1146/annurev.clinpsy.4.022007.141216
Leon AC, Fiedorowicz JG, Solomon DA, Li C, Coryell WH, Endicott J, Fawcett J, Keller MB (2014) Risk of suicidal behavior with antidepressants in bipolar and unipolar disorders. J Clin Psychiatry 75(7):720–727. doi:10.4088/JCP.13m08744
Leung JG (2014) Donepezil-induced mania. Consult Pharm 29(3):191–195. doi:10.4140/TCP.n.2014.191
Lloyd C, Miller PM (1997) The relationship of parental style to depression and self-esteem in adulthood. J Nerv Ment Dis 185(11):655–663
Luoma JB, Martin CE, Pearson JL (2002) Contact with mental health and primary care providers before suicide: a review of the evidence. Am J Psychiatry 159(6):909–916
Lyketsos CG, Corazzini K, Steele C (1995) Mania in Alzheimer's disease. J Neuropsychiatry Clin Neurosci 7(3):350–352
Lyness J, Conwell Y, Nelson J (1992) Suicide attempts in elderly psychiatric inpatients. J Am Geriatr Soc 40:320–324
Marchand WR, Wirth L, Simon C (2004) Quetiapine adjunctive and monotherapy for pediatric bipolar disorder: a retrospective chart review. J Child Adolesc Psychopharmacol 14(3):405–411. doi:10.1089/cap.2004.14.405
McClellan J (2005) Commentary: treatment guidelines for child and adolescent bipolar disorder. J Am Acad Child Adolesc Psychiatry 44(3):236–239. doi:10.1097/00004583-200503000-00007
McClellan J, Kowatch R, Findling RL, Work Group on Quality I (2007) Practice parameter for the assessment and treatment of children and adolescents with bipolar disorder. J Am Acad Child Adolesc Psychiatry 46(1):107–125. doi:10.1097/01.chi.0000242240.69678.c4
McClure EB, Treland JE, Snow J, Dickstein DP, Towbin KE, Charney DS, Pine DS, Leibenluft E (2005a) Memory and learning in pediatric bipolar disorder. J Am Acad Child Adolesc Psychiatry 44(5):461–469. doi:10.1097/01.chi.0000156660.30953.91
McClure EB, Treland JE, Snow J, Schmajuk M, Dickstein DP, Towbin KE, Charney DS, Pine DS, Leibenluft E (2005b) Deficits in social cognition and response flexibility in pediatric bipolar disorder. Am J Psychiatry 162(9):1644–1651. doi:10.1176/appi.ajp.162.9.1644

McCormack PL (2010) Olanzapine: in adolescents with schizophrenia or bipolar I disorder. CNS Drugs 24(5):443–452. doi:10.2165/11204430-000000000-00000

McDonald WM, Krishnan KR, Doraiswamy PM, Blazer DG (1991) Occurrence of subcortical hyperintensities in elderly subjects with mania. Psychiatry Res 40(4):211–220

Meinhard N, Kessing LV, Vinberg M (2014) The role of estrogen in bipolar disorder, a review. Nord J Psychiatry 68(2):81–87. doi:10.3109/08039488.2013.775341

Mendlewicz J (1976) The age factor in depressive illness: some genetic consideration. J Gerontol 31:300–303

Meyer TD, Kossmann-Bohm S, Schlottke PF (2004) Do child psychiatrists in Germany diagnose bipolar disorders in children and adolescents? Results from a survey. Bipolar Disord 6(5): 426–431. doi:10.1111/j.1399-5618.2004.00131.x

Mirchandani IC, Young RC (1993) Management of mania in the elderly: an update. Ann Clin Psychiatry 5(1):67–77

Mitchell PB, Loo CK, Gould BM (2010) Diagnosis and monitoring of bipolar disorder in general practice. Med J Aust 193(4 Suppl):S10–S13

Modai I, Bleich A, Gygielman G (1982) Masked depression: an ambiguous entity. Psychother Psychosom 37:235–240

Moller HJ (2006) Evidence for beneficial effects of antidepressants on suicidality in depressive patients: a systematic review. Eur Arch Psychiatry Clin Neurosci 256(6):329–343. doi:10.1007/s00406-006-0650-x

Monfort J (1995) The difficult elderly patient: curable hostile depression or personality disorder? Int Psychogeriatr 7:95–111

Monkman M (1987) Epidemiology of suicide. Epidemiol Rev 9:51–62

Morales OG, Henry ME, Nobler MS, Wassermann EM, Lisanby SH (2005) Electroconvulsive therapy and repetitive transcranial magnetic stimulation in children and adolescents: a review and report of two cases of epilepsia partialis continua. Child Adolesc Psychiatr Clin N Am 14(1):193–210, viii–ix. doi:10.1016/j.chc.2004.07.010, S1056-4993(04)00073-2 [pii]

Murphy E (1994) The course and outcome of depression in late life. In: Schneider L, Reynolds C, Lebowitz B, Friedhoff A (eds) Diagnosis and treatment of depression in late life: results of the NIH Consensus Development Conference. American Psychiatric Press, Washington, DC, pp 81–98

Musetti L, Perugi G, Soriani A, Rossi V, Cassano G (1989) Depression before and after age 65: a re-examination. Br J Psychiatry 155:330–336

Nazroo JY, Edwards AC, Brown GW (1997) Gender differences in the onset of depression following a shared life event: a study of couples. Psychol Med 27(1):9–19

Nelson J, Conwell Y, Kim K, Mazure C (1989) Age at onset in late life delusional depression. Am J Psychiatry 146:785–786

Ng B, Camacho A, Lara DR, Brunstein MG, Pinto OC, Akiskal HS (2008) A case series on the hypothesized connection between dementia and bipolar spectrum disorders: bipolar type VI? J Affect Disord 107(1–3):307–315. doi:10.1016/j.jad.2007.08.018

NIH (1992) Consensus development panel on depression in late life: diagnosis and treatment of depression in late life. JAMA 268:1018–1024

Nivoli AM, Murru A, Pacchiarotti I, Valenti M, Rosa AR, Hidalgo D, Virdis V, Strejilevich S, Vieta E, Colom F (2014) Bipolar disorder in the elderly: a cohort study comparing older and younger patients. Acta Psychiatr Scand. doi:10.1111/acps.12272

Nolen-Hoeksema S, Girgus JS (1994) The emergence of gender differences in depression during adolescence. Psychol Bull 115(3):424–443

Nolen-Hoeksema S, Larson J, Grayson C (1999) Explaining the gender difference in depressive symptoms. J Pers Soc Psychol 77(5):1061–1072

Nolen-Hoeksema S, Stice E, Wade E, Bohon C (2007) Reciprocal relations between rumination and bulimic, substance abuse, and depressive symptoms in female adolescents. J Abnorm Psychol 116(1):198–207. doi:10.1037/0021-843X.116.1.198, 2007-01891-019 [pii]

Nordstrom P, Samuelsson M, Asberg M, Traskman-Bendz L, Aberg-Wistedt A, Nordin C, Bertilsson L (1994) CSF 5-HIAA predicts suicide risk after attempted suicide. Suicide Life Threat Behav 24(1):1–9

Olie E, Seyller M, Beziat S, Loftus J, Bellivier F, Bougerol T, Azorin JM, Gard S, Kahn JP, Passerieux C, Leboyer M, Etain B, Henry C, Courtet P (2014) Clinical and neuropsychological characteristics of euthymic bipolar patients having a history of severe suicide attempt. Acta Psychiatr Scand. doi:10.1111/acps.12326

Ozcan NK, Boyacioglu NE, Enginkaya S, Dinc H, Bilgin H (2014) Reproductive health in women with serious mental illnesses. J Clin Nurs 23(9–10):1283–1291. doi:10.1111/jocn.12332

Ozerdem A, Tunca Z, Cimrin D, Hidiroglu C, Ergor G (2014) Female vulnerability for thyroid function abnormality in bipolar disorder: role of lithium treatment. Bipolar Disord 16(1):72–82. doi:10.1111/bdi.12163

Pampallona S, Bollini P, Tibaldi G, Kupelnick B, Munizza C (2004) Combined pharmacotherapy and psychological treatment for depression: a systematic review. Arch Gen Psychiatry 61(7):714–719

Parker G, Fletcher K, McCraw S, Synnott H, Friend P, Mitchell PB, Hadzi-Pavlovic D (2014) Screening for bipolar disorder: does gender distort scores and case-finding estimates? J Affect Disord 162:55–60. doi:10.1016/j.jad.2014.03.032

Parmelee P, Kleban M, Lawton M, Katz I (1991) Depression and cognitive change among institutionalized aged. Psychol Aging 6:504–511

Parmelee P, Kalz I, Lawton M (1992) Depression and mortality among institutionalized aged. J Gerontol Psychol Sci 47:P3–P10

Pathak S, Findling RL, Earley WR, Acevedo LD, Stankowski J, Delbello MP (2013) Efficacy and safety of quetiapine in children and adolescents with mania associated with bipolar I disorder: a 3-week, double-blind, placebo-controlled trial. J Clin Psychiatry 74(1):e100–e109. doi:10.4088/JCP.11m07424

Philibert RA, Richards L, Lynch CF, Winokur G (1997) The effect of gender and age at onset of depression on mortality. J Clin Psychiatry 58(8):355–360

Phillips DL, Segal BE (1969) Sexual status and psychiatric symptoms. Am Sociol Rev 34(1):58–72

Pike A, Plomin R (1996) Importance of nonshared environmental factors for childhood and adolescent psychopathology. J Am Acad Child Adolesc Psychiatry 35(5):560–570

Prakash O, Kumar CN, Shivakumar PT, Bharath S, Varghese M (2009) Clinical presentation of mania compared with depression: data from a geriatric clinic in India. Int Psychogeriatr 21(4):764–767. doi:10.1017/S1041610209009466

Rabins R, Pearlson G, Aylward E, Kumar A, Dowell K (1991) Cortical magnetic resonance imaging changes in elderly inpatients with major depression. Am J Psychiatry 148:617–620

Rapp S, Parisi S, Walsh D (1988) Psychological dysfunction and physical health among elderly medical inpatients. J Consult Clin Psychol 56:851–855

Rej S, Butters MA, Aizenstein HJ, Begley A, Tsay J, Reynolds CF 3rd, Mulsant BH, Gildengers A (2014) Neuroimaging and neurocognitive abnormalities associated with bipolar disorder in old age. Int J Geriatr Psychiatry 29(4):421–427. doi:10.1002/gps.4021

Reynolds C (1992) Treatment of depression in special populations. J Clin Psychiatry 53(suppl 9):45–53

Rihmer Z (2007) Suicide risk in mood disorders. Curr Opin Psychiatry 20(1):17–22

Rihmer Z, Akiskal H (2006) Do antidepressants t(h)reat(en) depressives? Toward a clinically judicious formulation of the antidepressant-suicidality FDA advisory in light of declining national suicide statistics from many countries. J Affect Disord 94:3–13

Rihmer Z, Pestality P (1999) Bipolar II disorder and suicidal behavior. Psychiatr Clin North Am 22(3):667–673, ix–x

Rihmer Z, Barsi J, Arato M, Demeter E (1990) Suicide in subtypes of primary major depression. J Affect Disord 18(3):221–225

Rihmer Z, Belso N, Kiss K (2002) Strategies for suicide prevention. Curr Opin Psychiatr 15:83–87

Rihmer Z, Gonda X, Fountoulakis KN (2009) Suicide prevention programs through education in the frame of healthcare. Psychiatr Hung 24(6):382–387

Rihmer Z, Gonda X, Rihmer A, Fountoulakis KN (2010) Suicidal and violent behaviour in mood disorders: a major public health problem. A review for the clinician. Int J Psychiatry Clin Pract 14(2):88–94. doi:10.3109/13651501003624712

Roesler TA, McKenzie N (1994) Effects of childhood trauma on psychological functioning in adults sexually abused as children. J Nerv Ment Dis 182(3):145–150

Sackheim H, Prohonik I, Moeller J et al (1993) Regional cerebral blood flow in mood disorders II. Comparison of major depression and Alzheimer's disease. J Nucl Med 34:1090–1101

Sajatovic M, Blow F (2007) Bipolar disorder in later life. The Johns Hopkins University Press, Baltimore

Sajatovic M, Chen P (2011) Geriatric bipolar disorder. Psychiatr Clin North Am 34(2):319–333, vii. doi:10.1016/j.psc.2011.02.007

Sala R, Strober MA, Axelson DA, Gill MK, Castro-Fornieles J, Goldstein TR, Goldstein BI, Ha W, Liao F, Iyengar S, Yen S, Hower H, Hunt J, Dickstein DP, Ryan ND, Keller MB, Birmaher B (2014) Effects of comorbid anxiety disorders on the longitudinal course of pediatric bipolar disorders. J Am Acad Child Adolesc Psychiatry 53(1):72–81. doi:10.1016/j.jaac.2013.09.020

Salloway S, Malloy P, Kohn R, Gillard E, Duffy J, Rogg J, Tung G, Richardson E, Thomas C, Westlake R (1996) MRI and neuropsychological differences in early- and late-life-onset geriatric depression. Neurology 46(6):1567–1574

Samuelsson M, Jokinen J, Nordstrom AL, Nordstrom P (2006) CSF 5-HIAA, suicide intent and hopelessness in the prediction of early suicide in male high-risk suicide attempters. Acta Psychiatr Scand 113(1):44–47

Saunders EF, Nazir R, Kamali M, Ryan KA, Evans S, Langenecker S, Gelenberg AJ, McInnis MG (2014) Gender differences, clinical correlates, and longitudinal outcome of bipolar disorder with comorbid migraine. J Clin Psychiatry 75(5):512–519. doi:10.4088/JCP.13m08623

Saxena S, Fleischmann A (2014) WHO launches the first world suicide report. Lancet (in press)

Schaffer A, Sinyor M, Reis C, Goldstein BI, Levitt AJ (2014) Suicide in bipolar disorder: characteristics and subgroups. Bipolar Disord. doi:10.1111/bdi.12219

Schenkel LS, Chamberlain TF, Towne TL (2014) Impaired theory of mind and psychosocial functioning among pediatric patients with type I versus type II bipolar disorder. Psychiatry Res 215(3):740–746. doi:10.1016/j.psychres.2013.10.025

Seida JC, Schouten JR, Boylan K, Newton AS, Mousavi SS, Beaith A, Vandermeer B, Dryden DM, Carrey N (2012) Antipsychotics for children and young adults: a comparative effectiveness review. Pediatrics 129(3):e771–e784. doi:10.1542/peds.2011-2158

Shah A, De T (1998) Documented evidence of depression in medical and nursing case-notes and its implications in acutely ill geriatric inpatients. Int Psychogeriatr 10(2):163–172

Shulman KI (1997) Disinhibition syndromes, secondary mania and bipolar disorder in old age. J Affect Disord 46(3):175–182

Shulman K, Post F (1980) Bipolar affective disorder in old age. Br J Psychiatry 136:26–32

Shulman KI, Tohen M, Satlin A, Mallya G, Kalunian D (1992) Mania compared with unipolar depression in old age. Am J Psychiatry 149(3):341–345

Snowdon J (1991) A retrospective case-note study of bipolar disorder in old age. Br J Psychiatry 158:485–490

Sondergard L, Lopez AG, Andersen PK, Kessing LV (2007) Continued antidepressant treatment and suicide in patients with depressive disorder. Arch Suicide Res 11(2):163–175

Steffens DC, Krishnan KR (1998) Structural neuroimaging and mood disorders: recent findings, implications for classification, and future directions. Biol Psychiatry 43(10):705–712

Stone K (1989) Mania in the elderly. Br J Psychiatry 155:220–224

Suwalska A, Lojko D (2014) Sex dependence of cognitive functions in bipolar disorder. Scientific World Journal 2014:418432. doi:10.1155/2014/418432

Tariot PN, Podgorski CA, Blazina L, Leibovici A (1993) Mental disorders in the nursing home: another perspective. Am J Psychiatry 150(7):1063–1069

Teixeira AM, Kleinman A, Zanetti M, Jackowski M, Duran F, Pereira F, Lafer B, Busatto GF, Caetano SC (2014) Preserved white matter in unmedicated pediatric bipolar disorder. Neurosci Lett 579:41–45. doi:10.1016/j.neulet.2014.06.061

Tidemalm D, Haglund A, Karanti A, Landen M, Runeson B (2014) Attempted suicide in bipolar disorder: risk factors in a cohort of 6,086 patients. PLoS One 9(4):e94097. doi:10.1371/journal.pone.0094097

Tiihonen J, Lonnqvist J, Wahlbeck K, Klaukka T, Tanskanen A, Haukka J (2006) Antidepressants and the risk of suicide, attempted suicide, and overall mortality in a nationwide cohort. Arch Gen Psychiatry 63(12):1358–1367

Tohen M, Shulman KI, Satlin A (1994) First-episode mania in late life. Am J Psychiatry 151(1):130–132

Tohen M, Kryzhanovskaya L, Carlson G, Delbello M, Wozniak J, Kowatch R, Wagner K, Findling R, Lin D, Robertson-Plouch C, Xu W, Dittmann RW, Biederman J (2007) Olanzapine versus placebo in the treatment of adolescents with bipolar mania. Am J Psychiatry 164(10):1547–1556. doi:10.1176/appi.ajp.2007.06111932

Tondo L, Baldessarini RJ, Hennen J, Minnai GP, Salis P, Scamonatti L, Masia M, Ghiani C, Mannu P (1999) Suicide attempts in major affective disorder patients with comorbid substance use disorders. J Clin Psychiatry 60(Suppl 2):63–69; discussion 75–76, 113–116

Tondo L, Isacsson G, Baldessarini R (2003) Suicidal behaviour in bipolar disorder: risk and prevention. CNS Drugs 17(7):491–511

Tsapakis EM, Soldani F, Tondo L, Baldessarini RJ (2008) Efficacy of antidepressants in juvenile depression: meta-analysis. Br J Psychiatry 193(1):10–17. doi:10.1192/bjp.bp.106.031088, 193/1/10 [pii]

Umamaheswari V, Avasthi A, Grover S (2014) Risk factors for suicidal ideations in patients with bipolar disorder. Bipolar Disord 16(6):642–651. doi:10.1111/bdi.12179

Uradhyaya A, Abou-Saleh M, Wilson K, Grime S, Critchley M (1990) A study of depression in old age using SPECT. Br J Psychiatry 157(suppl 9):76–81

Usala T, Clavenna A, Zuddas A, Bonati M (2008) Randomised controlled trials of selective serotonin reuptake inhibitors in treating depression in children and adolescents: a systematic review and meta-analysis. Eur Neuropsychopharmacol 18(1):62–73. doi:10.1016/j.euroneuro.2007.06.001, S0924-977X(07)00125-3 [pii]

Vaillant G, Orav J, Meyer S, McCullough Vaillant L, Roston D (1996) Late-life consequences of affective spectrum disorder. Int Psychogeriatr 8:13–32

Van Gerpen MW, Johnson JE, Winstead DK (1999) Mania in the geriatric patient population: a review of the literature. Am J Geriatr Psychiatry 7(3):188–202

Van Meter AR, Moreira AL, Youngstrom EA (2011) Meta-analysis of epidemiologic studies of pediatric bipolar disorder. J Clin Psychiatry 72(9):1250–1256. doi:10.4088/JCP.10m06290

Vieta E, Benabarre A, Colom F, Gasto C, Nieto E, Otero A, Vallejo J (1997) Suicidal behavior in bipolar I and bipolar II disorder. J Nerv Ment Dis 185(6):407–409

Wagner KD, Redden L, Kowatch RA, Wilens TE, Segal S, Chang K, Wozniak P, Vigna NV, Abi-Saab W, Saltarelli M (2009) A double-blind, randomized, placebo-controlled trial of divalproex extended-release in the treatment of bipolar disorder in children and adolescents. J Am Acad Child Adolesc Psychiatry 48(5):519–532. doi:10.1097/CHI.0b013e31819c55ec

Weller RA, Weller EB, Tucker SG, Fristad MA (1986) Mania in prepubertal children: has it been underdiagnosed? J Affect Disord 11(2):151–154

Weyerer S, Hafner H, Mann A, Ames D, Graham N (1995) Prevalence and course of depression among elderly residential home admissions in Mannheim and Camden, London. Int Psychogeriatr 7:479–493

WHO (2014) Preventing suicide: a global imperative. World Health Organization, Geneva

Williamson G, Schulz R (1992) Pain, activity restriction and symptoms of depression among community-residing elderly adults. J Gerontol 47:367–372

Williamson DE, Birmaher B, Anderson BP, al-Shabbout M, Ryan ND (1995) Stressful life events in depressed adolescents: the role of dependent events during the depressive episode. J Am Acad Child Adolesc Psychiatry 34(5):591–598

Wozniak J, Biederman J, Kiely K, Ablon JS, Faraone SV, Mundy E, Mennin D (1995) Mania-like symptoms suggestive of childhood-onset bipolar disorder in clinically referred children. J Am Acad Child Adolesc Psychiatry 34(7):867–876. doi:10.1097/00004583-199507000-00010

Yassa R, Nair NP, Iskandar H (1988) Late-onset bipolar disorder. Psychiatr Clin North Am 11(1):117–131

Yerevanian B, Koek R, Feusner J, Hwang S, Mintz J (2004) Antidepressants and suicidal behaviour in unipolar depression. Acta Psychiatr Scand 110:452–458

Young RC (1992) Geriatric mania. Clin Geriatr Med 8(2):387–399

Young RC (1997) Bipolar mood disorders in the elderly. Psychiatr Clin North Am 20(1):121–136

Young RC, Klerman GL (1992) Mania in late life: focus on age at onset. Am J Psychiatry 149(7):867–876

Zimmerman M, Martinez J, Young D, Chelminski I, Morgan TA, Dalrymple K (2014) Comorbid bipolar disorder and borderline personality disorder and history of suicide attempts. J Pers Disord 28(3):358–364. doi:10.1521/pedi_2013_27_122

Creativity and the Position of Bipolar Disorder in Popular Culture 20

20.1 Creativity

20.1.1 The Concept of Creativity

While the word 'creativity' is a word celebrated around the world and its essence is considered to be one of the most valuable properties of human nature, it is very difficult to define its meaning in an operationalized way. The word comes from the Latin verb *creo* (make, create, form) which in turn comes from the Greek word *χειρ* (khir = hand) and the verbs *χερεω* or *χρεω* (khereo or khreo = form or model with hands) (Jackson 1828). However, while the original meaning had to do with handcraft, the modern meaning has to do more with mental work.

There is not one specific universally accepted operationalized definition of creativity. There are many different approaches on the basis of different concepts, theoretical views and objective features. The earlier studies were based on the concept of 'genius' (Lombroso 1891; Ellis 1926; Galton 1892), but this is not the modern approach on the issue. The most reliable index of creativity would be 'creative accomplishments', but this idea is not practical since many ingenious people are not recognized as such until after many years or even after death. Although recognition is considered a key issue for the defining creativity (Csikszentmihalyi 1996), it is important to point out that recognition of creativity is not equivalent to creativity itself. Much debate is in place on this matter. At the end of the day, the common denominator of all definitions for creativity is novelty and originality, but they should be balanced against utility. Creativity in fact is considered as the development of novel solutions which are functional and not simply impressive (Runco 2004). The meaning of 'functional' is also open to interpretation since much creativity has to do with aesthetics and ideas rather than with practical solutions (Figs. 20.1, 20.2, and 20.3) (Andreasen 2008).

Important elements in this development of novel solutions are drive and motivation, but also external favourable factors including opportunities and resources are necessary. Central to creative thinking seems to be the ability for divergent thinking

K.N. Fountoulakis, *Bipolar Disorder: An Evidence-Based Guide to Manic Depression*, DOI 10.1007/978-3-642-37216-2_20

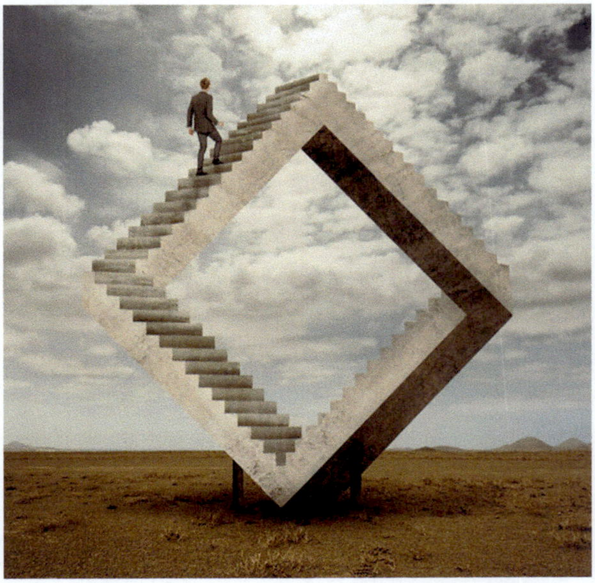

Fig. 20.1 An example of impossible geometry. Creativity demands unusual thought procedures and breaking of the rules of everyday life

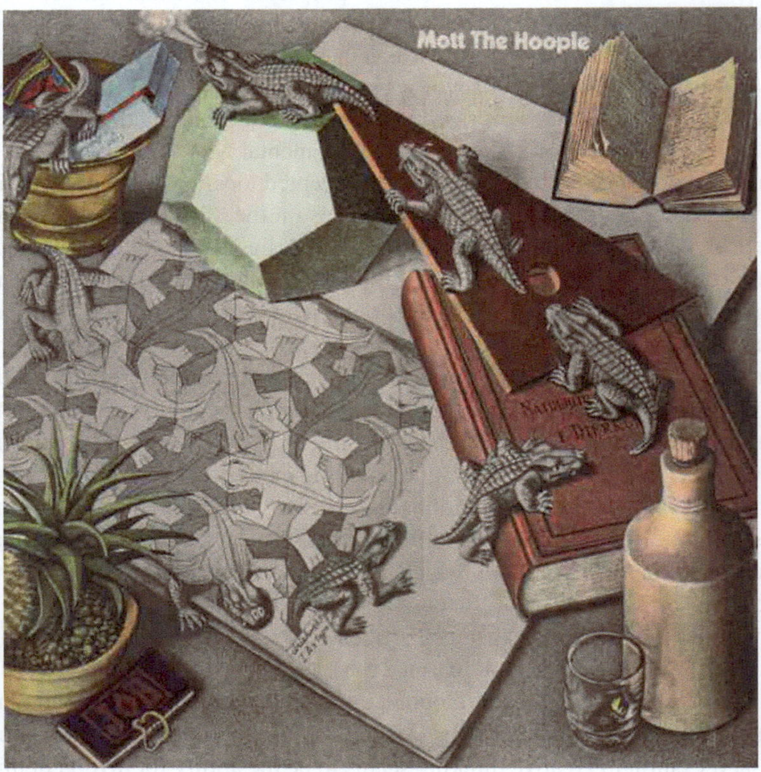

Fig. 20.2 A modified version of the drawing 'reptiles' by Maurits Cornelis Escher originally printed in 1943

Fig. 20.3 Hand with reflecting sphere by Maurits Cornelis Escher (1935)

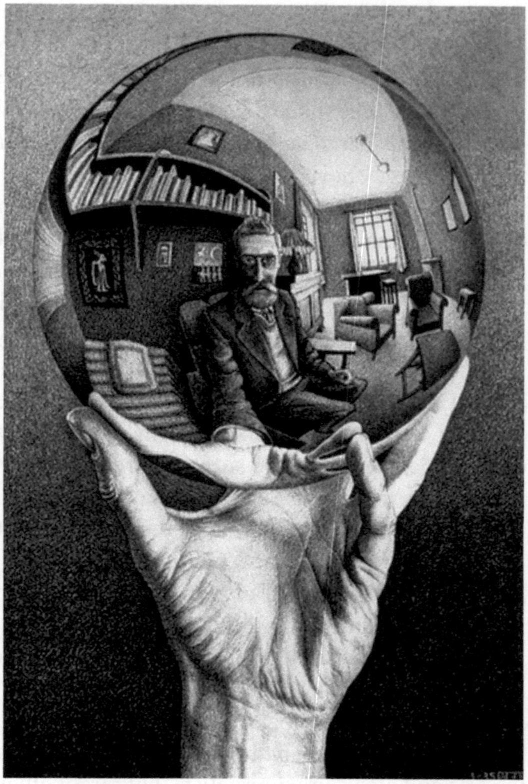

which refers to the ability to generate novel and variable solutions. On the contrary, convergent thinking refers to the ability to find the only one correct solution or answer. This is probably the reason why IQ scores are poor predictors of creativity (Terman et al. 1925–1959). In this frame, it is believed that creative thinking emerges from the ability to combine conceptually distinct associative elements in a novel manner (Mednick 1962) and from a willingness and flexibility to consider atypical and unusual associations (Eysenck and Furnham 1993), but at the same time from the coexisting ability to concentrate, complete the task and test the solution against reality. The presence of unusual combinations of talents might be an important factor in the way the concept of 'multiple intelligences' proposed (Gardner 1999).

Probably, the procedures which define creativity include both an insight-based 'unconscious' element and an analytical conscious element. The paradigms that can be found in the literature are often conflicting, but they seem to converge in the above.

20.1.2 The Philosophical and Journalistic Approach

The belief that there is a link between creativity and madness is so ancient that it is depicted in many myths of different cultures. A recurring theme in ancient myths is the gifted individual persecuted by the Gods. The coexistence of mental illness and creativity is positioned in this frame. For the first time, it is systematically mentioned and supported in the teachings of Socrates and the writings of Plato, but it was Aristotle who made the most important contribution. Technique and skills alone were not considered sufficient for a man to be creative; the gift of a different way of thinking was believed to be the key. So it seems that the essence of creativity was well understood since antiquity. Aristotle suggested that this difference in the way of thinking should be so profound that melancholia and even madness were necessary conditions. Along this line of thought, the book 'On the Sacred Disease' which is part of the Hippocratic Corpus attributes genius and talent to people suffering from epileptic fits and considers epilepsy a gift by the Gods.

Since then, there was much controversy on the issue. Probably there was some kind of naïve romanticization involved in the overemphasizing of this relationship between creativity and madness, fuelled at least partially by the lives of several eminent people who were suffering from BD. It is difficult to be sure of the kind of their illness today, after centuries have passed since their deaths; however, it seems that the list includes Martin Luther (1483–1546), Sir Isaac Newton (Fig. 20.4; 1642–1726), Lord George Gordon Byron (Fig. 20.5; 1788–1824) and Friedrich Nietzsche (1844–1900), among others. It is important to note the prevalence of neurosyphilis during these times, before the era of antibiotics. Many of those eminent people who eventually developed some type of mental disease were most probably suffering from the late stages of syphilitic infection rather than BD or schizophrenia. A number of well-known people today have announced or indirectly let be publically known that they are suffering from BD. Most of them are people in the arts and also some journalists, but rarely other types of successful career people make similar announcements. The reliability of these announcements remains questionable in the majority of cases. Two historical cases are rather beyond dispute: Virginia Woolf (Fig. 20.6; 1882–1941) and Ernest Hemingway (Fig. 20.7; 1899–1961).

Virginia Woolf was suffering from repeated mood episodes and eventually during a depressive episode with psychotic features, as she revealed in a note she left behind, on 28 March 1941 she filled her coat pockets with stones and committed suicide by falling into the river Ouse near her home. Her father was probably suffering from cyclothymia, while her whole family from the side of her father seemed to manifest some kind of mental problems with her half-sister suffering probably from childhood schizophrenia and one of her cousins having probably manic depression insanity. They both died in an asylum. Virginia Woolf experienced her first manic episode at the age of 13 which later turned into mixed and lasted at least 2 years. The second episode came at the age of 22 after the death of her father, and the descriptions suggest it was an agitated psychotic mania which lasted for several months. Probably depressive features were also present since she attempted suicide for the first time by launching herself off a first floor window. A third episode and a second attempt occurred at age 31, but it seems that after that and until her death, no overt episodes happened, although some kind of chronic subthreshold depression was present. Some descriptions are also suggestive of hypomanic periods and

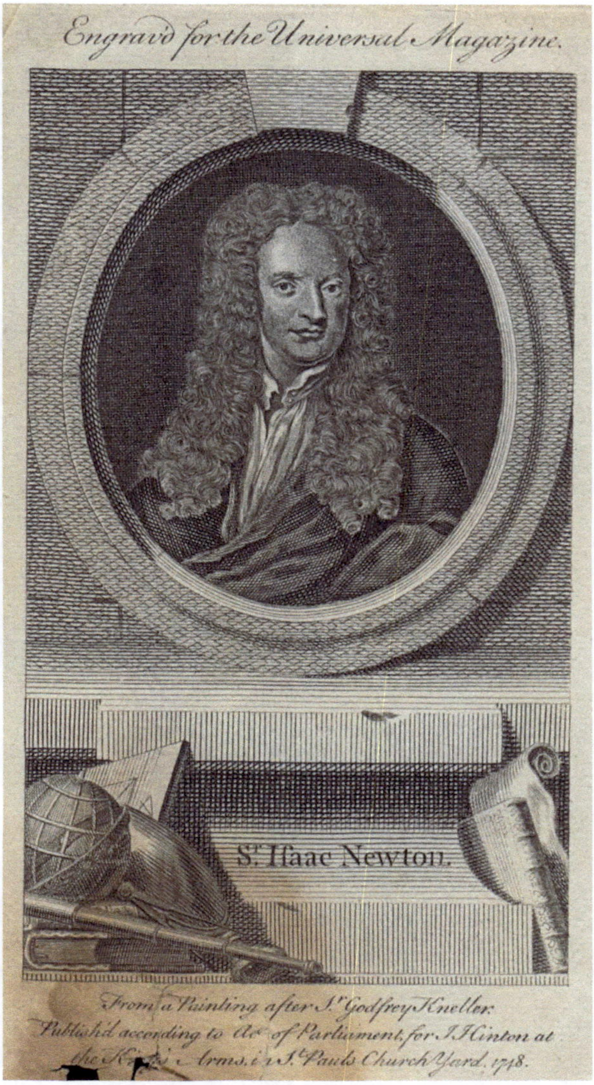

Fig. 20.4 Sir Isaac Newton (1642–1726)

cyclothymia. The symptomatology around the period of her death might suggest the presence of a hyperthymic episode, during which she completed writing her last book, followed by a major depressive episode with hallucinations which were giving her the command to kill herself (Koutsantoni 2012; Bond 1985).

Ernest Hemingway is a prominent figure in the international literature. He won the Nobel Prize in Literature in 1954. The study of his biography suggests that he was suffering from BD, alcohol abuse, traumatic brain injury and probably borderline and narcissistic personality traits. Biographies also suggest that his mother was dressing and treating him like a girl to a problematic degree and until he was relatively a grown kid (Fig. 20.8). Probably he experienced his first manic episode at the

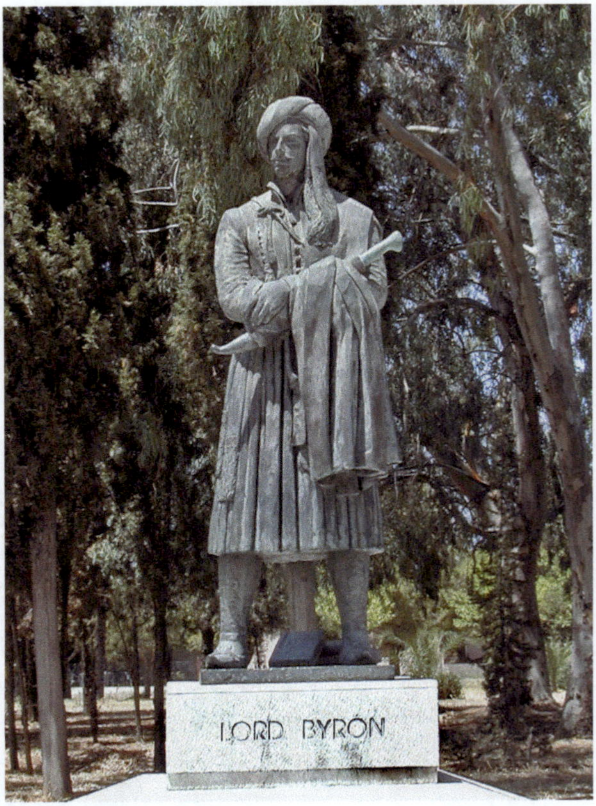

Fig. 20.5 George Gordon Byron (1788–1824) 6th Baron Byron, commonly known simply as Lord Byron. Lord Byron took active participation in the Greek revolution (1821) and died during it. The statue with Lord Byron wearing a local costume is positioned in the Park of Heroes of the revolution in the city of Messolonghi, Greece

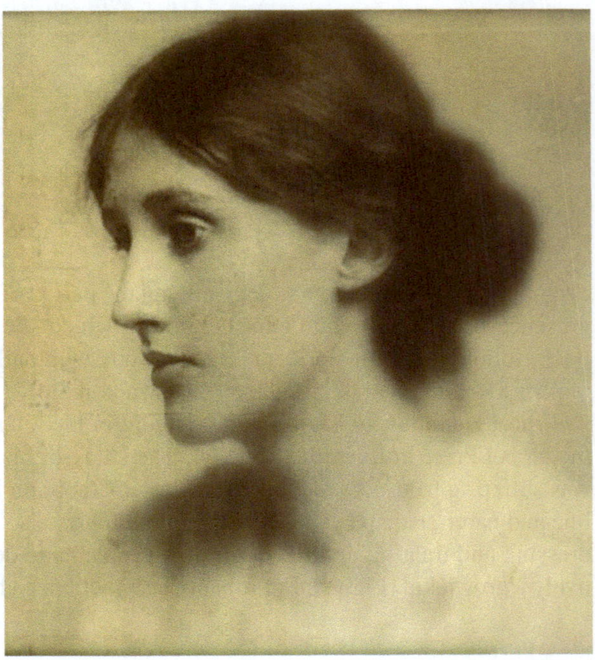

Fig. 20.6 Adeline Virginia Woolf (1882–1941)

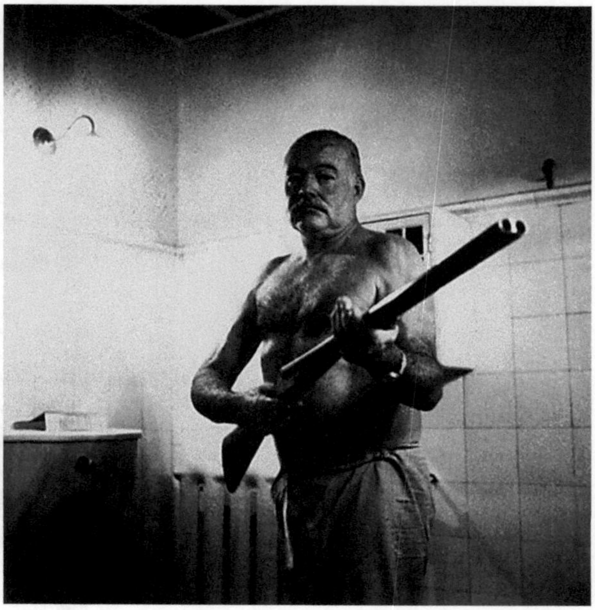

Fig. 20.7 Ernest Miller Hemingway (1899–1961) posing with the same rifle he used to take his life. One of the many photos in which Hemingway was posing in an extreme masculine way as hunter, fisherman or boxer

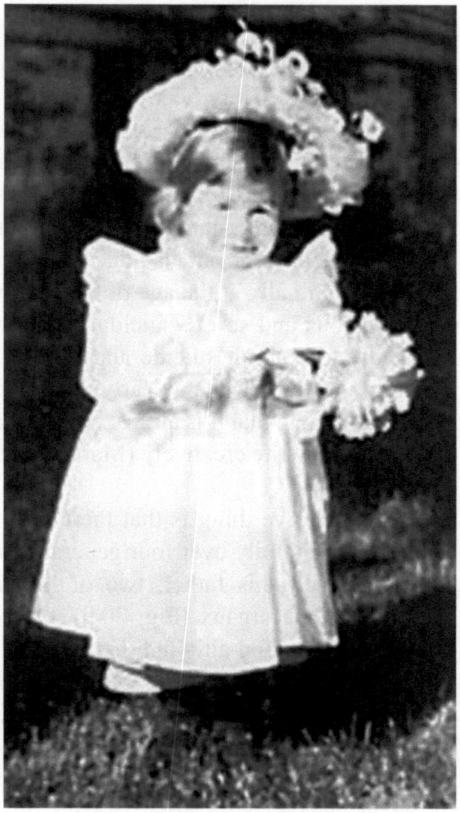

Fig. 20.8 Ernest Hemingway in a photo from 1901 at the age of 2. At that time, it was usual to dress also boys in girl's clothes with dress, probably for practical reasons. However, his mother went to extremes, specifically decorating him as a girl. Note the flower hat, unusual for a boy

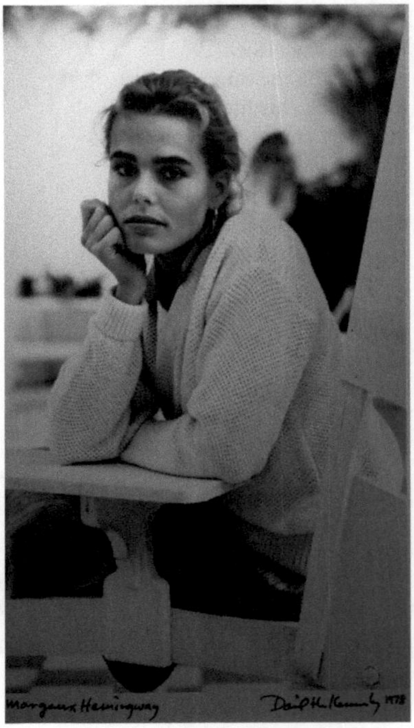

Fig. 20.9 Margaux Louise Hemingway (1954–1996)

age of 25 and the first major depressive episode (with mixed features) at the age of 36 although it is likely he was never free of subthreshold symptoms. A constant feature in his biographies is that his mood was continuously switching from megalomania to melancholy. Suicidal ideation probably arose in his late 20s. He suffered from concussion after a traffic accident at the age of 45. This was one of the two most severe in a number of head traumas he experienced in his life, due to a risk-taking behaviour but also due to alcohol abuse. The second one included skull fracture. Eventually at the age of 61, he developed severe depression with persecutory delusions and severe suicidal ideation. He was repeatedly hospitalized, tried repeatedly to commit suicide and treated with ECT. A few days after discharge, seemingly well, he woke up early in the morning and shot himself to the head. It is important to note that it is almost certain that during the last few years of his life, he was unable to write creatively (Martin 2006; Pearson 1997; Craig 1995; Yalom and Yalom 1971).

The impressive thing is that there have been five confirmed suicides in Ernest Hemingway's family over four generations, while another two are probable. These include himself, his father, two of his siblings (Ursula and Leicester) and his granddaughter Margaux (Fig. 20.9). One of his sisters, Marceline, was suffering from depression and although her death is considered to be due to natural causes, the family suspected suicide. Out of six siblings, three and possibly a fourth died of suicide. It is unclear whether his sun Gregory, who suffered from depression, had a sex change operation and died in 2001 as a transsexual named Gloria, actually committed suicide. From his granddaughters, Muffet is suffering from schizophrenia and Mariel has repeatedly announced publically that she is dealing with a number of mental problems. The third granddaughter Margaux suffered from depression, epilepsy, bulimia and alcoholism. She committed suicide on 1 July 1996, 1 day before the anniversary of her grandfather's suicide. Alcohol and drug abuse and reported sexual abuse seem to be widespread within the family. Also Ernest's second wife Pauline Pfeifer Hemingway was the sixth confirmed suicidal victim in the family (but not from the same bloodline).

Overall, the biographical research, as well as studies of living artists and writers, has provided insight into the relationship between creativity and BD. It seems that Emil Kraepelin and William James were right in pointing out that only the milder forms of insanity could be related to creativity, while the more severe forms have a devastating effect on the mental abilities of the patients. However, the research based on biographical information is severely flawed and methodologically problematic. It is clear that the vast majority of bipolar patients are not creative and the vast majority of creative people are not bipolar. Biographies report selective parts of the lives of selected people and thus are prone to bias. Thus, they can give only some hints for further research which will demand the utilization of large and well-designed population-based studies (Jamison 2011).

20.1.3 The Scientific Approach

20.1.3.1 Rates of BD in Creative Individuals

The traditional approach in the study of the relationship between creativity and mood disorders is the systematic study of biographical information and so far has provided data confirming the high rates of BD in a wide range of creative individuals, from poets to jazz musicians (Jamison 1993; Schildkraut et al. 1994; Post 1994; Ludwig 1992, 1995; Ellis 1926; Juda 1949; Akiskal 2012). However, as mentioned above, this method the study samples are convenient rather than representative, and the information are probably biased, incomplete and often inaccurate. It is impossible to extract data concerning the diagnosis on the basis of modern classification systems from studies of this kind which took place before the 1960s, while the composition of the control group remains a challenge.

There are only a few studies that utilized a rigorous methodology and included highly creative individuals using personal interviews in comparison to a noncreative control group. The majority of these studies have examined writers. Overall the results suggest that the rate of both unipolar and bipolar mood disorders is higher in creative individuals in comparison to controls (Jones et al. 2014).

Research data suggest that the rates of mood disorder and alcohol abuse are extremely high in writers with 80 % suffering from any type of mood disorder and 30 % suffering from BD-I or BD-II (Andreasen 1987). According to another study, it seems that a significant percentage of writes had received some kind of treatment with playwrights having the highest rate (63 %). More than half had received psychotherapy rather than medication, and this might reflect one of the biases inherent in this kind of studies because of the distinct preferences of the study participants. According to the same study, the poets was the subgroup which had the highest rate of medication treatment for mood disorder (33 %) and also the only group to have received treatment for mania (Jamison 1989). A third study reported high rates of both depression (56 %) and mania (19 %) in writers (Ludwig 1994).

Similar findings were reported concerning jazz musicians (Wills 2003), while an in-depth analysis of the lives and works of a number of jazz musicians from Memphis, Tennessee, suggested that the presence of cyclothymia was a decisive factor, while no overt BD was present in any of them. The suffering from all kinds of mood symptoms was clearly reflected in their songs (Akiskal 2012).

A large epidemiological study analysed interview data from the Epidemiologic Catchment Area Study and reported that individuals with BD were disproportionately concentrated in the most creative occupational categories. Of course having a creative occupation is different from being creative as a person; however, it should be considered a fair approximation (Tremblay et al. 2010). A more recent large, well-designed prospective population study also reported a disproportionately high rate of mental illness and especially BD in creative individuals (Kyaga et al. 2011), but further analysis restricted these findings to writers and not to persons with supposedly creative occupations (Kyaga et al. 2013).

20.1.3.2 Level of Creativity in BD Patients

From a different point of view, a study of non-eminent individuals, reported higher creativity scores in patients with BD and cyclothymia in comparison to controls (Richards et al. 1988). A second study confirmed the presence of these high creativity scores in BD patients (Rybakowski and Klonowska 2011), while a third one suggested these high scores are present even during an acute manic or mixed state at least in comparison to acute depression. This last study also suggested that creativity was correlated with executive function but not with IQ (Soeiro-de-Souza et al. 2011). However, since the validity of creativity scales is problematic, the meaning of these findings is open to interpretations.

The first study to show that children with BD or at high risk to develop BD have higher creativity than healthy control children was published in 2005 and reported that these children had an enhanced ability to experience and express dislike of simple and symmetric images, suggesting the presence of an increased access to negative affect. This trait could be both an advantage since it provides with affective energy for creative achievement, but it could also represent a vulnerability factor for the development of mood disorders (Simeonova et al. 2005). From a similar perspective, a prospective, 10-year, whole-population cohort study from Sweden reported that those who demonstrated excellent school performance were at a four times higher risk to develop BD in comparison to those who showed only an average level of performance. Persons with excellence in language or music were at a particularly increased risk. Interestingly, schizophrenia was associated with a decreased rate of excellence (MacCabe et al. 2010). Also, spirituality, empathy, creativity, realism and resilience were reported to be enhanced in BD patients (Galvez et al. 2011) as are sociability and verbal functioning (Higier et al. 2014).

It is interesting that the vast majority (82 %) of BD patients confirmed they were feeling being creative when hypomanic and were engaging in writing, painting, work or business ideas and art in general. The rates were similar for BD-I and BD-II. What is more interesting is that the effect of mania was not stable and often destructive, while hypomania was constantly correlated to improved focus and clarity of mind. All patients reported creative personality styles most often when free of major symptomatology (McCraw et al. 2013).

20.1.3.3 Creativity in Families of BD Probands

A number of studies support the concept that creativity and mental illness but especially BD co-segregate in families (Andreasen 1987; Richards et al. 1988; Jamison 2011).

The first study to report such a loading in families was published in 1987 and reported that the first-degree relatives of the writers were more likely to suffer from mood disorders, and they also were more likely to be creative in comparison to controls (Andreasen 1987). A second study reported higher creativity scores in the normal first-degree relatives of patients with BD or cyclothymia in comparison to controls (Richards et al. 1988) and another one reported that the children in bipolar families are more creative than control children (Simeonova et al. 2005).

Finally, Kyaga et al. reported that the non-affective first-degree relatives of people with BD and schizophrenia, but not of people with unipolar depression, were more likely than controls to hold creative jobs. The maternal or paternal type of relationship was not significant, but the familial distance was suggesting that a biological substrate is responsible for this cosegregation (Kyaga et al. 2011, 2013).

20.1.4 Possible Mediating Mechanisms Between Creativity and BD

As discussed in the respective chapters, mania especially when accompanied by psychotic features has a profound effect on the neurocognitive function. On the other hand, not only it is known that IQ and 'hard' neurocognition do not seem to strongly correlate with creativity, but also it is possible that in milder cases, the 'at the edge' lifestyle and peculiarities in thinking in combination with the experiencing of extreme emotions have a major role in the emergence and expression of creativity.

It is mild mania and especially hypomania which are related with creativity while the role of psychotic features is unknown. Just as a brief note, both Virginia Woolf and Ernest Hemingway were experiencing psychotic features. It is also important to note that most creative people do not suffer from any mental illness and most psychiatric patients are not creative. This holds true also concerning BD. The key issue is that the coexistence of BD and creativity is rather disproportional, especially in highly creative persons.

This puts forward the most vital question: Are some people eminent *because* they suffer from bipolar spectrum disorders? Or is the higher prevalence of the bipolar spectrum in certain groups of creative people the result of some kind of selection, that is, are people suffering from BD and related disorders more likely to choose certain jobs and lifestyles? It is important to stress that in order for creativity to flourish and give fruits, it needs great amounts of hard work, ability to concentrate and discipline, and to say it in other words, it needs some kind of obsessive personality-type traits.

A second important question is whether BD or some of its endophenotypes constitute an evolutionary advantage. Since studies have shown that this relationship is probably neurobiologically based (McNeil 1971), it is possible that mood disorders constitute the extreme manifestation of a pool of genes which also determines genius and creativity (Akiskal and Akiskal 2007), with cyclothymic features playing a major role (Vellante et al. 2011; Srivastava et al. 2010; Akiskal and Akiskal 2005) but moderated by obsessional traits (Akiskal et al. 2005). Isolated features probably related to this gene pool have been detected in a number of studies. For example, creative Harvard students had much lower inhibition scores in comparison to less creative students (Carson et al. 2003), while impulsivity in general has been linked with creativity (Baas et al. 2008).

One possible explanation in terms of neurocognitive function is that mania and hypomania increase associational fluency, divergent and combinatory thinking in a loose but extravagant and elaborated way, as well as cognitive flexibility accompanied by humour, flippancy and playfulness (Guilford 1957; Christensen et al. 1957; Henry et al. 1971; Pons et al. 1985; Levine et al. 1996; Shenton et al. 1987; Solovay et al. 1987; Baas et al. 2008; Strong et al. 2007). Other features of manic states including risk-taking, grandiosity, restlessness and discontent, illness-induced introspection and a need to make meaning of, or to ameliorate, suffering could be the pathways linking BD with creativity possibly with the mediating effect of temperament (Jamison 1993; Santosa et al. 2007). Additionally, impulsivity and openness to experience seem to be of importance (Strong et al. 2007; Baas et al. 2008).

The problematic definitions make interpretations difficult. In this case, both the concept of 'creativity' as well as the definitions of many neurocognitive abilities including IQ and executive function, suffer from vagueness. Thus, the understanding of the interplay between neurocognitive, perceptual, mood and behavioural changes related to altered mood states are of prime importance (Parker 2014; Jamison 1989). Probably creativity is not a trait feature of BD but rather fluctuates in concert with mood changes (Lovejoy and Steuerwald 1995).

20.1.5 The Effect of Treatment and Other Ethical Considerations

If BD and its clinical manifestations are related with creativity, then the obvious next question is whether successful treatment kills creativity especially in highly gifted individuals. Where there be a Virginia Woolf or a Nobel Laureate Ernest Hemingway if proper modern treatment was available at that time? What about the future? At some time in the (not so) near future, there might be prevention of BD in terms of genetic engineering or very early treatment. Will this have a direct effect on human culture with the extinction of a subgroup of people with high creativity but also suffering from BD? Is it ethical? Will treating or even eradicating one of the most devastating diseases human kind is currently struggling with come at a very high cost for humanity?

These are questions still open to debate, but the debate cannot be based on opinions or romantic assumptions in the dawn of the era of evidence-based psychiatry. On the other hand, such a debate will provide with valuable guidance on which aspects of treatment are especially unacceptable and problematic and which are those 'positive' features of bipolar disorders that should be preserved or protected.

One possible conclusion from the literature is that bipolar persons are most creative when their symptoms are under good control (Schou 1979; Jones et al. 2014; Andreasen and Glick 1988) and, as in the case of Hemingway, loss of creativity by passing the years and by accumulation of insults and eventually premature death can be avoided. Losing creative individuals is a tragedy for human society (Jamison 1993). The biography of Robert Lowell (1917–1977), which was a great American poet, suggests that he was more creative after he had started treatment with lithium (Andreasen 2008). However, some patients feel that medication blunts their neurocognitive abilities and destroys their creativity in addition to their longing for hypomanic or manic periods or even for their depressions (Pickering 1974).

It is of outmost importance that the therapist should be listening to the patients' worries and subjective experiences and should be willing and ready to work together with them to optimize the treatment effect and minimize the undesirable consequences (Murray and Johnson 2010).

20.2 The Place of BD in Popular Culture

BD together with schizophrenia has a prominent place in popular culture. On one hand, this has a negative face; the aggressive dark side of the disease is depicted and often issues like death and suicidality are used to provoke and stimulate (Fig. 20.10). On the other hand, BD has become together with depression some kind of fashion with many famous people declaring openly in the mass media that they suffer from these disorders. This is a status clearly better than that of schizophrenia which essentially is not yet accepted and carries a heavy negative stigma. Lists of famous people supposedly suffering from BD can be found in the internet, but for many of them, the information is weak and unreliable.

Below is a list of some of the most important films having BD as a main theme:

- *Running from Crazy* (2013) is a documentary film by director Barbara Kopple about the family of Nobel Prize-winning author Ernest Hemingway.
- Vincente Minnelli's *Lust for Life* (1956) starring Kirk Douglas and Anthony Quinn. The film is a biography of Vincent van Gogh, based on the novel by Irving Stone, with Kirk Douglas in the role of the tortured artistic genius.
- Graeme Clifford's *Frances* (1982) with Jessica Lange, Sam Shepard, and Kim Stanley. Jessica Lange has the role of the 1930s Hollywood star Frances Farmer who ended up in an asylum.

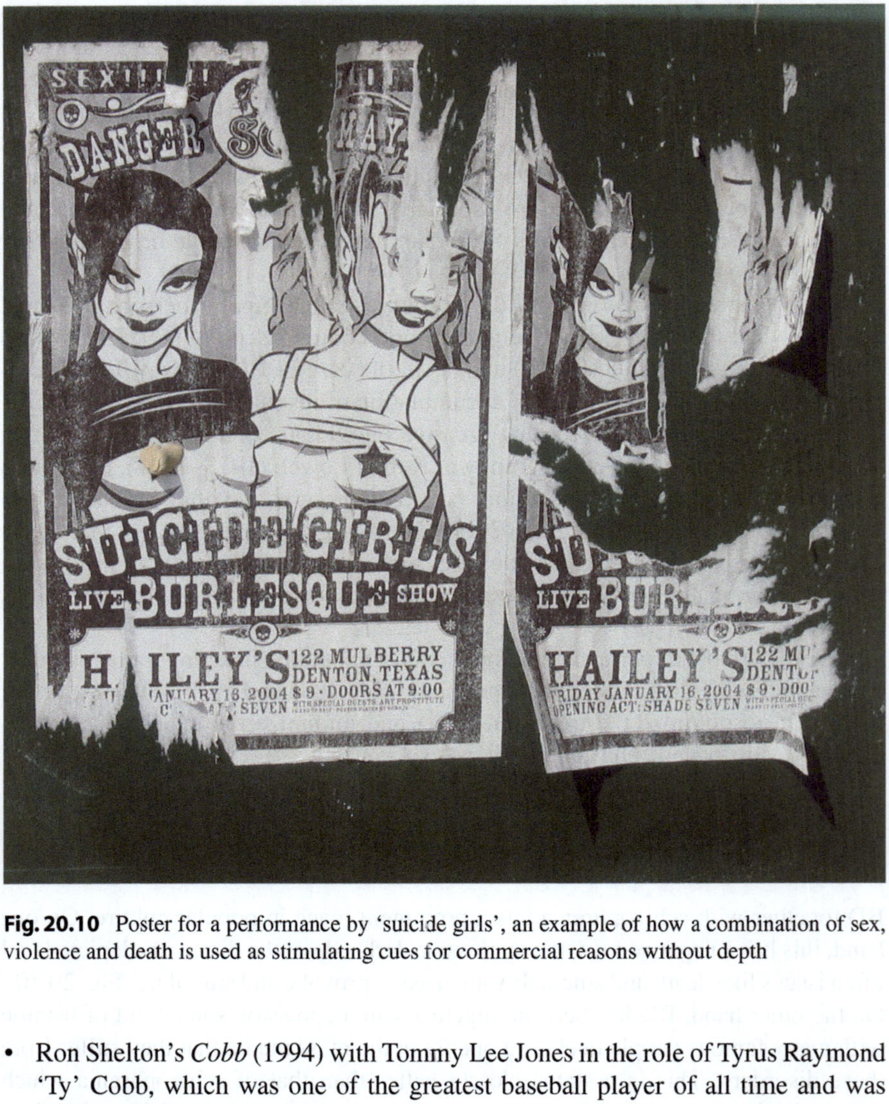

Fig. 20.10 Poster for a performance by 'suicide girls', an example of how a combination of sex, violence and death is used as stimulating cues for commercial reasons without depth

- Ron Shelton's *Cobb* (1994) with Tommy Lee Jones in the role of Tyrus Raymond 'Ty' Cobb, which was one of the greatest baseball player of all time and was treated with lithium
- Jeff Feuerzeig's *The Devil and Daniel Johnston* (2005) with Daniel Johnston, Matt Groening, Freddie Mercury and Thurston Moore. A complex documentary on Daniel Johnston's manic–depressive illness, creativity and family support.
- Irvin Kershner's *A Fine Madness* (1966) with Sean Connery and Joanne Woodward. Sean Connery has the role of genius poet Samson Shillitoe who is recommended lobotomy, in a movie full of pop culture clichés about 'madness' (Fig. 20.11).
- Mike Figgis' *Mr Jones* (1993) with Richard Gere, Lena Olin, Anne Bancroft and Bill Pullman. Richard Gere has the role of Mr. Jones who suffers from BD, and

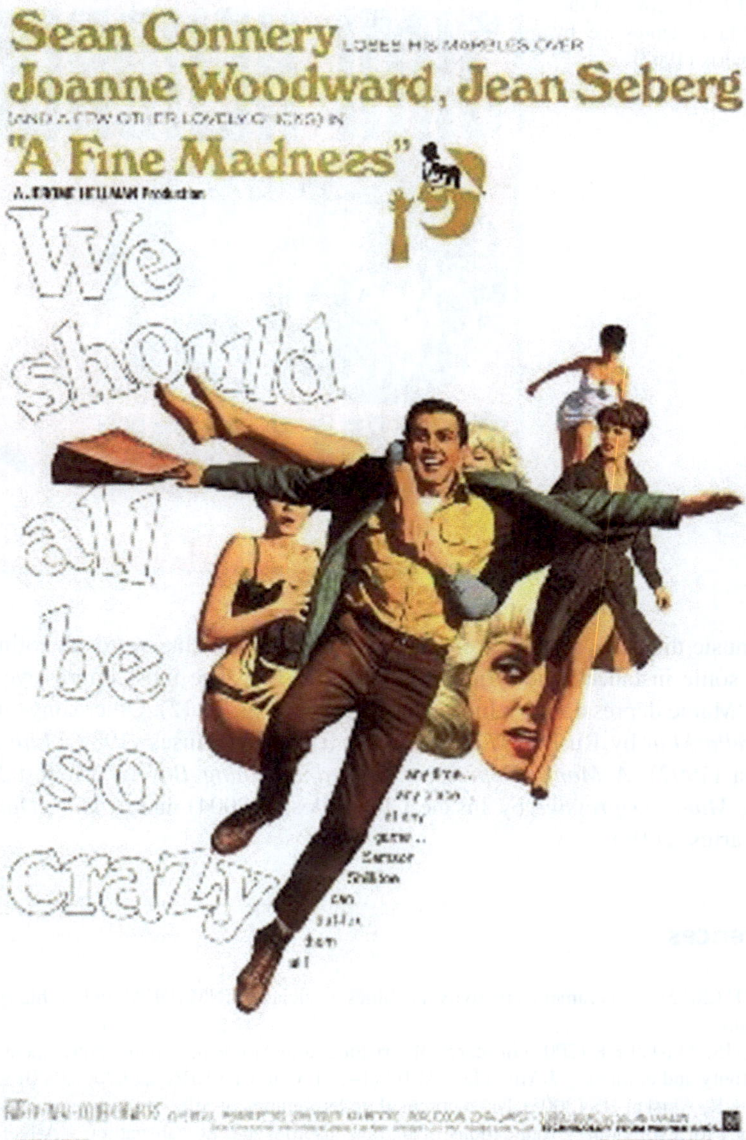

Fig. 20.11 The poster of the movie 'A fine madness' by Irvin Kershner with Sean Connery (1966)

Lena Olin has the role of the psychiatrist who eventually falls in love with him. Essentially, the film spins around a doctor–patient romance.

- Antonia Bird's *Mad Love* (1995) with Drew Barrymore, Joan Allen and Chris O'Donnell. Drew Barrymore has the role of Casey, who suffers from BD (though the film suggests only depression) with antisocial behaviour and severe suicidal thoughts. This is a film for teens, again full of clichés.

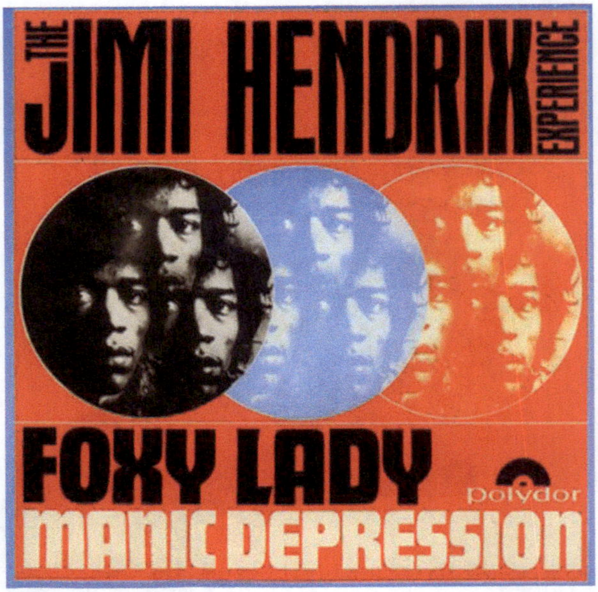

Fig. 20.12 The cover of the album 'Manic-depressive' by Jimi Hendrix (1967)

In music there are a number of songs and albums utilizing words denoting BD, and in some instances, the lyrics really refer to BD. The most impressive is the album 'Manic depression' by Jimi Hendrix (1967; Fig. 20.12). Other songs include *Cinderella Man* by Rush (1977), *Mania* by Throwing Muses (1989), *Lithium* by Nirvana (1992), *A Manic Depressive Named Laughing Boy* by Modest Mouse (1996), *Manic Depressive* by Insane Clown Posse (2004) and *Maniac Dance* by Stratovarius (2005).

References

Akiskal H (2012) Temperament, creativity and blues musicians. UNM IDEAS in Psychiatry Public Lecture

Akiskal HS, Akiskal KK (2007) In search of Aristotle: temperament, human nature, melancholia, creativity and eminence. J Affect Disord 100(1–3):1–6. doi:10.1016/j.jad.2007.04.013

Akiskal KK, Akiskal HS (2005) The theoretical underpinnings of affective temperaments: implications for evolutionary foundations of bipolar disorder and human nature. J Affect Disord 85(1–2):231–239. doi:10.1016/j.jad.2004.08.002

Akiskal KK, Savino M, Akiskal HS (2005) Temperament profiles in physicians, lawyers, managers, industrialists, architects, journalists, and artists: a study in psychiatric outpatients. J Affect Disord 85(1–2):201–206. doi:10.1016/j.jad.2004.08.003

Andreasen NC (1987) Creativity and mental illness: prevalence rates in writers and their first-degree relatives. Am J Psychiatry 144(10):1288–1292

Andreasen NC (2008) The relationship between creativity and mood disorders. Dialogues Clin Neurosci 10(2):251–255

Andreasen NC, Glick ID (1988) Bipolar affective disorder and creativity: implications and clinical management. Compr Psychiatry 29(3):207–217

Baas M, De Dreu CK, Nijstad BA (2008) A meta-analysis of 25 years of mood-creativity research: hedonic tone, activation, or regulatory focus? Psychol Bull 134(6):779–806. doi:10.1037/a0012815

Bond AH (1985) Virginia Woolf: manic-depressive psychosis and genius. An illustration of separation-individuation theory. J Am Acad Psychoanal 13(2):191–210

Carson SH, Peterson JB, Higgins DM (2003) Decreased latent inhibition is associated with increased creative achievement in high-functioning individuals. J Pers Soc Psychol 85(3): 499–506. doi:10.1037/0022-3514.85.3.499

Christensen PR, Guilford JP, Wilson RC (1957) Relations of creative responses to working time and instructions. J Exp Psychol 53(2):82–88

Craig RJ (1995) Contributions to psychohistory: XXIII. Hemingway "analyzed". Psychol Rep 76(3 Pt 2):1059–1079. doi:10.2466/pr0.1995.76.3c.1059

Csikszentmihalyi M (1996) Creativity: flow and the psychology of discovery and invention. Harper Collins, New York

Ellis H (1926) A study of British genius. Houghton-Mifflin, New York

Eysenck HJ, Furnham A (1993) Personality and the Barron-Welsh Art Scale. Percept Mot Skills 76(3 Pt 1):837–838. doi:10.2466/pms.1993.76.3.837

Galton F (1892) Hereditary genius. Macmillan and Company, London

Galvez JF, Thommi S, Ghaemi SN (2011) Positive aspects of mental illness: a review in bipolar disorder. J Affect Disord 128(3):185–190. doi:10.1016/j.jad.2010.03.017

Gardner H (1999) Intelligence reframed: multiple Intelligences for the twenty-first century. Basic Books, New York

Guilford JP (1957) Creative abilities in the arts. Psychol Rev 64(2):110–118

Henry GM, Weingartner H, Murphy DL (1971) Idiosyncratic patterns of learning and word association during mania. Am J Psychiatry 128(5):564–574

Higier RG, Jimenez AM, Hultman CM, Borg J, Roman C, Kizling I, Larsson H, Cannon TD (2014) Enhanced neurocognitive functioning and positive temperament in twins discordant for bipolar disorder. Am J Psychiatry. doi:10.1176/appi.ajp.2014.13121683

Jackson F (1828) An etymological dictionary of the Latin language. VALPY, London

Jamison K (1993) Touched with fire. Manic-depressive illness and the artistic temperament. The Free Press, New York

Jamison KR (1989) Mood disorders and patterns of creativity in British writers and artists. Psychiatry 52(2):125–134

Jamison KR (2011) Great wits and madness: more near allied? Br J Psychiatry 199(5):351–352. doi:10.1192/bjp.bp.111.100586

Jones S, Dodd A, Gruber J (2014) Development and validation of a new multidimensional measure of inspiration: associations with risk for bipolar disorder. PLoS One 9(3):e91669. doi:10.1371/journal.pone.0091669

Juda A (1949) The relationship between high mental capacity and psychic abnormalities. Am J Psychiatry 106:296–307

Koutsantoni K (2012) Manic depression in literature: the case of Virginia Woolf. Med Humanit 38(1):7–14. doi:10.1136/medhum-2011-010075

Kyaga S, Landen M, Boman M, Hultman CM, Langstrom N, Lichtenstein P (2013) Mental illness, suicide and creativity: 40-year prospective total population study. J Psychiatr Res 47(1):83–90. doi:10.1016/j.jpsychires.2012.09.010

Kyaga S, Lichtenstein P, Boman M, Hultman C, Langstrom N, Landen M (2011) Creativity and mental disorder: family study of 300,000 people with severe mental disorder. Br J Psychiatry 199(5):373–379. doi:10.1192/bjp.bp.110.085316

Levine J, Schild K, Kimhi R, Schreiber G (1996) Word associative production in affective versus schizophrenic psychoses. Psychopathology 29(1):7–13

Lombroso C (1891) The man of genius. Walter Scott, London

Lovejoy MC, Steuerwald BL (1995) Subsyndromal unipolar and bipolar disorders: comparisons on positive and negative affect. J Abnorm Psychol 104(2):381–384

Ludwig A (1995) The price of greatness: resolving the creativity and madness controversy. Guilford Press, New York

Ludwig AM (1992) Creative achievement and psychopathology: comparison among professions. Am J Psychother 46(3):330–356

Ludwig AM (1994) Mental illness and creative activity in female writers. Am J Psychiatry 151(11):1650–1656

MacCabe JH, Lambe MP, Cnattingius S, Sham PC, David AS, Reichenberg A, Murray RM, Hultman CM (2010) Excellent school performance at age 16 and risk of adult bipolar disorder: national cohort study. Br J Psychiatry 196(2):109–115. doi:10.1192/bjp.bp.108.060368

Martin CD (2006) Ernest Hemingway: a psychological autopsy of a suicide. Psychiatry 69(4): 351–361. doi:10.1521/psyc.2006.69.4.351

McCraw S, Parker G, Fletcher K, Friend P (2013) Self-reported creativity in bipolar disorder: prevalence, types and associated outcomes in mania versus hypomania. J Affect Disord 151(3):831–836. doi:10.1016/j.jad.2013.07.016

McNeil TF (1971) Prebirth and postbirth influence on the relationship between creative ability and recorded mental illness. J Pers 39(3):391–406

Mednick SA (1962) The associative basis of the creative process. Psychol Rev 69:220–232

Murray G, Johnson SL (2010) The clinical significance of creativity in bipolar disorder. Clin Psychol Rev 30(6):721–732. doi:10.1016/j.cpr.2010.05.006

Parker G (2014) The suprasensory world of bipolar II disorder. Am J Psychiatry 171(6):614–615. doi:10.1176/appi.ajp.2014.13121570

Pearson R (1997) Ernest Hemmingway and Sir William Osler. Med Health R I 80(6):195–199

Pickering G (1974) Creative malady. Oxford University Press, New York

Pons L, Nurnberger JI Jr, Murphy DL (1985) Mood-independent aberrancies in associative processes in bipolar affective disorder: an apparent stabilizing effect of lithium. Psychiatry Res 14(4):315–322

Post F (1994) Creativity and psychopathology. A study of 291 world-famous men. Br J Psychiatry 165(1):22–34

Richards R, Kinney DK, Lunde I, Benet M, Merzel AP (1988) Creativity in manic-depressives, cyclothymes, their normal relatives, and control subjects. J Abnorm Psychol 97(3):281–288

Runco MA (2004) Creativity. Annu Rev Psychol 55:657–687. doi:10.1146/annurev.psych.55.090902.141502

Rybakowski JK, Klonowska P (2011) Bipolar mood disorder, creativity and schizotypy: an experimental study. Psychopathology 44(5):296–302. doi:10.1159/000322814

Santosa CM, Strong CM, Nowakowska C, Wang PW, Rennicke CM, Ketter TA (2007) Enhanced creativity in bipolar disorder patients: a controlled study. J Affect Disord 100(1–3):31–39. doi:10.1016/j.jad.2006.10.013

Schildkraut JJ, Hirshfeld AJ, Murphy JM (1994) Mind and mood in modern art, II: depressive disorders, spirituality, and early deaths in the abstract expressionist artists of the New York school. Am J Psychiatry 151(4):482–488

Schou M (1979) Artistic productivity and lithium prophylaxis in manic-depressive illness. Br J Psychiatry 135:97–103

Shenton ME, Solovay MR, Holzman P (1987) Comparative studies of thought disorders. II. Schizoaffective disorder. Arch Gen Psychiatry 44(1):21–30

Simeonova DI, Chang KD, Strong C, Ketter TA (2005) Creativity in familial bipolar disorder. J Psychiatr Res 39(6):623–631. doi:10.1016/j.jpsychires.2005.01.005

Soeiro-de-Souza MG, Dias VV, Bio DS, Post RM, Moreno RA (2011) Creativity and executive function across manic, mixed and depressive episodes in bipolar I disorder. J Affect Disord 135(1–3):292–297. doi:10.1016/j.jad.2011.06.024

Solovay MR, Shenton ME, Holzman PS (1987) Comparative studies of thought disorders. I. Mania and schizophrenia. Arch Gen Psychiatry 44(1):13–20

Srivastava S, Childers ME, Baek JH, Strong CM, Hill SJ, Warsett KS, Wang PW, Akiskal HS, Akiskal KK, Ketter TA (2010) Toward interaction of affective and cognitive contributors to creativity in bipolar disorders: a controlled study. J Affect Disord 125(1–3):27–34. doi:10.1016/j.jad.2009.12.018

Strong CM, Nowakowska C, Santosa CM, Wang PW, Kraemer HC, Ketter TA (2007) Temperament-creativity relationships in mood disorder patients, healthy controls and highly creative individuals. J Affect Disord 100(1–3):41–48. doi:10.1016/j.jad.2006.10.015

Terman L, Cox C, Oden M, Burks B, Jensen D (1925–1959) Genetic studies of genius. Stanford University Press, Stanford

Tremblay CH, Grosskopf S, Yang K (2010) Brainstorm: occupational choice, bipolar illness and creativity. Econ Hum Biol 8(2):233–241. doi:10.1016/j.ehb.2010.01.001

Vellante M, Zucca G, Preti A, Sisti D, Rocchi MB, Akiskal KK, Akiskal HS (2011) Creativity and affective temperaments in non-clinical professional artists: an empirical psychometric investigation. J Affect Disord 135(1–3):28–36. doi:10.1016/j.jad.2011.06.062

Wills GI (2003) Forty lives in the bebop business: mental health in a group of eminent jazz musicians. Br J Psychiatry 183:255–259

Yalom ID, Yalom M (1971) Ernest Hemingway. A psychiatric view. Arch Gen Psychiatry 24(6):485–494

Index

K.N. Fountoulakis, *Bipolar Disorder: An Evidence-Based Guide to Manic Depression*, DOI 10.1007/978-3-642-37216-2

N

T

MIX
Papier aus verantwortungsvollen Quellen
Paper from responsible sources
FSC® C105338

If you have any concerns about our products,
you can contact us on
ProductSafety@springernature.com

In case Publisher is established outside the EU,
the EU authorized representative is:
Springer Nature Customer Service Center GmbH
Europaplatz 3, 69115 Heidelberg, Germany

Printed by Libri Plureos GmbH
in Hamburg, Germany